Shargel and Yu's

# Applied Biopharmaceutics and Pharmacokinetics

# Shargel and Yu's
# Applied Biopharmaceutics and Pharmacokinetics

**Eighth Edition**

## EDITORS

**Murray P. Ducharme, PharmD**
*President and CEO*
*Learn and Confirm, Inc.*
*Professeur Associé*
*Faculté de Pharmacie*
*University of Montreal*
*Montreal, Quebec*
*Canada*

**Leon Shargel, PhD, RPh**
*Applied Biopharmaceutics, LLC*
*Raleigh, North Carolina*
*Affiliate Professor, School of Pharmacy*
*Virginia Commonwealth University*
*Richmond, Virginia*
*Adjunct Professor, School of Pharmacy*
*University of Maryland*
*Baltimore, Maryland*

New York   Chicago   San Francisco   Athens   London   Madrid
Mexico City   Milan   New Delhi   Singapore   Sydney   Toronto

**Shargel and Yu's Applied Biopharmaceutics and Pharmacokinetics, Eighth Edition**

2  3  4  5  6  7  8  9    LCR    26  25  24  23  22

ISBN 978-1-260-14299-0
MHID 1-260-14299-X

This book was set in Minion Pro by KnowledgeWorks Global Ltd.
The editors were Michael Weitz and Peter J. Boyle.
The production supervisor was Richard Ruzycka.
Production management was provided by Deepanshu Manral, KnowledgeWorks Global Ltd.
Interior design by Mary McKeon.
The cover designer was W2 Design.

This book is printed on acid-free paper.

**Library of Congress Cataloging-in-Publication Data**

Names: Ducharme, Murray P., editor. | Shargel, Leon, 1941- editor. |
    Shargel, Leon, 1941- Applied biopharmaceutics & pharmacokinetics 2016.
Title: Shargel and Yu's applied biopharmaceutics and pharmacokinetics /
    editors, Murray P. Ducharme, Leon Shargel.
Other titles: Applied biopharmaceutics and pharmacokinetics
Description: Eighth edition. | New York : McGraw Hill, [2022] | Preceded by
    Applied biopharmaceutics & pharmacokinetics / Leon Shargel, Andrew B.C.
    Yu. Seventh edition. 2016. | Includes bibliographical references and index.
Identifiers: LCCN 2021049960 (print) | LCCN 2021049961 (ebook) | ISBN
    9781260142990 (hardcover ; alk. paper) | ISBN 9781260143003 (ebook)
Subjects: MESH: Pharmacokinetics | Biopharmaceutics | Models, Chemical |
    Drug Administration Routes
Classification: LCC RM301.5 (print) | LCC RM301.5 (ebook) | NLM QV 38 |
    DDC 615.7—dc23/eng/20211015
LC record available at https://lccn.loc.gov/2021049960
LC ebook record available at https://lccn.loc.gov/2021049961

McGraw Hill books are available at special quantity discounts to use as premiums and sales promotions, or for use in corporate training programs. To contact a representative please visit the Contact Us pages at www.mhprofessional.com.

# Contents

About the Editors ....................................................... *xiii*

Contributors ............................................................... *xv*

Preface ........................................................................ *xix*

Remarks by the New Editor .................................. *xxi*

## PART I

### Introduction to Biopharmaceutics and Pharmacokinetics ....................................... 1

## Chapter 1

### Introduction to Biopharmaceutics and Pharmacokinetics ...............................................3

*Leon Shargel and Murray P. Ducharme*

Drug Product Performance ...................................3

Biopharmaceutics .....................................................3

Pharmacokinetics ......................................................6

Pharmacodynamics ..................................................6

Clinical Pharmacokinetics ......................................7

Drug Exposure and Drug Response ................. 12

Toxicokinetics and Clinical Toxicology ........... 12

Measurement of Drug Concentrations ........... 13

Pharmacokinetic Models ..................................... 17

Computers in Pharmacokinetics ...................... 20

Chapter Summary .................................................. 21

Learning Questions ............................................... 22

Answers ...................................................................... 23

References ................................................................. 25

Bibliography ............................................................. 25

## Chapter 2

### Mathematical Fundamentals in Pharmacokinetics ..... 27

*Antoine Al-Achi*

Calculus ...................................................................... 27

Graphs ........................................................................ 29

Practice Problem .................................................... 31

Mathematical Expressions and Units ............. 32

Units for Expressing Blood Concentrations ............. 34

Measurement and Use of Significant Figures ............ 34

Practice Problem .................................................... 34

Practice Problem .................................................... 35

Rates and Orders of Processes ......................... 39

Chapter Summary .................................................. 42

Learning Questions ............................................... 42

Answers ...................................................................... 45

References ................................................................. 48

## Chapter 3

### Biostatistics ............................................................ 51

*Charles Herring, Antoine Al-Achi, and Abby Harris*

Variables ..................................................................... 51

Types of Data (Nonparametric Versus Parametric) ..... 52

Distributions ............................................................. 52

Measures of Central Tendency .......................... 53

Measures of Variability ......................................... 55

Hypothesis Testing ................................................ 59

Statistically Versus Clinically Significant Differences ..... 64

Clinical Case .............................................................. 64

Statistical Inference Techniques in Hypothesis Testing for Parametric Data ..... 65

Goodness of Fit ....................................................... 69

Statistical Inference Techniques for Hypothesis Testing with Nonparametric Data .......... 69

Controlled Versus Uncontrolled Studies ...... 72

Blinding ...................................................................... 73

Confounding ............................................................ 73

Validity ........................................................................ 74

Bioequivalence Studies ....................................... 74

Evaluation of Risk for Clinical Studies ............ 75

Chapter Summary .................................................. 77

Learning Questions ............................................... 77

Answers ...................................................................... 79

References ................................................................. 80

## PART II

### Fundamentals of Biopharmaceutics ......................... 83

## Chapter 4

### Physiologic Factors Related to Drug Absorption ........ 85

*Phillip M. Gerk*

Drug Absorption and Design of a Drug Product ...... 85

Route of Drug Administration ........................... 86

Nature of Cell Membranes .................................. 89

Passage of Drugs across Cell Membranes .................. 90

Drug Interactions in the Gastrointestinal Tract........100

Oral Drug Absorption ...............................................101

Oral Drug Absorption during
Drug Product Development...................................114

Methods for Studying Factors That
Affect Drug Absorption.........................................115

Effect of Disease States on Drug Absorption ..........118

Miscellaneous Routes of Drug Administration........120

Chapter Summary ....................................................121

Learning Questions..................................................122

Answers....................................................................123

References.................................................................124

Bibliography .............................................................126

## Chapter 5

### Drug Distribution and Protein Binding ......................129

*Craig K. Svensson*

Introduction .............................................................129

How Does a Drug Interact with
the Various Constituents in Blood? ......................130

How Does Drug Move from
Blood into Tissues?...............................................131

What Determines the Rate and Extent
of Drug Distribution into Various Tissues?............133

How Do Membrane Transporters
Influence Drug Distribution?.................................136

Do Drugs Distribute into Breast Milk?.....................138

Practice Problem ......................................................139

How Is the Extent of Drug Distribution
in the Body Measured? .........................................139

What Is the Effect of Plasma Protein Binding
and Tissue Binding on Drug Distribution? .............141

Practice Problem ......................................................142

How Is the Extent of Drug–Protein
Binding Measured? ...............................................142

Practice Problem ......................................................143

How Are the Kinetics of Drug–Protein
Binding Measured? ...............................................143

Practice Problems.....................................................144

How Are Binding Constants and
Binding Sites Determined Experimentally? ...........145

What Are the Primary Plasma
Proteins to Which Drugs Bind? .............................147

How Do Drug–Drug Protein
Binding Interactions Influence
Drug Distribution and Effect? ...............................149

Chapter Summary ....................................................149

References.................................................................150

## Chapter 6

### Physiology of Drug Elimination ....................................151

*Fang Wu, Murray P. Ducharme and Liang Zhao*

Introduction .............................................................151

Anatomy and Physiology of the Liver ......................151

Hepatic Enzymes Involved
in the Biotransformation of Drugs .......................153

Drug Biotransformation Reactions ..........................156

Pathways of Drug Biotransformation ......................156

Drug Interaction Example ........................................162

Clinical Example .......................................................168

First-Pass Effects ......................................................169

Biliary Excretion of Drugs ........................................169

Clinical Example .......................................................171

Role of Transporters in the
Elimination of Drugs from the Liver......................171

The Kidney and Renal Elimination ...........................172

Practice Problems.....................................................178

Chapter Summary ....................................................178

Learning Questions..................................................179

Answers....................................................................179

References.................................................................180

Bibliography .............................................................181

## Chapter 7

### Biopharmaceutic Considerations
in Drug Product Design and
*In Vitro* Drug Product Performance .............................183

*Maziar Kakhi, Poonam Delvadia,
and Sandra Suarez-Sharp*

Introduction .............................................................183

Biopharmaceutic Factors and
Rationale for Drug Product Design .......................184

Rate-Limiting Steps in Drug Absorption...................186

Physicochemical Properties of the Drug...................188

Influence of Excipients on
Drug Product Performance....................................192

Evaluation of Drug Product Performance.................194

Considerations in the Design and
Performance of Drug Products..............................221

Examples Related to the Design and
Perfomance of Drug Products ..............................224

Chapter Summary ....................................................234

Learning Questions..................................................235

Answers....................................................................235

References.................................................................236

Bibliography .............................................................241

## Chapter 8
### Drug Product Performance, *In Vivo*: Bioavailability and Bioequivalence ............................ 243
*Leon Shargel and Murray P. Ducharme*

Drug Product Performance .......................... 243
Purpose of Bioavailability and Bioequivalence Studies ............................... 243
Relative and Absolute Availability .................... 246
Practice Problem ................................... 248
Methods for Assessing Bioavailability and Bioequivalence ............................. 249
*In Vivo* Measurement of Active Moiety or Moieties in Biological Fluids .................... 250
Bioequivalence Studies Based on Pharmacodynamic Endpoints—*In Vivo* Pharmacodynamic Comparison ................... 252
Bioequivalence Studies Based on Clinical Endpoints—Clinical Endpoint Study ............ 253
*In Vitro* Studies ................................... 255
Other Approaches Deemed Acceptable (by the FDA) ........................ 256
Bioequivalence Studies Based on Multiple Endpoints ........................... 256
Bioequivalence Studies ............................ 256
Design and Evaluation of Bioequivalence Studies ........................... 256
Study Designs .................................... 264
Crossover Study Designs ........................... 265
Clinical Example .................................. 270
Clinical Example .................................. 271
Systemic Drug Exposure and Pharmacokinetic Evaluation of the Data ......... 271
The Partial AUC in Bioequivalence Analysis .......... 273
Bioequivalence Examples ........................... 275
Study Submission and Drug Review Process ......... 277
Bioequivalence for Specific Drugs and Drug Products ............................... 278
Waivers of *In Vivo* Bioequivalence Studies (Biowaivers) ............................. 281
The Biopharmaceutics Classification System .......... 283
Generic Biologics (Biosimilar Drug Products) .......... 285
Clinical Significance of Bioequivalence Studies ........................... 287
Special Concerns in Bioavailability and Bioequivalence Studies .................... 288
Chapter Summary ................................. 295
Learning Questions ................................ 295
Answers .......................................... 300
References ........................................ 302

## Chapter 9
### Modified-Release Drug Products and Drug Devices .............................. 305
*Hong Ding*

Modified-Release Drug Products and Conventional (Immediate-Release) Drug Products ................................... 305
Biopharmaceutic Factors ........................... 310
Dosage Form Selection ............................. 313
Advantages and Disadvantages of Extended-Release Products .................... 313
Kinetics of Extended-Release Dosage Forms .......... 315
Pharmacokinetic Simulation of Extended-Release Products .................... 317
Clinical Examples ................................. 319
Types of Extended-Release Products ................. 320
Considerations in the Evaluation of Modified-Release Products .................... 342
Evaluation of Modified-Release Products ............. 344
Evaluation of In Vivo Bioavailability Data ............ 346
Chapter Summary ................................. 347
Learning Questions ................................ 348
Answers .......................................... 349
References ........................................ 350
Bibliography ...................................... 354

## Chapter 10
### Targeted Drug Delivery Systems and Biotechnology Products ...................... 355
*Dhaval K. Shah, Zhe Li, and Donald E. Mager*

Introduction ...................................... 355
Biotechnology .................................... 356
Drug Carriers and Targeting ........................ 367
Targeted Drug Delivery ............................ 370
Pharmacokinetics of Biopharmaceuticals ............ 373
Chapter Summary ................................. 377
References ........................................ 377

## PART III
### Pharmacokinetic Principles .................... 381

## Chapter 11
### Introduction to Pharmacokinetic and Pharmacodynamic Models and Analyses ......... 383
*Murray P. Ducharme and Luciano Gama Braga*

Introduction ...................................... 383
The Different Methods for Calculating PK/PD ......... 384
Compartment Models .............................. 384
Noncompartmental Model .......................... 393

Physiologically-Based Pharmacokinetic Model ...... 393
Pharmacokinetic/Pharmacodynamic (PK/PD)
Model ........................................................................ 395
Chapter Summary .................................................... 396
References ................................................................. 396

**Chapter 12**
One-Compartment Open Model:
Intravenous Bolus Administration ...................... 399
*Kayleigh Wight, Philippe Colucci,*
*and Murray P. Ducharme*
Introduction ............................................................. 399
Calculations of Pharmacokinetic
Parameters ............................................................... 401
Clinical Utility of the
One-Compartment Model ....................................... 405
Chapter Summary .................................................... 407
Learning Questions .................................................. 407
Answers ..................................................................... 408
References ................................................................. 409
Bibliography ............................................................. 409

**Chapter 13**
Multicompartment Models:
Intravenous Bolus Administration ...................... 411
*Shabnam N. Sani and Rodney C. Siwale*
Two-Compartment Open Model ............................ 415
Clinical Application ................................................. 420
Practice Problem ..................................................... 422
Practical Focus ......................................................... 422
Practice Problem ..................................................... 424
Practical Focus ......................................................... 425
Three-Compartment Open Model ......................... 427
Clinical Application ................................................. 428
Clinical Application ................................................. 429
Determination of Compartment Models ............... 429
Practical Focus ......................................................... 430
Clinical Application ................................................. 430
Clinical Example ...................................................... 431
Practical Problem .................................................... 432
Clinical Application ................................................. 433
Practical Application ............................................... 434
Clinical Application ................................................. 435
Chapter Summary .................................................... 435
Learning Questions .................................................. 436
Answers ..................................................................... 438
References ................................................................. 441
Bibliography ............................................................. 441

**Chapter 14**
Intravenous Infusion ............................................. 443
*HaiAn Zheng*
Introduction ............................................................. 443
One-Compartment Model Drugs ........................... 444
Infusion Method for Calculating
Patient Elimination Half-Life ................................. 447
Loading Dose Plus IV
Infusion—One-Compartment Model ..................... 448
Practice Problems .................................................... 450
Estimation of Drug Clearance
and $V_D$ from Infusion Data ................................... 452
Intravenous Infusion of
Two-Compartment Model Drugs ........................... 453
Practical Focus ......................................................... 454
Chapter Summary .................................................... 456
Learning Questions .................................................. 456
Answers ..................................................................... 458
Bibliography ............................................................. 461

**Chapter 15**
Pharmacokinetic Calculations for
Drug Elimination and Clearance ......................... 463
*Murray P. Ducharme, Fang Wu, and Liang Zhao*
Drug Elimination ..................................................... 463
Clinical Importance of Drug Clearance ................. 463
Practice Problem ..................................................... 464
Principles of Clearance Calculations ..................... 464
Clearance Models .................................................... 466
The Compartmental Approach ............................... 467
Relationship between Rate Constants,
Volumes of Distribution and Clearances ............... 469
The Noncompartmental Approach ......................... 471
Practice Problem ..................................................... 478
Practice Problem ..................................................... 478
Integration of Compartmental and
Noncompartmental Approaches ............................ 479
The Physiologic Approach
Using the "Well-Stirred Model"
for Liver (and Other Organs) Clearance ................ 479
Clearance Predictions Based on the Fractions
Eliminated through the Kidney and Liver .............. 489
Practice Problem ..................................................... 489
Chapter Summary .................................................... 489
Learning Questions .................................................. 490
Answers ..................................................................... 492
References ................................................................. 495
Bibliography ............................................................. 495

## Chapter 16
### Pharmacokinetics of Drug Absorption.......................497
*Corinne Seng Yue and Dina Al-Numani*

Introduction .................................................................497

Relationship between Absorption
and Elimination Processes Following
Oral Drug Administration ...........................................498

Drug Absorption Processes—General Concepts......499

Zero-Order Drug Absorption .....................................500

Clinical Application—Transdermal
Drug Delivery..............................................................501

First-Order Drug Absorption .....................................501

Equations Describing Concentration–Time
Profiles Following Drug Absorption .........................502

Clinical Application ....................................................504

Practice Problem .........................................................504

Methods for Calculating Pharmacokinetic Parameters
Describing Drug Absorption ......................................506

Practice Problem .........................................................507

Relationship between Absorption Rate and
Bioavailability Parameters (AUC, $C_{max}$, $T_{max}$) .............509

Chapter Summary .......................................................511

Learning Questions.....................................................512

Answers........................................................................513

References....................................................................515

Bibliography ...............................................................516

Appendix A ..................................................................516

Appendix B ..................................................................518

## Chapter 17
### Multiple-Dosage Regimens ...........................521
*Rodney C. Siwale and Shabnam N. Sani*

Drug Accumulation ....................................................522

Clinical Example .........................................................525

Repetitive Intravenous Injections..............................526

Intermittent Intravenous Infusion ............................531

Clinical Example .........................................................532

Estimation of $K$ and $V_D$ of
Aminoglycosides in Clinical Situations......................533

Multiple-Oral-Dose Regimen ....................................534

Loading Dose..............................................................536

Dosage Regimen Schedules ......................................537

Clinical Example .........................................................538

Practice Problems........................................................538

Chapter Summary .......................................................541

Learning Questions.....................................................541

Answers........................................................................542

References....................................................................545

Bibliography ...............................................................545

## Chapter 18
### Nonlinear Pharmacokinetics...........................547
*Leon Shargel and Murray P. Ducharme*

Saturable Enzyme
Elimination Processes ................................................550

Practice Problem.........................................................550

Practice Problem.........................................................551

Drug Elimination by Capacity-Limited
Pharmacokinetics: One-Compartment Model,
IV Bolus Injection ......................................................552

Practice Problems........................................................554

Clinical Focus ..............................................................561

Drugs Distributed as
One-Compartment Model and
Eliminated by Nonlinear Pharmacokinetics..............561

Clinical Focus ..............................................................562

Chronopharmacokinetics and
Time-Dependent Pharmacokinetics...........................563

Clinical Focus ..............................................................564

Bioavailability of Drugs That
Follow Nonlinear Pharmacokinetics...........................565

Nonlinear Pharmacokinetics
Due to Drug–Protein Binding ....................................565

Dose-Dependent Pharmacokinetics ..........................570

Chapter Summary .......................................................571

Learning Questions.....................................................571

Answers........................................................................572

References....................................................................574

Bibliography ...............................................................575

## Chapter 19
### Empirical Models, Mechanistic Models, Statistical Moments, and Noncompartmental PK/PD Analyses .................................................577
*Corinne Seng Yue, Philippe Colucci,
and Murray P. Ducharme*

Noncompartmental Analysis.....................................577

Model Development
Considerations............................................................584

Empirical Models ........................................................585

Mechanistic Models....................................................589

Comparison of Different Approaches .......................603

Selection of Pharmacokinetic Models ......................605

Chapter Summary .......................................................606

Learning Questions.....................................................607

Answers........................................................................607

References....................................................................608

Bibliography ...............................................................611

**Chapter 20**

**Applications of Software Packages in Pharmacokinetics** ...............................613

*Philippe Colucci, Corinne Seng Yue, and Murray P. Ducharme*

Introduction ..............................................613

Software Applications..............................613

Overview of the Different Approaches in Software Packages ..............................614

Software Packages.....................................617

Chapter Summary .....................................635

Learning Questions....................................649

Answers......................................................649

References..................................................650

Bibliography ..............................................650

**PART IV**

**Pharmacodynamics and Clinical Pharmacokinetics** .......................... 653

**Chapter 21**

**Pharmacogenetics, Drug Metabolism, Transporters, and Individualization of Drug Therapy** ......................................655

*Brianne Raccor and Michael L. Adams*

Genetic Polymorphisms.............................656

Phase II Enzymes.......................................665

Transporters .............................................666

Glossary.....................................................668

Chapter Summary .....................................668

Answers......................................................669

References..................................................670

**Chapter 22**

**Relationship between Pharmacokinetics and Pharmacodynamics** ...............................673

*Mathangi Gopalakrishnan, Vipul Kumar Gupta, and Manish Issar*

Pharmacokinetics and Pharmacodynamics..............673

Relationship of Dose to Pharmacologic Response ...........................678

Relationship between Dose and Duration of Activity ($t_{eff}$), Single IV Bolus Injection...........................680

Practice Problem........................................680

Effect of Both Dose and Elimination Half-Life on the Duration of Activity.............681

Effect of Elimination Half-Life on Duration of Activity ..............................681

Substance Abuse Potential .......................682

Drug Tolerance and Physical Dependency..............682

Hypersensitivity and Adverse Response ..................683

Biological Markers (Biomarkers)................684

Types of Pharmacodynamic Response ......686

Chapter Summary .....................................708

Learning Questions....................................709

Answers......................................................712

References..................................................714

**Chapter 23**

**Application of Pharmacokinetics to Clinical Situations** .........................................717

*Dana R. Bowers and Vincent H. Tam*

Medication Therapy Management..............717

Individualization of Drug Dosage Regimens...........718

Therapeutic Drug Monitoring....................718

Clinical Example ........................................726

Clinical Example ........................................728

Design of Dosage Regimens......................728

Conversion from Intravenous Infusion to Oral Dosing ..............................730

Determination of Dose..............................731

Practice Problems......................................731

Effect of Changing Dose and Dosing Interval on $C_{max(ss)}$, $C_{min(ss)}$, and $C_{av(ss)}$ ........732

Determination of Frequency of Drug Administration...............................733

Determination of Both Dose and Dosage Interval ..............................733

Practice Problem........................................733

Determination of Route of Administration ..............734

Dosing in Specific Populations .................735

Pharmacokinetics of Drug Interactions.....................735

Inhibition of Drug Metabolism, Monoamine Oxidase (MAO), Drug Metabolism, Drug Absorption, and Biliary Excretion .....................739

Altered Renal Reabsorption due to Changing Urinary pH ......................741

Practical Focus ..........................................741

Effect of Food on Drug Disposition...........741

Adverse Viral Drug Interactions................742

Population Pharmacokinetics....................742

Clinical Example 1 .....................................745

Clinical Example 2 .....................................747

Practice Problem........................................747

Regional Pharmacokinetics ......................748

Chapter Summary .....................................749

Learning Questions....................................749

Answers..................................................751
References..............................................753
Bibliography ..........................................755

## Chapter 24
## Application of Pharmacokinetics and Pharmacodynamics to Aging, Obese, and Pediatric Patients...........................757

*Brian R. Overholser, Michael B. Kays, and Kevin M. Sowinski*

Introduction .........................................757
Application of Pharmacokinetics to Older Adults ......................................757
Application of Pharmacokinetics to the Obese Patient..............................765
Application of Pharmacokinetics to Pediatric Patients...............................773
Learning Questions................................779
Answers..................................................781
References..............................................782

## Chapter 25
## Dose Adjustment in Renal and Hepatic Diseases..............................787

*Yuen Yi Hon and Murray P. Ducharme*

Renal Impairment..................................787
Pharmacokinetic Considerations.............788
General Approaches for Dose Adjustment in Renal Disease ...........789
Measurement of the Kidney's Glomerular Filtration Rate .....................791
Serum Creatinine Concentration and Creatinine Clearance ....................792
Practice Problems ..................................794
Dose Adjustment in Patients with Renal Impairment........................797
Practice Problem ....................................805
Practice Problem ....................................805
Extracorporeal Removal of Drugs............807
Practice Problem ....................................809
Clinical Example ....................................811
Effect of Hepatic Disease on Pharmacokinetics................................813
Practice Problem ....................................815
Chapter Summary ..................................820
Learning Questions................................820
Answers..................................................821
References..............................................826
Bibliography ..........................................827

## PART V
## Biopharmaceutics and Pharmacokinetics in Drug Product Development ...........................829

## Chapter 26
## Biopharmaceutical Aspects of the Active Pharmaceutical Ingredient and Pharmaceutical Equivalence ...............831

*Changquan Calvin Sun, Andrew B.C. Yu, and Leon Shargel*

Introduction .........................................831
Pharmaceutical Alternatives...................836
Practice Problem ....................................837
Changes to an Approved NDA or ANDA ...839
Size, Shape, and Other Physical Attributes of Generic Tablets and Capsules ............841
How Prevalent Is the Therapeutic Nonequivalence of a Generic Product?.....841
The Future of Pharmaceutical Equivalence and Therapeutic Equivalence ..............842
Complex Drug Products...........................843
Biosimilar Drug Products.........................844
Historical Perspective.............................844
Chapter Summary ..................................845
Learning Questions................................845
Answers..................................................846
References..............................................847

## Chapter 27
## Rational Drug Product Development, Quality, and Performance...........................849

*Trupti Dixit, and Leon Shargel*

Risks from Medicines..............................849
Risk Assessment.....................................853
Drug Product Quality and Drug Product Performance........................853
Pharmaceutical Development ..................853
Excipient Effect on Drug Product Performance.......859
Practical Focus .......................................859
Quality Control and Quality Assurance .....861
Practical Focus .......................................861
Types of Quality Risk..............................861
Risk Management....................................865
Scale-Up and Postapproval Changes........866
Practical Focus .......................................868
Product Quality Problems .......................869
Postmarketing Surveillance.....................869
Glossary.................................................870

Chapter Summary .................................................871
Learning Questions.............................................871
Answers ...............................................................872
References ...........................................................872
Bibliography .......................................................873

**Chapter 28**
FDA-Approved Novel Dosage Forms ...........................875
*Ziyaur Rahman, Naseem A. Charoo,*
*Mohammad T.H. Nutan, and Mansoor A. Khan*
Introduction .......................................................875
Regulatory Pathway for New, Novel,
and Drug–Device Combination Products.................876
New and Novel Dosage Forms ..........................877
Drug–Device Combination Products .........................889
Chapter Summary .................................................908
Learning Questions.............................................908
Answers ...............................................................909
References ...........................................................910

**Chapter 29**
Clinical Development and Therapeutic
Equivalence of Generic Drugs
and Biosimilar Products .........................................913
*Murray P. Ducharme, and Deniz Ozdin*
Introduction .......................................................913
Bioequivalence ...................................................914
Interchangeability, Substitution,
and Switchability Notions ..................................916
Documentation Showing Establishment
of Bioequivalence and Interchangeability
of Generic Products .............................................916
Approval of Generic Products............................919
Filing of Generic Submissions in the
United States, Canada, and the European Union.......919
The Different "Generic" Terms ...........................921
Regulatory Requirements for
Generic Submissions in the
United States, Canada, and Europe.....................921
Clinical Pharmacology Basis Linking PK
Equivalence Studies with Presumed
Equivalent Safety and Efficacy.............................924

Statistical Evaluation of
Bioequivalence Metrics .......................................927
PK Equivalence Clinical Study
Requirements for FDA, HC, and EMA....................929
Equivalence Requirements for Products
That Are Not Intended to Act Via the
Systemic Circulation ("Locally Acting")...............935
Equivalence Requirements for
Biological Products ("Biosimilars")......................935
Chapter Summary .................................................940
Answers ...............................................................941
References ...........................................................942
Bibliography .......................................................944

**Chapter 30**
Pharmacokinetics and Pharmacodynamics
in Clinical Drug Product Development ......................945
*Murray P. Ducharme, Olga Ponomarchuk,*
*Dana Bakir, Deniz Ozdin, and Leon Shargel*
Introduction .......................................................945
Overview of the Drug Development Process...........946
Overview of the Drug Submission
Pathways in the United States,
the European Union, and Canada .......................946
Essential PK/PD Knowledge
for a New Drug Submission .................................948
Practical Problem ...............................................949
Practical Problems .............................................950
Practical Problem ...............................................952
Practical Problem ...............................................955
Clinical Problem .................................................960
Pre-Submission Scientific
Meetings with Regulators ..................................974
Phase IV Studies ................................................974
Chapter Summary .................................................976
References ...........................................................977
Bibliography .......................................................978
Glossary...............................................................979
Index...................................................................983

# About the Editors

**Murray P. Ducharme, PharmD,** has 30 years of academic, clinical, and industrial experience in pharmacometrics, infectious diseases, drug metabolism, and clinical drug and biological development. Murray has an undergraduate Pharmacy degree and a graduate diploma in Hospital Pharmacy from the University of Montreal, Canada, and a graduate PharmD degree from the College of Pharmacy and Allied Health Professions of Wayne State University in Michigan. He has presented more than 300 seminars and posters internationally and published more than 150 abstracts, manuscripts and book chapters in clinical pharmacology. He has been involved in thousands of clinical trials as a PI or sub-PI, and has served as an expert consultant in the drug development field for dozens of pharmaceutical companies located in the United States, Europe, Africa, Asia, or Canada. Murray has directed the work of 8 PhD candidates, 6 post-doctoral fellows, and 11 MSc candidates at the University of Montreal. He has trained thousands of pharmacy students in PK/PD and infectious diseases and has given special workshops and training sessions to regulatory agencies and pharmaceutical companies in Canada, United States, Asia, Middle-East, Africa, and Europe. Murray was elected as a Fellow of the American College of Clinical Pharmacy in 2000 and nominated as a Fellow of the American College of Clinical Pharmacology in 2001. Since 2012, Murray also serves as a Core Member of the Health Canada Scientific Advisory Committee on Pharmaceutical Sciences and Clinical Pharmacology.

**Leon Shargel, PhD,** is manager and founder of Applied Biopharmaceutics LLC, a pharmaceutical consulting company. Dr. Shargel holds academic appointments as Affiliate Professor, School of Pharmacy, Virginia Commonwealth University and Adjunct Associate Professor of Pharmacy, University of Maryland. He has varied experience in both academia and the pharmaceutical industry. Dr. Shargel has been a member or chair of numerous national committees responsible for state formulary issues, biopharmaceutics and bioequivalence issues and institutional review boards. In addition, he was a member of the USP Biopharmaceutics Expert Committee and was the generic drug industry representative on the FDA Pharmaceutical Sciences Advisory Committee. Dr. Shargel received a BS in Pharmacy from the University of Maryland and a PhD in Pharmacology from the George Washington University Medical Center. He is a registered pharmacist and has over 200 publications including several leading textbooks in pharmacy. He is a member of various professional societies including the American Association Pharmaceutical Scientists (AAPS), American Pharmacists Association (APhA) and the American Society for Pharmacology and Experimental Therapeutics (ASPET). Dr. Shargel has also published children's stories and is active in adult literacy programs.

# Contributors

**Michael L. Adams, PharmD, PhD**
Dean and Professor of Pharmaceutical Sciences
College of Pharmacy and Health Sciences
Campbell University
Buies Creek, North Carolina
*Chapter 21*

**Antoine Al-Achi, PhD**
Professor
College of Pharmacy and Health Sciences
Campbell University
Buies Creek, North Carolina
*Chapters 2, 3*

**Dina Al-Numani, MSc**
Senior Clinical Pharmacology Scientist
Learn and Confirm Inc.
St-Laurent, Quebec, Canada
*Chapter 16*

**Dana Bakir, MSc**
PhD candidate
Faculté de Pharmacie, University of Montreal
Learn and Confirm Inc.
St-Laurent, Quebec, Canada
*Chapter 30*

**Dana R. Bowers, PharmD, BCPS (AQ-ID), BCIDP**
Clinical Assistant Professor—Pharmacotherapy
College of Pharmacy and Pharmaceutical Sciences
Washington State University
Yakima, Washington
*Chapter 23*

**Naseem A. Charoo, PhD**
Principle Scientist
Zeino Pharma FZ LLC,
Dubai Science Park
Dubai, United Arab Emirates
*Chapter 28*

**Philippe Colucci, MSc, PhD**
Vice-President, Clinical Pharmacology
   and Operations
Learn and Confirm Inc.
St-Laurent, Quebec, Canada
*Chapters 12, 19, 20*

**Poonam Delvadia, PhD**
Silver Spring, Maryland
*Chapter 7*

**Hong Ding, PhD**
Chemist
Silver Spring, Maryland
*Chapter 9*

**Trupti Dixit, PhD**
Director, Combination Product Program
   Management
Parenteral Center of Excellence (PCoE)
Pfizer Inc
Lake Forest, Illinois
*Chapter 27*

**Murray P. Ducharme, PharmD, FCCP, FCP**
President and CEO, Learn and Confirm Inc.
St-Laurent, Quebec, Canada
Professeur Associé, Faculté de Pharmacie
Université de Montréal, Quebec, Canada
*Chapters 1, 6, 8, 11, 12, 15, 18, 19, 20, 29, 30*

**Luciano Gama Braga, PhD**
Clinical Research Scientist
Learn and Confirm Inc.
St-Laurent, Quebec, Canada
*Chapter 11*

**Phillip M. Gerk, PharmD, PhD**
Professor and Vice Chair
Department of Pharmaceutics
Virginia Commonwealth University
MCV Campus
School of Pharmacy
Richmond, Virginia
*Chapter 4*

**Mathangi Gopalakrishnan, MPharm, PhD**
Assistant Professor
Center for Translational Medicine
School of Pharmacy, University of Maryland
Baltimore, Maryland
*Chapter 22*

**Vipul Kumar Gupta, PhD**
Senior Director
DMPK, Bioanalysis and Clinical Pharmacology
Spero Therapeutics
Cambridge, Massachusetts
*Chapter 22*

**Abby Harris, PharmD**
PGY2 Critical Care Pharmacy Resident
Novant Health Forsyth Medical Center
*Chapter 3*

**Charles Herring, PharmD, BCPS, CPP**
Associate Professor
Campbell University
College of Pharmacy and Health Sciences
Clinical Pharmacist Practitioner
Adult Medicine Team
Winston-Salem, North Carolina
*Chapter 3*

**Yuen Yi Hon, PharmD, BCOP**
Clinical Analyst
Division of Rare Diseases and Medical Genetics
Office of Rare Diseases, Pediatrics, Urologic and
    Reproductive Medicine
Office of New Drugs
Center for Drug Evaluation
    and Research
Food and Drug Administration
Silver Spring, Maryland
*Chapter 25*

**Manish Issar, PhD**
Assistant Professor of Pharmacology
College of Osteopathic Medicine of the Pacific
Western University of Health Sciences
Pomona, California
*Chapter 22*

**Maziar Kakhi, PhD**
Formerly: AVL-List GmbH
Graz, Austria
Bayer AG, Leverkusen, Germany
Currently: US Food and Drug Administration
Silver Spring, Maryland
*Chapter 7*

**Michael B. Kays, PharmD**
Associate Professor of Pharmacy Practice
Department of Pharmacy Practice
College of Pharmacy, Purdue University
West Lafayette and Indianapolis, Indiana
*Chapter 24*

**Mansoor A. Khan, RPh, PhD**
Professor and Vice Dean
Irma Lerma Rangel College of Pharmacy
Texas A&M University
College Station, Texas
*Chapter 28*

**Zhe Li, PhD**
Senior Clinical Pharmacologist
Clinical Pharmacology and
    Pharmacometrics (CPPM)
AbbVie, Inc.
North Chicago, Illinois
*Chapter 10*

**Donald E. Mager, PharmD, PhD, FCP**
Professor and Vice Chair
Department of Pharmaceutical Sciences
University at Buffalo
School of Pharmacy and Pharmaceutical
    Sciences
Buffalo, New York
*Chapter 10*

**Mohammad T.H. Nutan, PhD**
Associate Professor
Irma Lerma Rangel College of Pharmacy
Texas A&M University
Kingsville, Texas
*Chapter 28*

**Brian R. Overholser, PharmD**
Professor of Pharmacy Practice
Department of Pharmacy Practice
College of Pharmacy, Purdue University
West Lafayette and Indianapolis, Indiana
*Chapter 24*

**Deniz Ozdin, BPharm, MSc, PhD**
Pharmacometrician
Syneos Health
Montréal, Canada
*Chapters 29, 30*

**Olga Ponomarchuk, PhD**
Clinical Research Scientist
Learn and Confirm Inc.
St-Laurent, Quebec, Canada
*Chapter 30*

**Brianne Raccor, PhD**
College of Pharmacy and Health Sciences
Campbell University
Buies Creek, North Carolina
*Chapter 21*

**Ziyaur Rahman, PhD**
Associate Professor
Irma Lerma Rangel College of Pharmacy
Texas A&M University
College Station, Texas
*Chapter 28*

**Shabnam N. Sani, MSc, PharmD, PhD**
Senior Manager, Clinical Pharmacology
Deciphera Pharmaceuticals, LLC
Waltham, Massachusetts
*Chapters 13, 17*

**Corinne Seng Yue, BPharm, MSc, PhD**
Vice-President, Clinical Pharmacology
    and Pharmacometrics
Learn and Confirm Inc.
St-Laurent, Quebec, Canada
*Chapters 16, 19, 20*

**Dhaval K. Shah, PhD**
Associate Professor
Department of Pharmaceutical Sciences
University at Buffalo, SUNY
Buffalo, New York
*Chapter 10*

**Leon Shargel, PhD, RPh**
Manager and Founder
Applied Biopharmaceutics, LLC
Raleigh, North Carolina
Affiliate Professor
School of Pharmacy
Virginia Commonwealth University
Richmond, Virginia
*Chapters 1, 8, 18, 26, 27, 30*

**Rodney C. Siwale, PhD, MSc**
Associate Professor of Pharmacy
Wingate University School of Pharmacy
Levine College of Health Sciences
515 N Main Street
Wingate, North Carolina
*Chapters 13, 17*

**Kevin M. Sowinski, PharmD**
Professor of Pharmacy Practice
Department of Pharmacy Practice
College of Pharmacy, Purdue University
West Lafayette and Indianapolis, Indiana
*Chapter 24*

**Sandra Suarez-Sharp, PhD**
Formerly Master Biopharmaceutics Reviewer,
    CDER, FDA
Vice President, Regulatory Affairs
Simulations Plus, Inc.
Lancaster, California
*Chapter 7*

**Changquan Calvin Sun, PhD**
Professor of Pharmaceutics
University of Minnesota
Department of Pharmaceutics
College of Pharmacy
Minneapolis, Minnesota
*Chapter 26*

**Craig K. Svensson, PharmD, PhD**
Dean Emeritus and Professor of Medicinal
    Chemistry and Molecular Pharmacology
Purdue University College of Pharmacy
Adjunct Professor of Pharmacology and Toxicology
Indiana University School of Medicine
West Lafayette, Indiana
*Chapter 5*

**Vincent H. Tam, PharmD**
Professor
Department of Pharmacy Practice
    and Translational Research
University of Houston College of Pharmacy
Houston, Texas
*Chapter 23*

**Kayleigh Wight, DEC**
Administrative Coordinator
    and Research Associate
Learn and Confirm Inc.
St-Laurent, Quebec, Canada
*Chapter 12*

**Fang Wu, PhD**
Senior Pharmacologist
Silver Spring, Maryland
*Chapters 6, 15*

**Andrew B.C. Yu, PhD**
Registered Pharmacist
Formerly senior reviewer, CDER, FDA
Associate Professor, Pharmaceutics
Albany College of Pharmacy
Albany, New York
*Chapter 26*

**Liang Zhao, PhD**
Supervisory Pharmacologist
Silver Spring, Maryland
*Chapters 6, 15*

**HaiAn Zheng, PhD**
Associate Professor
Department of Pharmaceutical Sciences
Albany College of Pharmacy and Health Sciences
Albany, New York
*Chapter 14*

# Preface

Biopharmaceutics and pharmacokinetics play a key role in the development of safer and more efficacious drug products. Application of these concepts makes possible better and more successful drug therapy in patients, allowing individualizing dosage regimens and improving therapeutic outcomes. Biopharmaceutic and pharmacokinetic principles are essential in the development of new and novel dosage forms.

Scientific developments and innovations in biopharmaceutics and pharmacokinetics have expanded exponentially since publication of the first edition in 1980. The first edition was based on a collaboration of two colleagues who saw a need to provide students with supplementary material to a pharmacy course. The *objectives* of the first edition were to:

1. Define the basic concepts in biopharmaceutics and pharmacokinetics.
2. Use raw data and derive the pharmacokinetic models and parameters that best describe the process of drug absorption, distribution, and elimination.
3. Critically evaluate biopharmaceutic studies involving drug product equivalency and unequivalency.
4. Design and evaluate dosage regimens of drugs using pharmacokinetic and biopharmaceutic parameters.
5. Detect potential clinical pharmacokinetic problems and apply basic pharmacokinetic principles to solve them.

These basic objectives have been incorporated into each subsequent edition of this textbook. Due to the expansion of knowledge in this discipline, the authors saw a need for an edited edition that would include experts from academia, pharmaceutical research, and regulatory affairs. As editors of this edition, we kept the original objectives, starting with fundamental concepts followed by a holistic integrated approach that can be applied to practice. The contributors were tasked to provide objectives for each chapter that were commensurate with the overall objectives.

The publication of the eighth edition of *Shargel and Yu's Applied Biopharmaceutics and Pharmacokinetics* embodies more than four decades of scientific developments in the field. In planning for the eighth edition, we realized the need to organize the chapters in a more logical sequence starting with introductory and fundamental principles, developing these basic concepts and then applying these concepts to clinical situations. The new edition ends with a discussion of biopharmaceutics and pharmacokinetics in drug product development.

The eighth edition represents the collective contribution of experts with intimate knowledge and experience in the selected subject areas. Each chapter was written to include practical applications of the theoretical material. Frequently asked questions are included to provide a discussion of overall concepts. Practice problems, clinical examples and learning questions are included in each chapter to show how these concepts relate to practical situations.

This textbook remains unique in teaching basic concepts that may be applied to understanding complex issues that are essential for understanding drug development and safe and efficacious drug therapy. The primary audience is pharmacy students enrolled in pharmaceutical science courses in pharmacokinetics and biopharmaceutics. This text fulfills course work offered in separate or combined courses in these subjects. Secondary audiences for this textbook are research, technological and development scientists in pharmaceutics, biopharmaceutics, and pharmacokinetics.

We would like to acknowledge the contributions of Andrew B.C. Yu, PhD. Dr. Yu provided valuable expertise in the writing of the first six editions and in editing the seventh edition of this textbook. Dr. Yu's input helped with the success of this textbook. As the first author, I would also like to acknowledge the input of our new editor, Murray Ducharme, PharmD. Dr. Ducharme has provided substantial guidance and expertise in organizing and editing this new eighth edition of *Shargel and Yu's Applied Biopharmaceutics and Pharmacokinetics*.

We are grateful to our contributors, readers, colleagues and students for their helpful feedback and support throughout the years.

**Leon Shargel, PhD**
**Murray P. Ducharme, PharmD**

# Remarks by the New Editor

Leon Shargel was a name that I was very familiar with, when in 1999 I had the pleasure of meeting him for the first time at a Pharmaceutical Industry meeting. I am not sure if it was at the Annual AAPS meeting or if it was at what was then a national US generic industry meeting (National Association of Pharmaceutical Manufacturers (NAPM)), but I thought I was meeting a "giant" at the time, being extremely familiar with the textbook "Applied Biopharmaceutics and Pharmacokinetics" as I possessed personally all of the previous editions and I was recommending this particular textbook to all my pharmacy students when teaching the two graduate PK courses at the University of Montreal. Leon came to talk to me and was genuinely interested in what I was doing and what I was thinking from a PK point of view on a wide variety of topics, not just asking me complicated questions (which I was expecting) but also what felt to me at the time to be very simple and already "addressed" questions. I was too "star-struck" at the time to fully understand his thinking and rationale for asking me this range of questions, and for considering my opinion when at the time I had evolved academically, yes, but I was quite a junior in the industrial and regulatory field. Of course, now I know that whatever we think has been fully addressed and is "known," is never really fully addressed and known. Science evolves all the time and one has to pick the "brain" of others to make sure that one's understanding of things is always large enough and one always remains open scientifically to controversial and differing opinions. We have always stayed in touch on at least a yearly basis since then, and it was a pleasant shock again when he proposed to me to join him for this new edition of what I consider to be the "bible" in the field. Through Leon, I have got to know Andy, who is as humble, open-minded and interesting scientifically. Leon and Andy, thank you so much for allowing me to contribute to your great book!

Being the "new kid on the block" I had a few ideas for change, and appropriately as the "wise elders" that they are, Leon and Andy have agreed to some while respectfully disagreeing on others but have been the "open minded" scientists that I have come to respect. Some of the changes that we are presenting in this edition come from the realization that the teaching and understanding of PK/PD does not come from a "silo" approach where everything is known academically or clinically, or in industry, or by regulators. It has to be at the forefront of these three areas where they each contribute. A good PK/PD scientist does not only need to know the academic and clinical side of PK, but also has to understand the Industry and regulatory side. This is a big change from the early editions of this textbook and of the others that populate this space. I hope you will like this edition as much as we liked putting it together.

**Murray P. Ducharme**
Montreal, Canada

Shargel and Yu's

# Applied Biopharmaceutics and Pharmacokinetics

PART I

# Introduction to Biopharmaceutics and Pharmacokinetics

# Introduction to Biopharmaceutics and Pharmacokinetics

Leon Shargel and Murray P. Ducharme

## CHAPTER OBJECTIVES

- Define biopharmaceutics and pharmacokinetics.
- Define drug product performance and discuss how biopharmaceutics can affect drug product performance.
- Describe how pharmacokinetic studies relate to clinical efficacy and drug toxicity.
- Discuss how clinical pharmacokinetics is used to develop drug dosage regimens in patients.
- Define a pharmacokinetic model and the assumptions that are used in developing a pharmacokinetic model.
- Discuss how the prescribing information or approved labeling for a drug helps the practitioner to recommend an appropriate dosage regimen for a patient.

## DRUG PRODUCT PERFORMANCE

Drugs are substances intended for use in the diagnosis, cure, mitigation, treatment, or prevention of disease. Drugs are given in a variety of dosage forms or *drug products* such as solids (tablets, capsules), semisolids (ointments, creams), solutions, suspensions, emulsions, etc, for systemic or local therapeutic activity. Drug products are drug delivery systems that release and deliver drug to the site of action to produce the desired therapeutic effect and minimize adverse toxicity. Drug products should be designed to meet the patient's individual requirements including palatability, convenience, compliance, and safety.

*Drug product performance* is defined as the release of the drug substance from the drug product either for local drug action or for absorption into the plasma for systemic drug activity. Advances in pharmaceutical technology and manufacturing have improved the quality of drug products and improved drug delivery.

## BIOPHARMACEUTICS

*Biopharmaceutics* examines the relationship of the physical and chemical properties of the drug, the dosage form (drug product) in which the drug is formulated, and the route of administration for the delivery of the drug to the site of action. In pharmacokinetics, *bioavailability* (F) is the fraction of the administered dose of a drug that reaches the systemic circulation. Bioavailability is a formulation parameter that enables clinicians to consider the proportion of the dose that will be systemically absorbed in the patient when changing dosage forms of the same drug. For example, the extent of systemic drug absorption (*drug exposure*) should be the same when changing from an intravenous (IV) drug formulation in a stabilized patient during hospitalization to an oral tablet formulation of the same drug when the patient is discharged. In regulatory science, *bioavailability* is defined as both the rate and extent of drug that reaches systemic circulation or to the site of action. The US FDA defines *bioequivalence* as "the absence of a significant difference in the rate and extent to which the active ingredient or active moiety in pharmaceutical equivalents or pharmaceutical alternatives becomes available at the site of drug action when administered at the same molar dose under similar conditions in an appropriately designed study." Bioequivalence is a critical component for the approval of drug products, whether they are new or generic drug products. Regulatory agencies such as the US Food and Drug Administration (FDA) define *bioavailability* more broadly as both the rate and extent to which the active ingredient or active moiety is absorbed from a drug product and becomes available at the site of drug action.

Other regulatory agencies, such as Health Canada (HC) and the European Medicines Agency (EMA) define bioavailability and bioequivalence slightly different than the US FDA. All regulatory agencies consider bioavailability as an important quantitative measurement of *drug product performance*. In this book, *bioavailability* (F) is considered in its pharmacokinetic definition as the fraction or percentage of the administered dose that reaches the systemic circulation.

When comparing formulations, *bioavailability* is defined as a measure of the rate and extent of drug that reaches the systemic circulation, and bioequivalence is a comparison bioavailability study of two or more formulations of the same drug. *Bioequivalence* compares drug product performance and determines whether there is a difference in extent of systemic drug exposure (Chapter 8). Strict statistical tests are used to evaluate the results in bioequivalence studies to determine whether formulations of the same drug (eg, brand drug product versus generic drug product) are bioequivalent.

*Relative bioavailability* ($F_{rel}$) compares the extent of drug exposure between two or more drug formulations using the area under the curve (AUC) as the metric but does not consider the rate of drug exposure.

The importance of the drug substance (active pharmaceutical ingredient) and the drug formulation on drug release, drug absorption, and distribution to the site of action is described as a sequence of events that precede elicitation of a drug's therapeutic effect. A general scheme describing this dynamic relationship is illustrated in Fig. 1-1.

First, the drug product is administered to the patient. The drug product may be given by route of oral, IV, subcutaneous, transdermal, topical, inhalation, or another route of administration. Then, the drug is released from the dosage form. A fraction of the drug is absorbed from the site of administration into either the surrounding tissue for local action (as with topical ointments) or into the body (as with oral dosage forms), or both. Finally, the drug reaches the site of action. A *pharmacodynamic response* results when the drug concentration at the site of action reaches or exceeds the *minimum effective concentration* (MEC). The suggested dosing regimen, including starting dose, maintenance dose, dosage form, and dosing interval, is determined in clinical trials prior to drug approval. The suggested dosage regimen provides the drug concentrations at the site of action that are therapeutically effective in most patients.

Historically, pharmaceutical scientists evaluated the relative drug availability in the body after giving a drug product by different routes of administration and then comparing the observed pharmacologic, clinical, or toxic responses. For example, isoproterenol hydrochloride, a β-adrenoreceptor agonist, causes an increase in heart rate when given intravenously but has no observable effect on the heart

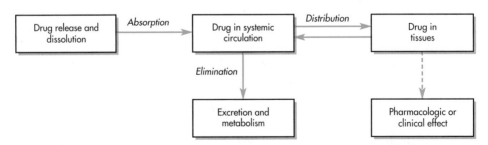

FIGURE 1-1 • Scheme demonstrating the dynamic relationship between the drug, the drug product, and the pharmacologic effect.

when given orally at the same dose level. This observation showed the importance of the route of drug administration on the systemic availability of the drug. In this example, isoproterenol is more systemically available after IV administration compared to oral administration. The development of analytical methods for measuring drugs in biological tissues allows the quantitative measurement of plasma drug concentrations at various times after drug product is given to the patient. The ability to measure the time course of drug concentrations in the body yields objective data that relate the drug dosage regimen to the therapeutic effect and adverse events.

Bioavailability of a drug from a drug product can vary depending upon the physical and chemical properties of the drug, the type of drug product that contains the drug, the formulation of the drug product, and the manufacturing process for making the drug product. Depending upon the therapeutic objective, the drug product can be designed so that the rate of exposure from a drug product at the intended site of action is rapid, delayed, or prolonged. These differences in the rate and extent of drug exposure will affect the therapeutic effectiveness and safety of the drug product. The study of biopharmaceutics allows the pharmaceutical scientist to rationally develop a drug product that improves drug safety, efficacy, and patient compliance. These topics are discussed more fully in later chapters.

The US FDA approves all drug products to be marketed in the United States. Pharmaceutical manufacturers perform extensive research and development studies prior to approval of a new drug product. The manufacturer of a new drug product must submit a *New Drug Application* (NDA) to the FDA, whereas a generic drug pharmaceutical manufacturer must submit an *Abbreviated New Drug Application* (ANDA) (Chapters 8 and 29). Both new and generic drug product manufacturers must demonstrate that the drug product is safe and efficacious before the products can be approved by the FDA and made available to consumers.

Biopharmaceutics provides the scientific basis for drug product design and drug product development. Each step in the manufacturing process may potentially affect the safety and drug product performance of the finished dosage form. The most important steps in the manufacturing process are termed

*critical manufacturing variables* (Chapter 27). Some of the more important biopharmaceutic considerations in drug product design are listed in Table 1-1. A detailed discussion of drug product design is found in Chapter 7. Knowledge of physiologic factors necessary for designing oral products is discussed in Chapter 4. The quality of the active pharmaceutical ingredient and the formulation of the drug product are discussed in later chapters. Many finished drug products and their ingredients are imported into the United States and other countries due to globalization

**TABLE 1-1 •** Biopharmaceutic Considerations in Drug Product Design

| Items | Considerations |
|---|---|
| Therapeutic objective | Drug may be intended for rapid relief of symptoms, slow extended action given once per day, or longer for chronic use; some drugs may be intended for local action or systemic action |
| Drug (active pharmaceutical ingredient, API) | Physical and chemical properties of API, including solubility, polymorphic form, particle size; impurities |
| Route of administration | Oral, topical, parenteral, transdermal, inhalation, etc |
| Drug dosage and dosage regimen | Large or small drug dose, frequency of doses, patient acceptance of drug product, patient compliance |
| Type of drug product | Orally disintegrating tablets, immediate release tablets, extended release tablets, transdermal, topical, parenteral, implant, etc |
| Excipients | Although very little pharmacodynamic activity, excipients may affect drug product performance including release of drug from drug product |
| Method of manufacture | Variables in manufacturing processes, including weighing accuracy, blending uniformity, release tests, and product sterility for parenterals |

of the pharmaceutical industry. Each country has its own regulatory agency for the approval of drug products (Chapter 29). It is important that pharmacists understand the relationship between the drug dosage form and the testing procedures that ensure the safety, efficacy, and quality of the drug product.

The study of biopharmaceutics is based on fundamental scientific principles and experimental methodology. Studies in biopharmaceutics use both *in vitro* and *in vivo* methods. *In vitro* methods are procedures employing test apparatus and equipment without involving laboratory animals or humans. *In vivo* methods are more complex studies involving human subjects or laboratory animals. These methods must be able to assess the impact of the physical and chemical properties of the drug, drug stability, and large-scale production of the drug and drug product on the biologic performance of the drug.

In summary, biopharmaceutics involves factors that influence (1) the design of the drug product, (2) stability of the drug product and active pharmaceutical ingredient, (3) the manufacture of the drug product, (4) the release of the drug from the drug product, and (5) the bioavailability of the drug. The pharmacist must understand these complex relationships to objectively choose the most appropriate drug product for therapeutic success.

## PHARMACOKINETICS

*Pharmacokinetics* describes the movement of drug in the body. It is the study of the kinetics of drug absorption, distribution, and elimination (metabolism and excretion). Pharmacokinetics can quantitatively characterize and predict the time course of drug action using mathematical models and statistics. The quantitative characterization of drug concentrations in the body with respect to time by pharmacokinetics is important for the determination of the drug dose and the dosing regimen needed to obtain the proper therapeutic objective in each patient.

The study of pharmacokinetics involves both experimental and theoretical approaches. The experimental aspect of pharmacokinetics involves the development of biologic sampling techniques, analytical methods for the measurement of drugs and metabolites, and procedures that facilitate data collection and manipulation. The theoretical aspect

of pharmacokinetics involves the development of pharmacokinetic models and computer simulations that predict drug disposition after drug administration. The application of statistics is an integral part of pharmacokinetic studies. Statistical methods are used for pharmacokinetic parameter estimation and data interpretation ultimately for the purpose of designing and predicting optimal dosing regimens for individuals or groups of patients. Statistical methods are applied to pharmacokinetic models to determine data error and structural model deviations. Mathematics and computer techniques also form the theoretical basis of many pharmacokinetic methods.

## PHARMACODYNAMICS

The interrelationship of pharmacokinetics and pharmacodynamics is important in the development of a new drug to ensure the safety and efficacy of the drug in patients. Pharmacokinetics examines the movement of drugs in the body and predicts the time course of drug concentrations in the body, whereas *pharmacodynamics* relates the drug concentration in the body to the therapeutic effect and possible adverse events.

Pharmacodynamics studies the biochemical and physiological effects of drugs on the body. The interaction of a drug molecule with a receptor causes the initiation of a sequence of molecular events resulting in a pharmacologic or toxic response. Pharmacodynamics examines the molecular interaction of the drug at a receptor site and the resulting physiologic effect. Furthermore, pharmacodynamics along with pharmacokinetics considers the relationship between changing drug concentrations and the resulting physiologic response. For example, pharmacodynamics studies how a drug interacts quantitatively with a drug receptor to produce a response (effect). Receptors are the molecules within cells or on cell membranes that interact with specific drugs to produce a pharmacological effect in the body.

The pharmacodynamic (or pharmacologic) effect can be the desired therapeutic response and/or the undesired side effects (adverse events). For many drugs, the pharmacodynamic effect is drug dose or drug concentration related. Higher drug doses produce higher drug concentrations in the body, more drug at the receptor site, and a more intense pharmacodynamic effect up to a maximum effect. It is desirable that side effects and/or toxicity of drugs occur at higher drug concentrations than the drug concentrations needed for the therapeutic effect. Unfortunately, unwanted side effects often occur concurrently with the therapeutic doses. The relationship between pharmacodynamics and pharmacokinetics is discussed in Chapter 22.

## CLINICAL PHARMACOKINETICS

*Clinical pharmacokinetics* utilizes the application of biopharmaceutics, pharmacokinetics, and pharmacodynamics to achieve optimum drug therapy in the individual patient (Chapter 23). Proper drug therapy is dependent upon the therapeutic objective of the drug in the patient and involves the selection of the appropriate drug, the route of drug administration, the drug product, the drug dose, the dosage regimen, and various patient factors. Clinical pharmacokinetics considers the pharmacokinetics and pharmacodynamics of drugs in disease states and covariates such as pathophysiology, age, gender, weight, body mass index, renal and hepatic function, and genetic and ethnic differences that may affect the outcome of drug therapy (Chapters 24 and 25). Clinical pharmacokinetics must consider patient compliance, cost of medication, drug–drug interactions, patient diet, and the use of dietary supplements that may affect therapeutic efficacy. After drug administration, clinical pharmacokinetics may need to follow patient outcomes through therapeutic drug monitoring.

Due to intra- and interindividual variations, the recommended dose may result in either a subtherapeutic (drug concentration below the MEC) or an adverse response (drug concentrations above the *minimum toxic concentration,* MTC). In these cases, the clinical pharmacist will need to suggest an adjustment to the dosing regimen or in a few cases, suggest another drug in the same therapeutic category. The clinical pharmacist uses therapeutic strategies based on known pharmacokinetics, the patient's disease state, and patient-specific considerations.

### New Drug Application

Prior to drug product approval, the pharmaceutical manufacture submits an NDA. The NDA describes the ingredients of the drug product, formulation of the drug product, manufacturing process, results of animal and human studies, drug safety, efficacy, packaging, and labeling.

The goals of the NDA are to provide enough information to permit the FDA reviewer to reach the following key decisions[1]:

- Whether the drug is safe and effective in its proposed use(s), and whether the benefits of the drug outweigh the risks.
- Whether the drug's proposed labeling (package insert) is appropriate based on the data submitted, and what it should contain.
- Whether the methods used in manufacturing the drug and the controls used to maintain the drug's quality are adequate to preserve the drug's identity, strength, quality, and purity.

### Prescription Drug Label

During the clinical phases of drug development process, patients are enrolled in clinical trials to determine the safety and efficacy of the drug and to determine the optimum dosing regimens that will provide the best therapeutic response. Along with safety and efficacy data and other patient information, the FDA approves a label that becomes the *Patient Package Insert* (PPI). The prescription information is developed by manufacturers, approved by the FDA, and dispensed with each prescription drug product. The approved labeling recommends the proper starting dosage regimens for the general patient population and may have additional recommendations for special populations of patients that need an adjusted dosage regimen. These recommended dosage regimens produce the desired pharmacologic response in the majority of the anticipated patient population.

In 2013, the FDA redesigned the format of the prescribing information necessary for safe and effective use of the drugs and biological products (FDA Guidance for Industry, 2013). This design was developed to make information in prescription drug labeling easier for health care practitioners to access and read. The practitioner can use the prescribing

---

[1]US FDA, New Drug Application: https://www.fda.gov/drugs/types-applications/new-drug-application-nda

information to make prescribing decisions. The labeling includes three sections:

- *Highlights of Prescribing Information (Highlights)*— contains selected information from the Full Prescribing Information (FPI) that health care practitioners most commonly reference and consider most important. In addition, highlights may contain any boxed warnings that give a concise summary of all of the risks described in the Boxed Warning section in the FPI.
- *Table of Contents (Contents)*—lists the sections and subsections of the FPI.
- *Full Prescribing Information (FPI)*—contains the detailed prescribing information necessary for safe and effective use of the drug.

An example of the Highlights of Prescribing Information and Table of Contents for Nexium (esomeprazole magnesium) delayed release capsules appears in Tables 1-2A and 1-2B. The prescribing information sometimes referred to as the approved label or the package insert may be found at the FDA website, Drugs@FDA (http://www.accessdata.fda.gov/scripts/cder/drugsatfda/). Prescribing information is updated periodically as new information becomes available. The prescribing information contained in the label recommends dosage regimens for the average patient from data obtained from clinical trials. The indications and usage section are those indications that the FDA has approved and that have been shown to be effective in clinical trials.

On occasion, a practitioner may want to prescribe the drug to a patient drug for a *non-approved use* or indication. The pharmacist must decide if there is sufficient evidence for dispensing the drug for a non-approved use (off-label indication). The decision to dispense a drug for a *non-approved indication* may be difficult and is often made with consultation of other health professionals.

## Clinical Pharmacology

*Pharmacology* is the study of drugs and includes the mechanism of drug action, pharmacokinetics, pharmacodynamics, pharmacotherapeutics, and toxicology. The application of pharmacology in clinical medicine is referred to as *clinical pharmacology*. The approved prescription drug label provides important

clinical study information in Table 1-2B under Section 12, *Clinical Pharmacology* and includes 12.1 Mechanism of Action, 12.2 Pharmacodynamics, 12.3 Pharmacokinetics, and 12.4 Microbiology.

## Pharmacogenetics and Pharmacogenomics

Variations in drug response have been observed for most drugs. This variability in drug response is primarily due to the patient's heredity.[2] With development of genetic methods, *personalized medicine* is used to make treatment decisions for the individual patient based on genetic or other biomarker information. *Pharmacogenetics* is the study of variability in drug response due to heredity. *Pharmacogenomics* is often used interchangeably with pharmacogenetics but includes the study of the genetic basis of disease and the pharmacodynamic impact of the drug in the patient (Chapter 21). Studies during drug development have shown the presence of genetically controlled polymorphisms of drug-metabolizing enzymes, drug transporters, and drug receptors. Pharmacogenetics and pharmacogenomics are important in new drug development and are based on our increasing ability to characterize all genes in the human genome.

## Relationship of Drug Concentrations to Drug Response

Initiation of drug therapy starts with the manufacturer's recommended dosage regimen that is part of the approved drug label. The recommended dose includes the drug dose and frequency of doses (eg, 100 mg every 8 hours). The dosage regimen in the approved drug label is the dosage regimen that was found to be safe and efficacious in most of the patients that were enrolled in clinical trials performed by the drug manufacturer. Due to individual variation that may be due to genetic differences, pathophysiology (eg, renal disease, hepatic disease), age, and other factors, the suggested starting dose may need to be modified accordingly (Chapters 23, 24, 25). Even with the best dose estimates, the recommended

---

[2]Although heredity is a major factor in patient drug response, environmental and other factors such as pathophysiology of the patient, drug–drug interactions, age, and smoking may also affect drug response.

## TABLE 1-2A • Highlights of Prescribing Information for Nexium (Esomeprazole Magnesium)

**These highlights do not include all the information needed to use NEXIUM safely and effectively. See full prescribing information for NEXIUM.**

NEXIUM® (esomeprazole magnesium) delayed-release capsules, for oral use
NEXIUM® (esomeprazole magnesium) for delayed-release oral suspension
Initial US Approval: 1989 (omeprazole)

················································RECENT MAJOR CHANGES·····················································

Warnings and Precautions, Fundic Gland Polyps (5.12)

06/2018

··················································INDICATIONS AND USAGE·······················································

NEXIUM is a proton pump inhibitor indicated for the following:
• Treatment of gastroesophageal reflux disease (GERD). (1.1)
• Risk reduction of NSAID-associated gastric ulcer. (1.2)
• *H. pylori* eradication to reduce the risk of duodenal ulcer recurrence. (1.3)
• Pathological hypersecretory conditions, including Zollinger-Ellison syndrome. (1.4)

··············································DOSAGE AND ADMINISTRATION····················································

| Indication | Dose | Frequency |
|---|---|---|
| **Gastroesophageal Reflux Disease (GERD)** | | |
| Adults | 20 mg or 40 mg | Once daily for 4 to 8 weeks |
| 12 to 17 years | 20 mg or 40 mg | Once daily for up to 8 weeks |
| 1 to 11 years | 10 mg or 20 mg | Once daily for up to 8 weeks |
| 1 month to less than 1 year: 2.5 mg, 5 mg, or 10 mg (based on weight). Once daily, up to 6 weeks for erosive esophagitis (EE) due to acid-mediated GERD only. | | |
| **Risk Reduction of NSAID-Associated Gastric Ulcer** | | |
| 20 mg or 40 mg | | Once daily for up to 6 months |
| **H. pylori Eradication** *(Triple Therapy):* | | |
| NEXIUM | 40 mg | Once daily for 10 days |
| Amoxicillin | 1000 mg | Twice daily for 10 days |
| Clarithromycin | 500 mg | Twice daily for 10 days |
| **Pathological Hypersecretory Conditions** | | |
| 40 mg | | Twice daily |
| See full prescribing information for administration options (2) | | |
| Patients with severe liver impairment—do not exceed dose of 20 mg (2) | | |

··············································DOSAGE FORMS AND STRENGTHS···················································

• NEXIUM Delayed-Release Capsules: 20 mg and 40 mg (3)
• NEXIUM For Delayed-Release Oral Suspension: 2.5 mg, 5 mg, 10 mg, 20 mg, and 40 mg (3)

··················································CONTRAINDICATIONS········································

Patients with known hypersensitivity to proton pump inhibitors (PPIs) (angioedema and anaphylaxis have occurred) (4)

*(Continued)*

**TABLE 1-2A** • Highlights of Prescribing Information for Nexium (Esomeprazole Magnesium) *(Continued)*

····················································· WARNINGS AND PRECAUTIONS ·····················································

- Gastric Malignancy: In adults, symptomatic response does not preclude the presence of gastric malignancy. Consider additional follow-up and diagnostic testing (5.1)
- Acute Interstitial Nephritis: Observed in patients taking PPIs (5.2)
- *Clostridium difficile*-Associated Diarrhea: PPI therapy may be associated with increased risk (5.3)
- Bone Fracture: Long-term and multiple daily dose PPI therapy may be associated with an increased risk for osteoporosis-related fractures of the hip, wrist or spine (5.4)
- Cutaneous and Systemic Lupus Erythematosus: Mostly cutaneous; new onset or exacerbation of existing disease; discontinue NEXIUM and refer to specialist for evaluation (5.5)
- Interaction with Clopidogrel: Avoid concomitant use of NEXIUM (5.6)
- Cyanocobalamin (Vitamin B-12) Deficiency: Daily long-term use (eg, longer than 3 years) may lead to malabsorption or a deficiency of cyanocobalamin (5.7)
- Hypomagnesemia: Reported rarely with prolonged treatment with PPIs (5.8)
- Interaction with St. John's Wort or Rifampin: Avoid concomitant use of NEXIUM (5.9, 7.3)
- Interactions with Diagnostic Investigations for Neuroendocrine Tumors: Increased chromogranin A (CgA) levels may interfere with diagnostic investigations for neuroendocrine tumors; temporarily stop NEXIUM at least 14 days before assessing CgA levels (5.10, 12.2)
- Interaction with Methotrexate: Concomitant use with PPIs may elevate and/or prolong serum concentrations of methotrexate and/or its metabolite, possibly leading to toxicity; with high dose methotrexate administration, consider temporary withdrawal of NEXIUM (5.11, 7.7)
- Fundic Gland Polyps: Risk increases with long-term use, especially beyond one year; use the shortest duration of therapy (5.12)

····················································· ADVERSE REACTIONS ·····················································

Most common adverse reactions (6.1):
- Adults (≥18 years) (incidence ≥1%) are headache, diarrhea, nausea, flatulence, abdominal pain, constipation, and dry mouth
- Pediatric (1 to 17 years) (incidence ≥2%) are headache, diarrhea, abdominal pain, nausea, and somnolence
- Pediatric (1 month to less than 1 year) (incidence 1%) are abdominal pain, regurgitation, tachypnea, and increased ALT

**To report SUSPECTED ADVERSE REACTIONS, contact AstraZeneca at 1-800-236-9933 or FDA at 1-800-FDA-1088 or www.fda.gov/medwatch.**

····················································· DRUG INTERACTIONS ·····················································

- May affect plasma levels of antiretroviral drugs – use with atazanavir and nelfinavir is not recommended; if saquinavir is used with NEXIUM, monitor for toxicity and consider saquinavir dose reduction (7.1)
- May interfere with drugs for which gastric pH affects bioavailability (eg, ketoconazole, iron salts, erlotinib, digoxin, and mycophenolate mofetil); patients treated with NEXIUM and digoxin may need to be monitored for digoxin toxicity (7.2)
- Combined inhibitor of CYP2C19 and 3A4 may raise esomeprazole levels (7.3)
- Clopidogrel: NEXIUM decreases exposure to the active metabolite of clopidogrel (7.3)
- May increase systemic exposure of cilostazol and an active metabolite; consider dose reduction (7.3)
- Tacrolimus: NEXIUM may increase serum levels of tacrolimus (7.5)
- Methotrexate: NEXIUM may increase serum levels of methotrexate (7.7)

*See 17 for PATIENT COUNSELING INFORMATION and Medication Guide*

## TABLE 1-2B • Full Prescribing Information: Contents* for Nexium (Esomeprazole Magnesium)

1. **INDICATIONS AND USAGE**
   1.1 Treatment of Gastroesophageal Reflux Disease (GERD)
   1.2 Risk Reduction of NSAID-Associated Gastric Ulcer
   1.3 *Helicobacter pylori* Eradication to Reduce the Risk of Duodenal Ulcer Recurrence
   1.4 Pathological Hypersecretory Conditions Including Zollinger-Ellison Syndrome
2. **DOSAGE AND ADMINISTRATION**
3. **DOSAGE FORMS AND STRENGTHS**
4. **CONTRAINDICATIONS**
5. **WARNINGS AND PRECAUTIONS**
   5.1 Presence of Gastric Malignancy
   5.2 Acute Interstitial Nephritis
   5.3 *Clostridium difficile*-Associated Diarrhea
   5.4 Bone Fracture
   5.5 Cutaneous and Systemic Lupus Erythematosus
   5.6 Interaction with Clopidogrel
   5.7 Cyanocobalamin (Vitamin B-12) Deficiency
   5.8 Hypomagnesemia
   5.9 Interaction with St. John's Wort or Rifampin
   5.10 Interactions with Diagnostic Investigations for Neuroendocrine Tumors
   5.11 Interaction with Methotrexate
   5.12 Fundic Gland Polyps
6. **ADVERSE REACTIONS**
   6.1 Clinical Trials Experience
   6.2 Postmarketing Experience
7. **DRUG INTERACTIONS**
   7.1 Interference with Antiretroviral Therapy
   7.2 Drugs for which Gastric pH can Affect Bioavailability
   7.3 Effects on Hepatic Metabolism/Cytochrome P-450 Pathways
   7.5 Tacrolimus
   7.6 Combination Therapy with Clarithromycin
   7.7 Methotrexate
8. **USE IN SPECIFIC POPULATIONS**
   8.1 Pregnancy
   8.2 Lactation
   8.4 Pediatric Use
   8.5 Geriatric Use
10. **OVERDOSAGE**
11. **DESCRIPTION**
12. **CLINICAL PHARMACOLOGY**
   12.1 Mechanism of Action
   12.2 Pharmacodynamics
   12.3 Pharmacokinetics
   12.4 Microbiology
13. **NONCLINICAL TOXICOLOGY**
   13.1 Carcinogenesis, Mutagenesis, Impairment of Fertility
   13.2 Animal Toxicology and/or Pharmacology
14. **CLINICAL STUDIES**
   14.1 Healing of Erosive Esophagitis
   14.2 Symptomatic Gastroesophageal Reflux Disease (GERD)
   14.3 Pediatric Gastroesophageal Reflux Disease (GERD)
   14.4 Risk Reduction of NSAID-Associated Gastric Ulcer
   14.5 *H. pylori* Eradication in Patients with Duodenal Ulcer Disease
   14.6 Pathological Hypersecretory Conditions Including Zollinger-Ellison Syndrome
16. **HOW SUPPLIED/STORAGE AND HANDLING**
17. **PATIENT COUNSELING INFORMATION**

*Sections or subsections omitted from the full prescribing information are not listed.*

dosage regimen drug may not provide the desired therapeutic outcome in an individual patient.

The measurement of plasma drug concentrations can confirm whether the drug dose was subtherapeutic due to the patient's individual pharmacokinetic profile (observed by low plasma drug concentrations) or was not responsive to drug therapy due to genetic difference in receptor response. In this case, the drug concentrations are in the therapeutic range but the patient does not respond to drug treatment. Figure 1-2 shows that the concentration of drug in the body can range from subtherapeutic to toxic. In contrast, some patients respond to drug treatment at lower drug doses that result in lower drug concentrations. Other patients may need higher drug concentrations to obtain a therapeutic effect, which requires higher drug doses. It is desirable that adverse drug responses occur at drug concentrations higher relative to the therapeutic drug concentrations. For many potent drugs, adverse effects can also occur close to the same drug concentrations as needed for the therapeutic effect.

## FREQUENTLY ASKED QUESTIONS

▶ Which is more closely related to drug response, the total drug dose administered or the concentration of the drug in the body?

▶ Why do individualized dosing regimens need to be determined for some patients?

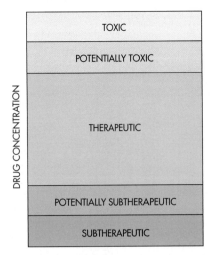

FIGURE 1-2 • Relationship of drug concentrations to drug response.

## DRUG EXPOSURE AND DRUG RESPONSE

*Drug exposure* refers to the dose (drug input into the body) and various measures of drug concentrations in plasma and other biological fluid (eg, $C_{max}$, $C_{min}$, $C_{ss}$, AUC) (FDA Guidance for Industry, 2003). *Drug response* refers to the pharmacologic effect of the drug. Drug response includes a broad range of endpoints or biomarkers including the clinically remote biomarkers (eg, receptor occupancy) (Chapter 22), a presumed mechanistic effect (eg, ACE inhibition), a potential or accepted surrogate (eg, effects on blood pressure, lipids, or cardiac output), and the full range of short-term or long-term clinical effects related to either efficacy or safety. For many drugs, there is a direct relationship of the drug exposure in the body as measured by the plasma drug concentration versus time profile and the drug response.

## TOXICOKINETICS AND CLINICAL TOXICOLOGY

*Toxicokinetics* is the application of pharmacokinetic principles to the design, conduct, and interpretation of drug safety evaluation studies (Leal et al, 1993) and the demonstration of dose-related exposure in animals. Toxicokinetic evaluation is a regulatory and scientific requirement in the drug development process. Toxicokinetic data aid in the interpretation of toxicologic findings in animals and extrapolation of the resulting data to humans. Toxicokinetic studies are performed in animals during preclinical drug development and may continue after the drug has been tested in clinical trials. The objective of toxicokinetics is to describe systemic drug exposure in animals and its relationship to dose level, drug concentrations, and the time course of the drug toxicity studies. These data may be used in the interpretation of toxicology findings and their relevance to clinical safety issues.

*Clinical toxicology* is the study of adverse effects of drugs and toxic substances (poisons) in the body. The pharmacokinetics of a drug in an overmedicated (intoxicated) patient may be very different from the pharmacokinetics of the same drug given in lower therapeutic doses. At very high doses, the drug concentration in the body may saturate enzymes involved in the absorption, biotransformation, or active renal secretion mechanisms, thereby changing the pharmacokinetics from linear to *nonlinear pharmacokinetics* (Chapter 18). Drugs frequently involved in toxicity cases include acetaminophen, salicylates, antihistamines, opiates, alcohol, stimulants, and street drugs.

Toxicologic and clinical efficacy studies provide information on the safety and effectiveness of the drug during development and in special patient populations such as subjects with renal and hepatic insufficiencies. The prescribed drug dosage regimen is based on the therapeutic objective after weighing the risks of favorable and unfavorable outcomes in the patient. For some potent drugs, the doses and dosing rate may need to be titrated in order to obtain the desired effect and be tolerated.

## MEASUREMENT OF DRUG CONCENTRATIONS

For most drugs, there is a relationship between the drug dose and the pharmacodynamic response of the drug (Chapter 22). A higher drug dose generally produces a greater pharmacodynamic response compared to a lower drug dose. Studies on variability of drug response in patients given similar drug doses show that drug concentrations (mg/L) in the body are more closely related to drug response compared to the amount (mg) of administered drug. The concentration of the drug at the receptor site is more consistently related to magnitude of the pharmacodynamic effect. The measurement of drug concentrations in the body at various time intervals after a given dose is the basis of pharmacokinetics.

Drug concentrations are measured in biologic samples, such as milk, saliva, plasma, urine, and other tissues. Sensitive, accurate, and precise analytical methods are available for the direct measurement of drugs in biologic matrices. Such analytical measurements must be validated so that accurate information is generated for pharmacokinetic and clinical drug monitoring. In general, chromatographic and mass spectrometric methods are most frequently employed for drug concentration measurement, because chromatography separates the drug from other related materials that may cause assay interference, and mass spectrometry allows detection of molecules or molecule fragments based on their mass-to-charge ratio.

### Sampling of Biologic Specimens

Only a few biologic specimens may be obtained safely from the patient to gain information as to the drug concentration in the body. *Invasive methods* include sampling blood, spinal fluid, synovial fluid, tissue biopsy, or any biologic material that requires parenteral or surgical intervention in the patient. In contrast, *noninvasive methods* include sampling of urine, saliva, feces, expired air, or any biologic material that can be obtained without parenteral or surgical intervention.

The measurement of drug and metabolite concentration in each of these biologic materials yields important information, such as the amount of drug retained in, or transported into, that region of the tissue or fluid, the likely pharmacologic or toxicologic outcome of drug dosing, and drug metabolite formation or transport. Analytical methods should be able to distinguish between protein-bound and nonprotein-bound (unbound) parent drug and each metabolite. In most cases, the unbound concentrations are the drug concentrations related to safety and efficacy (Chapter 5) The pharmacologically active species of the drug should be identified. Such distinctions between metabolites in each tissue and fluid are especially important for initial pharmacokinetic modeling of a drug.

### Drug Concentrations in Blood, Plasma, or Serum

Measurement of drug and metabolite concentrations (levels) in the blood, serum, or plasma is the most direct approach to assessing the pharmacokinetics of the drug in the body. *Whole blood* contains cellular elements including red blood cells, white blood cells, platelets, and various other proteins, such as albumin and globulins (Table 1-3). In general, *serum* or *plasma* is most commonly used for drug measurement. To obtain serum, whole blood is allowed to clot and the serum is collected from the supernatant after centrifugation. Plasma is obtained from the supernatant of centrifuged whole blood to which an anticoagulant, such as heparin, has been added. The protein content of serum and plasma is not the same. Plasma perfuses all the tissues of the body, including the cellular elements in the blood. Assuming that a drug in the plasma is in dynamic equilibrium with the tissues (including the cellular elements of whole blood), then

## TABLE 1-3 • Blood Components

| Blood Component | How Obtained | Components |
|---|---|---|
| Whole blood | Whole blood is generally obtained by venous puncture and contains an anticoagulant such as heparin or EDTA | Whole blood contains all the cellular and protein elements of blood |
| Serum | Serum is the liquid obtained from whole blood after the blood is allowed to clot and the clot is removed | Serum does not contain the cellular elements, fibrinogen, or the other clotting factors from the blood |
| Plasma | Plasma is the liquid supernatant obtained after centrifugation of non-clotted whole blood that contains an anticoagulant | Plasma is the noncellular liquid fraction of whole blood and contains all the proteins including albumin |

a change in the drug concentration in plasma will reflect a change in tissue drug concentrations. Drugs in the plasma are often bound to plasma proteins. The unbound (free) drug concentration in the plasma may be obtained by removing the protein-bound drug by ultrafiltration or dialysis. The total plasma drug concentration may be measured from unfiltered plasma. When interpreting plasma drug concentrations, it is important to understand what type of plasma drug concentration the data reflect.

### FREQUENTLY ASKED QUESTIONS

▶ Why are drug concentrations more often measured in plasma rather than whole blood or serum?

▶ What are the differences between bound drug, unbound drug, total drug, parent drug, and metabolite drug concentrations in the plasma?

### Plasma Drug Concentration–Time Curve

The plasma drug concentration (level)–time curve is generated from blood samples taken at various time intervals after the drug product is administered. The concentration of drug in each plasma sample is plotted on a graph against the corresponding time at which the blood sample was removed. After a single drug dose by an extravascular route (eg, oral), the drug is absorbed into the body and enters the general (systemic) circulation. Plasma drug concentrations will rise up to a maximum and then decline. Usually, drug absorption is more rapid than drug elimination. As the drug is being absorbed into the systemic circulation, the drug is distributed to all the tissues in the body and is also *simultaneously* being eliminated. Elimination of a drug can proceed by excretion, biotransformation, or a combination of both. Other elimination mechanisms may also be involved, such as elimination in the feces, sweat, or exhaled air.

The relationship between the drug level–time curve and various pharmacologic parameters for the drug is shown in Fig. 1-3. MEC and MTC represent the *minimum effective concentration* and *minimum toxic concentration* of drug, respectively. For some drugs, it is useful to know the concentration of drug that will just barely produce a pharmacologic effect (ie, MEC). Assuming the drug concentration

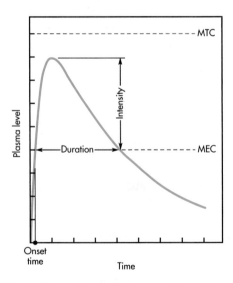

FIGURE 1-3 • Plasma drug level–time curve after oral administration of a drug.

in the plasma is in equilibrium with the tissues, the MEC reflects the minimum concentration of drug needed at the receptors to produce the desired pharmacologic effect. Similarly, the MTC represents the drug concentration needed to just barely produce a toxic effect. The *onset time* corresponds to the time required for the drug to reach the MEC. The *intensity* of the pharmacologic effect is proportional to the number of drug receptors occupied, which is reflected in the observation that higher plasma drug concentrations produce a greater pharmacologic response, up to a maximum. The *duration of drug action* is the difference between the onset time and the time for the drug to decline back to the MEC.

The *therapeutic window* is the concentrations between the MEC and the MTC. Drugs with a wide therapeutic window are generally considered safer than drugs with a narrow therapeutic window. Sometimes the term *therapeutic index* is used. This term refers to the ratio between the toxic and therapeutic doses.

The pharmacokineticist views the plasma drug concentration versus time curve somewhat differently. The pharmacokineticist describes the plasma drug concentration versus time curve using the terms *peak plasma level* ($C_{max}$), *time for peak plasma level* ($T_{max}$), and *area under the curve,* or AUC (Fig. 1-4).

The time for peak plasma level is the time of maximum drug concentration in the plasma and is a rough marker of average rate of drug absorption. The peak plasma level or maximum drug concentration is related to the dose, the rate constant for drug absorption, and the drug elimination rate constant. The AUC is related to the amount of drug absorbed systemically (bioavailable). These and other pharmacokinetic parameters are discussed in succeeding chapters.

---

### FREQUENTLY ASKED QUESTIONS

▶ At what time intervals should plasma drug concentration be taken in order to best predict drug response and side effects?

▶ What happens if plasma concentrations fall outside of the therapeutic window?

---

### Drug Concentrations in Tissues

Tissue biopsies are occasionally removed for diagnostic purposes, such as the verification of a malignancy. Usually, only a small sample of tissue is removed, making drug concentration measurement difficult. Drug concentrations in tissue biopsies may not reflect drug concentration in all parts of the tissue from which the biopsy material was removed. For example, if the tissue biopsy was for the diagnosis of a tumor within the tissue, the blood flow to the tumor cells may not be the same as the blood flow to other cells in this tissue. For many tissues, blood flow to one part of the tissues need not be the same as the blood flow to another part of the same tissue. The measurement of the drug concentration in tissue biopsy material may be used to ascertain if the drug reached the tissues and reached the proper concentration within the tissue. Generally, drug concentrations in tissues are not measured directly, but estimated by the use of pharmacokinetic models.

### Drug Concentrations in Urine and Feces

Measurement of drug in urine is an indirect method to ascertain the bioavailability of a drug. The rate and extent of drug excreted in the urine reflects the rate and extent of systemic drug absorption. Excreted drug urinary data can be used to clarify the percentage of the drug excreted via the renal route

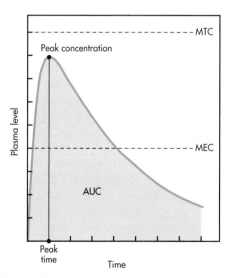

**FIGURE 1-4** • Plasma level–time curve showing peak time and concentration. The shaded portion represents the AUC (area under the curve).

versus other non-renal elimination routes (eg, hepatic metabolism). This data is pivotal information for the adjustment of drug dosages in patients with various levels of renal function. The use of urinary drug excretion measurements to establish various pharmacokinetic parameters is discussed in Chapter 16.

Measurement of drug in feces may reflect drug that has not been absorbed after an oral dose and/or may reflect drug that has been expelled by biliary secretion after being already systemically bioavailable. Fecal drug excretion is often performed in mass balance studies, in which the investigator attempts to account for the entire dose given to the patient. For a mass balance study, both urine and feces are collected and their drug content measured. Some solid oral dosage forms do not dissolve in the gastrointestinal tract but slowly release the drug from the dosage form. In this case, fecal collection is performed to recover the dosage form and then assayed for residual drug.

### Drug Concentrations in Saliva

Saliva drug concentrations have been reviewed for many drugs for therapeutic drug monitoring (Pippenger and Massoud, 1984). Because only free drug diffuses into the saliva, saliva drug levels tend to approximate free drug rather than total plasma drug concentration. The saliva/plasma drug concentration ratio is less than 1 for many drugs. The saliva/plasma drug concentration ratio is mostly influenced by the pKa of the drug and the pH of the saliva. Weak acid drugs and weak base drugs with pKa significantly different than pH 7.4 (plasma pH) generally have better correlation to plasma drug levels. The saliva drug concentrations taken after equilibrium with the plasma drug concentration generally provide more stable indication of drug levels in the body. Measurement of salivary drug concentrations as a therapeutic indicator should be used with caution and preferably as a secondary indicator.

### Forensic Drug Measurements

*Forensic science* is the application of science to personal injury, murder, and other legal proceedings. Drug measurements in tissues obtained at autopsy or in other bodily fluids such as saliva, urine, and blood may be useful if a suspect or victim has taken an overdose of a legal medication, has been poisoned, or has been using drugs of abuse such as opiates (eg, heroin, cocaine, or marijuana). The appearance of social drugs in blood, urine, and saliva drug analysis shows short-term drug abuse. These drugs may be eliminated rapidly, making it more difficult to prove that the subject has been using drugs of abuse. The analysis for drugs of abuse in hair samples by very sensitive assay methods, such as gas chromatography coupled with mass spectrometry, provides information regarding past drug exposure. A study by Cone et al (1993) showed that the hair samples from subjects who were known drug abusers contained cocaine and 6-acetylmorphine, a metabolite of heroin (diacetylmorphine).

### Significance of Measuring Plasma Drug Concentrations

The intensity of the pharmacologic or toxic effect of a drug is often related to the concentration of the drug at the receptor site, usually located in the tissue cells. Because most of the tissue cells are richly perfused with tissue fluids or plasma, measuring the plasma drug level is an objective method of monitoring the course of therapy.

Variations in the pharmacokinetics of drugs are quite common in patients. Monitoring the concentration of drugs in plasma ascertains that the calculated dose actually delivers the plasma level required for therapeutic effect. With some drugs, receptor expression and/or sensitivity in individuals varies, so monitoring of plasma levels is needed to distinguish the patient who is receiving too much of a drug from the patient who is supersensitive to the drug. Moreover, the patient's physiologic functions may be affected by disease, nutrition, environment, concurrent drug therapy, and other factors. Pharmacokinetic models allow more accurate interpretation of the relationship between plasma drug levels and pharmacologic response.

In the absence of pharmacokinetic information, plasma drug levels are relatively useless for dosage adjustment. For example, suppose a single blood sample from a patient was assayed and found to contain 10 $\mu$g/mL. According to the literature, the maximum safe concentration of this drug is 15 $\mu$g/mL. In order to apply this information properly, it is important to know when the blood sample was drawn, what dose of the drug was given, and the route of administration. If the proper information is available, the use of pharmacokinetic equations and models may describe the plasma level–time curve accurately and be used to modify dosing for the patient.

Monitoring of plasma drug concentrations allows for the adjustment of the drug dosage in order to optimize therapeutic drug regimens. When alterations in physiologic functions occur, monitoring plasma drug concentrations may provide a guide to the adequacy of the dosage regimen and whether the investigator needs to modify the drug dosage accordingly to the progress of the disease. Sound medical judgment and patient observation are most important. Therapeutic decisions should not be based solely on plasma drug concentrations.

In many cases, the *pharmacodynamic response* to the drug may be more important to measure than just the plasma drug concentration. For example, the electrophysiology of the heart, eg, an electrocardiogram (ECG), is important to assess patients medicated with cardiotonic drugs such as digoxin. For an anticoagulant drug, such as dicoumarol, prothrombin clotting time may indicate whether proper dosage was achieved. Most diabetic patients taking insulin will monitor their own blood or urine glucose levels.

For drugs that act irreversibly at the receptor site, plasma drug concentrations may not accurately predict pharmacodynamic response. Drugs used in cancer chemotherapy often interfere with nucleic acid or protein biosynthesis to destroy tumor cells. For these drugs, the plasma drug concentration may not relate directly to the pharmacodynamic response. In this case, other pathophysiologic parameters and side effects are monitored in the patient to prevent adverse toxicity. (Rodman and Evans, 1991)

## PHARMACOKINETIC MODELS

Drugs are in a dynamic state within the body. Drugs get absorbed into the body, distribute into and out of tissues, bind with plasma or cellular components, and are excreted by the kidneys and/or metabolized by the liver. The biologic nature of drug absorption, distribution, and elimination is complex, and drug events often happen simultaneously. Mathematical models use simplifying assumptions to reduce the complexity of these events, to better understand the relationship of drug concentrations in the body to drug response, to estimate a dosage regimen, and to predict the time course of drug action. The validity of the model is based on the choice of the underlying assumptions and whether these assumptions are valid.

A *model* is a hypothesis using mathematical terms to concisely describe quantitative relationships. A model can help explain experimental observations and to predict future observations (see Chapter 11). The predictive capability of a model lies in the validity of the assumptions and the development of mathematical function(s) that parameterizes the essential factors governing the kinetic process. The key parameters in a process are commonly estimated by fitting the model to the experimental data, known as *variables*. A *pharmacokinetic parameter* is a constant for the drug that is estimated from the experimental data. For example, estimated pharmacokinetic parameters such as the elimination rate constant, $k$, depend on the method of tissue sampling, the timing of the sample, drug analysis, and the predictive model selected.

A pharmacokinetic function relates an *independent variable* to a *dependent variable*, often through the use of parameters. For example, a pharmacokinetic model may predict the drug concentration in the liver 1 hour after an oral administration of a 20-mg dose. The independent variable is the time, and the dependent variable is the drug concentration in the liver. Based on a set of time-versus-drug concentration data, a model equation is derived to predict the liver drug concentration with respect to time. In this case, the drug concentration depends on the time after the administration of the dose, where the time–concentration relationship is defined by a pharmacokinetic parameter, $k$, the elimination rate constant.

Such mathematical models can be devised to simulate the rate processes of drug absorption, distribution, and elimination to describe and *predict* drug concentrations in the body as a function of time. Pharmacokinetic models are used to:

1. Predict plasma, tissue, and urine drug levels with any dosage regimen

2. Calculate the optimum dosage regimen for each patient individually

3. Estimate the possible accumulation of drugs and/or metabolites

4. Correlate drug concentrations with pharmacologic or toxicologic activity

5. Evaluate differences in the rate or extent of availability between formulations (bioequivalence)

6. Describe how changes in physiology or disease affect the absorption, distribution, or elimination of the drug

7. Explain drug interactions

Simplifying assumptions are made in pharmacokinetic models to describe a complex biologic system concerning the movement of drugs within the body. For example, most pharmacokinetic models assume that the plasma drug concentration reflects drug concentrations globally within the body. A model requires accurate data and valid assumptions.

A model may be empirically, physiologically, or compartmentally based. The model that simply interpolates the data and allows an empirical formula to estimate drug level over time is justified when limited information is available. *Empirical models are practical but not very useful in explaining the mechanism of the actual process by which the drug is absorbed, distributed, and eliminated in the body.* Examples of empirical models used in pharmacokinetics are described in Chapter 11 and other chapters.

Theoretically, an unlimited number of models may be constructed to describe the kinetic processes of drug absorption, distribution, and elimination in the body, depending on the degree of detailed information considered. More complex pharmacokinetic models have been developed due to the increase in computer power. However, the validity of these models must be examined (Chapter 11).

## Compartment Models

*Compartment-based models* are the simplest and most popular models used to describe the pharmacokinetics of a drug. For example, assume a drug is given by IV injection and that the drug dissolves (distributes) rapidly in the body fluids. In this case, the pharmacokinetic model assumes that the drug in the body dissolves in a volume of fluid that is rapidly equilibrated

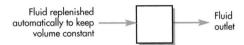

FIGURE 1-5 • Tank with a constant volume of fluid equilibrated with drug. The volume of the fluid is 1.0 L. The fluid outlet is 10 mL/min. The fraction of drug removed per unit of time is 10/1000, or 0.01 min$^{-1}$.

with the drug. The concentration of the drug in the body after a given dose is governed by two parameters: (1) the fluid volume of the body that will dilute the drug, and (2) the elimination rate of drug from the body. Though this model is perhaps an overly simplistic view of drug disposition in the human body, a drug's pharmacokinetic properties can frequently be described by a model called the *one-compartment open model* (Fig. 1-5). In the one-compartment body model, a fraction of the drug is continually eliminated as a function of time (Fig. 1-6). In pharmacokinetics, these parameters are assumed to be constant for a given drug. If drug concentrations in the body are determined at various time intervals following an IV dose, the volume of fluid in the body or compartment in which the drug is dissolved (apparent volume of distribution, $V_D$) and the rate constant for drug elimination, $k$, can be estimated.

MODEL 1. One-compartment open model, IV injection.

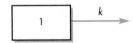

MODEL 2. One-compartment open model with first-order absorption.

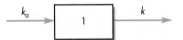

MODEL 3. Two-compartment open model, IV injection.

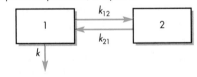

MODEL 4. Two-compartment open model with first-order absorption.

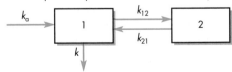

FIGURE 1-6 • Various compartment models.

In practice, pharmacokinetic parameters such as the elimination rate constant, $k$, and the apparent volume of distribution, $V_D$, are determined experimentally from collecting blood and measuring their plasma drug concentrations over various times after drug administration. The values for the plasma drug concentrations are the experimental observations, or *data*. The number of parameters needed to describe a model depends on the complexity of the kinetic process, the route of drug administration, and the data available. In general, as the number of parameters required to develop a model increases then the data needs to increase proportionally. Without sufficient data, the accurate estimation of these parameters becomes increasingly more difficult. Computer programs are used to facilitate parameter estimation for complex pharmacokinetic models. For parameter estimates to be valid, the number of data points should equal or exceed the number of parameters in the model.

Because a model is based on a hypothesis and simplifying assumptions, a certain degree of caution is necessary when relying totally on the pharmacokinetic model to predict drug action. If a simple model does not fit all the experimental observations accurately, a new, more elaborate model may be proposed and subsequently tested. Since limited data are generally available in most clinical situations, pharmacokinetic data should not replace sound judgment by the clinician. Appropriate drug therapy should be based on both the pharmacokinetic data and clinical observations.

Because of the vast complexity of the body, drug kinetics in the body is frequently simplified to be represented by one or more compartments that communicate reversibly with each other. A *compartment* is not a real physiologic or anatomic region but is considered a tissue or group of tissues that have similar blood flow and drug affinity. Within each compartment, the drug is considered to be uniformly distributed. Mixing of the drug within a compartment is rapid and homogeneous and is considered to be *well stirred*, so that the drug concentration in the compartment represents an average concentration, and each drug molecule has an equal probability of leaving the compartment. *Rate constants* are used to represent the overall rate processes of drug entry into and exit from the compartment. The model is an *open system* because drug can enter into or be eliminated from the system. Compartment models are often based on linear kinetic assumptions using linear differential equations.

A compartmental model provides a simple way of grouping all the tissues into one or more compartments where drugs move to and from the central or plasma compartment in a relatively homogeneous manner. The *mammillary model* is the most common compartment model used in pharmacokinetics. The mammillary model is a strongly connected system, because one can estimate the amount of drug in any compartment of the system after drug is introduced into a given compartment. In the one-compartment model, drug is both added to and eliminated from a central compartment. The *central compartment* is assigned to represent plasma and highly perfused tissues that rapidly equilibrate with drug. When an IV dose of drug is given, the drug enters directly into the central compartment. Elimination of drug occurs from the central compartment because the organs involved in drug elimination, primarily kidney and liver, are well-perfused tissues by cardiac blood flow.

In a *two-compartment model*, drug can move between the central or plasma compartment to and from the tissue compartment. Although the tissue compartment does not represent a specific tissue or group of tissues, mass balance accounts for the drug present in all the tissues. In this model, the total amount of drug in the body is the sum of drug present in the central compartment plus the drug present in the tissue compartment. Knowing the parameters of the one-compartment or the two-compartment model, the amount of drug left in the body and the amount of drug eliminated from the body can be estimated at any time. Compartmental models are particularly useful when little information is known about drug in tissues.

Several types of compartment models are described in Fig. 1-6. The pharmacokinetic rate constants are represented by the letter $k$. Compartment 1 represents the plasma or central compartment, and compartment 2 represents the tissue compartment. The diagram of models has three functions. The model (1) enables the pharmacokineticist to write differential equations to describe drug concentration changes in each compartment, (2) gives a visual representation of the rate processes, and (3) shows how many pharmacokinetic constants are necessary to describe the process adequately.

## EXAMPLE ▷ ▷ ▷

Two parameters are needed to describe model 1 (Fig. 1-6): the volume of the compartment and the elimination rate constant, $k$. In the case of model 4, the pharmacokinetic parameters consist of the volumes of compartments 1 and 2 and the rate constants—$k_a$, $k$, $k_{12}$, and $k_{21}$—for a total of six parameters.

In studying these models, it is important to know whether drug concentration data may be sampled directly from each compartment. For models 3 and 4 (Fig. 1-6), data concerning compartment 2 cannot be obtained easily because tissues are not easily sampled and may not contain homogeneous concentrations of drug. If the amount of drug absorbed and eliminated per unit time is obtained by sampling compartment 1, then the amount of drug contained in the tissue compartment 2 can be estimated mathematically. The appropriate mathematical equations for describing these models and evaluating the various pharmacokinetic parameters are given in subsequent chapters.

### Physiologic Based Pharmacokinetic Model (Flow Model)

*Physiologic based pharmacokinetic models* (PBPK), also known as blood flow or perfusion models, are pharmacokinetic models based on known anatomic and physiologic data. In contrast to the compartment model, the PBPK model includes individual organs or in some cases groups of organs and considers the blood flow to the organ and uptake of the drug by the organ. PBPK models use data that include tissues' drug concentrations and their respective blood flow. PBPK models are frequently used in describing drug distribution in animals, because tissue samples are available for assay. In contrast, tissue samples are not available for human subjects.

PBPK models assume an average set of blood flow and estimates of tissue drug concentrations. Drug uptake into organs is determined by blood flow to the organ and the binding of drug in these tissues. In the compartment model, a tissue volume of distribution is estimated indirectly. With the PBPK model, the actual tissue or organ volume is used. PBPK requires that each tissue volume in the body must be obtained and its drug concentration described. PBPK is a complex model and potentially predicts tissue drug concentrations better than the compartmental model. Unfortunately, much of the information required for adequately describing a PBPK model is experimentally difficult to obtain. In spite of this limitation, theoretically, the physiologic pharmacokinetic model may provide better insight into how physiologic factors may change drug distribution from one animal species to another. (Kawai, et al 1998) An example of a physiologic model is shown in Fig. 1-7. Physiological models are described in more detail in Chapters 11 and 19.

### FREQUENTLY ASKED QUESTIONS

▶ What are the reasons to use a multicompartment model instead of a physiologic model?

▶ What do the boxes in the mammillary model mean?

### Population Pharmacokinetic Models

Population pharmacokinetic models integrate relevant PK information across a range of doses and clinical studies to identify factors that can affect a drug's exposure. Statistical methods are used to predict drug response among patients in the population and quantify the variability in drug concentrations among individuals (Sheiner, et al 1982, Sheiner and Ludden 1992) (Chapters 11 and 23).

## COMPUTERS IN PHARMACOKINETICS

Mathematical models to describe rate processes have been used for over 100 years (Wagner, 1981). For example, Michaelis and Menten derived an equation for describing enzyme kinetics, later known as the Michaelis-Menten equation (Michaelis and Menten, 1913). In pharmacokinetics, this same equation is used to describe the elimination kinetics of ethanol, salicylate, phenytoin, and several other drugs. The solutions to these and other pharmacokinetic equations were tedious to solve manually. The development of computers and software packages has

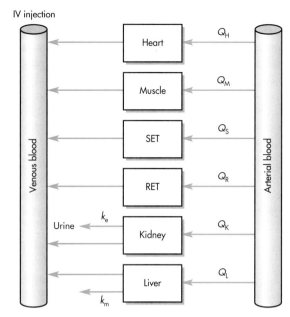

**FIGURE 1-7** • Pharmacokinetic model of drug perfusion. The *k*s represent kinetic constants: $k_e$ is the first-order rate constant for urinary drug excretion and $k_m$ is the rate constant for hepatic elimination. Each "box" represents a tissue compartment. Organs of major importance in drug absorption are considered separately, while other tissues are grouped as RET (rapidly equilibrating tissue) and SET (slowly equilibrating tissue). The size or mass of each tissue compartment is determined physiologically rather than by mathematical estimation. The concentration of drug in the tissue is determined by the ability of the tissue to accumulate drug as well as by the rate of blood perfusion to the tissue, represented by Q.

enabled the pharmacokineticist to process large data sets, develop more complicated models, solve complicated equations, make predictions, and develop simulations that would be difficult to solve manually.

Computer software packages use algorithms and equations to analyze experimental observations (data) and recommend an optimal pharmacokinetic model that can predict new data (Chapter 20). Computer simulations, sometimes termed *in silico*, can look at many different variables and predict multiple outcomes depending upon which assumptions are used in the model. *In silico* approaches in drug product development are used to predict human pharmacokinetic behavior of the experimental drug based on nonclinical (animal) studies. Some models, such as GastroPlus®, use anatomic, physiological, physical, and chemical descriptions to capture the behavior of the system being modeled (Chapter 20). The ability to run simulations for different scenarios can allow the investigator to make better decisions and potentially avoid performing expensive studies that fail to meet expectations.

## CHAPTER SUMMARY

*Drug product performance* is defined as the release of the drug substance from the drug product either for local drug action or for absorption into the plasma for systemic drug activity. *Biopharmaceutics* provides the scientific basis for drug product design and drug product performance. Biopharmaceutics examines the interrelationship of the physical/chemical properties of the drug, the type of drug product in which the drug is given, and the route of administration on the rate and extent of systemic drug absorption. *Pharmacokinetics* is the study movement of drug in the body and includes the kinetics of drug absorption, distribution, and elimination (ie, excretion and metabolism).

*Clinical pharmacokinetics* considers the applications of pharmacokinetics to drug therapy.

The quantitative measurement of drug concentrations in the plasma after dose administration is important to obtain relevant data of systemic drug exposure. The plasma drug concentration-versus-time profile provides the basic data from which various pharmacokinetic models can be developed that predict the time course of drug action, relates the drug concentration to the pharmacodynamic effect or adverse response, and enables the development of individualized therapeutic dosage regimens and new and novel drug delivery systems. Pharmacokinetic models and computer algorithms use simplifying assumptions to better understand the relationship of drug concentrations in the body to drug response.

## LEARNING QUESTIONS

1. What is the significance of the plasma level–time curve? How does the curve relate to the pharmacologic activity of a drug?

2. What is the purpose of pharmacokinetic models?

3. Draw a diagram describing a three-compartment model with first-order absorption and drug elimination from compartment 1.

4. The pharmacokinetic model presented in Fig. 1-8 represents a drug that is eliminated by renal excretion, biliary excretion, and drug metabolism. The metabolite distribution is described by a one-compartment open model. The following questions pertain to Fig. 1-8.

   a. How many parameters are needed to describe the model if the drug is injected intravenously (ie, the rate of drug absorption may be neglected)?

   b. Which compartment(s) can be sampled?

   c. What would be the overall elimination rate constant for elimination of drug from compartment 1?

   d. Write an expression describing the rate of change of drug concentration in compartment 1 ($dC_1/dt$).

5. Give two reasons for the measurement of the plasma drug concentration, $C_p$, assuming (a) the $C_p$ relates directly to the pharmacodynamic activity of the drug and (b) the $C_p$ does not relate to the pharmacodynamic activity of the drug.

6. Consider two biologic compartments separated by a biologic membrane. Drug A is found in compartment 1 and in compartment 2 in a concentration of $c_1$ and $c_2$, respectively.

   a. What possible conditions or situations would result in concentration $c_1 > c_2$ at equilibrium?

   b. How would you experimentally demonstrate these conditions given above?

   c. Under what conditions would $c_1 = c_2$ at equilibrium?

   d. The total amount of Drug A in each biologic compartment is $A_1$ and $A_2$, respectively. Describe a condition in which $A_1 > A_2$, but $c_1 = c_2$ at equilibrium.

   Include in your discussion how the physicochemical properties of Drug A or the biologic properties of each compartment might influence equilibrium conditions.

7. Why should a pharmacist read label revisions after a new drug is approved? Which part of the label do you expect mostly likely to be revised?

   a. The chemical structure of the drug

   b. The description section

   c. Adverse side effects

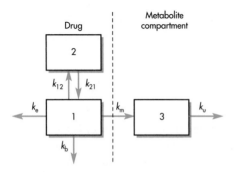

FIGURE 1-8 • Pharmacokinetic model for a drug eliminated by renal and biliary excretion and drug metabolism. $k_m$ = rate constant for metabolism of drug; $k_u$ = rate constant for urinary excretion of metabolites; $k_b$ = rate constant for biliary excretion of drug; and $k_e$ = rate constant for urinary drug excretion.

8. A pharmacist wishing to find if an excipient such as aspartame is in a product should look under which section in the SPL drug label?

   **a.** How supplied

   **b.** Patient guide

   **c.** Description

9. A pregnant patient is prescribed pantoprazole sodium (Protonix) delayed release tablets for erosive gastroesophageal reflux disease (GERD). Where would you find information concerning the safety of this drug in pregnant women?

## ANSWERS

### Frequently Asked Questions

*Why are drug concentrations more often measured in plasma rather than whole blood or serum?*

- Blood is composed of plasma and red blood cells (RBCs). Serum is the fluid obtained from blood after it is allowed to clot. Serum and plasma do not contain identical proteins. RBCs may be considered a cellular component of the body in which the drug concentration in the serum or plasma is in equilibrium, in the same way as with the other tissues in the body. Whole blood samples are generally harder to process and assay than serum or plasma samples. Plasma may be considered a liquid tissue compartment in which the drug in the plasma fluid equilibrates with drug in the tissues and cellular components.

*At what time intervals should plasma drug concentration be taken in order to best predict drug response and side effects?*

- The exact site of drug action is generally unknown for most drugs. The time needed for the drug to reach the site of action, produce a pharmacodynamic effect, and reach equilibrium are deduced from studies on the relationship of the time course for the drug concentration and the pharmacodynamic effect. Often, the drug concentration is sampled during the elimination phase after the drug has been distributed and reached equilibrium. For multiple-dose studies, both the peak and trough drug concentrations are frequently taken.

*What are the reasons to use a multicompartment model instead of a physiologic model?*

- Physiologic models are complex and require more information for accurate prediction compared to compartment models. Missing information in the physiologic model will lead to

bias or error in the model. Compartment models are more simplistic and they assume that both arterial and venous drug concentrations are similar. The compartment model accounts for a rapid distribution phase and a slower elimination phase. Physiologic clearance models postulate that arterial blood drug levels are higher than venous blood drug levels. In practice, only venous blood samples are obtained. Organ drug clearance is useful in the treatment of cancers and in the diagnosis of certain diseases involving arterial perfusion. Physiologic models are difficult to use for general application.

### Learning Questions

1. The plasma drug level–time curve describes the pharmacokinetics of the systemically absorbed drug. Once a suitable pharmacokinetic model is obtained, plasma drug concentrations may be predicted following various dosage regimens such as single oral and IV bolus doses, multiple-dose regimens, IV infusion, etc. If the pharmacokinetics of the drug relates to its pharmacodynamic activity (or any adverse drug response or toxicity), then a drug regimen based on the drug's pharmacokinetics may be designed to provide optimum drug efficacy. In lieu of a direct pharmacokinetic–pharmacodynamic relationship, the drug's pharmacokinetics describes the bioavailability of the drug including inter- and intrasubject variability; this information allows for the development of drug products that consistently deliver the drug in a predictable manner.

2. The purpose of pharmacokinetic models is to relate the time course of the drug in the body to

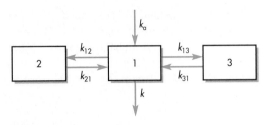

FIGURE A-1 •

its pharmacodynamic and/or toxic effects. The pharmacokinetic model also provides a basis for drug product design, the design of dosage regimens, and a better understanding of the action of the body on the drug.

3. (Figure A-1)

4. **a.** Nine parameters: $V_1$, $V_2$, $V_3$, $k_{12}$, $k_{21}$, $k_e$, $k_b$, $k_m$, $k_u$

   **b.** Compartment 1 and compartment 3 may be sampled.

   **c.** $k = k_b + k_m + k_e$

   **d.** $\dfrac{dC_1}{dt} = k_{21}C_2 - (k_{12} + k_m + k_e + k_b)C_1$

6.

| Compartment 1 | Compartment 2 |
|---------------|---------------|
| $C_1$ | $C_2$ |

**a.** $C_1$ and $C_2$ are the *total* drug concentration in each compartment, respectively. $C_1 > C_2$ may occur if the drug concentrates in compartment 1 due to protein binding (compartment 1 contains a high amount of protein or special protein binding), due to partitioning (compartment 1 has a high lipid content and the drug is poorly water soluble), if the pH is different in each compartment and the drug is a weak electrolyte (the drug may be more ionized in compartment 1), or if there is an active transport mechanism for the drug to be taken up into the cell (eg, purine drug). Other explanations for $C_1 > C_2$ may be possible.

**b.** Several different experimental conditions are needed to prove which of the above hypotheses is the most likely cause for $C_1 > C_2$. These

experiments may use *in vivo* or *in vitro* methods, including intracellular electrodes to measure pH *in vivo*, protein-binding studies *in vitro*, and partitioning of drug in chloroform/water *in vitro*, among others.

**c.** In the case of protein binding, the total concentration of drug in each compartment may be different (eg, $C_1 > C_2$) and, at the same time, the free (nonprotein-bound) drug concentration may be equal in each compartment—assuming that the free or unbound drug is easily diffusible. Similarly, if $C_1 > C_2$ is due to differences in pH and the nonionized drug is easily diffusible, then the nonionized drug concentration may be the same in each compartment. The total drug concentrations will be $C_1 = C_2$ when there is similar affinity for the drug and similar conditions in each compartment.

**d.** The total amount of drug, $A$, in each compartment depends on the volume, $V$, of the compartment and the concentration, $C$, of the drug in the compartment. Since the amount of drug ($A$) = concentration ($C$) times volume ($V$), any condition that causes the product, $C_1V_1 \neq C_2V_2$, will result in $A_1 \neq A_2$. Thus, if $C_1 = C_2$ and $V_1 \neq V_2$, then $A_1 \neq A_2$.

7. A newly approved NDA generally contains sufficient information for use labeled. However, as more information becomes available through postmarketing commitment studies, more information is added to the labeling, including Warnings and Precautions.

8. An excipient such as aspartame in a product is mostly found under the Description section, which describes the drug chemical structure and the ingredients in the drug product.

9. Section 8, Use in Specific Populations, reports information for geriatric, pediatric, renal, and hepatic subjects. This section will report dosing for pediatric subjects as well.

## REFERENCES

Cone EJ, Darwin WD, Wang W-L: The occurrence of cocaine, heroin and metabolites in hair of drug abusers. *Forensic Sci Int* **63**:55–68, 1993.

FDA Guidance for Industry: Exposure-Response Relationships—Study Design, Data Analysis, and Regulatory Applications, FDA, Center for Drug Evaluation and Research, April 2003 (http://www.fda.gov/cder/guidance/5341fnl.htm).

FDA Guidance for Industry: Labeling for Human Prescription Drug and Biological Products – Implementing the PLR Content and Format Requirements, February 2013.

Kawai R, Mathew D, Tanaka C, Rowland M: Physiologically based pharmacokinetics of cyclosporine. *J Pharmacol Exp Ther* **287**:457–468.

Leal M, Yacobi A, Batra VJ: Use of toxicokinetic principles in drug development: Bridging preclinical and clinical studies. In Yacobi A, Skelly JP, Shah VP, Benet LZ (eds). *Integration of Pharmacokinetics, Pharmacodynamics and Toxicokinetics in Rational Drug Development*. New York, Plenum Press, 1993, pp 55–67.

Michaelis L, Menten ML: Die Kinetik der Invertinwirkung. *Biochem Z* **49**:333–369, 1913.

Pippenger CE, Massoud N: Therapeutic drug monitoring. In Benet LZ, et al (eds). *Pharmacokinetic Basis for Drug Treatment*. New York, Raven, 1984, chap 21.

Rodman JH, Evans WE: Targeted systemic exposure for pediatric cancer therapy. In D'Argenio DZ (ed). *Advanced Methods of Pharmacokinetic and Pharmacodynamic Systems Analysis*. New York, Plenum Press, 1991, pp 177–183.

Sheiner LB, Beal SL: Bayesian individualization of pharmacokinetics. Simple implementation and comparison with non-Bayesian methods. *J Pharm Sci* **71**:1344–1348, 1982.

Sheiner LB, Ludden TM: Population pharmacokinetics/dynamics. *Annu Rev Pharmacol Toxicol* **32**:185–201, 1992.

Wagner, JG: History of pharmacokinetics. *Pharmacol Ther* **12**:537–562, 1981.

## BIBLIOGRAPHY

Benet LZ: General treatment of linear mammillary models with elimination from any compartment as used in pharmacokinetics. *J Pharm Sci* **61**:536–541, 1972.

Benowitz N, Forsyth R, Melmon K, Rowland M: Lidocaine disposition kinetics in monkey and man. *Clin Pharmacol Ther* **15**:87–98, 1974.

Bischoff K, Brown R: Drug distribution in mammals. *Chem Eng Med* **62**:33–45, 1966.

Tucker GT, Boas RA: Pharmacokinetic aspects of IV regional anesthesia. *Anesthesiology* **34**:538–549, 1971.

Bischoff K, Dedrick R, Zaharko D, Longstreth T: Methotrexate pharmacokinetics. *J Pharm Sci* **60**:1128–1133, 1971.

Chiou W: Quantitation of hepatic and pulmonary first-pass effect and its implications in pharmacokinetic study. I: Pharmacokinetics of chloroform in man. *J Pharm Biopharm* **3**:193–201, 1975.

Colburn WA: Controversy III: To model or not to model. *J Clin Pharmacol* **28**:879–888, 1988.

Cowles A, Borgstedt H, Gilles A: Tissue weights and rates of blood flow in man for the prediction of anesthetic uptake and distribution. *Anesthesiology* **35**:523–526, 1971.

Dedrick R, Forrester D, Cannon T, et al: Pharmacokinetics of 1-β-d-arabinofurinosulcytosine (ARA-C) deamination in several species. *Biochem Pharmacol* **22**:2405–2417, 1972.

Gerlowski LE, Jain RK: Physiologically based pharmacokinetic modeling: Principles and applications. *J Pharm Sci* **72**:1103–1127, 1983.

Gibaldi M: *Biopharmaceutics and Clinical Pharmacokinetics*, 3rd ed. Philadelphia, Lea & Febiger, 1984.

Gibaldi M: Estimation of the pharmacokinetic parameters of the two-compartment open model from post-infusion plasma concentration data. *J Pharm Sci* **58**:1133–1135, 1969.

Himmelstein KJ, Lutz RJ: A review of the applications of physiologically based pharmacokinetic modeling. *J Pharm Biopharm* **7**:127–145, 1979.

Lutz R, Dedrick RL: Physiologic pharmacokinetics: Relevance to human risk assessment. In Li AP (ed). *Toxicity Testing: New Applications and Applications in Human Risk Assessment*. New York, Raven, 1985, pp 129–149.

Lutz R, Dedrick R, Straw J, et al: The kinetics of methotrexate distribution in spontaneous canine lymphosarcoma. *J Pharm Biopharm* **3**:77–97, 1975.

Mallet A, Mentre F, Steimer JL, Lokiec F: Pharmacometrics: Nonparametric maximum likelihood estimation for population pharmacokinetics, with application to cyclosporine. *J Pharm Biopharm* **16**:311–327, 1988.

Metzler CM: Estimation of pharmacokinetic parameters: Statistical considerations. *Pharmacol Ther* **13**:543–556, 1981.

Montandon B, Roberts R, Fischer L: Computer simulation of sulfobromophthalein kinetics in the rat using flow-limited models with extrapolation to man. *J Pharm Biopharm* **3**:277–290, 1975.

Rescigno A, Beck JS: The use and abuse of models. *J Pharm Biopharm* **15**:327–344, 1987.

Ritschel WA, Banerjee PS: Physiologic pharmacokinetic models: Applications, limitations and outlook. *Meth Exp Clin Pharmacol* **8**:603–614, 1986.

Rowland M, Tozer T: *Clinical Pharmacokinetics—Concepts and Applications*, 3rd ed. Philadelphia, Lea & Febiger, 1995.

Rowland M, Thomson P, Guichard A, Melmon K: Disposition kinetics of lidocaine in normal subjects. *Ann NY Acad Sci* **179**:383–398, 1971.

Segre G: Pharmacokinetics: Compartmental representation. *Pharm Ther* **17**:111–127, 1982.

Tozer TN: Pharmacokinetic principles relevant to bioavailability studies. In Blanchard J, Sawchuk RJ, Brodie BB (eds). *Principles and Perspectives in Drug Bioavailability*. New York, S Karger, 1979, pp 120–155.

Wagner JG: Do you need a pharmacokinetic model, and, if so, which one? *J Pharm Biopharm* **3**:457–478, 1975.

Welling P, Tse F: *Pharmacokinetics*. New York, Marcel Dekker, 1993.

Winters ME: *Basic Clinical Pharmacokinetics*, 3rd ed. Vancouver, WA, Applied Therapeutics, 1994.

# 2

# Mathematical Fundamentals in Pharmacokinetics

Antoine Al-Achi

## CHAPTER OBJECTIVES[1]

- Algebraically solve mathematical expressions related to pharmacokinetics.

- Express the calculated and theoretical pharmacokinetic values in proper units.

- Represent pharmacokinetic data graphically using Cartesian coordinates (rectangular coordinate system) and semilogarithmic graphs.

- Use the least squares method to find the best fit straight line through empirically obtained data.

- Define various models representing rates and order of reactions and calculate pharmacokinetic parameters (eg, zero- and first-order) from experimental data based on these models.

---

[1]It is not the objective of this chapter to provide a detailed description of mathematical functions, algebra, or statistics. Readers who are interested in learning more about these topics are encouraged to consult textbooks specifically addressing these subjects.

## CALCULUS

Pharmacokinetic models consider drugs in the body to be in a dynamic state. Calculus is an important mathematical tool for analyzing drug movement quantitatively. Differential equations are used to relate the change in concentrations of drugs in various body organs over time. Integrated equations are frequently used to model the cumulative therapeutic or toxic responses of drugs in the body.

### Differential Calculus

Differential calculus is a branch of calculus that involves finding the rate at which a variable quantity is changing. For example, a specific amount of drug $X$ is placed in a beaker of water to dissolve. The rate at which the drug dissolves is determined by the rate of drug diffusing away from the surface of the solid drug and is expressed by the *Noyes–Whitney equation*:

The Noyes–Whitney equation may be written in two possible ways:

$$\frac{dX}{dt} = \frac{DA}{l}(C_1 - C_2)$$

where $X$ is the amount or mass (mg) of the solute dissolved at time $t$

$$\frac{dC}{dt} = \frac{DA}{l}(C_1 - C_2)$$

where C is the concentration (mg/L) of drug at time $t$

$$\text{Dissolution rate} = \frac{dC}{dt} = \frac{DA}{l}(C_1 - C_2)$$

where $d$ denotes a very small change; $C$ = concentration of drug $X$; $t$ = time; $D$ = diffusion coefficient; $A$ = effective surface area of drug; $l$ = length of diffusion layer; $C_1$ = surface concentration of drug in the diffusion layer; and $C_2$ = concentration of drug in the bulk solution.

The derivative $dC/dt$ may be interpreted as a change in $C$ (or a derivative of $C$) with respect to a change in $t$.

In pharmacokinetics, the amount or concentration of drug in the body is a variable quantity (dependent variable), and time is an independent variable. Thus, we consider the amount or concentration of drug to vary with respect to time.

# EXAMPLE ▷ ▷ ▷

The concentration $C$ of a drug changes as a function of time $t$:

$$C = f(t) \qquad (2.1)$$

Consider the following data:

| Time (hours) | Plasma Concentration of Drug C (μg/mL) |
|:---:|:---:|
| 0 | 12 |
| 1 | 10 |
| 2 | 8 |
| 3 | 6 |
| 4 | 4 |
| 5 | 2 |

The concentration of drug $C$ in the plasma is declining by a constant rate of 2 μg/mL for each hour of time. The rate of change in the concentration of the drug with respect to time (ie, the derivative of $C$) may be expressed as

$$\frac{dC}{dt} = 2\,\mu g/mL/h$$

Here, $f(t)$ is a mathematical equation that describes how $C$ changes, expressed as

$$C = 12 - 2t \qquad (2.2)$$

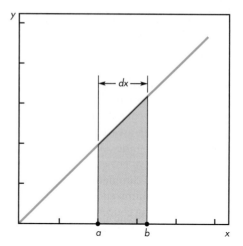

FIGURE 2-1 • Integration of $y = ax$ or $\int ax \cdot dx$.

## Integral Calculus

Integration is the reverse of differentiation and is considered the summation of $f(x) \cdot dx$; the integral sign $\int$ implies summation. For example, given the function $y = ax$, plotted in Fig. 2-1, the integration is $\int ax \cdot dx$. Compare Fig. 2-1 to a second graph (Fig. 2-2), where the function $y = Ae^{-x}$ is commonly observed after an intravenous bolus drug injection. The integration process is actually a summing up of the small individual pieces under the graph. When $x$ is specified and is given boundaries from $a$ to $b$, then the expression becomes a definite integral, that is, the summing up of the area from $x = a$ to $x = b$.

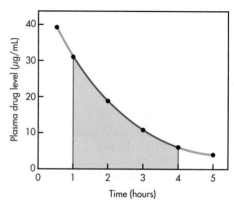

FIGURE 2-2 • Graph of the elimination of drug from the plasma after a single IV injection.

A *definite integral* of a mathematical function is the sum of individual areas under the graph of that function. There are several reasonably accurate numerical methods for approximating an area. These methods can be programmed into a computer for rapid calculation. The *trapezoidal rule* is a numerical method frequently used in pharmacokinetics to calculate the area under the plasma drug concentration-versus-time curve, called the *area under the curve* (AUC). For example, Fig. 2-2 shows a curve depicting the elimination of a drug from the plasma after a single intravenous injection. For most drugs, the plasma drug concentrations decline exponentially in the body. The drug plasma levels and the corresponding time intervals plotted in Fig. 2-2 are as follows:

| Time (hours) | Plasma Drug Level (µg/mL) |
|---|---|
| 1.0 | 30.3 |
| 2.0 | 18.4 |
| 3.0 | 11.1 |
| 4.0 | 6.77 |
| 5.0 | 4.10 |

## Area under the Curve (AUC)

The AUC is used in pharmacokinetics as a measure for amount of drug in the body. The *trapezoidal rule* is used to estimate the AUC and does not depend upon the shape of the plasma drug concentration versus time curve.

The area between time intervals is the area of a trapezoid and can be calculated with the following formula:

$$[AUC]_{t_{n-1}}^{t_n} = \frac{C_{n-1} + C_n}{2}(t_n - t_{n-1}) \qquad (2.3)$$

where [AUC] = area under the curve, $t_n$ = time of observation of drug concentration $C_n$, and $t_{n-1}$ = time of prior observation of drug concentration corresponding to $C_{n-1}$.

To obtain the AUC from 1 to 5 hours in Fig. 2-2, each portion of this area must be summed. The AUC between 1 and 2 hours is calculated by proper substitution into Equation 2.3:

$$[AUC]_{t_1}^{t_2} = \frac{30.3 + 18.4}{2}(2-1) = 24.35 \ \mu g \cdot h/mL$$

Similarly, the AUC between 2 and 3 hours is calculated as 14.8 µg · h/mL, the AUC between 3 and 4 hours is calculated as 8.9 µg · h/mL, and that between 4 and 5 hours is 5.44 µg · h/mL. The total AUC between 1 and 5 hours is obtained by adding the AUC values together (24.4 + 14.8 + 8.9 + 5.4) = 53.5 µg · h/mL.

The total area under the plasma drug level–time curve from time zero to infinity (Fig. 2-2) is obtained by summation of each individual area between each pair of consecutive data points using the trapezoidal rule. The value on the $y$ axis when time equals 0 is estimated by back extrapolation of the data points using a log linear plot (ie, log $y$ vs $x$). The last plasma level–time curve is extrapolated to $t = \infty$. In this case, the residual area $[AUC]_{t_n}^{t_\infty}$ is calculated as follows:

$$[AUC]_{t_n}^{t_\infty} = \frac{C_{pn}}{k} \qquad (2.4)$$

where $C_{pn}$ = last observed plasma concentration at $t_n$ and $k$ = slope obtained from the terminal portion of the curve.

The trapezoidal rule written in its full form to calculate the AUC from $t = 0$ to $t = \infty$ is as follows:

$$[AUC]_0^\infty = \Sigma[AUC]_{t_{n-1}}^{t_n} + \frac{C_{pm}}{k}$$

This numerical method of obtaining the AUC is fairly accurate if sufficient data points are available. As the number of data points increases, the trapezoidal method of approximating the area becomes more accurate.

The trapezoidal rule assumes a linear or straight-line function between data points. If the data points are spaced widely, then the normal curvature of the line will cause a greater error in the area estimate.

---

**FREQUENTLY ASKED QUESTIONS**

▶ What are the units for logarithms?

▶ What is the difference between a common log and a natural log (ln)?

---

## GRAPHS

The construction of a curve or straight line by plotting observed or experimental data on a graph is an important method of visualizing relationships between variables. By general custom, the values of

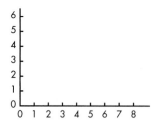

FIGURE 2-3 • Rectangular coordinates.

the independent variable ($x$) are placed on the horizontal line in a plane, or on the abscissa ($x$ axis), whereas the values of the dependent variable are placed on the vertical line in the plane, or on the ordinate ($y$ axis). The values are usually arranged so that they increase linearly or logarithmically from left to right and from bottom to top.

In pharmacokinetics, time is the independent variable and is plotted on the abscissa ($x$ axis), whereas drug concentration is the dependent variable and is plotted on the ordinate ($y$ axis). Two types of graphs or graph papers are usually used in pharmacokinetics. These are Cartesian or rectangular coordinate (Fig. 2-3) and semilogarithmic graph or graph paper (Fig. 2-4). Semilogarithmic allows placement of the data at logarithmic intervals so that the numbers need not be converted to their corresponding log values prior to plotting on the graph.

## Curve Fitting

Fitting a curve to the points on a graph implies that there is some sort of relationship between the variables $x$ and $y$, such as dose of drug versus pharmacologic effect (eg, lowering of blood pressure). Moreover, when using curve fitting, the relationship is not confined to isolated points but is a continuous function of $x$ and $y$. In many cases, a hypothesis is made concerning the relationship between the variables $x$ and $y$. Then, an empirical equation is formed that best describes the hypothesis. This empirical equation must satisfactorily fit the experimental or observed data. If the relationship between $x$ and $y$ is linearly related, then the relationship between the two can be expressed as a straight line.

Physiologic variables are not always linearly related. However, the data may be arranged or transformed to express the relationship between the variables as a straight line. Straight lines are very useful for accurately *predicting* values for which there are no experimental observations.

## Linear Regression/Least Squares Method

This method is often encountered and used in clinical pharmacy studies to construct a linear relationship between an independent variable (also known as the input factor or the $x$ factor) and a dependent variable (commonly known as an output variable, an outcome, or the $y$ factor). In pharmacokinetics, the relationship between the plasma drug concentrations versus time can be expressed as a linear function. Because of the availability of computing devices (computer programs, scientific calculators, etc), the development of a linear equation has indeed become a simple task.

The values of the slope and the $y$ intercept may be positive, negative, or zero. A positive linear relationship has a positive slope, and a negative slope belongs to a negative linear relationship (Gaddis and Gaddis, 1990; Munro, 2005).

The strength of the linear relationship is assessed by the correlation coefficient ($r$). The value of $r$ is positive when the slope is positive, and it is negative when the slope is negative. When $r$ takes the value of either $+1$ or $-1$, a perfect linear relationship exists between the variables. A zero value for the slope (or for $r$) indicates that there is no linear relationship existing between $y$ and $x$ (Fig. 2-5). In addition to $r$, the coefficient of determination ($r^2$) is often computed to express how much variability in the outcome is explained by the input factor. For example, if $r$ is 0.90, then $r^2$ equals to 0.81. This means that the input variable explains 81% of the variability observed in $y$. It should be

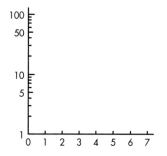

FIGURE 2-4 • Semilog coordinates.

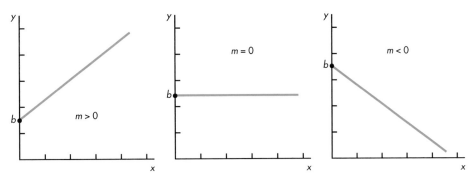

FIGURE 2-5 • Graphic demonstration of variations in slope (*m*).

noted, however, that a high correlation between the two variables does not necessarily mean causation. For example, the passage of time is not really the cause for the drug concentration in the plasma to decrease. Rather it is the physiological distribution and the elimination functions that cause the level of the drug to decrease over time (Gaddis and Gaddis, 1990; Munro, 2005).

The linear regression/least squares method assumes, for simplicity, that there is a linear relationship between the variables. If a linear line deviates substantially from the data, it may suggest the need for a nonlinear regression model. Nonlinear regression models are complex mathematical procedures that are best performed with a computer program.

## PRACTICE PROBLEM

Plot the following data and obtain the equation for the line that best fits the data by (a) using a ruler and (b) using the method of least squares. Data can be plotted manually or by using a computer spreadsheet program such as Microsoft Excel.

| x (mg) | y (hours) | x (mg) | y (hours) |
|--------|-----------|--------|-----------|
| 1 | 3.1 | 5 | 15.3 |
| 2 | 6.0 | 6 | 17.9 |
| 3 | 8.7 | 7 | 22.0 |
| 4 | 12.9 | 8 | 23.0 |

### Solution

Many computer programs have a regression analysis, which fits data to a straight line by least squares. In the least squares regression, the slope $m$ and the $y$ intercept $b$ are calculated so that the average sum of the deviations squared is minimized (ie, $\Sigma(y_i - y_{Line})^2 =$ minimum). (A deviation is the distance between the observed value and the predicted value from the linear equation.)

The following graph was obtained by using a Microsoft Excel spreadsheet and calculating a regression line (sometimes referred to as a trendline in the computer program):

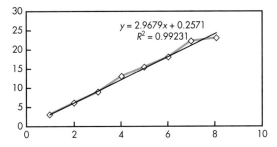

Therefore, the linear equation that best fits the data is

$$y = 2.97x + 0.257$$

Although an equation for a straight line is obtained by the least squares procedure, the reliability of the values should be ascertained. A correlation coefficient, $r$, is a useful statistical term that indicates the relationship of the $x,y$ data fit to a straight line. For a perfect linear relationship between $x$ and $y$, $r = \pm 1$. Usually, $|r| \geq 0.95$ demonstrates good evidence or a strong correlation that there is a linear relationship between $x$ and $y$.

### Problems of Fitting Points to a Graph

When $x$ and $y$ data points are plotted on a graph, a relationship between the $x$ and $y$ variables is sought. Linear relationships are useful for predicting values for the dependent variable $y$, given values for the independent variable $x$.

The *linear regression* calculation using the least squares method is used for calculating a straight line through a given set of points. However, it is important to realize that, when using this method, one has already assumed that the data points are related linearly. Indeed, for three points, this linear relationship may not always be true. As shown in Fig. 2-6, Riggs (1963) calculated three different curves that fit the data accurately. Generally, one should consider the *law of parsimony*, which broadly means "keep it simple"; that is, if a choice between two hypotheses is available, choose the simpler relationship.

If a linear relationship exists between the $x$ and $y$ variables, one must be careful as to the estimated value for the dependent variable $y$, assuming a value for the independent variable $x$. *Interpolation*, which means filling the gap between the observed data on a graph, is usually safe and assumes that the trend between the observed data points is consistent and predictable. In contrast, the process of *extrapolation* means predicting new data beyond the observed data, and assumes that the same trend obtained between two data points will extend in either direction beyond the last observed data points. The use of extrapolation may be erroneous if the regression line no longer follows the same trend beyond the measured points.

Graphs should always have the axes (abscissa and ordinate) properly labeled with units. For example, the amount of drug on the ordinate ($y$ axis) is given in milligrams and the time on the abscissa ($x$ axis) is given in hours. The equation that best fits the points on this curve is the equation for a straight line, or $y = mx + b$. Because the slope $m = \Delta y / \Delta x$, the units for the slope should be milligrams per hour (mg/h). Similarly, the units for the $y$ intercept $b$ should be the same units as those for $y$, namely, milligrams (mg).

## MATHEMATICAL EXPRESSIONS AND UNITS

*Mathematics* is a basic science that helps to explain relationships among variables. For an equation to be valid, the units or dimensions must be constant on both sides of the equation. Many different units are used in pharmacokinetics, as listed in Table 2-1. For an accurate equation, both the integers and the units must balance. For example, a common expression for total body clearance is

$$Cl_T = kV_d \tag{2.5}$$

After insertion of the proper units for each term in the above equation from Table 2-1,

$$\frac{\text{mL}}{\text{h}} = \frac{1}{\text{h}}\text{mL}$$

Thus, the above equation is valid, as shown by the equality mL/h = mL/h.

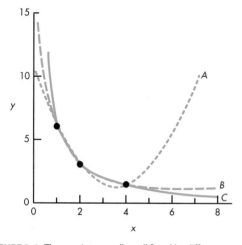

**FIGURE 2-6** • Three points equally well fitted by different curves. The parabola, $y = 10.5 - 5.25x + 0.75x^2$ (*curve A*); the exponential, $y = 12.93e^{-1.005}x + 1.27$ (*curve B*); and the rectangular hyperbola, $y = 6/x$ (*curve C*) all fit the three points (1,6), (2,3), and (4,1.5) perfectly, as would an infinite number of other curves. (Reproduced with permission from Riggs DS: The Mathematical Approach to Physiological Problems. Baltimore, MA: Williams & Wilkins; 1963.)

## TABLE 2-1 • Common Units Used in Pharmacokinetics

| Parameter | Symbol | Unit | Example |
|-----------|--------|------|---------|
| Rate | $\dfrac{dD}{dt}$ | $\dfrac{\text{Mass}}{\text{Time}}$ | mg/h |
| | $\dfrac{dC}{dt}$ | $\dfrac{\text{Concentration}}{\text{Time}}$ | ug/mL/h |
| Zero-order rate constant | $K_0$ | $\dfrac{\text{Concentration}}{\text{Time}}$ | µg/mL/h |
| | | $\dfrac{\text{Mass}}{\text{Time}}$ | mg/h |
| First-order rate constant | $k$ | $\dfrac{1}{\text{Time}}$ | 1/h or h⁻¹ |
| Drug dose | $D_0$ | Mass | mg |
| Concentration | $C$ | $\dfrac{\text{Mass}}{\text{Volume}}$ | µg/mL |
| Plasma drug concentration | $Cp$ | $\dfrac{\text{Drug}}{\text{Volume}}$ | µg/mL |
| Volume | $V$ | Volume | mL or L |
| Area under the curve | AUC | Concentration × time | µg · h/mL |
| Fraction of drug absorbed | $F$ | No units | 0 to 1 |
| Clearance | $Cl$ | $\dfrac{\text{Volume}}{\text{Time}}$ | mL/h |
| Half-life | $t_{1/2}$ | Time | H |

An important rule in using equations with different units is that the units may be added or subtracted if they are alike but divided or multiplied if they are different. When in doubt, check the equation by inserting the proper units. For example,

$$\text{AUC} = \frac{FD_0}{kV_D} = \text{concentration} \times \text{time} \quad (2.6)$$

$$\frac{\mu g}{mL}h = \frac{1\,mg}{h^{-1}L} = \frac{\mu g \cdot h}{mL}$$

Certain terms have no units. These terms include logarithms and ratios. Percent may have no units and is expressed mathematically as a decimal between 0 and 1 or as 0% to 100%, respectively. On occasion, percent may indicate mass/volume, volume/volume, or mass/mass. Table 2-1 lists common pharmacokinetic parameters with their symbols and units.

A constant is often inserted in an equation to quantify the relationship of the dependent variable to the independent variable. For example, *Fick's law of diffusion* relates the rate of drug diffusion, $dQ/dt$, to the change in drug concentration, $C$, the surface area of the membrane, $A$, and the thickness of the membrane, $h$. In order to make this relationship an equation, a diffusion constant $D$ is inserted:

$$\frac{dQ}{dt} = \frac{DA}{h} \times \Delta C \quad (2.7)$$

To obtain the proper units for $D$, the units for each of the other terms must be inserted:

$$\frac{mg}{h} = \frac{D\,(cm^2)}{cm} \times \frac{mg}{cm^3}$$

$$D = cm^2 / h$$

The diffusion constant $D$ must have the units of area/time or cm$^2$/h if the rate of diffusion is in mg/h.

## UNITS FOR EXPRESSING BLOOD CONCENTRATIONS

Various units have been used in pharmacology, toxicology, and the clinical laboratory to express drug concentrations in blood, plasma, or serum. Drug concentrations or drug levels should be expressed as mass/volume. The expressions mcg/mL, $\mu$g/mL, and mg/L are equivalent and are commonly reported in the literature. Drug concentrations may also be reported as mg% or mg/dL, both of which indicate milligrams of drug per 100 mL (1 deciliter) of blood. Two older expressions for drug concentration occasionally used in veterinary medicine are the terms ppm and ppb, which indicate the number of parts of drug per one million parts of blood (ppm) or per one billion parts of blood (ppb), respectively. One ppm is equivalent to 1.0 $\mu$g/mL. The accurate interconversion of units is often necessary to prevent confusion and misinterpretation.

## MEASUREMENT AND USE OF SIGNIFICANT FIGURES

Every measurement is performed within a certain degree of accuracy, which is limited by the instrument used for the measurement. For example, the weight of freight on a truck may be measured accurately to the nearest 0.5 kg, whereas the mass of drug in a tablet may be measured to 0.001 g (1 mg). Measuring the weight of freight on a truck to the nearest milligram is not necessary and would require a very costly balance or scale to detect a change in a milligram quantity.

*Significant figures* are the number of accurate digits in a measurement. If a balance measures the mass of a drug to the nearest milligram, measurements containing digits representing less than 1 mg are inaccurate. For example, in reading the weight or mass of a drug of 123.8 mg from this balance, the 0.8 mg is only approximate; the number is therefore rounded to 124 mg and reported as the observed mass.

For practical calculation purposes, all figures may be used until the final number (answer) is obtained. However, the answer should retain only the number of significant figures in the least accurate initial measurement.

## PRACTICE PROBLEM

When a patient swallows a tablet containing 325 mg of aspirin (ASA), the tablet comes in contact with the contents of the gastrointestinal tract and the ASA is released from the tablet. Assuming a constant amount of the drug release over time ($t$), the rate of drug release is expressed as:

$$\text{Rate of drug (ASA) release (mg / min)} = \frac{d(\text{ASA})}{dt}$$

$$= k_0$$

where $k_0$ is a rate constant.

Integration of the rate expression above gives Equation 2.8:

$$\text{Amount of ASA released (mg)} = at + b \quad (2.8)$$

The symbol $a$ represents the slope (equivalent to $k_0$), $t$ is time, and $b$ is the $y$ intercept. Assuming that time was measured in minutes, the following mathematical expression is obtained representing Equation 2.8:

$$\text{Amount of ASA released (mg)} = 0.86t - 0.04 \quad (2.9)$$

To calculate the amount of ASA released at 180 seconds, the following algebraic manipulations are needed:

1. Convert 180 seconds to minutes: 3 minutes.
2. Replace $t$ in Equation 2.9 by the value 3.
3. Solve the equation for the amount of ASA released.

$$\text{Amount of ASA released (mg)} = 0.86(3) - 0.04$$
$$= 2.54 \text{ mg}$$

A pharmacist is interested in learning the time needed for 90% of ASA to be released from the tablet. To answer her inquiry the following steps are taken:

1. Calculate the amount of ASA in milligrams representing 90% of the drug present in the tablet.

2. Replace the value found in step (1) in Equation 2.9 and solve for time ($t$):

90% of 325 = (0.9) (325 mg) = 292.5 mg

292.5 mg = 0.86$t$ − 0.04

292.5 + 0.04 = 0.86$t$

Dividing both sides of the equation by 0.86:

(292.5 + 0.04)/0.86 = (0.86$t$)/0.86

340.2 minutes = $t$

Or it takes 5.7 hours for this amount of ASA (90%) to be released from the tablet.

The above calculations show that this tablet releases the drug very slowly over time and it may not be useful in practice when the need for the drug is more immediate. It should also be emphasized that only the amount of the drug released and soluble in the GI juices is available for absorption. If the drug precipitates out in the GI tract, it will not be absorbed by the GI mucosa. It is also assumed that the unabsorbed portion of the drug in the GI tract is considered to be "outside the body" because its effect cannot be exerted systematically.

To calculate the amount of ASA that was immediately released from the tablet upon contact with gastric juices, the time in Equation 2.9 is set to the value zero:

Amount of ASA released (mg) = 0.86(0) − 0.04
Amount of ASA released (mg) = −0.04 mg

Since an amount released cannot be negative, this indicates that no amount of ASA is released from the tablet instantly upon coming in touch with the juices. Equation 2.9 may be represented graphically using Cartesian or rectangular coordinates (Fig. 2-7).

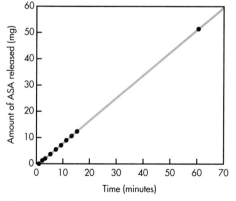

FIGURE 2-7 • Amount of ASA released versus time (minutes) plotted on Cartesian coordinates.

## PRACTICE PROBLEM

Briefly, $C_{max}$ is the maximum drug concentration in the plasma and $T_{max}$ is the time associated with $C_{max}$ (see Fig. 1-4, Chapter 1). First-order elimination rate constant signifies the fraction of the drug that is eliminated per unit time. The biological half-life of the drug is the time needed for 50% of the drug to be eliminated. The AUC term or the area under the drug plasma concentration-versus-time curve reflects the extent of absorption from the site of administration. The term AUMC is the area under the moment curve, whereas MRT is the mean residence time, which is estimated from the ratio of AUMC(0–infinity)/AUC(0–infinity). These pharmacokinetic terms are discussed in more details throughout this textbook.

Table 2-X shows pharmacokinetic data obtained from a study conducted in rabbits following administration of various formulations of rectal suppositories containing ASA (600 mg each). Various formulations were prepared in a suppository base made of a mixture of gelatin and glycerin. Formulation Fas9 had the same composition as Fs9 with the exception that Fas9 contained ASA in the form of nanoparticles, whereas Fs9 had ASA in its free form (so did formulations Fs2, Fs4, and Fs11, but varied in their gelatin/glycerin composition). The authors concluded that the incorporation of ASA in the form of nanoparticles increased the $T_{max}$. The other pharmacokinetic parameters taken together indicate that nanoparticles produced a sustained-release profile of ASA when given in this dosage form. In this study, the plasma concentration was expressed in "micrograms per milliliter." If the $\mu g/mL$ were not specified, it would have been difficult to compare the results from this study with other similar studies. It is imperative, therefore, that pharmacokinetic parameters such as $C_{max}$ be properly defined by units.

Expressing the $C_{max}$ value by equivalent units is also possible. For example, converting $\mu g/mL$ to mg/dL follows these steps:

1. Convert micrograms (also written as mcg) to milligrams.

2. Convert milliliters to deciliters:

Since:

1 mg = 1000 $\mu g$, then 31.86 $\mu g/mL$ = 0.03186 mg/mL

**TABLE 2-X •** Pharmacokinetics Data Obtained from a Study Conducted on Rabbits Following Administration of Various Formulations of Rectal Suppositories Containing Aspirin (600 mg each)

| Pharmacokinetic Parameters | Fs2 | Fs4 | Fs9 | Fs11 | Fas9 |
|---|---|---|---|---|---|
| $C_{max}$ ($\mu$g/mL) | 34.93 ± 0.60 | 31.16 ± 1.04 | 32.66 ± 1.52 | 35.33 ± 0.57 | 31.86 ± 0.41 |
| $T_{max}$ (hours) | 1 ± 0.01 | 1 ± 0.03 | 1 ± 0.06 | 1 ± 0.09 | 6 ± 0.03 |
| Elimination rate constant ($h^{-1}$) | 0.14 ± 0.02 | 0.19 ± 0.06 | 0.205 ± 0.03 | 0.17 ± 0.01 | 0.133 ± 0.004 |
| Half-life (hours) | 1.88 ± 0.76 | 1.9 ± 1.19 | 1.43 ± 0.56 | 1.99 ± 0.24 | 5.11 ± 0.15 |
| AUC (0–t) | 127.46 ± 8.9 | 126.62 ± 2.49 | 132.11 ± 3.88 | 127.08 ± 1.95 | 260.62 ± 4.44 |
| AUC (0–infinity) (ng·h/mL) | 138.36 ± 13.87 | 131.61 ± 0.27 | 136.89 ± 4.40 | 133.07 ± 2.97 | 300.48 ± 24.06 |
| AUMC (0–t) (ng·h²/mL) | 524.51 ± 69.64 | 516.04 ± 28.25 | 557.84 ± 16.25 | 501.29 ± 26.65 | 2006.07 ± 38.00 |
| AUMC (0–infinity) (ng·h²/mL) | 382.09 ± 131.45 | 237.74 ± 64.37 | 232.93 ± 28.16 | 257.71 ± 30.04 | 1494.71 ± 88.21 |
| MRT (hours) | 2.45 ± 0.36 | 2.31 ± 0.80 | 1.41 ± 0.31 | 2.95 ± 0.17 | 8.23 ± 0.06 |

*Reproduced with permission from Ravi SV, Dachinamoorthi D, Chandra Shekar KB: A comparative pharmacokinetic study of aspirin suppositories and aspirin nanoparticles loaded suppositories, 2012 Clinic Pharmacol Biopharm 1(3):105.*

1 dL = 100 mL, then 31.86 $\mu$g/mL = 3186 $\mu$g/dL We have to divide the value of $C_{max}$ by 1000 and multiply it by 100. The net effect is to divide the number by 10, or (31.86) (100/1000) = 3.19 mg/dL.

Expressing the $C_{max}$ value 34.93 $\mu$g/mL in nanograms per microliter (ng/$\mu$L) is done as follows:

1. Convert the number of micrograms to nanograms.
2. Convert milliliters to microliters:

1 $\mu$g = 1000 ng, or 34.93 $\mu$g/mL = 34,930 ng/mL 1 mL = 1000 $\mu$L, or 34.93 $\mu$g/mL = 0.03493 $\mu$g/$\mu$L As 34.93 was multiplied and divided by the same number (1000), the final answer is 34.93 ng/$\mu$L.

Express the $C_{max}$ value 35.33 $\mu$g/mL in %w/v (this is defined as the number of grams of ASA in 100 mL plasma).

(35.33 $\mu$g/mL)(100 mL) = 3533 $\mu$g/dL = 3.533 mg/dL = 0.0035 g/dL, or 0.0035% w/v (This means that there is 0.0035 g of ASA in every 100 mL plasma.)

The data ($T_{max}$, $C_{max}$) represent a maximum point on the plasma drug level-versus-time curve. This point reflects *the rate of absorption* of the drug from its site of administration. Another pharmacokinetic measure obtained from the same curve is the AUC. It reflects *the extent of absorption* for a drug from the site of administration into the circulation. The general format for the AUC units is ([amount][time]/ [volume]). Together, the rate and extent of absorption refers to the bioavailability of the drug from the site of administration. The term *absolute bioavailability* is used when the reference route of administration is the intravenous injection (ie, the IV route). If the reference route is different from the intravenous route, then the term *relative bioavailability* is used. The value for the AUC (0 to +∞) following the administration of Fs2, Fs4, and Fas9 was 138.36, 131.61, and 300.48 ng·h/mL, respectively (Ravi Sankar et al, 2012). The origin of the AUC units is based on the *trapezoidal rule*. The *trapezoidal rule* is a numerical method frequently used in pharmacokinetics to calculate the area under the plasma drug concentration-versus-time curve, called the AUC. This rule computes the average concentration value of each consecutive concentration and multiplies them by the difference in their time values. To compute the AUC (0 to time *t*), the sum of all these products is calculated. For example, AUC(0–*t*) = 127.46 ng·h/mL can be written as 127.46 (ng/mL)(h).

To convert 260.62 ng·h/mL to $\mu$g·h/mL, divide the value by 1000 (recall that 1 $\mu$g is 1000 ng). Therefore, the AUC value becomes 0.26 $\mu$g·h/mL.

Expressing the AUC (0 to +∞) value 300.48 ng·h/mL in ng·min/mL can be accomplished by dividing 300.48 by 60 (1 hour is 60 min). Thus, the AUC value becomes 5.0 ng·min/mL.

Consider the following data:

| Plasma Concentration (ng/L) | Time (hours) | AUC (ng·h/L) |
| --- | --- | --- |
| 0 | 0 | 0 |
| 0.05 | 1 | 0.025 |
| 0.10 | 2 | 0.075 |
| 0.18 | 3 | 0.140 |
| 0.36 | 5 | 0.540 |
| 0.13 | 7 | 0.490 |
| 0.08 | 9 | 0.210 |

To compute the AUC value from initial to 9 hours, sum up the values under the AUC column above (0.025 + 0.075 + … + 0.210 = 1.48 ng·h/L).

To convert the AUC value 1.48 ng·h/L to mg·min/dL, use the following steps:

1. Divide the value by $10^6$ to convert the nanograms to milligrams.

2. Divide the value by 60 to convert the hours to minutes.

3. Divide the value by 10 to convert the liters to deciliters.

$$AUC = (1.48)/[(10^6)(60)(10)]$$ (2.10)

$$= 2.47 \times 10^{-9}\,mg \cdot min/dL$$

Figure 2-8 represents the data in a rectangular coordinate–type graph. Time is placed on the $x$ axis (*the abscissa*) and plasma concentration is placed on the $y$ axis (*the ordinate*). The highest point on the graph can simply be determined by spotting it on the graph. Note that the plasma concentration declines *exponentially* from the apex point on the curve over time. Figure 2-9 shows the exponential portion of the graph on its own.

## Exponential and Logarithmic Functions

These two mathematical functions are related to each other. For example, the pH of biological fluids

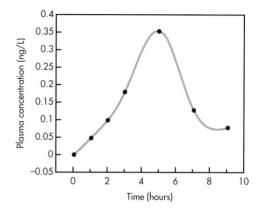

FIGURE 2-8 · Plasma concentration (ng/L)-versus-time (hours) curve plotted on Cartesian coordinates.

(eg, plasma or urine) can influence all pharmacokinetic aspects including drug dissolution/release *in vitro* as well as systemic absorption, distribution, metabolism, and excretion. Since most drugs are either weak bases or weak acids, the pH of the biological fluid determines the degree of ionization of the drug and this in turn influences the pharmacokinetic profile of the drug. The pH scale is a logarithmic scale:

$$pH = -log[H_3O^+] = log(1/[H_3O^+])$$ (2.11)

where the symbol "log" is the *logarithm to base 10*. The *natural logarithm* has the symbol "ln," which is the logarithm to base $e$ (the value of $e$ is approximately 2.71828). The two functions are linked by the following expression:

$$ln\,x = 2.303\,log\,x$$ (2.12)

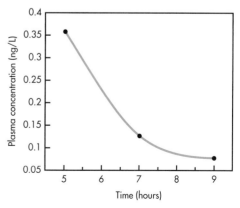

FIGURE 2-9 · The exponential decline in plasma concentration over time portion in Fig. 2-8.

The concentration of hydronium ions $[H_3O^+]$ can be calculated from Equation 2.13 as follows:

$$[H_3O^+] = 10^{-pH} \qquad (2.13)$$

For example, the pH of a patient's plasma is 7.4 at room temperature. Therefore, the hydronium ion concentration in plasma is:

$$[H_3O^+] = 10^{-7.4} = 3.98 \times 10^{-8} \text{ M}$$

The value $(4.0 \times 10^{-8})$ is the *antilogarithm* of 7.4. With the availability of scientific calculators and computers, these functions can be easily calculated.

Oftentimes, converting plasma concentrations to logarithmic values and plotting the logarithmic values against time would convert an exponential relationship to a linear function between the two variables. Consider, for example, Fig. 2-9. When the concentration values are converted to logarithmic values, the graph now becomes linear (Fig. 2-10). This same linear function may be obtained by plotting the *actual* values of the plasma concentration versus time using a semilogarithmic graph (Fig. 2-11). The following equation represents the straight line:

$$\ln (\text{Plasma concentration}) = 0.77 - 0.38 \text{ Time (hours)} \qquad (2.14)$$

The slope of the line is (−0.38). Thus,

$$\text{Slope} = -0.38 = -k_1$$

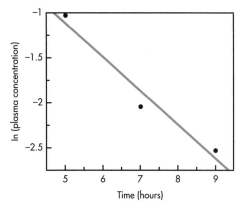

FIGURE 2-10 • In (Plasma concentration)-versus-time curve plotted on Cartesian coordinates.

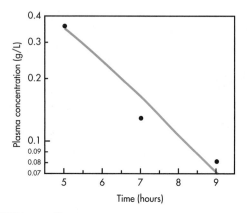

FIGURE 2-11 • Plasma concentration-versus-time curve using a semilogarithmic graph.

Multiplying both sides of the equation by (−1) results in:

$$k_1 = 0.38 \text{ h}^{-1}$$

where $k_1$ is *the first-order elimination rate constant.* The units for this constant are reciprocal time, such as $h^{-1}$ or $1/h$. The value $0.38 \text{ h}^{-1}$ means that 38% of the concentration remaining of the drug in plasma is eliminated every hour.

Using Equation 2.12, Equation 2.14 can be converted to the following expression:

$$2.303 [\log (\text{Plasma concentration})] = 0.77 - 0.38 \text{ Time (hours)}$$

Dividing both sides of the equation by 2.303:

$$2.303 [\log (\text{Plasma Concentration})]/2.303 = [0.77 - 0.38 \text{ Time (hours)}]/2.303 \qquad (2.15)$$

$$\log (\text{Plasma concentration}) = 0.334 - 0.17 \text{ Time (hours)}$$

Equation 2.15 is mathematically equivalent to Equation 2.14.

The value 0.77 in Equation 2.14 equals $(\ln C_0)$, where $C_0$ is the initial concentration of the drug in plasma. Thus,

$$\ln C_0 = 0.77$$

$$C_0 = e^{0.77} = 2.16 \text{ ng/L}$$

Once $k_1$ is known, the AUC from the last data point to $t_{-infinity}$ can be calculated as follows:

$$AUC = C_{Last}/k_1 \qquad (2.16)$$

Applying Equation 2.16 on the data used to obtain the AUC value in Equation 2.10 results in the following value:

$$AUC = 0.08/0.38 = 0.21 \text{ ng·h/L}$$

and the total AUC ($t = 0$ to $t =$ infinity):

$$AUC_{Total} = 1.48 + 0.21 = 1.69 \text{ ng·h/L}$$

The following rules may be useful in handling exponential and logarithmic functions. For this, if $m$ and $n$ are positive, then for the real numbers $q$ and $s$ (Howard, 1980):

**Exponent rules:**

1. $m^0 = 1$
2. $m^1 = m$
3. $m^{-1} = 1/m^1$
4. $m^q/m^s = m^{q-s}$
5. $(m^q)(m^s) = m^{q+s}$
6. $(m^q)^s = m^{qs}$
7. $(m^q/n^q) = (m/n)^q$
8. $(m^q)(n^q) = (mn)^q$

If $z$ is any positive number other than 1 and if $z^y = x$, then following logarithmic rules apply:
   **Logarithm rules:**

1. $y = \log_z x$ ($y$ is the logarithm to the base $z$ of $x$)
2. For $x > 1$, then $\log_e x = \ln x$ (where $e$ is approximately 2.71828)
3. $\log_z x = (\ln x/\ln z)$
4. $\log_z mn = \log_z m + \log_z n$
5. $\log_q (m/n) = \log_q m - \log_q n$
6. $\log_z (1/m) = -\log_z m$
7. $\ln e = 1$
8. For $z = 10$, then $\log_z 1 = 0$
9. $\log_z m^h = h \log_z m$
10. For $z = 10$, then $(2.303) \log_z x = \ln x$

## RATES AND ORDERS OF PROCESSES

Oftentimes, a process such as drug absorption or drug elimination may be described by the *rate* by which the process proceeds. The rate of a process, in turn, may be defined in terms of specifying its *order*. In pharmacokinetics, two orders are of importance, the *zero order* and the *first order*.

### Zero-Order Process

The rate of a zero-order process is one that proceeds over time ($t$) independent from the concentration of the drug ($c$). The negative sign for the rate indicates that the concentration of the drug decreases over time.

$$-dc/dt = k_0 \qquad (2.17)$$
$$dc = -k_0 \, dt$$
$$c = c_0 - k_0 t$$
$$c = -k_0 t + c_0 \qquad (2.18)$$

where $c_0$ is the initial concentration of the drug at $t = 0$ and $k_0$ is the zero-order rate constant. The units for $k_0$ are concentration per unit time (eg, [mg/mL]/h) or amount per unit time (eg, mg/h).

For example, calculate the zero-order rate constant ([ng/mL]/min) if the initial concentration of the drug is 200 ng/mL and that at $t = 30$ minutes is 35 ng/mL.

$$c = c_0 - k_0 \, t$$
$$35 = 200 - k_0 (30)$$
$$-k_0 = (35 - 200)/30 = -5.5$$
$$k_0 = 5.5 \, (\text{ng/mL})/\text{min}$$

When does the concentration of drug equal to 100 ng/mL?

$$100 = 200 - 5.5t$$
$$(100 - 200)/5.5 = -t$$
$$-18.2 = -t$$
$$t = 18.2 \text{ min}$$

In pharmacokinetics, the time required for one-half of the drug concentration to disappear is known as $t_{1/2}$. Thus, for this drug the $t_{1/2}$ is 18.2 minutes.

In general, $t_{1/2}$ may be calculated as follows for a zero-order process:

$$c = c_0 - k_0 t$$

$$(0.5c_0) = c_0 - k_0 t_{1/2}$$

$$(0.5c_0) - c_0 = -k_0 t_{1/2}$$

$$-0.5c_0 = -k_0 t_{1/2}$$

$$t_{1/2} = (0.5c_0)/k_0 \qquad (2.19)$$

Applying Equation 2.19 to the example above should yield the same result:

$$t_{1/2} = (0.5c_0)/k_0$$

$$t_{1/2} = (0.5)(200)/5.5 = 18.2 \text{ min}$$

A plot of $x$ versus time on rectangular coordinates produces a straight line with a slope equal to $(-k_0)$ and a $y$ intercept as $c_0$. In a zero-order process the $t_{1/2}$ is not constant and depends upon the initial amount or concentration of drug.

## First-Order Process

The rate of a first-order process is dependent upon the concentration of the drug:

$$-dc/dt = k_1 c$$

$$-dc/c = k_1 dt$$

$$C = C_0 e^{-kt} \qquad (2.20)$$

$$ln\, c = ln\, c_0 - k_1 t \qquad (2.21)$$

While the rate of the process is a function of the drug concentration, the $t_{1/2}$ is not. Figure 2-12A contrasts the zero-order and the first-order decline in the plasma drug concentration over time using a Cartesian plot. The same data may be linearized by plotting them on a semilogarithmic graph. Natural logarithmic or logarithm of base 10 can be used for this transformation (note that ln C = 2.3 log C) (Equation 2.12).

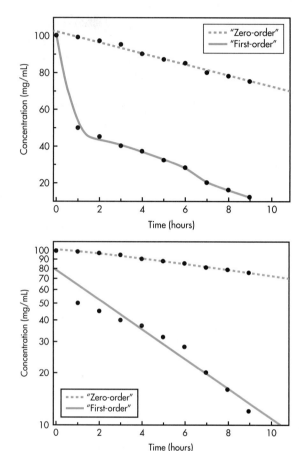

FIGURE 2-12 • **(A)** Zero-order versus first-order plots: plasma concentration-versus-time curve plotted on Cartesian coordinates. Note the appearance of the exponential decline of the plasma drug concentration over time for the "first-order" graph. **(B)** Linear transformation of the first-order graph in A: plasma concentration-versus-time curve plotted using a semilogarithmic graph. Note the transformation of the exponential decline shown in A for the "first-order" to a linear one.

$$ln\, c = ln\, c_0 - k_1 t$$

$$ln\,(0.5\, c_0) = ln\, c_0 - k_1 t_{1/2}$$

$$ln\,(0.5\, c_0) - ln\, c_0 = -k_1 t_{1/2}$$

$$ln\,(0.5c_0 /c_0) = -k_1 t_{1/2}$$

$$ln\, 0.5/-k_1 = t_{1/2}$$

$$t_{1/2} = -0.693/-k_1$$

$$t_{1/2} = 0.693/k_1 \qquad (2.22)$$

**TABLE 2-2 •** Comparison of Zero- and First-Order Reactions

|  | Zero-Order Reaction | First-Order Reaction |
|---|---|---|
| Equation | $-dC/dt = k_0$ | $-dC/dt = kC$ |
|  | $C = -k_0 t + C_0$ | $C = C_0 e^{-kt}$ |
| Rate constant— units | (mg/L)/h | 1/h |
| Half-life, $t_{1/2}$ (units = time) | $t_{1/2} = 0.5C/k_0$ (not constant) | $t_{1/2} = 0.693/k$ (constant) |

Unlike a zero-order rate process, the $t_{1/2}$ for a first-order rate process is always a constant, independent of the initial drug concentration or amount (Table 2-2, Fig. 2-13).

A plot between ln $c$ versus $t$ produces a straight line. A semilogarithmic graph also produces a straight line between $c$ and $t$. The units of the first-order rate constant ($k_1$) are in reciprocal time.

For a drug with $k_1 = 0.04$ h$^{-1}$, find $t_{1/2}$.

$$t_{1/2} = 0.693/k_1$$

$$t_{1/2} = 0.693/0.04 = 17.3 \text{ hours}$$

The value 0.04 h$^{-1}$ for the first-order rate constant indicates that 4% of the drug disappears every hour.

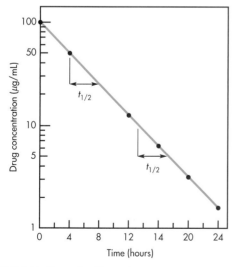

FIGURE 2-13 • The $t_{1/2}$ in a first-order rate process is a constant.

Calculate the time needed for 70% of the drug to disappear.

$$\ln c = \ln c_0 - k_1 t$$

$$\ln (0.3 \, c_0) = \ln c_0 - k_1 t$$

$$\ln (0.3 \, c_0) - \ln c_0 = -k_1 t$$

$$\ln 0.3 / -k_1 = t$$

$$t = -1.2 / -0.04 = 30 \text{ hours}$$

The value 30 hours may be written as $t_{30} = 30$ hours (it is $t_{30}$ because 70% of the drug is eliminated).

### Determination of Order

Graphical representation of experimental data provides a visual relationship between the $x$ values (generally time) and the $y$ axis (generally drug concentrations). Much can be learned by inspecting the line that connects the data points on a graph. The relationship between the $x$ and $y$ data will determine the order of the process, data quality, basic kinetics, and number of outliers, and provide the basis for an underlying pharmacokinetic model. To determine the order of reaction, first plot the data on a rectangular graph. If the data appear to be a curve rather than a straight line, the reaction rate for the data is non-zero order. In this case, plot the data on a semilog graph. If the data now appear to form a straight line with good correlation using linear regression, then the data likely follow first-order kinetics. This simple graph interpretation is true for one-compartment, IV bolus (Chapter 4). Curves that deviate from this format are discussed in other chapters in terms of route of administration and pharmacokinetic model.

### FREQUENTLY ASKED QUESTIONS

▶ How is the rate and order of reaction determined graphically?

▶ What is the difference between a rate and a rate constant?

## CHAPTER SUMMARY

Pharmacokinetic calculations require basic skills in mathematics. Although the availability of computer programs and scientific calculators facilitate pharmacokinetic calculations, the pharmaceutical scientist should be familiar with fundamental rules pertaining to calculus. The construction of a curve or straight line by plotting observed or experimental data on a graph is an important method of visualizing relationships between variables. The linear regression calculation using the least squares method is used for calculation of a straight line through a given set of points. However, it is important to realize that, when using this method, one has already assumed that the data points are related linearly. For all equations, both the integers and the units must balance. The rate of a process may be defined in terms of specifying its order. In pharmacokinetics, two orders are of importance, the *zero order* and the *first order*. Mathematical skills are important in pharmacokinetics in particular and in pharmacy in general.

## LEARNING QUESTIONS

1. Plot the following data on both semilogarithmic graph paper and standard rectangular coordinates.

| Time (minutes) | Drug A (mg) |
|---|---|
| 10 | 96.0 |
| 20 | 89.0 |
| 40 | 73.0 |
| 60 | 57.0 |
| 90 | 34.0 |
| 120 | 10.0 |
| 130 | 2.5 |

   a. Does the decrease in the amount of drug *A* appear to be a zero-order or a first-order process?

   b. What is the rate constant $k$?

   c. What is the half-life $t_{1/2}$?

   d. Does the amount of drug *A* extrapolate to zero on the *x* axis?

   e. What is the equation for the line produced on the graph?

2. Plot the following data on both semilogarithmic graph paper and standard rectangular coordinates.

| Time (minutes) | Drug A (mg) |
|---|---|
| 4 | 70.0 |
| 10 | 58.0 |

| Time (minutes) | Drug A (mg) |
|---|---|
| 20 | 42.0 |
| 30 | 31.0 |
| 60 | 12.0 |
| 90 | 4.5 |
| 120 | 1.7 |

Answer questions **a, b, c, d,** and **e** as stated in Question 1.

3. A pharmacist dissolved a few milligrams of a new antibiotic drug into exactly 100 mL of distilled water and placed the solution in a refrigerator (5°C). At various time intervals, the pharmacist removed a 10-mL aliquot from the solution and measured the amount of drug contained in each aliquot. The following data were obtained:

| Time (hours) | Antibiotic ($\mu$g/mL) |
|---|---|
| 0.5 | 84.5 |
| 1.0 | 81.2 |
| 2.0 | 74.5 |
| 4.0 | 61.0 |
| 6.0 | 48.0 |
| 8.0 | 35.0 |
| 12.0 | 8.7 |

   a. Is the decomposition of this antibiotic a first-order or a zero-order process?

   b. What is the rate of decomposition of this antibiotic?

**c.** How many milligrams of antibiotics were in the original solution prepared by the pharmacist?

**d.** Give the equation for the line that best fits the experimental data.

**4.** A solution of a drug was freshly prepared at a concentration of 300 mg/mL. After 30 days at 25°C, the drug concentration in the solution was 75 mg/mL.

**a.** Assuming first-order kinetics, when will the drug decline to one-half of the original concentration?

**b.** Assuming zero-order kinetics, when will the drug decline to one-half of the original concentration?

**5.** How many half-lives $(t_{1/2})$ would it take for 99.9% of any initial concentration of a drug to decompose? Assume first-order kinetics.

**6.** If the half-life for decomposition of a drug is 12 hours, how long will it take for 125 mg of the drug to decompose by 30%? Assume first-order kinetics and constant temperature.

**7.** Exactly 300 mg of a drug is dissolved into an unknown volume of distilled water. After complete dissolution of the drug, 1.0-mL samples were removed and assayed for the drug. The following results were obtained:

| Time (hours) | Concentration (mg/mL) |
|---|---|
| 0.5 | 0.45 |
| 2.0 | 0.3 |

Assuming zero-order decomposition of the drug, what was the original volume of water in which the drug was dissolved?

**8.** For most drugs, the overall rate of drug elimination is proportional to the amount of drug remaining in the body. What does this imply about the kinetic order of drug elimination?

**9.** A single cell is placed into a culture tube containing nutrient agar. If the number of cells doubles every 2 minutes and the culture tube is completely filled in 8 hours, how long does it take for the culture tube to be only half full of cells?

**10.** Cunha (2013) reported the following: "…CSF levels following 2 g of ceftriaxone are approximately 257 mcg/mL, which is well above the minimal inhibitory concentration (MIC) of even highly resistant (PRSP) in CSF…" What is the value of 257 mcg/mL in mg/mL?

**11.** Refer to Question 10 above; express the value 257 mcg/mL in mcg/dL.

**12.** The following information was provided by Steiner et al (2013):

*ACT-335827 hydrobromide (Actelion Pharmaceuticals Ltd., Switzerland) was freshly prepared in 10% polyethylene glycol 400/0.5% methylcellulose in water, which served as vehicle (Veh). It was administered orally at 300 mg/kg based on the weight of the free base, in a volume of 5 mL/kg, and administered daily 2 h before the onset of the dark phase.*

How many milligrams of ACT-335827 hydrobromide would be given orally to a 170-g rat?

**13.** Refer to Question 12; how many milliliters of drug solution would be needed for the 170-g rat?

**14.** Refer to Question 12; express 0.5% methylcellulose (%w/v) as grams in 1 L solution.

**15.** The $t_{1/2}$ value for aceclofenac tablet following oral administration in Wistar male rats was reported to be 4.35 hours (Shakeel et al, 2009). Assuming a first-order process, what is the elimination rate constant value in hours$^{-1}$?

**16.** Refer to Question 15; express the value of $t_{1/2}$ in minutes.

**17.** Refer to Question 15; the authors reported that the relative bioavailability of aceclofenac from a transdermally applied gel is 2.6 folds higher compared to that of an oral tablet. The following equation was used by the authors to calculate the relative bioavailability:

$$F\% \ \{[(AUC \ sample)(Dose \ oral)]/ \\ [(AUC \ oral)(Dose \ sample)]\}*100 \qquad (2.23)$$

where AUC/Dose sample is for the gel and AUC/Dose oral is for the tablet. F% is the relative bioavailability expressed in percent. If oral and transdermal doses were the same, calculate AUC sample given AUC oral of 29.1 $\mu g \cdot h/mL$. What are the units for AUC sample in (mg·day/mL)?

**18.**

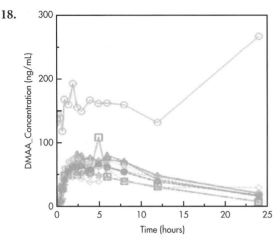

DMAA_Concentration vs Time
- 1
- 2
- 3
- 4
- 5
- 6
- 7
- 8
- Mean

The above figure (from Basu Sarkar et al, 2013) shows the plasma concentration–time profile of DMAA (1,3-dimethylamylamine) in eight men following a single oral dose of the DMAA (25 mg).

What type of graph paper is the above graph? (Semilogarithmic or rectangular?)

**19.** Refer to Question 18; what are the $C_{max}$ and $T_{max}$ values for subject #1? (subject #1) occurred at $T_{max}$ of _____ hour.

**20.** Refer to Question 18; what is the average $C_{max}$ value for all eight subjects? Please use the correct units for your answer.

**21.** Refer to Question 18; what are the units for AUC obtained from the graph?

**22.** Refer to Question 18; for subject #3, the $C_{max}$ value is approximately 105 ng/mL. Express this concentration in %w/v.

**23.** Consider the following graph (Figure 2a in the original article) presented in Schilling et al (2013):

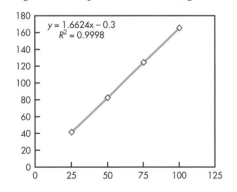

The equation in the graph is that for the standard curve generated for progesterone using a high-performance liquid chromatography method. In the equation, $y$ is the area under the curve of progesterone peak and $x$ represents the concentration of the drug in $\mu$g/mL. Using this equation, predict the AUC for a drug concentration of 35 $\mu$g/mL.

**24.** Refer to Question 23; predict the concentration of progesterone (mg/L) for a peak area (AUC) of 145.

**25.** Consider the following function $dc/dt = 0.98$ with $c$ and $t$ being the concentration of the drug and time, respectively. This equation can also be written as _____.

**a.** $x = x_0 - 0.98\,t$

**b.** $x = 0.98 - t$

**c.** $x = x_0 + 0.98\,t$

**d.** $x = t/0.98$

**26.** Warner et al (2009) reported the value of the terminal half-life of isavuconazole in plasma to be 3.41 h in mice. Assuming a first-order kinetics, estimate the elimination rate constant (min$^{-1}$) of the drug.

## ANSWERS

### Learning Questions

**1.** **a.** Zero-order process (Fig. A-1).

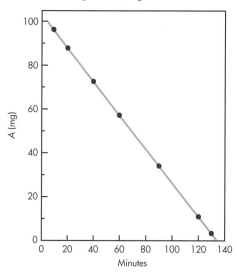

FIGURE A-1 •

**b.** Rate constant, $k_0$:
**Method 1**
Values obtained from the graph (see Fig. A-1):

| $t$ (minutes) | $A$ (mg) |
|---------------|----------|
| 40            | 70       |
| 80            | 41       |

$$-k_0 = \text{slope} = \frac{\Delta Y}{\Delta X} = \frac{y_2 - y_1}{x_2 - x_1}$$

$$-k_0 = \frac{41 - 71}{80 - 40}$$

$$k_0 = 0.75 \text{ mg} / \text{min}$$

Notice that the negative sign shows that the slope is declining.
**Method 2**
By extrapolation:

$$A_0 = 103.5 \text{ at } t = 0; A = 71 \text{ at } t = 40 \text{ min}$$

$$A = k_0 t + A_0$$

$$71 = -40k_0 + 103.5$$

$$k_0 = 0.81 \, mg / \text{min}$$

Notice that the answer differs in accordance with the method used.

**c.** $t_{1/2}$
For zero-order kinetics, the larger the initial amount of drug $A_0$, the longer the $t_{1/2}$.
**Method 1**

$$t_{1/2} = \frac{0.5 A_0}{k_0}$$

$$t_{1/2} = \frac{0.5(103.5)}{0.78} = 66 \text{ min}$$

The value of 0.78 for $k_0$ is the average of 0.75 and 0.81 mg/min.
**Method 2**
The zero-order $t_{1/2}$ may be read directly from the graph (see Fig. A-1):

$$\text{At } t = 0, \, A_0 = 103.5 \text{ mg}$$

$$\text{At } t_{1/2}, \, A = 51.8 \text{ mg}$$

Therefore, $t_{1/2} = 66$ min.

**d.** The amount of drug, $A$, does extrapolate to zero on the $x$ axis.

**e.** The equation of the line is

$$A = -k_0 t + A_0$$

$$A = -0.78t + 103.5$$

**2.** **a.** First-order process (Fig. A-2).

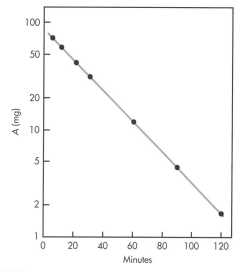

FIGURE A-2 •

**b.** Rate constant, $k$:

**Method 1**

Obtain the first-order $t_{1/2}$ from the semilog graph (see Fig. A-2):

| $t$ (minutes) | $A$ (mg) |
|---|---|
| 30 | 30 |
| 53 | 15 |

$$t_{1/2} = 23 \text{ min}$$

$$k = \frac{0.693}{t_{1/2}} = \frac{0.693}{23} = 0.03 \text{ min}^{-1}$$

**Method 2**

$$\text{Slope} = \frac{-k}{2.3} = \frac{\log Y_2 - \log Y_1}{X_2 - X_1}$$

$$k = \frac{-2.3(\log 15 - \log 30)}{53 - 30} = 0.03 \text{ min}^{-1}$$

**c.** $t_{1/2} = 23$ min (see Method 1 above).

**d.** The amount of drug, $A$, does not extrapolate to zero on the $x$ axis.

**e.** The equation of the line is

$$\log A = -\frac{kt}{2.3} + \log A_0$$

$$\log A = -\frac{0.03t}{2.3} + \log 78$$

$$A = 78e^{-0.03t}$$

On a rectangular plot, the same data show a curve (not plotted).

**3.  a.** Zero-order process (Fig. A-3).

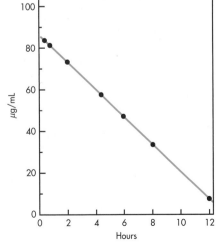

FIGURE A-3 ·

**b.** $k_0 = \text{slope} = \dfrac{\Delta Y}{\Delta X}$

Values obtained from the graph (see Fig. A-3):

| $t$ (hours) | $C$ ($\mu$g/mL) |
|---|---|
| 1.2 | 80 |
| 4.2 | 60 |

It is always best to plot the data. Obtain a regression line (ie, the line of best fit), and then use points $C$ and $t$ from that line.

$$-k_0 = \frac{60 - 80}{4.2 - 1.2}$$

$$k_0 = 6.67 \ \mu\text{g/mL/h}$$

**c.** By extrapolation:

At $t_0$, $C_0 = 87.5 \ \mu$g/mL.

**d.** The equation (using a ruler only) is

$$A = -k_0 t + A_0 = -6.67t + 87.5$$

A better fit to the data may be obtained by using a linear regression program. Linear regression programs are available on spreadsheet programs such as Excel.

**4.  Given:**

| $C$ (mg/mL) | $t$ (days) |
|---|---|
| 300 | 0 |
| 75 | 30 |

**a.**  $\log C = -\dfrac{kt}{2.3} + \log C_0$

$$\log 75 = -\frac{30k}{2.3} + \log 300$$

$$k = 0.046 \text{ days}^{-1}$$

$$t_{1/2} = \frac{0.693}{k} = \frac{0.693}{0.046} = 15 \text{ days}$$

**b. Method 1**

$$300 \text{ mg/mL} = C_0 \text{ at } t = 0$$

$$75 \text{ mg/mL} = C \text{ at } t = 30 \text{ days}$$

225 mg/mL = difference between initial and final drug concentration

$$k_0 = \frac{225 \text{ mg/mL}}{30 \text{ days}} = 7.5 \text{ mg/mL/d}$$

The time, $t_{1/2}$, for the drug to decompose to one-half $C_0$ (from 300 to 150 mg/mL) is calculated by (assuming zero order):

$$t_{1/2} = \frac{150 \text{ mg/mL}}{7.5 \text{ mg/mL/day}} = 20 \text{ days}$$

### Method 2

$$C = -k_0 t + C_0$$
$$75 = -30k_0 + 300$$
$$k_0 = 7.5 \text{ mg/mL/d}$$

At $t_{1/2}$, $C = 150 \text{ mg/mL}$

$$150 = -7.5t_{1/2} + 300$$
$$t_{1/2} = 20 \text{ days}$$

### Method 3

A $t_{1/2}$ value of 20 days may be obtained directly from the graph by plotting $C$ against $t$ on rectangular coordinates.

5. Assume the original concentration of drug to be 1000 mg/mL.

### Method 1

| mg/mL | No. of Half-Lives | mg/mL | No. of Half-Lives |
|---|---|---|---|
| 1000 | 0 | 15.6 | 6 |
| 500 | 1 | 7.81 | 7 |
| 250 | 2 | 3.91 | 8 |
| 125 | 3 | 1.95 | 9 |
| 62.5 | 4 | 0.98 | 10 |
| 31.3 | 5 | | |

99.9% of 1000 = 999
Concentration of drug remaining = 0.1% of 1000
1000 − 999 = 1 mg/mL
It takes approximately 10 half-lives to eliminate all but 0.1% of the original concentration of drug.

### Method 2

Assume any $t_{1/2}$ value:

$$t_{1/2} = \frac{0.693}{k}$$

Then

$$k = \frac{0.693}{t_{1/2}}$$

$$\log C = \frac{-kt}{2.3} + \log C_0$$

$$\log 1.0 = \frac{-kt}{2.3} + \log 1000$$

Substituting $0.693/t_{1/2}$ for $k$:

$$\log 1.0 = \frac{-0.693\,t}{2.3 \times t_{1/2}} + \log 1000$$

$$t = 9.96\,t_{1/2}$$

6. $t_{1/2} = 12\text{h}$

$$k = \frac{0.693}{t_{1/2}} = \frac{0.693}{12} = 0.058\text{h}^{-1}$$

If 30% of the drug decomposes, 70% is left. Then 70% of 125 mg = (0.70)(125) = 87.5 mg

$$A_0 = 125 \text{ mg}$$
$$A = 87.5 \text{ mg}$$
$$k = 0.058 \text{ h}^{-1}$$

$$\log A = -\frac{kt}{2.3} + \log A_0$$

$$\log 87.5 = -\frac{0.058t}{2.3} + \log 125$$

$$t = 6.1 \text{ hours}$$

7. Immediately after the drug dissolves, the drug degrades at a constant, or zero-order rate. Since concentration is equal to mass divided by volume, it is necessary to calculate the initial drug concentration (at $t = 0$) to determine the original volume in which the drug was dissolved. From the data, calculate the zero-order rate constant, $k_0$:

$$-k_0 = \text{slope} = \frac{\Delta Y}{\Delta X} = \frac{0.45 - 0.3}{2.0 - 0.5}$$

$$k_0 = 0.1 \text{ mg/mL/h}$$

Then calculate the initial drug concentration, $C_0$, using the following equation:

$$C = -k_0 t + C_0$$

At $t = 2$ hours,

$$0.3 = -0.1(2) + C_0$$
$$C_0 = 0.5 \text{ mg/mL}$$

Alternatively, at $t = 0.5$ hour,

$$0.45 = -0.1(0.5) - C_0$$
$$C_0 = 0.5 \text{ mg/mL}$$

Since the initial mass of drug $D_0$ dissolved is 300 mg and the initial drug concentration $C_0$ is 0.5 mg/mL, the original volume may be calculated from the following relationship:

$$C_0 = \frac{D_0}{V}$$

$$0.5 \text{ mg/mL} = \frac{300 \text{ mg}}{V}$$

$$V = 600 \text{ mL}$$

**8.** First order.

**9.** The volume of the culture tube is not important. In 8 hours (480 minutes), the culture tube is completely full. Because the doubling time for the cells is 2 minutes (ie, one $t_{1/2}$), then in 480 minutes less 2 minutes (478 minutes), the culture tube is half full of cells.

**10. b.** Since 1 mg = 1000 $\mu$g, then (257 $\mu$g/mL)/1000 = 0.257 mg/mL.

**11. c.** Since 1 dL = 100 mL, then (257 $\mu$g/mL) $\times$ 100 = 25,700 $\mu$g/dL.

**12. a.** Since 1 kg = 1000 g, then (170 g)/1000 = 0.17 kg.

The oral dose was 300 mg/kg; therefore, for 0.17 kg rat, (0.17 kg)(300 mg)/1 kg = 51 mg.

**13. c.** The volume given was 5 mL/kg. For 0.17 kg rat, (0.17 kg)(5 mL)/1 kg = 0.85 mL.

**14. d.** 0.5% of methylcellulose (% w/v) means 0.5 g of methylcellulose in 100 mL solution, or 5 g of methylcellulose in 1 L solution.

**15. b.** $k_{el} = 0.693/t_{1/2} = 0.693/4.35 = 0.16 \text{ h}^{-1}$

**16. b.** 4.35 hours $\times$ 60 min/h = 261 minutes.

**17. c.** $F\% = \{[(\text{AUC sample})(\text{Dose oral})]/[(\text{AUC oral})(\text{Dose sample})]\} * 100$

$F\% = [(\text{AUC sample})/\text{AUC oral}] * 100$
2.6 folds higher = 260%
260 = [AUC sample]/29.1] * 100
AUC sample = 75.66 $\mu$g·h/mL = 0.07566 mg·h/mL = 1.8 mg·day/mL

**18. b.** A rectangular coordinate graph.

**19. d.** According to the figure, the highest plasma concentration for subject #1 occurred at 24 hours.

**20. b.** From the graph, the average $C_{max}$ was between 50 and 100 ng/mL.

**21. c.** It is (concentration units) $\times$ (time) = (ng/mL) $\times$ (hours) = (ng·h/mL).

**22. c.** 105 ng/mL = 10,500 ng/100 mL
= 10.5 $\mu$g/100 mL = 0.0105 mg/100 mL
= 0.0000105 g/100 mL.

**23. c.** $y = 1.6624 \times -0.3$
$y = 1.6624 (35) - 0.3 = 57.9 = \text{AUC}$

**24. a.** $y = 1.6624 \times -0.3$
$145 = 1.6624 \times -0.3$
$x = 87.4 \mu\text{g/mL} = 87.4 \text{ mg/L}$

**25. c.** $dc/dt = 0.98$
$$dc = 0.98 \, dt$$
$$\int dc = 0.98 \int dt$$
$$c = c_0 + 0.98t$$

**26.** $k_{el} = 0.693/t_{1/2(el)} = 0.693/3.42 = 0.20 \text{ h}^{-1}$; or 0.2/60 = 0.0034 min$^{-1}$

## REFERENCES

Basu Sarkar A, Kandimalla A, Dudley R: Chemical stability of progesterone in compounded topical preparations using PLO Transdermal Cream™ and HRT Cream™ base over a 90-day period at two controlled temperatures. *J Steroids Horm Sci* 4:114, 2013. doi:10.4172/2157-7536.1000114. (© 2013 Basu Sarkar A, et al. This is an open-access article distributed under the terms of the Creative Commons Attribution License, which permits unrestricted use, distribution, and reproduction in any medium, provided the original author and source are credited.)

Cunha AB: Repeat lumbar puncture: CSF lactic acid levels are predictive of cure with acute bacterial meningitis. *J Clin Med* 2(4):328–330, 2013. doi:10.3390/jcm2040328. (© 2013 by MDPI [http://www.mdpi.org]. Reproduction is permitted.)

Gaddis LM, Gaddis MG: Introduction to biostatistics: Part 6, Correlation and regression. *Ann Emerg Med* 19(12):1462–1468, 1990.

Howard A: Chapter 7: Logarithm and exponential functions. In *Calculus with Analytical Geometry*. John Wiley and Sons, pp 486–563, 1980.

Munro HB: *Statistical Methods for Health Care Research*. Lippincott Williams & Wilkins, 2005, Philadelphia, PA.

Ravi Sankar V, Dachinamoorthi D, Chandra Shekar KB: A comparative pharmacokinetic study of aspirin suppositories and aspirin nanoparticles loaded suppositories. *Clinic Pharmacol Biopharm* 1:105, 2012. doi:10.4172/2167-065X.1000105. (© 2012 Ravi Sankar V, et al. This is an open-access article distributed under the terms of the Creative Commons Attribution License, which permits unrestricted use, distribution, and reproduction in any medium, provided the original author and source are credited.)

Riggs DS: The Mathematical Approach to Physiological Problems. Baltimore, Williams & Wilkins, 1963.

Schilling et al: Physiological and pharmacokinetic effects of oral 1,3-dimethylamylamine administration in men. *BMC Pharmacol Toxicol* **14**:52, 2013. (© 2013 Schilling et al; licensee BioMed Central Ltd. This is an open-access article distributed under the terms of the Creative Commons Attribution License [http://creativecommons.org/licenses/by/2.0], which permits unrestricted use, distribution, and reproduction in any medium, provided the original work is properly cited.)

Shakeel F, Mohammed SF, Shafiq S: Comparative pharmacokinetic profile of aceclofenac from oral and transdermal application. *J Bioequiv Availab* **1**:013–017, 2009. doi:10.4172/jbb.1000003. (Permission granted under open access: The author[s] and copyright holder[s] grant to all users a free, irrevocable, worldwide, perpetual right of access and a license to copy, use, distribute, transmit, and display the work publicly and to make and distribute derivative works in any digital medium for any responsible purpose, subject to proper attribution of authorship, as well as the right to make small number of printed copies for their personal use.)

Steiner MA, Sciarretta C, Pasquali A, Jenck F: The selective orexin receptor 1 antagonist ACT-335827 in a rat model of diet-induced obesity associated with metabolic syndrome. *Front Pharmacol* **4**:165, 2013. doi: 10.3389/fphar.2013.00165. (© 2013 Steiner MA, et al. This is an open-access article distributed under the terms of the Creative Commons Attribution License [CC BY]. The use, distribution, or reproduction in other forums is permitted, provided the original author[s] or licensor is credited and that the original publication in this journal is cited, in accordance with accepted academic practice. No use, distribution, or reproduction is permitted which does not comply with these terms.)

Warner PA, Sharp A, Parmar A, Majithiya J, Denning DW, Hope WW. Pharmacokinetics of a novel triazole, Isavuconazole: Mathematical modeling, importance of tissue concentrations, and impact of immune status on antifungal effect. *Antimicrob Agents Chemother* **53**(8):3453–3461, 2009.

# Biostatistics

Charles Herring, Antoine Al-Achi, and Abby Harris

## CHAPTER OBJECTIVES

- Describe basic statistical methodology and concepts
- Describe how basic statistical methodology may be used in pharmacokinetic and pharmacodynamics study designs
- Describe how basic statistical methodology may be used in critically evaluating data
- Describe how basic statistical methodology may be used to help minimize error, bias, and confounding, and therefore promote safe and efficacious drug therapy
- Provide examples of how basic statistical methodology may be used for study design and data evaluation

## VARIABLES[1]

Several types of variables will be discussed throughout this text. A *random variable* is "a variable whose observed values may be considered as outcomes of an experiment and whose values cannot be anticipated with certainty before the experiment is conducted" (Herring, 2015). There are two types of random variables: discrete and continuous. *Discrete variables* are also known as counting or nonparametric variables (Glasner, 1995). *Continuous variables* are also known as measuring or parametric variables (Glasner, 1995). We will explore this further in the next section, but a basic example of a discrete variable would be hospitalization or death. Was the patient hospitalized: yes or no? Did the patient die: yes or no? Whereas a continuous variable would be something like drug concentration since these have a consistent difference between data points; the difference between 1 mcg/mL and 6 mcg/mL is the same as the difference between 2 mcg/mL and 7 mcg/mL. The difference for both is 5 mcg/mL.

An *independent variable* is defined as the "intervention or what is being manipulated" in a study (eg, the drug or dose of the drug being evaluated) (Herring, 2015). "The number of independent variables determines the category of statistical methods that are appropriate to use" (Herring, 2015). A *dependent variable* is the "outcome of interest within a study." In bioavailability and bioequivalence studies, examples include the maximum concentration of the drug in circulation, the time to reach that maximum level, and the area under the curve (AUC) of drug level-versus-time curve. These are "the outcomes that one intends to explain or estimate" (Herring, 2015). There may be multiple dependent (ie, outcome)

---

[1]Quick Stats: Basics for Medical Literature Evaluation, 5th ed. was utilized for the majority of this chapter (Herring, 2015). In order to discuss basic statistics, some background terminology must be defined.

variables. For example, in a study determining the half-life ($t_{1/2}$), clearance, and plasma protein binding of a new drug following an oral dose, the independent variable is the oral dose of the new drug. The dependent variables are the $t_{1/2}$, clearance, and plasma protein binding of the drug because these variables "depend upon" the oral dose given.

## TYPES OF DATA (NONPARAMETRIC VERSUS PARAMETRIC)

There are two types of *nonparametric* data, nominal and ordinal. For *nominal* data, numbers are purely arbitrary or without regard to any order or ranking of severity (Gaddis and Gaddis, 1990a; Glasner, 1995). Nominal data may be either dichotomous or categorical. Dichotomous (aka binary) nominal data evaluate yes/no questions. For example, patients lived or died, were hospitalized or were not hospitalized. Examples of categorical nominal data would be things like tablet color or blood type; there is no order or inherent value for nominal, categorical data.

*Ordinal* data are also nonparametric and categorical, but unlike nominal data, ordinal data are scored on a continuum, without a consistent level of magnitude of difference between ranks (Gaddis and Gaddis, 1990a; Glasner, 1995). Examples of ordinal data include a pain scale, New York Heart Association heart failure classification, cancer staging, bruise staging, military rank, or Likert-like scales (poor/fair/good/very good/excellent) (Gaddis and Gaddis, 1990a; DeYoung, 2005).

*Parametric* data (these occur when the distribution of the data is normal—has a bell-shaped curve) are utilized in biopharmaceutics and pharmacokinetic research more so than are the aforementioned types of nonparametric data, since the majority of the pharmacokinetics variables are parametric. Parametric data are also known as "continuous" or "measuring" data or variables. There is an order and consistent level of magnitude of difference between data units. As in the example above, the difference between 1 mcg/mL and 6 mcg/mL is the same as the difference between 2 mcg/mL and 7 mcg/mL. The difference for both is 5 mcg/mL.

There are two types of parametric data: interval and ratio. Both interval and ratio scale parametric data have a predetermined order to their numbering and a consistent level of magnitude of difference between the observed data units (Gaddis and Gaddis, 1990a; Glasner, 1995). However, for interval scale data, there is no absolute zero; examples include temperature in degrees Celsius or Fahrenheit (Gaddis and Gaddis, 1990a; Glasner, 1995). For ratio scale data, there is an absolute zero; examples include temperature in Kelvin, drug concentrations, plasma glucose, heart rate, blood pressure, distance, and time (Gaddis and Gaddis, 1990a; Glasner, 1995). Although the specific definitions of these two types of parametric data are listed above, their definitions are somewhat academic since all parametric data utilize the same statistical tests. In other words, regardless of whether the parametric data are interval or ratio scale, the same tests are used to detect statistical differences. Variables that are interval or ratio in nature are known as continuous variables. Examples of parametric data include plasma protein binding, the maximum concentration of the drug in the circulation, the time to reach that maximum level, the AUC of drug level-versus-time curve, drug clearance, and elimination $t_{1/2}$.

---

**FREQUENTLY ASKED QUESTIONS**

▶ Is it appropriate to degrade parametric data to nonparametric data for data analysis?

▶ What occurs if this is done?

---

### Data Scale Summary Example

In pharmacokinetic studies, researchers may be interested in testing the difference in the oral absorption of a generic versus a branded form of a drug. In this case, "generic or branded" is a nominal scale-type variable, whereas expressing the "rate of absorption" numerically is a parametric-type scale (Gaddis and Gaddis, 1990a; Ferrill and Brown 1994; Munro, 2005).

## DISTRIBUTIONS

*Normal distributions* (see Fig. 3-1) are "symmetrical on both sides of the mean" and are sometimes termed as a bell-shaped curve, Gaussian curve, curve of error, or normal probability curve (Shargel et al, 2012).

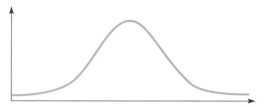

FIGURE 3-1 • Normal distribution—also known as (aka) bell-shaped curve, Gaussian curve, curve of error, or normal probability curve.

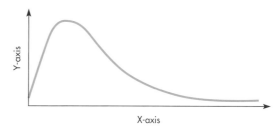

FIGURE 3-3 • Positive skew: cluster of data on the low end of the X-axis.

An example of normally distributed data includes drug elimination half-lives in a specific population, as would be the case in a sample of men with normal renal (kidney) and hepatic (liver) function, whereas we would not expect a normal distribution of half-lives if a data set included men with varying states of abnormal renal and hepatic function. As will be discussed later in this chapter, parametric statistical tests like the *t*-test and various types of analysis of variance (ANOVA) are utilized for normally distributed data.

Sometimes in bioequivalence or pharmacokinetic studies, a bimodal distribution (see Fig. 3-2) is noted. In this case, two peaks of cluster or areas of high frequency occur. For example, a medication that is acetylated at different rates in humans would be a "bimodal distribution, indicating two populations consisting of fast acetylators and slow acetylators" (Gaddis and Gaddis, 1990a; Glasner, 1995; Shargel et al, 2012).

*Skewed distributions* occur when data are not normally distributed and tail off to either the high or the low end of measurement units. A *positive skew* (see Fig. 3-3) occurs when data cluster on the low end of the *x* axis (Gaddis and Gaddis, 1990a; Glasner, 1995). For example, the *x* axis could be the income of patients seen in an inner-city emergency department (ED), the cost of generic medications, or the number

of prescribed medications in patients younger than 30 years of age.

A *negative skew* (see Fig. 3-4) occurs when data cluster on the high end of the *x* axis (Gaddis and Gaddis, 1990a; Glasner, 1995). For example, the *x* axis could be the income of patients seen in an ED of an affluent area, cost of brand name medications, or number of prescribed medications in patients older than 60 years of age. Most, if not all, of the pharmacokinetic variables are expected to have skewed distributions (positive or negative) with small sample sizes. However, presence of minor skewness in data does not mean that data are unmanageable.

*Kurtosis* (see Fig. 3-5) occurs when data cluster on both ends of the *x* axis such that the graph tails upward (ie, clusters on both ends of the graph). For example, the J-curve of hypertension treatment: with the J-curve, mortality increases if blood pressure is either too high or too low (Glasner, 1995).

## MEASURES OF CENTRAL TENDENCY

There are several *measures of central tendency* that are utilized in biopharmaceutical and pharmacokinetic research. The most common one is the *arithmetic mean*, or average. It is the "sum of all values

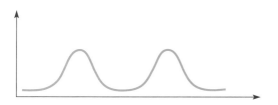

FIGURE 3-2 • Bimodal distribution: 2 peaks of cluster, or areas of high frequency.

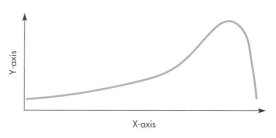

FIGURE 3-4 • Negative skew: cluster of data on the high end of the X-axis.

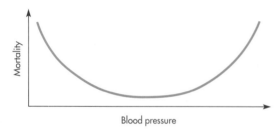

FIGURE 3-5 • Kurtosis: when each end of the graph tails up and clusters on both ends of the X-axis.

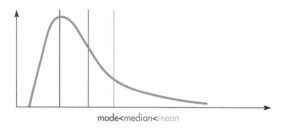

FIGURE 3-7 • Positively skewed data (Reproduced with permission from Glasner AN: High Yield Biostatistics. Philadelphia, PA: Williams & Wilkins; 1995).

divided by the total number of values." It is used for parametric data and is affected by outliers or extreme values which "deviate far from the majority of the data" (Gaddis and Gaddis, 1990b; Shargel et al, 2012). Mu ($\mu$) is the population mean and $X$-bar ($\bar{X}$) is the sample mean (Gaddis and Gaddis, 1990b).

*Median* is also known as the 50th percentile, the second quartile, or the mid-most point (Gaddis and Gaddis, 1990b). It is "the point above which or below which half of the data points in a distribution lie" (Gaddis and Gaddis, 1990b). It is not affected by outliers and may be used for ordinal and parametric data (Gaddis and Gaddis, 1990b). Median is used when outliers exist, when a data set spans a wide range of values, or "when continuous data are not normally distributed" (Gaddis and Gaddis, 1990b; DeYoung, 2005).

*Mode* is the most common value; it is the value occurring most frequently in a data set (Gaddis and Gaddis, 1990b). Mode is not affected by outliers and may be used for nominal, ordinal, or parametric data (Gaddis and Gaddis, 1990b). However, the mode is not helpful when a data set contains a large (or wide) range of infrequently occurring values (Gaddis and Gaddis, 1990b).

For normally distributed data (see Fig. 3-6), mean, median, and mode are the same. For positively skewed data, the mode is less than the median and the median is less than the mean (see Fig. 3-7). For negatively skewed data, the mode is greater than the median and the median is greater than the mean (Gaddis and Gaddis, 1990b; Glasner, 1995) (see Fig. 3-8).

**Log Transformation of Data** Although measures of central tendency do not describe variability or spread of data, based upon a data set's mean, median, and mode values, one can determine if the data are normally distributed or skewed when no graphical representation is provided. Due to small sample size, sometimes data may not be normally distributed such that it looks skewed (see Table 3-1 and Fig. 3-9). *Logarithmic transformation* may be used to make skewed data appear more normally distributed (see Table 3-2 and Fig. 3-10).

One point to note here is that the mean of logarithmic transformed values, when converting it back to its regular scale (ie, taking the antilog value), would produce the *geometric mean* rather than the arithmetic mean. Discussions of geometric mean are beyond the scope of this chapter. Other types of transformation to normality are also used in statistics

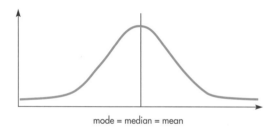

FIGURE 3-6 • Normally distributed data (Reproduced with permission from Glasner AN: High Yield Biostatistics. Philadelphia, PA: Williams & Wilkins; 1995).

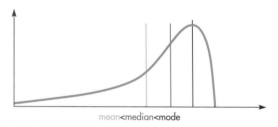

FIGURE 3-8 • Negatively skewed data (Reproduced with permission from Glasner AN: High Yield Biostatistics. Philadelphia, PA: Williams & Wilkins; 1995).

| TABLE 3-1 • Concentration Versus Time | |
|---|---|
| Time (hrs) | Concentration (mg/dL) |
| 0 | 0 |
| 1 | 20 |
| 2 | 7.65785772 |
| 3 | 2.932139243 |
| 4 | 1.122695257 |
| 5 | 0.429872027 |
| 6 | 0.164594941 |
| 7 | 0.063022232 |
| 8 | 0.024130764 |
| 9 | 0.009239498 |
| 10 | 0.003537738 |
| 11 | 0.001354575 |
| 12 | 0.000518657 |
| 13 | 0.00019859 |
| 14 | 7.60387E-05 |
| 15 | 2.91147E-05 |

| TABLE 3-2 • Log(Concentration) Versus Time | |
|---|---|
| Time (hrs) | Log(Concentration) (mg/dL) |
| 0 | 0 |
| 1 | 1.301029996 |
| 2 | 0.884107293 |
| 3 | 0.46718459 |
| 4 | 0.050261888 |
| 5 | −0.366660815 |
| 6 | −0.783583517 |
| 7 | −1.20050622 |
| 8 | −1.617428923 |
| 9 | −2.034351625 |
| 10 | −2.451274328 |
| 11 | −2.868197031 |
| 12 | −3.285119733 |
| 13 | −3.702042436 |
| 14 | −4.118965138 |
| 15 | −4.535887841 |

if logarithmic transformation does not produce the desired results.

In summary, measures of central tendency provide information regarding the center of data and help in determining normality versus skewing. However, these measures are unable to describe variability or spread of data and may be misleading. This brings us to our next topic, measures of variability (Herring, 2015).

## MEASURES OF VARIABILITY

Measures of variability describe data spread and, in the case of *confidence intervals (CIs)*, can help one infer statistical significance (Gaddis and Gaddis, 1990b).

*Range* is the interval between lowest and highest values (Gaddis and Gaddis, 1990b; Glasner, 1995). Range only considers extreme values, so it is affected

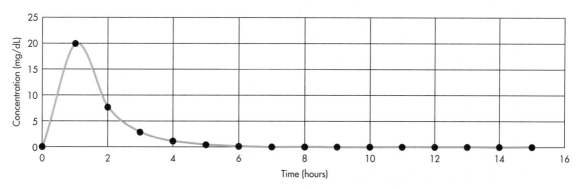

FIGURE 3-9 • Concentration versus time curve.

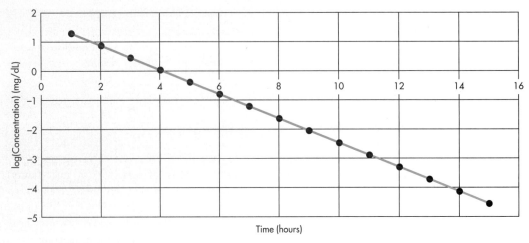

**FIGURE 3-10** • Log(Concentration) versus time curve.

by outliers (Gaddis and Gaddis, 1990b). Range is descriptive only, so it is not used to infer statistical significance (Gaddis and Gaddis, 1990b). Since the sample does not include the total population, the sample is very unlikely to find the population's maximum and minimum values of the variable being studied. Thus, the sample's range is expected to be a poor representation of the population's range. *Interquartile range* is the interval between the 25th and 75th percentiles (Gaddis and Gaddis, 1990b). Since the interquartile range does not include the bottom 25th percent of data (ie, the bottom extreme values) or the top 25th percent of data (ie, the top extreme values), it is not affected by outliers and, along with the median, is used for ordinal scale data (Gaddis and Gaddis, 1990b).

*Variance* is deviation from the mean, expressed as the square of the units used. The value of the variance is the square of the standard deviation (SD). "As sample size (*n*) increases, variance decreases" (Herring, 2015). Sample variance equals the sum of (mean − data point) squared, divided by $n - 1$.

$$\text{Variance} = \frac{\Sigma(\overline{X} - X)^2}{n-1} \qquad (3.1)$$

*Standard deviation (SD)* is the square root of variance (Gaddis and Gaddis, 1990b; Glasner, 1995). SD estimates the degree of data scatter around the sample mean. Approximately 68% of data lie within ±1 SD of the mean and 95% of data lie within ±2 SD

of the mean (Gaddis and Gaddis, 1990b; Glasner, 1995). SD is only meaningful when data are normally or near-normally distributed and therefore is only applicable to parametric data (Gaddis and Gaddis, 1990b; Glasner, 1995). Sigma (σ) is the population SD and *S* is the sample SD (Glasner, 1995).

$$SD = \sqrt{\text{Variance}} \qquad (3.2)$$

"*Coefficient of variation (or relative standard deviation)* is another measure used when evaluating dispersion from one data set to another. The coefficient of variation is the SD expressed as a percentage of the mean. This is useful in comparing the relative difference in variability between two or more samples, or which group has the largest relative variability of values from the mean" (Herring, 2015). The smaller the coefficient of variation, the less the variability in the data set. For example, if there are two different drug formulations, one may vary from the mean AUC concentration by 5%, and another formulation may vary by 11%. The formulation that varies by 5% has less variation relative to its mean AUC.

$$\text{Coefficient of variation} = 100 \times SD/\overline{X} \qquad (3.3)$$

*Standard error of the mean (SEM)* is the SD divided by the square root of *n* (Gaddis and Gaddis, 1990b; Glasner, 1995). The larger *n* is, the smaller SEM is (Gaddis and Gaddis, 1990b; Glasner, 1995).

Also, as can be noted by the calculation, SEM is always a smaller value than the SD value.

The variability for the distribution of means (also known as the Y-bar population) is estimated by the SEM. The SEM helps to estimate how well a sample represents the population from which it was drawn (Glasner, 1995). However, since the SEM is always smaller than SD, the SEM should *not* be used as a measure of variability when publishing a study; doing so is misleading because it makes the data look less variable, and therefore, better. The only purpose of SEM is to calculate CIs, which contain an estimate of the true population value from which the sample was drawn (Gaddis and Gaddis, 1990b).

$$SEM = SD/\sqrt{n} \qquad (3.4)$$

*Confidence interval (CI)* is a method of estimating the range of values likely to include the true value of a population parameter (Gaddis and Gaddis, 1990b). In medical literature, a 95% CI is most frequently used. The 95% CI is a range of values that, "if the entire population could be studied, 95% of the time the true population value would fall within the CI estimated from the sample" (Gaddis and Gaddis, 1990b). For a 95% CI, 5 times out of 100, the true population parameter may *not* lie within the CI. For a 97.5% CI, 2.5 times out of 100, the true population parameter may *not* lie within the CI. Therefore, a 97.5% CI is more likely to include the true population value than a 95% CI (Gaddis and Gaddis, 1990b). The range of values is wider for a 97.5% CI than a 95% CI. A 97.5% CI will be wider than a 95% CI because a 97.5% CI will contain more data than a 95% CI. For example, let's say that in a data set, the 97.5% CI ranged from 1 to 20 and the 95% CI ranged from 4 to 14. Since the range of values for the 97.5% CI is wider than for the 95% CI, there is more confidence that the true population mean is within the 97.5% CI than the 95% CI.

The true strength of a CI is that it is both descriptive and inferential; descriptive meaning it describes the variability of the data and inferential meaning that it provides the ability to determine statistical significance. "All values contained in the CI are statistically possible" (Herring, 2015). However, the closer the point estimate lies to the middle of the CI, the more likely the point estimate represents the population.

For example, if a point estimate and 95% CI for drug clearance are 3 L/h (95% CI: 1.5–4.5 L/h), all values including and between 1.5 and 4.5 L/h are statistically possible. However, a CI value that is closer to the sample's point estimate of 3 L/h would be a more accurate representation of the studied population; a value of 2.5 L/h is a more accurate representation of the studied population than a value of 1.6 L/h since 2.5 L/h is closer to the sample's point estimate of 3 L/h than is 1.6 L/h. As seen in this example, CI shows the degree of certainty (or uncertainty) in each comparison in an easily interpretable way. So there is a higher degree of certainty in CI values that lie closer to the point estimate.

In addition, CIs make it easier to assess clinical significance and are less likely to mislead one into thinking that non-significantly different sample values imply equal population values.

$$95\% \, CI = \overline{X} \pm 1.96 \, (SEM) \qquad (3.5)$$

Significance of CIs depends upon the objective of the trial being conducted or evaluated.

In superiority trials (ie, trials that test if one drug is superior to another drug), all values within a CI are statistically possible. For *differences* like differences in $t_{1/2}$, differences in AUC, differences in blood pressure (BP), differences in cholesterol, relative risk reductions/increases (RRR/RRI), or absolute risk reductions/increases (ARR/ARI), if the CI includes zero (0), then the results are not statistically significant (NSS). In the case of a 90% CI, if the CI includes zero (0) for these types of data, it can be interpreted as a $p > 0.10$. In the case of a 95% CI, if the CI includes zero (0) for these types of data, it can be interpreted as a $p > 0.05$. In the case of a 97.5% CI, if the CI includes zero (0) for these types of data, it can be interpreted as a $p > 0.025$.

Let us employ the example of a 95% CI since this is most commonly used. In a study evaluating BP lowering with a new medication relative to placebo, average BP change (95% CI) is −10 mm Hg (0 to −18 mm Hg) (see Fig. 3-11). In this example, although the point estimate demonstrates a 10 mm Hg decrease in average BP, the 95% CI, which includes all statistically possible values, includes zero (0). Since the 95% CI includes zero (0), all values within the 95% CI do not demonstrate a BP decrease and it is statistically

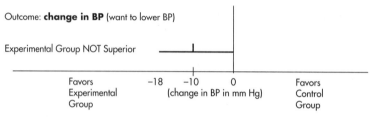

FIGURE 3-11 • Superiority Trial Table.

possible that there is zero (0) mm Hg BP lowering (no change in BP) with this new medication. Therefore, the 10 mm Hg average BP decrease is NSS.

This would also be the case if the average BP change (95% CI) were $^-10$ mm Hg ($^+5$ to $^-18$ mm Hg) since, again, the 95% CI includes zero (0) (see Fig. 3-12). In this example, not only is it statistically possible that there is zero (0) BP lowering (no change in BP), but it is also statistically possible that there is a 5 mm Hg BP increase with using this new BP medication. Therefore, again, the point estimate 10 mm Hg average BP decrease is NSS.

Using this same example, what if the average BP change (95% CI) were $^-10$ mm Hg ($^-4$ to $^-18$ mm Hg)? See Fig. 3-13. In this example, not only does the point estimate demonstrate a 10 mm Hg decrease in average BP, but also all values within the 95% CI demonstrate a BP decrease, the least being a 4 mm Hg BP decrease and the most being an 18 mm Hg BP decrease. Therefore, in this example, the point estimate 10 mm Hg average BP decrease is statistically significant since the 95% CI excludes zero (0).

In these scenarios, the 95% CI not only measures variability, but also infers whether any measured differences are statistically significant, so this is why CIs are descriptive and inferential as mentioned earlier in the chapter.

Batty et al (1995) found that the concomitant administration of ciprofloxacin with theophylline in nine healthy subjects significantly reduced the oral clearance of theophylline by $-7.73$ ml kg$^{-1}$ on average (95% CI $-2.79$ to $-12.66$) (Batty et al, 1995). Since zero (0) was not found in the CI, this reduction in the oral clearance was statistically significant.

For superiority trials, since all values within a CI are statistically possible, for *ratios* like relative risk (RR), odds ratio (OR), or hazards ratio (HR), if the CI includes one (1.0), then the results are NSS. See "Evaluation of Risk for Clinical Studies" section of this chapter for clarification of RR, OR, and HR. In the case of a 90% CI, if the CI includes one (1.0) for these types of data, it can be interpreted as a $p > 0.10$. In the case of a 95% CI, if the CI includes one (1.0) for these types of data, it can be interpreted as a $p > 0.05$. In the case of a 97.5% CI, if the CI includes one (1.0) for these types of data, it can be interpreted as a $p > 0.025$. Again, let us employ the example of a 95% CI since this is most commonly used.

In a study evaluating the ability of a new antibiotic formulation to attain goal maximum concentration ($C_{max}$; ie, RR of attaining goal $C_{max}$) relative to the current standard of care formulation, RR (95% CI) was 1.2 (1.0 to 1.6) (see Fig. 3-14). In this example, although the point estimate demonstrates a 20% (RR 1.20) relative increase in attainment of goal $C_{max}$, the 95% CI, which includes all statistically possible values, includes one (1.0). Since the 95% CI includes one (1.0), all values within the 95% CI

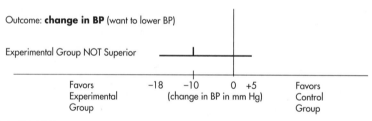

FIGURE 3-12 • Superiority Trial Table.

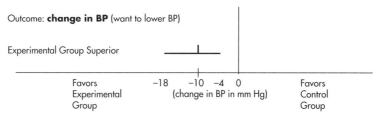

FIGURE 3-13 • Superiority Trial Table.

do not demonstrate an increase in the attainment of goal $C_{max}$ and it is statistically possible that there is no improvement in attaining goal $C_{max}$ with this new formulation. Said another way, although the point estimate demonstrates a 20% increase (RR 1.20) in attainment of goal $C_{max}$, the 95% CI values range from no increase (RR 1.0) to a 60% (RR 1.6) increase in attainment of goal $C_{max}$ relative to the standard formulation. Therefore, the 20% relative increase in attainment of goal $C_{max}$ is NSS.

This would also be the case if the RR (95% CI) were 1.2 (0.7 to 1.6) since, again, the 95% CI includes one (1.0) (see Fig. 3-15). In this example, not only is it possible that there is no increase, but it is also possible that there is a 30% relative decrease (RR 0.7) in attainment of goal $C_{max}$ with the new formulation. Therefore, the 20% relative increase (RR 1.2) in attainment of goal $C_{max}$ is not statistically significant.

Using this same new formulation example, what if the RR (95% CI) were 1.2 (1.1 to 1.4)? See Fig. 3-16. In this example, not only does the point estimate demonstrate a 20% increase in attainment of goal $C_{max}$, but also all values within the 95% CI demonstrate an increase in attainment of goal $C_{max}$, the least being a 10% increase and the most being a 40% increase. Therefore, in this example, the 20%

increase in attainment of goal $C_{max}$ with the new formulation is statistically significant since the 95% CI excludes one (1.0). As in the prior scenarios, in these scenarios, the 95% CI not only measures variability, but also infers whether any measured differences are statistically significant.

Sato et al. studied the efficacy and safety of arbekacin, an antibiotic that is used in Japan for the treatment of methicillin-resistant *Staphylococcus aureus* (MRSA), in 174 MRSA patients. The probability of cure/improvement rose when the $C_{max}$ of the drug was increased from 7.9 to 12.5 micrograms/mL. An OR of 6.7 (95% CI 1.1 to 39) was computed for this effect. Since the value of one (1.0) was not included in the 95% CI for the OR, the observed OR of 6.7 was statistically significant (Sato et al, 2006).

## HYPOTHESIS TESTING

For superiority trials (eg, when testing if a new drug is superior to placebo), the *null hypothesis* ($H_0$) states that no difference exists between studied populations (Gaddis and Gaddis, 1990c). For superiority trials, the *alternative hypothesis* ($H_1$) states that a difference does exist between studied populations (Gaddis and Gaddis, 1990c).

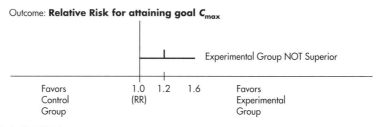

FIGURE 3-14 • Superiority Trial Table.

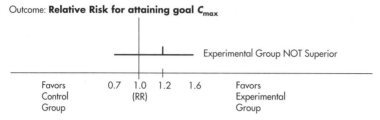

FIGURE 3-15 • Superiority Trial Table.

$H_0$ (aka $\mu_0$ when evaluating mean differences): There is no difference in the AUC for drug formulation A relative to formulation B.

$H_1$ (aka $H_a$ or $\mu_a$ when evaluating mean differences): There *is* a difference in AUC for drug formulation A relative to formulation B.

$H_1$ (aka $H_a$ or $\mu_a$ when evaluating mean differences) is sometimes directional. For example,

$H_1$ (aka $H_a$ or $\mu_a$ when evaluating mean differences): We expect AUC for drug formulation A to be 25% higher than that of formulation B.

$H_0$ is tested instead of $H_1$ because there are an infinite number of alternative hypotheses. It would be impossible to calculate the required statistics for each of the infinite number of possible magnitudes of difference between population samples $H_1$ hypothesizes (Gaddis and Gaddis, 1990c). $H_0$ is used to determine "if any observed differences between groups are due to chance alone" or sampling variation.

*Statistical significance* is tested (*hypothesis testing*) to indicate if $H_0$ should be rejected or not rejected (Gaddis and Gaddis, 1990c). For superiority trials, if $H_0$ is "rejected," this means a statistically significant difference between groups exists (results unlikely due to chance) (Gaddis and Gaddis, 1990c). For superiority trials, if $H_0$ is "not rejected," this means no statistically significant difference exists

(Gaddis and Gaddis, 1990c). However, "failing to reject $H_0$ is not sufficient to conclude that groups are equal" (DeYoung, 2005). Furthermore, conclusion of any statistical analysis cannot be reached with 100% certainty due to *statistical errors (type 1 and type 2)*.

A *type 1 error* occurs if one rejects the $H_0$ when, in fact, the $H_0$ is true (Gaddis and Gaddis, 1990c). For superiority trials, this is when one concludes there is a difference between treatment groups, when in fact no difference exists (Gaddis and Gaddis, 1990c).

*Alpha (α)* is *defined* as the probability of making a type 1 error (Gaddis and Gaddis, 1990c). When α level is set *a priori* (or before the trial), the $H_0$ is rejected when $p \leq \alpha$ (Gaddis and Gaddis, 1990c). By convention, an acceptable α is usually 0.05 (5%), which means that 1 time out of 20, a type 1 error will be committed. This is a consequence that investigators are willing to accept and is denoted in trials as a $p \leq 0.05$ (Gaddis and Gaddis, 1990c). So, the *p*-value is the calculated chance that a type 1 error has occurred (Gaddis and Gaddis, 1990c). In other words, it tells us the likelihood of obtaining a statistically significant result if $H_0$ were true (ie, a statistically significant difference detected when there truly was not a difference). "At $p = 0.05$, the likelihood is 5%. At $p = 0.10$, the likelihood is 10%" (Herring, 2015). A $p \leq \alpha$ means the observed treatment difference is statistically significant. However, statistical significance does not

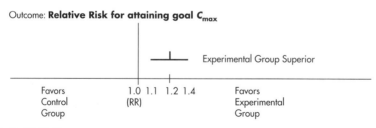

FIGURE 3-16 • Superiority Trial Table.

indicate the size or direction of the difference. The size of the *p*-value is not related to the importance of the result (Gaddis and Gaddis, 1990f; Berensen, 2000). Smaller *p*-values simply mean that "chance" is less likely to explain observed differences (Gaddis and Gaddis, 1990f; Berensen, 2000).

A *type 2 error* occurs if one accepts the $H_0$ when in fact, the $H_0$ is false (Gaddis and Gaddis, 1990c). For superiority trials, one may conclude there is no difference between treatment groups, when in fact, a difference does exist. *Beta (β)* is the probability of making a type 2 error (Gaddis and Gaddis, 1990c). By convention, an acceptable β is 0.2 (20%) or less (Gaddis and Gaddis, 1990c).

Regardless of the trial design, α and β are interrelated (Gaddis and Gaddis, 1990c). All other variables being held constant, α and β are inversely related (Gaddis and Gaddis, 1990c). As α is decreased, β is increased, and as α is increased, β is decreased (ie, as risk for a type 1 error is increased, risk for a type 2 error is decreased and vice versa) (Gaddis and Gaddis, 1990c). The most common use of β is in calculating the approximate sample size required for a study to keep α and β acceptably small (Gaddis and Gaddis, 1990c).

*Power* is the ability of an experiment to detect a statistically significant difference between samples, when in fact, a significant difference truly exists (Gaddis and Gaddis, 1990c). Thus, the power of the test is defined as the probability of rejecting a null hypothesis when it is false (ie, one of the alternative hypotheses is true). In addition, power is the complement of type 2 error (β). Accordingly, as the power increases,

β decreases. Said another way, power is the probability of making a correct decision when $H_0$ is false.

$$\text{Power} = 1 - \beta \qquad (3.6)$$

As stated in the section on type 2 error risk, by convention, an acceptable β is 0.2 (20%) or less; therefore, most investigators set up their studies, and their sample sizes, based upon an estimated power of at least 80%.

For superiority trials, inadequate power may cause one to conclude that no difference exists when in fact, a difference does exist. As described above, this would be a type 2 error (Gaddis and Gaddis, 1990c). Since power is related to β, power is an issue only if one accepts the $H_0$. In this case, there are only two possibilities: either a type 2 error or there truly was not a difference (see Table 3-3). For example, when evaluating two medications, with regard to blood pressure lowering, if no difference is detected, then power may be an issue. In other words, there may not be enough power (collected data) to detect a difference.

---

### FREQUENTLY ASKED QUESTIONS

▶ For a superiority trial, if a statistically significant difference were detected, is there any way that the study was underpowered?

▶ Asked another way, for a superiority trial, if a statistically significant difference were detected, is there any way a type 2 error could have occurred?

---

In the opposite scenario, if one rejects the $H_0$, there is no way that one could have made a type 2 error;

## TABLE 3-3 • Type 1 and Type 2 Error for Superiority Trials

| | Reality | |
|---|---|---|
| | Difference Exists (H₀ False) | No Difference Exists (H₀ True) |
| **Decision From Stat Test** | | |
| Difference Found (Reject H₀) | Correct No error | Incorrect **Type 1** error (false positive) |
| No Difference Found (Accept H₀) | Incorrect **Type 2** error (false negative) | Correct No error |

*Modified with permission from Gaddis GM, Gaddis ML. Introduction to biostatistics: Part 3, Sensitivity, specificity, predictive value, and hypothesis testing, Ann Emerg Med 1990 May;19(5):591-597.*

the only two possibilities in this case are that there was a type 1 error or there truly was a difference. Again, see Table 3-3. In the same blood pressure study example as listed above, if a difference is detected, then power cannot be an issue; there were enough data to detect a difference so there would not be a need to collect more data. An exception to this general rule would be if one wanted to decrease data variability or spread. For example, if one wanted to narrow the 95% CI or SD, increasing power by increasing sample size could help.

*Delta (Δ)* (also known as effect size) is a measure of the degree of difference between tested population samples (Gaddis and Gaddis, 1990c). For parametric data, the value of Δ is the ratio of the clinical difference expected to be observed in the study to the SD of the variable:

$$\Delta = (\mu_a - \mu_0)/SD \qquad (3.7)$$

where $\mu_a$ is the alternative hypothesis value expected for the mean and $\mu_0$ is the null hypothesis value for the mean.

*One-tailed versus two-tailed tests:* A one-tailed test is used whenever the hypothesis is directional (ie, it contains words that imply a direction, such as increase or decrease). When one is attempting to find *any* difference between the averages of the groups, then a two-tailed test is used. It is easier to show a statistically significant difference with a *one-tailed test* than with a *two-tailed test*, because with a one-tailed test, a statistical test result must *not* vary as much from the mean to achieve significance at any level of α chosen (Gaddis and Gaddis, 1990c) (see Fig. 3-17).

However, most reputable journals require that investigators perform statistics based upon a two-tailed test even if it innately makes sense that a difference would only occur unidirectionally.

For research purposes, power calculations are generally used to determine the required sample size when designing a study (ie, prior to the study). Power calculations are generally based upon the *primary* endpoint of the study and, as is depicted in the examples below, the *a priori* (prespecified) α, β, Δ, SD, and whether a one-tailed or two-tailed design is used.

### Parametric Data Sample Size/Power Examples

A parametric test (*t*-test or ANOVA) is applicable to interval and ratio scale variables. Parametric tests require the distribution of the outcome to be normally distributed (ie, has a bell-shape curve). A study's *a priori* parameters help determine the required sample size. In other words, the preset α, β, Δ, SD, and tailing (one-tailed versus two-tailed) affect sample size required for a study (Drew R, discussions and provisions).

A larger SD will require a larger sample size, since a large SD means there is a large variation in the data. As discussed in the section above, a one-tailed test requires a smaller sample size to detect differences between groups than a two-tailed test (Drew R, discussions and provisions). If all *a priori* parameters are held constant, a one-tailed test has more *power* to reject the null hypothesis than a two-tailed test (see Table 3-4).

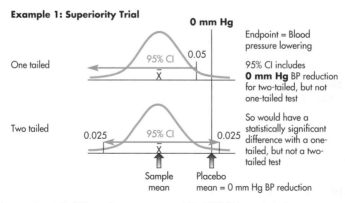

FIGURE 3-17 • One tailed versus two tailed (the red arrows represent the 95% CI boundaries).

| TABLE 3-4 • One-Tailed Versus Two-Tailed Sample Size Requirements | | | | | |
|---|---|---|---|---|---|
| **Differences** | | **Statistical Limits** | | **Sample Size** | |
| SD | Δ (%) | α | β | One-tailed | Two-tailed |
| 1 (68% of data) | 10 | 0.05 | 0.20 | 1237 | 1570 |
| 2 (95% of data) | 10 | 0.05 | 0.20 | 4947 | 6280 |

| TABLE 3-6 • How Changing Beta (β) Affects Sample Size Requirements | | | | | |
|---|---|---|---|---|---|
| **Differences** | | **Statistical Limits** | | **Sample Size** | |
| SD | Δ (%) | α | β | One-tailed | Two-tailed |
| 2 (95% of data) | 10 | 0.05 | 0.10 | 6852 | 8406 |
| 2 (95% of data) | 10 | 0.05 | 0.20 | 4947 | 6280 |

Decreasing the acceptable type 1 ($\alpha$) statistical error risk increases the required sample size (Drew R, discussions and provisions). An easy way to remember this is that, in general, more data, if collected correctly, decreases risk for any type of error (see Table 3-5).

Decreasing the acceptable type 2 ($\beta$) statistical error risk will also increase the required sample size (see Table 3-6). Power = $1 - \beta$, so a larger sample size is required for smaller $\beta$ and higher power (Drew R, discussions and provisions).

Larger differences ($\Delta$) are easier to detect and therefore require a smaller sample size. (Drew R, discussions and provisions) (see Table 3-7).

An example for estimating the sample size for a study would be as follows:

$\alpha = 0.05$
$\beta = 0.20$
$\Delta = 0.25$
$SD = 2.0$

Statistical test = two-sided $t$-test
Single sample

From a statistics table, the total sample size needed for this study is *128, or 64 in each group*. This also indicates that the investigators are interested in *detecting* a clinically meaningful difference of 0.50 unit:

$$\Delta = (\mu_a - \mu_0) / SD$$
$$0.25 = (\mu_a - \mu_0) / 2.0$$
$$(\mu_a - \mu_0) = (2.0) \times (0.25) = 0.50 \text{ unit}$$

For the researchers to significantly detect the difference of 0.50 units, they would need a total sample size of 128 patients, or 64 in each group. This test would have an estimated power of 80% (since $\beta = 0.20$) and a confidence level of 95% (since $\alpha = 0.05$). It is important to reemphasize here that the smaller the value for $\Delta$, the greater would be the sample size needed for the study.

| TABLE 3-5 • How Changing Alpha (α) Affects Sample Size Requirements | | | | | |
|---|---|---|---|---|---|
| **Differences** | | **Statistical Limits** | | **Sample Size** | |
| SD | Δ (%) | α | β | One-tailed | Two-tailed |
| 2 (95% of data) | 10 | 0.05 | 0.20 | 4947 | 6280 |
| 2 (95% of data) | 10 | 0.10 | 0.20 | 3607 | 4947 |

| TABLE 3-7 • How Differences in Delta (Δ) Affect Sample Size Requirements | | | | | |
|---|---|---|---|---|---|
| **Differences** | | **Statistical Limits** | | **Sample Size** | |
| SD | Δ (%) | α | β | One-tailed | Two-tailed |
| 2 (95% of data) | 10 | 0.05 | 0.20 | 4947 | 6280 |
| 2 (95% of data) | 20 | 0.05 | 0.20 | 1237 | 1570 |

## STATISTICALLY VERSUS CLINICALLY SIGNIFICANT DIFFERENCES

*Statistically significant differences* may or may not translate into *clinically significant differences* and vice versa (Gaddis and Gaddis, 1990c). To demonstrate this, let's review some examples, starting with two examples of studies producing statistically significant results.

Grapefruit juice inhibits enzymatic activity of the liver for some medications such that their clearance is decreased and elimination $t_{\frac{1}{2}}$ becomes longer. Current data support that consistent grapefruit consumption statistically *and* clinically significantly decreases clearance and prolongs the elimination $t_{\frac{1}{2}}$ of some medications by more than 50%. This may lead to statistically and clinically significant increases in $C_{max}$ and AUC, and therefore, increased therapeutic and adverse effects that are clinically meaningful (eg, intolerable central nervous system [CNS] depression, hepatic damage, renal dysfunction, gastrointestinal intolerance, etc.).

For other medications, grapefruit consumption may decrease clearance and therefore increase $t_{\frac{1}{2}}$ by less than 5%. In this case, if enough data were collected, one could detect a statistically significant 5% or less decrease in clearance and increase in $t_{\frac{1}{2}}$. However, excluding narrow therapeutic index medications, this would not likely be clinically significant. In other words, one would not expect an increase in $C_{max}$ and AUC that would produce clinically meaningful increases in therapeutic and adverse effects. (eg, no change in CNS depression or risk for hepatic, renal, or gastrointestinal damage, etc.).

In other cases, non-statistically significant differences may be clinically significant. A non-statistically significant difference is more likely to be accepted as being clinically significant in the instance of safety issues (such as adverse effects) than for endpoint improvements (such as greater likelihood to attain goal $C_{max}$). Remember that studies are generally powered based upon the *primary* endpoint rather than *secondary* endpoints like adverse effects. Many times this translates into a lack of power to detect statistically significant differences between groups regarding adverse effects. For example, a study may detect an increase in the risk of the *secondary* safety endpoint invasive cancer without detecting a difference in the *primary* endpoint. The investigators may calculate that 83 patients would need to be treated with the drug to possibly cause one invasive cancer case (see NNH calculation under the "Evaluation of Risk for Clinical Studies" section of this chapter). In this case, although the study was underpowered for the *secondary* safety endpoint of invasive cancer such that the difference detected was not statistically significant, this may very well be clinically meaningful to clinicians, patients, and families, leading to the decision to avoid using this study medication until an appropriately conducted and powered study is completed. This is because statistical significance helps minimize the risk that clinically significant differences are due to chance alone.

In another example, suppose a study was conducted to examine the response rate for a drug in two different populations. The response rates are 55% and 72% for groups 1 and 2, respectively. This difference in response rate is 17% (72 − 55 = 17%) with a 95% CI of −3% to 40%, $p = 0.17$. Let's also further assume that the minimum clinically acceptable difference in response rate for the particular disease is 15%. Although these results are not statistically significant, since the response rate is 17% (which is greater than 15%), it may very well be clinically meaningful enough to lead investigators to conduct another, more adequately powered study. Or, if prior study data were supportive of these results (prior probability), the results may be believable enough to affect how clinicians choose to treat the two different populations.

As demonstrated throughout these examples, when evaluating statistical and clinical significance, one must consider a number of factors, including the study's design, power, population, associated risks, prior probability, and cost effectiveness of the treatment (Gaddis and Gaddis, 1990f).

## CLINICAL CASE

AB is a 33-year-old patient who has been taking carbamazepine for prevention of seizures for 3 years. She has been tolerating her currently prescribed carbamazepine product well and has been seizure free for 2 years. She was informed by her physician that there is a new carbamazepine product available that provides better absorption. She asks you about the new formulation regarding cost and benefit. The new product copay is twice the price of the currently prescribed product. You find the pharmaceutical company's research noting that the new product provides a longer $t_{max}$: 1 hour longer. You also note that the $C_{max}$ is 6.2 versus 5.95 mg/L and the AUC is 296 versus 292 mg h/L for the new and current products, respectively. Per the drug manufacturer, all $p$-values were statistically significant at $p < 0.05$. What recommendation will you make to your patient? In your opinion, are these statistically significantly differences clinically meaningful such that your patient should change to the new carbamazepine product?

**Answer**

Although enough data were collected to detect statistically significant differences among the parameters of $t_{max}$, $C_{max}$, and AUC, these differences were so small that they would not be expected to be clinically meaningful. In other words, they would not be expected to affect the therapeutic benefit or adverse event risk for this patient in a clinically meaningful way.

## STATISTICAL INFERENCE TECHNIQUES IN HYPOTHESIS TESTING FOR PARAMETRIC DATA

*Parametric statistical methods* (*t*-test and *ANOVA*) are used for analyzing normally distributed, parametric data (Gaddis and Gaddis, 1990d). Parametric data include interval and ratio data, but since the same parametric tests are used for both, knowing the differences between these is solely academic. Parametric tests are more powerful and more flexible than nonparametric tests (Gaddis and Gaddis, 1990d). Also, more information about data is generated from parametric tests (Gaddis and Gaddis, 1990d).

The *t*-test (*aka Student's t*-test) is the method of choice when making a single comparison between two groups. An *un-paired t*-test (also known as a non-paired or pooled *t*-test) is used when observations between groups are independent as in the case of a parallel study (ie, there is no crossover in the treatments such that every subject is assigned to a group and receives a single treatment) (see Fig. 3-18). In Fig. 3-18, $E_{xp}$ represents the experimental group and $C_{trl}$ represents the control group.

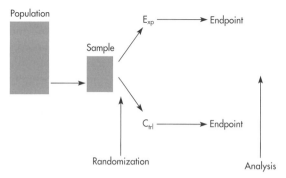

FIGURE 3-18 • Parallel design.

A *paired t*-test is used when observations between groups are dependent, as would be the case in a pretest/posttest study or a crossover study (ie, when every subject enrolled in the study receives all the treatments, but at different periods of time) (Gaddis and Gaddis, 1990d) (see Fig. 3-19). Initially in a crossover study design, group A receives the experimental drug ($E_{xp}$) while group B receives the control ($C_{trl}$: placebo or gold standard treatment). After a washout period, group A receives the control ($C_{trl}$) and group B receives the experimental drug ($E_{xp}$). It is very important to ensure adequate time for washout to prevent carryover effects.

However, when making either multiple comparisons between two groups or a single comparison between multiple groups, type 1 error risk increases if utilizing a *t*-test. For example, when rolling dice, think of rolling ones on both dice (also known as "snake eyes") as being a type 1 error. For each roll of the dice, there is a 1 in 36 chance (2.78%) of rolling snake eyes. For each statistical analysis, we generally accept a 1 in 20 chance (5%) of a type 1 error. Although the chance for snake eyes is the same for

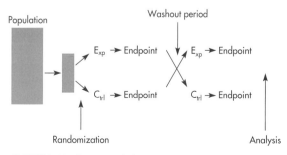

FIGURE 3-19 • Crossover design.

each roll and the chance for type 1 error is the same for each analysis, increasing the number of rolls and analyses increases the opportunity for snake eyes and type 1 errors, respectively. Said another way, the more times one rolls the dice, the more opportunity one has to roll snake eyes. It's the same with statistical testing. The more times one performs a statistical test on a particular data set, the more likely one is to commit a type 1 error.

An example of multiple comparisons of two groups is a trial evaluating chlorthalidone versus placebo for the primary endpoint of change in blood pressure. The trial was evaluated without making type 1 error risk corrections. There were other evaluated endpoints (including potassium concentration, serum creatinine, BUN:SCr ratio, calcium concentration, and others), and the authors did not control for these additional comparisons. There were a total of 20 comparisons including the primary endpoint of change in blood pressure. We can actually calculate the increased risk for type 1 error. If the original $\alpha$ level were $p = 0.05$, the corrected $\alpha$ would be $1 - (1 - 0.05)^{20} = 0.64$. Therefore, if the original $p$-value threshold of 0.05 were used, there would be a 64% chance of inappropriately rejecting the null hypothesis (ie, committing a type 1 error) for at least one of the 20 comparisons (Gaddis and Gaddis, 1990d).

As an example of a single comparison of multiple groups for which the authors and/or statisticians did not make type 1 error risk corrections, a trial evaluated the difference in cholesterol among four lipid-lowering medications. With four groups, there were six paired comparisons. If the original $\alpha$ level were $p = 0.05$, the corrected $\alpha$ would be $1 - (1 - 0.05)^6 = 0.26$. Therefore, if the original $p$-value threshold of 0.05 were used, there would be a 26% chance of inappropriately rejecting the null hypothesis (type 1 error) for at least one of the six comparisons (Gaddis and Gaddis, 1990d).

Investigators should make their best effort to keep the type 1 error risk $\leq 5\%$ (ie, $\leq 0.05$). The best way of doing so for multiple comparisons is by avoiding unnecessary comparisons or analyses, using the appropriate statistical test(s) for multiple comparisons, and using an alpha spending function for interim analyses. However, if investigators fail to do so, there is a crude method for adjusting the preset $\alpha$ level based upon the number of comparisons

being made: the *Bonferroni* correction. This simply divides the preset $\alpha$ level by the number of comparisons being made (Gaddis and Gaddis, 1990d). This estimates the $\alpha$ level that is required to reach statistical significance (Gaddis and Gaddis, 1990d). However, Bonferroni is very conservative as the number of comparisons increases. A less conservative and more accepted way of minimizing type 1 error risk for multiple comparisons with parametric data is through utilization of one of several types of *ANOVA*, which is a parametric test that compares two or more groups simultaneously.

Unlike *t*-test, *ANOVA* holds $\alpha$ level (type 1 error risk) constant when comparing more than two groups (Gaddis and Gaddis, 1990d). ANOVA tests for statistically significant difference(s) among a group's collective values (Gaddis and Gaddis, 1990d). Another way of stating this is that ANOVA analyzes intra- and intergroup variability instead of the means of the groups (Gaddis and Gaddis, 1990d). ANOVA involves calculation of an *F-ratio*, which answers the question, "is the variability between the groups large enough in comparison to the variability of data within each group to justify the conclusion that two or more of the groups differ?" (Gaddis and Gaddis, 1990d).

The most commonly used *ANOVA is for independent (aka un-paired) samples* as is the case for a parallel design.

A *one-way ANOVA* is used if there are no confounders (variables other than the one being studied that influence study results) and at least three independent un-paired samples. For example, if investigators wanted to evaluate the excretion rate (percent of dose excreted unchanged in the urine) in subjects who used different blood pressure medications, a one-way ANOVA can be used if (1) each sample were independent (ie, a parallel design), (2) there were at least three samples (ie, at least three different blood pressure medications), and (3) the experimental groups differed in only *one* factor, which, for this case, would be the type of blood pressure drug being used (ie, there were no differences between the groups with regard to confounding factors like age, gender, kidney function, plasma protein binding, etc).

*Multifactorial ANOVAs* include any type of ANOVA that controls for at least one confounder for at least two independent (un-paired) samples as is the case for a parallel design (see Table 3-8).

## TABLE 3-8 • Common Tests for Parametric Data Analysis

| | Parallel Design | | Crossover or Pre-Post Design | |
|---|---|---|---|---|
| | 2 Independent Samples | ≥ 3 Independent Samples | 2 Related Samples | ≥ 3 Related Samples |
| No confounders[1] | Student's *t*-test (unpaired) | 1-way ANOVA | Paired *t*-test | Repeated measures ANOVA |
| 1 confounder[1] | 2-way ANOVA | 2- ANOVA | 2-way repeated measures ANOVA | 2-way repeated measures ANOVA |
| ≥ 2 confounders[1] | ANCOVA (aka ANACOVA) | ANCOVA (aka ANACOVA) | Repeated measures regression | Repeated measures regression |

[1]Herring C: *Quick Stats: Basics for Medical Literature Evaluation*, 5th ed. Ann Arbor, MI, XanEdu Publishing, 2015.
*Reproduced with permission from Herring C: Quick Stats: Basics for Medical Literature Evaluation, 5th ed. Ann Arbor, MI: XanEdu Publishing; 2015.*

A *2-way ANOVA* is a multifactorial ANOVA that is used if there is one identifiable confounder and at least two independent (aka un-paired) samples (see Table 3-8). For example, if investigators wanted to evaluate the excretion rate (percent of dose excreted unchanged in the urine) of different blood pressure medications, they could use a 2-way ANOVA if (1) each sample were independent (ie, a parallel design), (2) there were at least two samples (ie, at least two different blood pressure medications), and (3) the experimental groups differed in only *two* factors, which for this case would be the type of blood pressure drug being used and one confounding variable (eg, differences between the groups' renal function).

Other types of multifactorial ANOVAs include *analyses of covariance (ANACOVA or ANCOVA)* (see Table 3-8). These are used if there are at least two confounders for at least two independent (un-paired) samples as is the case for a parallel design. These include the *3-way ANOVA, 4-way ANOVA*, etc.

A *3-way ANOVA* is used if there are two identifiable confounders and at least two independent (aka un-paired) samples (see Table 3-8). For example, if investigators wanted to evaluate the excretion rate (percent of dose excreted unchanged in the urine) of different blood pressure medications, they could use a 3-way ANOVA if (1) each sample were independent (ie, a parallel design), (2) there were at least two samples (ie, at least two different blood pressure medications), and (3) the experimental groups differed in *three* factors, which for this case would be the type of blood pressure drug being used and two

confounding variables (eg, differences between the groups' renal function and plasma protein binding).

A *4-way ANOVA* is used if there are three identifiable confounders and at least two independent (aka un-paired) samples (see Table 3-8). For example, if investigators wanted to evaluate the excretion rate (percent of dose excreted unchanged in the urine) of different blood pressure medications, they could use a 4-way ANOVA if (1) each sample were independent (ie, a parallel design), (2) there were at least two samples (ie, at least two different blood pressure medications), and (3) the experimental groups differed in *four* factors, which for this case would be the type of blood pressure drug being used and three confounding variables (eg, differences between the groups' renal function, plasma protein binding, and average patient age).

There are also *ANOVAs for related (aka paired, matched, or repeated) samples* as is the case for a crossover design (see Table 3-8). These include the *repeated measures ANOVA*, which is used if there are no confounders and at least three related (aka paired) samples. For example, if investigators wanted to evaluate the bioavailability of different cholesterol-lowering medications to determine $C_{max}$, they could use a *repeated measures ANOVA* if (1) each subject served as his/her own control (ie, a crossover design), (2) there were at least three samples (ie, at least three different cholesterol medications), and (3) the experimental groups differed in only *one* factor, which for this case would be the type of cholesterol drug being used (ie, there were no identified confounders like fluctuations in renal function, administration times, etc).

A second type of ANOVA for related (aka paired, matched, or repeated) samples is the *2-way repeated measures ANOVA*, which is used if there is one identifiable confounder and at least two related (aka paired) samples (see Table 3-8). For example, if investigators wanted to evaluate the bioavailability of different cholesterol-lowering medications to determine $C_{max}$, they could use a *2-way repeated measures ANOVA* if (1) each subject served as his/her own control (ie, a crossover design), (2) there were at least two samples (ie, at least two different cholesterol medications), and (3) the experimental groups differed in only *two* factors, which for this case would be the type of cholesterol drug being used and one confounding variable (eg, fluctuations in renal function).

Beyond that, *repeated measures regression analysis* is used if there are two or more related (aka paired) samples and two or more confounders (see Table 3-8). For example, if investigators wanted to evaluate the bioavailability of different cholesterol-lowering medications to determine $C_{max}$, they could use a *repeated measures regression analysis* if (1) each subject served as his/her own control (ie, a crossover design), (2) there were at least two samples (ie, at least two different cholesterol medications), and (3) the experimental groups differed in *at least three* factors, which for this case would be the type of cholesterol drug being used and at least two confounding variables (eg, fluctuations in renal function and administration times).

ANOVA will indicate if differences exist between groups but will not indicate where these differences exist. For example, if an investigator is interested in comparing the volume of distribution of a drug among various species, both clearance and the elimination rate constant must be considered. Clearance and the elimination rate constant may be species dependent (ie, rats versus dogs versus humans), and thus they are expected to produce different outcomes (ie, volumes of distribution). However, a statistically significant ANOVA does not point to where these differences exist. To find where the differences lie, *post hoc* (after analysis) multiple comparison methods must be performed.

*Multiple comparison methods* are types of *post hoc* tests that help determine which groups in a statistically significant ANOVA analysis differ (Gaddis and Gaddis, 1990d). These methods are based upon the *t*-test but have built-in corrections to keep α level constant when >1 comparison is being made. In other words, these help control for type 1 error rate for multiple comparisons (Gaddis and Gaddis, 1990d).

Examples include (1) *least significant difference,* which controls individual type 1 error rate for each comparison, (2) *layer (aka stepwise) methods,* which gradually adjust the type 1 error rate and include *Newman-Keuls* and *Duncan,* and (3) *experiment-wise methods,* which hold type 1 error rate constant for a set of comparisons and include *Dunnett,* which tests for contrasts with a control only; *Dunn,* which tests for small number of contrasts; *Tukey,* which tests for a large number of contrasts when no more than two means are involved; and *Scheffe,* which tests for a large number of contrasts when more than two means are involved (Gaddis and Gaddis, 1990d).

Sometimes, otherwise parametric data are not normally distributed (ie, are skewed) such that aforementioned parametric testing methods, *t*-test and the various types of ANOVA, would be inaccurate for data analysis. In these cases, investigators can logarithmically transform the data to normalize data distribution such that *t*-test or ANOVA can be used for data analysis (Shargel et al, 2012).

When performing statistical analyses of subgroup data sets, the term *interaction* or *p for interaction* is often seen (Shargel et al, 2012). *P for interaction (aka p-value for interaction)* simply detects heterogeneity or differences among subgroups. A significant *p* for interaction generally ranges from 0.05 to 0.1 depending on the analysis. In other words, if a subgroup analysis finds a *p* for interaction <0.05 (or <0.1 for smaller studies) for $t_{1/2}$ by male versus female patients, then there is *possibly* a significant difference in $t_{1/2}$ based upon gender. This difference may be worth investigating in future analyses. Just as with other types of subgroup analyses, *p* for interaction solely detects hypothesis-generating differences. However, if multiple similar studies are available, a properly performed meta-analysis may help answer the question of gender and $t_{1/2}$ differences.

### Pharmacokinetic Study Example Incorporating Parametric Statistical Testing Principles

The $t_{1/2}$ of phenobarbital in a population is 5 days with a standard deviation of 0.5 days. A clinician observed that patients who consumed orange juice

2 hours prior to dosing with phenobarbital had a reduction in their $t_{1/2}$ by 10%. To test this hypothesis, the clinician selected a group of 9 patients who were already taking phenobarbital and asked them to drink a glass of orange juice 2 hours prior to taking the medication. The average calculated $t_{1/2}$ value from this sample of 9 patients was 4.25 days. The clinician has to decide from the results obtained from the study whether orange juice consumption decreases the value of $t_{1/2}$. Assuming that alpha was 0.05 (5%), there are several ways to reach the conclusion. Based on the null hypothesis [$H_0$ ($\mu_0$ when evaluating mean differences)], "drinking orange juice 2 hours prior to taking phenobarbital *does not* affect $t_{1/2}$ of the drug." Remember that $H_0$ states that there is no difference whether orange juice was or was not consumed; the $t_{1/2}$ of phenobarbital does not differ. The conclusion of the test is written with respect to $H_0$. An alternative hypothesis is that "orange juice *lowers* the $t_{1/2}$ value of phenobarbital." The alternative hypothesis has the symbol of $H_1$ or $H_a$ ($\mu_a$ when evaluating mean differences).

## GOODNESS OF FIT

*Goodness of fit* (GOF) in pharmacokinetic data analysis is an important concept to assure the reliability of proposed pharmacokinetic models. GOF is a way to describe the "agreement between the model and the observed data" (Anonymous, 2003). This is done by plotting the residuals (RES; the difference between observed and predicted values) versus predicted (PRED) data points. In addition to this plot, GOF analysis includes other plots such as PRED versus observed (OBS) or PRED versus time (Brendel et al, 2007). GOF methodology is often used in population pharmacokinetic studies. For example, the pharmacokinetic profile of the antiretroviral drug nelfinavir and its active metabolite M8 was investigated with the aim of optimizing treatment in a pediatric population (Hirt et al, 2006). The authors used GOF in their assessment of the proposed pharmacokinetic models to compare the population predicted versus the observed nelfinavir and M8 concentrations. The GOF methodology can also refer to how well the empirical data fit a distribution, such as the normal distribution. One of the main requirements of applying parametric methods on continuous scale data

(interval and ratio) is that the observed distribution fits the normal distribution. When the data do not fit the normal distribution, then the investigator can use nonparametric statistical methods for the analysis.

## STATISTICAL INFERENCE TECHNIQUES FOR HYPOTHESIS TESTING WITH NONPARAMETRIC DATA

*Nonparametric statistical methods* are used for analyzing data that are not normally distributed and cannot be defined as parametric data (Gaddis and Gaddis, 1990e). For *nominal data*, the most common tests for proportions and frequencies include *chi-square* ($\chi^2$) and *Fisher's exact*. These tests are "used to answer questions about rates, proportions, or frequencies" (Gaddis and Gaddis, 1990e). *Fisher's exact* test is only used for very small data sets ($N \leq 20$) and when the *predicted* count in one of the cells is zero (0). *Chi-square* ($\chi^2$) is used for all others. For matrices that are larger than $2 \times 2$, $\chi^2$ tests will detect difference(s) between groups but will not indicate where the difference(s) lie(s) (Gaddis and Gaddis, 1990e). To find this, *post hoc* tests are needed. These *post hoc* tests should only be performed if the $\chi^2$ test is statistically significant. Doing otherwise will increase type 1 error risk. Also, if the post-hoc test does not protect against an increase in $\alpha$ for multiple test comparisons, then Bonferroni correction (or another multiple comparison $\alpha$ correction) should be applied to protect against an increase in type 1 error.

For *ordinal data*, the most appropriate test depends upon the number of groups being compared, the number of comparisons being made, and whether the study is of parallel or crossover design. The most commonly used ordinal tests are *Mann–Whitney U*, *Wilcoxon Rank Sum*, *Kolmogorov–Smirnov*, *Wilcoxon Signed Rank*, *Kruskal–Wallis*, and *Friedman*.

The procedure for utilizing all of these tests is very similar to the example provided in the parametric data testing section:

1. State the null and alternate hypotheses at a given alpha value.

2. Calculate test statistics (a computed value for Chi-square or *z*, depending on the test being used).

3. Compare the calculated value with a tabulated value.

4. Build a confidence interval on the true proportion that is expected in the population.

5. Make a decision whether or not to reject the null hypothesis.

Many statistical software programs perform the above tests or other similar tests found in the literature. Computer programs calculate a $p$-value for the test to determine whether or not the results are statistically significant. This is, of course, accomplished by comparing the computed $p$-value with a predetermined $\alpha$ value. In the practice of pharmacokinetics, it is recommended to have computer software for calculating pharmacokinetic parameters and another software program for statistical analyses of experimental data.

## Linear Regression and Correlation (Least Squares Method)

Statistical testing is also applicable to the linear least squares method (Gaddis and Gaddis, 1990f; Ferrill and Brown, 1994). This method allows us to generate a linear relationship between two variables, $x$ and $y$, the independent and dependent variables, respectively. This linear relationship will have a slope and a $y$ intercept. In statistical analysis of this linear equation, the analysis focuses on whether the slope of the line is different from zero, as a slope of zero means that no linear relationship exists between the variables $x$ and $y$. To that end, testing for the *significance* of the slope requires the use of a *Student's t*-test; a statistically *significant* test is when the $H_0$ is rejected. The $t$-test uses a bell-shaped distribution. The mean of the $t$-distribution is zero, and its standard deviation is a function of the sample size (or the degrees of freedom). The larger the sample size, the closer the value of the standard deviation is to 1. With the advances in computer technology and the availability of software programs that readily calculate these statistics, the function of the researcher is to enter the data in a computer database, calculate the slope, and find the $p$-value associated with the slope. If the $p$-value is less than $\alpha$, then the slope is considered statistically

significantly different from zero. Otherwise, do not reject the null hypothesis and the slope is not considered statistically significantly different from zero. Similar analyses can be done on the $y$ intercept using a $t$-test. For the significance of the regression coefficient ($r$), a critical value is obtained from statistics tables at a given degrees of freedom ($n - 2$), a two- or one-tailed test, and a selected $\alpha$ value. If the observed $r$ value equals or exceeds the critical value, then $r$ is significant (ie, reject $H_0$ of $r = 0$); otherwise, $r$ is statistically insignificant. For example, a calculated $r$ value of 0.75 is computed based on 30 pairs of $x$ and $y$ values. The following calculations are taken in the analysis:

1. State the null hypothesis and alternate hypothesis:

   $H_0$: $r = 0$

   $H_1$: $r$ is not equal to zero

   Two-tailed test

2. State the alpha value:

   $\alpha = 0.05$

3. Find the critical value of $r$ (tables for this may be found in statistical textbooks):

   Degrees of freedom = $n - 2 = 30 - 2 = 28$

   Critical value = 0.361

4. Since the calculated value ($r = 0.75$) is greater than 0.361, then the null hypothesis is rejected at the given $\alpha$ level of 5% (ie, with 95% confidence)

5. A linear relationship exists between variables $x$ and $y$

Another way to test the significance of $r$ is to build a confidence interval on the true value of $r$ in the population. If the CI contains the value of zero (0), then do not reject the null hypothesis ($H_0$: the true value of $r$ in the population is zero); otherwise, reject $H_0$ and declare that $r$ is statistically significantly different from zero (this indicates that a linear relationship exists between the variables $x$ and $y$). For example, if the 95% CI were [0.54, 0.88], it would not contain the value zero (0), so the null hypothesis would be rejected and one would conclude that $r$ is statistically significant.

## Accuracy Versus Precision

"*Accuracy* refers to the closeness of the observation to the actual or true value. *Precision (or reproducibility)* refers to the closeness of repeated measurements" (Shargel et al, 2012) (see Fig. 3-20).

Two distributions may have exactly the same mean, yet their variability about the mean may be totally different. Precision is a term that is evaluated by one of the measures used to estimate the variability associated with a mean value. Among the measures that can represent precision are the range, the standard deviation, or the coefficient of variation. Suppose that the maximum plasma concentration mean ($C_{max}$) (± 1 standard deviation) for drug A were 200 µg/mL (± 10 µg/mL) and for drug B were 250 µg/mL (± 12.5 µg/mL). Suppose also that the expected $C_{max}$ value following administration of the two drugs were 210 µg/mL. In term of accuracy, the drug A value would be more accurate than that of drug B (the value 200 is closer to 210 than the value 250 is). With respect to precision, both drugs have the same precision based on the coefficient of variation (CV = [S.D./Mean] × 100; $CV_A$ = [10/200] × 100 = 5%; $CV_B$ = [12.5/250] × 100 = 5%). Note that the use of standard deviation in this case would not be the correct measure because the mean values for the two drugs are different (Sokal, 1981).

### Error Versus Bias

*Error* occurs when *non-systematic* mistakes are made and these neither under- nor overestimate effect size consistently (Drew, 2003). This is sometimes referred to as random error. An example would be if a non-weighted coin were tossed 10 times, it may land on the same side 6 or 7 times; this may lead one to conclude that the probability of landing on that particular side is 60% to 70% (Drew, 2003). However, *bias* refers to *systematic* errors or flaws in study design that consistently either under- or overestimate effect size, leading to incorrect results (Drew, 2003). Using the coin example, bias would be if a coin were weighted such that it would systematically (consistently) land on a particular side 80% of the time. In other words, bias is "error with direction" leading to systematic (consistent) under- or overestimation of effect size (Drew, 2003). There are many types of bias. *Selection bias* occurs when investigators select included and/or excluded samples or data. *Diagnostic or detection bias* can occur when outcomes are detected more or less frequently. For example, this can be from changes in the sensitivity of instruments used to detect drug concentrations.

A. Observed data are precise, but NOT accurate

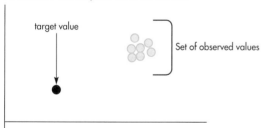

B. Observed data are NOT precise, but accurate

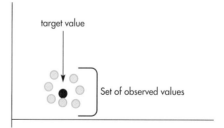

C. Observed data are BOTH precise and accurate

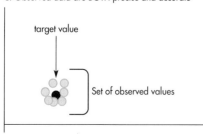

D. Observed data are NEITHER precise nor accurate

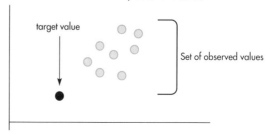

FIGURE 3-20 • A–D.

*Observer or investigator bias* may occur when an investigator favors one sample over another. This is most problematic with "open" or unblinded study designs. *Misclassification bias* may occur when samples are inappropriately classified and may bias in favor of one group over another or in favor of finding no difference between the groups. Bias can also occur when there is a significant dropout rate or loss to follow-up such that data collection is incomplete. *Channeling bias* is sometimes called *confounding by indication* and can occur when one group or sample is "channeled" into receiving one treatment over another.

*Bias is minimized* through a combination of proper study design, methods, and analysis. Proper analysis *cannot* "de-flaw" a study with poor design or methodology (DeYoung, 2000). There are several means of minimizing bias. *Randomization* is sometimes referred to as allocation. In this process, samples are divided into groups by chance alone such that potential confounders are divided equally among the groups and bias is minimized. Doing so helps ensure that all within a studied sample have an equal and independent opportunity of being selected as part of the sample. This can be carried a step further in that once the subject has been selected for a sample, he/she has an equal opportunity of being selected for any of the study arms. An example of *simple randomization* would be drawing numbers from a hat. Its advantage is that it is simple. Its disadvantage is that if a study were stopped early, there is no assurance of similar numbers of subjects in each group at any given point in time. *Block randomization* involves randomizing subjects into small groups called blocks. These blocks generally range from 4 to 20 subjects. Block randomization is advantageous in that there are nearly equal numbers of subjects in each group at any point during a study. Therefore, if a study is stopped early, equal comparisons and more valid conclusions can be made.

Other means of minimizing bias include (DeYoung, 2000, 2005; Drew, 2003):

1. Utilizing objective study endpoints
2. Proper and accurate means of defining exposures and endpoints
3. Accurate and complete sources of information
4. Proper controls to allow investigators to minimize outside influences when evaluating treatments or exposures
5. Proper selection of study subjects, which would require proper inclusion and exclusion criteria
6. Minimizing loss of data
7. Appropriate statistical tests for data analysis
8. Blinding as described later in this chapter
9. *Matching*, which involves either
   a. identifying characteristics that are a potential source of bias and matching controls based upon those characteristics (this is called propensity score matching)
   b. estimating subject prognoses that are a potential source of bias and matching controls based upon those prognoses (this is called prognostic score matching or disease-risk score matching)

## CONTROLLED VERSUS UNCONTROLLED STUDIES

*Uncontrolled studies* do not utilize a control group such that outside influences may affect study results. Using *controls* helps minimize bias when study groups are kept as similar as possible and outside influences are minimized. Ideally, groups will differ only in the factor being studied. There are many types of controls. "Utilizing a *placebo control* is not always practical or ethical, but in placebo control studies one or more groups receive(s) active treatment(s) while the control group receives a placebo" (Drew, 2003). *Historical control* studies are generally less expensive to perform but this design introduces problems with diagnostic, detection, and procedure biases. In these, "data from a group of subjects receiving the experimental drug or intervention are compared to data from a group of subjects previously treated during a different time period, perhaps in a different place" (Herring, 2015). *Crossover control* is very efficient at minimizing bias while maximizing power when used appropriately. It does this by allowing each subject to serve as his/her own control, thereby minimizing differences between subjects in each group and doubling the sample size. Initially, group A receives the experimental drug while group B receives the control (placebo or gold standard treatment). After a washout period of sufficient length, group A receives the control and group B receives the experimental drug. *Standard treatment (aka active treatment) control* is very practical and ethical. The control group receives "standard" treatment while the other group(s) receives experimental treatment(s). This type of control is used when the investigator wishes to demonstrate that the experimental treatment(s) is/are equally efficacious, non-inferior, or superior to "standard" treatment.

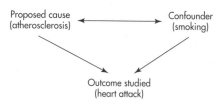

FIGURE 3-21 • Confounding example 1.

## BLINDING

*Blinding* limits investigators' treating or assessing one group differently from another. It is especially important if there is any degree of subjectivity associated with the outcome(s) being assessed. However, it is expensive and time consuming. There are several types of blinding, but we will only discuss the three most common forms. In a *single-blind* study, someone, usually the subject, but in rare cases it may be the investigator, is unaware of what treatment or intervention the subject is receiving. In a *double-blind* study, neither the investigator nor the subject is aware of what treatment or intervention the subject is receiving. In a *double-dummy* study, if one is comparing two different dosage forms (eg, intranasal sumatriptan versus injectable sumatriptan) and doesn't want the patient or investigator to know in which group a patient is participating, then one group would receive intranasal sumatriptan and a placebo injection and the other group would receive intranasal placebo and a sumatriptan injection. Another example of when this would be useful would be for a trial evaluating a tablet versus an inhaler. It should be noted that some trials that claim to be blinded are not. For example, a medication may have a distinctive taste, physiologic effect, or adverse effect that un-blinds patients and/or investigators.

## CONFOUNDING

*Confounding* occurs when variables other than the one(s) being studied influence(s) study results. Confounding variables are difficult to detect sometimes and are linked to study outcome(s) and may be linked to hypothesized cause(s). As discussed in more detail later in this chapter, *validity* of a study depends upon how well investigators minimize the influence of confounders (DeYoung, 2000).

For example, atherosclerosis and myocardial infarction (MI); there is an association between atherosclerosis and smoking, smoking and risk for an MI, and atherosclerosis and risk for an MI. The proposed cause is atherosclerosis, and the potential confounder is smoking (see Fig. 3-21).

Another example of confounding is the relationship between fasting blood glucose (FBG) in patients being treated for diabetes with medication (see Fig. 3-22). One confounder of FBG is diet. For example, dietary cinnamon consumption can lower blood glucose. If patients regularly consume cinnamon, FBG could be lowered beyond the patient's diabetic medication's capabilities. In this case, although cinnamon may not affect the proposed cause (type of diabetes medication that is being used), it very well may affect FBG concentrations, possibly resulting in biased results by augmenting the diabetes drug's FBG-lowering effect, and therefore affecting its pharmacodynamic profile. In general, many dietary supplements may interfere with drugs' action(s). Therefore, it is important that subjects disclose their use of these prior to the start of pharmacokinetic studies (Al-Achi, 2008).

As with bias, confounding is minimized through the combination of proper study design and methodology, including randomization, proper inclusion and exclusion criteria, and matching if appropriate. However, unlike bias, confounding may also be minimized through proper statistical

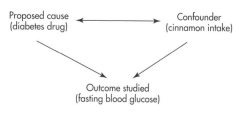

FIGURE 3-22 • Confounding example 2.

analysis. *Stratification* separates subjects into non-overlapping groups called strata, where specific factors (eg, gender, ethnicity, race, smoking status, weight, diet, etc) are evaluated for any influence on study results (DeYoung, 2000). However, stratification has limits (Herring, 2015). As one stratifies, subgroup sample sizes decrease, so one's ability to detect meaningful influences in each subgroup will also decrease.

*Multivariate (or multiple) regression analysis (MRA)* is a possible solution (DeYoung, 2000). With MRA, "multiple predictor variables (aka independent variables) can be used to predict outcomes (aka dependent variables)" (Herring, 2015). For example, both the national cholesterol and hypertension guidelines utilize MRA to help establish atherosclerotic cardiovascular disease (ASCVD) risk for patients based upon population data. A patient's ASCVD risk is the dependent variable because its estimate "depends upon" several independent variables. The independent variables include gender, race, age, total cholesterol, HDL-cholesterol, smoking status, systolic blood pressure, and whether a patient is being treated for hypertension or has diabetes. All of these independent variables are used to help predict a patient's ASCVD risk. Similar factors to those listed above can influence a multitude of pharmacokinetic parameters as well.

As previously discussed, various types of ANOVAs help account for confounding: multivariate ANOVAs for un-paired data, and two-way repeated measures ANOVA for paired data (see Table 3-8).

## VALIDITY

*Internal validity* addresses how well a study is conducted: if appropriate methods are used to minimize bias and confounding and ensure that exposures, interventions, and outcomes are measured correctly (DeYoung, 2000). This includes ensuring the study accurately tests and measures what it claims to test and measure (DeYoung, 2000; Anonymous, 2003). Internal validity directly affects external validity; without internal validity, a study has no external validity. Presuming internal validity, *external validity* addresses the application of study findings to other groups, patients, systems, or the general population (DeYoung, 2000; Drew, 2003). "A high degree of internal validity is often achieved at the expense of external validity" (Drew, 2003). For example, excluding diabetic hypertensive patients from a study may provide very clean statistical endpoints. However, clinicians who treat mainly diabetic hypertensive patients may be unable to utilize the results from such a trial (Drew, 2003).

---

**FREQUENTLY ASKED QUESTION**

▶ Are there any types of statistical tests that can be used to correct for a lack of internal validity?

---

## BIOEQUIVALENCE STUDIES

"Statistics have wide application in bioequivalence studies for the comparison of drug bioavailability for two or more drug products. The FDA has published Guidance for Industry for the statistical determination of bioequivalence (1992, 2001) that describes the comparison between a test (T) and reference (R) drug product. These trials are needed for approval of new or generic drugs. If the drug formulation changes, bioequivalence studies may be needed to compare the new drug formulation to the previous drug formulation. For new drugs, several investigational formulations may be used at various stages, or one formulation with several strengths must show equivalency by extent and rate (eg, $2 \times 250$-mg tablet vs $1 \times 500$-mg tablet, suspension vs capsule, immediate-release vs extended-release product). The blood levels of the drug are measured for both the new and the reference formulation. The derived pharmacokinetic parameters, such as $C_{max}$ and AUC, must meet accepted statistical criteria for the two drugs to be considered bioequivalent. In bioequivalence trials, a 90% confidence interval of the ratio of the mean of the new formulation to the mean of the old formulation (Test/Reference) is calculated. That confidence interval needs to be completely within 0.80–1.25 for the drugs to be considered bioequivalent (see above for logarithmic transformation under the "Measures of Central Tendency" section of this chapter). Adequate power should be built into the design and validated methods used for analysis of the samples. Typically, both the rate (reflected by $C_{max}$) and the extent (AUC) are tested. The ANOVA may also reveal any sequence effects, period effects, treatment effects, or inter- and intrasubject variability. Because of the small subject population usually employed in bioequivalence studies, the true distribution of the data, ie, normal distribution or skewed distribution, is not known. The ANOVA is based on parametric testing and uses log-transformed data to make an inference about the difference of the two groups."

(Shargel et al, 2012).

## EVALUATION OF RISK FOR CLINICAL STUDIES

*Risk calculations* estimate the magnitude of association between exposure and outcome (DeYoung, 2000). These effect measurers are mainly used for nominal outcomes, but in rare cases may be applied to ordinal outcomes. The following calculations for cohort studies and randomized controlled trials (RCTs) are the same, but nomenclature is different. For a cohort study, the exposed group is referred to as such. For an RCT, the exposed group may be referred to as the interventional, experimental, or treatment group. For a cohort study, the unexposed group is referred to as such. For an RCT, the unexposed group is referred to as the control group. For the following examples, the subscript "E" will refer to the exposed or experimental (treatment, interventional) group and the subscript "C" will refer to the unexposed or control group.

*Absolute risk (AR)* is simply another term for incidence. It is the number of *new cases* that occur during a specified time period divided by the number of subjects initially followed to detect the outcome(s) of interest during that time period (Gaddis and Gaddis, 1990c).

$$AR = \frac{\text{Number who develop the outcome of interest during a specified time period}}{\text{Number initially followed to detect the outcome of interest}} \quad (3.8)$$

*Absolute risk reduction (ARR) and absolute risk increase (ARI)* are measures of the absolute incidence differences in the event rate between the studied groups. Absolute differences are more meaningful than relative differences in outcomes when

evaluating clinical trials (DeYoung, 2005). For negative outcomes like death, ARR would be a good thing to see since one wants risk for death to be reduced. With death, ARI would be bad, for the same reason. However, for outcomes like clinical cure or clearing of infection, ARI would be good to see since one wants risk for clinical cure or clearing of infection to increase. ARR would be bad for the same reason.

$$ARR \text{ (or } ARI) = AR_C - AR_E \quad (3.9)$$

*Numbers needed to treat (NNT)* is the reciprocal of the ARR or ARI, depending upon the outcome of interest (DeYoung, 2000, Herring, 2015). The term NNT would be used when a positive outcome like reduction in the risk of death or increase in the risk for clinical cure or clearing of infection is detected. The term NNH would be used when a negative outcome like increase in risk of death or decrease in risk for clinical cure or clearing of infection is detected.

$$NNT \text{ (or } NNH) = \frac{1}{ARR \text{ (or } ARI)} \quad (3.10)$$

For example, if a study were to detect an increase in the risk of death for a particular medication, the terminology would be NNH. This study may detect death in 2.2% of patients taking study medication and 1% of those in the control group over an average follow-up of 2 years. Since numbers needed to harm (NNH) = 1/ARI = 1/0.012 = 83, one would need to treat approximately 83 patients with the study medication over the average follow-up of 2 years to harm 1 patient by possibly causing 1 death.

However, if the outcome for another study were clearing of infection and the study detected clearing of infection in 2.2% of patients taking the study medication and 1% of those in the control group over an average follow-up, the terminology would be NNT since clearing of infection is a good thing. One would need to treat approximately 83 patients with the study medication over an average follow-up of 2 years to help clear 1 patient's infection.

These calculations help in understanding the magnitude of an intervention's effectiveness (DeYoung, 2000). A weakness of these is that they "assume baseline risk is the same for all patients or that it is unrelated to relative risk" (DeYoung, 2000).

Although rarely seen, "confidence intervals (CIs) may be calculated for NNT and NNH" (DeYoung, 2005).

*Relative risk (RR)* compares the AR (incidence) of the experimental group to that of the control group (DeYoung, 2000). It is simply a ratio of the AR for the experimental or exposed group to the AR of the control or unexposed group. RR is sometimes called *risk ratio, rate ratio,* or *incidence rate ratio.*

$$RR = \frac{AR_E}{AR_C} \qquad (3.11)$$

*Relative risk differences* are sometimes presented in studies, and these estimate the relative percentage of baseline risk that is changed between the exposed or experimental group and the unexposed or control group. The relative risk difference is termed *relative risk reduction (RRR)* or *relative risk increase (RRI)*. For negative outcomes like death, RRR would be good since one wants risk for death to be reduced. With death, RRI would be bad, for the same reason. However, for outcomes like clinical cure or clearing of infection, RRI would be good since one wants risk for clinical cure or clearing of infection to increase. RRR would be bad for the same reason.

RRR and RRI can be calculated in two different ways:

$$RRR \text{ (or RRI)} = 1 - RR \qquad (3.12)$$

or

$$RRR \text{ (or RRI)} = \frac{ARR \text{ (or ARI)}_E}{AR_C} \qquad (3.13)$$

Using the example we used above, if a study were to detect an increase in the risk of death for a particular medication, the terminology would be NNH. This study may detect death in 2.2% of patients taking study medication and 1% of those in the control group over an average follow-up of 2 years. The unadjusted RR (95% CI) would be:

$$AR_E/AR_C = 2.2\%/1\% = 0.022/0.01 = 2.2.$$

We could then calculate RRI.

$$RRI = 1 - RR = 1 - 2.2 = -1.2, \text{ or } 120\%$$

If we had detected a decrease in death rate, the term would be RRR rather than RRI.

*Hazard ratio (HR)* is used with Cox proportional hazards regression analysis. It is used when a study is evaluating the length of time required for an outcome of interest to occur (Katz, 2003). HR is often used similarly to RR and is a reasonable estimate of RR as long as adequate data are collected and outcome incidence is <15% (Katz, 2003; Shargel et al, 2012). However, whereas RR only represents the probability of having an event between the beginning and the end of a study, HR can represent the probability of having an event *during a certain time interval* between the beginning and the end of the study (DeYoung, 2005).

*Odds ratio (OR)* is mainly used in case-control studies as an estimate of RR. Since these studies identify cases/controls based upon outcomes (diseases) rather than exposure (risk factors), and since the time between exposure and outcome cannot be estimated accurately, incidence cannot be calculated, and therefore RR cannot be calculated. This is why the calculation for OR is used to estimate RR. OR is fairly accurate in estimating RR as long as disease incidence is <15%, which is usually the case since case-control studies evaluate potential risk factors for rare diseases (Katz, 2003). In addition, OR is sometimes reported for RCTs utilizing logistic or multivariate regression analysis simply because these analyses automatically calculate OR. They do so because regression analysis is utilized to adjust for confounding and adjustments are easier to perform with OR than with RR (De Muth, 2006). OR is presented differently for case-control studies than for RCTs. For RCTs, OR is presented in the same way as RR. For example, in an RCT evaluating an association of an intervention and death rate, an OR of 0.75 would be reported as patients receiving the intervention were 25% less likely to have died than controls. Since case-control studies identify patients based upon disease rather than intervention, OR is presented differently than for an RCT; it compares the odds that a case was exposed to a risk factor to the odds that a control was exposed to a risk factor. For example, in a case-control study evaluating an association of a rare type of cancer and exposure to pesticides, an OR of 1.5 would be reported as cases (those with the rare cancer) were 50% more likely, or 1.5 times as likely, to have been exposed to pesticides than controls. CIs should always be provided for RR, OR, and HR.

These above calculations and principles are commonly utilized for interpreting data in FDA-approved package inserts. For example, in the Coreg® (carvedilol) package insert, there are several major studies that are presented. The COPERNICUS trial evaluated carvedilol's efficacy against that of placebo for patients with severe systolic dysfunction heart failure over a median of 10 months (GlaxoSmith-Kline, 2008). The primary endpoint of mortality occurred in 190 out of 1133 patients taking placebo and 130 out of 1156 patients taking carvedilol. This means that the AR for patients taking placebo was 190/1133 = 0.17 or 17% and the AR for patients taking carvedilol was 130/1156 = 0.11 or 11%. The RR would be 0.11/0.17 or 11%/17% = 0.65 or 65%. RRR would be 1 − 0.65 = 0.35 or 35%. Therefore, patients treated with carvedilol were 35% less likely to die

than were patients treated with placebo. However, sometimes RR and RRR can be deceptive, so one should always calculate the ARR or ARI and NNT or NNH. In this case, carvedilol improved the death rate, so one would calculate ARR and NNT. The ARR is simply the difference between the AR of each agent: 17% − 11% = 6% or 0.17 − 0.11 = 0.06. NNT is the reciprocal of ARR, so 1/0.06 = 17. Therefore, since the median follow-up of this trial was 10 months, one would need to treat 17 patients for 10 months with carvedilol rather than placebo to prevent 1 death.

## FREQUENTLY ASKED QUESTION

▶ Which is more important: relative or absolute difference?

## CHAPTER SUMMARY

Statistical applications are vital in conducting and evaluating biopharmaceutical and pharmacokinetic research. Utilization includes, but is not limited to, studies involving hypothesis testing, finding ways to improve a product, its safety, or performance. Proper statistics are required for experimental running, data collection, analysis, and interpretation results, allowing decision making throughout these pro-cesses. (Durham and Turner, 2008; Shagel et al, 2012)

In this chapter, we have presented very basic, practical principles in hopes of guiding the reader throughout the research process. For readers who are interested in learning about this topic in more depth, we recommend statistics textbooks or online resources and/or taking a research-based statistics course at the college or university of their choosing.

## LEARNING QUESTIONS

1. The following data represent the concentration of vitamin C in infant urine:

| Age (months) | Gender | Conc. (ng/mL) |
|---|---|---|
| 1 | F | 2.7 |
| 3 | F | 2.8 |
| 4 | M | 2.9 |
| 6 | M | 2.9 |
| 7 | M | 2.3 |
| 9 | M | 2.3 |
| 12 | F | 1.5 |

| Age (months) | Gender | Conc. (ng/mL) |
|---|---|---|
| 15 | F | 1.1 |
| 16 | M | 1.3 |
| 17 | F | 1.3 |
| 18 | F | 1.1 |
| 24 | F | 1.5 |
| 25 | F | 1.0 |
| 29 | M | 0.4 |
| 30 | F | 0.2 |

The column for **concentration (ng/mL)** refers to the concentration of vitamin C in infant urine. Calculate the **arithmetic** mean for vitamin C in the urine.

2. Refer to Question 1. Find the standard deviation for the concentration of vitamin C in urine for the male infants.

3. Refer to Question 1. Find the coefficient of variation (%) value for the variable age.

4. Refer to Question 1. Consider the following graph representing the data:

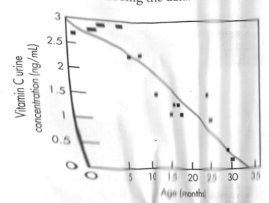

Based on the above graph, the value for the correlation coefficient is most likely _____.

5. Refer to Questions 1 and 4. The older the infant, the _____ the concentration of vitamin C.

6. The p-value associated with the slope of the line in Question 4 is less than 0.0001 (p<0.0001). For α of 5%, the slope is statistically _____.

7. Find the slope value for the graph in Question 4.

8. The following results were presented by Chin KH, Sathyyasurya DR, Abu Saad H, Jan Mohamed HJB: Effect of ethnicity, dietary intake and physical activity on plasma adiponectin concentrations among Malaysian patients with type 2 diabetes mellitus. (*Int J Endocrinol Metab* 11(3):16–174, 2013. DOI:10.5812/ijem.8298. Copyright © 2013, Research Institute for Endocrine Sciences and Iran Endocrine Society; Licensee Kowsar Ltd. This is an Open Access article distributed under the terms of

|  | Malay | Chinese | Indian |
|---|---|---|---|
| Adiponectin (µg/mL) | 6.85 (4.66) | 6.21 (3.62) | 4.98 (2.22) |

*Data from Chin KH, Sathyasurya DR, Abu Saad H, et al: Effect of ethnicity, dietary intake and physical activity on plasma adiponectin concentrations among malaysian patients with type 2 diabetes mellitus. Int J Endocrinol Metab Summer 2013;11(3):167–174.*

The concentration of adiponectin (a protein produced by adipocytes) in plasma is reported in Malaysian patients with three different ethnicities. The values in the table above are given as arithmetic mean (standard deviation). The significance of adiponectin plasma concentrations that its plasma levels correlate well with the clinical response to administered insulin in patients with type 2 diabetes. Referring to the results above, which group of patients is more variable with respect to its mean than the other two groups?

9. Which statistics did you use in answering Question 8?

10. Investigators were comparing two doses of perform anticoagulant for prevention investigation. They calculate that a sample combemembers (20 in each arm) will be needed 400 subjects difference (based upon an alpha of 0.05 how a dif0.20). They predict that given the patient beta population, approximately 50% of subjects will dropout of the study. Based upon the dropout rate, how many subjects will be needed in each treatment arm?

11. A superiority trial evaluating the doses of a new cholesterol medication was performed comparing AUC. There were 200 patients in this trial and differences were statistically significant. Was this study underpowered?

12. A study is planned to evaluate differences in $t_{1/2}$ ($t_{1/2}$) of three different metoprolol formulations. The investigators plan to include 150 subjects (50 in each arm) to reach statistical significance based upon a beta of 0.20 and alpha of 0.05. Which statistical test would be the most appropriate? (Hint: Assume no confounders.)

13. If you conduct a pharmacokinetic study that utilizes appropriate methodology and a broad population base for inclusion, how will this affect the strength of internal and external validity?

14. Investigators wish to study the differences in patients with subtherapeutic concentrations of vancomycin via two different delivery systems. The results from this 2-week study are listed below:

| | New (Experimental) Formulation (E) ($n = 55$) | Standard of Care (Control) Formulation (C) ($n = 62$) |
|---|---|---|
| Subtherapeutic vancomycin concentrations | 35 | 17 |

How should these results be reported?

## ANSWERS

### Learning Questions

1. The arithmetic mean for vitamin C in infant urine is 1.69 ng/mL. Recall that the arithmetic mean is the numerical sum of all the observations divided by their number.

2. The standard deviation of vitamin C in urine for male infants is 0.98 ng/mL. Alternatively, Equation 3.2 may be used for this calculation.

3. The coefficient of variation (%) for age is (SD/mean) × 100 = (9.49/14.4) × 100 = 66%

4. The slope of the line depicted in the graph is negative. Therefore, the correlation coefficient must be a negative value.

5. A negative linear relationship was observed between age of infants and the concentration of vitamin C in urine. Thus, the vitamin C concentration in urine in older infants is lower than that found in younger infants.

6. Since $p$-value is less than 0.05, the results were statistically significant.

7. The slope of the line is negative. The value of the slope may be obtained by a scientific calculator or by a spreadsheet such as Excel.

8. The coefficient of variation (%) for Malay, Chinese, and Indian patients was 68.03%, 58.29%, and 44.58%, respectively. Recall that CV (%) = (SD/mean) × 100. Since Malay patients had the highest CV (%) value, the adiponectin plasma concentrations were more variable with respect to its mean than the other two values.

9. The coefficient of variation (%).

10. Sample size (corrected for drop-outs)

$$= \frac{\text{Number of patients}}{1 - \% \text{ of expected drop-outs}}$$

200 in each arm/(1 − 0.5) = 200/0.5 = 400 in each treatment arm. If the question had been asked how many total subjects would be needed (ie, both arms), the answer would have been 400/(1 − 0.5) = 400/0.5 = 800.

11. Power is associated with beta: power = 1 − beta. Beta is the risk of committing a type 2 error. (See Table 3-3.) For superiority trials, if a statistically significant difference is detected, a type 2 error could not occur. Therefore, the trial was not underpowered. With this scenario, there are only two possibilities: either (1) the findings were correct or (2) a type 1 error occurred.

12. Differences in $t_{1/2}$ are parametric data since they are scored on a continuum and there is a consistent level of magnitude of difference between data units. Since there are three metoprolol formulations being evaluated, and no identified

confounders, a 1-way ANOVA is appropriate. If there were only two groups and no identified confounders, a *t*-test would be appropriate.

13. Utilizing appropriate methodology helps increase internal validity. Including a broad population helps increase external validity.

14. There are several ways the results could be reported. $AR_E = 35/55 = 0.64$ or 64%, $AR_C = 17/62 = 0.27$ or 27%, $ARI = AR_C - AR_E = 0.27 - 0.64 = -0.37$ or 37%, so there was a 37% absolute risk increase in having subtherapeutic vancomycin concentrations in those patients receiving the new (experimental) formulation A relative to those patients receiving the standard of care (control) formulation B. Since having subtherapeutic concentrations is a bad thing, we will use the terminology of NNH. NNH = 1/0.37 = 2.7. If using scientific rounding, 3 patients over 2 weeks. In other words, one would need to treat 3 patients over 2 weeks with the new (experimental) formulation rather than the standard of practice (control) formulation to cause one episode of a subtherapeutic vancomycin concentration.

Some would argue that to be more conservative with NNT and NNH estimates, when calculating NNT, the number should always be rounded up, and when calculating NNH, the number should always be rounded down. In this case, since NNH is 2.7, rounding down would give the estimate that one would need to treat 2 patients over 2 weeks with the new (experimental) formulation rather than the standard of practice (control) formulation to cause one episode of a subtherapeutic vancomycin concentration. Since RR = 35/55 divided by 17/62 = approximately $0.64/0.27 = 2.3$, the results could also be reported as those utilizing the new (experimental) formulation A were 2.3 times as likely to have subtherapeutic vancomycin concentrations as those being given the standard of practice (control) formulation B. Since RRI = 1 − RR = 1 − 2.3 = −1.3, another way of explaining the results would be that those utilizing the new (experimental) formulation A were 130% more likely to have subtherapeutic vancomycin concentrations than those being given the standard of care (control) formulation B.

## REFERENCES

Anonymous: SOP 13: Pharmacokinetic data analysis. *Onkologie* 26(suppl 6):56–59, 2003.

Al-Achi, A: *An Introduction to Botanical Medicines: History, Science, Uses, and Dangers.* Westport, CT, Praeger Publishers, 2008.

Batty KT1, Davis TM, Ilett KF, Dusci LJ, Langton SR: The effect of ciprofloxacin on theophylline pharmacokinetics in healthy subjects. *Br J Clin Pharmacol* 39(3):305–311, 1995.

Berensen NM: Biostatistics review with lecture for the MUSC/VAMC BCPS study group. Charleston, SC, July 17, 2000.

Brendel K, Dartois C, Comets E, et al: Are population pharmacokinetic-pharmacodynamic models adequately evaluated? A survey of the literature from 2002 to 2004. *Clin Pharmacokinet* 46(3):221–234, 2007.

De Muth JE: In Chow SC (ed). *Basic Statistics and Pharmaceutical Statistical Applications,* 2nd ed. Boca Raton, London, New York, Chapman & Hall/CRC, Taylor & Francis Group, 2006.

DeYoung GR: Clinical Trial Design (handout). 2000 Updates in Therapeutics: The Pharmacotherapy Preparatory Course, 2000.

DeYoung GR: *Understanding Statistics: An Approach for the Clinician. Science and Practice of Pharmacotherapy PSAP Book 5,* 5th ed. Kansas City, MO, American College of Clinical Pharmacy, 2005.

Drew R: Clinical Research Introduction (handout). Drug Literature Evaluation/Applied Statistics Course. Campbell University School of Pharmacy, 2003.

Drew R: Discussions and provisions. circa 2003.

Durham TA, Turner JR: *Introduction to Statistics in Pharmaceutical Clinical Trials.* London, UK, Pharmaceutical Press, RPS Publishing, 2008.

Ferrill JM, Brown LD: Statistics for the nonstatistician: A systematic approach to evaluating research reports. *US Pharmacist* July:H-3-H-16, 1994.

Gaddis ML, Gaddis GM: Introduction to biostatistics: Part 1, Basic concepts. *Ann Emerg Med* 19(1):86–89, 1990a.

Gaddis ML, Gaddis GM: Introduction to biostatistics: Part 2, Descriptive statistics. *Ann Emerg Med* 19(3):309–315, 1990b.

Gaddis ML, Gaddis GM: Introduction to biostatistics: Part 3, Sensitivity, specificity, predictive value, and hypothesis testing. *Ann Emerg Med* 19(5):591–597, 1990c.

Gaddis ML, Gaddis GM: Introduction to biostatistics: Part 4, Statistical inference techniques in hypothesis testing. *Ann Emerg Med* 19(7):820–825, 1990d.

Gaddis ML, Gaddis GM: Introduction to biostatistics: Part 5, Statistical inference techniques for hypothesis testing with nonparametric data. *Ann Emerg Med* 19(9):1054–1059, 1990e.

Gaddis ML, Gaddis GM: Introduction to biostatistics: Part 6, Correlation and regression. *Ann Emerg Med* 19(12):1462–1468, 1990f.

Glasner AN: *High Yield Biostatistics*. Philadelphia, PA, Williams & Wilkins, 1995.

GlaxoSmithKline. Coreg CR [package insert], https://www.gsksource.com/gskprm/htdocs/documents/COREG-CR-PI-PIL.PDF. Research Triangle Park, NC, 2008.

Goyvaerts H: Statistics for Non-Statisticians (handout). Presentation for ABEMEP, May 22, 2002.

Herring C: *Quick Stats: Basics for Medical Literature Evaluation*, 5th ed. Ann Arbor, MI, XanEdu Publishing, 2015.

Hirt D, Urien S, Jullien V, et al: Age-related effects on nelfinavir and M8 pharmacokinetics: A population study with 182 children. *Antimicrob Agents Chemother* 50(3):910–916, 2006.

Katz MH: Multivariable analysis: A primer for readers of medical research. *Annal Internal Med* 138:644–650, 2003.

Munro HB: *Statistical Methods for Health Care Research*. Lippincott Williams & Wilkins, Philadelphia, PA, 2005.

Sato R, Tanigawara Y, Kaku M, Aikawa N, Shimizu K: Pharmacokinetic-pharmacodynamic relationship of arbekacin for treatment of patients infected with methicillin-resistant *Staphylococcus aureus*. *Antimicrob Agents Chemother* 50(11): 3763–3769, 2006.

Shargel L, Wu-Pong S, Yu A: *Statistics. Applied Biopharmaceutics and Pharmacokinetics*, 6th ed. New York, NY, McGraw-Hill, 2012, Appendix.

Sokal R, Rohlf JF: *Biometry*, 2nd ed. New York, W.H. Freeman and Company, 1981.

## PART II

# Fundamentals of Biopharmaceutics

# 4 Physiologic Factors Related to Drug Absorption

Phillip M. Gerk

## CHAPTER OBJECTIVES

- Define passive and active drug absorption.
- Explain how Fick's law of diffusion relates to passive drug absorption.
- Calculate the percent of drug nonionized and ionized for a weak acid or weak-base drug using the Henderson–Hasselbalch equation and explain how this may affect drug absorption.
- Define transcellular and paracellular drug absorption and explain using drug examples.
- Describe the anatomy and physiology of the GI tract and explain how stomach emptying time and GI transit time can alter the rate and extent of drug absorption.
- Explain the effect of food on GI physiology and systemic drug absorption.
- Describe the various transporters and how they influence the pharmacokinetics of drug disposition in the GI tract.
- Explain the pH-partition hypothesis and how gastrointestinal pH and the $pK_a$ of a drug may influence systemic drug absorption. Describe how drug absorption may be affected by a disease that causes changes in intestinal blood flow and/or motility.
- List the major factors that affect drug absorption from oral and non-oral routes of drug administration.
- Describe various methods that may be used to study oral drug absorption from the GI transit.

## DRUG ABSORPTION AND DESIGN OF A DRUG PRODUCT

Major considerations in the design of a drug product include the therapeutic objective, the application site, and systemic drug absorption from the application site. If the drug is intended for systemic activity, the drug should ideally be completely and consistently absorbed from the application site. In contrast, if the drug is intended for local activity, then systemic absorption from the application should be minimal to prevent systemic drug exposure and possible systemic side effects. For extended-release drug products, the drug product should remain at or near the application site and then slowly release the drug for the desired period of time. The systemic absorption of a drug is dependent on (1) the physicochemical properties of the drug, (2) the nature of the drug product, and (3) the anatomy and physiology of the drug absorption site. Thus, the rate and extent to which a drug gets from the site of administration to the blood will depend on its release from the dosage form into physiologic fluids, the permeability of the drug through the tissues in the absorption site, and any degradation or metabolism of the drug that may occur before reaching the blood.

In order to develop a drug product that elicits the desired therapeutic objective, the pharmaceutical scientist must have a thorough understanding of the biopharmaceutic properties of the drug and drug product and the physiologic and pathologic factors affecting drug absorption from the application site. A general description of drug absorption, distribution, and elimination is shown in Fig. 4-1. Pharmacists must also understand the relationship of drug dosage to therapeutic efficacy and adverse reactions and the potential for drug–drug and drug–nutrient interactions. This chapter will focus on the anatomic and physiologic considerations for the

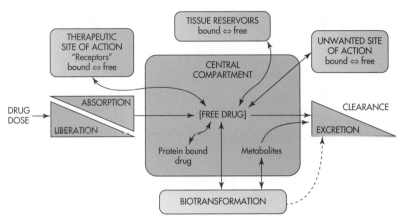

FIGURE 4-1 • The interrelationship of the absorption, distribution, binding, metabolism, and excretion of a drug and its concentration at its sites of action. (Reproduced with permission from Brunton LL, Hilal-Dandan R, Knollmann BC: Goodman & Gilman's Pharmacological Basis of Therapeutics, 13th ed. New York, NY: McGraw Hill; 2018.)

systemic absorption of a drug, whereas Chapters 7 to 8 will focus on the biopharmaceutic aspects of the drug and drug-product design, including considerations in manufacturing and performance tests. Since the major route of drug administration is the oral route, major emphasis in this chapter will be on gastrointestinal (GI) drug absorption.

## ROUTE OF DRUG ADMINISTRATION

Drugs may be given by parenteral, enteral, inhalation, intranasal, transdermal (percutaneous), or intranasal route for systemic absorption. Each route of drug administration has certain advantages and disadvantages. Characteristics of the more common routes of drug administration are listed in Table 4-1. The systemic availability and onset of drug action are affected by blood flow at the administration site, the physicochemical characteristics of the drug and the drug product, and any pathophysiologic condition at the absorption site. After a drug is systemically absorbed, drug distribution and clearance follow normal physiological conditions of the body. Drug distribution and clearance are not usually altered by the drug formulation but may be altered by pathology, genetic polymorphism, and drug–drug interactions, as discussed in other chapters.

Many drugs are not administered orally because of insufficient systemic absorption from the GI tract.

The diminished oral drug absorption may be due to drug instability in the GI tract, drug degradation by the digestive enzymes in the intestine, high hepatic clearance (first-pass effect), and efflux transporters such as P-glycoprotein resulting in poor and/or erratic systemic drug availability. Some orally administered drugs, such as cholestyramine and others (Table 4-2), are not intended for systemic absorption but may be given orally for local activity in the GI tract. However, some oral drugs such as mesalamine and balsalazide that are intended for local activity in the GI tract may also have a significant amount of systemic drug absorption. Small, highly lipid-soluble drugs such as nitroglycerin and fentanyl that are subject to high first-pass effects if swallowed may be given by buccal or sublingual routes to bypass degradation in the GI tract and/or first-pass effects. Insulin is an example of protein peptide drug generally not given orally due to degradation and inadequate absorption in the GI tract.

Biotechnology-derived drugs (see Chapter 10) are usually given by the parenteral route because they are too labile in the GI tract to be administered orally. For example, erythropoietin and human growth hormone (somatropin) are administered intramuscularly, and insulin is given subcutaneously or intramuscularly. Subcutaneous injection results in relatively slow absorption from the site of administration compared to intravenous injection, which provides immediate delivery to the plasma. Pathophysiologic conditions

## TABLE 4-1 • Common Routes of Drug Administration

| Route | Bioavailability | Advantages | Disadvantages |
|---|---|---|---|
| **Parenteral Routes** | | | |
| Intravenous bolus (IV) | Complete (100%) systemic drug absorption. Instant bioavailability. | Drug is given for immediate effect. | Increased chance for adverse reaction. Possible anaphylaxis. |
| Intravenous infusion (IV inf) | Complete (100%) systemic drug absorption. Rate of drug absorption controlled by infusion rate. | Plasma drug levels more precisely controlled. May inject large fluid volumes. May use drugs with poor lipid solubility and/or irritating drugs. | Requires skill in insertion of infusion set. Tissue damage at site of injection (infiltration, necrosis, or sterile abscess). |
| Subcutaneous (SC) injection | Prompt from aqueous solution. Slow absorption from repository formulations. | Generally, used for insulin injection. | Rate of drug absorption depends on blood flow and injection volume. Insulin formulation can vary from short to intermediate and long acting. |
| Intradermal injection | Drug injected into surface area (dermal) of skin. | Often used for allergy and other diagnostic tests, such as tuberculosis. | Some discomfort at site of injection. |
| Intramuscular (IM) injection | Rapid from aqueous solution. Slow absorption from nonaqueous (oil) solutions. | Easier to inject than IV injection. Larger volumes may be used compared to SC solutions. | Irritating drugs may be very painful. Different rates of absorption depending on muscle group injected and blood flow. |
| Intra-arterial injection | 100% of solution is absorbed. | Used in chemotherapy to target drug to organ. | Drug may also distribute to other tissues and organs in the body. |
| Intrathecal injection | 100% of solution is absorbed. | Drug is directly injected into cerebrospinal fluid (CSF) for uptake into brain. | Careful injection skill required. |
| Intraperitoneal injection | In laboratory animals (eg, rat) drug absorption resembles oral absorption. | Used more in small laboratory animals. Less common injection in humans. Used for renally impaired patients on peritoneal dialysis who develop peritonitis. | Drug absorption via mesenteric veins to liver, may have some hepatic clearance prior to systemic absorption. |
| **Enteral Routes** | | | |
| Buccal or sublingual (SL) | Rapid absorption from lipid soluble drugs. | No "first-pass" effects. Buccal route may be formulated for local prolonged action, eg, adhere to the buccal mucosa with some antifungal. Buccal is different from SL, which is usually placed under tongue. | Some drugs may be swallowed. Not for most drugs or drugs with high doses. |

*(Continued)*

## TABLE 4-1 • Common Routes of Drug Administration (*Continued*)

| Route | Bioavailability | Advantages | Disadvantages |
|---|---|---|---|
| Oral (PO) | Absorption may vary. Generally, slower absorption rate compared to IV bolus or IM injection. | Safest and easiest route of drug administration. May use immediate-release and modified-release drug products. | Some drugs may have erratic absorption, be unstable in the gastrointestinal tract, or be metabolized by liver prior to systemic absorption. |
| Rectal (PR) | Absorption may vary from suppository. More reliable absorption from enema (solution). | Useful when patient cannot swallow medication. Used for local and systemic effects. | Absorption may be erratic. Suppository may migrate to different position. Some patient discomfort. |
| **Other Routes** | | | |
| Transdermal | Slow absorption, rate may vary. Increased absorption with occlusive dressing. | Transdermal delivery system (patch) is easy to use. Used for lipid-soluble drugs with low dose and low molecular weight (MW). | Some irritation by patch or drug. Permeability of skin variable with condition, anatomic site, age, and gender. Type of cream or ointment base affects drug release and absorption. |
| Inhalation and intranasal | Rapid absorption. Total dose absorbed is variable. | May be used for local or systemic effects. | Particle size of drug determines anatomic placement in respiratory tract. May stimulate cough reflex. Some drug may be swallowed. |

## TABLE 4-2 • Drugs Given Orally for Local Drug Activity in the Gastrointestinal Tract

| Drug | Example | Comment |
|---|---|---|
| Cholestyramine | Questran | Cholestyramine resin is the chloride salt of a basic anion exchange resin, a cholesterol-lowering agent. Cholestyramine resin is hydrophilic but insoluble in water and not absorbed from the digestive tract. |
| Balsalazide disodium | Colazal | Balsalazide disodium is a prodrug that is enzymatically cleaved in the colon to produce mesalamine, an anti-inflammatory drug. Balsalazide disodium is intended for local action in the treatment of mildly to moderately active ulcerative colitis. Balsalazide disodium and its metabolites are absorbed from the lower intestinal tract and colon. |
| Mesalamine[a] delayed-release tablet | Asacol HD tablet | Asacol HD delayed-release tablets have an outer protective coat and an inner coat, which dissolves at pH 7 or greater, releasing mesalamine in the terminal ileum for topical anti-inflammatory action in the colon. |
| Mesalamine controlled-release capsule | Pentasa capsule | Pentasa capsule is an ethylcellulose-coated, controlled-release capsule formulation of mesalamine designed to release therapeutic quantities of mesalamine throughout the gastrointestinal tract. |

[a]Also referred to as 5-aminosalicylic acid or 5-ASA. Although mesalamine is indicated for local anti-inflammatory activity in the lower GI tract, mesalamine is systemically absorbed from the GI tract.

such as burns will increase the permeability of drugs across the skin compared with normal intact skin. Currently, pharmaceutical research is being directed to devise approaches for the oral absorption of various protein drugs such as insulin (Dhawan et al, 2009). Recently, inhaled insulin was approved for use by the FDA but the product was discontinued by the manufacturer because of poor patient and physician acceptance of this new route of administration. Biotechnology-derived drugs are discussed more fully in Chapter 10.

When a drug is administered by an extravascular route of administration (eg, oral, topical, intranasal, inhalation, rectal), the drug must first be absorbed into the systemic circulation and then diffuse or be transported to the site of action before eliciting biological and therapeutic activity. The general principles and kinetics of absorption from these extravascular sites follow the same principles as oral dosing, although the physiology of the site of administration differs.

## NATURE OF CELL MEMBRANES

Many drugs administered by extravascular routes are intended for local effect. Other drugs are designed to be absorbed from the site of administration into the systemic circulation. For systemic drug absorption, the drug may cross cellular membranes. After oral administration, drug molecules must cross the intestinal epithelium by going either through or between the epithelial cells to reach the systemic circulation. The permeability of a drug at the absorption site into the systemic circulation is intimately related to the molecular structure and properties of the drug and to the physical and biochemical properties of the cell membranes. Once in the plasma, the drug may act directly or may have to cross biological membranes to reach the site of action. Therefore, biological membranes potentially pose a significant barrier to drug delivery.

*Transcellular absorption* is the process of drug movement across a cell. Some polar molecules may not be able to traverse the cell membrane but instead go through gaps or *tight junctions* between cells, a process known as *paracellular drug diffusion*. Figure 4-2 shows the difference between the two

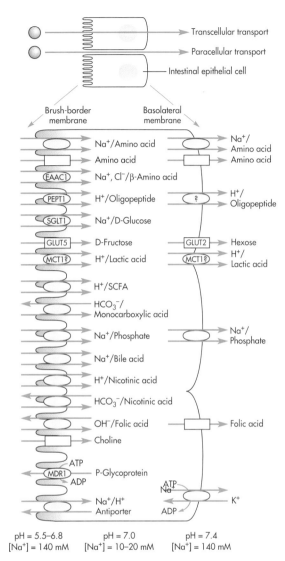

**FIGURE 4-2 •** Summary of intestinal epithelial transporters. Transporters shown by square and oval shapes demonstrate active and facilitated transporters, respectively. Names of cloned transporters are shown with square or oval shapes. In the case of active transporters, arrows in the same direction represent symport of substance and the driving force. Arrows going in the reverse direction mean the antiport. (Reproduced with permission from Tsuji A, Tamai I. Carrier-mediated intestinal transport of drugs, Pharm Res 1996 Jul;13(7):963-977.) Note that BCRP and MRP2 are positioned similarly to MDR1 (P-glycoprotein).

processes. Some drugs are probably absorbed by a mixed mechanism involving multiple processes.

Membranes are major structures in cells, surrounding the entire cell (plasma membrane) and acting as a boundary between the cell and the interstitial fluid. In addition, membranes enclose most of the cell organelles (eg, the mitochondrion membrane). Functionally, cell membranes are semipermeable partitions that act as selective barriers to the passage of molecules. Water, some selected small molecules, and lipid-soluble molecules pass readily through such membranes, whereas highly charged molecules and large molecules, such as proteins and protein-bound drugs, do not.

The transmembrane movement of drugs is influenced by the composition and structure of the plasma membranes. Cell membranes are generally thin, approximately 70–100 Å in thickness. Cell membranes are composed primarily of phospholipids in the form of a bilayer interdispersed with carbohydrates and protein groups. There are several theories as to the structure of the cell membrane. The *lipid bilayer* or *unit membrane theory*, originally proposed by Danielli and Davson (1935) and reviewed by Danielli and Davson (1952), considers the plasma membrane to be composed of two layers of phospholipid between two surface layers of proteins, with the hydrophilic "head" groups of the phospholipids facing the protein layers and the hydrophobic "tail" groups of the phospholipids aligned in the interior. The lipid bilayer theory explains the observation that lipid-soluble drugs tend to penetrate cell membranes more easily than polar molecules. However, the bilayer cell membrane structure does not account for the diffusion of water, small-molecular-weight molecules such as urea, and certain charged ions.

The *fluid mosaic model*, proposed by Singer and Nicolson (1972), explains the transcellular diffusion of polar molecules (Lodish, 1979). According to this model, the cell membrane consists of globular proteins embedded in a dynamic fluid, lipid bilayer matrix (Fig. 4-3). These proteins provide a pathway for the selective transfer of certain polar molecules and charged ions through the lipid barrier. As shown in Fig. 4-3, transmembrane proteins are interdispersed throughout the membrane. Two types of pores of about 10 nm and 50–70 nm were inferred to be present in membranes based on capillary membrane transport studies (Pratt and Taylor, 1990). These small pores provide a channel through which water, ions, and dissolved solutes such as urea may move across the membrane.

Membrane proteins embedded in the bilayer serve special purposes. These membrane proteins function as structural anchors, receptors, ion channels, or transporters to transduce electrical or chemical signaling pathways that facilitate or prevent selective actions. In contrast to simple bilayer structure, membranes are highly ordered and compartmented (Brunton, 2011). Indeed, many early experiments on drug absorption or permeability using isolated gut studies were proven not valid because the membrane proteins and electrical properties of the membrane were compromised in many epithelial cell membranes, including those of the GI tract.

## PASSAGE OF DRUGS ACROSS CELL MEMBRANES

There are several mechanisms by which drugs may pass through cell membranes. Passive (simple) diffusion does not involve any energy or transporter protein. Carrier-mediated transport involves a protein which facilitates the movement of the drug across the membrane, either with or without an energy source. Active transport is a special case of carrier-mediated transport, in which an energy source is used to drive the transport process. These different types of transport will each be discussed further in the following sections.

### Passive Diffusion

Theoretically, a lipophilic drug may pass through the cell or go around it. If the drug has a low molecular weight and is lipophilic, the lipid cell membrane is not a barrier to drug diffusion and absorption. *Passive diffusion* is the process by which molecules spontaneously diffuse from a region of higher concentration to a region of lower concentration. This process is *passive* because no external energy is expended. In Fig. 4-4, drug molecules move forward and back across a membrane. If the two sides have the same drug concentration, forward-moving drug molecules are balanced by molecules moving back, resulting in no net transfer of drug. When one side is higher in drug concentration at any given time, the number of forward-moving drug molecules will be higher than the number of backward-moving molecules; the net result will be a transfer of molecules

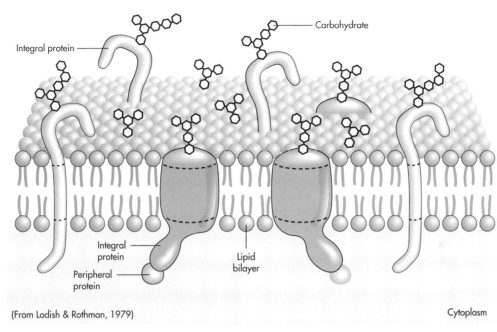

*(From Lodish & Rothman, 1979)*

**FIGURE 4-3 •** Model of the plasma membrane including proteins and carbohydrates as well as lipids. Integral proteins are embedded in the lipid bilayer; peripheral proteins are merely associated with the membrane surface. The carbohydrate consists of monosaccharides, or simple sugars, strung together in chains attached to proteins (forming glycoproteins) or to lipids (forming glycolipids). The asymmetry of the membrane is manifested in several ways. Carbohydrates are always on the exterior surface and peripheral proteins are almost always on the cytoplasmic, or inner, surface. The two lipid monolayers include different proportions of the various kinds of lipid molecules. Most important, each species of integral protein has a definite orientation, which is the same for every molecule of that species. (Lodish and Rothman, 1979.)

to the alternate side downstream from the concentration gradient, as indicated in the figure by the big arrow. The rate of transfer is called *flux* and is represented by a vector to show its direction in space. The tendency of molecules to move in all directions is natural because molecules possess kinetic energy and constantly collide with one another in space. Only left and right molecule movements are shown in Fig. 4-4, because movement of molecules in other directions will not result in concentration changes due to the limitation of the container wall.

Passive diffusion is the major absorption process for most drugs. The driving force for passive diffusion is higher drug concentrations, typically on the mucosal side compared to the blood (serosal) side as in the case of oral drug absorption. According to *Fick's law of diffusion*, drug molecules diffuse from a region of high drug concentration to a region of low drug concentration.

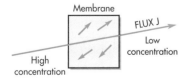

**FIGURE 4-4 •** Passive diffusion of molecules. Molecules in solution diffuse randomly in all directions. As molecules diffuse from left to right and vice versa (small arrows), a net diffusion from the high-concentration side to the low-concentration side results. This results in a net flux (*J*) to the right side. Flux is measured in mass per unit time (eg, ng/min).

$$\frac{dQ}{dt} = \frac{DAK}{h}(C_{GI} - C_p) \qquad (4.1)$$

where $dQ/dt$ = rate of diffusion, $D$ = diffusion coefficient, $A$ = surface area of membrane, $K$ = lipid–water partition coefficient of drug in the biologic membrane that controls drug permeation, $h$ = membrane thickness, and $C_{GI} - C_p$ = difference between the concentrations of drug in the GI tract and in the plasma.

Because the drug distributes rapidly into a large volume after entering the blood, the concentration of drug in the blood initially is quite low with respect to the concentration at the site of drug absorption. For example, a drug is usually given in milligram doses so that the drug concentration at the absorption site maybe in mg/mL, whereas plasma drug concentrations are often in the microgram-per-milliliter or nanogram-per-milliliter range. If the drug is given orally, then $C_{GI} \gg C_p$. A large concentration gradient is maintained until most of the drug is absorbed, thus driving drug molecules from the GI tract into the plasma.

Given Fick's law of diffusion, several other factors may influence the rate of passive diffusion of drugs. For example, the degree of lipid solubility of the drug influences the rate of drug absorption. The partition coefficient, $K$, represents the lipid–water partitioning of a drug across a membrane such as the mucosa. Drugs that are more lipid soluble have a larger K value. The surface area, $A$, of the membrane also influences the rate of absorption. Drugs may be absorbed from most areas of the GI tract. However, the duodenal area of the small intestine shows the most rapid drug absorption, due to such anatomic features as villi and microvilli, which provide a large surface area. These villi are less abundant in other areas of the GI tract.

The thickness of the membrane, $h$, is generally a constant[1] for any particular absorption site. Drugs usually diffuse very rapidly through capillary plasma membranes in the vascular compartments, in contrast to diffusion through plasma membranes of capillaries in the brain. In the brain, the capillaries are densely lined with glial cells, so a drug diffuses slowly into the brain as if a thick lipid membrane exists. The term *blood–brain barrier* is used to describe the slow diffusion of water-soluble molecules across capillary plasma membranes into the brain. However, in certain disease states such as meningitis, these membranes may be disrupted or become more permeable to drug diffusion.

The diffusion coefficient, $D$, is a constant for each drug and is defined as the amount of a drug that diffuses across a membrane of a given unit area per unit time when the concentration gradient is unity.

The dimensions of $D$ are area per unit time—for example, cm²/sec.

Because $D$, $A$, $K$, and $h$ are constants under usual conditions for absorption, a combined constant $P$ or permeability coefficient may be defined.

$$P = \frac{DAK}{h} \tag{4.2}$$

Furthermore, in Equation 4.1 the drug concentration in the plasma, $C_p$, is extremely small compared to the drug concentration in the GI tract, $C_{GI}$. If $C_p$ is negligible and $P$ is substituted into Equation 4.1, the following relationship for Fick's law is obtained:

$$\frac{dQ}{dt} = P(C_{GI}) \tag{4.3}$$

Equation 4.3 is an expression for a first-order process. In practice, the extravascular absorption of most drugs tends to be a first-order absorption process. Moreover, because of the large concentration gradient between $C_{GI}$ and $C_p$, the rate of drug absorption is usually more rapid than the rate of drug elimination.

Many drugs have both lipophilic and hydrophilic chemical substituents. Those drugs that are more lipid soluble tend to traverse cell membranes more easily than less lipid-soluble or more water-soluble molecules. For drugs that act as weak electrolytes, such as weak acids and bases, the extent of ionization influences the drug's diffusional permeability. The ionized species of the drug contains a charge and is more water soluble than the nonionized species of the drug, which is more lipid soluble. The extent of ionization of a weak electrolyte will depend on both the $pK_a$ of the drug and the pH of the medium in which the drug is dissolved. *Henderson and Hasselbalch* used the following expressions pertaining to weak acids and weak bases to describe the relationship between $pK_a$ and pH:
For weak acids,

$$\text{Ratio} = \frac{[\text{Salt}]}{[\text{Acid}]} = \frac{[A^-]}{[HA]} = 10^{(pH - pk_a)} \tag{4.4}$$

For weak bases,

$$\text{Ratio} = \frac{[\text{Base}]}{[\text{Salt}]} = \frac{[RNH_2]}{[RNH_3^+]} = 10^{(pH - pk_a)} \tag{4.5}$$

With Equations 4.4 and 4.5, the proportion of free acid or free base existing as the nonionized species

---

[1] The thickness of the membrane is generally a constant. However, under certain pathological conditions such as meningitis, drugs penetrate into the brain more quickly or in the case of burns, drugs can permeate through the skin more easily.

may be determined at any given pH, assuming the $pK_a$ for the drug is known. For example, at a plasma pH of 7.4, salicylic acid ($pK_a$ = 3.0) exists mostly in its ionized or water-soluble form, as shown below:

$$\text{Ratio} = \frac{[\text{Salt}]}{[\text{Acid}]} = 10^{(7.4-3.0)}$$

$$\log \frac{[\text{Salt}]}{[\text{Acid}]} = 7.4 - 3.0 = 4.4$$

$$\frac{[\text{Salt}]}{[\text{Acid}]} = 2.51 \times 10^4$$

In a simple system, the total drug concentration on either side of a membrane should be the same at equilibrium, assuming Fick's law of diffusion is the only distribution factor involved. For diffusible drugs, such as nonelectrolyte drugs or drugs that do not ionize, the drug concentrations on either side of the membrane are the same at equilibrium. However, for electrolyte drugs or drugs that ionize, the total drug concentrations on either side of the membrane are not equal at equilibrium if the pH of the medium differs on respective sides of the membrane. For example, consider the concentration of salicylic acid ($pK_a$ = 3.0) in the stomach (pH 1.2) as opposed to its concentration in the plasma (pH 7.4) (Fig. 4-5). According to the Henderson–Hasselbalch equation (Equation 4.4) for weak acids, at pH 7.4 and at pH 1.2, salicylic acid exists in the ratios that follow. In the plasma, at pH 7.4

$$\text{Ratio} = \frac{[\text{RCOO}^-]}{[\text{RCOOH}]} = 2.51 \times 10^4$$

In gastric juice, at pH 1.2

$$\text{Ratio} = \frac{[\text{RCOO}^-]}{[\text{RCOOH}]} = 10^{(1.2-3.0)} = 1.58 \times 10^{-2}$$

The total drug concentration on either side of the membrane is determined as shown in Table 4-3.

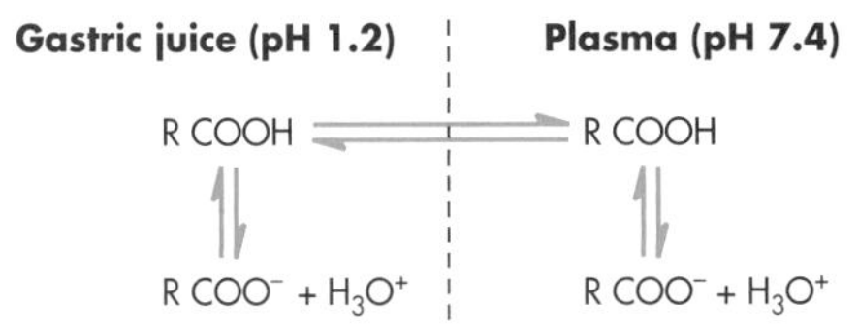

FIGURE 4-5 • Model for the distribution of an orally administered weak electrolyte drug such as salicylic acid.

**TABLE 4-3** • Relative Concentrations of Salicylic Acid as Affected by pH

| Drug | Gastric Juice (pH 1.2) | Plasma (pH 7.4) |
| --- | --- | --- |
| RCOOH | 1.0000 | 1 |
| RCOO⁻ | 0.0158 | 25,100 |
| Total drug concentration | 1.0158 | 25,101 |

Thus, the pH affects distribution of salicylic acid (RCOOH) and its salt (RCOO⁻) across cell membranes. It is assumed that the acid, RCOOH, is freely permeable and the salt, RCOO⁻, is not permeable across the cell membrane. In this example, the total concentration of salicylic acid at equilibrium is approximately 25,000 times greater in the plasma than in the stomach (see Table 4-3). These calculations can also be applied to weak bases, using Equation 4.5.

According to the *pH-partition hypothesis*, if the pH on one side of a cell membrane differs from the pH on the other side of the membrane, then (1) the drug (weak acid or base) will ionize to different degrees on respective sides of the membrane; (2) the total drug concentrations (ionized plus nonionized drug) on either side of the membrane will be unequal; and (3) the compartment in which the drug is more highly ionized will contain the greater total drug concentration. For these reasons, a weak acid (such as salicylic acid) will be more rapidly absorbed from the stomach (pH 1.2) than a weak base (such as quinidine).

Another factor that can influence drug concentrations on either side of a membrane is a particular *affinity* of the drug for a tissue component, which prevents the drug from moving freely back across the cell membrane. For example, a drug such as dicumarol binds to plasma protein, and digoxin binds to tissue protein. In each case, the protein-bound drug does not move freely across the cell membrane. Drugs such as chlordane are very lipid soluble and will partition into adipose (fat) tissue. In addition, a drug such as tetracycline might form a complex with calcium in the bones and teeth. Finally, a drug may concentrate in a tissue due to a specific uptake or active transport process. Such processes have been demonstrated for iodide in thyroid tissue, potassium in the intracellular water, and certain catecholamines into adrenergic storage sites. Such drugs may have a higher total drug concentration on the side where binding occurs, yet the free drug concentration that diffuses across cell membranes will be the same on both sides of the membrane.

Instead of diffusing into the cell, drugs can also diffuse into the spaces around the cell as an absorption mechanism. In *paracellular drug absorption*, drug molecules smaller than 500 MW diffuse through the tight junctions, or spaces between intestinal epithelial cells. Generally, paracellular drug absorption is very slow, being limited by tight junctions between cells. For example, if mannitol is dosed orally, it would be absorbed minimally through this route; mannitol has very, very low oral bioavailability.

## Carrier-Mediated Transport

*Enterocytes* are simple columnar epithelial cells that line the intestinal walls in the small intestine and colon. They express various drug transporters, are connected by tight junctions, and often play an important role in determining the rate and extent of drug absorption. Uptake transporters move drug molecules into the blood and increase plasma drug concentration, whereas efflux transporters move drug molecules back into the gut lumen and reduce systemic drug absorption. These cells also express some drug-metabolizing enzymes, and can contribute to presystemic drug metabolism (Doherty and Charman, 2002).

Theoretically, a lipophilic drug may either pass through the cell or go around it. If the drug has a low molecular weight and is lipophilic, the lipid cell membrane is not a barrier to drug diffusion and absorption. In the intestine, drugs and other molecules can go through the intestinal epithelial cells by either diffusion or a carrier-mediated mechanism. Numerous specialized carrier-mediated transport systems are present in the body, especially in the intestine for the absorption of ions and nutrients required by the body.

### Active Transport

Active transport is a carrier-mediated transmembrane process that plays an important role in the GI absorption and in urinary and biliary secretion of many drugs and metabolites. A few lipid-insoluble

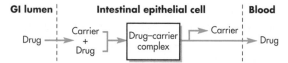

FIGURE 4-6 • Hypothetical carrier-mediated transport process.

drugs that resemble natural physiologic metabolites (such as 5-fluorouracil) are absorbed from the GI tract by this process. Active transport is characterized by the ability to transport drug against a concentration gradient—that is, from regions of low drug concentrations to regions of high drug concentrations. Therefore, this is an energy-consuming system. In addition, active transport is a specialized process requiring a carrier that binds the drug to form a carrier–drug complex that shuttles the drug across the membrane and then dissociates the drug on the other side of the membrane (Fig. 4-6).

The carrier molecule may be highly selective for the drug molecule. If the drug structurally resembles a natural substrate that is actively transported, then it is likely to be actively transported by the same carrier mechanism. Therefore, drugs of similar structure may compete for sites of adsorption on the carrier. Furthermore, because only a fixed number of carrier molecules are available, all the binding sites on the carrier may become saturated if the drug concentration gets very high. A comparison between the rate of drug absorption and the concentration of drug at the absorption site is shown in Fig. 4-7. Notice that for a drug absorbed by passive diffusion, the rate of absorption increases in a linear relationship to drug

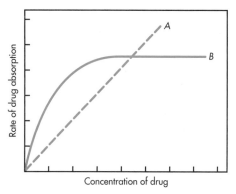

FIGURE 4-7 • Comparison of the rates of drug absorption of a drug absorbed by passive diffusion (line *A*) and a drug absorbed by a carrier-mediated system (line *B*).

concentration (first-order rate). In contrast, for drugs that are absorbed by a carrier-mediated process, the rate of drug absorption increases with drug concentration until the carrier molecules are completely saturated. At higher drug concentrations, the rate of drug absorption remains constant, or zero order, as expected in Michaelis-Menten kinetics.

Several transport proteins are expressed in the intestinal epithelial cells (Suzuki and Sugiyama, 2000; Takano et al, 2006) (Fig. 4-8). Although some transporters facilitate absorption, other transporters such as P-gp may effectively inhibit drug absorption. P-gp (also known as MDR1), an energy-dependent, membrane-bound protein, is an *efflux transporter* that mediates the secretion of compounds from inside the cell back out into the intestinal lumen, thereby limiting overall absorption (see Chapter 21). Thus, drug absorption may be reduced or increased by the presence or absence of efflux proteins. The role of efflux proteins is generally believed to be a defense mechanism for the body to excrete and reduce drug accumulation.

P-gp is expressed also in other tissues such as the blood–brain barrier, liver, and kidney, where it limits drug penetration into the brain, mediates biliary drug secretion, and mediates renal tubular drug secretion, respectively. Efflux pumps are present throughout the body and are involved in transport of a diverse group of hydrophobic drugs, natural products, and peptides. Many drugs and chemotherapeutic agents, such as cyclosporin A, verapamil, terfenadine, fexofenadine, and most HIV-1 protease inhibitors, are substrates of P-gp (see Chapter 21). In addition, individual genetic differences in intestinal absorption may be the result of genetic differences in P-gp and other transporters.

### Facilitated Diffusion

Facilitated diffusion is also a carrier-mediated transport system, differing from active transport in that the drug moves along a concentration gradient (ie, moves from a region of high drug concentration to a region of low drug concentration). Therefore, this system does not require energy input. However, because this system is carrier mediated, it is saturable and structurally selective for the drug and shows competition kinetics for drugs of similar structure. In terms of drug absorption, facilitated diffusion seems to play a very minor role.

### Transporters and Carrier-Mediated Intestinal Absorption

Various carrier-mediated systems (transporters) are present at the intestinal brush border and basolateral membrane for the absorption of specific ions and nutrients essential for the body (Tsuji and Tamai, 1996). Both influx and efflux transporters are present in the brush border and basolateral membrane that will increase drug absorption (influx transporter) or decrease drug absorption (efflux transporter).

**Uptake transporters.** For convenience, *influx transporters* were referred to as those that enhance absorption as uptake transporters and those that cause drug outflow as *efflux transporters*. However, this concept is too simple and inadequate to describe the roles of many transporters that have bidirectional efflux and other functions related to their location

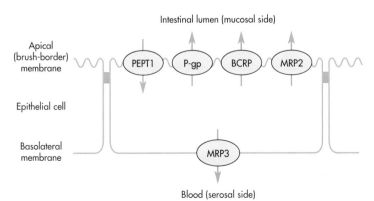

**FIGURE 4-8** • Localization of efflux transporters and PEPT1 in intestinal epithelial cell. (Reproduced with permission from Takano M, Yumoto R, Murakami T. Expression and function of efflux drug transporters in the intestine. Pharmacol Ther 2006 Jan;109(1-2):137–161.)

in the membrane. Recent progress has been made in understanding the genetic role of membrane transporters in drug safety and efficacy. In particular, more than 400 membrane transporters in two major superfamilies—ATP-binding cassette (ABC) and solute carrier (SLC)—have been annotated in the human genome. Many of these transporters have been cloned, characterized, and localized in the human body including the GI tract. The subject was reviewed by The International Transporter Consortium (ITC) (Giacomini, 2010).

Many drugs are absorbed by carrier systems because of the structural similarity to natural substrates or simply because they encounter the transporters located in specific part of the GI tract (Table 4-4). The small intestine expresses a variety of uptake transporters (see Fig. 4-2) for amino acids, peptides, hexoses, organic anions, organic cations, nucleosides, and other nutrients (Tsuji and Tamai, 1996; Giacomini, 2010). Among these uptake (absorptive) transporters are the intestinal oligopeptide transporter, or di-/tripeptide transporter, PEPT1 has potential for enhancing intestinal absorption of peptide drugs. The expression and function of PEPT1 (gene symbol *SLC15A1*) are now well analyzed for this application. Proteins given orally are digested in the GI tract to produce a variety of short-chain peptides; these di- and tripeptides could be taken up by enterocytes and the proton/peptide cotransporter (PepT1) localized on the brush-border membrane. These uptake transporters are located at the brush border as well as in the basolateral membrane to allow efficient absorption of essential nutrients into the body. Uptake transporters such as those for hexoses and amino acids also favor absorption (see arrows as shown in Fig. 4-7).

**Efflux transporters.** Many of the efflux transporters in the GI tract are membrane proteins located strategically in membranes to protect the body from influx of undesirable compounds. A common example is MDR1 or P-gp (alias), which has the gene symbol *ABCB1*. P-gp is an example of the ABC subfamily. MDR1 is one of the many proteins known as *multidrug-resistance-associated protein*. It is important in pumping drugs out of cells and causing treatment resistance in some cell lines (see Chapter 21).

P-gp has been identified in the intestine and reduces apparent intestinal epithelial cell permeability from lumen to blood for various lipophilic or cytotoxic drugs. P-gp is highly expressed on the apical surface of superficial columnar epithelial cells of the ileum and colon, and expression decreases proximally into the jejunum, duodenum, and stomach. Takano et al (2006) reported that P-gp is present in various human tissues

## TABLE 4-4 • Intestine Transporters and Examples of Drugs Transported

| Transporter | Examples | |
|---|---|---|
| Amino acid transporter | Gabapentin | D Cycloserine |
| | Methyldopa | Baclofen |
| | L-dopa | |
| Oligopeptide transporter | Cefadroxil | Cephradine |
| | Cefixime | Ceftibuten |
| | Cephalexin | Captopril |
| | Lisinopril | Thrombin inhibitor |
| Phosphate transporter | Fostomycin | Foscarnet |
| Bile acid transporter | S3744 | |
| Glucose transporter | p-Nitrophenyl-β-d-glucopyranoside | |
| P-glycoprotein efflux | Etoposide | Vinblastine |
| | Cyclosporin A | |
| Monocarboxylic acid transporter | Salicylic acid | Benzoic acid |
| | Pravastatin | |

*Data from Tsuji A, Tamai I. Carrier-mediated intestinal transport of drugs, Pharm Res 1996 Jul;13(7):963–977.*

and ranked as follows: (1) adrenal medulla (relative level to that in KB-3-1 cells, >500-fold); (2) adrenal (160-fold); (3) kidney medulla (75-fold); (4) kidney (50-fold); (5) colon (31-fold); (6) liver (25-fold); (7) lung, jejunum, and rectum (20-fold); (8) brain (12-fold); (9) prostate (8-fold); and so on, including skin, esophagus, stomach, ovary, muscle, heart, and kidney cortex. The widespread presence of P-gp in the body appears to be related to its defensive role in effluxing drugs and other xenobiotics out of different cells and vital body organs. This transporter is sometimes called an efflux transporter while others are better described as "influx" proteins. P-gp has the remarkable ability to efflux drug out of many types of cells including endothelial lumens of capillaries. The expression of P-gp is often triggered in many cancer cells making them drug resistant due to drug efflux.

For many GI transporters, the transport of a drug is often bidirectional (Fig. 4-9), and whether the transporter causes drug absorption or exsorption depends on which direction the flux dominates with regard to a particular drug at a given site. An example of how P-gp affects drug absorption can be seen with the drug digoxin. P-gp is present in the liver and the GI tract. In Caco-2 cells and other model systems, P-gp is known to efflux drug out of the enterocyte. Digoxin was previously known to have erratic/incomplete absorption or bioavailability problems. While reported bioavailability issues were attributed to formulation or other factors, it is also now known that knocking out the P-gp gene in mice increases bioavailability of the drug. In addition, human P-gp genetic polymorphisms occur. Hoffmeyer et al (2000) demonstrated that a polymorphism in exon 26 (C3435T) resulted in reduced intestinal P-gp, leading to increased oral bioavailability of digoxin

in the subject involved. However, direct determination of P-gp substrate *in vivo* is not always readily possible. Most early determinations are done using *in vitro* cell assay methods, or *in vivo* studies involving a cloned animal with the gene knocked out such as the P-gp, a knock-out (KO) mouse, for example, P-gp (−/−), which is the most sensitive method to identify P-gp substrates. Changes in the expression of P-gp may be triggered by diseases or other drugs, contributing to variability in P-gp activity and variable plasma drug concentrations after a given dose is administered. Results from *in vitro* and preclinical (animal) studies may need to be verified through clinical drug–drug interaction studies to establish the role of P-gp in the oral bioavailability of a drug.

The breast cancer resistance protein (BCRP; gene symbol *ABCG2*) is like P-gp in that it is also found in many important fluid barrier layers, including the intestine, liver, kidney, and brain. BCRP also transports many drugs out of cells, working (like P-gp) to keep various compounds out of the body (by decreasing their absorption) or helping to eliminate them. Drugs transported by BCRP include many anticancer drugs (methotrexate, irinotecan, mitoxantrone), statins (rosuvastatin), as well as nitrofurantoin and various sulfated metabolites of drugs and endogenous compounds. The FDA requires all investigational new drugs to be tested for their potential activity as substrates of both P-gp and BCRP, and also recommends determining if they are inhibitors (Huang and Zhang, 2012).

### FREQUENTLY ASKED QUESTIONS

▶ What is the effect of intestinal P-gp on the blood level of the substrate drug digoxin when a substrate inhibitor (ketoconazole) is present?

▶ According to the diagram in Fig. 4-9, in which direction is P-gp pumping the drug? Is P-gp acting as an efflux transporter in this diagram?

▶ Why is it too simple to classify transporters based on an "absorption" and "exsorption" concept?

▶ Would a drug transport process involving ABC transporter be considered a passive or active transport process?

▶ How does a transporter influence the level of drug within the cell?

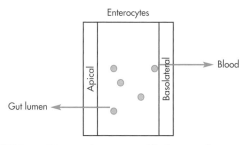

FIGURE 4-9 • Diagram showing possible directional movement of a substrate drug by a transporter.

P-gp affects the bioavailability of many substrate drugs listed in Table 4-5. P-gp inhibitors should be carefully evaluated before coadministration with a P-gp substrate drug. Other transporters are also present in the intestines (Tsuji and Tamai, 1996). For example, many oral cephalosporins are absorbed through amino acid transporters. Cefazolin, a parenteral-only cephalosporin, is not available orally because it cannot be absorbed to a significant degree through this mechanism.

## FREQUENTLY ASKED QUESTIONS

▶ The bioavailability of an antitumor drug is provided in the package insert. Why is it important to know whether the drug is an efflux transporter substrate or not?

▶ Can the expression of efflux transporter in a cell change as the disease progresses?

▶ Why is blockade of efflux transporter efflux of a drug, its glucuronide, or sulfate metabolite into the bile clinically important?

## TABLE 4-5 • Reported Substrates of P-gp—A Member of ATP-Binding Cassette (ABC) Transporters

Acebutolol, acetaminophen, actinomycin d, h-acetyldigoxin, amitriptyline, amprenavir, apafant, asimadoline, atenolol, atorvastatin, azidopine, azidoprocainamide methiodide, azithromycin

Benzo(a)pyrene, betamethasone, bisantrene, bromocriptine, bunitrolol, calcein-AM

Camptothecin, carbamazepine, carvedilol, celiprolol, cepharanthin, cerivastatin, chloroquine, chlorpromazine, chlorothiazide, clarithromycin, colchicine, corticosterone, cortisol, cyclosporin A

Daunorubicin (daunomycin), debrisoquine, desoxycorticoster one, dexamethasone, digitoxin

Digoxin, diltiazem, dipyridamole, docetaxel, dolastatin 10, domperidone, doxorubicin (adriamycin)

Eletriptan, emetine, endosulfan, erythromycin, estradiol, estradiol-17h-d-glucuronide, etoposide (VP-16)

Fexofenadine, gf120918, grepafloxacin

Hoechst 33342, hydroxyrubicin, imatinib, indinavir, ivermectin

Levofloxacin, loperamide, losartan, lovastatin

Methadone, methotrexate, methylprednisolone, metoprolol, mitoxantrone, monensin

Morphine, $_{99m}$tc-sestamibi

N-desmethyltamoxifen, nadolol, nelfinavir, nicardipine, nifedipine, nitrendipine, norverapamil

Olanzapine, omeprazole

PSC-833 (valspodar), perphenazine, prazosin, prednisone, pristinamycin IA, puromycin

Quetiapine, quinidine, quinine

Ranitidine, reserpine

Rhodamine 123, risperidone, ritonavir, roxithromycin

Saquinavir, sirolimus, sparfloxacin, sumatriptan,

Tacrolimus, talinolol, tamoxifen, taxol (paclitaxel), telithromycin, terfenadine, timolol, toremifene

Tributylmethylammonium, trimethoprim

Valinomycin, vecuronium, verapamil, vinblastine

Vincristine, vindoline, vinorelbine

*Adapted with permission from Takano M, Yumoto R, Murakami T. Expression and function of efflux drug transporters in the intestine. Pharmacol Ther 2006 Jan;109(1–2):137–161.*

## Clinical Examples of Transporter Impact

Multidrug resistance (MDR) to cancer cells has been linked to efflux transporter proteins such as P-gp that can efflux or pump out chemotherapeutic agents from the cells (Sauna et al, 2001). Paclitaxel (Taxol) is an example of coordinated metabolism, efflux, and triggering of hormone nuclear receptor to induce efflux protein (Fig. 4-10). P-gp (see MDR1 in Fig. 4-2) is responsible for 85% of paclitaxel excretion back into the GI tract (Synold et al, 2001). Paclitaxel activates the pregnane X receptor (also known as PXR, or alternatively as steroid X receptor [SXR]), which in turn induces MDR1 transcription and P-gp expression, resulting in even further excretion of paclitaxel into the intestinal fluid. Paclitaxel also induces CYP3A4 and CYP2C8 transcription, resulting in increased paclitaxel metabolism. Thus, in response to a xenobiotic challenge, PXR can induce both a first line of defense (intestinal excretion) and a backup system (hepatic drug inactivation) that limits exposure to potentially toxic compounds. In contrast to paclitaxel, docetaxel is a closely related antineoplastic agent that does not activate PXR but has a much better absorption profile.

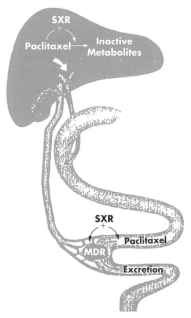

FIGURE 4-10 • Mechanism of coordinated efflux and metabolism of paclitaxel by PXR (SXR). (Reproduced with permission from Synold TW, Dussault I, Forman BM. The orphan nuclear receptor SXR coordinately regulates drug metabolism and efflux. Nat Med 2001 May;7(5):584–590.)

Mutations of other transporters, particularly those involved in reuptake of serotonin, dopamine, and gamma-aminobutyric acid (GABA), are presently being studied with regard to clinically relevant changes in drug response. Pharmacogenetic variability in these transporters is an important consideration in patient dosing. When therapeutic failures occur, the following questions should be asked: (1) Is the drug a substrate for P-gp and/or CYP3A4? (2) Is the drug being coadministered with anything that inhibits P-gp and/or CYP3A4? For example, grapefruit juice and many drugs can affect drug metabolism and oral absorption.

### Vesicular Transport

Vesicular transport is the process of engulfing particles or dissolved materials by the cell. Pinocytosis and phagocytosis are forms of vesicular transport that differ by the type of material ingested. *Pinocytosis* refers to the engulfment of small solutes or fluid, whereas *phagocytosis* refers to the engulfment of larger particles or macromolecules, generally by macrophages. *Endocytosis* and *exocytosis* are the processes of moving specific macromolecules into and out of a cell, respectively.

During pinocytosis, phagocytosis, or transcytosis, the cell membrane invaginates to surround the material and then engulfs the material, incorporating it inside the cell (Fig. 4-11). Subsequently, the cell membrane containing the material forms a vesicle or vacuole within the cell. *Transcytosis* is the process by which various macromolecules are transported across the interior of a cell. In transcytosis, the vesicle fuses with the plasma membrane to release the encapsulated material to another side of the cell. Vesicles are employed to intake the macromolecules on one side of the cell, draw them across the cell, and eject them on the other side. Transcytosis (sometimes referred to as vesicular transport) is the proposed process for the absorption of orally administered Sabin polio vaccine and various large proteins.

*Pinocytosis* is a cellular process that permits the active transport of fluid from outside the cell through the membrane surrounding the cell into the inside of the cell. In pinocytosis, tiny incuppings called caveolae (little caves) in the surface of the cell close and

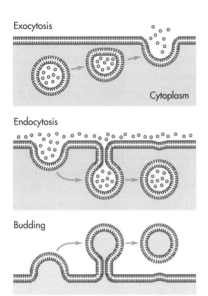

Exocytosis

Cytoplasm

Endocytosis

Budding

FIGURE 4-11 • Diagram showing exocytosis and endocytosis.

then pinch off to form pinosomes, little fluid-filled bubbles, that are free within the cytoplasm of the cell.

An example of *exocytosis* is the transport of a protein such as insulin from insulin-producing cells of the pancreas into the extracellular space. The insulin molecules are first packaged into intracellular vesicles, which then fuse with the plasma membrane to release the insulin outside the cell.

### Pore (Convective) Transport

Very small molecules (such as urea, water, and sugars) are able to cross cell membranes rapidly, as if the membrane contained channels or pores. Although such pores have never been directly observed by microscopy, the model of drug permeation through aqueous pores is used to explain renal excretion of drugs and the uptake of drugs into the liver.

A certain type of protein called a *transport protein* may form an open channel across the lipid membrane of the cell (see Fig. 4-2). Small molecules including drugs move through the channel by diffusion more rapidly than at other parts of the membrane.

### Ion-Pair Formation

Strong electrolyte drugs are highly ionized or charged molecules, such as quaternary nitrogen compounds with extreme $pK_a$ values. Strong electrolyte drugs

maintain their charge at all physiologic pH values and penetrate membranes poorly. When the ionized drug is linked with an oppositely charged ion, an *ion pair* is formed in which the overall charge of the pair is neutral. This neutral drug complex diffuses more easily across the membrane. For example, the formation of ion pairs to facilitate drug absorption has been demonstrated for propranolol, a basic drug that forms an ion pair with oleic acid, and quinine, which forms ion pairs with hexylsalicylate (Nienbert, 1989).

An interesting application of ion pairs is the complexation of amphotericin B and DSPG (distearoylphosphatidylglycerol) in some amphotericin B/liposome products. Ion pairing may transiently alter distribution, reduce high plasma free drug concentration, and reduce renal toxicity.

## DRUG INTERACTIONS IN THE GASTROINTESTINAL TRACT

Many agents (drug or chemical substances) may have dual roles as substrate and/or inhibitor between CYP3A4 and P-glycoprotein, P-gp. Simultaneous administration of these agents results in an increase in the oral drug bioavailability of one or both of the drugs. Various drug–drug and drug–nutrient interactions involving oral bioavailability have been reported in human subjects (Thummel and Wilkinson, 1998; Di Marco et al, 2002; von Richter et al, 2004).

Many commonly used medications (eg, dextromethorphan hydrobromide) and certain food groups (eg, grapefruit juice) are substrates both for the efflux transporter, P-gp, and for the CYP3A enzymes involved in biotransformation of drugs (see Chapter 21). Grapefruit juice also affects drug transport in the intestinal wall. Certain components of grapefruit juice (such as naringin and bergamottin) are responsible for the inhibition of P-gp and CYP3A. Di Marco et al (2002) demonstrated the inhibitory effect of grapefruit and Seville orange juice on the pharmacokinetics of dextromethorphan. Using dextromethorphan as the substrate, these investigators showed that grapefruit juice inhibits both CYP3A activity as well as P-gp resulting in an increased bioavailability of dextromethorphan. Grapefruit juice has been shown to increase the oral bioavailability of many drugs, such as cyclosporine or saquinavir, by inhibiting intestinal metabolism.

Esomeprazole (Nexium) and omeprazole (Prilosec°) are proton pump inhibitors that inhibit gastric acid secretion, resulting an increased stomach pH. Esomeprazole and omeprazole may interfere with the absorption of drugs where gastric pH is an important determinant of bioavailability (eg, ketoconazole, iron salts, and digoxin). Both esomeprazole and omeprazole are extensively metabolized in the liver by CYP2C19 and CYP3A4. The prodrug clopidogrel (Plavix) inhibits platelet aggregation entirely due to an active metabolite. Coadministration of clopidogrel with omeprazole, an inhibitor of CYP2C19, reduces the pharmacological activity of clopidogrel if given either concomitantly or 12 hours apart.

The dual effect of a CYP isoenzyme and a transporter on drug absorption is not always easy to determine or predict based on pharmacokinetic studies alone. A well-studied example is the drug digoxin. Digoxin is minimally metabolized (CYP3A4), orally absorbed (Suzuki and Sugiyama, 2000), and a substrate for P-gp based on:

1. Human polymorphism single-nucleotide polymorphism (SNP) in exon 26 (C3435T) results in a reduced intestinal expression level of P-gp, along with increased oral bioavailability of digoxin.

2. Ketoconazole increases the oral bioavailability and shortens mean absorption time from 1.1 to 0.3 hour. Ketoconazole is a substrate and inhibitor of P-gp; P-gp can subsequently influence bioavailability. The influence of P-gp is not always easily detected unless studies are designed to investigate its presence.

For this analysis, a drug is given orally and intravenously before and after administration of an inhibitor drug. The AUC of the drug is calculated for each case. For example, ketoconazole causes an increase in the oral bioavailability of the immunosuppressant tacrolimus from 0.14 to 0.30, without affecting hepatic bioavailability (0.96–0.97) (Suzuki and Sugiyama, 2000). Since hepatic bioavailability is similar, the increase in bioavailability from 0.14 to 0.30 is the result of ketoconazole suppression on P-gp.

Mouly and Paine (2003) reported P-gp expression determined by Western blotting along the entire length of the human small intestine. They found that relative P-gp levels increased progressively from the proximal to the distal region. von Richter et al (2004) measured P-gp as well as CYP3A4 in paired human small intestine and liver specimens obtained from 15 patients. They reported that much higher levels of both P-gp (about seven times) and CYP3A4 (about three times) were found in the intestine than in the liver, suggesting the critical participation of intestinal P-gp in limiting oral drug bioavailability.

The concept of drug–drug interactions has received increased attention in recent years, as they may be responsible for many drug therapy-induced medical problems (Johnson et al, 1999).

---

### FREQUENTLY ASKED QUESTIONS

▶ Animal studies are not definitive when extrapolated to humans. Why are animal studies or in vitro transport studies in human cells often performed to decide whether a drug is a P-gp substrate?

▶ How would you demonstrate that digoxin metabolism is solely due to hepatic extraction and not due to intestinal extraction since both CYP3A4 and P-gp are present in the intestine in larger amounts?

---

## ORAL DRUG ABSORPTION

The oral route of administration is the most common and popular route of drug dosing. The oral dosage form must be designed to account for extreme pH ranges, the presence or absence of food, degradative enzymes, varying drug permeability in the different regions of the intestine, and motility of the GI tract. In this chapter we will discuss intestinal variables that affect absorption; dosage-form considerations are discussed in Chapters 7–10.

### Anatomic and Physiologic Considerations

The normal physiologic processes of the alimentary canal may be affected by diet, contents of the GI tract, hormones, the visceral nervous system, disease, and drugs. Thus, drugs given by the enteral route for systemic absorption may be affected by the anatomy, physiologic functions, and contents of the alimentary tract. Moreover, the physical, chemical, and pharmacologic properties of the drug and the formulation of the drug product will also affect systemic drug absorption from the alimentary canal.

The *enteral system* consists of the alimentary canal from the mouth to the anus (Fig. 4-12). The major physiologic processes that occur in the GI system are secretion, digestion, and absorption. Secretion includes the transport of fluid, electrolytes, peptides, and proteins into the lumen of the alimentary canal. Enzymes in saliva and pancreatic secretions are also involved in the digestion of carbohydrates and proteins. Other secretions, such as mucus, protect the linings of the lumen of the GI tract. *Digestion* is the breakdown of food constituents into smaller structures in preparation for absorption. Food constituents are mostly absorbed in the proximal area (duodenum) of the small intestine. The process of absorption is the entry of constituents from the lumen of the gut into the body. Absorption may be considered the net result of both lumen-to-blood and blood-to-lumen transport movements.

Drugs administered orally pass through various parts of the enteral canal, including the oral cavity, esophagus, and various parts of the GI tract. Residues eventually exit the body through the anus with the feces. The total transit time, including gastric emptying, small intestinal transit, and colonic transit, ranges from 0.4 to 5 days (Kirwan and Smith, 1974). The small intestine, particularly the duodenum area, is the most important site for drug absorption. Small intestine transit time (SITT) ranges from 3 to 4 hours for most healthy subjects. If absorption is not completed by the time a drug leaves the small intestine, absorption may be erratic or incomplete.

The small intestine is normally filled with digestive juices and liquids, keeping the lumen contents fluid. In contrast, the fluid in the colon is reabsorbed, and the lumenal content in the colon is either semisolid or solid, making further drug dissolution and absorption erratic and difficult. The lack of the solubilizing effect of the chyme and digestive fluid contributes to a less favorable environment for drug absorption.

### Oral Cavity

Saliva is the main secretion of the oral cavity, and it has a pH of about 7. Saliva contains ptyalin (salivary amylase), which digests starches. Mucin, a glycoprotein that lubricates food, is also secreted and may interact with drugs. About 1500 mL of saliva is secreted per day.

The oral cavity can be used for the buccal absorption of lipid-soluble drugs such as fentanyl citrate (Actiq®) and nitroglycerin, also formulated for sublingual routes. Recently, orally disintegrating tablets (ODTs) have become available. These ODTs, such as aripiprazole (Abilify Discmelt®), rapidly disintegrate in the oral cavity in the presence of saliva. The resulting fragments, which are suspended in the saliva, are swallowed and the drug is then absorbed from the GI tract. A major advantage for ODTs is that the drug may be taken without water. In the case of the antipsychotic drug, aripiprazole, a nurse may give the drug in the form of an ODT (Abilify Discmelt) to a schizophrenic patient. The nurse can easily ascertain that the drug was taken and swallowed.

### Esophagus

The esophagus connects the pharynx and the cardiac orifice of the stomach. The pH of the fluids in the esophagus is between 5 and 6. The lower part of the esophagus ends with the esophageal sphincter,

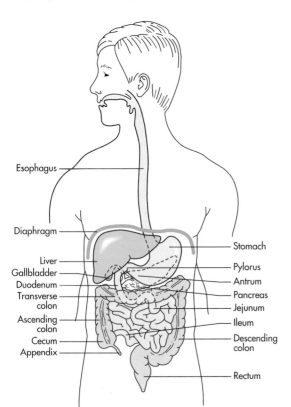

Esophagus

Diaphragm

Liver
Gallbladder
Duodenum
Transverse colon
Ascending colon
Cecum
Appendix

Stomach
Pylorus
Antrum
Pancreas
Jejunum
Ileum
Descending colon

Rectum

FIGURE 4-12 • Gastrointestinal tract.

## TABLE 4-6 • Fasting physiologic pH values of the human gastrointestinal tract

| Stomach | Small intestine | | Large intestine | | Rectum | Reference |
|---|---|---|---|---|---|---|
| 1 to 2.5 | Proximal | 6.6 (0.5) | Caecum | 6.4 (0.4) | | Evans 1988 |
| | Terminal Ileum | 7.5 (0.4) | Left Colon | 7.0 (0.7) | | |
| Highly Acidic | Duodenum | 6 | Caecum | 5.7 | 6.7 | Fallingborg 1999 |
| | Terminal Ileum | 7.4 | | | | |
| | Duodenum | 7.0 (0.4) | | | | Moreno 2006 |
| | Jejunum | 6.8 (0.4) | | | | |
| 1.7 to 4.7 | Proximal | 5.9 to 6.3 | Colon | 5 to 8 | | Koziolek 2015 |
| | Distal | 7.4 to 7.8 | | | | |

Note: pH values are provided as either a range or mean (SD).

which prevents acid reflux from the stomach. Tablets or capsules may lodge in this area, causing local irritation. Very little drug dissolution occurs in the esophagus.

### Stomach

The stomach is innervated by the vagus nerve. However, local nerve plexus, hormones, mechano-receptors sensitive to the stretch of the GI wall, and chemoreceptors control the regulation of gastric secretions, including acid and stomach emptying. The pH values of the stomach under fasting and fed conditions are listed in Tables 4-6 and 4-7. Stomach acid secretion by parietal cells is stimulated by gastrin and histamine. Gastrin is released from G cells, mainly in the antral mucosa and also in the duodenum. Gastrin release is regulated by stomach distention (swelling) and the presence of peptides and amino acids. A substance known as intrinsic factor enhances vitamin B-12 (cyanocobalamin) absorption. Various gastric enzymes, such as pepsin, which initiates protein digestion, are secreted into the gastric lumen to initiate digestion.

Basic drugs are solubilized rapidly in the presence of stomach acid. Mixing is intense and pressurized in the antral part of the stomach, a process of breaking down large food particles described as *antral milling*. Food and liquid are emptied by opening the pyloric sphincter into the duodenum. Stomach emptying is influenced by the food content and osmolality. Fatty acids and mono- and diglycerides delay gastric emptying (Hunt and Knox, 1968). High-density foods generally are emptied from the stomach more slowly. The relation of gastric emptying time to drug absorption is discussed more fully in the next section.

Factors affecting stomach pH are listed in Table 4-8. Increased stomach pH may cause a drug interaction with enteric-coated drug products (eg, diclofenac enteric-coated tablets, Voltaren). The enteric coating does not dissolve in acid pH in the stomach. The release of drug from an enteric-coated drug product can be delayed in the stomach until it reaches the higher pH of the intestine. If the stomach pH is too high, the enteric-coated drug product may release the drug in the stomach, thus causing irritation to the stomach.

## TABLE 4-7 • pH Values of gastrointestinal fluid, by stage of digestion

| | Simulated gastric fluid | Simulated intestinal fluid |
|---|---|---|
| Fasting | 1.6 | 6.5 |
| Fed | | |
| early | 6.4 | 6.5 |
| middle | 5 | 5.8 |
| late | 3 | 5.4 |

Data from Jantratid E, Janssen N, Reppas C, Dressman JB. Dissolution media simulating conditions in the proximal human gastrointestinal tract: an update, Pharm Res 2008 Jul;25(7):1663–1676.

**TABLE 4-8** • Factors Affecting Human Gastric Acid Secretion and Stomach pH

| Stimulating Acid Secretion (Decreasing pH) | Inhibiting Acid Secretion (Increasing pH) |
|---|---|
| Digestion phase: cephalic | Digestion phase: intestinal |
| Digestion phase: gastric | |
| Food: protein | Food: fats |
| | Food: carbohydrates |
| Drinks: tea | Drugs: histamine receptor antagonists |
| Drinks: coffee | Drugs: proton pump inhibitors |
| Drinks: milk | |
| Drinks: ethanol | Achlorhydria |

Data from Khanna MU, Abraham P. Determinants of acid secretion, Assoc Physicians India 1990 Sep;38 Suppl 1:727–730.

A few fat-soluble, acid-stable drugs may be absorbed from the stomach by passive diffusion. Ethanol is completely miscible with water, easily crosses cell membranes, and is efficiently absorbed from the stomach. Ethanol is more rapidly absorbed from the stomach in the fasting state compared to the fed state (Levitt et al, 1997).

### Duodenum

A common duct from both the pancreas and the gallbladder enters into the duodenum. The duodenal pH is about 6–6.5 (see Tables 4-6 and 4-7), because of the presence of bicarbonate that neutralizes the acidic chyme emptied from the stomach. The duodenum pH is optimum for enzymatic digestion of protein and peptide-containing food. Pancreatic juice containing enzymes is secreted into the duodenum from the bile duct. Trypsin, chymotrypsin, and carboxypeptidase are involved in the hydrolysis of proteins into amino acids. Amylase is involved in the digestion of carbohydrates. Pancreatic lipase secretion hydrolyzes fats into fatty acid. The complex fluid medium in the duodenum helps dissolve many drugs with limited aqueous solubility.

The duodenum is the major site for passive drug absorption due to both its anatomy, which creates a high surface area, and high blood flow (see Fig. 4-13). The duodenum is a site where many ester prodrugs are hydrolyzed during absorption. Proteolytic enzymes in the duodenum degrade many protein drugs preventing adequate absorption of protein drugs.

### Jejunum

The jejunum is the middle portion of the small intestine, between the duodenum and the ileum. Digestion of protein and carbohydrates continues after addition of pancreatic juice and bile in the duodenum. This portion of the small intestine generally has fewer contractions than the duodenum and is preferred for *in vivo* drug absorption studies.

### Ileum

The ileum is the terminal part of the small intestine. This site also has fewer contractions than the duodenum and may be blocked off by catheters with an inflatable balloon and perfused for drug absorption studies. The pH is about 7, with the distal part as high as pH 8. Due to the presence of bicarbonate secretion, acid drugs will dissolve in the ileum. Bile secretion helps dissolve fats and hydrophobic drugs. The ileocecal valve separates the small intestine from the colon.

### Colon

The colon lacks villi and has limited drug absorption due to lack of large surface area, blood flow, and the more viscous and semisolid nature of the lumen contents. The colon is lined with mucin that functions as lubricant and protectant. The pH in this region is 5.5–7 (Shareef et al, 2003). A few drugs, such as theophylline and metoprolol, are absorbed in this region. Drugs that are absorbed well in this region are good candidates for an oral sustained-release dosage form. The colon contains both aerobic and anaerobic microorganisms that may metabolize some drugs. For example, L-dopa and lactulose are metabolized by enteric bacteria. Crohn's disease affects the colon and thickens the bowel wall. The microflora also become more anaerobic. Absorption of clindamycin and propranolol is increased,

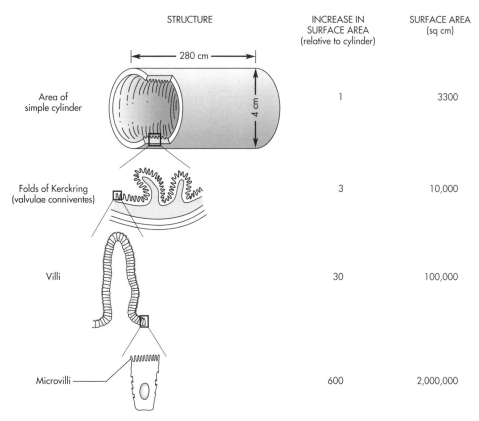

| STRUCTURE | INCREASE IN SURFACE AREA (relative to cylinder) | SURFACE AREA (sq cm) |
|---|---|---|
| Area of simple cylinder | 1 | 3300 |
| Folds of Kerckring (valvulae conniventes) | 3 | 10,000 |
| Villi | 30 | 100,000 |
| Microvilli | 600 | 2,000,000 |

**FIGURE 4-13** • Three mechanisms for increasing surface area of the small intestine. The increase in surface area is due to folds of Kerkring, villi, and microvilli. (Reproduced with permission from Wilson TH: Intestinal Absorption. Philadelphia, PA: Saunders; 1962.)

whereas other drugs have reduced absorption with this disease (Rubinstein et al, 1988). A few delayed-release drug products such as mesalamine (Asacol tablets, Pentasa capsules) have a pH-sensitive coating that dissolves in the higher pH of the lower bowel, releasing the mesalamine to act locally in Crohn's disease. Balsalazide disodium capsules (Colazal), also used in Crohn's disease, is a prodrug containing an azo group that is cleaved by anaerobic bacteria in the lower bowel to produce mesalamine (5-aminosalicylic acid or 5-ASA), an anti-inflammatory drug.

### Rectum

The rectum is about 15 cm long, ending at the anus. In the absence of fecal material, the rectum has a small amount of fluid (approximately 2 mL) with a pH of about 7. The rectum is perfused by the superior, middle, and inferior hemorrhoidal veins. The inferior hemorrhoidal vein (closest to the anal sphincter)

and the middle hemorrhoidal vein feed into the vena cava and back to the heart, thus bypassing the liver and avoiding hepatic first-pass effect. The superior hemorrhoidal vein joins the mesenteric circulation, which feeds into the hepatic portal vein and then to the liver.

The small amount of fluid present in the rectum has virtually no buffer capacity; as a consequence, the dissolving drug(s) or even excipients can have a determining effect on the existing pH in the anorectal area. Drug absorption after rectal administration may be variable, depending on the placement of the suppository or drug solution within the rectum. A portion of the drug dose may be absorbed via the lower hemorrhoidal veins, from which the drug feeds directly into the systemic circulation; some drugs may be absorbed via the superior hemorrhoidal vein, which feeds into the mesenteric veins to the hepatic portal vein to the liver, and be metabolized before systemic absorption. Thus some of the variability in drug absorption following rectal administration may occur due to variation in the site of absorption within the rectum.

## Factors Affecting Drug Absorption in the Gastrointestinal Tract

Drugs may be absorbed by passive diffusion from all parts of the alimentary canal including sublingual, buccal, GI, and rectal absorption. For most drugs, the optimum site for drug absorption after oral administration is the upper portion of the small intestine or duodenum region. The unique anatomy of the duodenum provides an immense surface area for the drug to diffuse passively (Fig. 4-13). The large surface area of the duodenum is due to the presence of valve-like folds in the mucous membrane on which are small projections known as *villi.* These villi contain even smaller projections known as *microvilli,* forming a brush border. In addition, the duodenal region is highly perfused with a network of capillaries, which helps maintain a concentration gradient from the intestinal lumen and plasma circulation.

### *Gastrointestinal Motility*

Once a drug is given orally, the exact location and/ or environment of the drug product within the GI tract is difficult to discern. GI motility tends to move the drug through the alimentary canal, so the drug may not stay at the absorption site. For drugs given orally, an anatomic *absorption window* may exist within the GI tract in which the drug is efficiently absorbed. Drugs contained in a nonbiodegradable controlled-release dosage form should be completely released into this absorption window to be absorbed before the movement of the dosage form into the large bowel.

The transit time of the drug in the GI tract depends on the physicochemical and pharmacologic properties of the drug, the type of dosage form, and various physiologic factors. Movement of the drug within the GI tract depends on whether the alimentary canal contains recently ingested food (digestive or fed state) or is in the fasted or interdigestive state (Fig. 4-14 and Table 4-9). During the fasted or interdigestive state, alternating cycles of activity known as the *migrating motor complex* (MMC) act as a propulsive movement that empties the upper GI tract to the cecum. Initially, the alimentary canal is quiescent. Then, irregular contractions followed by regular contractions with high amplitude (housekeeper waves) push any residual contents distally or farther down the alimentary canal. In the fed state, the MMC is replaced by irregular contractions, which have the effect of mixing intestinal contents and advancing the intestinal stream toward the colon in short segments (Table 4-6). The pylorus and ileocecal valves prevent regurgitation or movement of food from the distal to the proximal direction.

### *Gastric Emptying Time*

Anatomically, a swallowed drug rapidly reaches the stomach. Eventually, the stomach empties its contents into the small intestine. Because the duodenum has the greatest capacity for the absorption of drugs from the GI tract, a delay in the gastric emptying time

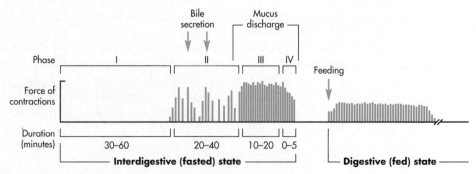

**FIGURE 4-14 •** A pictorial representation of the typical motility patterns in the interdigestive (fasted) and digestive (fed) state. (Reproduced with permission from Yacobi A, Halperin-Walega E: Oral Sustained Release Formulations: Design and Evaluation. New York, NY: Pergamon; 1988.)

| TABLE 4-9 • Characteristics of the Motility Patterns in the Fasted Dog | | |
|---|---|---|
| **Phase** | **Duration** | **Characteristics** |
| **Fasted State** | | |
| I | 30–60 min | Quiescence |
| II | 20–40 min | • Irregular contractions<br>• Medium amplitude but can be as high as phase III<br>• Bile secretion begins<br>• Onset of gastric discharge of administered fluid of small volume usually occurs before that of particle discharge<br>• Onset of particle and mucus discharge may occur during the later part of phase II |
| III | 5–15 min | • Regular contractions (4–5 contractions/min) with high amplitude<br>• Mucus discharge continues<br>• Particle discharge continues |
| IV | 0–5 min | • Irregular contractions<br>• Medium descending amplitude<br>• Sometimes absent |
| **Fed State** | | |
| One phase only | As long as food is present in the stomach | • Regular, frequent contractions<br>• Amplitude is lower than phase III<br>• 4–5 contractions/min |

Reproduced with permission from Yacobi A, Halperin-Walega E: Oral Sustained Release Formulations: Design and Evaluation. New York, NY: Pergamon; 1988.

for the drug to reach the duodenum will slow the rate and possibly the extent of drug absorption, thereby prolonging the onset time for the drug. Some drugs, such as penicillin, are unstable in acid and decompose if stomach emptying is delayed. Other drugs, such as aspirin, may irritate the gastric mucosa during prolonged contact.

A number of factors affect gastric emptying time. Some factors that tend to delay gastric emptying include consumption of meals high in fat, cold beverages, and anticholinergic drugs (Burks et al, 1985; Rubinstein et al, 1988). Liquids and small particles less than 1 mm are generally not retained in the stomach. These small particles are believed to be emptied due to a slightly higher basal pressure in the stomach over the duodenum. Different constituents of a meal empty from the stomach at different rates. Feldman et al (1984) observed that 10 oz of liquid soft drink, scrambled egg (digestible solid), and a radio-opaque marker (undigestible solid) were 50% emptied from the stomach in 30 minutes,

154 minutes, and 3–4 hours, respectively. Thus, liquids are generally emptied faster than digested solids from the stomach (Fig. 4-15).

Large particles, including tablets and capsules, are delayed from emptying for 3–6 hours by the presence of food in the stomach. Indigestible solids empty very slowly, probably during the interdigestive phase, a phase in which food is not present and the stomach is less motile but periodically empties its content due to housekeeper wave contraction (Fig. 4-16).

### Intestinal Motility

Normal peristaltic movements mix the contents of the duodenum, bringing the drug particles into intimate contact with the intestinal mucosal cells. The drug must have a sufficient time (*residence time*) at the absorption site for optimum absorption. In the case of high motility in the intestinal tract, as in diarrhea, the drug has a very brief residence time and less opportunity for adequate absorption.

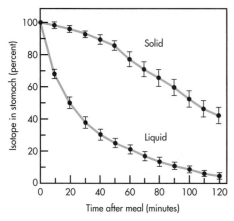

FIGURE 4-15 • Gastric emptying of a group of normal subjects using the dual-isotope method. The mean and 1 SE of the fraction of isotope remaining in the stomach are depicted at various time intervals after ingestion of the meal. Note the exponential nature of liquid emptying and the linear process of solid emptying. (Reproduced with permission from Minami H, McCallum RW. The physiology and pathophysiology of gastric emptying in humans, Gastroenterology 1984 Jun;86(6):1592–1610.)

The average normal SITT was about 7 hours as measured in early studies using indirect methods based on the detection of hydrogen after an oral dose of lactulose (fermentation of lactulose by colon bacteria yields hydrogen in the breath). Newer studies using gamma scintigraphy have shown SITT to be about 3–4 hours. Thus a drug may take about 4–8 hours to pass through the stomach and small intestine during the fasting state. During the fed state, SITT may take 8–12 hours. For modified-release or

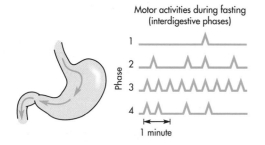

FIGURE 4-16 • Motor activity responsible for gastric emptying of indigestible solids. Migrating myoelectric complex (MMC), usually initiated at proximal stomach or lower esophageal sphincter, and contractions during phase 3 sweep indigestible solids through open pylorus. (Reproduced with permission from Minami H, McCallum RW. The physiology and pathophysiology of gastric emptying in humans, Gastroenterology 1984 Jun;86(6):1592–1610.)

controlled-dosage forms, which slowly release the drug over an extended period of time, the dosage form must stay within a certain segment of the intestinal tract so that the drug contents are released and absorbed before loss of the dosage form in the feces. Intestinal transit is discussed further in relation to the design of sustained-release products in Chapter 9.

In one study reported by Shareef et al (2003), utilizing a radio-opaque marker, mean mouth-to-anus transit time was 53.3 hours. The mean colon transit time was 35 hours, with 11.3 hours for the right (ascending transverse portion), 11.4 hours for the left (descending and portion of the transverse), and 12.4 hours for the rectosigmoid colon. Dietary fiber has the greatest effect on colonic transit. Dietary fiber increases fecal weight, partly by retaining water and partly by increasing bacterial mass (Shareef et al, 2003).

### Perfusion of the Gastrointestinal Tract

The blood flow to the GI tract is important in carrying absorbed drug to the systemic circulation. A large network of capillaries and lymphatic vessels perfuse the duodenal region and peritoneum. The splanchnic circulation receives about 28% of the cardiac output and is increased after meals. This high degree of perfusion helps to maintain a concentration gradient favoring absorption. Once the drug is absorbed from the small intestine, it enters via the mesenteric vessels to the hepatic-portal vein and goes to the liver prior to reaching the systemic circulation. Any decrease in mesenteric blood flow, as in the case of congestive heart failure, will decrease the rate of drug removal from the intestinal tract, thereby reducing the rate of drug bioavailability (Benet et al, 1976).

### Absorption through the Lymphatic System

The role of the lymphatic circulation in drug absorption is well established. Lipophilic drugs may be absorbed through the lacteal or lymphatic vessels under the microvilli. Absorption of drugs through the lymphatic system bypasses the liver and avoids the first-pass effect due to liver metabolism, because the lymphatic vessels drain into the vena cava rather than the hepatic-portal vein. The lymphatics are important in the absorption of dietary lipids and may be partially responsible for the absorption of some lipophilic drugs. Many poorly water-soluble drugs are soluble in oil and lipids, which may dissolve in chylomicrons and be absorbed systemically via the lymphatic system. Bleomycin or aclarubicin were prepared in chylomicrons to improve oral absorption through the lymphatic system (Yoshikawa et al, 1983, 1989). Other drugs that can be significantly absorbed through the lymphatic system include halofantrine, certain testosterone derivatives, temarotene, ontazolast, vitamin D-3, and the pesticide DDT. Notably, as the trend in drug development is to produce more highly potent lipophilic drugs, targeting of the lymphatic system is receiving increased attention. In such efforts, the formulation of lipid excipients plays a very dramatic role in the success of lymphatic targeting (Yanez et al, 2011).

### Effect of Food on Gastrointestinal Drug Absorption

The presence of food in the GI tract can affect the bioavailability of the drug from an oral drug product (Table 4-10). Digested foods contain amino acids, fatty acids, and many nutrients that may affect intestinal pH and solubility of drugs. The effects of food are not always predictable and can have clinically significant consequences. Some effects of food on the bioavailability of a drug from a drug product include (US Food and Drug Administration, Guidance for Industry, December 2002):

- Delay in gastric emptying
- Stimulation of bile flow
- A change in the pH of the GI tract
- An increase in splanchnic blood flow
- A change in luminal metabolism of the drug substance
- Physical or chemical interaction of the meal with the drug product or drug substance

Food effects on bioavailability are generally greatest when the drug product is administered shortly after a meal is ingested. The nutrient and caloric contents of the meal, the meal volume, and the meal temperature can cause physiologic changes in the GI tract in a way that affects drug product transit time, luminal dissolution, drug permeability, and systemic availability. In general, meals that are high in total calories and fat content are more likely to affect

GI physiology and thereby result in a larger effect on the bioavailability of a drug substance or drug product. The FDA recommends the use of high-calorie and high-fat meals to study the effect of food on the bioavailability and bioequivalence of drug products (FDA Guidance for Industry, 2002; see also Chapter 29).

The absorption of some antibiotics, such as penicillin and tetracycline, and certain hydrophilic drugs, is decreased with food, whereas other drugs, particularly lipid-soluble drugs such as griseofulvin, metaxalone, and metolazone, are better absorbed when given with food containing a high-fat content (Fig. 4-17). The presence of food in the GI lumen stimulates the flow of bile. Bile contains bile acids, which are surfactants involved in the digestion and solubilization of fats, and also increases the solubility of fat-soluble drugs through micelle formation. For some basic drugs (eg, cinnarizine) with limited aqueous solubility, the presence of food in the stomach stimulates hydrochloric acid secretion, which lowers the pH, causing more rapid dissolution of the drug and better absorption. Absorption of this basic drug is reduced when gastric acid secretion is reduced (Ogata et al, 1986).

Most drugs should be taken with a full glass (approximately 8 fluid oz or 250 mL) of water to ensure that drugs will wash down the esophagus and be more available for absorption. Generally, the bioavailability of drugs is better in patients in the fasted state and with a large volume of water (Fig. 4-18). The solubility of many drugs is limited, and sufficient fluid is necessary for dissolution of the drug. Some patients may be on several drugs that are dosed frequently for months. These patients are often nauseous and are reluctant to take a lot of fluid. For example, HIV patients with active viral counts may be on an AZT or DDI combination with one or more of the protease inhibitors, Invirase (Hoffmann-La Roche), Crixivan (Merck), or Norvir (Abbott) as well as HIV viral integrase inhibitors such as raltegravir, dolutegravir, or elvitegravir. Any complications affecting drug absorption can influence the outcome of these therapies. With antibiotics, unabsorbed drug may influence the GI flora. For drugs that cause GI disturbances, residual drug dose in the GI tract can potentially aggravate the incidence of diarrhea.

## TABLE 4-10 • The Effect of Food on the Bioavailability of Selected Drugs

| Drug | Food Effect |
|---|---|
| **Decreased bioavailability with food** | |
| Doxycycline hyclate delayed-release tablets | The mean $C_{max}$ and $AUC_{0-\infty}$ of doxycycline are 24% and 13% lower, respectively, following single-dose administration with a high-fat meal (including milk) compared to fasted conditions. |
| Atorvastatin calcium tablets | Food decreases the rate and extent of drug absorption by approximately 25% and 9%, respectively, as assessed by $C_{max}$ and AUC. |
| Clopidogrel bisulfate tablets | Clopidogrel is a prodrug and is metabolized to a pharmacologically active metabolite and inactive metabolites. The active metabolite $AUC_{0-24}$ was unchanged in the presence of food, while there was a 57% decrease in active metabolite $C_{max}$. |
| Naproxen delayed-release tablets | Naproxen delayed-release tablets are enteric-coated tablets with a pH-sensitive coating. The presence of food prolonged the time the tablets remained in the stomach. $T_{max}$ is delayed but peak naproxen levels, $C_{max}$ was not affected. |
| Alendronate sodium tablets | Bioavailability was decreased by approximately 40% when 10 mg alendronate was administered either 0.5 or 1 hour before a standardized breakfast. Alendronate must be taken at least one-half hour before the first food, beverage, or medication of the day with plain water only. Other beverages (including mineral water), food, and some medications are likely to reduce drug absorption. |
| Tamsulosin HCl capsules | Taking tamsulosin capsules under fasted conditions results in a 30% increase in bioavailability (AUC) and 40% to 70% increase in peak concentrations ($C_{max}$) compared to fed conditions. |
| **Increased bioavailability with food** | |
| Oxycodone HCl CR tablets | Food has no significant effect on the extent of absorption of oxycodone from OxyContin. However, the peak plasma concentration of oxycodone increased by 25% when an OxyContin 160-mg tablet was administered with a high-fat meal. |
| Metaxalone Tablets | A high-fat meal increased $C_{max}$ by 177.5% and increased AUC ($AUC_{0-t}$, $AUC_{\infty}$) by 123.5% and 115.4%, respectively. $T_{max}$ was delayed (4.3 h versus 3.3 h) and terminal $t_{1/2}$ was decreased (2.4 h versus 9.0 h). |
| Spironolactone tablets | Food increased the bioavailability of unmetabolized spironolactone by almost 100%. The clinical importance of this finding is not known. |
| **Food has very little effect on bioavailability** | |
| Gabapentin capsules | Food has only a slight effect on the rate and extent of absorption of gabapentin (14% increase in AUC and $C_{max}$). |
| Tramadol HCl tablets | Oral administration of Tramadol hydrochloride tablets with food does not significantly affect its rate or extent of absorption. |
| Digoxin tablets | When digoxin tablets are taken after meals, the rate of absorption is slowed, but the total amount of digoxin absorbed is usually unchanged. When taken with meals high in bran fiber, however, the amount absorbed from an oral dose may be reduced. |
| Bupropion HCl ER tablets | Food did not affect the $C_{max}$ or AUC of bupropion. |
| Methylphenidate HCl ER tablets (Concerta®) | In patients, there were no differences in either the pharmacokinetics or the pharmacodynamic performance of Concerta when administered after a high-fat breakfast. There is no evidence of dose dumping in the presence or absence of food. |
| Fluoxetine HCl capsules | Food does not appear to affect the systemic bioavailability of fluoxetine, although it may delay its absorption by 1 to 2 hours, which is probably not clinically significant. |
| Dutasteride soft gelatin capsules | Food reduces the $C_{max}$ by 10% to 15%. This reduction is of no clinical significance. |

*Food can affect bioavailability of the drug by affecting the rate and/or extent of drug absorption. In some cases, food may delay the $T_{max}$ for enteric-coated drugs due to a delay in stomach emptying time. For each drug, the clinical importance of the change in bioavailability due to food must be assessed.*

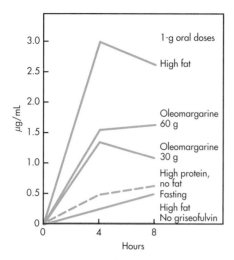

FIGURE 4-17 • A comparison of the effects of different types of food intake on the serum griseofulvin levels following a 1.0-g oral dose. (Reproduced with permission from Crounse RG: Human pharmacology of griseofulvin: the effect of fat intake on gastrointestinal absorption, J Invest Dermatol 1961 Dec;37:529–533.)

Some drugs, such as erythromycin, iron salts, aspirin, and nonsteroidal anti-inflammatory agents (NSAIDs), are irritating to the GI mucosa and are given with food to reduce this irritation. For these drugs, the rate of absorption may be reduced in the presence of food, but the extent of absorption may be the same and the efficacy of the drug is retained.

The GI transit time for enteric-coated and non-disintegrating drug products may also be affected by the presence of food. Enteric-coated tablets may stay in the stomach for a longer period of time because food delays stomach emptying. Thus, the enteric-coated tablet does not reach the duodenum rapidly, delaying drug release and systemic drug absorption. The presence of food may delay stomach emptying of enteric-coated tablets or nondisintegrating dosage forms for several hours. In contrast, since enteric-coated beads or microparticles disperse in the stomach, stomach emptying of the particles is less affected by food, and these preparations demonstrate more consistent drug absorption from the duodenum. Fine granules (smaller than 1–2 mm in size) and tablets that disintegrate are not significantly delayed from emptying from the stomach in the presence of food.

Food can also affect the integrity of the dosage form, causing an alteration in the release rate of the drug. For example, theophylline bioavailability from

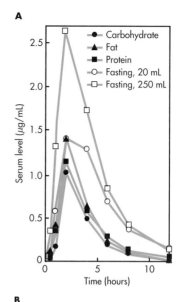

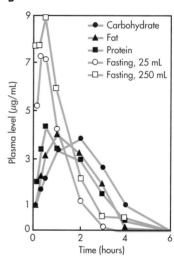

FIGURE 4-18 • Effect of water volume and meal on the bioavailability of erythromycin and aspirin (ASA). (**A.** Reproduced with permission from Welling PG, Huang H, Hewitt PF, et al: Bioavailability of erythromycin stearate: influence of food and fluid volume, J Pharm Sci 1978 Jun;67(6):764-766.**B**. Reproduced with permission from Koch PA, Schultz CA, Wills RJ, et al: Influence of food and fluid ingestion on aspirin bioavailability, J Pharm Sci 1978 Nov;67(11):1533–1535.)

Theo-24 controlled-release tablets is much more rapid when given to a subject in the fed rather than fasted state because of dosage form failures, known as *dose-dumping* (Fig. 4-19). This and other bioavailability studies with food led to the FDA requirement

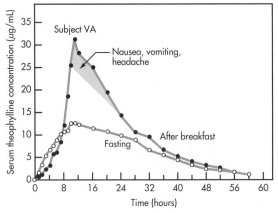

FIGURE 4-19 • Theophylline serum concentrations in an individual subject after a single 1500-mg dose of Theo-24 taken during fasting and after breakfast. The shaded area indicates the period during which this patient experienced nausea, repeated vomiting, or severe throbbing headache. The pattern of drug release during the food regimen is consistent with "dose-dumping." Reproduced with permission from Hendeles L, Weinberger M, Milavetz G, Hill M 3rd, Vaughan L. Food-induced "dose-dumping" from a once-a-day theophylline product as a cause of theophylline toxicity, Chest 1985 Jun;87(6):758–765.)

for most bioequivalence students to be performed in both fed and fasted subjects (see Chapter 29).

Food may enhance the absorption of a drug beyond 2 hours after meals. For example, the timing of a fatty meal on the absorption of cefpodoxime proxetil was studied in 20 healthy adults (Borin et al, 1995). The area under the plasma concentration–time curve and peak drug concentration was significantly higher after administration of cefpodoxime proxetil tablets with a meal and 2 hours after a meal relative to dosing under fasted conditions or 1 hour before a meal. The time to peak concentration was not affected by food, which suggests that food increased the extent but not the rate of drug absorption. These results indicate that absorption of cefpodoxime proxetil is enhanced with food or if the drug is taken closely after a heavy meal.

Timing of drug administration in relation to meals is often important. Pharmacists regularly advise patients to take a medication either 1 hour before or 2 hours after meals to avoid any delay in drug absorption.

Alendronate sodium (Fosamax®) is a bisphosphonate that acts as a specific inhibitor of osteoclast-mediated bone resorption used to prevent osteoporosis. Bisphosphonates are very soluble in water and their systemic oral absorption is greatly reduced in the presence of food. The approved labeling for alendronate sodium states that (Fosamax) "must be taken at least one-half hour before the first food, beverage, or medication of the day with plain water only."

Since fatty foods may delay stomach emptying time beyond 2 hours, patients who have just eaten a heavy, fatty meal should take these drugs 3 hours or more after the meal, whenever possible. Products that are used to curb stomach acid secretion are usually taken before meals, in anticipation of acid secretion stimulated by food. Famotidine (Pepcid) and cimetidine (Tagamet) are taken before meals to curb excessive acid production. In some cases, drugs are taken directly after a meal or with meals to increase the systemic absorption of the drug (eg, itraconazole, metaxalone) or with food to decrease gastric irritation of the drug (eg, ibuprofen). Many lipophilic drugs have increased bioavailability with food possibly due to formation of micelles in the GI tract and some lymphatic absorption.

Fluid volume tends to distend the stomach and speed up stomach emptying; however, a large volume of nutrients with high caloric content supersedes that faster rate and delays stomach emptying time. Reduction in drug absorption may be caused by several other factors. For example, tetracycline hydrochloride absorption is reduced by milk and food that contains calcium, due to tetracycline chelation. However, significant reduction in absorption may simply be the result of reduced dissolution due to increased pH. Coadministration of sodium bicarbonate raises the stomach pH and reduces tetracycline dissolution and absorption (Barr et al, 1971).

Ticlopidine (Ticlid®) is an antiplatelet agent that is commonly used to prevent thromboembolic disorders. Ticlopidine has enhanced absorption after a meal. The absorption of ticlopidine was compared in subjects who received either an antacid or food or were in a control group (fasting). Subjects who received ticlopidine 30 minutes after a fatty meal had an average increase of 20% in plasma concentrations over fasting subjects, whereas antacid reduced ticlopidine plasma concentrations by approximately the same amount. There was a higher incidence of GI complaint in the fasting group. Many other drugs have reduced GI side effects when taken with food. The decreased GI side effects associated with food consumption may greatly improve tolerance and compliance in patients.

## Double-Peak Phenomenon

Some drugs, such as ranitidine, cimetidine, and dipyridamole, after oral administration produce a blood concentration curve consisting of two peaks (Fig. 4-20). This double-peak phenomenon is generally observed after the administration of a single dose to fasted patients. The rationale for the double-peak phenomenon has been attributed to variability in stomach emptying, variable intestinal motility, presence of food, enterohepatic recycling, or failure of a tablet dosage form.

The double-peak phenomenon observed for cimetidine (Oberle and Amidon, 1987) may be due to variability in stomach emptying and intestinal flow rates during the entire absorption process after a single dose. For many drugs, very little absorption occurs in the stomach. For a drug with high water solubility,

dissolution of the drug occurs in the stomach, and partial emptying of the drug into the duodenum will result in the first absorption peak. A delay in stomach emptying results in a second absorption peak as the remainder of the dose is emptied into the duodenum.

In contrast, ranitidine (Miller, 1984) produces a double peak after both oral or parenteral (IV bolus) administration. Ranitidine is apparently concentrated in the bile within the gallbladder from the general circulation after IV administration. When stimulated by food, the gallbladder contracts and bile-containing drug is released into the small intestine. The drug is then reabsorbed and recycled (enterohepatic recycling).

Tablet integrity may also be a factor in the production of a double-peak phenomenon. Mellinger and Bohorfoush (1966) compared a whole tablet or a crushed tablet of dipyridamole in volunteers and showed that a tablet that does not disintegrate or incompletely disintegrates may have delayed gastric emptying, resulting in a second absorption peak.

## Presystemic Metabolism in the Intestine and Liver

The human intestine expresses several drug-metabolizing enzymes, including CYPs, UGTs, and SULTs (Ho 2017) (Table 4-11). Although the protein expression levels are much lower than those in the liver, the time a given drug molecule is exposed to an intestinal enzyme may be higher, due to lower blood flow and very high surface area. Thus, some drugs can undergo significant presystemic metabolism in the intestine before they even get to the liver. In fact, for some drugs undergoing phase 2 metabolism, the intestine's contribution to first-pass metabolism is even greater than that of the liver (Mizuma 2008; Mizuma 2009).

The absolute oral bioavailability (F) is determined by several factors. First, a drug's solubility and permeability, which determine the extent to which it gets absorbed (fraction absorbed, Fa). Thus, a drug with problematic solubility or permeability may have a low Fa. Next, the drug needs to escape metabolism in the intestine; the fraction of the dose escaping metabolism in the gut is Fg. To finally reach systemic circulation, the drug needs to get past the liver without being extracted; the fraction of dose escaping the

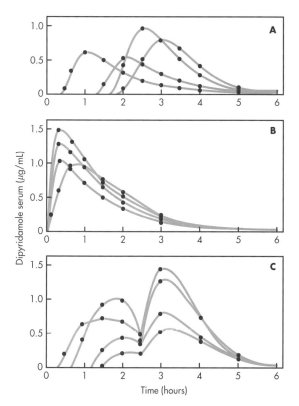

FIGURE 4-20 • Serum concentrations of dipyridamole in three groups of four volunteers each. **A.** After taking 25 mg as tablet intact. **B.** As crushed tablet. **C.** As tablet intact 2 hours before lunch. (Reproduced with permission from Mellinger TJ, Bohorfoush JG: Blood levels of dipyridamole (Persantin) in humans. *Arch Int Pharmacodynam Ther* 1966 163:471–480)

**TABLE 4-11 •** Intestinal Enzymes and Transporters Affecting Selected Compounds

| Drug | Enzyme(s) | Efflux Transporter | Uptake Transporter |
|---|---|---|---|
| Atorvastatin | CYP3A4, UGT1A1/3 | P-gp, BCRP | OATP1B1/1B3/2B1 |
| Ethinylestradiol | CYP3A4, SULT1E1, UGT1A1 | MRP2/3, BCRP | OATP1B1/1B3/2B1 |
| Ezetimibe | UGT1A1/3 | P-gp, BCRP, MRP2/3 | OATP1B1 |
| Gemfibrozil | UGT2B7 | MRP2/3/4 | OATP1B1 |
| Irinotecan | CES1, UGT1A1/6 | BCRP, MRP2 | OATP1B1 |
| Morphine | UGT2B7 | P-gp, MRP2/3 | |
| Mycophenylate mofetil | UGT1A9 | P-gp, MRP2/3 | OATP1B3 |
| Raloxifene | UGT1A1/8/10 | P-gp, MRP2/3 | OATP1B1/1B3 |
| Resveratrol | UGT1A1/9, SULT1A1 | BCRP, MRP2/3 | OATP1B1/1B3/2B1 |

Data from Müller J, Keiser M, Drozdzik M, Oswald S. Expression, regulation and function of intestinal drug transporters: an update, Biol Chem 2017 Feb 1; 398(2):175–192.
For each compound, the phase 2 metabolites are substrates for the efflux transporters in the intestine, and/or the uptake and efflux transporters in the liver.

liver is Fh. So the absolute oral bioavailability is the product of each of these processes: $F = F_a * F_g * F_h$. Notably, variability in these factors increases as they get further from 1. Thus, drugs with low oral bioavailability quite often also have highly variable bioavailability. High interpatient and intrasubject variability is not overcome through increased doses. By understanding and quantitating each of these factors and the processes they involve, F can be predicted or explained and enables the biopharmaceutical scientist to know the expected problems with drug bioavailability.

## ORAL DRUG ABSORPTION DURING DRUG PRODUCT DEVELOPMENT

### Prediction of Oral Drug Absorption

During the screening of new chemical entities for possible therapeutic efficacy, some drugs might not be discovered due to lack of systemic absorption after oral administration. Lipinski et al (2001) reviewed the chemical structure of many orally administered drugs and published the Rule of Five. During drug screening, the *"Rule of Five"* predicts that poor drug absorption or permeation is more likely when: (1) there are more than five hydrogen-bond (H-bond) donors, (2) there are more than 10 H-bond acceptors, (3) the molecular weight is greater than 500, and (4) the calculated log $P$ (Clog $P$)[2] is greater than 5

(or Mlog $P$ > 4.15). The rule is based on molecular computation and simulation and the effect of hydrophobicity, hydrogen bond, molecular size, and other relevant factors in assessing absorption using computational methods. The method is not applicable to drugs whose absorption involves transporters. These rules were developed to avoid types of chemical structures during early drug development that are unlikely to have adequate bioavailability. These rules have been modified by others (Takano et al, 2006). Rules for drug molecules that would improve the chance for oral absorption would include:

- Molecular weight ≤500 Da
- Not more than five *H-bond* donors (*nitrogen* or *oxygen atoms* with one or more *hydrogen atoms*) (O–H or N–H group)
- Not more than 10 *H-bond* acceptors (*nitrogen* or *oxygen atoms*)
- An octanol–water partition coefficient, log $P$ ≤ 5.0

These rules only help predict adequate drug absorption and do not predict adequate pharmacodynamic activity. Moreover, some chemical structures do not

---

[2]Log P, this is measure of lipophilicity and is the partition coefficient of a molecule between an aqueous and lipophilic phases, usually octanol and water.

follow the above rules, but may have good therapeutic properties.

Burton et al (2002) reviewed the difficulty in predicting drug absorption based only on physicochemical activity of drug molecules and discussed other factors that can affect oral drug absorption. Burton et al state that drug absorption is a complex process dependent upon drug properties such as solubility and permeability, formulation factors, and physiological variables, including regional permeability differences, pH, mucosal enzymology, and intestinal motility, among others. These investigators point out that intestinal drug absorption, permeability, fraction absorbed, and, in some cases, even bioavailability are not equivalent properties and cannot be used interchangeably. Often these properties are influenced by the nature of the drug product and physical and chemical characteristics of the drug.

Software programs, such as GastroPlus™, have recently been developed to predict oral drug absorption, pharmacokinetics, and pharmacodynamic drugs in human and preclinical species. Simulation programs may use physicochemical data, such as molecular weight, $pK_a$, solubility at various pH, log $P$/log $D$, type of dosage form, *in vitro* inputs such as dissolution, permeability/Caco-2, CYP metabolism (gut/liver), transporter rates, and *in vivo* inputs such as drug clearance and volume of distribution.

## METHODS FOR STUDYING FACTORS THAT AFFECT DRUG ABSORPTION

### Biorelevant Drug Dissolution Studies

Before a drug molecule can be absorbed, it must be released from the dosage form into physiologic fluids. Much progress has been made in recent years regarding the simulation of physiologic fluids involved in drug dissolution, especially for the GI tract. Fluids in the human stomach, small intestine, and colon have been characterized for their chemical and enzymatic content and physicochemical characteristics under both fasting and fed conditions. Many studies have been performed regarding simulated (artificial) GI fluids and their relevance to *in vivo* drug absorption (Fuchs 2015). These studies formed the basis of new compendial recommendations on drug dissolution testing, providing recipes for media

to be used (USP-NF 2019). Such efforts make drug development and drug product performance testing more biorelevant.

### Gamma Scintigraphy to Study Site of Drug Release

Gamma scintigraphy is a technique commonly used to track drug dosage form movement from one region to another within the GI tract after oral administration. Gamma scintigraphy also has many research applications and is widely used for formulation studies, such as the mechanism of drug release from a hydrophilic matrix tablet (Abrahamsson et al, 1998). Generally, a nonabsorbable radionuclide that emits gamma rays is included as marker in the formulation. In some studies, two radiolabels may be used for simultaneous detection of liquid and solid phases. One approach is to use labeled technetium ($Tc^{99m}$) in a capsule matrix to study how a drug is absorbed. The image of the capsule breaking up in the stomach or the GI tract is monitored using a gamma camera. Simultaneously, blood levels or urinary excretion of the drug may be measured. This study can be used to correlate residence time of the drug in a given region after capsule breakup to drug absorption. The same technique is used to study drug absorption mechanisms in different regions of the GI tract before a drug is formulated for extended release.

Gamma scintigraphy has been used to study the effect of transit time on the absorption of theophylline (Sournac et al, 1988). *In vitro* drug release characteristics were correlated with total GI transit time. The results showed a significant correlation between the *in vitro* release of theophylline and the percent of the total amount of theophylline absorbed *in vivo*. This study illustrates the importance of gamma scintigraphy for the development of specialized drug dosage forms.

### Markers to Study Effect of Gastric and GI Transit Time on Absorption

Many useful agents are available that may be used as tools to study absorption and understand the mechanism of the absorptive process. For example, mannitol has a concentration-dependent effect on small intestinal transit. Adkin et al (1995) showed that small concentrations of mannitol included in a pharmaceutical formulation could lead to reduced uptake of many drugs absorbed exclusively from the small intestine. No significant differences between the gastric emptying times of the four solutions of different concentrations tested were observed.

Similarly, Hebden et al (1999) demonstrated that codeine slowed GI transit, decreased stool water content, and diminished drug absorption when compared to controls. The results indicated that stool water content may be an important determinant in colonic drug absorption. In contrast, the sugar lactulose accelerated GI transit, increased stool water content, and enhanced drug absorption from the distal gut. Quinine absorption was greater when given with lactulose compared to no lactulose.

Riley et al (1992) studied the effects of gastric emptying and GI transit on the absorption of several drug solutions (furosemide, atenolol, hydrochlorothiazide, and salicylic acid) in healthy subjects. These drugs may potentially be absorbed differently at various sites in the GI system. Subjects were given 20 mg oral metoclopramide or 60 mg oral codeine phosphate to slow gastric emptying. The study showed that gastric emptying time affects the absorption of salicylic acid, but not that of furosemide, hydrochlorothiazide, or atenolol. *In vivo* experiments are needed to determine the effect of changing transit time on drug absorption.

## Remote Drug Delivery Capsules

Drug absorption *in vivo* may be studied either directly by an intubation technique that directly takes samples from the GI tract or remotely with a special device, such as the Heidelberg capsule. The *Heidelberg capsule* (Barrie, 1999) is a device used to determine the pH of the stomach. The capsule contains a pH sensor and a miniature radio transmitter (invented by H. G. Noeller and used at Heidelberg University in Germany decades ago). The capsule is about 2 cm × 0.8 cm and can transmit data to outside after the device is swallowed and tethered to the stomach. Other, newer telemetric methods may be used to take pictures of various regions of the GI tract.

An interesting *remote drug delivery capsule* (RDDC) with electronic controls for noninvasive regional drug absorption study was reported by Parr et al (1999). This device was used to study absorption of ranitidine hydrochloride solution in 12 healthy male volunteers. Mean gastric emptying of the RDDC was 1.50 hours, and total small intestine transit was 4.79 hours. The capsule was retrieved from the feces at 30.25 hours. The onset of ranitidine serum levels depended on the time of capsule activation and the site of drug release.

## Osmotic Pump Systems

The osmotic pump system is a drug product that contains a small hole from which dissolved drug is released (pumped out) at a rate determined by the rate of entrance of water from the GI tract across a semipermeable membrane due to osmotic pressure (see Chapter 9). The drug is either mixed with an osmotic agent or located in a reservoir. Osmotic pump systems may be used to study drug absorption in different parts of the GI tract because the rate of drug release is constant (zero order) and generally not altered by the environment of the GI tract. The constant rate of drug release provides relatively constant blood concentrations.

## In Vivo *GI Perfusion Studies*

In the past, segments of guinea pig or rat ileums were cut and used to study drug absorption; however, we now know that many of the isolated preparations were not viable shortly after removal, making the absorption data collected either invalid or difficult to evaluate. In addition, the differences among species make it difficult to extrapolate animal data to humans.

*GI perfusion* is an *in vivo* method used to study absorption and permeability of a drug in various segments of the GI tract. A tube is inserted from the mouth or anus and placed in a specific section of the GI tract. A drug solution is infused from the tube at a fixed rate, resulting in drug perfusion of the desired GI region. The jejunal site is peristaltically less active than the duodenum, making it easier to intubate, and therefore it is often chosen for perfusion studies. Perfusion studies in other sites such as the duodenum, ileum, and even the colon have also been performed by gastroenterologists and pharmaceutical scientists.

Lennernas et al (1992, 1995) have applied perfusion techniques in humans to study permeability in the small intestine and the rectum. These methods yield direct absorption information in various segments of the GI tract. The regional jejunal perfusion method was reported to have great potential for mechanistic evaluations of drug absorption.

Buch and Barr (1998) evaluated propranolol HCl in the proximal and distal intestine in humans ($n = 7$ subjects) using direct intubation. Propranolol HCl is a beta blocker that has high inter- and intrasubject variability in absorption and metabolism. These investigators showed that propranolol was better absorbed from a solution in the distal region of the intestine. This study is difficult to relate to the propranolol extended-release oral products for which differences in drug release rates and GI transit time may also influence inter- and intrasubject variability in bioavailability.

More recently, balloon-isolated jejunal drug administration has been used to determine the absorption characteristics of (-)epicatechin, vitamin E, and vitamin E acetate (Actis-Goretta et al, 2013). The current efforts to determine intestinal regional drug absorption have been recently reviewed, and data generated from these studies will be useful to refine models for predicting drug absorption (Lennernas, 2014).

### Intestinal Permeability to Drugs

Drugs that are completely absorbed ($F > 90\%$) after oral administration generally demonstrate high permeability in *in vitro* models. Previously, poor drug absorption was mostly attributed to poor dissolution, slow diffusion, degradation, or poor intestinal permeation. Modern technology has shown that poor or variable oral drug bioavailability among individuals is also the result of individual genetic differences in intestinal absorption (see Chapter 21). Interindividual differences in membrane proteins, ion channels, uptake transporters, and efflux pumps (such as P-glycoprotein, P-gp) that mediate directional transport of drugs and their metabolites across biological membranes can change the extent of drug absorption, or even transport to the site of action elsewhere in the body. It is now clear that the behavior of drugs in the body is the result of an intricate interplay between these receptors, drug transporters, and the drug-metabolizing systems. This insight provides another explanation for erratic drug absorption beyond poor formulation and first-pass metabolism.

Alternative methods to study intestinal drug permeability include *in vivo* or *in situ* intestinal perfusion in a suitable animal model (eg, rats), and/or *in vitro* permeability methods using excised intestinal tissues, or monolayers of suitable epithelial cells such as Caco-2 cells. In addition, the physicochemical characterization of a drug substance (eg, oil–water partition coefficient) provides useful information to predict a drug's permeability.

### Caco-2 Cells for In Vitro *Permeability Studies*

Although *in vivo* studies yield much definitive information about drug permeability in humans, they are tedious and costly to perform. The *Caco-2* cell line is a human colon adenocarcinoma cell line that differentiates in culture and resembles the epithelial lining of the human small intestine. The permeability of the cellular monolayer may vary with the stage of cell growth and the cultivation method used. However, using monolayers of Caco-2 cells under controlled conditions, the permeability of a drug may be determined. Caco-2 cells can also be used to study interactions of drugs with the transporter P-gp discussed below.

Drug permeability using the Caco-2 cell line has been suggested as an *in vitro* method for passively transported drugs. In some cases, the drug permeability may appear to be low due to efflux of drugs via membrane transporters such as P-gp. Permeability studies using the Caco-2 cell line have been suggested as a method for classifying the permeability of a drug according to the Biopharmaceutics Classification System, BCS (Tolle-Sander and Polli, 2002; US Food and Drug Administration, Guidance 2003, August 2002; Sun and Pang, 2007). The main purpose of the BCS is to identify a drug as having high or low permeability or solubility as predictors of systemic drug absorption from the GI tract (see Chapter 8).

### Drug Transporters

Many methods are available to study the actions of drug transporters in the GI tract. In addition to Caco-2 cells, there are several commercially available expression systems to study various transporters, including those required by the FDA in drug development. These systems include transporters recombinantly expressed in insect, frog, or mammalian cells. Also, the plasma membranes of some of these expression systems can also be isolated, providing membrane vesicle preparations that are devoid of drug-metabolizing activity.

### Determinations of Artificial Membrane Permeability

To accelerate early determinations of factors involved in drug absorption, permeability and solubility of a novel drug candidate are determined early in the drug development process. Permeability of drug candidates may be determined using high-throughput screening techniques, such as the parallel artificial membrane permeability assay (PAMPA). In this technique, artificial lipid membranes are supported on a filter between two fluid compartments, one of which contains the drug candidate. The rate of appearance into the opposite compartment is then measured to determine the permeability of the compound. Several models and variations of this approach are available, and investigators should pay attention particularly to the lipid composition of the artificial membranes as well as other experimental details. Notably, the PAMPA can only predict simple diffusional permeability, which does not involve uptake or efflux transporters (Avdeef et al, 2007).

## EFFECT OF DISEASE STATES ON DRUG ABSORPTION

Drug absorption may be affected by any disease that causes changes in (1) intestinal blood flow, (2) GI motility, (3) stomach emptying time, (4) gastric pH that affects drug solubility, (5) intestinal pH that affects the extent of ionization, (6) the permeability of the gut wall, (7) bile secretion, (8) digestive enzyme secretion, or (9) alteration of normal GI flora. Some factors may dominate, while other factors sometimes cancel the effects of one another. Pharmacokinetic studies comparing subjects with and without the disease are generally necessary to establish the effect of the disease on drug absorption.

Patients in an advanced stage of *Parkinson's disease* may have difficulty swallowing and greatly diminished GI motility.

*Patients on tricyclic antidepressants* (imipramine, amitriptyline, and nortriptyline) and antipsychotic drugs (phenothiazines) with anticholinergic side effects may have reduced GI motility or even intestinal obstructions. Delays in drug absorption, especially with slow-release products, have occurred.

*Achlorhydric patients* may not have adequate production of acids in the stomach; stomach HCl is essential for solubilizing insoluble free bases. Many weak-base drugs that cannot form soluble salts will remain undissolved in the stomach when there is no hydrochloric acid present and are therefore unabsorbed. Salt forms of these drugs are not helpful because the free base readily precipitates out due to the weak basicity.

Dapsone, itraconazole, and ketoconazole may also be less well absorbed in the presence of achlorhydria. In patients with acid reflux disorders, proton pump inhibitors, such as omeprazole, render the stomach achlorhydric, which may also affect drug absorption. Coadministering orange juice, colas, or other acidic beverages can facilitate the absorption of some medications requiring an acidic environment.

*HIV–AIDS patients* are prone to a number of GI disturbances, such as decreased gastric transit time, diarrhea, and achlorhydria. Rapid gastric transit time and diarrhea can alter the absorption of orally administered drugs. Achlorhydria may or may not decrease absorption, depending on the acidity needed for absorption of a specific drug. Indinavir, for example, requires a normal acidic environment for absorption. The therapeutic window of indinavir is extremely narrow, so optimal serum concentrations are critical for this drug to be efficacious.

*Congestive heart failure* (CHF) *patients* with persistent edema have reduced splanchnic blood flow and develop edema in the bowel wall. In addition, intestinal motility is slowed. The reduced blood flow to the intestine and reduced intestinal motility result in a decrease in drug absorption. For example, furosemide (Lasix), a commonly used loop diuretic, has erratic and reduced oral absorption in patients with CHF and a delay in the onset of action.

*Crohn's disease* is an inflammatory disease of the distal small intestine and colon. The disease is accompanied by regions of thickening of the bowel wall, overgrowth of anaerobic bacteria, and sometimes obstruction and deterioration of the bowel. The effect on drug absorption is unpredictable, although impaired absorption may potentially occur because of reduced surface area and thicker gut wall for diffusion. For example, higher plasma propranolol concentration has been observed in patients with Crohn's disease after oral administration of propranolol. Serum α-1-acid glycoprotein levels are increased in Crohn's disease patients and may affect the protein binding and distribution of propranolol in the body and result in higher plasma concentrations.

*Celiac disease* is an inflammatory disease affecting mostly the proximal small intestine. Celiac disease is caused by sensitization to *gluten*, a viscous protein found in cereals and grains. Patients with celiac disease generally have an increased rate of stomach emptying and increased permeability of the small intestine. Cephalexin absorption appears to be increased in celiac disease, although it is not possible to make general predictions about these patients. Other intestinal conditions that may potentially affect drug absorption include corrective surgery involving peptic ulcer, antrectomy with gastroduodenostomy, and selective vagotomy.

Recently, hypoxemia and hypovolemia have been shown to have adverse effects on the intestinal microvilli (Harrois et al, 2013). Since the microvilli are important for many aspects of drug absorption, patients with significant blood loss, hypoxemia, or intestinal ischemia may be reasonably expected to have altered drug oral absorption. Caregivers may need to consider non-enteral routes of drug administration.

## Drugs That Affect Absorption of Other Drugs

Anticholinergic drugs in general may reduce stomach acid secretion. Propantheline bromide is an anticholinergic drug that may also slow stomach emptying and motility of the small intestine. Tricyclic antidepressants and phenothiazines also have anticholinergic side effects that may cause slower peristalsis in the GI tract. Slower stomach emptying may cause delay in drug absorption.

Metoclopramide is a drug that stimulates stomach contraction, relaxes the pyloric sphincter, and, in general, increases intestinal peristalsis, which may reduce the effective time for the absorption of some drugs and thereby decrease the peak drug concentration and the time to reach peak drug concentration. For example, digoxin absorption from a tablet is reduced by metoclopramide but increased by an anticholinergic drug, such as propantheline bromide. Allowing more time in the stomach for the tablet to dissolve generally helps with the dissolution and absorption of a poorly soluble drug but would not be helpful for a drug that is not soluble in stomach acid.

Antacids should not be given with cimetidine, because antacids may reduce drug absorption. Antacids containing aluminum, calcium, or magnesium may complex with drugs such as tetracycline, ciprofloxacin, and indinavir, resulting in a decrease in drug absorption. To avoid this interaction, antacids should be taken 2 hours before or 6 hours after drug administration.

Proton pump inhibitors such as omeprazole (Prilosec), lansoprazole (Prevacid˚), pantoprazole (Protonix˚), and others decrease gastric acid production, thereby raising gastric pH. These drugs may interfere with drugs for which gastric pH affects bioavailability (eg, ketoconazole, iron salts, ampicillin esters, and digoxin) and enteric-coated drug products (eg, aspirin, diclofenac) in which the pH-dependent enteric coating may dissolve in the higher gastric pH and release drug prematurely ("dose-dumping").

Cholestyramine is a nonabsorbable ion-exchange resin for the treatment of hyperlipidemia. Cholestyramine binds warfarin, thyroxine, and loperamide, similar to activated charcoal, thereby reducing absorption of these drugs.

## Nutrients That Interfere with Drug Absorption

Many nutrients substantially interfere with the absorption or metabolism of drugs in the body (Anderson, 1988; Kirk, 1995). The effect of food on bioavailability was discussed earlier. Oral drug–nutrient interactions are often drug specific and can result in either an increase or a decrease in drug absorption.

Absorption of calcium in the duodenum is an active process facilitated by vitamin D, with calcium absorption as much as four times more than that in vitamin D deficiency states. It is believed that a calcium-binding protein, which increases after vitamin D administration, binds calcium in the intestinal cell and transfers it out of the base of the cell to the blood circulation.

Grapefruit juice often increases bioavailability, as observed by an increase in plasma levels of many drugs that are substrates for cytochrome P-450 (CYP) 3A4 (see Chapter 21). Grapefruit juice contains various flavonoids such as naringin and furanocoumarins such as bergamottin, which inhibit certain cytochrome P-450 enzymes involved in drug metabolism (especially CYP3A4). In this case, the observed increase in the plasma drug–blood levels is due to decreased presystemic elimination in the GI tract and/or liver. Indirectly, the amount of drug absorbed systemically from the drug product is increased. Grapefruit juice can also block drug efflux by inhibiting P-gp for some drugs.

## MISCELLANEOUS ROUTES OF DRUG ADMINISTRATION

For systemic drug absorption, the oral route is the easiest, safest, and most popular route of drug administration. Alternate routes of drug administration have been used successfully to improve systemic drug absorption or to localize drug effects in order to minimize systemic drug exposure and adverse events. Furthermore, enteral drug administration (through nasogastric tubes and the like) may be necessary in patients incapable of swallowing medications but requiring chronic dosing. In such cases, oral liquid (solutions, suspensions, or emulsions) may be administered; some of these may require extemporaneous compounding. Increasingly popular nonparenteral alternatives to oral drug delivery for systemic drug absorption include nasal, inhalation, and transdermal drug delivery. Nasal, inhalation, and topical drug delivery may also be used for local drug action (Mathias and Hussain, 2010).

### Nasal Drug Delivery

Nasal drug delivery may be used for either local or systemic effects. Because the nasal region is richly supplied with blood vessels, nasal administration is also useful for systemic drug delivery. However, the total surface area in the nasal cavity is relatively small,

retention time in the nasal cavity is generally short, and some drugs may be swallowed. The swallowed fraction of the dose would have all the disadvantages of oral route, including low oral bioavailability and undesirable taste, as seen with sumatriptan nasal spray (Imitrex). These factors may limit the nose's capacity for systemic delivery of drugs requiring large doses. Surfactants are often used to increase systemic penetration, although the effect of chronic drug exposure on the integrity of nasal membranes must also be considered. In general, a drug must be sufficiently lipophilic to cross the membranes of the nasal epithelium in order to be absorbed. Small molecules with balanced lipophilic and hydrophilic properties tend to be absorbed more easily. This observation poses a challenge for nasal delivery of larger molecules such as proteins and peptides, which would benefit from delivery routes that avoid the degradative environment of the intestine. Dosage forms intended for nasal drug delivery include nasal drops, nasal sprays, aerosols, and nebulizers (Su and Campanale, 1985).

Depending on the metabolic absorption, and chemical profile of the drug, some drugs are rapidly absorbed through the nasal membrane and can deliver rapid therapeutic effect. Various hormones and insulin have been tested for intranasal delivery. In some cases, the objective is to improve availability, and in other cases, it is to reduce side effects. Vasopressin and oxytocin are older examples of drugs marketed as intranasal products. In addition, many opioids are known to be rapidly absorbed from the nasal passages and can deliver systemic levels of the drug almost as rapidly as an intravenous injection (Dale et al, 2002). A common problem with nasal drug delivery is the challenge of developing a formulation with nonirritating ingredients. Many surfactants that facilitate absorption tend to be moderately or very irritating to the nasal mucosa.

Intranasal corticosteroids for treatment of allergic and perennial rhinitis have become more popular since intranasal delivery is believed to reduce the total dose of corticosteroid required. A lower dose also leads to minimization of side effects such as growth suppression. This logic has led to many second-generation corticosteroids such as beclomethasone dipropionate, budesonide, flunisolide, fluticasone propionate, mometasone furoate, and triamcinolone acetonide that are being considered or developed for intranasal delivery (Szefler, 2002). However, the potential for growth suppression in children varies. In one study, beclomethasone dipropionate reduced growth in children, but mometasone furoate nasal spray used for 1 year showed no signs of growth suppression. Overall, the second-generation corticosteroids are given by nasal delivery to cause minimal systemic side effects (Szefler, 2002).

### Inhalation Drug Delivery

Inhalation drug delivery may also be used for local or systemic drug effects. The lung has a potential absorption surface of some 70 m², a much larger surface than the small intestine or nasal passages. When a substance is inhaled, it is exposed to membranes of the mouth or nose, pharynx, trachea, bronchi, bronchioles, alveolar sacs, and alveoli. The lungs and their associated airways are designed to remove foreign matter from the highly absorptive peripheral lung surfaces via mucociliary clearance. However, if compounds such as aerosolized drug can reach the peripheral region of the lung, absorption can be very efficient.

Particle (droplet) size and velocity of application control the extent to which inhaled substances penetrate into airway spaces. Optimum size for deep airway penetration of drug particles is 3–5 μm. Large particles tend to deposit in upper airways, whereas very small molecules (<3 *μ*m) are exhaled before absorption can occur. Most inhalation devices deliver approximately 10% of the administered dose to the lower respiratory tract. A number of devices such as spacers (to reduce turbulence and improve deep inhalation) have been developed to increase lung delivery. An *in vitro* device useful to measure the particle size emitted from an aerosol or a mechanically produced fine mist is the cascade impactor.

Recombinant human insulin for inhalation (Exubera*) was approved by the FDA, demonstrating the viability of this delivery route even for large biological drugs. Insulin inhalation was withdrawn from the United States market in 2007 due to lack of consumer demand for the product.

### Topical and Transdermal Drug Delivery

*Topical drug delivery* is generally used for local drug effects at the site of application. Dosing is dependent upon the concentration of the drug in the topical product (eg, cream, ointment) and the total surface area applied. Drug may be applied as an ointment or cream to the skin or various mucous membranes such as intravaginally. Even though the objective is to obtain a local drug effect, some of the drugs may be absorbed systemically.

*Transdermal* products are generally used for systemic drug absorption. For transdermal drug delivery, the drug is incorporated into a transdermal therapeutic system or patch, but it may be incorporated into an ointment as well (see Chapter 7). The advantages of transdermal delivery include continuous release of drug over a period of time, low presystemic clearance, and good patient compliance.

Other routes of drug administration are discussed elsewhere and in Chapter 7.

---

### FREQUENTLY ASKED QUESTIONS

▶ What is an "absorption window"?

▶ Why are some drugs orally absorbed better with food, whereas the oral absorption of other drugs are slowed or decreased by food?

▶ What type of food is expected to have the greatest effect on GI pH and GI transit time?

▶ Are drugs that are administered as an oral solution completely absorbed from the GI tract?

▶ What factors influence drug absorption?

---

## CHAPTER SUMMARY

Oral systemic drug absorption is a complex process dependent upon many physiologic and biopharmaceutic factors including (1) the physicochemical properties of the drug, (2) the nature of the drug product, (3) the anatomy and physiology of the drug absorption site, and (4) the type and amount of food or other drugs present in the gut. Most drugs are passively absorbed as described by Fick's law of diffusion, which depends upon maintaining a concentration gradient within the GI tract and the plasma. Drug absorption is often a first-order process depending on rate of drug release and dissolution from the dosage form and drug permeability at the absorption site. Orally administered drugs may not be efficiently absorbed all along the GI tract. The duodenum affords the optimum area for absorption due to the high surface area and blood flow. Several substrate-specific transporters may be the dominant factor responsible for bioavailability of some drugs. These drugs are absorbed by active transport, which is a carrier-mediated process that requires energy and transports the drug against a concentration gradient. Active drug absorption may be saturable depending on the carrier protein involved and is often site specific. Influx and efflux transporters in the GI tract influence systemic drug absorption. A well-known class of transporters in the GI tract is known as the ABC family. MDR1 (alias P-gp) is an example. P-gp reduces drug absorption by effluxing the drug out of the enterocytes and back into the gut lumen. When the absorption process becomes saturated, the rate of drug absorption no longer follows a first-order process. Many efflux transporters in the GI and other parts of the body are now recognized, and their presence and quantity are genetically expressed and may be activated by certain diseases, such as cancer. P-glycoprotein is a common efflux transporter in the GI tract, which may be inhibited by coadministered drugs and nutrients leading to enhanced systemic absorption. In addition to normal GI and physiologic factors such as stomach emptying time, small intestine transit time, local pH, content of the GI tract, presystemic metabolism, and drug dosage form factors jointly influence systemic drug absorption.

Biopharmaceutic factors such as drug aqueous solubility, permeability of cell membranes, the degree of ionization, molecular size, particle size, and nature of the dosage form will also affect systemic drug absorption from the absorption site. The prediction of drug absorption based on physicochemical activity of drug molecules and other factors have been attempted during drug screening and discovery and using computer simulations. The rate and extent of drug absorption is greatly dependent on routes of administration. Parenteral, inhalation, transdermal, and intranasal routes all present physiologic and biopharmaceutic issues that must be understood in order to develop an optimum formulation that is consistently absorbed systemically. Various methods are used to study drug absorption depending on the route involved. Gamma scintigraphy and marker methods are used to study stomach emptying time and GI transit time. GI perfusion methods are used to determine the influence of transporters and the effect of presystemic clearance and regional drug absorption.

## LEARNING QUESTIONS

1. A recent bioavailability study in adult human volunteers demonstrated that after the administration of a single enteric-coated aspirin granule product given with a meal, the plasma drug levels resembled the kinetics of a sustained-release drug product. In contrast, when the product was given to fasted subjects, the plasma drug levels resembled the kinetics of an immediate-release drug product. Give a plausible explanation for this observation.

2. The aqueous solubility of a weak-base drug is poor. In an intubation (intestinal perfusion) study, the drug was not absorbed beyond the jejunum. Which of the following would be the correct strategy to improve drug absorption from the intestinal tract?

   a. Give the drug as a suspension and recommend that the suspension be taken on an empty stomach.

   b. Give the drug as a hydrochloride salt.

   c. Give the drug with milk.

   d. Give the drug as a suppository.

3. What is the primary reason that protein drugs such as insulin are not given orally for systemic absorption?

4. Which of the following statements is true regarding an acidic drug with a $pK_a$ of 4?

   a. The drug is more soluble in the stomach when food is present.

   b. The drug is more soluble in the duodenum than in the stomach.

   c. The drug is more soluble when dissociated.

5. Which region of the GI tract is most populated by bacteria? What types of drugs might affect the GI flora?

6. Discuss methods by which the first-pass effect (presystemic absorption) may be circumvented.

7. Misoprostol (Cytotec, GD Searle) is a synthetic prostaglandin E1 analog. According to the manufacturer, the following information was obtained when misoprostol was taken with an antacid or high-fat breakfast:

| Condition | $C_{max}$ (pg/mL) | $AUC_{0-24\ hour}$ (pg·h/mL) | $t_{max}$ (minutes) |
|---|---|---|---|
| Fasting | $811 \pm 317^a$ | $417 \pm 135$ | $14 \pm 8$ |
| With antacid | $689 \pm 315$ | $349 \pm 108^b$ | $20 \pm 14$ |
| With high-fat breakfast | $303 \pm 176^b$ | $373 \pm 111$ | $64 \pm 79^b$ |

[a]Results are expressed as the mean ± SD (standard deviation).
[b]Comparisons with fasting results statistically significant, $p < 0.05$.

What is the effect of antacid and high-fat breakfast on the bioavailability of misoprostol? Comment on how these factors affect the rate and extent of systemic drug absorption.

8. A given drug is completely absorbed but extensively metabolized by the intestinal epithelium (91%) followed by extensive hepatic extraction (71%). What is the expected overall oral bioavailability?

## ANSWERS

### Learning Questions

1. In the presence of food, undissolved aspirin granules larger than 1 mm are retained up to several hours longer in the stomach. In the absence of food, aspirin granules are emptied from the stomach within 1–2 hours. When the aspirin granules empty into the duodenum slowly, drug absorption will be as slow as with a sustained-release drug product. Enteric-coated aspirin granules taken with an evening meal may provide relief of pain for arthritic patients late into the night.

2. The answer is **b**. A basic drug formulated as a suspension will depend on stomach acid for dissolution as the basic drug forms a hydrochloric acid (HCl) salt. If the drug is poorly soluble, adding milk may neutralize some acid so that the drug may not be completely dissolved. Making an HCl salt rather than a suspension of the base ensures that the drug is soluble without being dependent on stomach HCl for dissolution.

3. Protein drugs are generally digested by proteolytic enzymes present in the GI tract and, therefore, are not adequately absorbed by the oral route. Protein drugs are most commonly given parenterally. Other routes of administration, such as intranasal and rectal administration, have had some success or are under current investigation for the systemic absorption of protein drugs.

4. The answer is **c**. Raising the pH of an acid drug above its $pK_a$ will increase the dissociation of the drug, thereby increasing its aqueous solubility.

5. The large intestine is most heavily populated by bacteria, yeasts, and other microflora. Some drugs that are not well absorbed in the small intestine are metabolized by the microflora to products that are absorbed in the large bowel. For example, drugs with an azo link (eg, sulfasalazine) are cleaved by bacteria in the bowel and the cleaved products (eg, 5-aminosalicylic acid and sulfapyridine) are absorbed. Other drugs, such as antibiotics (eg, tetracyclines), may destroy the bacteria in the large intestine, resulting in an overgrowth of yeast (eg, *Candida albicans*) and leading to a yeast infection. Destruction of the microflora in the lower bowel can also lead to cramps and diarrhea.

6. First-pass effects are discussed more fully in Chapter 12. Alternative routes of drug administration such as buccal, inhalation, sublingual, intranasal, and parenteral will bypass the first-pass effects observed after oral drug administration.

7. Although antacid statistically decreased the extent of systemic drug absorption ($p < .05$) as shown by an $AUC_{0-4\,h}$ of 349 ± 108 pg·h/mL, compared to the control (fasting) $AUC_{0-4\,h}$ value of 417 ± 135 pg·h/mL, the effect of antacid is not clinically significant. A high-fat diet decreased the rate of systemic drug absorption, as shown by a longer $t_{max}$ value (64 minutes) and lower $C_{max}$ value (303 pg/mL).

8. Complete absorption means that $F_a = 1$; also, 91% intestinal metabolism means $F_g = 1 - 0.91 = 0.09$; and 71% hepatic extraction means $F_h = 1 - 0.71 = 0.29$. Since $F = F_a * F_g * F_h$, then $F = 1 * 0.09 * 0.29 = 0.026$. This means the absolute oral bioavailability in this case would be 2.6%, which of course is very low.

## REFERENCES

Abrahamsson B, Alpsten M, Bake B, et al: Drug absorption from nifedipine hydrophilic matrix extended release (ER) tablet—Comparison with an osmotic pump tablet and effect of food. *J Controlled Release* (Netherlands) 52:301–310, 1998.

Adkin DA, Davis SS, Sparrow RA, et al: Effect of different concentrations of mannitol in solution on small intestinal transit: Implications for drug absorption. *Pharm Res* 12:393–396, 1995.

Actis-Goretta L, Lévèques A, Giuffrida F, et al: Elucidation of (-)-epicatechin metabolites after ingestion of chocolate by healthy humans. *Free Radic Biol Med* 53:787–795, 2013.

Alberts B, Bray D, Lewis J, et al: *Molecular Biology of the Cell*. New York, Garland, 1994.

Anderson KE: Influences of diet and nutrition on clinical pharmacokinetics. *Clin Pharm* 14:325–346, 1988.

Barr WH, Adir J, Garrettson L: Decrease in tetracycline absorption in man by sodium bicarbonate. *Clin Pharmacol Ther* 12:779–784, 1971.

Avdeef A, Bendels S, Di L, et al: PAMPA—critical factors for better predictions of absorption. *J Pharm Sci* 96:2893–2909, 2007.

Barrie S: Heidelberg pH capsule gastric analysis. In Pizzorno JE, Murray MT (eds). *Textbook of Natural Medicine*, 2nd ed. London, Churchill Livingstone, 1999, Chap 16.

Benet LZ, Greither A, Meister W: Gastrointestinal absorption of drugs in patients with cardiac failure. In Benet LZ (ed). *The Effect of Disease States on Drug Pharmacokinetics*. Washington, DC, American Pharmaceutical Association, 1976, Chap 3.

Borin MT, Driver MR, Forbes KK: Effect of timing of food on absorption of cefpodoxime proxetil. *J Clin Pharmacol* 35(5):505–509, 1995.

Brunton L, Chabner B, Knollman B: *Goodman & Gilman's The Pharmacological Basis of Therapeutics*, 12th ed. New York, McGraw-Hill, 2011.

Buch A, Barr WH: Absorption of propranolol in humans following oral, jejuna and ileal administration. *Pharm Res* 15(6):953–957, 1998.

Burks TF, Galligan JJ, Porreca F, Barber WD: Regulation of gastric emptying. *Fed Proc* 44:2897–2901, 1985.

Burton PS, Goodwin JT, Vidimar TJ, Amore BM: Predicting drug absorption: How nature made it a difficult problem. *J Pharmacol Exp Ther* 303(3):889–895, 2002.

Buxton IAO, Benet LZ: Pharmacokinetics: Dynamics of drug absorption, distribution, metabolism, and elimination. In *Goodman & Gilman's Pharmacological Basis of Therapeutics*. New York, McGraw-Hill, 2011, Chap 2.

Crounse RG: Human pharmacology of griseofulvin: The effect of fat intake on gastrointestinal absorption. *J Invest Dermatol* 37:529–533, 1961.

Dale O, Hoffer C, Sheffels P, Kharasch ED: Disposition of nasal, intravenous, and oral methadone in healthy volunteers. *Clin Pharmacol Therapeut* 72:536–545, 2002.

Danielli JF, Davson H: A contribution to the theory of permeability of thin films. *Journal of Cellular and Comparative Physiology* 5(4):495–508, 1935.

Danielli JF, Davson H: *The Permeability of Natural Membranes*. Cambridge, UK, Cambridge University Press, 1952.

Dhawan S, Chopra S, Kapil R, Kapoor D: Novel approaches for oral insulin delivery. *Pharm Tech* 33(7), 2009.

Di Marco MP, Edwards DJ, Irving IW, Murray P, Ducharme WP: The effect of grapefruit juice and Seville orange juice on the pharmacokinetics of dextromethorphan: The role of gut CYP3A and P-glycoprotein. *Life Sci* 71:1149–1160, 2002.

Doherty MM, Charman WN: The mucosa of the small intestine: How clinically relevant as an organ of drug metabolism? *Clin Pharmacokinet* 41(4):235–253, 2002.

Fallingborg J. Intraluminal pH of the human gastrointestinal tract. *Dan Med Bull* 46(3):183-196, 1999.

FDA Guidance for Industry: Food-Effect Bioavailability and Fed Bioequivalence Studies, 2002.

Feldman M, Smith HJ, Simon TR: Gastric emptying of solid radioopaque markers: Studies in healthy and diabetic patients. *Gastroenterology* 87:895–902, 1984.

Fuchs, A., M. Leigh, B. Kloefer and J. B. Dressman (2015). "Advances in the design of fasted state simulating intestinal fluids: FaSSIF-V3." *Eur J Pharm Biopharm* 94: 229-240.

GastroPlus™, Simulations Plus, Inc. (www.simulations-plus.com/Products.aspx?grpID=3&cID=16&pID=11).

Giacomini KM: The International Transporter Consortium Membrane transporters in drug development. *Nat Rev Drug Discov* 9:216–236, 2010.

Harrois A, Baudry N, Huet O, et al: Synergistic deleterious effect of hypoxemia and hypovolemia on microcirculation in intestinal villi. *Crit Care Med* 41(11):e376–384, 2013.

Hebden JM, et al: Stool water content and colonic drug absorption: Contrasting effects of lactulose and codeine. *Pharm Res* 16:1254–1259, 1999.

Hendeles L, Weinberger M, Milavetz G, et al: Food induced dumping from "once-a-day" theophylline product as cause of theophylline toxicity. *Chest* 87:758–785, 1985.

Hoffmeyer S, Burke O, von Richter O: Functional polymorphism of the human multidrug-resistance gene: Multiple sequence variations and correlation of one allele with P-glycoprotein expression and activity in vivo. *Proc Natl Acad Sci U S A* 97(7):3473–3478, 2000.

Ho, M.-C. D., N. Ring, K. Amaral, U. Doshi and A. P. Li (2017). "Human enterocytes as an in vitro model for the evaluation of intestinal drug metabolism: Characterization of drug-metabolizing enzyme activities of cryopreserved human enterocytes from twenty-four donors." *Drug Metab Dispos* 45(6): 686.

Huan SM, Zhang L: Drug Interaction Studies. http://www.fda.gov/downloads/drugs/guidancecomplianceregulatoryinformation/guidances/ucm292362.pdf. Accessed [2/23/2012]

Hunt JN, Knox M: Regulation of gastric emptying. In Code CF (ed). *Handbook of Physiology. Section 6: Alimentary Canal.* Washington, DC, American Physiological Society, 1968, pp 1917–1935.

Jantratid E, Janssen N, Reppas C, Dressman JB: Dissolution media simulating conditions in the proximal human gastrointestinal tract: An update. *Pharmaceut Res* 25(7):1663, 2008.

Jantratid, E., N. Janssen, C. Reppas and J. B. Dressman (2008). "Dissolution Media Simulating Conditions in the Proximal Human Gastrointestinal Tract: An Update." *Pharmaceutical Research* 25(7): 1663.

Johnson MD, Newkirk G, White JR Jr: Clinically significant drug interactions. *Postgrad Med* 105(2):193–195, 200, 205–206 passim, 1999.

Khanna MU, Abraham P: Determinants of acid secretion. *J Assoc Physicians India* 38(Suppl 1):727–730, 1990.

Kirk JK: Significant drug-nutrient interactions. *Am Fam Physician* 51:1175–1182, 1185, 1995.

Kirwan WO, Smith AN: Gastrointestinal transit estimated by an isotope capsule. *Scand J Gastroenterol* 9:763–766, 1974.

Koziolek M, Grimm M, Becker D, et al: Investigation of pH and temperature profiles in the GI tract of fasted human subjects using the Intellicap® system. *J Pharmaceut Sci* 104(9):2855–2863, 2015.

Lennernas H, Ahrenstedt O, Hallgren R, et al: Regional jejunal perfusion, a new in vivo approach to study oral drug absorption in man. *Pharm Res* 9:1243–1251, 1992.

Lennernas H, Falgerholm U, Raab Y, et al: Regional rectal perfusion: New in vivo approach to study rectal drug absorption in man. *Pharm Res* 12:426–432, 1995.

Lennernas H: Human in vivo regional intestinal permeability: Importance for pharmaceutical drug development. *Mol Pharm* 11:12–23, 2014.

Levitt DL, Li R, Demaster EG, Elson M, Furne J, Levitt DG: Use of measurements of ethanol absorption from stomach and intestine to assess human ethanol metabolism. *Am J Physiol Gastrointest Liver Physiol* 273:G951–G957, 1997 (http://ajpgi.physiology.org/cgi/content/full/273/4/G951).

Lipinski CA, Lombardo F, Dominy BW, Feeney PJ: Experimental and computational approaches to estimate solubility and permeability in drug discovery and development settings. *Adv Drug Del Rev* 46(1–3):3–26, 2001.

Lodish HF, Rothman JE: The assembly of cell membranes. *Sci Am* 240:48–63, 1979.

Mathias NR, Hussain MA: Non-invasive systemic drug delivery: Developability considerations for alternate routes of administration. *J Pharm Sci* 9:1–20, 2010.

Mellinger TJ, Bohorfoush JG: Blood levels of dipyridamole (Persantin) in humans. *Arch Int Pharmacodynam Ther* 163:465–480, 1966.

Miller R: Pharmacokinetics and bioavailability of ranitidine in humans. *J Pharm Sci* 73:1376–1379, 1984.

Minami H, McCallum RW: The physiology and pathophysiology of gastric emptying in humans. *Gastroenterology* 86:1592–1610, 1984.

Mizuma, T. (2008). "Assessment of presystemic and systemic intestinal availability of orally administered drugs using in vitro and in vivo data in humans: intestinal sulfation metabolism impacts presystemic availability much more than systemic availability of salbutamol, SULT1A3 substrate." *J Pharm Sci* 97(12): 5471-5476.

Mizuma, T. (2009). "Intestinal glucuronidation metabolism may have a greater impact on oral bioavailability than hepatic glucuronidation metabolism in humans: a study with raloxifene, substrate for UGT1A1, 1A8, 1A9, and 1A10." *Int J Pharm* 378(1-2): 140-141.

Moreno, MP de la Cruz, Oth M, S Deferme F, et al: Characterization of fasted-state human intestinal fluids collected from duodenum and jejunum. *J Pharm Pharmacol* 58(8):1079–1089, 2006.

Mouly S, Paine MF: P-glycoprotein increases from proximal to distal regions of human small intestine. *Pharm Res* 20(10):1595–1599, 2003.

Muller J, Keiser M, Drozdzik M, Oswald S: Expression, regulation and function of intestinal drug transporters: an update. *Biol Chem* 398(2):175–192, 2017.

Nienbert R: Ion pair transport across membranes. *Pharm Res* 6:743–747, 1989.

Oberle RL, Amidon GL: The influence of variable gastric emptying and intestinal transit rates on the plasma level curve of cimetidine: An explanation for the double-peak phenomenon. *J Pharmacokinet Biopharmacol* 15:529–544, 1987.

Ogata H, Aoyagi N, Kaniwa N, et al: Gastric acidity dependent bioavailability of cinnarizine from two commercial capsules in healthy volunteers. *Int J Pharm* 29:113–120, 1986.

Parr AF, Sandefer EP, Wissel P, et al: Evaluation of the feasibility and use of a prototype remote drug delivery capsule (RDDC) for noninvasive regional drug absorption studies in the GI tract of man and beagle dog. *Pharm Res* 16:266–271, 1999.

Pratt P, Taylor P (eds): *Principles of Drug Action: The Basis of Pharmacology*, 3rd ed. New York, Churchill Livingstone, 1990, p 241.

Riley SA, Sutcliffe F, Kim M, et al: Influence of gastrointestinal transit on drug absorption in healthy volunteers. *Br J Clin Pharm* 34:32–39, 1992.

Rubinstein A, Li VHK, Robinson JR: Gastrointestinal–physiological variables affecting performance of oral sustained release dosage forms. In Yacobi A, Halperin-Walega E (eds). *Oral Sustained Release Formulations: Design and Evaluation*. New York, Pergamon, 1988, Chap 6.

Sauna ZE, Smith MM, Muller M, Kerr KM, Ambudkar SV: The mechanism of action of multidrug-resistance-linked P-glycoprotein. *J Bioener Biomembr* 33:481–491, 2001.

Shareef MA, Ahuja A, Ahmad FJ, Raghava S: Colonic drug delivery: An updated review. *AAPS PharmSci* 5:161–186, 2003.

Singer SJ, Nicolson GL: The fluid mosaic model of the structure of cell membranes. *Science* 175:720–731, 1972.

Sournac S, Maublant JC, Aiache JM, et al: Scintigraphic study of the gastrointestinal transit and correlations with the drug absorption kinetics of a sustained release theophylline tablet. Part 1. Administration in fasting state. *J Controll Release* 7:139–146, 1988.

Su KSE, Campanale KM: Nasal drug delivery systems requirements, development and evaluations. In Chien YW (ed). *Transnasal Systemic Medications*. Amsterdam, Elsevier Scientific, 1985, pp 139–159.

Sun H, Pang KS: Permeability, transport, and metabolism of solutes in Caco-2 cell monolayers: A theoretical study. *Drug Metab Disp*, 36(1):102–123, 2007.

Suzuki H, Sugiyama Y: Role of metabolic enzymes and efflux transporters in the absorption of drugs from the small intestine. *Eur J Pharm Sci* 12:3–12, 2000.

Synold TW, Dussault I, Forman BM: The orphan nuclear receptor SXR coordinately regulates drug metabolism and efflux. *Nature Med* 7(5):584–590, 2001.

Szefler SJ: Pharmacokinetics of intranasal corticosteroids. *J Allergy Clin Immunol* 108:S26–S31, 2002.

Takano M, Yumoto R, Murakami T: Expression and function of efflux drug transporters in the intestine. *Pharmacol Therapeut* 109:137–161, 2006.

Thummel K, Wilkinson GR: In vitro and in vivo drug interactions involving human CYP3A. *Annu Rev Pharmacol Toxicol* 38:389–430, 1998.

Tolle-Sander S, Polli JE: Method considerations for Caco-2 permeability assessment in the biopharmaceutics classification system. *Pharmacopoeial Forum* 28:164–172, 2002.

Tsuji A, Tamai I: Carrier-mediated intestinal transport of drugs. *Pharm Res* 13(7):963–977, 1996.

US Food and Drug Administration: *FDA Guidance for Industry: Waiver of In Vivo Bioavailability and Bioequivalence Studies for Immediate-Release Solid Oral Dosage Forms Based on a Biopharmaceutics Classification System*, August 2002.

US Food and Drug Administration: *FDA Guidance for Industry: Food-Effect Bioavailability and Fed Bioequivalence Studies*, December 2002.

von Richter O, Burk O, Fromm MF, Thon KP, Eichelbaum M, Kivisto KT: Cytochrome P450 3A4 and P-glycoprotein expression in human small intestinal enterocytes and hepatocytes: A comparative analysis in paired tissue specimens. *Clin Pharmacol Ther* 75:172–183, 2004.

Welling PG, et al: Bioavailability of erythromycin state: Influence of food and fluid volume. *J Pharm Sci* **67**(6):764–766, June 1978

Wilson TH: *Intestinal Absorption*. Philadelphia, Saunders, 1962.

Yanez, J. A., S. W. Wang, I. W. Knemeyer, M. A. Wirth and K. B. Alton (2011). "Intestinal lymphatic transport for drug delivery." *Adv Drug Deliv Rev* **63**(10-11): 923–942.

Yoshikawa H, Muranishi S, Sugihira N, Seaki H: Mechanism of transfer of bleomycin into lymphatics by bifunctional delivery system via lumen of small intestine. *Chem Pharm Bull* 31:1726–1732, 1983.

Yoshikawa H, Nakao Y, Takada K, et al: Targeted and sustained delivery of aclarubicin to lymphatics by lactic acid oligomer microsphere in rat. *Chem Pharm Bull* 37:802–804, 1989.

## BIBLIOGRAPHY

Berge S, Bighley L, Monkhouse D: Pharmaceutical salts. *J Pharm Sci* 66:1–19, 1977.

Blanchard J: Gastrointestinal absorption, II. Formulation factors affecting bioavailability. *Am J Pharm* 150:132–151, 1978.

Davenport HW: *Physiology of the Digestive Tract*, 5th ed. Chicago, Year Book Medical, 1982.

Evans, D. F., G. Pye, R. Bramley, A. G. Clark, T. J. Dyson and J. D. Hardcastle (1988). "Measurement of gastrointestinal pH profiles in normal ambulant human subjects." *Gut* 29(8): 1035–1041.

Eye IS: A review of the physiology of the gastrointestinal tract in relation to radiation doses from radioactive materials. *Health Phys* 12:131–161, 1966.

Houston JB, Wood SG: Gastrointestinal absorption of drugs and other xenobiotics. In Bridges JW, Chasseaud LF (eds). *Progress in Drug Metabolism*, Vol 4. London, Wiley, 1980, Chap 2.

Leesman GD, Sinko PJ, Amidon GL: Stimulation of oral drug absorption: Gastric emptying and gastrointestinal motility. In Welling PW, Tse FLS (eds). *Pharmacokinetics: Regulatory, Industry, Academic Perspectives*. New York, Marcel Dekker, 1988, Chap 6.

Mackowiak PA: The normal microbial flora. *N Engl J Med* 307:83–93, 1982.

Martonosi AN (ed): *Membranes and Transport*, Vol 1. New York, Plenum, 1982.

McElnay JC: Buccal absorption of drugs. In Swarbick J, Boylan JC (eds). *Encyclopedia of Pharmaceutical Technology*, Vol 2. New York, Marcel Dekker, 1990, pp 189–211.

Palin K: Lipids and oral drug delivery. *Pharm Int* 272–275, November 1985.

Palin K, Whalley D, Wilson C, et al: Determination of gastric-emptying profiles in the rat: Influence of oil structure and volume. *Int J Pharm* 12:315–322, 1982.

Pisal DS, Koslowski MP, Balu-Iyer SV: Delivery of therapeutic proteins. *J Pharm Sci* 99(5):2557–2575, 2010.

Welling PG: Interactions affecting drug absorption. *Clin Pharmacokinet* 9:404–434, 1984.

Welling PG: Dosage route, bioavailability and clinical efficacy. In Welling PW, Tse FLS (eds). *Pharmacokinetics: Regulatory, Industry, Academic Perspectives.* New York, Marcel Dekker, 1988, Chap 3.

Welling PG: Absorption of drugs. In Swarbrick J, Boylan JC (eds). *Encyclopedia of Pharmaceutical Technology.* New York, Marcel Dekker, 2002, pp 8–22.

Welling PG: Drug bioavailability and its clinical significance. In Bridges KW, Chasseaud LF (eds). *Progress in Drug Metabolism,* Vol 4. London, Wiley, 1980, Chap 3.

Wilson TH: *Intestinal Absorption.* Philadelphia, Saunders, 1962.

# 5 Drug Distribution and Protein Binding

Craig K. Svensson

## CHAPTER OBJECTIVES

- Explain the importance of drug distribution in determining drug effect.

- Identify barriers to the distribution of drugs into tissues.

- Describe the dynamic of drug binding to constituents in blood and the impact on drug distribution in the body.

- Provide a concise statement of the free drug hypothesis.

- Describe the effects of membrane transporters on drug distribution into select tissues, such as the brain.

- Differentiate between the various methods to quantify the distribution of drugs in the body.

- Predict the effects of changes in protein binding on drug distribution.

- Describe the factors that alter the protein binding of drugs to albumin and $\alpha_1$-acid glycoprotein.

- Describe the primary methods to determine plasma and serum protein binding of drugs.

- Determine drug binding constants from *in vitro* data.

- Predict the probable clinical impact of protein binding displacement interactions.

## INTRODUCTION

Drugs are rarely administered or applied directly to their site of action. Even topical application commonly targets sites *under* or *within*, rather than *on* the skin. Hence, after a drug passes barriers to gain entry into the body, it must move from the entry site to the anatomical location(s) where the pharmacologic effect will occur. Unlike a guided missile, drug molecules do not home in on their desired site of action (though scientists are working to develop such drug products). Rather, they are subject to dynamic forces within the body similar to those that govern the movement of endogenous substances such as electrolytes and hormones. The extent and speed of this movement through the body—referred to as *distribution*—plays a critical role in drug effect.

Consider the case of anesthetic drugs. Patients receiving such drugs move through two stages prior to entering a level of central nervous system (CNS) depression known as surgical anesthesia (Wilson, 1981). The first stage (known simply as Stage I) produces analgesia. In Stage II, patients exhibit excitement and may vocalize delirium (though they will not remember this since the anesthetic produces amnesia). A patient's respiration, heart rate, and blood pressure increase during this stage. Stage III is the desired state—surgical anesthesia. Obviously, it is best to move through Stage II and into Stage III as rapidly as possible. The speed at which an anesthetic moves from the blood into the brain is the key determinant of the speed of progression through these stages and into surgical anesthesia. Thus, the best anesthetic agents for induction of anesthesia are those which rapidly distribute into the brain.

This example illustrates the importance of understanding drug distribution for the rational use of drugs. This chapter reviews the basic concepts of drug distribution, describes how drug distribution in the body can be measured, and discusses the effects of one of the most important factors influencing drug distribution—protein binding.

## HOW DOES A DRUG INTERACT WITH THE VARIOUS CONSTITUENTS IN BLOOD?

Blood traverses through arteries, capillaries, and veins, delivering oxygen and important nutrients to body tissues and removing cellular waste products. Circulating blood is also the primary delivery system for moving drugs from the site of administration to other parts of the body. But drug in the blood is not like a chemical dissolved in solution. A freshly collected blood sample may appear to the naked eye to be a simple dark red fluid. In fact, as described in Chapter 1, blood is a complex heterogeneous mixture of water, cells, macromolecules, and other constituents. The dynamic movement of drug *within* this complex mixture is the first phase of distribution. What happens to the drug during this phase has a marked influence on the rate and extent of drug distribution into other body tissues.

Approximately 55% of blood volume is comprised of plasma, while the remainder consists of three cell types: red blood cells (RBCs), white blood cells, and platelets (Barrett et al, 2016). Plasma consists of water (91%), proteins (7%), electrolytes,

nutrients, lipids, dissolved gases (eg, $CO_2$), and waste products (eg, urea). RBCs are the largest non-plasma component, making up almost 44% of total blood volume (or >99% of the cellular component). Based on their relative proportions in whole blood, the amount of drug in or bound to white blood cells, platelets, and lipids is quantitatively insignificant and can be ignored unless they are an important site of action for a specific drug (such as agents that alter platelet aggregation). Hence, when considering drug distribution within blood, one need only account for plasma water, plasma proteins, and RBCs. The dynamic movement of drug among these constituents is illustrated in Fig. 5-1.

It is important to recognize that drug molecules are not static in terms of where in the blood they reside. A drug molecule moves from being associated with free water to being bound to a plasma protein such as albumin or $\alpha_1$-acid glycoprotein. This binding is usually reversible, and drug molecules move back and forth between being bound and free (or unbound). If a small molecule (defined as <900 daltons) possesses the appropriate physicochemical characteristics, it may also cross the membrane of RBC. This is also a reversible process. Some drugs bind extensively within or on the surface of RBC.

Drug concentration can be measured in all three types of fluid that can be fractionated after the collection of a blood sample (whole blood, plasma, or serum). Serum differs from plasma in that it is

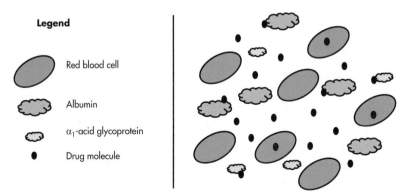

**Legend**

Red blood cell

Albumin

$\alpha_1$-acid glycoprotein

Drug molecule

FIGURE 5-1 • Movement of drug within blood. This diagram illustrates that drug in the blood is distributed among those drug molecules found freely in plasma water, those bound to plasma proteins (primarily albumin and/or $\alpha_1$-acid glycoprotein) and those moving into red blood cells. In the diagram, drug molecules overlapping with proteins represent drug bound to protein, while those within the sphere of a red blood cell represent drug that is either bound to the surface of the cell or has diffused into the cell.

devoid of clotting factors. If blood is collected in a tube without an anticoagulant, coagulation begins almost immediately upon removal of the blood from a vein. Sometimes silica particles or thrombin are contained in the tubes for clinical specimens to speed clotting after sample collection. Centrifugation of the sample will yield an upper layer of serum, while the lower layer contains cells and clotting factors. In contrast, blood collected into a tube with anticoagulant and separated with centrifugation yields an upper layer of plasma. Numerous specimen tubes are available containing different anticoagulants. These include EDTA (usually marked by a purple stopper on the tube), sodium citrate (light blue), lithium/sodium heparin (green), or sodium fluoride (grey or black). The anticoagulant used (and therefore tube choice) depends on what type of analytical tests will be performed on the sample. Regardless, the anticoagulated blood can be mixed and sampled to measure whole blood or centrifuged to provide plasma. Importantly, the drug concentration may not be the same in these three samples, and therefore the pharmacokinetics determined from these measurements may differ. When drug is extensively bound to RBC, measurement of drug in whole blood may be preferred.

When drug first enters the blood, it will be in the unbound state. Eventually, and usually quite rapidly, an equilibrium will be achieved between the various blood compartments. This dynamic equilibrium of drug in blood can be described as a simple mass balance relationship

$$D_{RBC} \leftrightarrow D_{up} \leftrightarrow D_b \qquad (5.1)$$

where $D_{RBC}$ is the amount of drug in or bound to RBC, $D_{up}$ is the amount of drug unbound in plasma water, and $D_b$ is the amount of drug bound to plasma protein. Note that only free drug moves into red blood cells. Thus, the total amount of drug in blood ($D_T$) is given as

$$D_T = D_{RBC} + D_{up} + D_b \qquad (5.2)$$

This dynamic relationship can also be expressed in terms of concentration

$$C_{RBC} \leftrightarrow C_{up} \leftrightarrow C_b \qquad (5.3)$$

where $C_{RBC}$ is the drug concentration in RBC, $C_{up}$ is the concentration of unbound drug in plasma water, and $C_b$ is the concentration of drug bound to plasma protein. If the amount of plasma protein decreases due to disease, less drug will be bound to plasma protein and the equilibrium will be shifted to the left of Equation 5.3.

## HOW DOES DRUG MOVE FROM BLOOD INTO TISSUES?

While drug moves around the body *within* the blood, the process of leaving circulating blood and entering tissues is critical for drug action. As capillary membranes usually only allow the passage of small molecules, drug bound to plasma proteins or within RBCs remains within the blood compartment and is inaccessible to the site of action. In addition, drug within tissue may bind to non-specific sites (ie, sites in the tissue that do not stimulate the pharmacologic effect). The overall equilibrium of drug in the body is illustrated in Fig. 5-2.

The processes by which drugs transverse capillary membranes into the tissue include passive diffusion and hydrostatic pressure. Passive diffusion is the main process by which most drugs cross cell membranes. *Passive diffusion* is the process by which drug molecules move from an area of high concentration to an area of low concentration. Passive diffusion is described by *Fick's law of diffusion*:

$$\text{Rate of drug diffusion } \frac{dQ}{dt} = \frac{-DKA(C_p - C_t)}{h} \qquad (5.4)$$

where $C_p - C_t$ is the difference between the drug concentration in the plasma ($C_p$) and in the tissue ($C_t$); $A$ is the surface area of the membrane; $h$ is the thickness of the membrane; $K$ is the lipid–water partition coefficient; and $D$ is the diffusion constant. The negative sign denotes net transfer of drug from inside the capillary lumen into the tissue and extracellular spaces. Diffusion is spontaneous and temperature dependent. Diffusion is distinguished from blood flow–initiated mixing, which involves hydrostatic pressure.

*Hydrostatic pressure* represents the pressure gradient between the arterial end of the capillaries

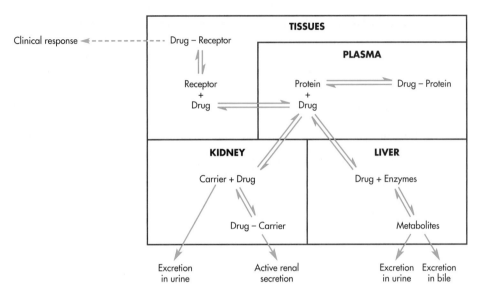

**FIGURE 5-2 •** Equilibrium of drug in the body. Unbound drug is in equilibrium between the plasma and tissues, including the site of action. Free (unbound) drug penetrates cell membranes, distributing into various tissues, including those involved in elimination of the drug (such as the kidney and liver). If a drug is displaced from plasma protein it can be more readily eliminated and also access the site of action to interact with drug receptors.

entering the tissue and the venous capillaries leaving the tissue. Hydrostatic pressure is responsible for penetration of water-soluble drugs into spaces between endothelial cells and possibly into lymph. In the kidneys, high arterial pressure creates a filtration pressure that allows small drug molecules to be filtered in the glomerulus of the renal nephron.

The fraction of drug bound to a specific receptor is usually very small compared to the amount that is free or bound to nonspecific sites in tissue. Hence, receptor binding has a negligible impact on the overall pharmacokinetics of a drug. An exception to this general rule is target-mediated drug disposition. This is an unusual phenomenon in which drug binds with very high affinity to its target site such that this binding influences the pharmacokinetic characteristics of the molecule in the body. This is most commonly seen after low doses of monoclonal antibodies.

Importantly, at distribution equilibrium, the concentration of unbound drug in tissue will be the same as that seen in blood. However, extensive binding of drug to nonspecific sites in tissue may result in a total tissue concentration (bound + unbound) much greater than the total concentration in blood. In this situation, most of the dose of a drug in the body will be in the tissues once equilibrium has been achieved. In contrast, for a drug with extensive plasma protein binding and negligible tissue binding, most of the dose will be in the blood. Similarly, a compound with a high molecular weight or high polarity that is unable to cross cell membranes may only reside in the blood.

This dynamic movement of drug between bound and unbound state underscores the importance of factors that alter binding to plasma proteins or tissue sites. Consider a drug (Drug 1) which does not enter red blood cells and is 99% bound to albumin. In this scenario, only 1% of drug is unbound in blood and therefore readily available for crossing capillary membranes and distributing into tissues. If a second drug is added (Drug 2) that displaces Drug 1 from albumin such that only 95% of Drug 1 remains bound, the fraction of unbound drug has increased 5-fold (to 5%). This enables significantly more drug to leave the blood compartment and enter tissues.

It is important to note that an increasing portion of therapeutic agents on the market are large molecules, such as monoclonal antibodies. These protein therapeutics are too large to cross the RBC membrane. In addition, they do not usually associate with plasma proteins. Thus, they exist solely in the unbound state in blood. Exceptions to this would be monoclonal antibodies with target antigens in the bloodstream (eg, rituximab in leukemia or lymphoma).

The dynamic illustrated in Fig. 5-2 provides the foundation for a fundamental principle in pharmacology—the *free drug hypothesis*. This hypothesis posits that only free drug exhibits pharmacologic activity. Hence, when considering the pharmacokinetics of a drug, the important component to measure/determine is the free drug concentration. There are numerous lines of experimental evidence supporting the free drug hypothesis.

Figure 5-3 provides an example of a common experiment supporting the free drug hypothesis. This study evaluated the ability of the antiviral drug ritonavir to inhibit the activity of human immunodeficiency virus (HIV) in cells in the presence or absence of human serum (which would contain serum proteins like albumin). These data show that higher concentrations of total drug are needed to achieve the same level of inhibition in the presence of human serum compared to the concentration needed in the absence of serum. This indicates that the presence of serum proteins to which ritonavir binds reduces its ability to inhibit the virus. Studies *in vivo* have also supported the principle that it is the free drug concentration that is able to access sites of action. Hence, measurements of total drug concentration in the presence of drug interactions, for example, can mislead investigators as to the clinical significance of changes in drug concentrations. Drug interactions resulting in changes in total drug concentration but no change in the free concentration do not result in changes in drug effect and therefore do not necessitate a change in drug dosing.

Though free drug concentration measurement is most relevant, its use in clinical settings is limited due to the increased cost and technical demands compared to measurement of total drug. Since the latter is most commonly measured, it is important to recognize those situations in which total drug concentration measurements may be misleading due to expected, but unmeasured, changes in unbound drug concentration.

## WHAT DETERMINES THE RATE AND EXTENT OF DRUG DISTRIBUTION INTO VARIOUS TISSUES?

Protein binding is not the only factor influencing the ability of drugs to cross biological membranes and enter tissues. As discussed in Chapter 4, there are numerous processes by which drugs cross membranes—including passive diffusion, facilitated diffusion, and membrane transporters. Thus, molecular size and shape, charge, and lipophilicity are each important in determining the rate and extent of distribution into and out of tissues. Some drugs are substrates for efflux transporters and are efficiently removed so that the drug never achieves a significant concentration in the tissue. For example, a number of drugs are efficiently removed from the brain by p-glycoprotein (p-gp) and are therefore not effective agents to treat diseases of the brain.

While Fig. 5-2 portrays the blood and tissue compartments as static for simplicity, a more realistic picture accounts for the constant perfusion of blood into and out of any given tissue (see Fig. 5-4).

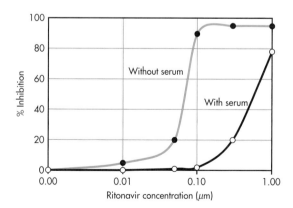

**FIGURE 5-3** • Effect of human serum on the inhibition of human immunodeficiency virus (HIV) replication by ritonavir. Adding human serum, which contains proteins, causes a shift to the right in the concentration-response curve for ritonavir. This is consistent with the principle that only free drug is able to exert a pharmacologic effect.

KY is a 24-year-old pregnant woman who presents with a hot and painful left calf. Diagnostic studies reveal she has a deep vein thrombosis. This places her at risk for developing a life-threatening pulmonary embolus. Thus, it is decided that anticoagulant therapy should be initiated immediately. There are two relatively inexpensive options for treatment: warfarin or low molecular weight heparin (LMWH). Warfarin is a small molecule given orally that readily crosses the placental barrier and its use has been associated with birth defects. In contrast, LMWH is a highly polar compound requiring subcutaneous injections, but does not readily cross the placenta and has not been associated with fetal abnormalities. Though oral therapy is generally preferred over parenteral administration, in this case, LMWH would be a better choice to reduce the risk to the developing child. This case illustrates how a knowledge of the physicochemical determinants of drug distribution can be used in evaluating therapeutic options.

When the unbound drug concentration in blood perfusing a tissue is high, the concentration gradient between blood and tissue results in a net movement of drug into the tissue. As drug is eliminated and the concentration in the circulating blood declines, the concentration gradient drives net movement of drug from tissue into blood. This dynamic equilibrium means that drug will not perpetually remain in tissue after administration—except in the unusual case of irreversible binding of drug to tissue proteins. The movement of monoclonal antibodies and other macromolecules out of blood and into tissues is largely driven by pressure gradients and not the concentration gradient (ie, by convection and not by diffusion).

Blood flow–facilitated drug distribution is rapid and efficient, but requires pressure. As blood pressure gradually decreases when arteries branch into the small arterioles, the speed of flow slows and diffusion into the interstitial space becomes diffusion or concentration driven and facilitated by the large surface area of the capillary network. The average

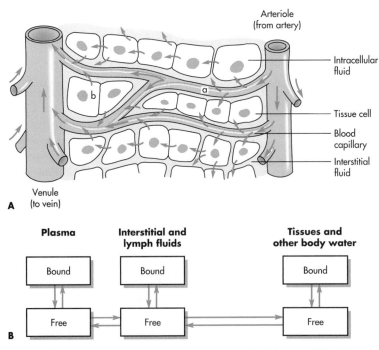

**FIGURE 5-4** • Diffusion of drug into and out of perfused tissues. **A.** Tissue is perfused by arterial blood containing drug. Unbound drug can diffuse into interstitial space and into tissues. Drug can also move out of tissues and be removed via the venous return. **B.** Model of drug equilibrium in plasma, interstitial fluids, and tissue.

pressure of the blood capillary is higher (+18 mm Hg) than the mean tissue pressure (−6 mm Hg), resulting in a net total pressure of 24 mm Hg higher in the capillary over the tissue. This pressure difference is offset by an average osmotic pressure in the blood of 24 mm Hg, pulling the plasma fluid back into the capillary. Thus, on average, the pressures in the tissue and most parts of the capillary are equal, with no net flow of water.

At the arterial end, as the blood newly enters the capillary (Fig. 5-4A), the pressure of the capillary blood is slightly higher (about 8 mm Hg) than that of the tissue, causing fluid to leave the capillary and enter the tissues. This pressure is called *hydrostatic* or *filtration pressure*. This filtered fluid (filtrate) is later returned to the venous capillary (Fig. 5-4B) due to a lower venous pressure of about the same magnitude. The lower pressure of the venous blood compared with the tissue fluid is termed as *absorptive pressure*. A small amount of fluid returns to the circulation through the lymphatic system.

The perfusion of tissues/organs in the body varies (Table 5-1). Some tissues (eg, brain and heart) are highly perfused, while others are more poorly perfused (eg, bone and fat). For example, as noted in Table 5-1 (last column), the average blood flow to the brain is 55 mL/100 g tissue/min. Muscle has a perfusion rate less than 10% of this value (3 mL/100 g tissue/min). This can have a dramatic influence on the time course of drug in various tissues after administration.

Figure 5-5 illustrates the concept with the varied time course of thiopental in key tissue groups in the body.

Thiopental is highly lipophilic and rapidly crosses biological membranes. Consequently, the rate-limiting step for its entry into any specific tissue is the perfusion rate of the tissue. In addition, the perfusion rate will determine how rapidly thiopental is removed from a tissue. The initial rapid decline of drug in blood after administration (occurring in seconds) shown in Fig. 5-5 is the result of distribution of thiopental into the brain and other highly perfused visceral tissues, reaching peak amounts within 1 minute following an intravenous bolus injection. Thiopental concentration in the brain then rapidly declines as the amount of drug in lean tissues (eg, muscle) increases—reaching peak

## TABLE 5-1 • Blood flow to various tissues in the body.

| Tissue | Percent Body Weight | Percent Cardiac Output | Blood Flow (mL/100 g tissue/min) |
|---|---|---|---|
| Adrenals | 0.02 | 1 | 550 |
| Kidneys | 0.4 | 24 | 450 |
| Thyroid | 0.04 | 2 | 400 |
| Liver | | | |
| Hepatic | 2.0 | 5 | 20 |
| Portal | | 20 | 75 |
| Portal-drained viscera | 2.0 | 20 | 75 |
| Heart (basal) | 0.4 | 4 | 70 |
| Brain | 2.0 | 15 | 55 |
| Skin | 7.0 | 5 | 5 |
| Muscle (basal) | 40.0 | 15 | 3 |
| Connective tissue | 7.0 | 1 | 1 |
| Fat | 15.0 | 2 | 1 |

Data from Spector WS: Handbook of Biological Data. *Philadelphia, PA: Saunders; 1956; Glaser O: Medical Physics, Vol 11. Chicago, IL: Year Book Publishers; 1950; Butler TC: Proc First International Pharmacological Meeting, Vol 6. Philadelphia, PA: Pergamon Press; 1962.*

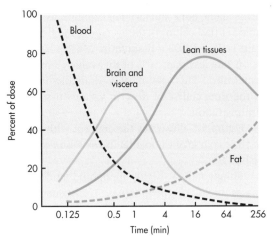

FIGURE 5-5 • Distribution of thiopental into tissues. Thiopental enters highly perfused tissues rapidly, with movement into poorly perfused tissue more slowly. Note that time axis is on a log scale and not linear.

amount in these tissues within 30 minutes of intravenous administration. Thiopental distributes considerably more slowly to poorly perfused tissue such as fat. Importantly, the initial reduction in blood concentration after administration is not due to elimination of the drug from the body, rather it is caused by movement of drug from blood into the highly perfused tissues. In addition, the short duration of action of thiopental as a CNS depressant is not a result of rapid metabolism. Rather, it is caused by redistribution of the drug from the brain and other highly perfused tissues into more poorly perfused tissues (Price, 1960). Thus, variance in the rate of tissue perfusion is the primary reason for the difference in timing of peak drug concentration in various tissues and the offset of pharmacologic effect. This example also illustrates why the time of peak drug concentration of a drug in circulating blood may occur sooner than the peak pharmacologic effect.

When there are significant differences in the rate of distribution into various tissues for a drug, complex pharmacokinetic models are often needed to describe the time course of drug in the body. If distribution occurs rapidly to all tissues to which a drug will distribute, the one-compartment open model shown in Fig. 1-6 of Chapter 1 often suffices to characterize the pharmacokinetics. In contrast, when drug distributes more slowly into one or more tissues (as is the case with thiopental), a more complex model (eg, the two-compartment open model shown in Fig. 1-6) may be necessary to accurately characterize the disposition of a drug. Figure 5-5 also illustrates the fact that the ability to detect and characterize this complex distribution is dependent on how quickly and frequently blood samples are taken. In the absence of early blood samples, the initial distribution phase would go undetected.

## HOW DO MEMBRANE TRANSPORTERS INFLUENCE DRUG DISTRIBUTION?

As discussed in Chapter 4, many membranes express transporters that are able to move drug molecules across membranes at a rate and to an extent far exceeding passive diffusion. These transporters can be key in determining how much drug distributes into specific tissues. There are two tissue barriers where this is especially important: the blood–brain barrier and the placenta. By their composition, both tissues normally impede the diffusion of many substances into the respective regions they protect. These regions are sometimes referred to as *privileged* sites of distribution—regions in the body where the penetration of drugs is substantially limited.

There are four distinct barriers regulating the entry of substances into various regions of the brain: the cerebral vasculature (blood–brain barrier), the choroid plexus (blood–cerebrospinal fluid barrier), the pia arachnoid (brain–cerebrospinal fluid barrier), and the neuroepedyma (cerebrospinal fluid–brain barrier) (Stolp et al, 2013). The gaps between cells in the first three of these barriers are miniscule and are referred to as tight junctions—meaning the movement of drug between these cells is essentially nonexistent. During development, the junctions in the neuroepedyma are also tight, though significant gaps in neuroepedymal junctions in adulthood exist that allow easier diffusion of substances from cerebral spinal fluid to brain.

A consequence of these tight junctions is that only lipophilic compounds can penetrate these barriers via diffusion. However, there are numerous molecules that are essential for brain cell survival that lack the lipophilicity needed to cross these membranes, including amino acids and glucose. Such molecules cross these barriers through membrane transporters. The diversity of transporters moving solutes from blood into cerebral endothelial cells is illustrated in Fig. 5-6. Drug molecules with similar structures can also move across the membranes by these transporters.

A knowledge of these transporters is essential for developing drugs that will distribute into the brain. For example, one approach to treating patients with Parkinson disease is to increase the amount of dopamine in the substantia nigra region of the brain, but dopamine does not cross the blood–brain barrier. In contrast, levodopa is transported across the blood–brain barrier via the amino acid membrane transporter. Once it distributes into the CNS, levodopa undergoes metabolic conversion to dopamine via a decarboxylase in the brain. Through this means, an effective treatment for Parkinson disease was developed, and levodopa is widely used to manage this degenerative neurological disease.

In addition to influx transporters, there are also efflux transporters on the cell surface of these CNS barriers. Efflux transporters have the ability to efficiently remove compounds that have entered into the cell (either through diffusion or an influx transporter). The efficiency of this efflux may be so high that therapeutic concentrations of the drug in the CNS cannot be achieved. Figure 5-7 illustrates the profound effect of two efflux transporters, P-gp and breast cancer resistance protein, on an experimental compound (Fig. 5-7, left). In animals with these two efflux transporters, essentially no compound is detected in the brain. Animals lacking these two transporters (through a process by which the genes for these transporters are knocked out) show extensive accumulation of the drug in the brain (Fig. 5-7, right). This experiment demonstrates that the experimental compound penetrates the brain well, but that its removal by efflux transporters is so efficient that measurable concentrations of the drug are not achieved in brain.

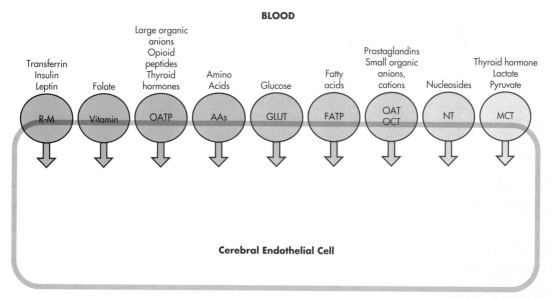

FIGURE 5-6 • Diversity of influx membrane transporters in cerebral endothelial cells. Many different transporters on the surface of endothelial cells transport various solutes across the membrane that otherwise would be unable to enter brain tissue. Most of the transporters illustrated represent families of transporters, not a single protein, with up to six different transporters in the family being expressed on the cell surface. The cerebral endothelial cell is highly populated with membrane transporters. Abbreviations: R-M = receptor-mediated transport; OATP = organic anion transporting polypeptides; AAs = amino acid transporters; GLUT = glucose transporters; FATP = fatty acid transport protein; OAT = organic anion transporters; OCT = organic cation transporters; NT = nucleoside transporters; MCT = monocarboxylate transporters.

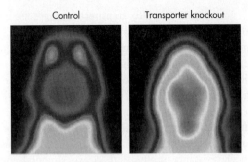

Control          Transporter knockout

FIGURE 5-7 • Effect of efflux membrane transporters on CNS penetration of drug in mice. Control mice were administered an experimental compound and the distribution into tissue monitored by positron emission tomography. The distribution of the experimental compound is shown in light shaded grey at the lower portion of the figure on the left. Note the lack of entry into the upper portion of the image, which represents the brain. In contrast, drug is highly concentrated in brain (light grey and darker central portion of the figure on the right) in animals lacking p-glycoprotein and breast cancer resistance protein (transporter knockout). Modified with permission from Kawamura K, Yamasaki T, Konno F, et al: Evaluation of limiting brain penetration related to P-glycoprotein and breast cancer resistance protein using [(11)C]GF120918 by PET in mice, Mol Imaging Biol. 2011 Feb;13(1):152-160.

This has important implications for drug design. If an experimental molecule does not penetrate the brain, analogs can be developed with the physicochemical characteristics necessary to enter the brain. In contrast, if low brain concentrations are due to efflux of the drug, it must either be administered in combination with a drug to inhibit these efflux transporters or analogs developed that are not substrates for these transporters.

Similar to the blood–brain barrier, membrane transporters in the placenta regulate the movement of many solutes from maternal blood to fetal blood. It is generally best to limit the entry of drugs into the circulation of the developing child. For this reason, there is concern about administering agents that inhibit efflux transporters (eg, p-gp) to pregnant women, as this may increase fetal exposure to some drugs and environmental chemicals.

## DO DRUGS DISTRIBUTE INTO BREAST MILK?

Another special area of concern regarding the distribution of drugs is their entry into breast milk. Lactating women who require drug therapy understandably express concern about whether the drug they are taking will reach their nursing child. Studies have found that most women consume one or more medications during the first week after childbirth, so this is an obvious issue for women who are also breast feeding. A simple rule of thumb is that any drug capable of entering the CNS is also capable of entering breast milk. For most drugs, the amount that will be ingested by the nursing child through this route is clinically insignificant. There are, however, notable exceptions. Importantly, the risk to the neonate is not simply a function of the dose they receive through milk ingestion, but also depends on their ability to eliminate the drug, thereby preventing accumulation to toxic concentrations (Ito, 2018).

The distribution of drug from blood into breast milk is governed by the same variables influencing entry into other tissues (lipophilicity, charge, substrate for membrane transporters, etc). A complicating factor is that breast milk changes in composition over time. Early in lactation, the fat and protein content of breast milk are similar. Over the first week, the fat content will nearly double, while the protein content decreases by 50% or more (Ballard and Morrow, 2013). This means that protein binding in breast milk will be expected to change over time, which will change the fraction of drug in the unbound state. In addition, the initial pH of breast milk is equivalent to that of plasma, but rapidly becomes more acidic over the first few days of lactation (Morriss et al, 1986). After 3 months, breast milk slowly returns to a pH equivalent to plasma pH. This may change the ionization of drug within breast milk over time. The dynamic composition of breast milk means that the partitioning of drugs from blood to breast milk may also change over time.

One way to quantify the distribution of drugs into breast milk is to calculate the milk to plasma ratio (M/P). While the M/P is often used to estimate drug exposure through breast milk, it is important to recognize that this ratio is time dependent. The peak concentration of drug in breast milk usually occurs later than the peak concentration in blood, simply due to the time required for distribution into milk to occur. Therefore, the timing of simultaneous collection of blood and milk is critical in using this parameter to estimate infant drug exposure. In addition, as noted previously, the changes in breast milk composition over time mean the M/P may change over the months of lactation.

## PRACTICE PROBLEM

Measuring the M/P for a specific drug enables the expected amount of drug a nursing child will ingest to be estimated. Assume a drug for which the M/P is 5 and the average maternal plasma concentration is 0.1 mg/L. Assuming the child averages 750 mL of breast milk per day, what is the approximate daily dose of the drug received by the nursing infant?

### Solution

Knowing the M/P and plasma concentration, you can calculate the average concentration of drug in breast milk ($C_M$) as

$$C_M = C_p \cdot \text{M/P} = 0.1 \text{ mg/L} \cdot 5 = 0.5 \text{ mg/L}$$

The daily dose of drug to which the infant is exposed is given as

$$\text{Dose} = C_M \cdot \text{Volume of milk consumed} = 0.5 \text{ mg/L}$$
$$\cdot 0.75 \text{ L} = 0.375 \text{ mg}$$

## HOW IS THE EXTENT OF DRUG DISTRIBUTION IN THE BODY MEASURED?

As discussed in preceding sections, the extent of distribution of drug in the body has important clinical implications. The extent of distribution has a major effect on the concentration of drug that is measured in blood (or other vascular fluids, such as plasma). For these reasons, methods to quantify the extent of distribution have practical use.

Consider the simple case of a beaker into which an unknown amount of water is added. Assume 10 mg of a drug is added to this water. After mixing to create a homogenous solution, a sample is taken and the concentration of drug measured to be 10 mg/L. The volume of liquid in the beaker can be determined using the relationship:

$$\text{Volume} = \text{amount/concentration} \qquad (5.5)$$

$$\text{Volume} = (10 \text{ mg})/(10 \text{ mg/L}) = 1 \text{ L}$$

| Extracellular | | Intracellular |
|---|---|---|
| Vascular | Extravascular | |
| **3 L** **4% BW** | **9 L** **13% BW** | **28 L** **41% BW** |

FIGURE 5-8 • Components of total body water. Values shown represent averages for 70-kg male. Abbreviations: L = liters; BW = body weight.

Similarly, we could theoretically determine the volume of body fluid into which a drug is distributed if we knew the amount of drug in the body and measured its concentration. For example, Fig. 5-8 illustrates the various components of total body water. If a drug distributed solely in vascular water, the volume that the drug would appear to be distributed into, termed the *apparent volume of distribution* ($V_D$), would be 3 L. In this case, a 100-mg dose of a drug would yield an initial concentration of 33.3 mg/L. In contrast, a drug distributing throughout extracellular

### CASE STUDY

TJ is a 55-year-old 70 kg male presenting to the emergency department (ED) in acute ventricular tachycardia. The attending physician elects to initiate therapy with lidocaine to treat this acute arrhythmia. Lidocaine is to be administered as an intravenous bolus with the goal of achieving an initial concentration of 2.0 mg/L. The ED pharmacist consults reference material that indicates the average $V_D$ for lidocaine is 1.0 L/kg. Based on this information, she is able to calculate the initial dose (called the loading dose) needed to achieve the target concentration. Specifically, the estimated $V_D$ for this patient can be calculated as 70 kg × 1.0 L/kg = 70 L. Since

$$\text{Volume} = \text{amount/concentration} \qquad (5.5)$$
$$V_D = \text{Dose}/C^0$$

where $C^0$ is the initial concentration immediately after the dose. Rearranging to solve for dose

$$\text{Dose} = C^0 \cdot V_D = 2 \text{ mg/L} \cdot 70 \text{ L} = 140 \text{ mg}$$

Thus, an initial dose of 140 mg would be administered, followed by a constant intravenous infusion to maintain arrhythmia suppression.

water would have a $V_D$ of 12 L, yielding an initial concentration of 8.3 mg/L, while a drug distributing throughout total body water would have a $V_D$ of 40 L and yield an initial concentration of 2.5 mg/L. It is apparent that the more extensively a drug distributes throughout the body, the lower the initial concentration after a given dose.

Many drugs bind to various tissues and the distribution of the drug is not limited to body water. The effects of this binding can be seen in the illustration of Fig. 5-9. Extensive tissue binding results in a calculated $V_D$ much larger than the true volume in which the drug is distributed. Hence, if we calculate $V_D$ by the dose and concentration after drug has distributed into all tissues into which it will distribute, many drugs have a calculated $V_D$ much larger than total body water. This is the reason the term is referred to as the *apparent volume of distribution*. $V_D$ does not represent a true volume of physiologic fluid. It represents the volume of fluid that would be necessary to achieve the concentration following a given dose of drug. Figure 5-10 shows the volume of distribution for a number of drugs. Note that all of the drugs have a $V_D$ greater than the volume of plasma—which means

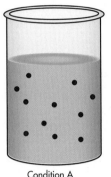
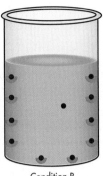

Condition A                    Condition B

**FIGURE 5-9** • Effect of tissue binding on the calculated volume of distribution for a drug. Condition A: 10 mg of drug is added to a beaker containing an unknown amount of fluid. The measured concentration from a sample of the fluid is 10 mg/L, yielding a $V_D$ of 1 L. Condition B: The same volume of fluid is added to a beaker coated with antibody to the drug, with the antibody irreversibly immobilized onto the sides of the beaker. When 10 mg of drug is added, most of the drug is bound to the antibody. Sampling the fluid only detects unbound drug and yields a concentration of 1 mg/L. In this case, the apparent $V_D$ is 10 L. The actual amount of fluid is the same as condition A (1 L), but the binding of drug to an inaccessible component (antibody bound to the sides of the beaker) makes it appear that the drug is dissolved in a much larger volume.

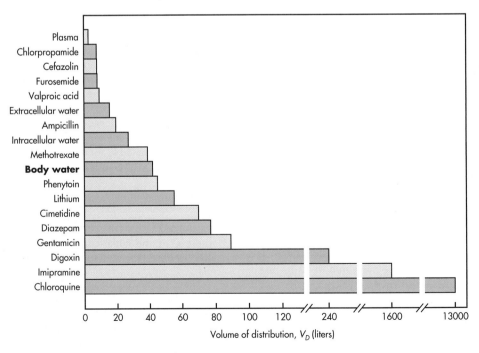

**FIGURE 5-10** • Volume of distribution of common drugs.

that a portion of the drug distributes into tissues. Some drugs, such as digoxin and chloroquine, have a $V_D$ several times the volume of total body water. This indicates these compounds are extensively bound in tissue and, at any given time after a dose, most of the drug is located in the tissues not in the circulation.

There are significant clinical implications when a drug has a high degree of tissue binding yielding a very large $V_D$. For example, when a patient overdoses on a drug, there are interventions (such as hemodialysis and hemoperfusion) that may reduce the amount of drug in the body more quickly than the body can eliminate the drug. However, since these interventions only remove drug from blood, they are of little clinical value for a drug for which most of the dose is in the tissue and $V_D$ is many times larger than total body water.

## WHAT IS THE EFFECT OF PLASMA PROTEIN BINDING AND TISSUE BINDING ON DRUG DISTRIBUTION?

The effects of both plasma protein binding and tissue binding on drug distribution can be better appreciated through a more quantitative characterization of the $V_D$. The total drug in the body ($D_T$) can be determined at any time as

$$D_T = V_p C_p + V_t C_t \qquad (5.6)$$

where $V_p$ and $V_t$ are the volumes of plasma and tissue, respectively, while $C_p$ and $C_t$ are the concentration of drug in plasma and tissue, respectively. At equilibrium, the unbound concentrations of drug in plasma ($C_{up}$) and tissue ($C_{ut}$) are equal and:

$$C_p f_u = C_t f_{ut} \qquad (5.7)$$

where $f_u$ and $f_{ut}$ are the unbound fraction of drug in plasma and tissue, respectively. Solving Equation 5.7 to solve for $C_t$ yields

$$C_t = C_p (f_u / f_{ut}) \qquad (5.8)$$

Substituting Equation 5.8 for $C_t$ in Equation 5.6:

$$D_T = V_p C_p + V_t [C_p (f_u / f_{ut})] \qquad (5.9)$$

Multiplying both sides of Equation 5.9 by $1/C_p$ yields

$$D_T / C_p = V_p + V_t (f_u / f_{ut}) \qquad (5.10)$$

Since $D_T / C_p = V_D$,

$$V_D = V_p + V_t (f_u / f_{ut}) \qquad (5.11)$$

Equation 5.11 defines the relationship between plasma volume, tissue volume, the unbound fraction in plasma, and the unbound fraction in tissue. For example, if the fraction unbound in plasma ($f_u$) increases (ie, a decrease in plasma protein binding occurs), while tissue binding ($f_{ut}$) does not change, the $V_D$ will increase. The relationship between protein binding and apparent volume of distribution is illustrated in Fig. 5.11. Similarly, if tissue binding increases (ie, $f_{ut}$ decreases), $V_D$ will also increase. In both situations, a larger fraction of drug will exist in the tissue at equilibrium.

Equation 5.11 is a simplistic and easy to understand view of the relationship between plasma

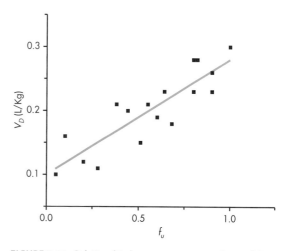

FIGURE 5-11 • Relationship between apparent volume of distribution and fraction of drug unbound in plasma. The graph shown is based on data from a series of antimicrobial agents, with each data point representing a different agent. The line drawn is the simple regression line of the data. Data from Calop J: *Pharmacie Clinique et Thérapeutique*. Paris: Editions Masson; 2008.

protein binding, plasma volume, tissue binding, tissue volume, and apparent volume of distribution. In reality, tissues have different affinities for drugs, and therefore different $f_{ut}$ values. A more comprehensive equation describing $V_D$ would be

$$V_D = V_p + \Sigma V_{ti}(f_u/f_{uti}) \qquad (5.12)$$

where $V_{ti}$ = tissue volume of the $i^{th}$ organ or tissue and $f_{uti}$ = unbound fraction of drug in the $i^{th}$ organ or tissue. Hence, while Equation 5.11 and Fig. 5-11 provide helpful conceptual insight, it is important to recognize that the relationship between $V_D$ and tissue binding can be quite complex and nonlinear.

## PRACTICE PROBLEM

Drug A and drug B have $V_D$ values of 20 and 100 L, respectively. Both drugs have a $V_p$ of 4 L and a $V_t$ of 10 L, and they are 60% bound to plasma protein. What is the fraction of tissue binding of the two drugs?

### Solution

**Drug A**
Applying Equation 5.11,

$$V_D = V_p + V_t(f_u/f_{ut}) \qquad (5.11)$$

Because drug A is 60% bound, the drug is 40% free, or $f_u = 0.4$.

$$20 = 4 + 10\left(\frac{0.4}{f_{ut}}\right)$$

$$f_{ut} = \frac{4}{16} = 0.25$$

The fraction of drug bound to tissues is $1 - 0.25 = 0.75$ or 75%.

**Drug B**

$$100 = 4 + 10\left(\frac{0.4}{f_{ut}}\right)$$

$$f_{ut} = 0.042$$

The fraction of drug bound to tissues is $1 - 0.042 = 0.958$ or 95.8%.

In this problem, the percent free (unbound) drug for drug A in tissue is 25% and the percent free drug for drug B is 4.2% in plasma fluid. Drug B is more highly bound to tissue, which results in a larger apparent volume of distribution. This approach assumes a pooled tissue group because it is not possible from the data given to identify the specific tissue or group of tissues to which the drug is bound.

## HOW IS THE EXTENT OF DRUG–PROTEIN BINDING MEASURED?

The preceding discussion points to the importance of methods to determine drug–protein binding in both research and clinical settings. While many methods are available to directly measure free drug concentration or to separate free and bound drug, the two most commonly used techniques are equilibrium dialysis and ultrafiltration. Equilibrium dialysis is illustrated in Fig. 5-12. With this method, free drug equilibrates across a semipermeable membrane, allowing measurement of both free and total drug concentration in the two compartments. While highly accurate, this approach

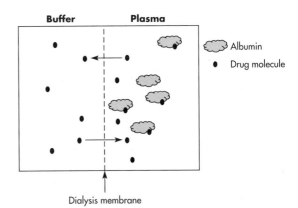

FIGURE 5-12 • Equilibrium dialysis. The apparatus consists of a cell with two compartments separated by a semipermeable membrane. The compartment on the left contains buffer with a pH of 7.4, while a plasma sample is added to the compartment on the right. The semipermeable membrane allows passage of free drug between the compartments, but large molecules and protein-bound drug are confined to the compartment on the right. After equilibrium is achieved, a sample is withdrawn from both sides and drug concentration measured. This allows determination of the unbound fraction of drug for a given concentration in plasma.

requires equilibrium to be achieved, which may take 4 to 6 hours. In addition, it is important to assure that drug does not bind to elements of the dialysis equipment, such as the dialysis membrane and dialysis cell. Such nonspecific binding can profoundly alter estimates of the fraction unbound. Equilibrium dialysis is the most common method used by the pharmaceutical industry to measure the plasma protein binding of drugs under development (Di et al, 2017). High throughput equilibrium devices have been developed that allow the technique to be deployed in 96-well plates, greatly increasing sample size for each experiment.

A more rapid approach with clinical utility is ultrafiltration. A typical ultrafiltration device is shown in Fig. 5-13. These devices can be micronized to allow for very small sample volumes, as well as utilizing specialized 96-well plates. This method utilizes centrifugal force to drive plasma water through a semipermeable membrane that excludes drug bound to plasma proteins. The ultrafiltrate represents the free drug concentration. Measurements with this technique can be obtained much more quickly than with equilibrium dialysis. The method is often used for drugs that are highly protein bound, unstable in buffer, and/or exhibit significant binding to dialysis components.

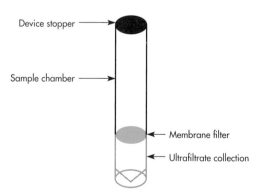

**FIGURE 5-13** • Typical ultrafiltration device for determination of free drug concentration. A plasma sample from a patient receiving the drug of interest is placed in the sample chamber. After stoppering, the entire device is placed in an ultracentrifuge. Centrifugal force is used to push serum water, which will contain free drug, across the membrane filter and into the ultrafiltrate collection cup. The drug content in the ultrafiltrate can then be measured and reflects the free drug concentration.

## PRACTICE PROBLEM

A blood sample is obtained from a patient on a drug to determine the $f_u$. After centrifugation, plasma is obtained and subjected to ultrafiltration. The concentration in plasma is found to be 3.6 mg/L, while that in the ultrafiltrate is 1.2 mg/L. From this data, determine the $f_u$ for this experimental agent.

### Solution

Since $C_{up} = f_u C_p$, we can solve for fraction unbound as

$$f_u = C_{up}/C_p = (1.2 \text{ mg/L})/(3.6 \text{ mg/L}) = 0.3$$

## HOW ARE THE KINETICS OF DRUG–PROTEIN BINDING MEASURED?

As stated previously, the binding of drug to plasma protein is a dynamic process. There has been considerable interest among researchers to quantify this process as a way of comparing drugs or proteins—in much the same way that affinity for target receptors can be used to compare various drug molecules. The kinetics of reversible drug–protein binding can be described by the *law of mass action*, as follows:

Protein + drug ⇔ drug–protein complex

or

$$[P] + [D] \Leftrightarrow [PD] \tag{5.13}$$

From Equation 5.13 and the law of mass action, an association constant ($K_a$, also called the affinity constant), can be expressed as the ratio of the molar concentration of the product and the molar concentration of the reactants. This equation assumes only one binding site per protein molecule.

$$K_a = \frac{[PD]}{[P][D]} \tag{5.14}$$

The extent of formation of the drug–protein complex formed depends on the association binding constant, $K_a$, and the magnitude of $K_a$ yields information on the degree of drug–protein binding. Drugs strongly bound to protein have a very large $K_a$ and exist mostly as the drug–protein complex. With such drugs, a large dose may be needed to obtain a therapeutic concentration of free drug.

Experimentally, both the free drug [D] and the protein-bound drug [PD], as well as the total protein concentration ([P] + [PD]), may be determined. To study the binding behavior of drugs, a determinable ratio r is defined, as follows:

$$r = \frac{\text{moles of drug bound}}{\text{total moles of protein}}$$

Since the moles of drug bound is given by [PD] and the total moles of protein is given by [P] + [PD], this equation becomes

$$r = \frac{[PD]}{[PD]+[P]} \tag{5.15}$$

According to Equation 5.14, $[PD] = K_a [P] [D]$. Substituting of this equivalent into Equation 5.15 gives

$$r = \frac{K_a[P][D]}{K_a[P][D]+[P]}$$
$$\tag{5.16}$$
$$r = \frac{K_a[D]}{1+K_a[D]}$$

This equation describes the simplest situation, in which 1 mole of drug binds to 1 mole of protein in a 1:1 complex. This case assumes only one independent binding site for each molecule of drug. If there are n identical independent binding sites per protein molecule, then the following equation is used:

$$r = \frac{nK_a[D]}{1+K_a[D]} \tag{5.17}$$

Binding affinity can also be expressed in terms of the dissociation binding constant, $K_d$, which is $1/K_a$. In this case, Equation 5.17 reduces to

$$r = \frac{n[D]}{K_d + [D]} \tag{5.18}$$

Protein molecules are usually much larger than drug molecules and may contain more than one type of binding site for the drug. If there is more than one type of binding site and the drug binds independently to each binding site with its own association constant, then Equation 5.18 becomes

$$r = \frac{n_1 K_1[P]}{1 + K_1[D]} + \frac{n_2 K_2[P]}{1 + K_2[D]} + \cdots \tag{5.19}$$

where the numerical subscripts represent different types of binding sites, the Ks represent the binding constants, and the ns represent the number of binding sites per molecule of albumin or other plasma protein.

These equations assume that each drug molecule binds to the protein at an independent binding site, and the affinity of a drug for one binding site does not influence binding to other sites, but this is not always true. Drug–protein binding sometimes exhibits *cooperativity*. For these drugs, the binding of the first drug molecule at one site on the protein molecule influences the successive binding of other drug molecules. The binding of oxygen to hemoglobin is an example of binding cooperativity. In this case, the binding of one oxygen molecule to hemoglobin results in structural changes making binding of the second, third, and fourth molecules of oxygen easier (or higher affinity). Drug–protein binding kinetics can provide valuable information on the proper therapeutic use of the drug, as well as predictions of possible drug interactions.

## PRACTICE PROBLEMS

1. How is r related to the fraction of drug bound ($f_u$), a term that is often of clinical interest?

### Solution

r is the ratio of the number of moles of drug bound to the number of moles of albumin (or other plasma protein to which the drug binds). r determines the fraction of drug binding sites that are occupied. $f_u$ is the fraction of drug which is free in the plasma. The value of $f_u$ is often assumed to be fixed. However, $f_u$ may change as drug concentration increases, especially with drugs that have therapeutic concentrations close to $K_d$.

2. At maximum drug binding, the number of binding sites is n (see Equation 5.19). The drug disopyramide has a $K_d = 1 \times 10^{-6}$ M/L. How close to saturation is the drug when the free drug concentration is $1 \times 10^{-6}$ M/L?

### Solution

Substitution for $[D] = 1 \times 10^{-6}$ M/L and $K_d = 1 \times 10^{-6}$ M/L in Equation 5.19 gives

$$r = \frac{n}{2}$$

when n = 1 and the unbound (free) drug concentration is equal to $K_d$, the protein binding of the drug is half-saturated.

# HOW ARE BINDING CONSTANTS AND BINDING SITES DETERMINED EXPERIMENTALLY?

While $f_u$ is the most important parameter for characterizing protein binding for clinical purposes, researchers often find a more exacting quantification of protein binding to be necessary when probing the mechanisms of drug binding, drug–drug interactions, and disease-induced changes.

### In Vitro Methods When the Protein Concentration is Known

A plot of the ratio of $r$ (moles of drug bound per mole of protein) versus free drug concentration $[D]$ is shown in Fig. 5-14. Equation 5.18 shows that as drug concentration increases, the number of moles of drug bound per mole of protein becomes saturated and plateaus. Thus, drug protein binding resembles a *Langmuir* adsorption isotherm. Because of nonlinearity in drug–protein binding, Equation 5.18 is often rearranged for estimating $n$ and $K_a$.

The values for the association constants and the number of binding sites can be obtained by various graphic methods. The reciprocal of Equation 5.16 gives the following equation:

$$\frac{1}{r} = \frac{1 + K_a[D]}{nK_a[D]}$$

$$\frac{1}{r} = \frac{1}{nK_a[D]} + \frac{1}{n} \qquad (5.20)$$

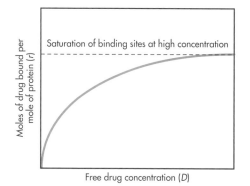

FIGURE 5-14 • Graphical representation of Equation 5.18, showing saturation of protein at high drug concentrations.

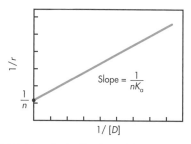

FIGURE 5-15 • Hypothetical binding of drug to protein. The line was obtained with the double reciprocal equation.

A graph of $1/r$ versus $1/[D]$ is called a *double reciprocal plot*. The $y$ intercept is $1/n$ and the slope is $1/nK_a$. From this graph (Fig. 5-15), the number of binding sites may be determined from the $y$ intercept, and the association constant may be determined from the slope, if the value for $n$ is known.

If the graph of $1/r$ versus $1/[D]$ does not yield a straight line, this suggests that the drug–protein binding process is probably more complex. Equation 5.18 assumes one type of binding site and no interaction among the binding sites. Frequently, Equation 5.20 is used to estimate the number of binding sites and binding constants.

Another graphic technique, called the *Scatchard plot*, is a rearrangement of Equation 5.18. The Scatchard plot spreads the data to allow a better line for the estimation of the binding constants and number of binding sites. From Equation 5.18, we obtain

$$r = \frac{nK_a[D]}{1 + K_a[D]}$$

$$r + rK_a[D] = nK_a[D]$$

$$r = nK_a[D] - rK_a[D] \qquad (5.21)$$

$$\frac{r}{D} = nK_a - rK_a$$

A graph of $r/[D]$ versus $r$ yields a straight line with the intercepts and slope shown in Figs. 5-16 and 5-17.

Some drug–protein binding data produce Scatchard graphs that are curved (Figs. 5-18 and 5-19). The curves are thought to represent the summation of two straight lines that collectively form the curve. The binding of salicylic acid to albumin

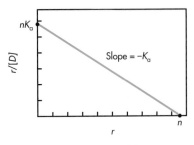

**FIGURE 5-16 •** Hypothetical binding of drug to protein. The line was obtained with the Scatchard equation.

is an example of this type of drug–protein binding in which there are at least two different independent binding sites ($n_1$ and $n_2$), each with its own independent association constant ($k_1$ and $k_2$). Equation 5.19 best describes this type of drug–protein interaction.

### In Vivo Methods When the Protein Concentration is Unknown

Reciprocal and Scatchard plots cannot be used if the exact nature and amount of protein in the experimental system are unknown. The percent of drug bound is often used to describe the extent

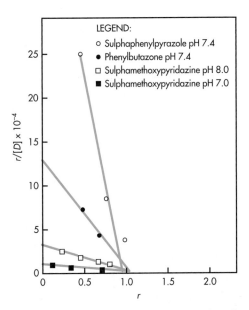

**FIGURE 5-17 •** Graphical determination of the number of binding sites and association constants for interaction of sulfonamides and phenylbutazone with albumin. (Reproduced with permission from Binns TB: Absorption and Distribution of Drugs. Baltimore, MA: Williams & Wilkins; 1964.)

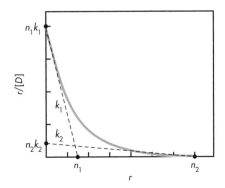

**FIGURE 5-18 •** Hypothetical binding of drug to protein. The $ks$ represent independent binding constants and the $ns$ represent the number of binding sites per molecule of protein.

of drug–protein binding in the plasma. The fraction of drug bound, $\beta$, can be determined experimentally and is equal to the ratio of the molar concentration of bound drug $[D_\beta]$ and the total protein concentration $[P_T]$ in the plasma, as follows:

$$\beta = \frac{[D_\beta]}{[P_T]} \qquad (5.22)$$

The value of the association constant ($K_a$) can be determined—even though the nature of the plasma

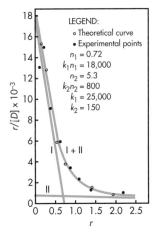

**FIGURE 5-19 •** Binding curves for salicylic acid to crystalline bovine serum albumin. Curve I shows binding for one class of binding sites, with $n_1 = 0.72$, $k_1 = 25,000$. Curve II shows binding for a second class, with $n_2 = 5.3$, $k_2 = 150$. The sum of the two curves (I + II) represents the experimentally observed Scatchard plot. (Reproduced with permission from LaDu BN, Mandel HG, Way EL: Fundamentals of Drug Metabolism and Drug Disposition. Baltimore, MA: Williams & Wilkins; 1971.)

proteins binding the drug is unknown—by rearranging Equation 5.22 into Equation 5.23:

$$r = \frac{[D_\beta]}{[P_T]} = \frac{nK_a[D]}{1 + K_a[D]} \qquad (5.23)$$

where $[D_\beta]$ is the bound drug concentration, $[D]$ is the free drug concentration, and $[P_T]$ is the total protein concentration. Rearranging this equation gives the following expression, which is analogous to the Scatchard equation:

$$\frac{[D_\beta]}{[D]} = nK_a[P_T] - K_a[D_\beta] \qquad (5.24)$$

The concentrations of both free and bound drug may be measured experimentally, and a graph obtained by plotting $[D_\beta]/[D]$ versus $[D_\beta]$ will yield a straight line for which the slope is the apparent association constant $K_a$. Equation 5.24 shows that the ratio of bound to free drug is influenced by the affinity constant, $K_a$, the protein concentration $[P_T]$ (which may change during disease states), and the drug concentration in the body.

The values for $n$ and $K_a$ give a general estimate of the affinity and binding capacity of the drug, as plasma contains a complex mixture of proteins. The drug–protein binding in plasma may be influenced by competing substances such as ions, free fatty acids, drug metabolites, and other drugs. Measurements of drug–protein binding should be obtained over a wide drug concentration range, because at high drug concentrations, saturation of high affinity, low-capacity binding sites might occur.

### Relationship between Protein Concentration and Drug Concentration in Drug–Protein Binding

The drug concentration, protein concentration, and association (affinity) constant ($K_a$) influence the fraction of drug bound (Equation 5.22). With a constant concentration of protein, only a certain number of binding sites are available for a drug. At low drug concentrations, most of the drug may be bound to the protein, whereas at high drug concentrations, the protein-binding sites may become saturated, with a consequent increase in the free drug concentration (Fig. 5-20).

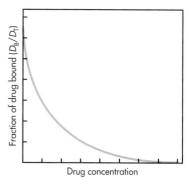

**FIGURE 5.20** · Fraction of drug bound versus drug concentration at constant protein concentration.

To demonstrate the relationship of the drug concentration, protein concentration, and $K_a$, the following expression can be derived from Equations 5.22 and 5.23.

$$\beta = \frac{1}{1 + ([D])/n[P_T] + (1/nK_a[P_T])} \qquad (5.25)$$

From Equation 5.25, both the free drug concentration $[D]$ and the total protein concentration $[P_T]$ have important effects on the fraction of drug bound. Any factors that suddenly increase the fraction of free drug concentration in the plasma will cause a change in the pharmacokinetics of the drug.

Because protein binding is nonlinear in most cases, the percent of drug bound depends on the concentrations of both the drug and proteins in the plasma. As previously noted, the concentration of protein may change with disease, affecting the percent of drug bound. As the protein concentration increases, the percent of drug bound increases to a maximum. The shapes of the curves are determined by the association constant of the drug–protein complex and the drug concentration. The effect of protein concentration on drug binding is shown in Fig. 5-21.

## WHAT ARE THE PRIMARY PLASMA PROTEINS TO WHICH DRUGS BIND?

While many different proteins are present in plasma, only two are quantitatively relevant in terms of binding to drugs: albumin and α₁-acid glycoprotein.

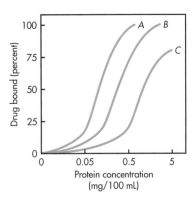

**FIGURE 5-21** • Effect of protein concentration on the percentage of drug bound. A, B, and C represent hypothetical drugs with decreasing binding affinity.

A comparison of these two proteins and their role in drug binding is presented in Table 5-2. Drugs bind to these proteins in a noncovalent, reversible manner. The binding interactions between drugs and proteins are most often governed by hydrogen bonding or hydrophobic interactions.

Albumin is the most abundant protein in plasma, and it plays a critical role in sustaining plasma oncotic pressure—which determines the movement of plasma water into or out of tissues. It also

**TABLE 5-2** • Comparison of the Two Major Plasma-Binding Proteins

|  | Albumin | $\alpha_1$-acid glycoprotein |
|---|---|---|
| Molecular weight | 66 kDa | ~42 kDa |
| Normal concentration | 3.5–5 g/dL | 0.04–0.1 g/dL |
| Types of drug that bind | Acidic and neutral drugs | Mostly basic, but some acidic and neutral drugs |
| Number of important binding sites | 2 | 1 |
| Effect of disease | Liver and renal disease, as well as burns decrease levels | Inflammatory diseases and trauma increase levels |

binds a wide variety of acidic drugs. While eight different binding sites on albumin have been identified, there are two primary high affinity binding sites (Bohnert and Gan, 2013). These are often referred to as the warfarin binding site (also known as Sudlow Site I) and the benzodiazepine binding site (also known as Sudlow Site II), based on early agents used in experiments to analyze these binding sites.

$\alpha_1$-acid glycoprotein (AAG), also known as orosomucoid, has considerably lower concentrations in plasma than albumin. AAG is a member of the class of acute phase proteins that increase in inflammatory conditions. The concentration of this protein may increase 2- to 5-fold in various diseases or trauma. This can have profound implications for the binding of basic drugs (eg, lidocaine), as well as some acidic (eg, phenytoin) and neutral drugs (eg, progesterone). Consider the simple relationship between drug, protein, and drug-protein complex:

$$Drug + Protein \Leftrightarrow Drug\text{-}Protein$$

In addition, the total protein concentration ($P_T$) is the sum of protein to which drug is bound ($P_b$) and free protein ($P_u$, protein with no drug bound):

$$P_T = P_u + P_b \qquad (5.26)$$

The fraction of protein unoccupied ($fu_p$) is given as

$$fu_p = P_u / P_T \qquad (5.27)$$

As described previously, the affinity of the drug for protein ($K_a$) is a function of bound drug ($C_b$), unbound drug ($C_u$), and $P_u$, such that

$$K_a = C_b/(C_u \bullet P_u) \qquad (5.28)$$

Since the unbound concentration is $f_u \bullet C_p$ and the bound concentration is $(1 - f_u) \bullet C_p$, substitution of equivalents into Equation 5.28 yields

$$f_u = 1/(1 + K_a \bullet fu_p \bullet P_T) \qquad (5.29)$$

Thus, an increase in AAG ($P_T$) as a consequence of traumatic injury will result in a decrease in the $f_u$ of a drug bound to this protein and may, under certain circumstances, require a change in dose or dosing interval.

Though there may be as many as seven binding sites on AAG, one high-affinity site is primarily responsible for binding basic drugs. Importantly, stereoisomers of drugs often bind to either albumin or AAG with different affinities. This means that the free concentrations of stereoisomers can differ significantly. Since the pharmacologic potencies of stereoisomers can also differ, stereospecific assays for determination of free drug concentration must be developed to precisely characterize the effects of changes in protein binding on both pharmacokinetics and pharmacodynamics.

## HOW DO DRUG–DRUG PROTEIN BINDING INTERACTIONS INFLUENCE DRUG DISTRIBUTION AND EFFECT?

In the same manner that different drugs may compete with one another for binding to receptors, drugs may compete for binding to albumin or AAG. Early drug–drug protein-binding interaction studies provided evidence for multiple binding sites on albumin. In particular, while some drugs displaced warfarin from albumin, the same drugs did not show a similar interaction with diazepam. This suggested that warfarin and diazepam bind to different sites on albumin—an inference subsequently confirmed by many studies. Table 5-3 provides examples of drugs that bind to each of the two high affinity binding sites on albumin. Additional binding sites are responsible for the binding of drugs such as amitriptyline, probenecid, and digitoxin. Recognizing the commonality of binding sites is important in predicting the potential for drug–drug protein binding interactions. For example, while salicylate would be expected to displace warfarin and valproate from albumin, it would not exhibit a similar interaction with diazepam.

**TABLE 5-3 • Examples of Binding of Drugs to the Two Primary High Affinity Binding Sites on Human Serum Albumin**

| Sudlow Site I | Sudlow Site II |
| --- | --- |
| Warfarin | Diazepam |
| Indomethacin | Ibuprofen |
| Salicylate | Halothane |
| Furosemide | Propofol |
| Valproate | Naproxen |
| Clofibrate | Diclofenac |

The consequence of altered fraction unbound arising from drug–drug protein binding displacement interactions can be seen in Fig. 5-11. If Drug B displaces Drug A from albumin, resulting in an increase in $f_u$, the $V_D$ will increase proportional to the increase in $f_u$. Hence, the protein binding interaction will result in more drug distributing into tissues.

The impact of drug–drug protein-binding interactions on free drug concentration and drug effect during multiple dose administration requires considerations related to the elimination of the drug and route of administration—topics discussed in later chapters. In general, however, protein binding displacement interactions during chronic administration do not require alterations in the dosing regimen, because drug clearance will also increase with the change in $f_u$ resulting in no change in the free drug concentration. For this reason, protein-binding displacement interactions, through readily demonstrated *in vitro*, are rarely clinically significant. Further discussion of the impact of drug–drug protein-binding interactions and free drug concentrations is provided in Chapters 15 and 23.

## CHAPTER SUMMARY

The concepts presented in this chapter illustrate the importance of understanding the process and variables affecting drug distribution for the rational use of drugs. The significance of the physicochemical characteristics of drugs as determinants of their movement within and out of blood and into various tissues has been repeatedly demonstrated through experimental studies. Additionally, differences in blood perfusion rates of various organs are critical in governing the speed at which a drug achieves its therapeutic concentration in the sites of action. Among factors that determine the extent of drug distribution into various tissues, plasma protein binding is most relevant. As only free drug is pharmacologically active, factors influencing free drug concentration must be understood for optimal development of dosing regimens and assessment of drug–drug interactions as well as changes in pharmacokinetics in the presence of various diseases.

A key factor that influences free drug concentration after multiple dosing is the mechanism and extent of drug elimination—the subject to which we turn in the next chapter.

## REFERENCES

Ballard O, Morrow AL: Human milk composition: Nutrients and bioactive factors. *Pediatr Clin North Am* **60**:49, 2013.

Barrett KE, Barman SM, Boitano S, Brooks HL: Blood as a circulatory fluid & the dynamics of blood & lymph flow. In Barrett KE, Barman SM, Boitano S, Brooks HL (eds). *Ganong's Review of Medical Physiology*, 25th ed. New York, NY, McGraw-Hill Education, 2016, Chapter 31.

Bohnert T, Gan LS: Plasma protein binding: From discovery to development. *J Pharm Sci* **102**:2953, 2013.

Di L, Breen C, Chambers R, et al: Industry perspective on contemporary protein-binding methodologies: Considerations for regulatory drug-drug interaction and related guidelines on highly bound drugs. *J Pharm Sci* **106**:3442, 2017.

Ito S: Opioids in breast milk: Pharmacokinetic principles and clinical implications. *J Clin Pharmacol* **58**:S151, 2018.

Morriss FH, Jr, Brewer ED, Spedale SB, et al: Relationship of human milk pH during course of lactation to concentrations of citrate and fatty acids. *Pediatrics* **78**:458, 1986.

Price HL: A dynamic concept of the distribution of thiopental in the human body. *Anesthesiology* **21**:40, 1960.

Stolp HB, Liddelow SA, Sa-Pereira I, Dziegielewska KM, Saunders NR: Immune responses at brain barriers and implications for brain development and neurological function in later life. *Front Integr Neurosci* **7**:61, 2013.

Wilson F: Stages of anesthesia. In Burton VW, Davies AH, Kilpatrick A, et al. *Essential Accident and Emergency Care*. Berlin, Springer, Dordrecht, 1981, p 201.

# 6

# Physiology of Drug Elimination

Fang Wu, Murray P. Ducharme and Liang Zhao

## CHAPTER OBJECTIVES

- Describe the pathways for drug elimination in the body.
- Describe the role of hepatic blood flow and drug protein binding on hepatic elimination.
- Describe the biotransformation of drugs in the liver and which enzymatic processes are considered "phase I reactions" and "phase II reactions."
- List the organs involved in drug elimination and the significance of each.
- Discuss the relationship between metabolic pathways and enzyme polymorphisms on inter-subject variability and drug–drug interactions.
- Describe how the exposure of a drug is changed when coadministered with another drug that shares the same metabolic pathway.
- Define first-pass metabolism.
- Use urine data to calculate fraction of drug excreted and metabolized.
- Describe biliary drug excretion and define enterohepatic drug elimination.
- Discuss the reasons why bioavailability is variable and can be less than 100%.
- Describe BDDCS—Biological Drug Disposition Classification System.
- Describe the processes for renal drug excretion and explain which renal excretion process predominates in the kidney for a specific drug.

## INTRODUCTION

The decline from peak plasma concentrations after drug administration results from drug elimination or removal by the body. The elimination of most drugs from the body involves the processes of both metabolism (biotransformation) and renal excretion. The liver and kidney are the two major drug eliminating organs in the body, though drug elimination can also occur almost anywhere in the body. For many drugs, the principal site of metabolism is the liver. However, other tissues or organs, especially those tissues associated with portals of drug entry into the body, may also be involved in drug metabolism. These sites include the lung, skin, gastrointestinal mucosal cells, microbiological flora in the distal portion of the ileum, and large intestine. The kidney may also be involved in certain drug metabolism reactions.

In this chapter, we will see how drugs are eliminated from the body. Non-endogenous drugs are viewed as foreign substances (xenobiotics) by the body, which will then be eliminated as efficiently as possible. In a simplifying scheme, hydrosoluble drugs can be readily excreted from the body by the kidney, while liposoluble drugs are generally transformed by the liver into either relatively small molecular weight metabolites that are more water soluble and can then be excreted by the kidney, or into larger MW metabolites such as conjugates that will then be excreted via the bile and eventually in the feces. We will provide a review of the liver and of its importance in the metabolism of drugs. We will then also discuss biliary excretion, and finally renal elimination.

## ANATOMY AND PHYSIOLOGY OF THE LIVER

The liver is the major organ responsible for drug metabolism and where enzymes are of utmost importance in transforming drugs. However, intestinal tissues, lungs, kidney, and skin also contain appreciable amounts of biotransformation enzymes, as reflected by human data (Table 6-1a). Metabolism may also occur in other tissues to a lesser degree depending on drug properties and route of drug administration. The expressions of biotransformation enzymes are found to be different across species (Table 6-1b).

The liver is both a synthesizing and an excreting organ. The basic anatomical unit of the liver is the liver lobule, which contains parenchymal cells in a network of interconnected lymph and blood vessels. The liver consists of large right and left lobes that merge in the middle. The liver is perfused by blood from the hepatic artery; in addition, the large hepatic portal vein that collects blood from various segments of the GI tract also perfuses the liver (Fig. 6-1). The hepatic artery carries oxygen to the liver and accounts for about 25% of the liver blood supply. The hepatic portal vein carries nutrients to the liver and accounts for about 75% of liver blood flow. The terminal branches of the hepatic artery and portal vein fuse within the liver and mix with the large vascular capillaries known as *sinusoids* (Fig. 6-2). Blood leaves the liver via the hepatic vein, which empties into the

## TABLE 6-1A • Total RNA Source Information and Values for Human /β-Actin and representative P450 mRNAs in Various Tissues

| CYP<br>Pool size<br>Age<br>Sex Race | Liver | Fetal Liver | Small Intestine | Kidney | Adrenal Gland | Lung | Brain | Prostate | Testis | Uterus | Placenta |
|---|---|---|---|---|---|---|---|---|---|---|---|
| Pool Size | 2 | 63 | 11 | 8 | 67 | 5 | 1 | 47 | 19 | 10 | 3 |
| Age | 15, 35 | 23-40 weeks | 15-60 | 24-55 | 17-72 | 14-40 | 28 | 14-50 | 17-61 | 15-77 | 23-31 |
| Gender | F, M | F, M | F, M | F, M | F, M | F, M | M | M | M | F | F |
| Race | C | C | C | C | C | C | A | C | C | C | C |
| Cause of Death | Sudden Death | Spontaneous Abortion | Trauma | Trauma | Sudden Death | Sudden Death | Sudden Death | Sudden Death | Trauma | Trauma | No Death |
| β-actin | 0.0832 | 0.0678 | 0.331 | 0.0733 | 0.249 | 0.561 | 0.0848 | 0.275 | 0.103 | 0.394 | 0.337 |
| CYP1A1 | 0.0594 | 0.000272 | 0.00176 | 0.000239 | 0.00677 | 0.0679 | 0.000388 | 0.00465 | 0.00215 | 0.0201 | 0.00101 |
| CYP1A2 | 4.77 | BLQ | BLQ | 0.000021 | 0.00113 | 0.000119 | BLQ | 0.000740 | 0.00141 | 0.00193 | BLQ |
| CYP1B1 | 0.00578 | 0.000622 | 0.0128 | 0.0139 | 0.0144 | 0.0167 | 0.00174 | 0.104 | 0.0197 | 0.0413 | 0.00490 |
| CYP2A6/7 | 27.8 | 0.199 | 0.00193 | 0.00188 | 0.0105 | 0.0622 | 0.00867 | 0.00809 | 0.0187 | 0.0390 | 0.0231 |
| CYP2A6 | 27.5 | 0.184 | BLQ | BLQ | BLQ | 0.0708 | 0.00731 | BLQ | BLQ | 0.00447 | 0.000611 |
| CYP2A7 | 0.617 | 0.00908 | 0.00249 | BLQ | 0.000322 | 0.000063 | 0.000619 | 0.000646 | 0.000600 | 0.00295 | 0.00131 |
| CYP2B6 | 1.46 | 0.0675 | 0.0537 | 0.0797 | 0.00178 | 0.456 | 0.00162 | 0.00558 | 0.00485 | 0.00796 | 0.000920 |
| CYP2C8 | 10.2 | 0.226 | 0.0166 | 0.00660 | 0.0364 | 0.00481 | 0.00214 | 0.00197 | 0.0720 | 0.000444 | BLQ |
| CYP2C9 | 3.11 | 0.0245 | 0.188 | 0.00295 | 0.000493 | 0.000334 | 0.000622 | 0.000111 | 0.000072 | 0.000592 | 0.000149 |
| CYP2C18 | 5.31 | 0.0188 | 1.41 | 0.00174 | BLQ | 0.0122 | 0.00148 | BLQ | 0.0240 | 0.0197 | 0.00425 |
| CYP2C19 | 0.187 | 0.000152 | 0.0303 | 0.0000148 | 0.000030 | 0.000038 | 0.000014 | 0.000001 | 0.000033 | 0.000037 | 0.000015 |
| CYP2D6 | 0.559 | 0.0238 | 0.0265 | 0.00607 | 0.00603 | 0.00651 | 0.00224 | 0.00875 | 0.224 | 0.00712 | 0.00613 |
| CYP2E1 | 53.8 | 0.419 | 0.220 | 0.0115 | 0.0178 | 0.0173 | 0.0189 | 0.0280 | 0.0302 | 0.0318 | 0.00485 |

*Abbreviations: BLQ, below the limit of quantification; F, female; M, male; C, Caucasian; A, Asian. Data are expressed as the ratio of β-actin or CYP mRNA to GAPDH mRNA. Experiments were performed in triplicate.*

*Data from Nishimura M, Yaguti H, Yoshitsugu H, et al: Tissue distribution of mRNA expression of human cytochrome P450 isoforms assessed by high-sensitivity real-time reverse transcription PCR, Yakugaku Zasshi. 2003 May;123(5):369-375.*

**TABLE 6-1B •** CYP Enzymes of the Major Drug-Metabolizing CYP Family in Human, Rat, Mouse, Dog, and Monkey

| Family | Subfamily | Human | Mouse | Rat | Dog | Monkey |
|---|---|---|---|---|---|---|
| CYP1 | A | 1A1, 1A2 | 1A1, 1A2 | 1A1, 1A2 | 1A1, 1A2 | 1A1, 1A2 |
| | B | 1B1 | 1B1 | 1B1 | 1B1 | 1B1 |
| CYP2 | A | 2A6, 2A7, 2A13 | 2A4, 2A5, 2A12, 2A22 | 2A1, 2A2, 2A3 | 2A13, 2A25 | 2A23, 2A24 |
| | B | 2B6, 2B7 | 2B9, 2B10 | 2B1, 2B2, 2B3 | 2B11 | 2B17 |
| | C | 2C8, 2C9, 2C18, 2C19 | 2C29, 2C37, 2C38, 2C39, 2C40, 2C44, 2C50, 2C54, 2C55 | 2C6, 2C7*, 2C11*, 2C12*, 2C13*, 2C22, 2C23 | 2C21, 2C41 | 2C20, 2C43 |
| | D | 2D6, 2D7, 2D8 | 2D9, 2D10, 2D11, 2D12, 2D13, 2D22, 2D26, 2D34, 2D40 | 2D1, 2D2, 2D3, 2D4, 2D5, 2D18 | 2D15 | 2D17[†], 2D19[†], 2D29[†], 2D30[†] |
| | E | 2E1 | 2E1 | 2E1 | 2E1 | 2E1 |
| CYP3 | A | 3A4, 3A5, 3A7, 3A43 | 3A11, 3A13, 3A16, 3A25, 3A41, 3A44 | 3A1/3A23, 3A2*, 3A9*, 3A18*, 3A62 | 3A12, 3A26 | 3A8 |

*Gender difference.
†Strain specific.
Data from Martignoni M, Groothuis GM, de Kanter R. Species differences between mouse, rat, dog, monkey and human CYP-mediated drug metabolism, inhibition and induction, Expert Opin Drug Metab Toxicol 2006 Dec;2(6):875–894.

vena cava (see Fig. 6-1). The liver also secretes bile acids within the liver lobes, which flow through a network of channels and eventually empty into the common bile duct (Figs. 6-2 and 6-3). The common bile duct drains bile and biliary excretion products from both lobes into the gallbladder.

Although the principal sites of liver metabolism are the hepatocytes, drug transporters are also present in the hepatocyte besides CYP enzymes. Transporters can efflux drug either into or out of the hepatocytes, thus influencing the rate of metabolism. In addition, drug transporters are also present in the bile canaliculi which can eliminate drug by efflux.

Drug metabolism in the liver has been shown to be *flow* and *site dependent*. Some enzymes are reached only when blood flow travels from a given direction. The quantity of enzymes involved in metabolizing drug is not uniform throughout the liver. Consequently, changes in blood flow can greatly affect the fraction of drug metabolized. Clinically, hepatic diseases, such as cirrhosis, can cause tissue fibrosis, necrosis, and hepatic shunt, resulting in changing blood flow and changing bioavailability of drugs (see Chapter 25). For this reason, and in part because of genetic differences in enzyme levels among different subjects and environmental factors, the half-lives of drugs eliminated by drug metabolism are generally very variable.

## HEPATIC ENZYMES INVOLVED IN THE BIOTRANSFORMATION OF DRUGS

### Mixed-Function Oxidases

The liver is the major site of drug metabolism, and the type of metabolism is based on the reaction involved. Oxidation, reduction, hydrolysis, and conjugation are the most common reactions,

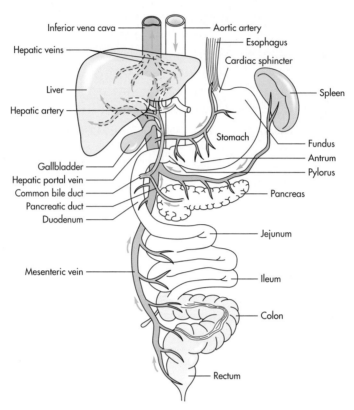

**FIGURE 6-1** • The large hepatic portal vein that collects blood from various segments of the GI tract also perfuses the liver.

as discussed under phase I and phase II reactions in the next two sections. The enzymes responsible for oxidation and reduction of drugs (*xenobiotics*) and certain natural metabolites, such as steroids, are monooxygenase enzymes known as *mixed-function*

*oxidases* (MFOs). The hepatic parenchymal cells contain MFOs in association with the *endoplasmic reticulum*, a network of lipoprotein membranes within the cytoplasm and continuous with the cellular and nuclear membranes. If hepatic

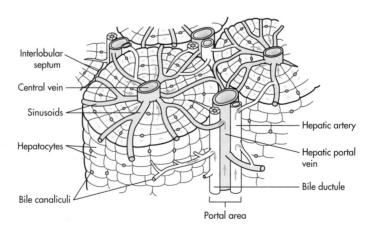

**FIGURE 6-2** • Intrahepatic distribution of the hepatic and portal veins.

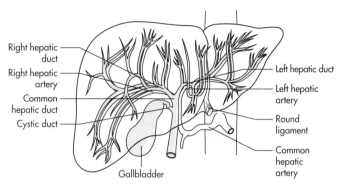

FIGURE 6-3 • Intrahepatic distribution of the hepatic artery, portal vein, and biliary ducts. (Reproduced with permission from Lindner HH. *Clinical Anatomy*. Norwalk, CT: Appleton & Lange, 1989.)

parenchymal cells are fragmented and differentially centrifuged in an ultracentrifuge, a microsomal fraction, or *microsome*, is obtained from the postmitochondrial supernatant. The microsomal fraction contains fragments of the endoplasmic reticulum.

The mixed-function oxidase enzymes are structural enzymes that constitute an electron-transport system that requires reduced NADPH ($NADPH_2$), molecular oxygen, CYP enzymes (formerly known as cytochrome P-450), NADPH–CYP enzyme reductase, and phospholipid. The phospholipid is involved in the binding of the drug molecule to the CYP enzyme and coupling the NADPH–CYP enzyme reductase to CYP enzyme. CYP enzyme is a heme protein with iron protoporphyrin IX as the prosthetic group. CYP enzyme is the terminal component of an electron-transfer system in the endoplasmic reticulum and acts as both an oxygen- and a substrate-binding locus for drugs and endogenous substrates in conjunction with a flavoprotein reductase, NADPH–CYP enzyme reductase. Many lipid-soluble drugs bind to CYP enzymes, resulting in oxidation (or reduction) of the drugs. CYP enzymes consist of closely related enzymes (*isozymes*) that differ somewhat in amino acid sequence and drug specificity (see Chapter 21). A general scheme for MFO drug oxidation is described in Fig. 6-4.

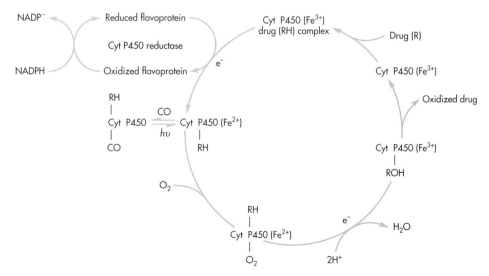

FIGURE 6-4 • Electron flow pathway in the microsomal drug-oxidizing system. (Reproduced with permission from Pratt WB, Taylor P: *Principles of Drug Action*, 3rd ed. New York, NY: Churchill Livingstone, 1990.)

In addition to the metabolism of drugs, the CYP monooxygenase enzyme system catalyzes the biotransformation of various endogenous compounds such as steroids. The CYP monooxygenase enzyme system is also located in other tissues such as kidney, GI tract, skin, and lungs.

A few enzymatic oxidation reactions involved in biotransformation do not include the CYP monooxygenase enzyme system. These include monoamine oxidase (MAO) that deaminates endogenous substrates including neurotransmitters (dopamine, serotonin, norepinephrine, epinephrine, and various drugs with a similar structure); alcohol and aldehyde dehydrogenase in the soluble fraction of liver are involved in the metabolism of ethanol and xanthine oxidase which converts hypoxanthine to xanthine and then to uric acid. Drug substrates for xanthine oxidase include theophylline and 6-mercaptopurine. Allopurinol used in the treatment of gout, is a substrate and inhibitor of xanthine oxidase and it delays the metabolism of substrates going through this pathway.

## DRUG BIOTRANSFORMATION REACTIONS

The hepatic biotransformation enzymes play an important role in the inactivation and subsequent elimination of drugs that are not easily cleared through the kidney. For these drugs—theophylline, phenytoin, acetaminophen, and others—there is a direct relationship between the rate of drug metabolism (*biotransformation*) and the elimination half-life for the drug.

For most biotransformation reactions, the metabolite of the drug is more polar than the parent compound. The conversion of a drug to a more polar metabolite enables the drug to be eliminated more quickly than if the drug remained lipid soluble. A lipid-soluble drug crosses cell membranes and is easily reabsorbed by the renal tubular cells, exhibiting a consequent tendency to remain in the body. In contrast, the more polar metabolite does not cross cell membranes easily, is filtered through the glomerulus, is not readily reabsorbed, and is more rapidly excreted in the urine.

Both the nature of the drug and the route of administration may influence the type of drug metabolite formed. For example, isoproterenol given orally forms a sulfate conjugate in the gastrointestinal mucosal cells, whereas after intravenous administration, it forms the 3-*O*-methylated metabolite via *S*-adenosylmethionine and catechol-*O*-methyltransferase. Azo drugs such as sulfasalazine are poorly absorbed after oral administration. However, the azo group of sulfasalazine is cleaved by the intestinal microflora, producing 5-aminosalicylic acid and sulfapyridine, which is absorbed in the lower bowel.

The biotransformation of drugs may be classified according to the pharmacologic activity of the metabolite or according to the biochemical mechanism for each biotransformation reaction. For most drugs, biotransformation results in the formation of a more polar metabolite(s) that is pharmacologically inactive and is eliminated more rapidly than the parent drug (Table 6-2).

For some drugs the metabolite may be pharmacologically active or produce toxic effects. *Prodrugs* are inactive and must be biotransformed in the body to metabolites that have pharmacologic activity. Initially, prodrugs were discovered by serendipity, as in the case of prontosil, which is reduced to the antibacterial agent sulfanilamide. More recently, prodrugs have been intentionally designed to improve drug stability, increase systemic drug absorption, or to prolong the duration of activity. For example, the antiparkinsonian agent levodopa crosses the blood–brain barrier and is then decarboxylated in the brain to L-dopamine, an active neurotransmitter. L-Dopamine does not easily penetrate the blood–brain barrier into the brain and therefore cannot be used as a therapeutic agent.

## PATHWAYS OF DRUG BIOTRANSFORMATION

Pathways of drug biotransformation may be divided into two major groups of reactions, phase I and phase II reactions. *Phase I*, or *asynthetic reactions*, include oxidation, reduction, and hydrolysis. *Phase II*, or *synthetic reactions*, include conjugations. A partial list of these reactions is presented in Table 6-3. In addition, a number of drugs that resemble natural biochemical molecules are able to utilize the metabolic

| TABLE 6-2 • Biotransformation Reactions and Pharmacologic Activity of the Metabolite | | |
|---|---|---|
| Reaction | | Example |
| **Active Drug to Inactive Metabolite** | | |
| Amphetamine | Deamination → | Phenylacetone |
| Phenobarbital | Hydroxylation → | Hydroxyphenobarbital |
| **Active Drug to Active Metabolite** | | |
| Codeine | Demethylation → | Morphine |
| Procainamide | Acetylation → | N-acetylprocainamide |
| Phenylbutazone | Hydroxylation → | Oxyphenbutazone |
| **Inactive Drug to Active Metabolite** | | |
| Hetacillin | Hydrolysis → | Ampicillin |
| Sulfasalazine | Azoreduction → | Sulfapyridine + 5-aminosalicylic acid |
| **Active Drug to Reactive Intermediate** | | |
| Acetaminophen | Aromatic → Hydroxylation | Reactive metabolite (hepatic necrosis) |
| Benzo[a]pyrene | Aromatic → Hydroxylation | Reactive metabolite (carcinogenic) |

pathways for normal body compounds. For example, isoproterenol is methylated by catechol O-methyl transferase (COMT), and amphetamine is deaminated by MAO. Both COMT and MAO are enzymes involved in the metabolism of noradrenaline.

## Phase I Reactions

Usually, phase I biotransformation reactions occur first and introduce or expose a functional group on the drug molecules. For example, oxygen is introduced into the phenyl group on phenylbutazone by aromatic hydroxylation to form oxyphenbutazone, a more polar metabolite. Codeine is demethylated to form morphine. In addition, the hydrolysis of esters, such as aspirin or benzocaine, yields more polar products, such as salicylic acid and p-aminobenzoic acid, respectively. For some compounds, such as acetaminophen, benzo[a]pyrene, and other drugs containing aromatic rings, reactive intermediates,

such as epoxides, are formed during the hydroxylation reaction. These aromatic epoxides are highly reactive and will react with macromolecules, possibly causing liver necrosis (acetaminophen) or cancer (benzo[a]pyrene). The biotransformation of acetaminophen (Fig. 6-5) demonstrates the variety of possible metabolites that may be formed. It should be noted that acetaminophen is also conjugated directly (phase II reaction, eg, glucuronidation and sulfation) without a preceding phase I reaction.

## Conjugation (Phase II) Reactions

Once a polar constituent is revealed or placed into the molecule, a phase II or conjugation reaction may occur. Common examples include the conjugation of salicylic acid with glycine to form salicyluric acid or glucuronic acid to form salicylglucuronide (see Fig. 6-5).

Conjugation reactions use conjugating reagents, which are derived from biochemical compounds

## TABLE 6-3 • Some Common Drug Biotransformation Reactions

| Phase I Reactions | Phase II Reactions |
|---|---|
| Oxidation | Glucuronide conjugation |
| Aromatic hydroxylation | Ether glucuronide |
| Side chain hydroxylation | Ester glucuronide |
| N-, O-, and S-dealkylation | Amide glucuronide |
| Deamination | |
| Sulfoxidation, N-oxidation | Peptide conjugation |
| N-hydroxylation | |
| Reduction | Glycine conjugation hippurate) |
| Azoreduction | |
| Nitroreduction | Methylation |
| Alcohol dehydrogenase | N-methylation |
| Hydrolysis | O-methylation |
| Ester hydrolysis | |
| Amide hydrolysis | Acetylation |
| | Sulfate conjugation |
| | Mercapturic acid synthesis |

involved in carbohydrate, fat, and protein metabolism. These reactions may include an active, high-energy form of the conjugating agent, such as uridine diphosphoglucuronic acid (UDPGA), acetyl CoA, 3'-phosphoadenosine-5'-phosphosulfate (PAPS), or S-adenosylmethionine (SAM), which, in the presence of the appropriate transferase enzyme, combines with the drug to form the conjugate. Conversely, the drug may be activated to a high-energy compound that then reacts with the conjugating agent in the presence of a transferase enzyme (Fig. 6-6). The major conjugation (phase II) reactions are listed in Tables 6-3 and 6-4.

Some of the conjugation reactions may have limited capacity at high drug concentrations, leading to nonlinear drug metabolism. In most cases, enzyme activity follows first-order kinetics with low drug (substrate) concentrations. At high doses, the drug concentration may rise above the Michaelis–Menten rate constant ($K_M$), and the reaction rate approaches zero order ($V_{max}$). Glucuronidation reactions have

a high capacity and may demonstrate nonlinear (saturation) kinetics at very high drug concentrations. In contrast, glycine, sulfate, and glutathione conjugations show lesser capacity and demonstrate nonlinear kinetics at therapeutic drug concentrations (Caldwell, 1980). The limited capacity of certain conjugation pathways may be due to several factors, including (1) limited amount of the conjugate transferase, (2) limited ability to synthesize the active nucleotide intermediate, or (3) limited amount of conjugating agent, such as glycine.

In addition, the N-acetylated conjugation reaction shows genetic polymorphism: for certain drugs, the human population may be divided into fast and slow acetylators. Finally, some of these conjugation reactions may be diminished or defective in cases of inborn errors of metabolism.

Glucuronidation and sulfate conjugation are very common phase II reactions that result in water-soluble metabolites being rapidly excreted in bile (for some high-molecular-weight glucuronides) and/or urine. Acetylation and mercapturic acid synthesis are conjugation reactions that are often implicated in the toxicity of the drug; they will now be discussed more fully.

### Acetylation

The acetylation reaction is an important conjugation reaction for several reasons. First, the acetylated product is usually less polar than the parent drug. The acetylation of such drugs as sulfanilamide, sulfadiazine, and sulfisoxazole produces metabolites that are less water soluble and that in sufficient concentration precipitate in the kidney tubules, causing kidney damage and crystalluria. In addition, a less polar metabolite is reabsorbed in the renal tubule and has a longer elimination half-life. For example, procainamide (elimination half-life of 3 to 4 hours) has an acetylated metabolite, N-acetylprocainamide, which is biologically active and has an elimination half-life of 6 to 7 hours. Last, the N-acetyltransferase enzyme responsible for catalyzing the acetylation of isoniazid and other drugs demonstrates a genetic polymorphism in patients with normal renal function. Two distinct subpopulations have been observed to inactivate isoniazid, including the "slow inactivators" and the "rapid inactivators" (Evans, 1968). Therefore, the former

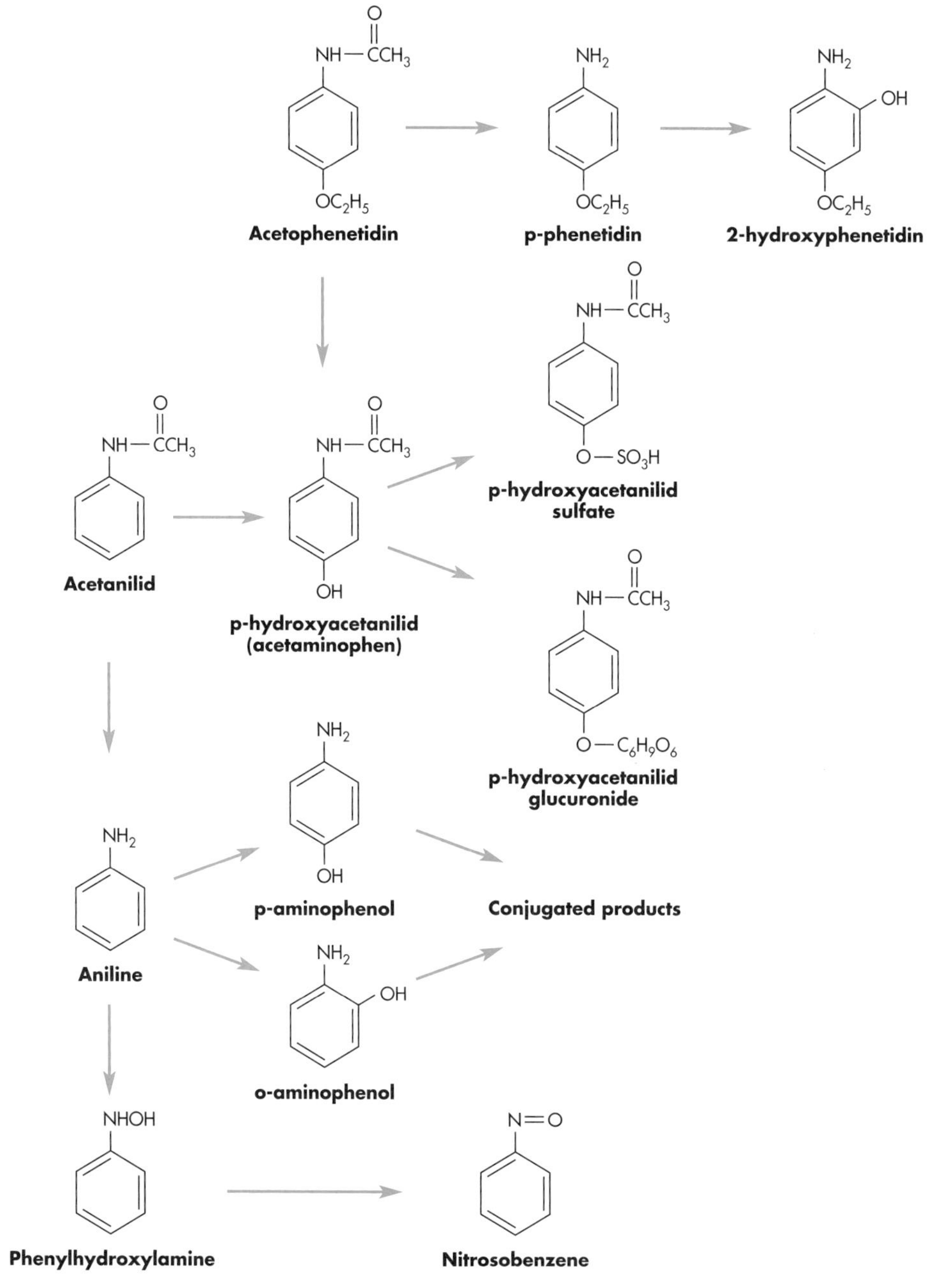

FIGURE 6-5 • Biotransformation of salicylic acid. (Reproduced with permission from Bridges JW, Chasseaud LF: *Progress in Drug Research*, vol 5. New York, NY: Wiley, 1980.)

group may demonstrate an adverse effect of isoniazid, such as encephalopathy, due to the longer elimination half-life and accumulation of the drug (Constantinescu et al, 2017).

### Glutathione and Mercapturic Acid Conjugation

Glutathione (GSH) is a tripeptide of glutamyl-cysteine-glycine that is involved in many important biochemical reactions. GSH is important in the

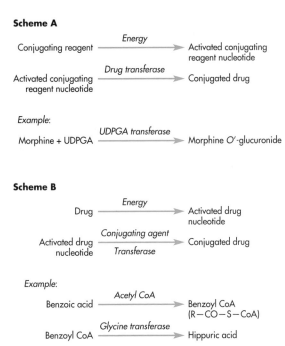

**Scheme A**

Conjugating reagent —(Energy)→ Activated conjugating reagent nucleotide

Activated conjugating reagent nucleotide —(Drug transferase)→ Conjugated drug

*Example:*

Morphine + UDPGA —(UDPGA transferase)→ Morphine O'-glucuronide

**Scheme B**

Drug —(Energy)→ Activated drug nucleotide

Activated drug nucleotide —(Conjugating agent / Transferase)→ Conjugated drug

*Example:*

Benzoic acid —(Acetyl CoA)→ Benzoyl CoA (R—CO—S—CoA)

Benzoyl CoA —(Glycine transferase)→ Hippuric acid

FIGURE 6-6 • General scheme for phase II reactions.

detoxification of reactive oxygen intermediates into nonreactive metabolites and is the main intracellular molecule for protection of the cell against reactive electrophilic compounds. Through the nucleophilic sulfhydryl group of the cysteine residue, GSH reacts nonenzymatically and enzymatically via the enzyme glutathione S-transferase, with reactive electrophilic oxygen intermediates of certain drugs, particularly aromatic hydrocarbons formed during oxidative biotransformation. The resulting GSH conjugates are precursors for a group of drug conjugates known as mercapturic acid (N-acetylcysteine) derivatives. The formation of a mercapturic acid conjugate is shown in Fig. 6-7.

The enzymatic formation of GSH conjugates is saturable. High doses of drugs such as acetaminophen (APAP) may form electrophilic intermediates and deplete GSH in the cell. The reactive intermediate covalently bonds to hepatic cellular macromolecules, resulting in cellular injury and necrosis. The suggested antidote for intoxication (overdose) of acetaminophen is the administration of N-acetylcysteine (Mucomyst), a drug molecule that contains available sulfhydryl (R–SH) groups.

## Metabolism of Enantiomers

Many drugs are given as mixtures of stereoisomers. Each isomeric form may have different pharmacologic actions and different side effects. For example, the natural thyroid hormone is *l*-thyroxine, whereas the synthetic *d* enantiomer, *d*-thyroxine, lowers cholesterol but does not stimulate basal metabolic rate like the *l* form. Since enzymes as well as drug receptors demonstrate stereoselectivity, isomers of drugs may show differences in biotransformation and pharmacokinetics (Tucker and Lennard, 1990).

## TABLE 6-4 • Phase II Conjugation Reactions

| Conjugation Reaction | Conjugating Agent | High-Energy Intermediate | Functional Groups Combined with |
|---|---|---|---|
| Glucuronidation | Glucuronic acid | UDPGA* | $-OH$, $-COOH$, $-NH_2$, SH |
| Sulfation | Sulfate | PAPS† | $-OH$, $-NH_2$ |
| Amino acid conjugation | Glycine‡ | Coenzyme A thioesters | $-COOH$ |
| Acetylation | Acetyl CoA | Acetyl CoA | $-OH$, $-NH_2$ |
| Methylation | $CH_3$ from S-adenosylmethionine | S-adenosylmethionine | $-OH$, $-NH_2$ |
| Glutathione (mercapturine acid conjugation) | Glutathione | Arene oxides, epoxides | Aryl halides, epoxides, arene oxides |

*UDPGA = uridine diphosphoglucuronic acid.
†PAPS = 3'-phosphoadenosine-5'-phosphosulfate.
‡Glycine conjugates are also known as hippurates.

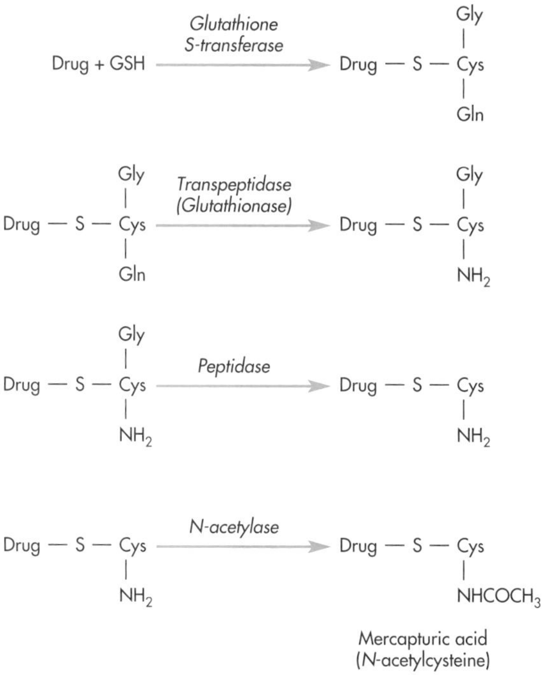

FIGURE 6-7 • Mercapturic acid conjugation.

With improved techniques for isolating mixtures of enantiomers, many drugs are now available as pure enantiomers. The rate of drug metabolism and the extent of drug protein binding are often different for each stereoisomer. For example, (S)-(+)disopyramide is more highly bound in humans than (R)-(−) disopyramide. Omeprazole, a proton pump inhibitor for the treatment of gastric acid–mediated disorders, is a racemic mixture of R-omeprazole and S-omeprazole (esomeprazole). Although both enantiomers are metabolized by CYP2C19 and CYP3A4, the contributions of these two enzymes to metabolism of the two enantiomers were different, with 73% and 27%, respectively, for esomeprazole and 98% and 2%, respectively, for R-omeprazole (Andersson and Weidolf, 2008). Besides being CYP2C19 substrates, both enantiomers are CYP2C19 inhibitors with different inhibition potency. *In vitro* studies have shown that esomeprazole is a time-dependent (irreversible) inhibitor (TDI) of CYP2C19 with weak reversible inhibition potency, and R-omeprazole is mainly a reversible inhibitor of CYP2C19 (Ogilvie et al, 2011). A list of common racemic drugs is given in Table 6-5.

### TABLE 6-5 • Common Drug Enantiomers

| | | |
|---|---|---|
| Atropine | Brompheniramine | Cocaine |
| Disopyramide | Doxylamine | Ephedrine |
| Propranolol | Nadolol | Verapamil |
| Tocainide | Propoxyphene | Morphine |
| Warfarin | Thyroxine | Flecainide |
| Ibuprofen | Atenolol | Salbutamol |
| Metoprolol | Terbutaline | Omeprazole |

### Regioselectivity

In addition to stereoselectivity, biotransformation enzymes may also be regioselective. In this case, the enzymes catalyze a reaction that is specific for a particular region in the drug molecule. For example, isoproterenol is methylated via COMT and SAM primarily in the meta position, resulting in a 3-O-methylated metabolite. Very little methylation occurs at the hydroxyl group in the para position.

### Species Differences in Hepatic Biotransformation Enzymes

The biotransformation activity of hepatic enzymes can be affected by a variety of factors (Table 6-6). During the early preclinical phase of drug development, drug metabolism studies attempt to identify

### TABLE 6-6 • Sources of Variation in Intrinsic Clearance

Genetic factors
    Genetic differences within population
    Racial differences among different populations
Environmental factors and drug interactions
    Enzyme induction
    Enzyme inhibition
Physiologic conditions
    Age
    Gender
    Diet/nutrition
    Pathophysiology
Drug dosage regimen
    Route of drug administration
    Dose-dependent (nonlinear) pharmacokinetics
Species

the major metabolic pathways of a new drug through the use of animal models. For most drugs, different animal species may have different metabolic pathways. For example, amphetamine is mainly hydroxylated in rats, whereas in humans and dogs it is largely deaminated. In many cases, the rates of metabolism may differ among different animal species even though the biotransformation pathways are the same. In other cases, a specific pathway may be absent in a particular species. A general consensus is that metabolite patterns and relative abundances display large interspecies differences. In addition, it is stressed that characterization of these patterns in experimental animals may be useful and sometimes necessary, because toxicity studies should preferably have been performed in a species that resembles humans as closely as possible with respect to kinetics and metabolism (Pelkonen et al, 2009). Generally, the researcher needs to find the best animal model that will be predictive of the metabolic profile in humans.

*In vitro* drug screening with human liver microsomes or with hepatocytes has helped confirm whether a given CYP enzyme is important in human drug metabolism. Preclinical animal models may also provide some supportive evidence. In recent years, it has been useful to simulate metabolism process virtually and predict drug interaction potential by *in silico* model approaches as described in FDA Guidance for Industry: In Vitro Drug Interaction Studies—Cytochrome P450 Enzyme- and Transporter-Mediated Drug Interactions, issued in 2020.

## DRUG INTERACTION EXAMPLE

Lovastatin (Mevacor®) is a cholesterol-lowering agent and was found to be metabolized by human liver microsomes to two major metabolites: $6'\beta$-hydroxy (Michaelis–Menten constant $[K_M]$: $7.8 \pm 2.7$ $\mu$M) and $6'$-exomethylene lovastatin ($K_M$, $10.3 \pm 2.6$ $\mu$M). $6'\beta$-Hydroxylovastatin formation in the liver was inhibited by the specific CYP3A inhibitors cyclosporine ($K_i$, $7.6 \pm 2.3$ $\mu$M), ketoconazole ($K_i$, $0.25 \pm 0.2$ $\mu$M), and troleandomycin ($K_i$, $26.6 \pm 18.5$ $\mu$M).

Hydroxylation of lovastatin is a phase I reaction and catalyzed by CYP3A enzymes. Ketoconazole and cyclosporine are CYP3A inhibitors and therefore affect lovastatin metabolism. Lovastatin is referred to

as a substrate. Substrate concentrations are expressed as [S], preferably in ($\mu$M). The Michaelis–Menten constant ($K_M$) of the enzyme is expressed in micromoles ($\mu$M) because most new drugs have different MW, making it easier to compare by expressing them in moles. Cyclosporine would be expected to produce a significant drug–drug interaction in the body based on a review of the $K_i$ values. In addition, an efflux transporter can deplete the drug before significant biotransformation occurs. Inhibition of efflux transporter would have the opposite effect. Thus, location (time and place) issues are important when drug–drug interaction involves a CYP and a transporter.

A systems biology approach that takes into account all aspects of Absorption, distribution, metabolism and excretion (ADME) processes integrated with pharmacogenetics is needed to properly address various pharmacokinetic, pharmacodynamic, and clinical issues of risk/benefit. The interplay among the various processes including influx and efflux transporters may sometimes overweigh any single process when complex drug–drug interactions are involved (FDA Guidance for Industry, 2020). For most drugs, metabolism has multiple pathways which are inherently complicated. Many pharmacodynamic drug actions in patients encounter the issue of responder and nonresponder due to differences in metabolism, which may be genetically defined or totally obscured. For example, the *CYP2C19* polymorphisms were found to be highly associated with clopidogrel variable responses. Poor metabolizers (based on *CYP2C19* genotype) had lower plasma concentration of clopidogrel active metabolite, which can cause attenuated platelets inhibition effect by clopidogrel (Amin et al, 2017). Therefore, the United States (US) Food and Drug Administration (FDA) requested a warning box in clopidogrel labeling Drugs@FDA, label for PLAVIX, 2021 recommending the genotyping of *CYP2C19* in order to prevent recurrence of cardiovascular events.

### Variation of Biotransformation Enzymes

Variation in metabolism may be caused by a number of biological and environmental variables (see Table 6-6). *Pharmacogenetics* is the study of genetic differences in pharmacokinetics and pharmacodynamics, including drug elimination (see Chapter 21). For example, the *N*-acetylation of isoniazid is genetically determined, with at least two identifiable groups, including rapid and slow acetylators (Evans et al, 1968). The difference is referred to as *genetic polymorphism*. Individuals with slow acetylation are prone to isoniazid-induced neurotoxicity. Procainamide and hydralazine are other drugs that are acetylated and demonstrate genetic polymorphism.

Another example of genetic differences in drug metabolism is glucose 6-phosphate-dehydrogenase deficiency, which is observed in approximately 10% of African Americans. A well-documented example of genetic polymorphism with this enzyme was observed with phenytoin (Wilkinson et al, 1989). Two phenotypes, extensive metabolizer (EM) and poor metabolizer (PM), were identified in the study population. The PM frequency in Caucasians was about 4% and in Japanese subjects was about 16%. Variation in metabolic rate was also observed with mephobarbital. The incidence of side effects was higher in Japanese subjects, possibly due to a slower oxidative metabolism. Variations in omeprazole metabolism due to genetic differences on CYP2C19 were also reported (Uno et al, 2007).

Besides genetic influence, the basal level of enzyme activity may be altered by environmental factors and exposure to chemicals. Shorter theophylline elimination half-life due to smoking was observed in smokers. Apparently, the aromatic hydrocarbons, such as benzopyrene, that are released during smoking stimulate the enzymes involved in theophylline metabolism. Young children are also known to eliminate theophylline more quickly. Phenobarbital is a potent inducer of a wider variety of hepatic enzymes. Polycyclic hydrocarbons such as 3-methylcholanthrene and benzopyrene also induce hepatic enzyme formation. These compounds are carcinogenic.

Hepatic enzyme activity may also be inhibited by a variety of agents including carbon monoxide, heavy metals, and certain imidazole drugs such as cimetidine. Enzyme inhibition by cimetidine may lead to higher plasma levels and longer elimination of coadministered phenytoin or theophylline. The physiologic condition of the host—including age, gender, nutrition, diet, and pathophysiology—also affects the level of hepatic enzyme activities.

## Genetic Variation of CYP Enzymes

The most important enzymes accounting for variation in phase I metabolism of drugs are the cytochrome (CYP) enzymes, which exist in many forms among individuals because of genetic differences (May, 1994; Tucker, 1994; Parkinson, 1996; see also Chapter 21). Initially, the CYP enzymes were identified according to the substrate that was biotransformed. Nowadays, the genes encoding many of these enzymes have been identified. Multiforms of CYP enzymes are classified into families (originally denoted by Roman numerals I, II, III, etc) and subfamilies (denoted by A, B, C, etc) based on the similarity of the amino acid sequences of the isozymes. If an isozyme amino acid sequence is 60% similar or more, it is placed within a family. Within the family, isozymes with amino acid sequences of 70% or more similarity are placed into a subfamily, and an Arabic number follows for further classification. Further information on the CYP enzymes including drug interactions, classification, table of substrates, inhibitors, and inducers have been published by Nelson (2009) and the US FDA Guidance for Industry, 2020. The CYP3A subfamily of CYP3 appears to be responsible for the metabolism of a large number of structurally diverse endogenous agents (eg, testosterone, cortisol, progesterone, estradiol) and xenobiotics (eg, nifedipine, lovastatin, midazolam, terfenadine, erythromycin).

The substrate specificities of the CYP enzymes appear to be due to the nature of the amino acid residues, the size of the amino acid side chain, and the polarity and charge of the amino acids (Negishi et al, 1996). The individual gene is denoted by an Arabic number (last number) after the subfamily. For example, CYP 1A2 (CYP1A2) is involved in the oxidation of caffeine and CYP2D6 is involved in the oxidation of drugs, such as codeine, propranolol, and dextromethorphan. The well-known CYP2D6 is responsible for debrisoquine metabolism among individuals showing genetic polymorphism. The vinca alkaloids used in cancer treatment have shown great inter- and intraindividual variabilities. CYP3A enzymes are known to be involved in the metabolism of vindesine, vinblastine, and other vinca alkaloids (Rahmani and Zhou, 1993). Failing to recognize variations in drug excretion in cancer chemotherapy may result in greater toxicity or even therapeutic failure.

There are now at least eight families of CYP enzymes known in humans and animals. CYP 1–3 are best known for metabolizing clinically useful drugs in humans. Variation in isozyme distribution and content in the hepatocytes may affect the hepatic excretion of a drug. The levels and activities of the CYP enzymes differ among individuals as a result of genetic and environmental factors. Clinically, it is important to look for evidence of unusual metabolic profiles in patients before dosing. Pharmacokinetic experiments using a "marker" drug such as the antipyrine or dextromethorphan may be used to determine if the hepatic ability at excreting drugs of the patient is significantly different from that of an average subject.

The metabolism of debrisoquin is polymorphic in the population, with some individuals having extensive metabolism (EM) and other individuals having poor metabolism (PM). Those individuals who are PM lack functional CYP2D6. In EM individuals, quinidine will block CYP2D6 so that genotypic EM individuals appear to be phenotypic PM individuals (Caraco et al, 1996). Some drugs metabolized by CYP2D6 are codeine, flecainide, dextromethorphan, imipramine, and other cyclic antidepressants that undergo ring hydroxylation. The inability to metabolize substrates for CYP2D6 results in increased plasma concentrations of the parent drug in PM individuals.

## Drug Interactions Involving Drug Metabolism

The enzymes involved in the metabolism of drugs may be altered by diet and the coadministration of other drugs and chemicals. *Enzyme induction* is a drug- or chemical-stimulated increase in enzyme activity, usually due to an increase in the amount of enzyme present. Enzyme induction usually requires some onset time for the synthesis of enzyme protein. For example, rifampin induction occurs within 2 days, while phenobarbital induction takes about 1 week to occur. Enzyme (eg, CYP3A) induction for carbamazepine becomes to be clinically significant after 3 to 5 days and is not complete for approximately 1 month or longer. It will also change every time the carbamazepine dose is adjusted, as it needs to be adjusted as it induces its own metabolism. Smoking can change the rate of metabolism of many cyclic antidepressant drugs (CAD) through enzyme induction (Toney and Ereshefsky, 1995). It was recently found that both marijuana and tobacco smoking induce cytochrome P450 (CYP) 1A2 through activation of the aromatic hydrocarbon receptor, and the induction effect between the two products is additive (Anderson and Chan, 2016). Agents that induce enzymes include aromatic hydrocarbons (such as benzopyrene, found in cigarette smoke), insecticides (such as chlordane), and drugs such as carbamazepine, rifampin, and phenobarbital. *Enzyme inhibition* may be due to substrate competition or due to direct inhibition of drug-metabolizing enzymes, particularly one of several of the CYP enzymes. Many widely prescribed antidepressants generally known as selective serotonin reuptake inhibitors (SSRIs) have been reported to inhibit the CYP2D6 system, resulting in significantly elevated plasma concentration of coadministered psychotropic drugs. Fluoxetine causes a 10-fold decrease in the elimination of imipramine and desipramine because of its inhibitory effect on hydroxylation (Toney and Ereshefsky, 1995).

A few clinical examples of enzyme inhibitors and inducers are listed in Table 6-7. Diet also affects drug-metabolizing enzymes. For example, plasma theophylline concentrations and theophylline clearance in patients on a high-protein diet are lower than in subjects whose diets are high in carbohydrates. Sucrose or glucose plus fructose decrease the activity of mixed-function oxidases, an effect related to a slower metabolism rate and a prolongation in hexobarbital sleeping time in rats. Chronic administration of 5% glucose was suggested to affect sleeping time in subjects receiving barbiturates. A decreased intake of fatty acids may lead to decreased basal MFO activities (Campbell, 1977) and affect the rate of drug metabolism.

The protease inhibitor saquinavir mesylate (Invirase®, Roche) has very low bioavailability—only about 4%. In studies conducted by Hoffmann-La Roche, the area under the curve (AUC) of saquinavir was increased to 150% when the volunteers took a 150-mL glass of grapefruit juice with the saquinavir, and then another 150-mL glass an hour later. Concentrated grapefruit juice increased the AUC up to 220%. Grapefruit juice, was found to be responsible for the inhibition of saquinavir metabolism by CYP3A4, present in the liver and the intestinal

## TABLE 6-7 • Examples of Drug Interactions Affecting Mixed Function Oxidase Enzymes

| Inhibitors of Drug Metabolism | Example | Result |
|---|---|---|
| Acetaminophen | Ethanol | Increased hepatotoxicity in chronic alcoholics |
| Cimetidine | Warfarin | Prolongation of prothrombin time |
| Erythromycin | Carbamazepine | Decreased carbazepine clearance |
| Fluoxetine | Imipramine (IMI) | Decreased clearance of CAD |
| Fluoxetine | Desipramine (DMI) | Decreased clearance of CAD |
| **Inducers of Drug Metabolism** | **Example** | **Result** |
| Carbamazepine | Acetaminophen | Increased acetaminophen metabolism |
| Rifampin | Methadone | Increased methadone metabolism, may precipitate opiate withdrawal |
| Phenobarbital | Dexamethasone | Decreased dexamethasone elimination half-life |
| Rifampin | Prednisolone | Increased elimination of prednisolone |

wall, which metabolizes saquinavir, resulting in an increase in its AUC. Ketoconazole and ranitidine (Zantac‡) may also increase the AUC of saquinavir by inhibition of the CYP enzymes. In contrast, rifampin greatly reduces the AUC of saquinavir, apparently due to enzymatic stimulation. Other drugs recently shown to have increased bioavailability when taken with grapefruit juice include several sedatives and the anticoagulant coumarin (Table 6-8). Increases in drug levels may be dangerous, and the pharmacokinetics of drugs with potential interactions should be closely monitored. More complete tabulations of CYP enzymes are available (Flockhart, 2021; Parkinson, 1996; Cupp and Tracy, 1998); some examples are given in Table 6-9.

### Auto-Inhibition or Auto-Induction and Time-Dependent Pharmacokinetics

Many drugs inhibit or enhance the activity of CYP enzymes and thereby change their own metabolism (*auto-inhibition* or *auto-induction*) or the metabolism of other compounds. When assessing inhibition or induction, the enzyme activity is usually measured before and after a period of treatment with the inhibiting or inducing agent. Thus, the inhibition or induction magnitude of various CYP enzymes is well known for several inhibiting or inducing agents.

The *time-dependent pharmacokinetics* have been described with a model where the production rates of the affected enzymes were reverse proportional or proportional to the amounts of the inhibiting or inducing agents and the time course of the inhibition or induction process was described by the turnover model. Examples of drugs with time-dependent pharmacokinetics are omeprazole and carbamazepine.

For new drugs, the potential for drug metabolism/interaction is studied *in vitro* and/or *in vivo* by

## TABLE 6-8 • Change in Drug Availability Due to Oral Coadministration of Grapefruit Juice

| Drug | Study |
|---|---|
| Triazolam | Hukkinen et al, 1995 |
| Midazolam | Kupferschmidt et al, 1995 |
| Cyclosporine | Yee et al, 1995 |
| Coumarin | Merkel et al, 1994 |
| Nisoldipine | Bailey DG et al, 1993a |
| Felodipine | Bailey DG et al, 1993b |
| Nitrendipine | Soons PA et al, 1991 |
| Saquinavir | James JS, 1995 |
| Simvastatin | Lilja JJ et al, 1998 |
| Atorvastatin | Reddy P et al, 2011 |
| Lovastatin | Kantola T et al, 1998 |

**TABLE 6-9 •** CYP Enzymes and Examples of Substrates, Inhibitors, and Inducers

| | |
|---|---|
| CYP1A2 | Substrates—amitriptyline, imipramine, theophylline (other enzymes also involved);<br>Sensitive index substrates—caffeine, tizanidine*;<br>induced by smoking<br>Fluvoxamine, cimetidine are inhibitors<br>Strong index inhibitors—fluvoxamine* |
| CYP2B6 | Substrates—cyclophosphamide, methadone |
| CYP2C9 | Metabolism of S-warfarin and tolbutamide by CYP2C9<br>Substrates—NSAIDs—ibuprofen, diclofenac<br>Sensitive index substrates—tolbutamide, S-warfarin* |
| CYP2C19 | Substrate—Omeprazole, S-mephenytoin, and propranolol<br>Sensitive index substrates—lansoprazole, omeprazole*<br>Diazepam (mixed), and imipramine (mixed)<br>Inhibitors: cimetidine, fluoxetine, and ketoconazole<br>Strong index inhibitors—fluvoxamine* |
| CYP2D6 | Many antidepressants, β-blockers are metabolized by CYP2D6<br>SRIIs, cimetidine are inhibitors<br>Substrates—amitriptyline, imipramine, fluoxetine, antipsychotics (haloperidol, thioridazine)<br>Sensitive index substrates—desipramine, dextromethorphan, nebivolol*<br>Inhibitors—paroxetine, fluoxetine, sertraline, fluvoxamine, cimetidine, haloperidol<br>Strong index inhibitors—fluvoxamine, paroxetine* |
| CYP2E1 | Substrates—acetaminophen, ethanol, halothane<br>Induced by INH and disulfiram |
| CYP3A4, 5, 7 | CYP3A subfamilies are the most abundant cytochrome enzymes in humans and include many key therapeutic and miscellaneous groups:<br>    Ketoconazole, atorvastatin, lovastatin<br>    Azithromycin, clarithromycin, amitriptyline<br>    Benzodiazepines—alprazolam, triazolam, midazolam<br>    Calcium blockers—verapamil, diltiazam<br>    Protease inhibitors—ritonavir, saquinavir, indinavir<br>Sensitive index substrates—midazolam, triazolam*<br>Strong index inhibitors—clarithromycin, itraconazole*<br>Strong Inducers—phenytoin, rifampin* |

Data from Flockhart (2003), Cupp and Tracy (1998), and Desta et al (2002).
*Examples based on FDA Guidance for Industry: In Vitro Drug Interaction Studies —Cytochrome P450 Enzyme- and Transporter-Mediated Drug Interactions (January, 2020) and FDA: Drug development and drug interactions |Tables of Substrates, Inhibitors and Inducers (https://www.fda.gov/drugs/drug-interactions-labeling/drug-development-and-drug-interactions-table-substrates-inhibitors-and-inducers).

identifying whether the drug is a substrate for the common CYP enzyme subfamilies (FDA Guidance for Industry, 1999, 2006, 2020). An understanding of the mechanistic basis of metabolic drug–drug interactions enables the prediction of whether the coadministration of two or more drugs may have clinical consequences affecting safety and efficacy. In practice, an investigational drug under development is coadministered with an approved drug (interacting drug), which utilizes similar CYP pathways.

Examples of substrates include (1) midazolam for CYP3A, (2) caffeine for CYP1A2, (3) repaglinide for CYP2C8, (4) warfarin for CYP2C9 (with the evaluation of S-warfarin), (5) omeprazole for CYP2C19, and (6) desipramine for CYP2D6. Additional examples of substrates, along with inhibitors and inducers of specific CYP enzymes, are available on the FDA's website on Drug Development and Drug Interactions.

Since metabolism usually occurs in the liver (some enzymes such as CYP3A4 are also important in gut metabolism), human liver microsomes provide a convenient way to study CYP enzyme metabolism. Microsomes are a subcellular fraction of tissue obtained by differential high-speed centrifugation. The key CYP enzymes are collected in the microsomal fraction. The CYP enzymes retain their activity for many years in microsomes or whole liver stored at low temperature. Hepatic microsomes can be obtained commercially, with or without prior phenotyping, for most important CYP enzymes. The cDNAs for the common CYPs have been cloned, and the recombinant human enzymatic proteins have been expressed in a variety of cells. These recombinant enzymes provide an excellent way to confirm results using microsomes. Pharmacokinetic endpoints recommended for assessment of the substrate are (1) exposure measures such as AUC, $C_{max}$, time to $C_{max}$ ($T_{max}$), and others as appropriate; and (2) pharmacokinetic parameters such as clearance, volumes of distribution, and half-lives (FDA Guidance for Industry, Clinical Drug Interaction Studies—Cytochrome P450 Enzyme- and Transporter-Mediated Drug Interactions, 2020). For metabolism induction studies, *in vivo* studies are more relied upon because enzyme induction may not be well predicted from *in vitro* results. Considerations in drug-metabolizing/interaction studies include (1) acute or chronic use of the substrate and/or interacting drug; (2) safety considerations, including whether a drug is likely to be a narrow therapeutic range (NTR) or non-NTR drug; (3) pharmacokinetic and pharmacodynamic characteristics of the substrate and interacting drugs; and (4) the need to assess induction as well as inhibition. The inhibiting/inducing drugs and the substrates should be dosed so that the exposures of both drugs are relevant to their clinical use.

## Transporter-Mediated Drug–Drug Interactions

Transporter-mediated interactions have been increasingly documented. Examples include the inhibition or induction of transport proteins, such as P-glycoprotein (P-gp), organic anion transporter (OAT), organic anion transporting polypeptide (OATP), organic cation transporter (OCT), multidrug resistance–associated proteins (MRP), and breast cancer–resistant protein (BCRP). Examples of transporter-based interactions include the interactions between digoxin and quinidine, fexofenadine and ketoconazole (or erythromycin), penicillin and probenecid, and dofetilide and cimetidine. Of the various transporters, P-gp is the most well understood and may be appropriate to evaluate during drug development. Table 6-10 lists some of the major human transporters and known substrates, inhibitors, and inducers.

Some hepatic transporters in the liver include P-gp and OATPs (Huang et al, 2009). When a transporter is known to play a major role in translocating drug in and out of cells and organelles within the liver, the simple hepatic clearance model that we will see in Chapter 15 may not adequately describe the pharmacokinetics of the drug within the liver. Micro constants may be needed to describe how the drug moves kinetically in and out within a group of cells or compartment. Canalicular transporters are present for many drugs. Biliary excretion should also be incorporated into the model as needed. For this reason, local drug concentration in the liver may be very high, leading to serious liver toxicity. Huang et al (2009) have discussed the importance of drug transporters, drug disposition, and how to study drug interaction for the new drugs.

Knowledge of drug transporters and CYPs can help predict whether many drug interactions have clinical significance. Pharmacists should realize that the combined effect of efflux and CYP inhibition can cause serious or even fatal adverse reaction due to severalfold increase in AUC or $C_{max}$. Impairment of bile flow, saturation of conjugation enzymes (phase II) such as glucuronide, and sulfate conjugate formation can lead to adverse toxicity.

## TABLE 6-10 • Major Human Transporters and Known Substrates, Inhibitors, and Inducers

| Gene | Protein Name | Tissue | Drug Substrate | Inhibitor | Inducer |
|------|-------------|--------|----------------|-----------|---------|
| ABCB1 | P-gp, MDR1 | Intestine, liver, kidney, brain, placenta, adrenal, testes | Digoxin, fexofenadine, indinavir, vincristine, colchicine, topotecan, paclitaxel | Ritonavir, cyclosporine, verapamil, erythromycin, ketoconazole, itraconazole, quinidine, elacridar (GF120918) LY335979 valspodar (PSC833) | Rifampin, St John's wort |
| ABCB4 | MDR3 | Liver | Digoxin, paclitaxel, vinblastine | | |
| ABCB11 | BSEP | Liver | Vinblastine | | |
| ABCC1 | MRP1 | Intestine, liver, kidney, brain | Adefovir, indinavir | | |
| ABCC2 | MRP2, CMOAT | Intestine, liver, kidney, brain | Indinavir, cisplatin | Cyclosporine | |
| ABCC3 | MRP3, CMOAT2 | Intestine, liver, kidney, placenta, adrenal | Etoposide, methotrexate, tenoposide | | |
| ABCC4 | MRP4 | | | | |
| ABCC5 | MRP5 | | | | |
| ABCC6 | MRP6 | Liver, kidney | Cisplatin, daunorubicin | | |
| ABCG2 | BCRP | Intestine, liver, breast, placenta | Daunorubicin, doxorubicin, topotecan, rosuvastatin, sulfasalazine | Elacridar (GFl20918), gefitinib | |
| SLCOIB1 | OATP1B1, OATP-C, OATP2 | Liver | Rifampin, rosuvastatin, methotrexate, pravastatin, thyroxine | Cyclosporine, rifampin | |
| SLCOIB3 | OATP1B3, OATP8 | Liver | Digoxin, methotrexate, rifampin, | | |
| SLCO2B1 | SLC21A9, OATP-B | Intestine, liver, kidney, brain | Pravastatin | | |
| SLC1OA1 | NTCP | Liver, pancreas | Rosuvastatin | | |

Reproduced with permission from FDA Guidance for Industry: In Vitro Metabolism and Transporter-Mediated Drug-Drug Interaction Studies (draft guidance, October 2017).

## CLINICAL EXAMPLE

Digoxin is an MDR1/P-gp substrate.

1.  Which of the following sites is important to influence on the plasma levels of digoxin after oral administration?

    a.  Hepatocyte (canalicular)

    b.  Hepatocyte (sinusoidal)

    c.  Intestinal enterocyte

2.  Ritonavir and quinidine are examples of P-gp inhibitors. What changes in AUC or $C_{max}$ would you expect for digoxin when coadministered with either one of these two inhibitors?

3.  Using your knowledge of drug transporters and their substrate inhibitors, can you determine whether the above change in digoxin plasma level is due to a change in metabolism or distribution?

## Solution

1. According to Table 6-10, MDR1 is an efflux transporter for digoxin in the liver (canaliculi) and intestine (enterocytes). Digoxin is also a substrate for MDR3, SLCO1B1, and other transporters. MDR1 is inhibited by quinidine and ritonavir.

2. Literature search shows that digoxin transport by P-gp occurs in the intestine and in the liver canaliculi and P-gp will interact with ritonavir or quinidine with coadministration (both are inhibitors of MDR1). Inhibition of efflux will increase the plasma level of digoxin. Other effects may also occur since most transport inhibitors are not 100% specific and may affect metabolism/disposition in other ways.

3. The package insert should be consulted on drug distribution and drug interaction. A pharmacist should realize that although either one of the two inhibitors can increase AUC of digoxin (by 1.5–2 *fold*) in this hypothetical case, in reality, a comprehensive evaluation of pharmacokinetics and pharmacodynamics of the drug doses involved and the medical profile of the patient is needed to determine if an interaction is clinically significant.

## TABLE 6-11 • Examples of Drugs Undergoing Enterohepatic Circulation and Biliary Excretion

| Enterohepatic Circulation | |
| --- | --- |
| Imipramine | |
| Indomethacin | |
| Morphine | |
| Pregnenolone | |
| **Biliary Excretion (intact or as metabolites)** | |
| Cefamandole | Fluvastatin |
| Cefoperazone | Lovastatin |
| Chloramphenicol | Moxalactam |
| Diazepam | Practolol |
| Digoxin | Spironolactone |
| Doxorubicin | Testosterone |
| Doxycycline | Tetracycline |
| Estradiol | Vincristine |

## FIRST-PASS EFFECTS

For some drugs, the route of administration affects the metabolic rate of the compound. For example, a drug given parenterally, transdermally, or by inhalation may distribute within the body prior to metabolism by the liver. In contrast, drugs given orally are normally absorbed in the duodenal segment of the small intestine and transported via the mesenteric vessels to the hepatic portal vein and then to the liver before entering the systemic circulation. Drugs that are highly metabolized by the liver or by the intestinal mucosal cells demonstrate poor systemic availability when given orally. This rapid metabolism of an orally administered drug before reaching the general circulation is termed *first-pass effect* or *presystemic elimination*.

First-pass effects may be suspected when there are relatively low concentrations of parent (or intact) drug in the systemic circulation after oral compared to intravenous administration. In such a case, the AUC for a drug given orally also is less than the AUC for the same dose of drug given intravenously. From experimental findings in animals, first-pass effects may be assumed if the intact drug appears in a cannulated hepatic portal vein but not in general circulation. The absolute bioavailability may reveal evidence of drug being removed due to hepatic first-pass effect (see Chapter 15 for details).

## BILIARY EXCRETION OF DRUGS

The biliary system of the liver is an important system for the secretion of bile and the excretion of drugs. Anatomically, the intrahepatic bile ducts join outside the liver to form the common hepatic duct (Fig. 6-8). The bile that enters the gallbladder becomes highly concentrated. The hepatic duct, containing hepatic bile, joins the cystic duct that drains the gallbladder to form the common bile duct. The common bile duct then empties into the duodenum. Bile consists primarily of water, bile salts, bile pigments, electrolytes, and, to a lesser extent, cholesterol and fatty acids. The hepatic cells lining the bile canaliculi are responsible for the production of bile. The production of bile appears to be an active secretion process. Separate active biliary secretion processes have been reported for organic

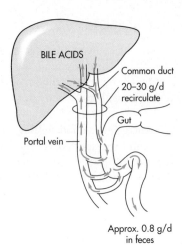

BILE ACIDS

Common duct
20–30 g/d
recirculate

Gut

Portal vein

Approx. 0.8 g/d
in feces

FIGURE 6-8 • Enterohepatic recirculation of bile acids and drug.

anions, organic cations, and for polar, uncharged molecules.

Drugs that are excreted mainly in the bile have MWs in excess of 500. Drugs with MWs between 300 and 500 are excreted both in urine and in bile. For these drugs, a decrease in one excretory route results in a compensatory increase in excretion via the other route. Compounds with MWs of less than 300 are excreted almost exclusively via the kidneys into urine.

In addition to relatively high MW, drugs excreted into bile usually require a strongly polar group. Many drugs excreted into bile are metabolites, very often glucuronide conjugates. Most metabolites are more polar than the parent drug. In addition, the formation of a glucuronide increases the MW of the compound by nearly 200, as well as increasing the polarity.

Drugs excreted into the bile include the digitalis glycosides, bile salts, cholesterol, steroids, and indomethacin (Table 6-11). Compounds that enhance bile production stimulate the biliary excretion of drugs normally eliminated by this route. Furthermore, phenobarbital, which induces many mixed-function oxidase activities, may stimulate the biliary excretion of drugs by two mechanisms: by an increase in the formation of the glucuronide metabolite and by an increase in bile flow. In contrast, compounds that decrease bile flow or pathophysiologic conditions that cause cholestasis decrease biliary

drug excretion. The route of administration may also influence the amount of the drug excreted into bile. For example, drugs given orally may be extracted by the liver into the bile to a greater extent than the same drugs given intravenously.

### Estimation of Biliary Clearance

In animals, bile duct cannulation allows both the volume of the bile and the concentration of drug in the bile to be measured directly using a special intubation technique that blocks off a segment of the gut with an inflating balloon. *Biliary clearance*, $CL_{biliary}$, is a measure of drug removal by biliary secretion (see Chapter 15 for CL calculations). $CL_{biliary}$ may be measured by monitoring the amount of drug secreted into the GI perfusate.

Assuming an average bile flow of 0.5 to 0.8 mL/min in humans, biliary excretion can be calculated if the bile concentration, $C_{bile}$, is known.

$$CL_{biliary} = \frac{\text{bile flow} \times C_{bile}}{C_p} \qquad (6.1)$$

Alternatively, using the perfusion technique, the amount of drug eliminated in bile is determined from the GI perfusate, and $CL_{biliary}$ may be calculated without the bile flow rate, as follows:

$$CL_{biliary} = \frac{\text{amount of drug secreted from bile per minute}}{C_p}$$

$$(6.2)$$

To avoid any complication of unabsorbed drug in the feces, the drug should be given by parenteral administration (eg, intravenously) during biliary determination experiments. The amount of drug in the GI perfusate recovered periodically may be determined. The extent of biliary elimination of digoxin has been determined in humans using this approach.

### Enterohepatic Circulation

A drug or its metabolite is secreted into bile and upon contraction of the gallbladder is excreted into the duodenum via the common bile duct. Subsequently, the drug or its metabolite may be excreted into the feces or the drug may be reabsorbed and become systemically available. The cycle in which the drug is absorbed, excreted into the bile, and reabsorbed is known as *enterohepatic circulation*. Some drugs excreted as a glucuronide conjugate become hydrolyzed in the gut back to the parent drug by the action of a $\beta$-glucuronidase enzyme present in the intestinal bacteria. In this case, the parent drug becomes available for reabsorption. Enterohepatic circulation results in a long half-life of parent drug. An example drug is obeticholic acid (OCA).

## Significance of Biliary Excretion

When a drug appears in the feces after oral administration, it is difficult to determine whether this presence of drug is due to biliary excretion or incomplete absorption. If the drug is given parenterally and then observed in the feces, one can conclude that some of the drug was excreted in the bile. Because drug secretion into bile is an active process, this process can be saturated with high drug concentrations. Moreover, other drugs may compete for the same carrier system.

Enterohepatic circulation after a single dose of drug is not as important as after multiple doses or a very high dose of drug. With a large dose or multiple doses, a larger amount of drug is secreted in the bile, from which drug may then be reabsorbed. This reabsorption process may affect the absorption and elimination rate constants. Furthermore, the biliary secretion process may become saturated, thus altering the plasma level–time curve.

Drugs that undergo enterohepatic circulation sometimes show a small secondary peak in the plasma drug–concentration curve. The first peak occurs as the drug in the GI tract is depleted; a small secondary peak then emerges as biliary-excreted drug is reabsorbed. In experimental studies involving animals, bile duct cannulation provides a means of estimating the amount of drug excreted through the bile. In humans, a less accurate estimation of biliary excretion may be made from the recovery of drug excreted through the feces. However, if the drug was given orally, some of the fecal drug excretion could represent unabsorbed drug.

## CLINICAL EXAMPLE

Leflunomide, an immunomodulator for rheumatoid arthritis, is metabolized to a major active metabolite and several minor metabolites. Approximately 48%

of the dose is eliminated in the feces due to high biliary excretion. The active metabolite is slowly eliminated from the plasma. In the case of serious adverse toxicity, the manufacturer recommends giving cholestyramine or activated charcoal orally to bind the active metabolite in the GI tract to prevent drug reabsorption and to facilitate drug elimination. The use of cholestyramine or activated charcoal reduces the plasma levels of the active metabolite by approximately 40% in 24 hours and by about 50% in 48 hours.

> ### FREQUENTLY ASKED QUESTIONS
>
> ▶ Please explain why many drugs with significant metabolism often have variable bioavailability.
>
> ▶ The metabolism of some drugs is affected more than others when there is a change in protein binding. Why?
>
> ▶ Give some examples that explain why the metabolic pharmacokinetics of drugs are important in patient care.

## ROLE OF TRANSPORTERS IN THE ELIMINATION OF DRUGS FROM THE LIVER

Patient variability and changes in the liver's ability to eliminate drugs may be due to (1) patient factors such as age and genetic polymorphism, (2) enzymatic induction or inhibition due to coadministered drugs, and (3) modification of influx and efflux transporters in the liver and the bile canaliculi. When a transporter is known to play a major role in translocating drug in and out of cells and organelles within the liver, the simple hepatic clearance model that we will see in Chapter 15 may not adequately describe the pharmacokinetics of the drug within the liver. Micro constants may be needed to describe how the drug moves kinetically in and out within a group of cells or compartment. Biliary excretion should also be incorporated into the model as needed. Since the development of the hepatic model is based on intrinsic clearance, much more information is now known about the interplay between transporters and strategically located CYP enzymes in the GI, the hepatocytes in various parts of the liver (see Figs. 6-2 and 6-3).

More elaborate models are now available to relate transporters to drug disposition. Huang et al (2009) discussed the importance of drug transporters, drug disposition, and how to study drug interaction of the new drugs. The interplay between transporters, drug permeability in GI, and hepatic drug extraction are important to the bioavailability and the extent of drug metabolism (see Chapter 15).

It appears that drugs may be classified in several classes to facilitate prediction of drug disposition. A drug substance is considered to be "highly permeable" when the extent of the absorption (parent drug plus metabolites) in humans is determined to be 90% of an administered dose based on a mass balance determination or in comparison to an intravenous reference dose. Drugs may be classified into four biopharmaceutical classification system (BCS) classes. With respect to oral bioavailability, Wu and Benet (2005) proposed categorizing drugs into the four classes based on solubility and permeability as criteria may provide significant new insights to predicting routes of elimination, effects of efflux, and absorptive transporters on oral absorption, when transporter–enzyme interplay will yield clinically significant effects such as low bioavailability and drug–drug interactions, the direction and importance of food effects, and transporter effects on post-absorption systemic levels following oral and intravenous dosing.

Figure 6-9 provides a good summary of how various physiologic and physiochemical factors influence drug disposition. For example, Class 1 drugs are not so much affected by transporters because absorption is generally good already due to high solubility and permeability. Class 2 drugs are very much affected by efflux transporters because of low solubility and high permeability. The limited amount of drug solubilized and absorbed could efflux back into the GI lumen due to efflux transporters, thus resulting in low plasma level. Further, efflux transporter may pump drug into bile if located in the liver canaliculi.

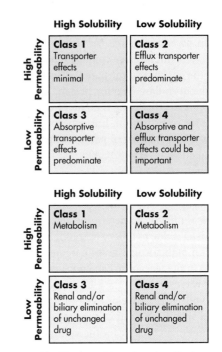

FIGURE 6-9 • Classification of Drugs Based on Biopharmaceutics Drug Disposition Classification System (BDDCS). (Data from Wu CY, Benet LZ. Predicting drug disposition via application of BCS: transport/absorption/ elimination interplay and development of a biopharmaceutics drug disposition classification system, *Pharm Res.* 2005 Jan;22(1):11–23.)

## THE KIDNEY AND RENAL ELIMINATION

The kidney is the main excretory organ for the removal of metabolic waste products and plays a major role in maintaining the normal fluid volume and electrolyte composition in the body. To maintain salt and water balance, the kidney excretes excess electrolytes, water, and waste products while conserving solutes necessary for proper body function. In addition, the kidney has two endocrine functions: (1) secretion of renin, which regulates blood pressure; and (2) secretion of erythropoietin, which stimulates red blood cell production.

### Anatomic Considerations

The kidneys are located in the peritoneal cavity. A general view is shown in Fig. 6-10 and a longitudinal view in Fig. 6-11. The outer zone of the kidney is called the *cortex*, and the inner region is called the *medulla*. The *nephrons* are the basic functional units, collectively responsible for the removal of metabolic waste and

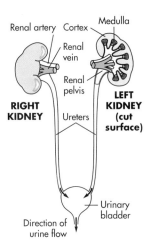

FIGURE 6-10 • The general organizational plan of the urinary system. (Reproduced with permission from Guyton AC: *Textbook of Medical Physiology*, 8th ed. Philadelphia, PA: Saunders; 1991.)

the maintenance of water and electrolyte balance. Each kidney contains 1 to 1.5 million nephrons. The *glomerulus* of each nephron starts in the cortex. *Cortical nephrons* have short *loops of Henle* that remain exclusively in the cortex; *juxtamedullary nephrons* have long loops of Henle that extend into the medulla (Fig. 6-12). The longer loops of Henle allow for a greater ability of the nephron to reabsorb water, thereby producing a more concentrated urine.

## Blood Supply

The kidneys represent about 0.5% of the total body weight and receive approximately 20% to 25% of the

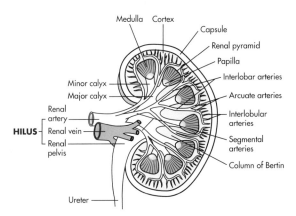

FIGURE 6-11 • Longitudinal section of the kidney, illustrating major anatomical features and blood vessels. (Reproduced with permission from West JB: *Best and Taylor's Physiological Basis of Medical Practice*, 11th ed. Baltimore, MA: Williams & Wilkins; 1985.)

cardiac output. The kidney is supplied by blood via the renal artery, which subdivides into the interlobar arteries penetrating within the kidney and branching farther into the afferent arterioles. Each afferent arteriole carries blood toward a single nephron into the glomerular portion of the nephron (*Bowman's capsule*). The filtration of blood occurs in the glomeruli in Bowman's capsule. From the capillaries (*glomerulus*) within Bowman's capsule, the blood flows out via the efferent arterioles and then into a second capillary network that surrounds the tubules (*peritubule capillaries* and *vasa recti*), including the loop of Henle, where some water is reabsorbed.

The *renal blood flow* (RBF) is the volume of blood flowing through the renal vasculature per unit of time. Renal blood flow exceeds 1.2 L/min or 1700 L/d. *Renal plasma flow* (RPF) is the renal blood flow minus the volume of red blood cells present. Renal plasma flow is an important factor in the rate of drug filtration at the glomerulus.

$$RPF = RBF - (RBF \times Hct) \qquad (6.3)$$

where Hct is the *hematocrit*.

Hct is the fraction of blood cells in the blood, about 0.45 or 45% of the total blood volume. The relationship of renal blood flow to renal plasma flow is given by a rearrangement of Equation 6.26:

$$RPF = RBF (1 - Hct) \qquad (6.4)$$

Assuming a hematocrit of 0.45 and a RBF of 1.2 L/min and using the above equation, RPF = $1.2 - (1.2 \times 0.45) = 0.66$ L/min or 660 mL/min, approximately 950 L/d. The average *glomerular filtration rate* (GFR) is about 120 mL/min in an average adult,[1] or about 20% of the RPF. The ratio GFR/RPF is the *filtration fraction*.

## Regulation of Renal Blood Flow

Blood flow to an organ is directly proportional to the arteriovenous pressure difference (*perfusion pressure*) across the vascular bed and indirectly proportional to the vascular resistance. The normal renal arterial pressure (Fig. 6-13) is approximately 100 mm Hg and falls to approximately 45 to 60 mm Hg in the

---

[1]GFR is often based on average body surface, 1.73 m². GFR is less in women and also decreases with age.

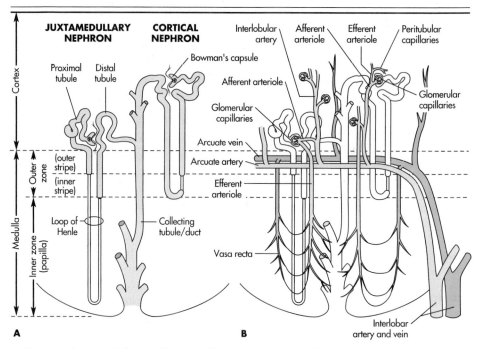

**FIGURE 6-12** • Cortical and juxtamedullary nephrons and their vasculature. (Reproduced with permission from West JB: *Best and Taylor's Physiological Basis of Medical Practice*, 11th ed. Baltimore, MA: Williams & Wilkins; 1985.)

glomerulus (glomerular capillary hydrostatic pressure). This pressure difference is probably due to the increasing vasculature resistance provided by the small diameters of the capillary network. Thus, the GFR is controlled by changes in the glomerular capillary hydrostatic pressure.

In the normal kidney, RPF and GFR remain relatively constant even with large differences in mean systemic blood pressure (Fig. 6-14). The term *autoregulation* refers to the maintenance of a

**FIGURE 6-13** • Approximate pressures at different points in the vessels and tubules of the functional nephron and in the interstitial fluid. (Reproduced with permission from Guyton AC: *Textbook of Medical Physiology*, 8th ed. Philadelphia, PA: Saunders; 1991.)

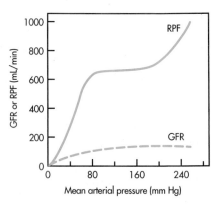

**FIGURE 6-14** • Schematic representation of the effect of mean arterial pressure on GFR and RPF, illustrating the phenomenon of autoregulation. (Reproduced with permission from West JB: *Best and Taylor's Physiological Basis of Medical Practice*, 11th ed. Baltimore, MA: Williams & Wilkins; 1985.)

constant blood flow in the presence of large fluctuations in arterial blood pressure. Because autoregulation maintains a relatively constant blood flow, the filtration fraction (GFR/RPF) also remains fairly constant in this pressure range.

## Glomerular Filtration and Urine Formation

A normal adult male subject has a GFR of approximately 120 mL/min. About 180 L of fluid per day is filtered through the kidneys. In spite of this large filtration volume, the average urine volume is 1 to 1.5 L. Up to 99% of the fluid volume filtered at the glomerulus is reabsorbed. Besides fluid regulation, the kidney also regulates the retention or excretion of various solutes and electrolytes (Table 6-12). With the exception of proteins and protein-bound substances, most small molecules are filtered through the glomerulus from the plasma. The filtrate contains some ions, glucose, and essential nutrients as well as waste products, such as urea, phosphate, sulfate, and other substances. The essential nutrients and water are reabsorbed at various sites, including the proximal tubule, loops of Henle, and distal tubules. Both active reabsorption and secretion mechanisms are involved. The urine volume is reduced, and the urine generally contains a high concentration of metabolic wastes and eliminated drug products. Advances

in molecular biology have shown that transporters such as P-gp and other efflux proteins are present in the kidney and can influence urinary drug excretion. Further, CYP enzymes are also present in the kidney and can impact drug clearance by metabolism.

## Renal Drug Excretion

Renal excretion is a major route of elimination for many drugs. Drugs that are nonvolatile, water soluble, have a low MW, or are slowly biotransformed by the liver are eliminated by renal excretion. The processes by which a drug is excreted via the kidneys may include any combination of the following:

- Glomerular filtration
- Active tubular secretion
- Tubular reabsorption

*Glomerular filtration* is a unidirectional process that occurs for most small molecules (MW < 500), including undissociated (nonionized) and dissociated (ionized) drugs. Protein-bound drugs behave as large molecules and do not get filtered at the glomerulus. The major driving force for glomerular filtration is the hydrostatic pressure within the glomerular capillaries. The kidneys receive a large blood supply (approximately 25% of the cardiac output)

## TABLE 6-12 • Quantitative Aspects of Urine Formation*

| Substance | PER 24 HOURS | | | | |
|---|---|---|---|---|---|
| | Filtered | Reabsorbed | Secreted | Excreted | Percent Reabsorbed |
| Sodium ion (mEq) | 26,000 | 25,850 | | 150 | 99.4 |
| Chloride ion (mEq) | 18,000 | 17,850 | | 150 | 99.2 |
| Bicarbonate ion (mEq) | 4,900 | 4,900 | | 0 | 100 |
| Urea (mM) | 870 | 460† | | 410 | 53 |
| Glucose (mM) | 800 | 800 | | 0 | 100 |
| Water (mL) | 180,000 | 179,000 | | 1000 | 99.4 |
| Hydrogen ion | | | Variable | Variable‡ | |
| Potassium ion (mEq) | 900 | 900§ | 100 | 100 | 100d |

*Quantity of various plasma constituents filtered, reabsorbed, and excreted by a normal adult on an average diet.
†Urea diffuses into, as well as out of, some portions of the nephron.
‡pH or urine is on the acid side (4.5–6.9) when all bicarbonate is reabsorbed.
§Potassium ion is almost completely reabsorbed before it reaches the distal nephron. The potassium ion in the voided urine is actively secreted into the urine in the distal tubule in exchange for sodium ion.
Data from Levine WG. Biliary excretion of drugs and other xenobiotics, Prog Drug Res. 1981;25:361–420.

via the renal artery, with very little decrease in the hydrostatic pressure.

*Glomerular filtration rate* (GFR) is measured by using a drug that is eliminated primarily by filtration only (ie, the drug is neither reabsorbed nor secreted). Clinically inulin and creatinine are often used for this purpose, although creatinine is also secreted. The clearance of inulin is approximately equal to the GFR, which is approximately equal to 120mL/min in an adult subject with normal renal function. The value for the GFR correlates fairly well with body surface area. Glomerular filtration of drugs is directly related to the free or nonprotein-bound drug concentration in the plasma. As the free drug concentration in the plasma increases, the glomerular filtration for the drug increases proportionately, thus increasing renal drug elimination for some drugs.

*Active tubular secretion* is an active transport process. As such, active renal secretion is a carrier-mediated system that requires energy input, because the drug is transported against a concentration gradient. The carrier system is capacity limited and may be saturated. Drugs with similar structures may compete for the same carrier system. Two active renal secretion systems have been identified, systems for (1) weak acids (OAT) and (2) weak bases (organic cation transporter, OCT). For example, probenecid competes with penicillin for the same carrier system (*weak acids*). Active tubular secretion rate is dependent on renal plasma flow. Drugs commonly used to measure active tubular secretion include *p*-amino-hippuric acid (PAH) and iodopyracet (Diodrast). These substances are both filtered by the glomeruli and secreted by the tubular cells. Active secretion is extremely rapid for these drugs, and practically all the drug carried to the kidney is eliminated in a single pass. The clearance for these drugs therefore reflects the *effective renal plasma flow* (ERPF), which varies from 425 to 650 mL/min. The ERPF is determined by both RPF and the fraction of drug that is effectively extracted by the kidney relative to the concentration in the renal artery.

For a drug that is excreted solely by glomerular filtration, the elimination half-life may change markedly in accordance with the binding affinity of the drug for plasma proteins. In contrast, drug protein binding has very little effect on the elimination half-life of the drug excreted mostly by active secretion.

Because drug protein binding is reversible, drug bound to plasma protein rapidly dissociates as free drug is secreted by the kidneys. For example, some of the penicillins are extensively protein bound, but their elimination half-lives are short due to rapid elimination by active secretion.

*Tubular reabsorption* occurs after the drug is filtered through the glomerulus, and can be an active or a passive process involving transporting back into the plasma. If a drug is completely reabsorbed (eg, glucose), then the value for the clearance of the drug is approximately zero. For drugs that are partially reabsorbed without being secreted, clearance values are less than the GFR of 120 mL/min.

The reabsorption of drugs that are acids or weak bases is influenced by the pH of the fluid in the renal tubule (ie, urine pH) and the $pK_a$ of the drug. Both of these factors together determine the percentage of dissociated (ionized) and undissociated (nonionized) drug. Generally, the undissociated species is more lipid soluble (less water soluble) and has greater membrane permeability. The undissociated drug is easily reabsorbed from the renal tubule back into the body. This process of drug reabsorption can significantly reduce the amount of drug excreted, depending on the pH of the urinary fluid and the $pK_a$ of the drug. The $pK_a$ of the drug is a constant, but the normal urinary pH may vary from 4.5 to 8.0, depending on diet, pathophysiology, and drug intake. In addition, the initial morning urine is generally more acidic and becomes more alkaline later in the day. Vegetable and fruit diets (alkaline residue diet[2]) result in higher urinary pH, whereas diets rich in protein result in lower urinary pH. Drugs such as ascorbic acid and antacids such as sodium carbonate may decrease (acidify) or increase (alkalinize) the urinary pH, respectively, when administered in large quantities. By far the most important changes in urinary pH are caused by fluids administered intravenously. Intravenous fluids, such as solutions of bicarbonate or ammonium chloride, are used in acid–base therapy to alkalinize or acidify the urine,

---

[2]The alkaline residue diet (also known as the alkaline ash diet) is a diet composed of foods, such as fruits and vegetables, from which the carbohydrate portion of the diet is metabolized in the body leaving an alkaline residue containing cations such as sodium, potassium, calcium, etc. These cations are excreted through the kidney and cause the urine to become alkaline.

| TABLE 6-13 • Effect of Urinary pH and pK$_a$ on the Ionization of Drugs | | |
|---|---|---|
| pH of Urine | Percent of Drug Ionized: pK$_a$3 | Percent of Drug Ionized: pK$_a$5 |
| 7.4 | 100 | 99.6 |
| 5 | 99 | 50.0 |
| 4 | 91 | 9.1 |
| 3 | 50 | 0.99 |

respectively. Excretion of these solutions may drastically change urinary pH and alter drug reabsorption and drug excretion by the kidney.

The percentage of ionized weak acid drug corresponding to a given pH can be obtained from the *Henderson–Hasselbalch equation.*

$$pH = pKa + \log \text{(ionized)/(nonionized)} \quad (6.5)$$

Rearrangement of this equation yields:

$$\text{(ionized)/(nonionized)} = 10^{pH-pKa} \quad (6.6)$$

Fraction of drug ionized

$$= [\text{ionized}]/([\text{ionized}] + [\text{nonionized}])$$
$$= (10^{pH-pKa}) / (1 + 10^{pH-pKa}) \quad (6.7)$$

The fraction or percent of weak acid drug ionized in any pH environment may be calculated with Equation 6.7. For acidic drugs with pK$_a$ values from 3 to 8, a change in urinary pH affects the extent of dissociation (Table 6-13). The extent of dissociation is more greatly affected by changes in urinary pH for drugs with a pK$_a$ of 5 than with a pK$_a$ of 3. Weak acids with pK$_a$ values of less than 2 are highly ionized at all urinary pH values and are only slightly affected by pH variations.

For a weak base drug, the Henderson–Hasselbalch equation is given as

$$pH = pKa + \log \text{(nonionized)/(ionized)} \quad (6.8)$$

and

$$\text{Percent of drug ionized} = (10^{pKa-pH})/(1 + 10^{pKa-pH}) \quad (6.9)$$

The greatest effect of urinary pH on reabsorption occurs for weak base drugs with pK$_a$ values of 7.5 to 10.5.

From the Henderson–Hasselbalch relationship, a concentration ratio for the distribution of a weak acid or basic drug between urine and plasma may be derived. The urine–plasma (*U/P*) ratios for these drugs are as follows.

For weak acids,

$$U/P = (1 + 10^{pH_{urine}-pKa})/(1 + 10^{pH_{plasma}-pKa}) \quad (6.10)$$

For weak bases,

$$U/P = (1 + 10^{pKa-pH_{urine}})/(1 + 10^{pKa-pH_{plasma}}) \quad (6.11)$$

For example, amphetamine, a weak base, will be reabsorbed if the urine pH is made alkaline and more lipid-soluble nonionized species are formed. In contrast, acidification of the urine will cause the amphetamine to become more ionized (form a salt). The salt form is more water soluble, less likely to be reabsorbed, and tends to be excreted into the urine more quickly. In the case of weak acids (such as salicylic acid), acidification of the urine causes greater reabsorption of the drug and alkalinization of the urine causes more rapid excretion of the drug.

In summary, renal drug excretion is a composite of passive filtration at the glomerulus, active secretion in the proximal tubule and passive reabsorption in the distal tubule (Table 6-14). Active secretion is

| TABLE 6-14 • Properties of Renal Drug Elimination Processes | | | | | |
|---|---|---|---|---|---|
| Process | Active/Passive Transport | Location in Nephron | Drug Ionization | Drug Protein Binding | Influenced by |
| Filtration | Passive | Glomerulus | Either | Only free drug | Protein binding |
| Secretion | Active | Proximal tubule | Mostly weak acids and weak bases | No effect | Competitive inhibitors |
| Reabsorption | Passive | Distal tubule | Nonionized | Not applicable | Urinary pH and flow |

an enzyme (transporter)-mediated process that is saturable. Although reabsorption of drugs is mostly a passive process, the extent of reabsorption of weak acid or weak base drugs is influenced by the pH of the urine and the degree of ionization of the drug. In addition, an increase in blood flow to the kidney, which may be due to diuretic therapy or large alcohol consumption, decreases the extent of drug reabsorption in the kidney and increases the rate of drug excreted in the urine.

### Clinical Application

Both sulfisoxazole (Gantrisin) tablets and the combination product, sulfamethoxazole/trimethoprim (Bactrim) tablets, are used for urinary tract infections. Sulfisoxazole and sulfamethoxazole are sulfonamides that are well absorbed after oral administration and are excreted in high concentrations in the urine. Sulfonamides are N-acetylated to a less water-soluble metabolite. Both sulfonamides and their corresponding N-acetylated metabolite are less water soluble in acid and more soluble in alkaline conditions. In acid urine, renal toxicity can occur due to precipitation of the sulfonamides in the renal tubules. To prevent crystalluria and renal complications, patients are instructed to take these drugs with a high amount of fluid intake and to keep the urine alkaline.

---

#### FREQUENTLY ASKED QUESTION

▶ Which renal elimination processes are influenced by protein binding?

---

### PRACTICE PROBLEMS

Let $pK_a = 5$ for an acidic drug. Compare the $U/P$ at urinary pH **(a)** 3, **(b)** 5, and **(c)** 7.

**Solution**

**a.** At pH = 3,

$$\frac{U}{P} = \frac{1+10^{3-5}}{1+10^{7.4-5}} = \frac{1.01}{1+10^{2.4}} = \frac{1.01}{252} = \frac{1}{252}$$

**b.** At pH = 5,

$$\frac{U}{P} = \frac{1+10^{5-5}}{1+10^{7.4-5}} = \frac{2}{1+10^{2.4}} = \frac{2}{252}$$

**c.** At pH = 7,

$$\frac{U}{P} = \frac{1+10^{7-5}}{1+10^{7.4-5}} = \frac{101}{1+10^{2.4}} = \frac{101}{252}$$

In addition to the pH of the urine, the rate of urine flow influences the amount of filtered drug that is reabsorbed. The normal flow of urine is approximately 1 to 2 mL/min. Nonpolar and nonionized drugs, which are normally well reabsorbed in the renal tubules, are sensitive to changes in the rate of urine flow. Drugs that increase urine flow, such as ethanol, large fluid intake, and methylxanthines (such as caffeine or theophylline), decrease the time for drug reabsorption and promote their excretion. Thus, forced diuresis through the use of diuretics may be a useful adjunct for removing excessive drug in an intoxicated patient, by increasing renal drug excretion.

---

## CHAPTER SUMMARY

The elimination of most drugs from the body involves the processes of both metabolism (biotransformation) and renal excretion. Drugs that are highly metabolized often demonstrate large intersubject variability in elimination half-lives and are dependent on the intrinsic activity of the biotransformation enzymes. Renal drug excretion is highly dependent on the GFR and blood flow to the kidney.

Hepatic clearance is influenced by hepatic blood flow, drug–protein binding, and intrinsic clearance.

The liver extraction ratio provides a direct measurement of drug removal from the liver after oral administration of a drug. Drugs that are metabolized by the liver enzymes follow Michaelis–Menten kinetics. At low drug concentrations the rate of metabolism is first order, whereas at very high drug concentrations, the rate of drug metabolism may approach zero-order pharmacokinetics. Phase I reactions are generally oxidation and reduction reactions and involve the mixed function oxidases or cytochrome enzymes. These enzymes may be altered by genetic and environmental factors. Phase II reactions are generally conjugation reactions such as the formation of glucuronide and sulfate conjugations. Cytochrome-mediated and acetylation reactions demonstrate polymorphic variability in humans.

First-pass effects or presystemic elimination may occur after oral drug administration in which some of the drugs may be metabolized or not absorbed prior to reaching the general circulation. Alternate routes of drug administration are often used to circumnavigate presystemic elimination. Large-MW, polar drugs may be eliminated by biliary drug excretion. Enterohepatic drug elimination occurs when the drug is secreted into the GI tract and then reabsorbed.

The role of transporters in hepatic excretion and bioavailability in addition to hepatic drug metabolism are important considerations when considering drug–drug interactions and oral drug absorption.

## LEARNING QUESTIONS

1. Why do elimination half-lives of drugs eliminated primarily by hepatic biotransformation demonstrate greater intersubject variability than those drugs eliminated primarily by glomerular filtration?

2. A new drug demonstrates high presystemic elimination when taken orally. From which of the following drug products would the drug be most bioavailable? Why?
   a. Aqueous solution
   b. Suspension
   c. Capsule (hard gelatin)
   d. Tablet
   e. Sustained release

3. For a drug that demonstrated presystemic elimination, would you expect qualitative and/or quantitative differences in the formation of metabolites from this drug given orally compared to intravenous injection? Why?

4. Pravastatin is a statin drug commonly prescribed. The package insert (approved labeling) states that, "The risk of myopathy during treatment with another HMG-CoA reductase inhibitor is increased with concurrent therapy with either erythromycin or cyclosporine." How does cyclosporine change the pharmacokinetics of pravastatin? Is pravastatin uptake involved? Pravastatin is 18% oral bioavailability and 17% urinary excreted.

## ANSWERS

### Learning Questions

1. The hepatic biotransformation of drugs involves many different enzymes and transporters, which are differently expressed among individuals. This creates significant inter-individual variability in the hepatic biotransformation of drugs. In contrast, humans with normal renal function will display a more consistent level of glomerular filtration.

2. High presystemic elimination usually refers to gut wall and hepatic first-pass metabolism and transport of drugs after their oral administration. The absorption of drugs (which is the passage of drugs through the gut wall) can be prevented by efflux transporters such as Pgp, while the abundantly present CYP3A enzymes in the gut wall will metabolize substrates into their metabolites before reaching the liver, where virtually all types of enzymes are present to further metabolize drugs before they can eventually reach the systemic circulation. All of the different proposed answers are oral pharmaceutical formulations, that would all be susceptible to presystemic elimination. A solution would be absorbed quicker than a suspension, which would be absorbed quicker than a capsule, a tablet, or a sustained release. A solution may have higher bioavailability if the products of other dosage forms have dissolution/release

issues, but all these formulations would be subject to presystemic elimination.

3. Yes we could expect qualitative and quantitative differences in the formation of metabolites because of the gut and hepatic first pass metabolism and transport that occurs after oral administration.

4. Erythromycin is a strong inhibitor of CYP3A enzymes and of the Pgp efflux transporter. Cyclosporin is an inhibitor of CYP3A enzymes and a strong inhibitor of the Pgp and OATP transporters. Pravastatin is a substrate of most OATP transporters within the liver, and of the efflux Pgp transporter in the gut wall, all transporters known to be inhibited by cyclosporin, resulting in huge increase in the overall bioavailability of pravastatin. Pravastatin has a low oral bioavailability (18%) due to the first pass gut and hepatic transport, and inhibition of these transport mechanisms by cyclosporin will result in much greater systemic concentrations of pravastatin, potentially resulting in hepatotoxicity and rhabdomyolysis.

## REFERENCES

Alvares AP, Pratt WB: Pathways of drug metabolism. In Pratt WB, Taylor P (eds). *Principles of Drug Action*, 3rd ed. New York, Churchill Livingstone, 1990, Chap 5.

Amin AM, Sheau Chin L, Azri Mohamed Noor D, Sk Abdul Kader MA, Kah Hay Y, Ibrahim B: The personalization of clopidogrel antiplatelet therapy: The role of integrative pharmacogenetics and pharmacometabolomics. *Cardiol Res Pract* 8062796, 2017.

Anderson GD, Chan LN: Pharmacokinetic drug interactions with tobacco, cannabinoids and smoking cessation products. *Clin Pharmacokinet.* 55(11):1353–1368, 2016.

Andersson T, Weidolf L: Stereoselective disposition of proton pump inhibitors. *Clin Drug Investig.* 28(5):263–279, 2008.

Bailey DG, Arnold JMO, Munoz C, Spence JD: Grapefruit juice–felodipine interaction: Mechanism, predictability, and effect of naringin. *Clin Pharm Ther* 53:637–642, 1993b.

Bailey DG, Arnold JMO, Strong HA, Munoz C, Spence JD: Effect of grapefruit juice and naringin on nisoldipine pharmacokinetics. *Clin Pharm Ther* 54:589–593, 1993a.

Caldwell J: Conjugation reactions. In Jenner P, Testa B (eds). *Concepts in Drug Metabolism*. New York, Marcel Dekker, 1980, Chap 4.

Campbell TC: Nutrition and drug-metabolizing enzymes. *Clin Pharm Ther* 22:699–706, 1977.

Caraco Y, Sheller J, Wood AJJ: Pharmacogenetic determination of the effects of codeine and prediction of drug interactions. *J Pharmacol Exp Ther* 278:1165–1174, 1996.

Cer RZ, Mudunuri U, Stephens R, Lebeda F: IC50-to-Ki: A web-based tool for converting IC50 to Ki values for inhibitors of enzyme activity and ligand binding. *Nucleic Acids Res* 37: Web Server issue W441–W445, 2009 (doi:10.1093/nar/gkp253).

Constantinescu SM, Buysschaert B, Haufroid V, Broly F, Jadoul M, Morelle J: Chronic dialysis, NAT2 polymorphisms, and the risk of isoniazid-induced encephalopathy - case report and literature review. *BMC Nephrol* 18(1):282–285, 2017.

Cupp MJ, Tracy TS: Cytochrome P-450: New nomenclature and clinical implications. *Am Family Physician* 57(1):107–116, January 1, 1998. http://www.aafp.org/afp/980101ap/cupp.html.

Desta Z, Xiaox, Shin JG, et al: Clinical significance of the cytochrome P450 2C19 genetic polymorphism. *Clin Pharmacokinet* 41(12):913–958, 2002.

Dow P: *Handbook of Physiology*, Vol 2, *Circulation*. Washington, DC, American Physiology Society, 1963, p 1406.

Drugs@FDA, Label for Plavix, 2021. https://www.accessdata.fda.gov/drugsatfda_docs/label/2021/020839s074lbl.pdf

Evans DAP: Genetic variations in the acetylation of isoniazid and other drugs. *Ann N Y Acad Sci* 151:723, 1968.

Evans DAP, Manley KA, McKusik VC: Genetic control of isoniazid metabolism in man. *Br Med J* 2:485, 1968.

FDA: Drug development and drug interactions |Tables of Substrates, Inhibitors and Inducers. https://www.fda.gov/drugs/drug-interactions-labeling/drug-development-and-drug-interactions-table-substrates-inhibitors-and-inducers. Content current as of 03/10/2020. Accessed in 2021.

FDA Guidance for Industry: In Vitro Drug Interaction Studies—Cytochrome P450 Enzyme- and Transporter-Mediated Drug Interactions, 2020. https://www.fda.gov/regulatory-information/search-fda-guidance-documents/vitro-drug-interaction-studies-cytochrome-p450-enzyme-and-transporter-mediated-drug-interactions

FDA Guidance for Industry: Clinical Drug Interaction Studies—Cytochrome P450 Enzyme- and Transporter-Mediated Drug Interactions, 2020. https://www.fda.gov/regulatory-information/search-fda-guidance-documents/clinical-drug-interaction-studies-cytochrome-p450-enzyme-and-transporter-mediated-drug-interactions

Flockhart DA: Drug Interactions: Cytochrome P450 Drug Interaction Table. Indiana University School of Medicine, 2021. http://medicine.iupui.edu/flockhart/. Accessed 2021.

Guyton AC: *Textbook of Medical Physiology*, 8th ed. Philadelphia, Saunders, 1991.

Huang S, Lesko L, Temple R: Adverse drug reactions and pharmacokinetic drug interactions. In Waldman SA, Terzic A (eds). *Fundamental Principles: Clinical Pharmacology, Pharmacology and Therapeutics: Principles to Practice*. New York, Elsevier, 2009, Chap 21.

Hucker HB, Kwan KC, Duggan DE: Pharmacokinetics and metabolism of nonsteroidal antiinflammatory agents. In Bridges JW, Chasseaud LF (eds). *Progress in Drug Research*, vol 5. New York, Wiley, 1980, Chap 3.

Hukkinen SK, Varhe A, Olkkola KT, Neuvonen PJ: Plasma concentrations of triazolam are increased by concomitant ingestion of grapefruit juice. *Clin Pharm Ther* **58**:127–131, 1995.

James JS: Grapefruit juice and saquinavir. *AIDS Treat News* **235**: 5–6, 1995.

Kantola T, Kivisto KT, Neuvonen PJ: Grapefruit juice greatly increases serum concentrations of lovastatin and lovastatin acid. *Clin Pharmacol Ther* **63**(4):397–402, 1998.

Kupferschmidt HH, Ha HR, Ziegler WH, Meier PJ, Krahenbuhl S: Interaction between grapefruit juice and midazolam in humans. *Clin Pharm Ther* **58**:20–28, 1995.

Lilja JJ, Kivisto KT, Neuvonen PJ: Grapefruit juice-simvastatin interaction: Effect on serum concentrations of simvastatin, simvastatin acid, and HMG-CoA reductase inhibitors. *Clin Pharmacol Ther*. **64**(5):477–483,1998.

Lindner HH: *Clinical Anatomy*. Norwalk, CT, Appleton & Lange, 1989.

May GD: Genetic differences in drug disposition. *J Clin Pharmacol* **34**:881–897, 1994.

Merkel U, Sigusch H, Hoffmann A: Grapefruit juice inhibits 7-hydroxylation of coumarin in healthy volunteers. *Eur J Clin Pharm* **46**:175–177, 1994.

Martignoni M, Groothuis GMM, de Kanter R: Species differences between mouse, rat, dog, monkey and human CYP-mediated drug metabolism, inhibition and induction. *Expert Opin Drug Metab Toxicol* **2**:875–894, 2006.

Negishi M, Tomohide U, Darden TA, Sueyoshi T, Pedersen LG: Structural flexibility and functional versatility of mammalian P-450 enzymes. *FASEB J* **10**:683–689, 1996.

Nelson DR: The cytochrome P450 homepage. *Human Genomics* **4**:59–65, 2009. http://drnelson.uthsc.edu/cytochromeP450.html.

Nishimura M, Yaguti H, Yoshitsugu H, Naito S, Satoh T: Tissue distribution of mRNA expression of human cytochrome P450 isoforms assessed by high-sensitivity real-time reverse transcription PCR. *Yakugaku Zasshi* **123**:369–375, 2003.

Ogilvie BW, Yerino P, Kazmi F, et al: The proton pump inhibitor, omeprazole, but not lansoprazole or pantoprazole, is a metabolism-dependent inhibitor of CYP2C19: Implications for coadministration with clopidogrel. *Drug Metab Dispos* **39**(11):2020–2033, 2011.

Parkinson A: Biotransformation of xenobiotics. In Klaassen, CD (ed). *Casarett & Doull's Toxicology*, 5th ed. New York, McGraw-Hill, 1996, Chap 6.

Pelkonen O, Tolonen A, Kojamo T, Turpeinen M, Raunio H: From known knowns to known unknowns: Predicting in vivo drug metabolites. *Bioanalysis* **1**(2):393–414, 2009.

Rahmani R, Zhou XJ: Pharmacokinetics and metabolism of vinca alkaloids. *Cancer Surv* **17**:269–281, 1993.

Reddy P, Ellington D, Zhu Y, et al: Serum concentrations and clinical effects of atorvastatin in patients taking grapefruit juice daily. *Br J Clin Pharmacol.* **72**(3):434–441, 2011.

Soons PA, Vogels BA, Roosemalen MC, et al: Grapefruit juice and cimetidine inhibit stereoselective metabolism of nitrendipine in humans. *Clin Pharmacol Ther* **50**(4):394–403, 1991.

Toney GB, Ereshefsky L: Cyclic antidepressants. In Schumacher GE (ed). *Therapeutic Drug Monitoring*. Norwalk, CT, Appleton & Lange, 1995, Chap 13.

Tucker GT: Clinical implications of genetic polymorphism in drug metabolism. *J Pharm Pharmacol* **46**(suppl):417–424, 1994.

Tucker GT, Lennard MS: Enantiomer-specific pharmacokinetics. *Pharmacol Ther* **45**:309–329, 1990.

Uno T, Niioka T, Hayakari M, Yasui-Furukori N, Sugawara K, Tateishi T: Absolute bioavailability and metabolism of omeprazole in relation to CYP2C19 genotypes following single intravenous and oral administrations. *Eur J Clin Pharmacol.* **63**(2):143–149, 2007.

West JB (ed): *Best and Taylor's Physiological Basis of Medical Practice*, 11th ed. Baltimore, Williams & Wilkins, 1985.

Wilkinson GR, Guengerich FP, Branch RA: Genetic polymorphism of S-mephenytoin hydroxylation. *Pharmacol Ther* **43**:53–76, 1989.

Wu CY, Benet LZ: Predicting drug disposition via application of BCS: Transport/absorption/elimination interplay and development of a biopharmaceutics drug disposition classification system. *Pharm Res* **22**:11–23, 2005.

Yee GC, Stanley DL, Pessa LJ, et al: Effect of grapefruit juice on blood cyclosporin concentration. *Lancet* **345**:955–956, 1995.

## BIBLIOGRAPHY

Anders MW: *Bioactivation of Foreign Compounds*. New York, Academic Press, 1985.

Ariens EJ: Racemic therapeutics–Problems all along the line. In Brown C (ed): *Chirality in Drug Design and Synthesis*. New York, Academic Press, 1990.

Balant LP, McAinsh JM: Use of metabolite data in the evaluation of pharmacokinetics and drug action. In Jenner P, Testa B (eds).

*Concepts in Drug Metabolism*. New York, Marcel Dekker, 1980, Chap 7.

Benet LZ: Effect of route of administration and distribution on drug action. *J Pharm Biopharm* **6**:559–585, 1978.

Bourne HR, von Zastrow M: Drug receptors and pharmacodynamics. In Katzung BG (ed). *Basic and Clinical Pharmacology,* 9th ed. New York, McGraw-Hill, 2004, Chap 2.

Brosen K: Recent developments in hepatic drug oxidation. *Clin Pharmacokinet* **18:**220, 1990.

Ducharme MP, Warbasse LH, Edwards DJ: Disposition of intravenous and oral cyclosporine after administration with grapefruit juice. *Clin Pharm Ther* **57:**485–491, 1995.

FDA Guidance for Industry: In Vitro Drug Interaction Studies—Cytochrome P450 Enzyme- and Transporter-Mediated Drug Interactions, 2020. https://www.fda.gov/regulatory-information/search-fda-guidance-documents/vitro-drug-interaction-studies-cytochrome-p450-enzyme-and-transporter-mediated-drug-interactions

FDA: Drug development and drug interactions |Tables of Substrates, Inhibitors and Inducers. https://www.fda.gov/drugs/drug-interactions-labeling/drug-development-and-drug-interactions-table-substrates-inhibitors-and-inducers. Content current as of 03/10/2020. Accessed in 2021.

Geroge CF, Shand DG, Renwick AG (eds): *Presystemic Drug Elimination*. Boston, Butterworth, 1982.

Gibaldi M, Perrier D: Route of administration and drug disposition. *Drug Metab Rev* **3:**185–199, 1974.

Gibson GG, Skett P: *Introduction to Drug Metabolism*, 2nd ed. New York, Chapman & Hall, 1994.

Glocklin VC: General considerations for studies of the metabolism of drugs and other chemicals. *Drug Metab Rev* **13:**929–939, 1982.

Gorrod JW, Damani LA: *Biological Oxidation of Nitrogen in Organic Molecules: Chemistry, Toxicology and Pharmacology*. Deerfield Beach, FL, Ellis Horwood, 1985.

Gray H: *Anatomy of the Human Body*, 30th ed. Philadelphia, Lea & Febiger, 1985, p 1495.

Harder S, Baas H, Rietbrock S: Concentration effect relationship of levodopa in patients with Parkinson's disease. *Clin Pharmacokinet* **29:**243–256, 1995.

Hildebrandt A, Estabrook RW: Evidence for the participation of cytochrome b5 in hepatic microsomal mixed-function oxidation reactions. *Arch Biochem Biophys* **143:**66–79, 1971.

Houston JB: Drug metabolite kinetics. *Pharmacol Ther* **15:**521–552, 1982.

Huang SM: New era in drug interaction evaluation: US Food and Drug Administration update on CYP enzymes, transporters, and the guidance process. *J Clin Pharmacol* **48:**662–670, 2008.

Jakoby WB: *Enzymatic Basis of Detoxification*. New York, Academic Press, 1980.

Jenner P, Testa B: *Concepts in Drug Metabolism*. New York, Marcel Dekker, 1980–1981.

Kaplan SA, Jack ML: Physiologic and metabolic variables in bioavailability studies. In Garrett ER, Hirtz JL (eds). *Drug Fate and Metabolism*, vol 3. New York, Marcel Dekker, 1979.

LaDu BL, Mandel HG, Way EL: *Fundamentals of Drug Metabolism and Drug Disposition*. Baltimore, Williams & Wilkins, 1971.

Lanctot KL, Naranjo CA: Comparison of the Bayesian approach and a simple algorithm for assessment of adverse drug events. *Clin Pharm Ther* **58:**692–698, 1995.

Levy RH, Boddy AV: Stereoselectivity in pharmacokinetics: A general theory. *Pharm Res* **8:**551–556, 1991.

Levine WG: Biliary excretion of drugs and other xenobiotics. *Prog Drug Res* **25:**361–420, 1981.

Morris ME, Pang KS: Competition between two enzymes for substrate removal in liver: Modulating effects due to substrate recruitment of hepatocyte activity. *J Pharm Biopharm* **15:**473–496, 1987.

Nies AS, Shand DG, Wilkinson GR: Altered hepatic blood flow and drug disposition. *Clin Pharmacokinet* **1:**135–156, 1976.

Pang KS, Rowland M: Hepatic clearance of drugs. 1. Theoretical considerations of a "well-stirred" model and a "parallel tube" model. Influence of hepatic blood flow, plasma, and blood cell binding and the hepatocellular enzymatic activity on hepatic drug clearance. *J Pharmacokinet Biopharmacol* **5:**625, 1977.

Papadopoulos J, Smithburger PL: Common drug interactions leading to adverse drug event in the intensive care unit: Management and pharmacokinetic considerations, *Crit Care Med* Jun: **35** (suppl 6),126–135, 2010.

Perrier D, Gibaldi M: Clearance and biologic half-life as indices of intrinsic hepatic metabolism. *J Pharmacol Exp Therapeut* **191:**17–24, 1974.

Plaa GL: The enterohepatic circulation. In Gillette JR, Mitchell JR (eds). *Concepts in Biochemical Pharmacology*. New York, Springer-Verlag, 1975, Chap 63.

Pratt WB, Taylor P: *Principles of Drug Action: The Basis of Pharmacology*, 3rd ed. New York, Churchill Livingstone, 1990.

Riddick DS, Ding X, Wolf RC, et al: NADPH-Cytochrome P450 oxidoreductase: Roles in physiology, pharmacology, and toxicology. *Drug Metab Dispos* **41:**12–23, 2013.

Roberts MS, Donaldson JD, Rowland M: Models of hepatic elimination: Comparison of stochastic models to describe residence time distributions and to predict the influence of drug distribution, enzyme heterogeneity, and systemic recycling on hepatic elimination. *J Pharm Biopharm* **16:**41–83, 1988.

Routledge PA, Shand DG: Presystemic drug elimination. *Annu Rev Pharmacol Toxicol* **19:**447–468, 1979.

Semple HA, Tam YK, Coutts RT: A computer simulation of the food effect: Transient changes in hepatic blood flow and Michaelis–Menten parameters as mediators of hepatic first-pass metabolism and bioavailability of propranolol. *Biopharm Drug Disp* **11:**61–76, 1990.

Shand DG, Kornhauser DM, Wilkinson GR: Effects of route administration and blood flow on hepatic drug elimination. *J Pharmacol Exp Therapeut* **195:**425–432, 1975.

Stoltenborg JK, Puglisi CV, Rubio F, Vane FM: High performance liquid chromatographic determination of stereoselective disposition of carprofen in humans. *J Pharm Sci* **70:**1207–1212, 1981.

Testa B, Jenner B: *Drug Metabolism: Chemical and Biochemical Aspects*. New York, Marcel Dekker, 1976.

Venot A, Walter E, Lecourtier Y, et al: Structural identifiability of "first-pass" models. *J Pharm Biopharm* **15:**179–189, 1987.

Wilkinson GR: Pharmacodynamics of drug disposition: Hemodynamic considerations. *Annu Rev Pharmacol* **15:**11–27, 1975.

Wilkinson GR: Pharmacodynamics in disease states modifying body perfusion. In Benet LZ (ed). *The Effect of Disease States on Drug Pharmacokinetics*. Washington, DC, American Pharmaceutical Association, 1976.

Wilkinson GR, Rawlins MD: *Drug Metabolism and Disposition: Considerations in Clinical Pharmacology*. Boston, MTP Press, 1985.

Williams RT: Hepatic metabolism of drugs. *Gut* **13:**579–585, 1972.

# 7

# Biopharmaceutic Considerations in Drug Product Design and *In Vitro* Drug Product Performance

Maziar Kakhi, Poonam Delvadia, and Sandra Suarez-Sharp

## CHAPTER OBJECTIVES

- Describe the biopharmaceutic factors affecting drug product design.

- Define the term "rate-limiting step" and discuss how the rate-limiting step relates to the bioavailability of a drug.

- Differentiate between the terms solubility and dissolution.

- Differentiate between the concept of drug absorption and bioavailability.

- Describe the various *in vitro* and *in vivo* tests commonly used to evaluate drug products.

- Describe the methods for comparing two dissolution profiles for similarity.

- List the compendial dissolution apparatus and provide examples of drug products for which these apparatus might be appropriate.

- Define sink conditions and explain why dissolution medium must maintain sink conditions.

- Define *in vitro–in vivo* correlation (IVIVC) and explain why a Level A correlation is the most important correlation for IVIVC.

- Define clinically relevant drug product specifications and describe the methods to establish them.

- Explain the biopharmaceutic classification system and how solubility, dissolution, and permeation apply to BCS classification.

- Provide a description of some common oral drug products and explain how biopharmaceutic principles may be used to formulate a product that will extend the duration of activity of the active drug.

## INTRODUCTION

*Biopharmaceutics* is the study of the physicochemical properties of both the drug substance and product and the *in vitro* quality attributes of the drug product as they relate to the bioavailability (BA) of the drug, with the goal of ensuring consistent drug product quality and the desired patient-centric therapeutic effect. BA refers to the rate and extent of appearance of active drug at the site of action. In practice, this is measured as the fraction of drug that reaches the systemic circulation.

Numerous routes of administration are available for drug products, such as ocular, nasal, pulmonary, transdermal, oral, rectal, vaginal, and parenteral (eg, intravenous, intra-arterial, intramuscular, intrathecal, subcutaneous). If the drug is given by an intravascular/intravenous (IV) route, systemic drug absorption is considered complete or 100% bioavailable, because the drug is placed directly into the general circulation. The choice of these routes is influenced by several factors which will be elaborated in this chapter. However, a salient consideration is the site of action for the drug to achieve its therapeutic objective. For systemically-acting drugs, the site of action is accessible via the systemic circulation and the drug must be absorbed to achieve a pharmacological response. Oral drug absorption involves the transport of the dissolved free drug through the gastrointestinal (GI) linings via passive and/or transporter-mediated pathways (Estudante et al, 2013). The passive route can be via a transcellular or paracellular mechanism depending on the hydrophilicity and size of the molecules (Lemmer and Hamman, 2013).

The site of absorption along the GI tract depends, *inter alia*, on the drug substance properties and how the drug product is formulated, as discussed further in this chapter. For absorption to be feasible, drug release (or *in vivo* dissolution) from the drug product into the gut lumen's fluids (juices) has to occur (with the exception of oral solutions, in which case the drug is already dissolved), and the dissolved free drug has to diffuse to the gut wall epithelia. As a point of definition in this text, it is understood that *dissolution* is a term traditionally employed to refer to the processes (including disintegration or capsule rupture) leading to the solvation of drug substance from orally administered immediate-release (IR) solid drug products. While this concept can be extended to cover other oral dosage forms, for non-oral dosage forms (eg, transdermal, topical, suppositories, liposomal delivery, etc), the term *drug release* has gained acceptance (Brown et al, 2011). While this distinction between drug release and dissolution may appear to be primarily semantic, suggesting that they can be employed interchangeably, it is important to note that the underlying mechanisms leading to the availability of drug for absorption are dependent on the nature of the formulation and its site of administration.

The extent of absorption can be further impacted by processes during GI transit (eg, drug substance degradation, precipitation, motility, gut wall metabolism). A further obstacle to systemic BA can be a result of first-pass metabolism. Additional drug disposition (ie, distribution and elimination) may occur in the systemic circulation and thus reduce the concentration of drug available to the target tissues. However, because the systemic blood circulation ultimately delivers therapeutically active drug to the tissues and to the drug's site of action, changes in BA will likely have an impact on the efficacy and safety of the drug product.

A drug product may also be designed to deliver the drug directly to the site of action before reaching the systemic circulation, which is often termed *locally acting* drug. In this instance, drug is designed to penetrate mainly no further than the local tissue where a therapeutic action is desired. Some examples of locally acting drug products in this class include ophthalmic, pulmonary, nasal, and transdermal drug products. It should be noted, however, that the pulmonary, nasal, and transdermal routes of administration can also be targeted for delivering drugs to the systemic circulation. Similar to systemic BA, local drug concentrations are strongly influenced by the physicochemical properties of the drug and the formulation *excipients* (inactive ingredients), which in turn impact the rate and extent of drug release from the drug product and permeation at the target site. It is noted, however, that the physiologies of the eye, lung, nose, and skin are all highly specialized and differentiated with respect to their permeation characteristics.

The rate of drug release and absorption is generally quantified by means of time to reach peak drug concentration ($T_{max}$) and peak drug concentration ($C_{max}$). The extent of drug release and absorption is represented by the area under the plasma concentration-time curve (AUC). Collectively, these parameters are important in determining the onset, intensity, and duration of drug action. Therefore, regardless of the intended site of drug action, biopharmaceutics aims to balance the extent of drug delivered from the drug product to achieve optimal therapeutic efficacy and safety for the patient.

## BIOPHARMACEUTIC FACTORS AND RATIONALE FOR DRUG PRODUCT DESIGN

In broad terms, the factors affecting drug BA may be related to the drug substance properties, the formulation of the drug product, and the biological characteristics of the patient. These are classified as drug and system properties, respectively, whereby "drug" encompasses both the drug substance and product physicochemical properties, of which the latter could comprise particle size distribution (PSD) of granules, water content, etc.

Drugs are usually formulated into finished dosage forms (ie, drug products) rather than given as pure chemical drug substances, which would be impractical for highly insoluble active pharmaceutical ingredients (APIs). These drug products include the active drug substance combined with selected excipients that make up the dosage form. *Excipients* are generally considered inert with respect to pharmacodynamic (PD) activity. However, excipients are important in the manufacture of the drug product (eg, for processability of a particular dosage form), and they provide functionality to the drug product with respect to drug release and dissolution (eg, surfactants and polymer carriers for amorphous solid dispersions, permeation enhancers). Drug disposition may also be influenced by the specific formulation of the drug, eg, encapsulated drug in liposome or microspheres may change the drug distribution and systemic clearance; addition of mannitol may change the renal clearance of the drug.

Some common dosage forms include liquids (eg, solutions and suspensions), tablets, capsules, injectables, suppositories, transdermal systems, and topical creams and ointments. When administered appropriately, these finished dosage forms or drug products achieve a specific therapeutic objective. The design of the dosage form, the formulation of the drug product, and the manufacturing process require a thorough understanding of the biopharmaceutic principles of drug delivery. Considerations in the design of a drug product to deliver the active drug with the desired BA characteristics and therapeutic objectives include the following:

- Physicochemical properties of the drug substance
- Route of drug administration, including the anatomic and physiologic nature of the application site
- Desired PD effect (eg, immediate or prolonged activity)
- Toxicologic properties of the drug substance and the excipients
- Effect of excipients and dosage form
- Manufacturing processes

As mentioned above, some drugs are intended for local therapeutic action at the site of administration. Systemic drug absorption is often undesirable for locally acting drugs because they are designed to have a direct PD action without affecting other body organs. For locally acting drugs, the general measures for quantifying BA, including the onset, intensity, and duration of drug action (ie, $T_{max}$, $C_{max}$, and AUC) from plasma concentration-time data, may not be practical because of the very limited systemic drug absorption. Locally acting drugs may be administered orally (eg, local GI effect) or applied topically to the skin, ear, nose, eye, mucous membranes, buccal cavity, throat, or rectum. A drug intended for local activity may also be given intravaginally, into the urethral tract, intranasally, or inhaled into the lungs. Examples of drugs used for local action include anti-infectives, antifungals, local anesthetics, antacids, astringents, vasoconstrictors, antihistamines, bronchodilators, and corticosteroids. Though systemic absorption is undesired, it may occur with locally acting drugs, and modifying the drug product design may help to mitigate systemic effects.

Each route of drug administration presents special biopharmaceutic considerations in drug product design. For example, the design of a vaginal tablet formulation for the treatment of a fungal infection must use ingredients compatible with vaginal anatomy and physiology. An eye medication requires special considerations for formulation pH, isotonicity, sterility, the need to minimize local irritation to the cornea, potential for drug loss from draining by tears, and residual systemic drug absorption.

A drug product may also be designed as a combination drug/device product to allow the drug formulation to be used in conjunction with a specialized medical device or packaging component. The following sources discuss the regulatory definitions of drug, devices and combination products: FDA Guidance (September 2017); Code of Federal Regulations (21CFR3.2); FDA, Is the Product a Medical Device? (2018). Combination drug products include:

- Aerosolized drug products. A drug solution or suspension may be formulated to work with a nebulizer or metered-dose inhaler for administration into the lungs. Both the physical characteristics of the delivery system and the formulation of the drug product can influence the droplet particle size and its distribution, the spray pattern, and plume geometry of the emitted dose, which may affect its *in vivo* performance.
- Drug-eluting stents. A drug–polymer coating may be applied to a cardiac stent for local delivery of antiproliferative drugs directly to diseased tissue during percutaneous coronary intervention to treat a blocked artery.

By choosing the route of drug administration carefully and properly designing the drug product, the BA of the active drug can be varied from rapid and complete absorption to a slow, sustained rate of absorption or even minimal absorption, depending on the therapeutic objective. In the latter case, examples include sucralfate oral formulations for treating duodenal ulcers, bile acid sequestrants such as colesevelam, and non-calcium-based phosphate binders (sevelamer hydrochloride, lanthanum carbonate and sucroferric oxyhydroxide).

Biopharmaceutic considerations often determine the ultimate dose and dosage form of a drug product, once preliminary clinical and toxicological studies have characterized therapeutically effective and unsafe dose levels (respectively). The strength of a dosage form for a systemically acting drug is often expressed in units of mass. Oral solutions, transdermal patches, and topical products (eg, ointment) express strength as mass rates or concentrations. The dose is based on the amount of drug that is absorbed systemically and dissolved in an apparent volume of distribution to produce a desired drug concentration at the target site. The therapeutic dose may also be adjusted based on the weight or surface area of the patient, to account for the differences in the apparent volume of distribution, which is expressed as mass per unit of body weight (mg/kg) or mass per unit of body surface area (mg/m$^2$). For many commercial drug products, the dose is determined based on average body weights and may be available in several dose strengths, such as 10-mg, 5-mg, and 2.5-mg tablets, to accommodate differences in body weight and possibly to titrate the dose in the patient.

---

### FREQUENTLY ASKED QUESTIONS

▶ How do excipients improve the manufacturing of an oral drug product?

▶ If excipients do not have PD activity, how do excipients affect the performance of the drug product?

---

## RATE-LIMITING STEPS IN DRUG ABSORPTION

In general, the slowest step in a series of kinetic processes is called the *rate-limiting step*, and drug absorption is the result of a succession of rate processes. The first step is the delivery of the drug product formulation to the region of the human body where absorption is targeted, and as discussed above, numerous routes of administration exist for drug delivery. For many topical drug products, this first step is simple and direct, but for aerosolized pulmonary drug products, effective delivery to the relevant areas in the lung can be challenging. Except for solution formulations, the next critical step involves the release of the drug substance from the formulation (eg, see below for more detail on solid oral IR tablets). After the drug is released, it is transported to the absorption site where it can undergo permeation through the local cellular structure. Even this seemingly last step in the absorption process can be further compartmentalized into additional kinetic steps depending on the complexity of the cellular tissue/membrane and our understanding of the mechanistic processes taking place therein. For non-locally acting drugs, further rate-dependent steps are required, *post absorption*, to deliver and make the active drug available at the site of therapeutic action. These steps can involve distribution, metabolism, renal extraction, and permeation.

For solid oral, IR tablets, which comprise the largest category of administered drug products, the rate processes described above can also include disintegration of the drug product (Fig. 7-1). Drug is released from the formulation by means of its diffusional movement through the wetted matrix and subsequent dissolution into an aqueous environment. In general, for drug products that are designed to slowly release the drug from the formulation, such as extended-release (ER) formulations, the release of the drug from these formulations is the rate-limiting step.

### Disintegration

*Disintegration* is the process by which the dosage form is progressively transformed into smaller drug product fragments, granules, or aggregates thereby providing significantly greater surface area-to-volume ratio for drug release to occur. Disintegration does not imply complete (or even any) dissolution of the drug. Not all solid oral dosage forms undergo disintegration. Examples of such formulation are troches, chewable tablets, liquid-filled soft gelatin capsules, and sustained release drug products such as osmotic pump, monolithic matrix, and reservoir matrix oral dosage forms. Disintegration is achieved through the addition of one or more disintegrants (eg, sodium

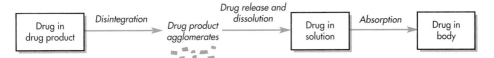

FIGURE 7-1 • Rate processes of drug bioavailability.

starch glycolate, crospovidone, microcrystalline cellulose) to the pool of other excipients (eg, diluent, binder, lubricant). Disintegrants are normally added before and/or after the granulation stage to achieve a target dissolution profile. They are generally understood to promote the drawing of surrounding liquid into the porous formulation through capillary action (wicking), thereby weakening the structural integrity of the dosage form. Swelling of the disintegrant is another mechanism of action which generates internal forces within the dosage form thereby facilitating its disintegration. Poor disintegration of a compressed tablet may be due to high compression of tablets without sufficient disintegrant.

To monitor consistent tablet disintegration *in vitro*, the United States Pharmacopeia (USP) specifies a disintegration test (Fig. 7-2) described in general chapter 701, USP (2018).

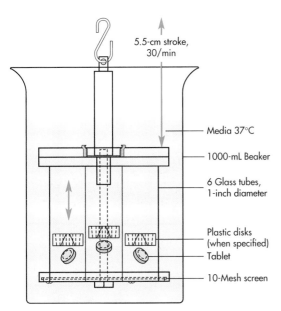

FIGURE 7-2 • USP disintegration testing apparatus. (Reproduced with permission from Hanson R, Gray V: *Handbook of Dissolution Testing*, 3rd ed. Hockessin, DE: Dissolution Technologies, Inc; 2004.)

Disintegration is defined therein as "that state in which any residue of the unit, except fragments of insoluble coating or capsule shell, remaining on the screen of the test apparatus or adhering to the lower surface of the disk, if used, is a soft mass having no palpably firm core."

As stated above, the disintegration test provides no information on the rate of dissolution of the active drug, even though it helps facilitate it. In general, the disintegration test serves as a component in the overall quality control of tablet manufacture. There has been some interest in using only the disintegration test in place of the dissolution test for some drug products. Disintegration testing can be used in lieu of dissolution testing provided the following ICH Q6A (1999) guidelines are met: (1) The product under consideration is rapidly dissolving (dissolution >80% in 15 minutes at pH 1.2, 4.0, and 6.8); (2) the drug product contains drugs that are highly soluble throughout the physiological range (dose/solubility volume <250 mL from pH 1.2 to 6.8); and (3) a relationship to dissolution has been established or when disintegration is shown to be more discriminating than dissolution and dissolution characteristics do not change on stability. By way of example, drug release cannot be practically characterized using *in vitro* dissolution (described in greater detail below) for highly soluble compounds formulated to disintegrate within a timeframe of a few seconds with complete dissolution taking place immediately thereafter. In these instances, disintegration is the rate-limiting step for absorption.

### Dissolution and Solubility

*Dissolution* is the process by which a solid drug substance becomes dissolved in a solvent over time. *Solubility* is the mass of solute that dissolves in a specific mass or volume of solvent at a given temperature (eg, 1 g of NaCl dissolves in 2.786 mL of water at 25°C). Solubility, by definition, is an *equilibrium* property, whereas dissolution is a *dynamic* property. In biologic systems, drug dissolution in an aqueous medium is an important prior condition for predicting systemic drug absorption. For IR drug products, *in vivo* dissolution can be a rate-limiting step for absorption particularly if the drug substance has a poor aqueous solubility. Under these circumstances, it is assumed that *in vitro* dissolution tests can be identified which, ideally, can be mapped to the *in vivo* dissolution and thus be used to quantitatively predict BA. Such a quantitative mapping, or relationship, is referred to as an *in vitro–in vivo* correlation (IVIVC). Ideally, such clinically relevant *in vitro* dissolution tests may also be used to discern formulation factors that affect drug BA. As per Title 21 CFR 314.50(d)(1)(ii)(a), dissolution testing is required for US Food and Drug Administration (FDA)-approved solid oral drug products.

Noyes and Whitney (1897) studied the rate of dissolution of two slightly soluble substances, benzoic acid and lead chloride in distilled water. They postulated that if the solid substances were surrounded by an indefinitely thin film of saturated solution from which diffusion takes place, the rate of dissolution would be proportional to the difference between the saturation solubility and the instantaneous bulk (well-stirred) concentration. The dissolved drug in the saturated solution, referred to interchangeably in the literature as the *stagnant*, *diffusion*, and *boundary layer*, diffuses to the bulk of the solvent from regions of high drug concentration to regions of low drug concentration (Fig. 7-3). Only at the solid surface is the relative fluid velocity zero; this is referred to as the no-slip condition in fluid mechanics.

In Fig. 7-3, the stagnant layer is depicted schematically and is not to scale with respect to the size of the drug particle. With increasing intensity of the hydrodynamic agitation in the bulk solvent, the diffusion layer forms an increasingly thin film around the solid drug particle allowing for more rapid dissolution. The overall rate of drug dissolution, as expressed by the *Noyes–Whitney equation* (Equation 7.1) takes the following form:

$$\frac{dC}{dt} = \frac{DA}{h}(C_s - C) \qquad (7.1)$$

where $dC/dt$ = rate of drug dissolution at time $t$, $D$ = diffusion coefficient, $A$ = surface area of the particle, $C_s$ = concentration of drug (equal to solubility of drug) in the stagnant layer, $C$ = concentration of drug in the bulk solvent, and $h$ = thickness of the stagnant layer.

The Noyes–Whitney equation shows that dissolution may be influenced by the physicochemical characteristics of the drug, the solvent the drug is dissolving in and the level of agitation in the bulk fluid medium. Furthermore, the temperature of the fluid medium (solvent) affects the equilibrium solubility of the drug and the diffusion coefficient of the drug in the fluid.

Factors that affect drug dissolution of a solid oral dosage form include (1) the physical and chemical nature of the active drug substance as noted above, (2) the nature of the excipients, (3) the method of manufacture, and (4) the dissolution test conditions. For this reason, the Noyes-Whitney equation cannot be used directly to make predictions of drug release from real formulations.

**FREQUENTLY ASKED QUESTIONS**

▶ What is meant by the rate-limiting step in drug BA from a solid oral drug product?

▶ What is the usual rate-limiting step for a poorly soluble and highly permeable drug (BCS 2)?

## PHYSICOCHEMICAL PROPERTIES OF THE DRUG

In addition to their effect on dissolution kinetics, the physical and chemical properties of the drug substance as well as the excipients are important

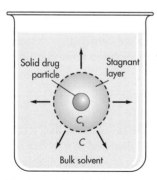

FIGURE 7-3 • Dissolution of a solid drug particle in a solvent. ($C_s$ = concentration of drug in the stagnant layer, $C$ = concentration of drug in the bulk solvent.)

considerations in the design of a drug product (Table 7-1). For example:

- The ability of a drug to exist in various crystal forms, referred to as *polymorphism*, may change the solubility of the drug. Also, the stability of each form is important because polymorphs may convert from one form to another.
- Moisture absorption may affect the physical structure as well as stability of the product.
- The partition coefficient may give some indication of the relative affinity of the drug for oil and water. A drug that has a high affinity for oil may have poor release and dissolution from the drug product in an aqueous environment.
- The compatibility of the excipients with the drug and sometimes trace elements in excipients may affect the stability of the product. It is important to have specifications of all raw materials.

- The stability of solutions is often affected by the pH of the vehicle; furthermore, because the pH in the stomach and gut is different, knowledge of the stability profile would help avoid or prevent degradation of the product during storage or after administration.
- The presence of impurities may depend upon the synthetic route for the active drug and subsequent purification. Impurities need to be "qualified" or tested for safety. Changes in the synthetic method may change the impurity profile.
- The presence of *chirality* may show that the isomers have differences in PD activity.

An additional, albeit not comprehensive, list of considerations can include:

- Intravenous solutions which are difficult to prepare with drugs that have poor aqueous solubility.
- Drugs that are physically or chemically unstable requiring special excipients, coatings, or manufacturing processes to protect the drug from degradation.
- Drugs with a potent PD response, such as estrogens and other hormones, penicillin antibiotics, cancer chemotherapeutic agents, and others, can cause adverse reactions to personnel who are exposed to these drugs during manufacture.

In the following sections, the relationship between the various physicochemical properties of the drug substance and its absorption will be presented in more detail.

## Solubility, pH, and Drug Absorption

The *solubility–pH profile* is a plot of the solubility of the drug at various physiologic pH values. In designing oral dosage forms, the formulator must consider that the natural pH environment of the GI tract varies from acidic in the stomach to slightly alkaline in the small intestine. A basic drug is more soluble in an acidic medium, forming a soluble salt. Conversely, an acid drug is more soluble in the intestine, forming a soluble salt in the more alkaline pH environment found there. The solubility–pH profile gives a first impression of the challenges to achieve complete dissolution for a dose of a drug in the stomach or in the small intestine.

**TABLE 7-1 • Physicochemical Properties for Consideration in Drug Product Design**

| Property | Potential Impact |
| --- | --- |
| $pK_a$ and pH profile | Stability and solubility of the final product |
| Particle size | Particle surface area of the drug and therefore the dissolution rate of the product |
| Polymorphism | Solubility and stability of the drug |
| Hygroscopicity | Physical structure and stability of the product |
| Partition coefficient | Relative affinity of the drug for oil and water |
| Excipient interaction | Stability of the drug product through interaction with trace elements |
| pH stability profile | Drug product degradation during storage or after administration |
| Impurity profile | Choice of synthetic route for the active drug and subsequent purification |
| Chirality | Differences in pharmacodynamic activity |

Solubility may be improved with the addition of an acidic or basic excipient(s). Solubilization of aspirin, for example, may be increased by the addition of an alkaline buffer. In the formulation of extended release (ER) drugs, buffering agents may be added to slow or modify the release rate of a fast-dissolving drug. Typically, the ER drug product of this type is non-disintegrating. The buffering agent is released slowly rather than rapidly so that the drug does not dissolve immediately in the surrounding GI fluid.

In addition to considering the potential for *in situ* salt formation at different pH values for ionizable drug substances, direct salt formation of the drug is a common approach for tailoring the dissolution rate, and consequently, drug absorption for many ionizable drugs. Salt formation may change the drug's physicochemical properties in many aspects, including its solubility, chemical stability, polymorphism, and manufacturability, all of which must be considered by the formulator during development. Also, the potential for converting from the salt form to the unionized drug form during drug product manufacturing must be considered for optimal drug product design.

### Stability, pH, and Drug Absorption

The *stability–pH profile* is a plot of the reaction rate constant for drug degradation versus pH. If drug decomposition occurs by acid or base catalysis, some prediction of degradation of the drug in the GI tract may be made. For example, erythromycin has a pH-dependent stability profile. In acidic medium, as in the stomach, erythromycin decomposition occurs rapidly, whereas in neutral or alkaline pH, the drug is relatively stable. Consequently, erythromycin tablets are coated with an acid-resistant film, which is referred to as enteric coating, to protect against acid degradation in the stomach. The knowledge of erythromycin stability subsequently led to the preparation of a less water-soluble erythromycin salt that is more stable in the stomach. The dissolution rate of erythromycin drug substance powder, without excipients, varied from 100% dissolved in 1 hour for the water-soluble version to less than 40% dissolved in 1 hour for the less water-soluble version. The slow-dissolving erythromycin drug substance also resulted in slow-dissolving drug

products formulated with the modified drug. Thus, in the erythromycin case, the dissolution rate of the powdered drug substance was a very useful *in vitro* tool for predicting BA problems of the resulting erythromycin product in the body.

### Particle Size and Drug Absorption

Dissolution kinetics is also affected by particle size. As previously described in the Noyes–Whitney dissolution model, the dissolution rate is proportional to the surface area of the drug. Dissolution takes place at the surface of the solute (drug), and thus, the greater the effective surface area per unit volume of drug, the better the water saturation, and the more rapid the rate of drug dissolution. The effective surface area of a drug is increased by a reduction in the particle size because there are more particles generated for a given volume. The geometric shape of the particle also affects the surface area, and, during dissolution, the surface is constantly changing. For dissolution calculations using the various models, however, the solute particle is usually assumed to retain its geometric shape.

Studies of particle physicochemical properties, such as hygroscopicity, morphology, and size, are especially important for drug substances that have low water solubility, particularly class II compounds, according to the Biopharmaceutical Classification System (BCS) (see Chapter 8) where release is often rate limiting for absorption. Consequently, there are many drugs that are active when administered intravenously but are not very effective when given orally because of poor oral absorption owing to the drug's poor aqueous solubility. Griseofulvin, nitrofurantoin, and many steroids are drugs with low aqueous solubility; reduction of the particle size by milling to a micronized form has improved the oral absorption of these drugs. A disintegrant may also be added to the formulation to ensure rapid disintegration of the tablet and release of the particles. The addition of surface-active agents may increase wetting as well as solubility of these drugs.

Sometimes micronization and varying the choice of excipient are not sufficient to overcome solubility-related BA problems. In these cases, the so-called *nanosizing*, ie, producing even smaller drug substance particles, may be beneficial. As compared with micronization, nanosized particles may be formulated for injection drug products (eg, nano-suspension) in addition to traditional oral dosage forms. It is possible that nanosized drug particles may not dissolve readily after IV administration and end up sequestered by the *reticuloendothelial system*. However, the nanoparticles will eventually dissolve, permeate through the cell membrane and diffuse into the cytoplasm, and contribute to overall systemic drug exposure.

## Polymorphism, Solvates, and Drug Absorption

*Polymorphism* refers to the arrangement of a drug substance in various crystal forms or polymorphs. In recent years, the term polymorph has been used frequently to describe polymorphs, solvates, amorphous forms, and desolvated solvates. *Amorphous forms* are noncrystalline forms, *solvates* are forms that contain a solvent (solvate) or water (hydrate), and *desolvated* solvates are forms that are made by removing the solvent from the solvate. Many drugs exist in an *anhydrous* state (no water of hydration) or in a hydrous state.

Drug products manufactured with polymorphs have the same chemical structure but different physical properties, such as different solubility, hygroscopicity, density, hardness, and compression characteristics. Some polymorphic crystals have much lower aqueous solubility than the amorphous (non-crystalline) forms, causing a product to be incompletely absorbed.

Chloramphenicol, for example, has several crystal forms, and when given orally as a suspension, the drug concentration in the body was found to be dependent on the percent of β-polymorph in the suspension (Aguiar et al, 1967). The β form is more soluble and better absorbed (Fig. 7-4). In general, the crystal form that has the lowest free energy is the most stable polymorph. A drug that exists as an amorphous form generally dissolves more rapidly than the same drug in a more structurally rigid crystalline form. Some polymorphs are *metastable* and may convert to a more stable form over time. A change in crystal form may cause problems in manufacturing the product. For example, a change in the crystal structure of the drug may cause cracking in a tablet (Yamaoka et al, 1982) or even prevent a granulation from being compressed into a tablet. Re-formulation of a product may be necessary if a new crystal form of a drug is used.

Some drugs interact with solvent during the manufacturing process to form a crystal called

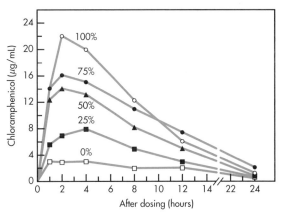

**FIGURE 7-4 •** Comparison of mean blood serum levels obtained with chloramphenicol palmitate suspensions containing varying ratios of α- and β-polymorphs, following single oral dose equivalent to 1.5 g chloramphenicol. Percentage polymorph β in the suspension. (Reproduced with permission from Aguiar AJ, Krc J Jr, Kinkel AW, et al: Effect of polymorphism on the absorption of chloramphenicol from chloramphenicol palmitate, *J Pharm Sci.* 1967 Jul;56(7):847-853.)

a *solvate*. Water may form special crystals with drugs called *hydrates*; for example, Allen et al (1978) reported that erythromycin hydrates have quite different solubility compared to the anhydrous form of the drug (Fig. 7-5).

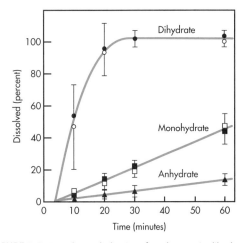

**FIGURE 7-5 •** Dissolution behavior of erythromycin dihydrate, monohydrate, and anhydrate in phosphate buffer (pH 7.5) at 37°C. (Reproduced with permission from Allen PV, Rahn PD, Sarapu AC, et al: Physical characterization of erythromycin: anhydrate, monohydrate, and dihydrate crystalline solids, *J Pharm Sci.* 1978 Aug;67(8):1087-93.)

## INFLUENCE OF EXCIPIENTS ON DRUG PRODUCT PERFORMANCE

*Excipients* are added to a formulation to provide certain functional properties to the drug and dosage form. Some of these functional properties of the excipients are used to improve the manufacturability of the dosage form, stabilize the drug against degradation, decrease gastric irritation, control the rate of drug absorption from the absorption site, increase drug BA, etc. Some of the excipients used in the manufacture of solid and liquid drug products are listed in Tables 7-2 and 7-3.

**TABLE 7-2** • Common Excipients Used in Solid Drug Products

| Excipient | Property in Dosage Form |
|---|---|
| Lactose | Diluent |
| Dibasic calcium phosphate | Diluent |
| Starch | Disintegrant, diluent, glidant |
| Microcrystalline cellulose | Disintegrant, diluent |
| Magnesium stearate | Lubricant, glidant |
| Stearic acid | Lubricant, emulsifying and solubilizing agent |
| Hydrogenated vegetable oil | Lubricant |
| Talc | Lubricant, glidant |
| Sucrose (solution) | Granulating/binding agent |
| Polyvinyl pyrrolidone (solution) | Granulating/binding agent |
| Hydroxypropylmethylcellulose | Tablet-coating agent, stabilizing agent |
| Titinium dioxide | Combined with dye as colored coating |
| Methylcellulose | Coating or granulating agent |
| Cellulose acetate phthalate | Enteric-coating agent |

**TABLE 7-3** • Common Excipients Used in Oral Liquid Drug Products

| Excipient | Property in Dosage Form |
|---|---|
| Sodium carboxymethyl cellulose | Suspending agent |
| Tragacanth | Suspending agent |
| Sodium alginate | Suspending agent |
| Xanthan gum | Thixotropic suspending agent |
| Veegum | Thixotropic suspending agent |
| Sorbitol | Sweetener |
| Alcohol | Solubilizing agent, preservative |
| Propylene glycol | Solubilizing agent |
| Methyl, propylparaben | Preservative |
| Sucrose | Sweetener |
| Polysorbates | Surfactant |
| Sesame oil | For emulsion vehicle |
| Corn oil | For emulsion vehicle |

Excipients in the drug product may also affect the dissolution kinetics of the drug, either by altering the medium in which the drug is dissolving or by reacting with the drug itself. For drug products where dissolution is rate-limiting, these effects in turn impact absorption and BA. Some of these general trends are presented in Table 7-4 for typical preparations. Other excipients include suspending agents that increase the viscosity of the drug vehicle and thereby diminish the rate of drug dissolution from suspensions. Tablet lubricants, such as magnesium stearate, may repel water and reduce dissolution when used in large quantities. Coatings, particularly shellac, will cross-link upon aging and decrease the dissolution rate.

Surfactants, on the other hand, may affect drug dissolution in an unpredictable fashion. Low concentrations of surfactants decrease the surface tension and increase the rate of drug dissolution, whereas higher surfactant concentrations tend to form micelles with the drug and thus decrease the dissolution rate.

| TABLE 7-4 • Effect of Excipients on the Pharmacokinetic Parameters of Oral Drug Products* | | | | |
|---|---|---|---|---|
| Excipients | Example | $k_a$ | $T_{max}$ | AUC |
| Disintegrants | Avicel, Explotab | ↑ | ↓ | ↑/– |
| Lubricants | Talc, hydrogenated vegetable oil | ↓ | ↑ | ↓/– |
| Coating agent | Hydroxypropylmethyl cellulose | – | – | – |
| Enteric coat | Cellulose acetate phthalate | ↓ | ↑ | ↓/– |
| Sustained-release agents | Methylcellulose, ethylcellulose | ↓ | ↑ | ↓/– |
| Sustained-release agents (waxy agents) | Castorwax, Carbowax | ↓ | ↑ | ↓/– |
| Sustained-release agents (gum/viscous) | Veegum, Keltrol | ↓ | ↑ | ↓/– |

*This may be concentration and drug dependent. ↑ = Increase, ↓ = decrease, – = no effect, $k_a$ = absorption rate coefficient, $T_{max}$ = time for peak drug concentration in plasma, AUC = area under the plasma drug concentration–time curve.

Some excipients, such as sodium bicarbonate, may change the pH of the medium surrounding the active drug substance. For example, aspirin is a weak acid and when formulated with sodium bicarbonate, a water-soluble salt in an alkaline medium is formed in which the drug rapidly dissolves. The term for this process is *dissolution in a reactive medium*. The solid drug dissolves rapidly in the reactive solvent surrounding the solid particle. However, as the dissolved drug molecules diffuse outward into the bulk solvent, the drug may precipitate out of solution with a very fine particle size (Chiou and Riegelman, 1971).

Excipients in a formulation may interact directly with the drug to form a water-soluble or water-insoluble complex. For example, if tetracycline is formulated with calcium carbonate, an insoluble complex of calcium tetracycline is formed that has a slow rate of dissolution and poor absorption.

Excipients may be added to the formulation to enhance the rate and extent of drug absorption or to delay or slow the rate of drug absorption (see Table 7-4). For example, excipients that increase the aqueous solubility of the drug generally increase the rate of dissolution and drug absorption. Excipients may increase the retention time of the drug in the GI tract and therefore increase the total amount of drug absorbed. Excipients may also act as carriers to increase drug diffusion across the intestinal wall. In contrast, certain excipients may create a barrier between the drug and body fluids that retard drug dissolution and thus reduce the rate or extent of drug absorption.

However, excipients may change the functionality (performance) of the drug substance and the BA of the drug from the dosage form. If used improperly in a formulation, the rate and extent of drug absorption may be affected. For example, magnesium stearate is a hydrophobic lubricant used to improve flowability of solid mixtures through processing equipment. Figures 7-6 and 7-7 show that an excessive quantity of magnesium stearate in the formulation retards drug dissolution *in vitro* and slows the rate and extent of drug absorption. In this instance, the lubricant level should be optimized to ensure that the target pharmacokinetic (PK) profile is realized. If a good understanding of the physicochemical properties and the clinical pharmacology

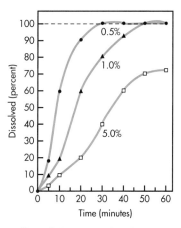

FIGURE 7-6 • Effect of lubricant on drug dissolution. Percentage of magnesium stearate in formulation.

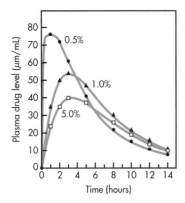

FIGURE 7-7 • Effect of lubricant on drug absorption. Percentage of magnesium stearate in formulation.

of the drug substance are available, a physiologically-based (mechanistic) absorption model may be leveraged to determine the optimal level of lubricant. Sometimes increasing the amount of disintegrant may overcome the retarding effect of lubricants on dissolution. However, with some poorly soluble drugs, even an increase in disintegrant level has little or no effect on drug dissolution because the fine drug particles are not wetted.

### FREQUENTLY ASKED QUESTIONS

▶ How can the solubility-pH profile of a drug substance be leveraged in drug product design?

▶ Why is it important to study the existence of various polymorphic forms of a drug substance?

▶ What are the typical excipients used in a tablet formulations?

## EVALUATION OF DRUG PRODUCT PERFORMANCE

### *In Vitro* Dissolution and Drug Release Testing

Dissolution and drug release tests are *in vitro* tests that measure the rate and extent of dissolution or release of the drug substance from a drug product, usually in an aqueous medium under specified conditions. *In vitro* dissolution testing provides useful information throughout the drug development process (Table 7-5).

The dissolution test is an important quality control procedure used to confirm batch-to-batch reproducibility. The dissolution test should exhibit

| TABLE 7-5 • Purpose of Dissolution and Drug Release Tests |
|---|
| Aid for formulation development and selection |
| Confirmation of batch-to-batch reproducibility |
| Demonstrate that the product performs consistently throughout its use period or shelf life |
| Establish IVIVC/IVIVR |
| Evaluate the biopharmaceutic implications of a minor/moderate product change (FDA Guidance, 1995) |

measured sensitivity to (or discriminate between) relevant changes in (1) the physicochemical characteristics of the drug, such as particle size, polymorphs, and surface area (Gray et al, 2001), (2) the drug product formulation, and/or (3) the manufacturing process that might affect drug release characteristics and consequently *in vivo* performance. Such a discriminating dissolution test is not only useful for the quality control of finished product but can provide valuable information during formulation development (ie, salt form selection, excipient selection, etc). Refer to the section below, "Discriminating Dissolution Test" for more information on this topic. The dissolution test can also be used for monitoring drug product stability. In this case, the dissolution test provides evidence that the product will perform consistently throughout its use period or shelf life. Dissolution and drug release tests can also be used as a measure of drug product performance, *in vitro*, if an appropriately defined link to product performance, *in vivo*, can be demonstrated. Such a clinically relevant dissolution method will uncover a formulation problem with the drug product that could result in a BA problem. Terms such as biorelevant, biopredictive, and clinically relevant dissolution testing are used interchangeably in several published articles. The reader is referred to a recent publication by Suarez-Sharp et al (2018) where a definition of several dissolution terminologies is provided.

Each dissolution method is specific for the drug product and its manufacturing strategy. When developing optimal dissolution parameters, a variety of conditions (ie, apparatus, media pH, etc) should be explored. The ultimate goal is to identify a dissolution test that is capable of distinguishing between acceptable and unacceptable drug formulations as observed by different drug dissolution rates under the same experimental conditions.

The dissolution test is typically a requirement for routine batch testing and qualification of certain scale-up and post-approval changes (SUPAC) for many marketed drug products. After a change is made to a formulation, the manufacturer needs to assess the potential effect of the change on the drug's BA. If the changes are deemed minor, the impact on its *in vivo* performance can be assessed by comparing the pre- and post-change product dissolution profile using the approved dissolution method or under different pH conditions. If differences exist between the dissolution profiles (the nature and magnitude of which will be described further on), an *in vivo* bioequivalence (BE) study may be performed (or required) to determine whether the observed difference *in vitro* translates into different PK *in vivo*, which could affect the safety and efficacy profile of the drug product. Major post-approval manufacturing changes require a BE study to support approval of the change. This BE study may be waived in the presence of an acceptable *in vitro–in vivo* correlation (see section "In Vitro-In Vivo Correlation" below), or, in general, be based on an established safe space (Suarez-Sharp et al, 2018).

## Development and Validation of Dissolution and Drug Release Tests

The USP dissolution tests are an *in vitro* performance tests applicable to many dosage forms such as tablets, capsules, transdermals, suppositories, suspensions, etc. The development and validation of dissolution tests is discussed in several USP general information chapters (eg, USP <711>, USP <1092>, USP <724>). The dissolution procedure requires a dissolution apparatus, dissolution medium, and test conditions that provide a method that is *discriminating* yet sufficiently rugged and reproducible for day-to-day operation and capable of being transferred between laboratories.

The choice of apparatus and dissolution medium is based on the physicochemical characteristics of the drug (including solubility, stability) and the type of formulation (such as immediate release, enteric coated, ER, rapidly dissolving, etc).

The development of an appropriate dissolution test requires the study of different agitation rates, media (including its volume and pH), and dissolution apparatus. The current USP-NF lists officially recognized dissolution apparatus (Table 7-6). For solid oral dosage forms, USP Apparatus 1 and Apparatus 2 are used most frequently.

Visual observations of the dissolution and disintegration behavior of the drug product are important markers of the manufacturing variables and should

## TABLE 7-6 • USP-NF and Non-USP-NF Dissolution Apparatus

| Apparatus* | Name | Agitation Method | Drug Product |
|---|---|---|---|
| Apparatus 1 | Rotating basket | Rotating stirrer | Tablets, capsules |
| Apparatus 2 | Paddle | Rotating stirrer | Tablets, capsules, modified drug products, suspensions |
| Apparatus 3 | Reciprocating cylinder | Reciprocation | Extended-release drug products |
| Apparatus 4 | Flow cell | Pump | Drug products containing low-water-soluble drugs |
| Apparatus 5 | Paddle over disk | Rotating stirrer | Transdermal drug products |
| Apparatus 6 | Cylinder | Rotating stirrer | Transdermal drug products |
| Apparatus 7 | Reciprocating disk | Reciprocation | Extended-release drug products |
| Rotating bottle | (Non-USP-NF) | Solid body rotation | Extended-release drug products (beads) |
| Diffusion cell (Franz) | (Non-USP-NF) | Magnetic capsule stirrer | Ointments, creams, transdermal drug products |

*USP-NF dissolution apparatus and Non-USP-NF dissolution apparatus.*

be recorded. These observations are particularly useful during dissolution method development and formulation optimization.

The size of the dissolution vessel may affect the rate and extent of dissolution. The usual medium volume is 500–1000 mL for apparatus 1 and 2. Drugs that are poorly water soluble may require use of a very large-capacity vessel (up to 2000 mL) to observe significant dissolution. In some cases, a surfactant (eg, sodium lauryl sulfate, Triton X-100, etc) may be added to the dissolution medium for water-insoluble drugs. *Sink conditions* is a term referring to an excess volume of medium (at least 3×) that allows the solid drug to dissolve continuously. If the drug solution becomes saturated, no further net drug dissolution will take place. According to the USP-NF, "the quantity of medium used should not be less than 3 times that needed to form a saturated solution of the drug substance." From a practical perspective, maintaining sink conditions ensures that dissolution is not influenced by the volume of medium, ie, the measurement reflects the unhindered release rate of drug from the formulation. In addition, sink conditions promote complete (100%) release of the nominal amount of drug from the formulation. Traditionally, it has been argued that dissolution rate-limited absorption implies that there is no buildup of drug concentration in the GI fluids, ie, the fluids function as a perfect sink (Gibaldi and Feldman, 1967). For drug products whose absorption is not necessarily dissolution-rate limited, it is questionable whether sink conditions are suitable for establishing a relationship between *in vitro* and *in vivo* (luminal) release. In other words, a dissolution test where non-sink conditions prevail could be more biopredictive of certain classes of drug formulations.

The shape of the dissolution vessel for apparatus 1 and 2 may be round- or flat-bottomed, although the compendial apparatus corresponds to the former configuration in which most studies have been conducted. Studies comparing the rate of dissolution of formulations of unspecified low- and high-solubility drug substances in flat- and round-bottomed vessels suggested no significant difference between them (Mirza et al, 2005). Experimental studies performed in USP apparatus 2 have demonstrated the sensitivity of dissolution to dosage form position inside the vessel (Qureshi and Shabnam, 2001; Baxter et al, 2005). The base of the round-bottomed apparatus 2 is understood to be a region of poor mixing resulting from solid body rotation (Bocanegra et al, 1990) which, in part, leads to the observation of "coning" for disintegrating tablets (Bai and Armenante, 2009). The presence of this coning region is a consequence of the shape of the vessel, the geometry of the stirrer blade, the verticality and centering of the stirrer shaft, and the lack of any baffles. From an engineering design perspective, "coning" would be undesirable if the goal were to achieve better dispersion. However, by the same token, the presence of a "coning" region is not in itself a reason for ruling out the value of USP (apparatus) 2, as evidenced by the vast amount of regulatory submissions which have specified this apparatus with dissolution results exhibiting low variability and a discriminating method.

The method of agitation (eg, impeller/shaft rotation speed, dips per minute, pump volume flow rates) and the degree thereof affect the hydrodynamics of the system, thereby influencing the dissolution rate. The degree of agitation must be controlled, and criteria differ among drug products. It has long been known (Hamlin et al, 1962) that increasing intensity of agitation can lead to a loss, discriminating ability of formulation factors. The temperature of the dissolution medium must be controlled. Most dissolution tests are performed at 37°C. However, for transdermal drug products, the recommended temperature is 32°C.

The nature of the dissolution medium will also affect the dissolution test. The solubility of the drug must be considered, as well as the total amount of drug in the dosage form. As pointed out above, sink conditions should be maintained. Which medium is best is determined through careful investigative studies. The dissolution medium in many USP dissolution tests is deaerated water or, if substantiated by the solubility characteristics of the drug or formulation, a buffered aqueous solution (typically pH 4–8) or dilute HCl may be used. The significance of deaeration of the medium should be determined. Various investigators have used 0.1 N HCl, phosphate buffer, simulated gastric fluid, water, and simulated intestinal fluid, depending on the nature of the drug product and the location in the GI tract where the drug is expected to dissolve.

The design of the dissolution apparatus, along with the other factors previously described, has a marked effect on the outcome of the dissolution test. No single apparatus and test can be used for all drug products. Each drug product must be considered individually with the dissolution test (method and limit(s)) that best correlates to *in vivo* BA to the extent feasible.

Usually, the dissolution test will state that a certain percentage of the labeled amount of drug product must dissolve within a specified period of time. In practice, the absolute amount of drug in the drug product may vary from tablet to tablet. Therefore, a prescribed number of tablets from each lot (eg, 12 units) are usually considered to get a representative dissolution rate for the batch.

---

### FREQUENTLY ASKED QUESTIONS

▶ How do excipients affect the dissolution kinetics of the drug?

▶ Why is it important to maintain sink conditions?

---

### Compendial Dissolution Methods

The USP-National Formulary (USP-NF) describes the official dissolution apparatus and includes information for performing dissolution tests on a variety of drug products including tablets, capsules, and other special products such as transdermal preparations. The selection of a particular dissolution method for a drug may be specified in the USP-NF monograph for a particular drug product or may be recommended by the FDA.[1] The USP-NF sets standards for dissolution and drug release tests of most drug products listed in USP monographs. Alternative dissolution methods, particularly the use of comparative dissolution rate profiles under various conditions, are often used during drug development to better understand the relationship of the formulation components and manufacturing process on drug release.

As stated above, the USP dissolution apparatus and the type of drug products that is often used with the apparatus are listed in Table 7-6. Dissolution profiles that show the drug dissolving too slowly or too rapidly may justify increasing or decreasing the rotational speed (Gray et al, 2001). The choice of apparatus for solid oral dosage forms is often Apparatus 1 (rotating basket) or Apparatus 2 (paddle) due to the ease of use, availability of the apparatus, and availability of automated methods. For USP Apparatus 1 (basket) and 2 (paddle), experimental and modeling studies suggest the importance of natural convection near the base of the vessel in which diffusion and the density difference between a saturated solution and pure dissolution medium are rate-determining factors (D'Arcy et al, 2006).

### Apparatus 1: Rotating Basket

The rotating basket apparatus (Apparatus 1) consists of a cylindrical basket held by a motor shaft. The basket holds the sample and rotates in a round flask containing the dissolution medium. The entire flask is immersed in a constant-temperature bath set at 37°C. Agitation is provided by rotating the basket. The rotating speed and the position of the basket must meet specific requirements set forth in the current USP. The most common rotating speed for the basket method is 50–100 rpm. A disadvantage of the rotating basket is that the formulation may clog to the 40-mesh screen.

### Apparatus 2: Paddle Method

The paddle apparatus (Apparatus 2) represents an unbaffled stirred tank configuration with a two-blade radial flow impeller (Fig. 7-8). The lack of baffles implies that solid body vortex motions can develop, which limit mixing efficiency throughout the vessel. Mixing conditions at the base of the vessel where the "coning effect" occurs can be improved by an axial (pitched-blade) impeller (Röst and Quist, 2003). The paddle is attached vertically to a variable-speed motor that rotates at a controlled speed. The tablet or capsule is normally placed at the base of the round-bottom dissolution vessel. The apparatus is housed in a constant-temperature water bath maintained at 37°C, similar to the rotating-basket method. The position

---

[1]The FDA provides information for many drug products on its website, https://www.accessdata.fda.gov/scripts/cder/dissolution/index.cfm (last accessed September 2019).

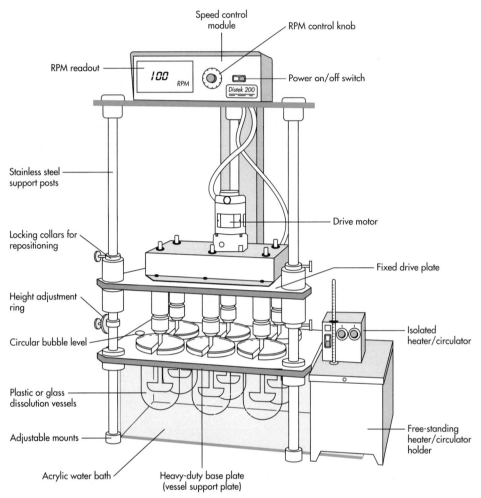

Speed control module

RPM control knob

RPM readout

*100* RPM

Distek 200

Power on/off switch

Stainless steel support posts

Drive motor

Locking collars for repositioning

Fixed drive plate

Height adjustment ring

Isolated heater/circulator

Circular bubble level

Plastic or glass dissolution vessels

Free-standing heater/circulator holder

Adjustable mounts

Acrylic water bath

Heavy-duty base plate (vessel support plate)

**FIGURE 7-8** • Typical setup for performing the USP dissolution test with the Distek 2000. The system is equipped with a height adjustment ring for easy adjustment of paddle height. (Reproduced with permission from Distek Inc, Somerset, NJ.)

and alignment of the paddle are specified in the USP. The paddle method is very sensitive to tilting. Improper alignment may drastically affect the dissolution results with some drug products. The most common operating speeds for Apparatus 2 are 50 or 75 rpm for solid oral dosage forms and 25 rpm for oral suspensions. A *sinker*, such as a few turns of platinum wire, may be used to prevent a capsule or tablet from floating. A sinker may also be used for film-coated tablets that stick to the vessel walls or to help position the tablet or capsule under the paddle (Gray et al, 2001).

The paddle apparatus has been subjected to several experimental and computational studies to map its detailed hydrodynamics (eg, Bocanegra et al, 1990; McCarthy et al, 2004; Baxter et al, 2005; Bai et al, 2007). These studies indicate that, as with most agitated tanks, the flow exhibits a highly non-uniform and time-dependent behavior with regions of poor mixing, notably at the base of the vessel directly under the axis of the impeller where the dosage form is normally located. However, despite these studies, if the apparatus is properly maintained and operated, and the dosage form's location along the vessel bottom is kept the same, the state of flow is sufficiently reproducible to ensure that hydrodynamic-induced variability is minimized.

## Apparatus 3: Reciprocating Cylinder

The reciprocating cylinder apparatus (Apparatus 3) consists of a set of cylindrical, flat-bottomed glass vessels equipped with reciprocating cylinders. Reciprocating agitation moves the dosage form up and down in the media. The agitation rate is generally 5–30 dpm (dips per minute). The reciprocating cylinder can be programmed for dissolution in various media for various times. The media can be changed easily. This apparatus may be used during drug product development to attempt to mirror pH changes and transit times in the GI tract such as starting at pH 1 and then pH 4.5 and then at pH 6.8.

## Apparatus 4: Flow-Through-Cell

The flow-through-cell apparatus (Apparatus 4) consists of a reservoir for the dissolution medium and a pump that forces dissolution medium through the cell holding the test sample. The apparatus can be operated in an "open" mode in which fresh dissolution medium is pumped through the dissolution vessel, or a "closed" mode in which the media are recirculated; sink conditions are best approximated in the open mode. The flow rate is the measure of the "degree of agitation" (or strain rate in this instance) and therefore critical to the drug release rate from the formulation. USP Chapter 711 specifies flow rates of 4, 8, and 16 mL/min. Until relatively recently, the flow being pumped through Apparatus 4 was required to be a pulsating flow with a frequency of 120±10 cycles (or pulses)/min provided the volumetric flow rate is limited to within ±5% of the average ("nominal") flow rate. Peristaltic and centrifugal pumps have not been recommended due to their poor control of the flow rate (Kakhi, 2009a). Dual piston reciprocating pumps, as used in HPLC applications, have been suggested as an alternative for constant, steady (non-pulsating) flow (Langenbucher et al, 1989). As described in Kakhi (2009a), it was unclear why a pulsating flow became the compendial standard. It has been suggested that this decision was influenced by the technical feasibility of the pumps at the time (1980s) and the apparent need to emulate the flow conditions with the established disintegration test (Langenbucher, private communuication, 2006).

Computational (Kakhi, 2009b; D'Arcy et al, 2010) and experimental studies (Shiko et al, 2011, Yoshida et al, 2015) have demonstrated that the flow structure in Apparatus 4 is complicated, particularly in the presence of pulsatile flow where reversed flow is predicted and observed; at low flow rates, natural convection appears to be an important factor too. This constitutes an important development because, originally, the device was understood to have "ideal" hydrodynamics (FIP, 1981). More recently, the major pharmacopeia (USP, European, and Japanese Pharmacopoeia) have harmonized on the use of a non-pulsating pump.

Apparatus 4 can be operated in "open column" (without 1 mm beads) and "packed column" modes, which traditionally have been referred to in the literature as the "turbulent mode" and "laminar mode," respectively. A comprehensive analysis of the flow regimes in the flow-through cell would suggest that the laminar/turbulent characterization is not justified (Kakhi, 2009a). For solid oral dosage forms being tested in the packed column mode, the sample can be placed in a tablet holder above the bed of beads, directly on top of the beads or within the packed bed.

A major advantage of the flow-through method is the easy maintenance of a sink condition for dissolution. A large volume of dissolution medium may also be used, and the mode of operation is easily adapted to automated equipment.

## Apparatus 5: Paddle-over-Disk

The USP-NF also lists a paddle-over-disk method for testing the release of drugs from transdermal products. Apparatus 5 uses the paddle and vessel assembly from Apparatus 2 with the addition of a stainless steel disk assembly designed for holding the transdermal system at the bottom of the vessel. The entire preparation is placed in a dissolution flask filled with specified medium maintained at 32°C and ideally with a pH adjusted from 5 to 6, reflecting physiological skin conditions (Siewart et al, 2003). The paddle is placed directly over the disk assembly. Samples are drawn midway between the surface of the dissolution medium and the top of the paddle blade at specified times. Matrix transdermal patches can be cut to size of the disk assembly.

### Apparatus 6: Cylinder

The cylinder method (Apparatus 6) for testing transdermal preparation is modified from the basket method (Apparatus 1). In place of the basket, a stainless-steel cylinder is used to hold the sample. The sample is mounted onto cuprophan (an inert porous cellulosic material) and the entire system adheres to the cylinder. Testing is maintained at 32°C. Apparatus 6 may be used for reservoir transdermal patches that cannot be cut smaller. Samples are drawn midway between the surface of the dissolution medium and the top of the rotating cylinder for analysis.

### Apparatus 7: Reciprocating Disk

The reciprocating disk method for testing transdermal products uses a motor drive assembly that reciprocates vertically. The samples are placed on disk-shaped holders using cuprophan supports. The test is also carried out at 32°C, and reciprocating frequency is about 30 cycles per minute.

## Alternative Methods of Dissolution Testing

### Rotating Bottle Method

The rotating bottle method was suggested in NF-XIII (National Formulary) but has become less popular since. The rotating bottle method was used mainly for ER beads. The equipment consists of a rotating rack that holds the sample drug products in bottles. The bottles are capped tightly and rotated in a 37°C temperature bath. At various times, the samples are removed from the bottle, decanted through a 40-mesh screen, and the residues are assayed. An equal volume of fresh medium is added to the remaining drug residues within the bottles and the dissolution test is continued. A dissolution test with pH 1.2 medium for 1 hour, pH 2.5 medium for the next 1 hour, followed by pH 4.5 medium for 1.5 hours, pH 7.0 medium for 1.5 hours, and pH 7.5 medium for 2 hours was recommended to simulate the condition of the GI tract. The main disadvantage is that this procedure is manual and tedious.

### Intrinsic Dissolution Method

The intrinsic dissolution test was originally conceived to study the dissolution behavior of an isotropic crystalline mass of a pure drug substance (Parrott et al, 1955). The intrinsic dissolution test can provide valuable insight in the early phases of drug development to determine which polymorphic forms can pose challenges to adequate absorption over the gastro-intestinal pH range, if drug absorption is primarily dissolution rate limited. Such an evaluation requires control of other material factors which affect dissolution rate, eg, particle size. Furthermore, it is reported that intrinsic dissolution testing requires only small quantities of material, which bears a significant economic benefit (Issa and Ferraz, 2011).

The configuration originally adapted by Wood et al (1965), involving a rotating disk system, has gained popularity and is described in USP <1087>. A compacted pellet is produced by compressing the test material with a benchtop tablet press in a cavity such that the test material is exposed on just one side to the dissolution medium. In one method, the basket method is adapted to test dissolution of powder by placing the powder in a disk attached with a clipper to the bottom of the basket. Intrinsic dissolution is usually expressed as mg/cm$^2$/min. For example, Kaplan (1972) reported that compounds with intrinsic dissolution rate above 1 mg/cm$^2$/min are usually not prone to dissolution rate limited absorption with 500 ml of dissolution media over a pH range of 1-7 at 37°C and stirring at 50 rpm.

### Diffusion Cells

Static and flow-through diffusion cells have been commonly used to characterize *in vitro* drug release and drug permeation kinetics from topically applied dosage forms (eg, ointment, gel, cream) or transdermal drug products. It should be noted that compendial apparatus, albeit with slight modifications, can be used too. The *Franz diffusion cell* is a commonly occurring configuration (Fig. 7-9) used with skin and synthetic membranes (Ueda et al, 2009; Chang et al, 2013). The source of skin may be human cadaver or animal skin (eg, hairless mouse skin). Cellulose acetate soaked in lipophilic acid is an example of synthetic membrane (Liebenberg et al, 2004). The drug product (eg, ointment) is placed on the skin surface and the drug permeates across the skin into a receptor fluid compartment that may be sampled at various times. The diffusion cell system is useful for comparing *in vitro* drug release profiles and

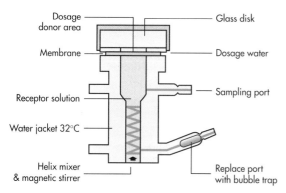

FIGURE 7-9 • The Franz diffusion cell. (Reproduced with permission from Hanson Research Corporation.)

skin permeation characteristics to aid in selecting an appropriate formulation that has optimum drug delivery.

### Dissolution Testing of Enteric-Coated Products

USP-NF lists two methods (Method A and Method B) for testing enteric-coated products. The latest revision of the USP-NF should be consulted for complete details of the methods.

Both methods require that the dissolution test be performed in the apparatus specified in the drug product monograph (usually Apparatus 1 or 2). The product is first studied with 0.1 N HCl for 2 hours and then the medium is changed to pH 6.8 buffer medium. The buffer stage generally runs for 45 minutes or for the time specified in the monograph. The objective is that no significant dissolution occurs in the acid phase (less than 10% for any sample unit), and a specified percentage of drug is released in the buffer phase. Dissolution acceptance criteria are defined in the individual drug monographs for commercial products. Appropriate criteria will need to be established for novel drugs formulated as enteric-coated drug products.

### Dissolution Approaches for Special Dosage Forms

Specialized dosage forms are being developed for improving patient compliance, to enhance therapeutic response, and for marketing exclusivity. Some of these dosage forms include osmotic capsules, orally disintegrating tablets, medicated chewing gums,

soft gelatin capsules containing drug dissolved in oil, nanomaterial, liposomal drug products, implants, intrauterine devices, transdermal drug products, and drug-eluting stents. For many of these dosage forms, compendial apparatus has been applied to evaluate their dissolution kinetics (Siewart et al, 2003). In the case of microsphere and nanoparticulate drug products, *in vitro* methods based on "sample and separate," continuous flow, and dialysis membrane have also gained popularity (D'Souza, 2014; Shen et al, 2016). Commonly reported "sample and separate" setups include Apparatus 1 (basket), Apparatus 2 (paddle), or vials. The continuous flow approach involves Apparatus 4 in closed loop mode.

### FREQUENTLY ASKED QUESTIONS

▶ Which dissolution apparatus are most often used for tablets and capsules?

▶ How does the intrinsic dissolution test differ from a conventional dissolution test and why is it useful?

▶ What is the "coning effect" in USP apparatus 2?

▶ Explain the difference between operating the flow-through cell in open and closed mode?

### Discriminating Dissolution Test

As mentioned at the start of the section "Evaluation of Drug Product Performance", the value of (*in vitro*) dissolution testing is its ability to assist in decision making to (1) ensure quality control through a linkage to batches used in pivotal clinical studies, (2) inform on batch-to-batch consistency, and (3) guide in formulation development. Dissolution testing measures the effect of formulation and physical properties of the API on the *in vitro* rate of drug solubilization. In addition, under certain circumstances (eg, presence of an adequate IVIVC) dissolution testing can serve as a surrogate for BE studies to assess the impact of some pre- and post-approval changes.

A discriminating (dissolution) method can be defined as being appropriately sensitive to manufacturing changes. "Appropriately sensitive" means the difference between cumulative dissolution profiles is quantitatively significant, as defined in the section "Dissolution Profile Comparisons." A discriminating method is able to differentiate drug products manufactured under target conditions versus drug products that are intentionally manufactured with meaningful variations (ie, ±10% to 20% change) to the specification ranges of the critical material attributes (CMAs) (eg, drug substance particle size, polymorphism) and critical process parameters (CPPs) (eg, tablet hardness, etc). A discriminating dissolution method is clearly a useful design tool to guide formulation development. The choice of experimental design to evaluate the CMAs and CPPs will depend on the design of the dosage form, the manufacturing process, and intrinsic properties of the API (Brown et al, 2004).

The term *over-discriminating dissolution method* implies that drug product batches, which have been shown to be bioequivalent based on clinical PK studies, exhibit significantly different *in vitro* dissolution profiles. Such a method is undesirable because batches with adequate performance might be otherwise rejected, thereby creating a burden for the pharmaceutical companies. However, if clinical data are available for product variants, an over-discriminating method may be leveraged to develop an *in vitro–in vivo* relationship (IVIVR)[2], which would allow for the setting of a clinically relevant drug product specification; see section below, "Approaches to Establish Clinically Relevant Drug Product Specifications." An under-discriminating method shows little to no sensitivity to changes in CMAs, CPPs, and critical formulation variables. As such, it is of little use for formulation development. The discriminating ability of such a method can be improved by setting drug product specifications very closely to the performance of the pivotal phase 3/biobatch. This approach, however, is likely to result in very tight drug product specifications. Dissolution acceptance criteria supported by clinical data (be it an IVIVR or IVIVC) may be wider than for non- or under-discriminating methods.

One should note that the discriminating ability is determined not only by the dissolution method settings

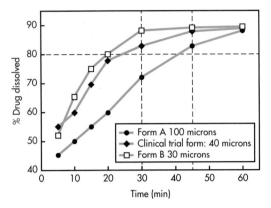

FIGURE 7-10 • Effect of particle size and drug release rate—importance of selecting the right specification-sampling time point and specification value to establish a discriminating dissolution method.

but also by the selected specification-sampling time point and specification value. Figure 7-10 illustrates the importance of selecting the right specification-sampling time point and specification value to establish a discriminating method. Batches A and B are commercial batches. The 40-micron batch corresponds to a pivotal Phase 3 clinical batch. The method seems sensitive to particle size changes; however, because batch A failed similarity testing (eg, $f_2$ statistical testing), then the dissolution acceptance criterion should be selected in a way that rejects this batch, increasing in this way the method's discriminating ability. Selecting a criterion of Q = 80% at 30 minutes fulfills this purpose. Note that setting a dissolution acceptance criterion to Q = 80% at 45 minutes may not be appropriate because it would be accepting a batch that does not have the same performance as that for the clinical batch. Selecting the wrong acceptance criterion (eg, overly permissive criterion), despite the method's intrinsic discriminating ability, renders the method not discriminating.

---

[2]An IVIVR is a qualitative link between the observed *in vivo* and *in vitro* performance of the drug product and can be used to define a safe space which will ensure BE with the target drug product. An IVIVC (discussed in more detail in the section In Vitro In Vivo Correlation) is a quantitative link developed to predict PK in order to assess whether BE is feasible or not.

---

## FREQUENTLY ASKED QUESTIONS

▶ Why is a discriminating dissolution test useful?

▶ What is the risk of an over-discriminating dissolution test?

▶ What is the risk of an under-discriminating dissolution test?

## Performance Verification Test and Mechanical Calibration

### The Need for Calibration

Analytical instruments require calibration so that there is confidence in the precision and accuracy of the measured quantity(ies). Unexplained and significant variability in these measurements can reduce credibility in the analytical technique. There are three principal sources of variability influencing *in vitro* dissolution testing: (1) the analyst, (2) the apparatus, and (3) the dosage form. The laboratory environment (eg, temperature, humidity, vibration) can also be considered a factor. The analytical procedure used to assay dissolved drug content is considered a separate test and requires its own thorough validation procedure. Studies designed to quantify the relative contribution of the sources of variability are referred to as gauge repeatability and reproducibility (R&R) studies. Repeatability is established by performing the same experiment under the same conditions of location, operator, procedure, and instrumentation. Reproducibility requires replication of the same work by another operator at a different location with another set of instruments. Gauge R&R data analyzed by Schuirmann (1980) concluded that the magnitude of within- and between-run variability was higher using the basket than the paddle apparatus, to the extent that computing a meaningful tolerance interval for results from the basket apparatus was not justified. Gao et al (2007a, 2007b) reported that the main contribution (70%) to variability is from the tablet, followed by apparatus vessel (25%) and analyst (5%). Deng et al (2008), in contrast, found that the apparatus assembly contributed the most to dissolution variability and that inherent tablet variability was low. The results summarized from the above gauge R&R studies referred to three different formulations of prednisone; therefore, a direct comparison is not straightforward.

The basic goal of the dissolution test, from a quality control perspective, is to characterize dosage form variability, and ultimately to assess manufacturing batch acceptability. It is therefore necessary to minimize the sources of variability related to analyst, apparatus, and laboratory environment. The following discussion is specific to USP Apparatus 1 (basket) and 2 (paddle) as they are the most widely used

in the pharmaceutical community and have been subjected to most of the scientific scrutiny in the field of dissolution testing. The numerous configurational factors influencing the *in vitro* release of drug from its formulation have been previously studied (eg, Cox et al, 1978, 1982; Cox and Furman, 1982). It is understood that these factors must be controlled so that precise, standardized technique and equipment generate reproducible results. There are two schools of thought on how to establish correct dissolution apparatus setup: chemical versus mechanical calibration. These approaches and their history are discussed below.

### Chemical Calibration

Chemical calibration involves the use of *reference standard (RS) tablets*, formerly known as "calibrator" tablets. In this discussion, the terminology "RS" and "calibrator" tablets will be used interchangeably. During a dissolution test under specifically defined conditions, the RS tablets' release behavior must fall within *a priori* determined acceptance limits to verify correct apparatus setup. The USP refers to this as a *Performance Verification Test* (PVT). PVT is recommended to be performed periodically, eg, twice a year (Gray et al, 1994).

USP began distributing calibrator tablets in 1978 for disintegrating 50-mg prednisone and non-disintegrating 300-mg salicylic acid formulations specifically for Apparatus 1 and 2 based in part on the results of an interlaboratory collaborative study undertaken in 1978 (Fusari et al, 1981; Cohen et al, 1990). Salicylic acid RS tablets were discontinued as part of the PVT and have not been available for purchase from USP since December 2009 because the prednisone RS tablet appeared to be sufficient (Hauck et al, 2009). The FDA also pursued the concept of a "performance standard" or calibrator to help assure reproducibility between different apparatus with the NCDA #1 and #2 prednisone formulations (Layloff, 1983). The NCDA #2 formulation was the basis of redesigned USP RS 10-mg prednisone formulation "Lot M" (Moore et al, 1996; Moore et al, 1997) and was introduced in 1999 (Foster and Brown, 2005).

The acceptance criteria for the USP RS tablets are based on results of collaborative studies (eg, Sarapu et al, 1980; Glasgow et al, 2008). These limits require reevaluation with new manufactured lots as determined by the results of the collaborative studies. With respect to stability, the dissolution characteristics of a particular manufacturing lot of USP RS tablets have also been observed to change with time as noted by official revisions to the limits. Regression analysis has been used to determine the valid use date for a particular lot (DeStefano et al, 2011; Hauck et al, 2013). More recently, the USP changed the acceptance criteria from a per-tablet approach to one based on the samples' (log transformed) geometric mean and coefficient of variation (Hauck et al, 2009). One of the proposed reasons for this modification was that, with the previous acceptance criteria limits, passing results might have occurred at the two extremes of the acceptance limits even though such results would have been suggestive of a problem with the assembly. As early as 1983, Cox et al stated that the official "per-tablet" ranges were too wide and showed considerable overlap such that the equipment could give identical results at 50 and 100 rpm and yet pass the requirements.

## Mechanical Calibration

Mechanical calibration relies on the use of diverse engineering techniques to ensure that the dissolution apparatus is correctly set up without requiring qualification by means of testing a dosage form. For example, it is known that if the shaft in Apparatus 2 is not properly centered and vertical, dissolution results can be significantly affected because of a modified hydrodynamic flow field at the base of the vessel. A centering device can be used to ensure the proper shaft alignment in the vessel. Studies using a two-point centering/verticality procedure demonstrated that 90% of the variance was due to tablets; in contrast, one-point centering resulted in 70% variability associated with the tablet and 30% with the vessel (Gao et al, 2007a). As stated earlier, the goal of dissolution testing is to analyze the variability of the sample tablets while minimizing operator and vessel variability. Therefore, the result with two-point centering suggests improved vessel setup.

USP Chapter 711 on dissolution provides tolerances for certain parameters relating to the dissolution vessel and its setup. Building on the Pharmaceutical Research and Manufacturers of America's

(PhRMA's) recommendations (Brown et al, 2009), the American Society for Testing and Materials (ASTM) approved in 2007 the standard E2503–07 (latest version, E2503-13 published in 2013). Compared to the pharmacopeial standard, E2503-13 provides a more detailed and stricter "enhanced" mechanical calibration procedure (Brown et al, 2009). For example, vessel centering and rotational speed tolerances in ASTM E2503-13 are tighter than in USP Chapter 711 and constitute recommendations made to USP over a decade before the appearance of ASTM E2503–07 (Moore et al, 1996).

## Chemical versus Mechanical Calibration

The difference of opinion regarding the value of chemical versus ("enhanced") mechanical calibration has a long history (eg, Cox et al, 1983; Skoug, 1994; Moore et al, 1995; McCormick, 1995; Gray and Foster, 1997; Oates, 1999; Mirza 2000; Commentaries in Dissolution Technologies, 2007; Brown et al, 2009). A pivotal set of studies identified that the USP RS tablets were not responsive to the critical parameters of the dissolution test, particularly by the paddle method (Cox et al, 1983; Moore et al, 1995). A significant milestone in this history was PhRMA's recommendation to include enhanced mechanical calibration testing on each dissolution bath and a reduction in reliance on the testing of USP RS tablets (PhRMA Subcommittee on Dissolution Calibration, 2000). Deng et al (2008) stated that USP's RS tablets are not a substitute for mechanical calibration; instead, both USP RS tablets and mechanical calibration are components of a well-designed PVT. The FDA Guidance on mechanical calibration (2010) recommends that an appropriately enhanced procedure for mechanical calibration can be applied to USP dissolution apparatus 1 and 2 *as an alternative procedure* to meet Current Good Manufacturing Practice calibration requirements.

In the literature, two traditional arguments for the continued use of calibrator tablets were the inability to measure dissolved gases in dissolution media (Moore et al, 1995) and the detection of significant vibration (Gray et al, 1994). Currently, USP 41/NF 36 Chapter 711 only provides a qualitative recommendation regarding acceptable levels of vibration, which limits its utility in a quantitative calibration process. However, instruments have been employed to quantify the influence of vibration on dissolution (Beyer and Smith, 1971; Fujiwara et al, 1997; Kaniwa et al, 1998; Vangani et al, 2007; Gao et al, 2009). Degassing of dissolution medium has been a well-documented standard practice for over four decades (Cox et al, 1978). Quantitative measurements of dissolved gases in dissolution media have also been reported (Gao et al, 2006).

Using a dosage form's release behavior to verify the overall correct setup of a dissolution apparatus appears to overlook the fact that a dissolution apparatus is required to provide a credible measure of a dosage form's release characteristics in the first place! Such a scenario can be likened to circular reasoning. Calibrator tablets (including NCDA #2) are real dosage forms manufactured using standard industry techniques. As such, they have an inherent lot-to-lot variability which obviously is not known *a priori*; if it were known *a priori*, there would be no need for dissolution testing. Consequently, the use of a dosage form as a true "reference standard" to qualify correct mechanical setup is questionable because there is currently no independent way of verifying the dosage form's "reference" qualification. Since nothing is known in the public domain about the composition and manufacture of the prednisone RS tablet formulations, the choice of these tablets as "ideal calibrators" cannot be studied properly.

Mechanical calibration allows for independent techniques (ie, not relying on the dissolution behavior of a dosage form) to *specifically address* critical aspects of the configurational setup known to influence dissolution results. A PVT test which fails cannot inform specifically on what went wrong. Therefore, a thorough *post-hoc* assessment of the apparatus setup (ie, mechanical calibration) and protocols would be necessary to eliminate, or at least determine, the root cause of the failure. Moreover, the basis of the PVT RS tablet is that if perturbations in the system are present (be it due to geometrical abnormalities/oversights, vibration, inadequate degassing, operator protocol, etc), the tablet's *in vitro* release profile will be sensitive to these perturbations. But what if two or more perturbations exist concurrently which could potentially cancel each other out such that the RS tablet shows release behavior within acceptance criteria?

## Meeting Dissolution Requirements

According to the Code of Federal Regulations (21CFR 314.50), a drug product application should include the specifications necessary to ensure the identity, strength, quality, purity, potency, and BA of the drug product, including, and acceptance criteria relating to, dissolution rate. For the selection of the dissolution acceptance criteria, the following points should be considered:

1. In the absence of IVIVR (eg, safe space), drug product acceptance criteria are based on the performance of the *biobatch*.[3] Dissolution data from registration batches should be used to make an assessment on the robustness of the in-process controls and control strategy. Trending or dissolution data from registration batches with disperse profiles should warrant risk mitigation strategies to avoid failing the dissolution acceptance criterion set based on the performance of the biobatches. A significant trend in the change in dissolution profile during stability should be justified with dissolution profile comparisons and *in vivo* data in those instances where the similarity testing fails.

2. Specifications should be established based on average *in vitro* dissolution data for each lot under study, equivalent to USP Stage 2 testing (ie, an average based on $n = 12$ dosage units).

3. For IR formulations, the last time point should be the time point where at least 80% of drug has been released. If the maximum amount released is less than 80%, the last time point should be the time when the plateau of the release profile has been reached. Percent release of less than 80% should be justified with data (eg, sink conditions information).

4. For ER formulations, a minimum of three time points is recommended to set the specifications. These time points should cover the early, middle, and late stages of the release profile. The last time point should be the time point where at least 80% of drug has been released. If the maximum amount released is less than 80%, the last time point should be the time when the plateau of the release profile has been reached.

---

[3]A biobatch is the finished drug product used in the pivotal clinical studies.

5. The dissolution acceptance criterion should be set in a way to ensure consistent performance from lot to lot, and this criterion should not allow the release of any lots with dissolution profiles outside those that were studied clinically.

The term Q means the amount of drug dissolved within a given time period established in the drug product specification table and is expressed as a percentage of label content. For example, a value of Q = 80% at 30 minutes means that the (arithmetic) mean percent dissolved of 12 units individually tested is at least 80% at the selected time point of 30 minutes. Note that when implementing dissolution as a quality control tool for batch release and stability analysis, the testing should follow the recommendations listed in the USP method <711>. For example, for Stage 1 testing of IR dosage forms, which considers the testing of six units, each unit must meet the criterion of not less than 85% at 30 minutes for a drug product whose acceptance criterion was set to Q = 80% at 30 minutes. Testing should continue through the three stages ($S_1$, $S_2$, $S_3$) unless the results conform at either Stage 1 or Stage 2 (Table 7-7).

## Problems of Variable Control in Dissolution Testing

As described above, various equipment and operating variables are associated with dissolution testing, and understanding the effects of operating conditions, and the geometric variables on the dissolution apparatus are critical to enhance the reliability of dissolution testing and to avoid product recalls.

Dissolution testing of solid formulations is a complex process involving various steps such as permeation of the surrounding liquid phase into the solid (ie, the wetting process), particle disintegration (depending on the formulation's composition), and solid–liquid mass transfer resulting in drug dissolved in solution. In the case of disintegration, the disperse agglomerates/particles can undergo erosion, suspension, and further particle wetting.

Depending on the particular dosage form involved, the equipment and operating variables may or may not exert a pronounced effect on the rate of dissolution of the drug or drug product. Variations may occur with the same type of equipment and procedure. The centering and alignment of the paddle is critical in the paddle method. Increased flow agitation results in higher shear stress distributions along the surfaces of dosage forms, which in turn bring about a higher dissolution rate. As a cautionary note, increased agitation is sometimes linked to the appearance of additional turbulence. However, it should be noted that compendial dissolution apparatus do not operate in a fully turbulent regime of flow. For example, at 50 or 100 rpm the paddle apparatus operates at an impeller Reynolds number (Re) of 6551 and 13,101 respectively. The laminar to turbulent transition for an agitated tank occurs at an impeller Reynolds number ranging from 1 to 10,000 (Tatterson, 1991). It is reported that the flow is still transitional at Re = 20,000 and a fully turbulent regime typically requires Re ≥ 300,000 (Machado et al, 2013). Furthermore, the impeller Re refers to conditions close to the paddle, and hence not reflective of what is occurring near the base of the dissolution vessel where the dosage form is located and where velocity magnitudes are considerably lower. At higher rotational speeds, increased velocity strain rates will, however, contribute to increased shear, thinner boundary layers, and faster dissolution, but not because of turbulence.

Wobbling and tilting due to worn equipment should be avoided, and a careful mechanical calibration procedure would screen for such effects. The basket method is less sensitive to the tilting

## TABLE 7-7 • Dissolution Acceptance

| Stage | Number Tested | Acceptance Criteria |
|---|---|---|
| $S_1$ | 6 | Each unit is not less than Q + 5% |
| $S_2$ | 6 | Average of 12 units ($S_1$ + $S_2$) is equal to or greater than Q, and no unit is less than Q – 15% |
| $S_3$ | 12 | Average of 24 units ($S_1$ + $S_2$ + $S_3$) is equal to or greater than Q, not more than 2 units are less than Q – 15%, and no unit is less than Q – 25% |

Adapted with permission from United States Pharmacopeia, 2004.

effect. However, the basket method is more sensitive to clogging due to gummy materials and to natural convection effects generated by temperature and/or concentration gradients. Pieces of small particles can also clog up the basket screen and create a local non-sink condition for dissolution. Furthermore, dissolved gas in the medium may form air bubbles on the surface of the dosage form unit and can affect dissolution in both the basket and paddle methods.

Several published articles are available describing high variability in dissolution results for dissolution apparatus calibrator tablets (Gray et al, 1994; Achanta et al, 1995; Qureshi and McGilveray, 1995; Qureshi and McGilveray, 1999). In contrast, Hamilton et al (1995) stated that since 1979 in a total of 17 different dissolution apparatus, the NCDA #2 exhibited remarkably little variation in results. The coefficient of variation (CV) of the mean results was 3.5%. They further reported results from a multi-laboratory collaborative study using NCDA #2 in which the pooled CV for individual runs was 10.8%. These values are notably lower than the variability from multi-laboratory collaborative studies reported, for example, in Qureshi and McGilveray (1995). The reasons for occurrences of high variability are numerous and can usually be traced to improper apparatus setup and/or analyst/procedural technique. Ultimately, the dosage form's real interaction with the dissolution apparatus is via the fluid behavior surrounding it, ie, the hydrodynamics. Small variations in the location of the tablet on the vessel bottom are known to significantly impact dissolution rates (Armenante and Muzzio, 2005; Qureshi and Shabnam, 2001). While it is understood that the location of the tablet in a highly non-uniform three-dimensional velocity field impacts dissolution, as in the case of the paddle apparatus, good laboratory practice would aim to minimize variability in tablet location. Positioning guides and manual placement have been used to control this source of variability (Gao et al, 2007b). This approach may not be feasible for all dosage forms and may require consideration of an alternative dissolution apparatus where variability as a result of spatial non-uniformity may prove less challenging, eg, a flow-through cell operated in a packed column mode (with 1-mm beads).

## Dissolution Profile Comparisons

Dissolution profile comparisons are used to assess the similarity of the dissolution characteristics of two formulations or different strengths of the same formulation. The results of such comparisons can impact:

- Formulation development for selecting a more optimal dissolution profile depending on the quality target product profile and the degree to which the dissolution method is known (or assumed) to be clinically relevant.

- Whether *in vivo* BA/BE studies are needed, if the dissolution method has been previously demonstrated to be predictive of clinical PK.

- Waiver of *in vivo* BA/BE studies for lower and/or higher strengths and demonstration of product strength equivalence.

- Manufacturing batch acceptability to ensure similar therapeutic performance of the drug product to the pivotal clinical batch. This assessment can be used to support certain types of post-approval changes.

The FDA guidances for IR and MR oral formulations, respectively SUPAC-IR (FDA, 1995) and SUPAC-MR (FDA Guidance for Industry, 1997c), provide recommendations to firms who intend, during the post-approval period, to change (a) the components or compositions; (b) the site of manufacture; (c) the scale-up/scale-down of manufacture; and/or (d) the manufacturing (process and equipment) of the drug product. For each type of change, these guidances list documentation (eg, dissolution testing, BE, etc) that should be provided to support the change depending on the level of impact the proposed change (Levels 1, 2, and 3) could have on the quality and *in vivo* performance of the drug product. Note that the principles listed in these guidances can also be applicable for formulation/manufacturing changes occurring during product development.

For Level 1 and Level 2 changes and some Level 3 changes such as manufacturing site change for an IR formulation, *in vivo* BE is not warranted; thus, dissolution profile comparisons either in the proposed/approved medium or in multimedia can support the change.

Dissolution profiles may be deemed similar by virtue of overall profile similarity and/or similarity at every dissolution sample time point. The FDA guidance on dissolution testing (FDA Guidance for Industry, 1997a) describes three statistical methods for the evaluation of similarity: (1) model-independent approach using a similarity factor; (2) model-independent multivariate confidence region procedure; and (3) model-dependent approach. The first approach is described below. Refer to the dissolution testing guidance for details on the other two approaches.

A model-independent approach, proposed by Moore and Flanner (1996), uses a *difference factor* ($f_1$) and a *similarity factor* ($f_2$) to compare dissolution profiles. The difference factor ($f_1$) calculates the percent (%) difference between the two curves.

$$f_1 = \left[ \left( \sum_{t=1}^{n} |R_t - T_t| \right) / \left( \sum_{t=1}^{n} R_t \right) \right] \times 100 \quad (7.2)$$

where $n$ is the number of time points, $R$ is the dissolution value of the reference batch at time $t$, and $T$ is the dissolution value of the test batch at time $t$. The dissolution value is the percent cumulative released, the fraction cumulative released (ie, the percent cumulative released normalized to unity), or any other choice of unit provided it is used consistently for $R_t$ and $T_t$. The difference factor ($f_1$) is zero when the test and reference profiles are identical and increases proportionally (in a linear 1:1 relationship) as a function of the average percent difference between the reference and test formulation data.

The *similarity factor* ($f_2$) is a logarithmic reciprocal square root transformation of the sum of squared error and is a measurement of the similarity in the percent (%) dissolution between the two curves.

$$f_2 = 50 \times \log \left[ \left( 1 + (1/n) \sum_{t=1}^{n} (R_t - T_t)^2 \right)^{-0.5} \times 100 \right] \quad (7.3)$$

where $n$ is the number of time points, $R$ is the dissolution value of the reference (pre-change) batch at time $t$, and $T$ is the dissolution value of the test (post-change) batch at time $t$ (Fig. 7-11). For $f_2$, the dissolution value at any given time point must be the percent cumulative released. The value of $f_2$ is 100

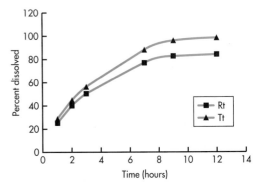

**FIGURE 7-11** • Dissolution of test and reference ER tablets. $R_t$ = reference and $T_t$ = test.

when the test and reference profiles are identical and approaches zero non-asymptotically (per a logarithmic decay curve) as the dissimilarity increases. In contrast to $f_1$, whose value remains positive, $f_2$ can become negative if the average difference between $R_t$ and $T_t$ is greater than or equal to 100%. A situation where $|R_t - T_t| \geq 100$ would be highly impractical and the difference in the release profiles would be visually self-evident.

The "fit factors", $f_1$ and $f_2$ (the term originally proposed in Moore and Flanner's publication) do not employ the data point at time zero, for which there is, by definition, zero dissolution. Both fit factors require the mean dissolution values at a given time point from the individual dissolution profiles.

The FDA Guidance for Industry (1997a) states that:

- For this calculation, three to four or more dissolution time points should be available.

- The dissolution measurements of the test and reference batches should be performed under exactly the same conditions.

- Only one measurement should be considered after 85% dissolution of both products. This requirement ensures that the computed values of $f_1$ and $f_2$ are not biased by data points suggestive of complete release which do not inform on the degree of difference between the profiles.

- The dissolution time points for both profiles must be the same in order to use the equations for $f_1$ and $f_2$. Depending on the experimental protocol, the data for test and reference may not conform with this requirement. In this case, interpolation is required to ensure data at the same time points are available.

- It can be shown that an $f_2$ value greater than 50 implies there is less than 10% difference between the two dissolution profiles. Consequently, $f_2$ values greater than 50 (50–100) are considered to ensure sameness or equivalence of the two curves and, thus, of the *in vitro* performance of the test (post-change) and reference (pre-change) products.

- To allow use of mean data, the percent coefficient of variation at the earlier time points (eg, 15 minutes) should not be more than 20%, and at other time points should not be more than 10%. If these criteria are not met, then other approaches such as multivariate approaches (refer to the dissolution guidance for details on these approaches) should be used to determine similarity. In addition, dissolution profile comparisons are not applicable when the dissolution/release characteristics are very fast achieving greater than or equal to 85% in 15 minutes.

## In Vitro–In Vivo Correlation

### Basic Concepts

ER formulations are designed to ensure that dissolution or release of the drug from the formulation is the rate-limiting step in the appearance of the drug into the systemic circulation. Under these circumstances, it may be possible to establish a quantitative linkage, referred to as an *in vitro–in vivo* correlation (IVIVC), between metrics characterizing the release of the drug *in vitro* and its release *in vivo*. The precise nature of these *in vitro* and *in vivo* metrics depends on the type, or "level" of IVIVC being considered, as discussed in the section "Categories of IVIVCs." Provided the IVIVC has been validated, it can be used to predict clinically relevant parameters from the drug formulation's *in vitro* release characteristics. An IVIVC can be a powerful design tool for formulation development during both pre- and post-market approval and can be used to justify regulatory flexibility for post-approval changes under specific circumstances.

An IVIVC should be developed with at least two or more formulations having different release characteristics. It is recommended that a correlation be established with three or more formulations (FDA Guidance for Industry,1997b). However, if the dissolution of the drug is independent of the dissolution conditions (such as apparatus agitation rate, pH, etc), then it is possible to establish such a correlation with only one formulation. When three formulations are used to develop the IVIVC (often labeled as "fast," "medium," and "slow"), it is important for the medium release to correspond to the to-be-marketed formulation. The formulations' *in vitro* and *in vivo* range of the release rates should be as wide as possible to allow for a meaningful interpolative analysis.

### Categories of IVIVCs

#### Level A Correlation

***Definition and Concepts*** A level A IVIVC is the highest level of correlation because it can predict either the complete time course of the percent (%) drug released *in vivo* ($f_r$), or the drug plasma concentration ($C_p$), from the percent (%) drug released *in vitro* ($f_d$). The quantity $f_r$ is often equated to the fraction of drug absorbed into the systemic circulation, $f_a$; this equivalence assumes very high permeability, and no gut wall and first-pass metabolism. In the following discussion, only $f_r$ will be referred to for conciseness with the understanding that $f_a$ could also be implied. Furthermore, the time derivative of $f_r$ (denoted as $\dot{f}_r$) is often referred to as the drug "input" rate; from a terminology perspective, the "release" from the formulation (embodied by the term $f_r$) corresponds to an "input" to the physiological system. Similarly, $\dot{f}_d$ represents the drug *in vitro* dissolution rate.

A level A correlation enables the *in vitro* dissolution test to become a meaningful and clinically relevant quality control tool that can predict *in vivo* drug product performance. For this reason, a validated and approved level A IVIVC can be used to support a waiver of *in vivo* BE studies required for certain major post-approval changes, such as a relocation of the manufacturing site (ie, for modified-release [MR] dosage forms), change of manufacturing process, formulation modification, and even product strength using the same formulation (FDA Guidance for Industry, 1997c). Despite the advantages of an IVIVC, it appears to be an underutilized tool in formulation development. It has been reported that the number of IVIVC studies seen in regulatory submissions per year is not increasing and the overall acceptance rate is about 40% (Suarez Sharp et al, 2016).

In the following subsections, the two main types of level A correlations are described together with the central concepts of convolution and deconvolution.

***One-Stage Methods*** One-stage IVIVC methods quantitatively map the *in vivo* metric $C_p(t)$, which is the measure of the PK response, to the *in vitro* metric $f_d(t)$, generated from an *in vitro* experiment, in one calculation step without having to calculate an intermediate *in vivo* input parameter ($f_r$ or $\dot{f}_r$). It should also be borne in mind that predictions of $C_p$ are directly verifiable against experimental observations, whereas currently, $f_r$ cannot be measured in a routinely accurate manner.

A one-stage IVIVC has been traditionally developed via a convolution approach (Gillespie, 1997). To understand this approach, the central concept of convolution requires clarification. The convolution integral is derived using the assumptions of linear superposition and time invariance (Finkelstein and Carson, 1985). Linearity implies that when a system's input is doubled, the output scales by the same factor. This is manifested in the concept of dose proportionality associated with linear PK and is often observed in clinical studies. Practical instances of non-linear PK do occur, for example involving saturable elimination kinetics or saturable active transport across a membrane. The linearity assumption underpinning the concept of convolution implies the principle of superposition, ie, if a subject is administered separate 3-mg and 5-mg doses, the resulting response is the additive response to each of the individual doses. Time invariance means that the system's response is unaffected by the timing of the input. In other words, if a subject is administered two doses of the same strength at times $t = 0$ and $t = 2$ hours respectively, the PK resulting from each administration is the same. Such a condition is violated, for example, when enterohepatic circulation occurs. The linearity and time-invariance assumptions relate to the "system" response, not the input (ie, absorption profile).

For example, a non-linear input function does not violate the underlying assumptions for it to be used in a convolution analysis. The convolution integral can be expressed as follows:

$$C_p(t) = \int_0^t g(t-\tau)\dot{f}_r(\tau)d\tau = \int_0^t g(t)\dot{f}_r(t-\tau)d\tau \quad (7.4)$$

In the above expression, the second integral is a result of the commutative property of convolution. The absorption of drug into the systemic circulation can be considered as a string of impulses occurring at different times. The above equation can be interpreted as stating that the response $C_p$ (ie, the plasma drug concentration–time profile) of the linear, time-invariant (LTI) system is the sum of the responses to these individual impulses. The function "$g$" is the "natural" response of the "system" to a disturbance from equilibrium. It is a system characteristic independent of the input (rate) function, $\dot{f}_r$. If the input $\dot{f}_r$ were a disturbance of very short duration (ideally a unit Dirac delta function), the response would be: $C_p(t) = g(t)$. For this reason, $g$ is referred to as the unit impulse response (UIR). In practical terms, the UIR represents the mathematical function, which describes how the "system" distributes, metabolizes, and eliminates drug *after* it has been absorbed.

The UIR is best characterized by administering an IV bolus to a subject and fitting the parameters associated with $g$ to the subject's measured PK response over time. In this manner, the subject's inherent disposition characteristics are being characterized and a measure of the inter-individual variability is being captured. It is noted, however, that very often IR formulations are also used to approximate $g(t)$. This is adequate provided the IR formulation's absorption time scale is significantly faster than that of the ER formulations. Alternatively, under the assumption of first-order absorption for an LTI process, described as a polyexponential profile, the UIR parameters fitted to the IR data can be "stripped" of the absorption phase resulting in a UIR with modified coefficients reflecting a hypothetical IV bolus administration (Kakhi et al, 2013).

In the one-stage direct convolution method, the *a priori* unknown input function $\dot{f}_r$ can be approximated by $\dot{f}_d$ in the simplest case. This corresponds to the assumption that *in vivo* input/release is equal to *in vitro* dissolution. A more complex relationship between $\dot{f}_r$ and $\dot{f}_d$ can be presumed entailing additional model parameters whose values would have to be estimated as part of the solution procedure (O'Hara et al, 2001). This representation of $\dot{f}_r$ as a function of $\dot{f}_d$ is the assumed IVIVC, and together with a representative UIR (ie, the $g(t)$ characterization), the plasma concentration–time profile can be predicted using the convolution integral. It is noted that in the ideal scenario, a linear, unity gradient relationship would be obtained between $\dot{f}_r$ and $\dot{f}_d$, but this is not a requirement. The correlation primarily needs to be robust and accurate, as discussed in more detail in the section "Validation of IVIVCs." Once the free parameters are estimated using an appropriately defined internal data set, the resulting IVIVC model can then be used to predict plasma concentrations from an *in vitro* dissolution profile based on the same dissolution method and type of formulation used to develop the IVIVC in the first place.

A major limitation of the one-stage, convolution-based approach, as defined by the strict use of the convolution integral defined above, is that it relies on the assumption of an LTI system. This constraint can be avoided by employing mass balance methods based on the solution of ordinary differential equations (ODEs) as expressed in classical compartmental PK theory (Gibaldi and Perrier, 1982). One such approach is described by Buchwald (2003) in which the drug absorption rate into the central compartment was modeled as a time-transformed linear function of the *in vitro* dissolution rate using a time-dependent multiplying factor that accounted for the variability of the *in vivo* absorption conditions as the drug moved along the GI tract. This time-dependent factor also included a cutoff parameter to emulate limited absorption window effects. The analysis was presented for averaged PK data, ie, interindividual variability was not considered. The introduction of the parameters related to Buchwald's (2003) method represents a compact way of representing complex physiologically based phenomena, which might otherwise not be well-understood. The weakness of such an approach is that it is difficult to relate model parameters (such as the aforementioned

time-dependent cutoff) defined to emulate physiological phenomena to actual physiological variables.

Another class of emerging one-stage IVIVC makes use of population PK approaches (Sheiner, 1984). These methods allow for a rigorous mathematical treatment of variability in the data, but their physiological relevance is limited compared to mechanistic absorption models (MAMs) described below in the context of two-stage methodologies. In a one-stage population PK-IVIVC, a mapping function is specified to link the *in vivo* input to the *in vitro* dissolution by means of mixed effects terms (Gaynor et al, 2011). The parameter estimation problem is treated by solvers suited to non-linear mixed effects (NLME) models, such as NONMEM (Boeckmann et al, 2017). The algorithmic basis for parameter estimation relies on the principle of maximum likelihood (Beal and Sheiner, 1982), The likelihood in this instance represents the probability of any observation given a model for predicting the observation.

***Two-Stage Methods*** Unlike the single-stage approach, which maps the *in vivo* metric $C_p(t)$ to the *in vitro* metric $f_d(t)$ in a single calculation step, the two-stage approach first calculates drug input, $f_r(t)$, and in the second step quantitatively characterizes the IVIVC by a regression analysis linking $f_r(t)$ to $f_d(t)$. The determination of $f_r(t)$ is referred to as "deconvolution," a mathematical operation described further below; however, as noted above with one-stage methods which do not involve a direct convolution (eg, the ODE-based approaches), several important classes of two-stage methods do not involve a strict deconvolution. Nevertheless, the term "deconvolution" is still used loosely to describe the first step of the analysis. The two-stage approach currently forms the basis of the majority of submitted regulatory IVIVCs (Suarez Sharp et al, 2016). Historically, the popularity of this approach is understandable because much effort has and still is being expended to develop clinically predictive *in vitro* dissolution tests. Based on this goal, it is natural to compare a percent absorbed *in vivo* profile with its proposed *in vitro* surrogate. The two-stage approach provides for an exploratory analysis of the relationship between $f_r(t)$ and $f_d(t)$. In this respect, a two-stage approach provides more insight compared to the one-stage because it examines the underlying $f_r(t)$

versus $f_d(t)$ relationship to better inform an appropriate selection for the proposed IVIVC function, even though there are no measurements to verify the accuracy of the $f_r(t)$ predictions. One drawback of the two-stage approach compared to the one-stage is that it does not directly predict the plasma time course, which is the metric of interest (Gillespie, 1997). However, the one-stage method requires an *a priori* guess for the mathematical form of the IVIVC, as explained in the previous section.

The first step of this "two-stage approach" involves the determination of the input function, and this is where the complexity resides. The purpose of "deconvolution" in PK systems analysis, regardless of its precise details, is to calculate *in vivo* release, $f_r(t)$, from the available clinical data. In the broader mathematical sense, deconvolution could involve the calculation of the UIR from the input and output (response) data (Gamel et al, 1973; Madden et al, 1996), however, for IVIVC analysis it is the UIR and $C_p(t)$ data which are known *a priori* through appropriate measurements.

Deconvolution, in the strictest sense, is the mathematical inverse of convolution. The convolution integral was introduced in the previous section. Thus, with $C_p(t)$ measured and $g(t)$ characterized by data generated after administration of an IV or IR formulation of the same drug substance, determining the input rate $\dot{f}_r$ is called deconvolution The fraction released, $f_r(t)$, can then be easily determined from $\dot{f}_r$ by integration. More formally, the Laplace transform of the convolution integral can be taken and then re-arranged explicitly to solve for $\dot{f}_r$, Qiu et al (2000):

$$\dot{f}_r(t) = L^{-1}\{\dot{f}_r(s)\} = L^{-1}\left\{\frac{\bar{C}_p(s)}{\bar{g}(s)}\right\} \qquad (7.5)$$

In the above, $L^{-1}$ denotes the inverse Laplace transform, $\bar{C}_p$ is the Laplace transform of $C_p$ and $s$ is a complex number frequency parameter. An analogous result can be obtained by means of a Fourier transform (Madden et al, 1996). Calculating the Laplace transform of the discrete datasets $C_p(t)$ and $g(t)$, and then further determining the inverse Laplace transform of its quotient can, in general, be mathematically intractable and/or fraught with numerical challenges (Vaughan and Dennis, 1978). Indeed, deconvolution is known to be an ill-conditioned

deterministic problem. "Ill conditioning" means that small perturbations in the output response (eg, due to measurement noise) give rise to large perturbations in the sought-after input (Ekstrom, 1973; Gamel et al, 1973). For this reason, the most commonly used deconvolution methods applied to analyze real PK data do not attempt a direct computation based on the mathematical inversion of convolution presented above. Instead, indirect approaches are sought, and these can be categorized as compartmental and non-compartmental methods.

One of the first level A IVIVCs described in the literature (Levy, 1964) employed a compartmental method known as a *Wagner-Nelson deconvolution* (Wagner and Nelson, 1963). This method is based on a single compartment mass balance and can be expressed as:

$$X_{abs}(t) = VC_p(t) + k_{el}V\int_0^t C_p(t^*)dt^* \qquad (7.6)$$

In the above equation, $X_{abs}(t)$ is the amount of drug absorbed at time $t$, $V$ is the volume of distribution, $k_{el}$ is the first-order elimination constant and the integral is simply the area under the curve at time $t$, $AUC(t)$. When determining the fraction of drug absorbed at a given time, defined as $X_{abs}(t)/X_{abs}$ ($t = \infty$), one is left with an expression involving $C_p(t)$, $AUC(t)$, and $k_{el}$, ie, the volume of distribution cancels out and only $k_{el}$ requires characterization. *Loo-Riegelman* deconvolution represents a two-compartment mass balance which can be mathematically expressed by the following expression (Loo and Riegelman, 1968):

$$X_{abs}(t) = V_1C_{p,1}(t) + k_{el}V_1\int_0^t C_p(t^*)dt^* + V_1C_{p,2}(t) \qquad (7.7)$$

The above equation states that the amount of drug absorbed, $X_{abs}(t)$, is the sum of the amounts present in the central and peripheral compartments ($V_1C_{p,1}(t)$ and $V_1C_{p,2}(t)$ respectively), and the amount eliminated through metabolism and excretion. It is presumed that drug concentration assays measure levels in compartment 1. The concentration in compartment 2 is defined with respect to the volume of distribution of compartment 1 and is an unknown. The Loo-Riegelman method employs a linearization of certain terms in the integration of the ODE for the mass balance in the peripherical compartment to obtain a closed-form approximation for $C_{p,2}(t)$. This deconvolution method requires characterization of $k_{el}$ and the intercompartmental rate constants, $k_{12}$ and $k_{21}$. Higher order compartmental kinetics can be envisaged to perform the appropriate deconvolution method, assuming the observed data conform to the model prescribed and the associated parameters (eg, intercompartmental rate constants) can be accurately identified.

Both the Wagner-Nelson and Loo-Riegelman methods are based on linear ODEs. Consequently, these approaches are only applicable to LTI systems. Stochastic deconvolution is a parameter estimation method embedded within an NLME population-PK formalism (Kakhi and Chittenden, 2013). In this approach, compartmental kinetics is coupled to an absorption rate coefficient modeled as a mixed effect whose random component is described by a Wiener process. Such an approach provides several advantages over traditional (non-physiologically based) methods of two-stage deconvolution, and one-stage convolution:

- It is not limited to LTI systems because an underlying PK model of arbitrary complexity relates the input to the output, similar to Buchwald's (2003) one-stage approach described above.

- It obviates the need for IR, IV, or oral solution data to determine the UIR, provided the PK data for the ER formulations are suitably sampled over time to adequately determine the disposition kinetics.

- The use of a population-PK framework allows for a mathematically rigorous treatment of the inter-subject and inter-occasion variability.

- Modeling the absorption rate coefficient as a mixed effect allows for a more flexible treatment of the potentially complex behavior of the absorption profile, as opposed to defining an abrupt cut-off time as in Buchwald's (2003) approach.

Stochastic deconvolution has been applied to analyze an IVIVC demonstrating that results comparable to numerical deconvolution (described below) can be obtained without the use of a UIR to characterize drug disposition kinetics (Kakhi et al, 2017).

A two-stage methodology can be combined with a physiologically-based or mechanistic absorption model (PBAM or MAM, respectively) to develop a "mechanistic IVIVC" (Kakhi and Lukacova, 2015; Kesisoglou et al, 2015; Mistry et al, 2016). A MAM is, mathematically speaking, a detailed system of ODEs used to describe a physiologically based multicompartmental model in which mass balances and physicochemical interactions are explicitly modeled. Since a system of ODEs is being employed, non-LTI system kinetics can be treated. MAMs can be used to investigate the effect of drug product manufacturing changes (eg, formulation and process changes) on the plasma concentration (Kesisoglou and Mitra, 2015). The MAM accounts for GI transit times, drug degradation, precipitation, passive and active transcellular transport across the apical and basolateral membranes, paracellular transport, gut wall, and first-pass metabolism. The MAM can be combined with a classical, compartmental PK model or with a physiologically-based PK (PBPK) model to account for drug disposition. In the PBPK description, a multicompartment, whole-body model describing systemic disposition is employed. In a two-stage mechanistic IVIVC, a MAM is used to first calculate $f_r(t)$. The procedure is referred to as a mechanistic deconvolution. In this procedure, an $f_r(t)$ relationship is presumed (eg, a Weibull function) which includes unknown parameters to be estimated. An initial guess for the profile is then proposed (eg, the observed *in vitro* dissolution of the formulation) and the presumed $f_r(t)$ is fitted to this initial guessed profile. By means of an iterative process, the to-be-estimated parameters of the drug release profile are then updated in an optimization where the objective function attempts to minimize the sum of the least-squares residual of the calculated and observed concentration-time data. In the second stage of the procedure, an IVIVC relationship linking the optimized $f_r(t)$ to $f_d(t)$ is proposed and its free parameters are estimated in a regression analysis.

*Non-compartmental*, or *model-independent*, approaches to deconvolution are generally referred to as numerical deconvolution and they are, to date, the most widely used class of methods to develop regulatory IVIVCs (Suarez-Sharp et al, 2016). The two-stage methods described above are technically not deconvolutions because they are not attempting to invert the convolution integral. Indeed, stochastic and mechanistic deconvolutions are not limited to LTI systems, but a strict deconvolution (and its inverse, the convolution) presumes LTI system kinetics. There are many numerical deconvolution algorithms in the scientific literature and their derivations are independent of any assumptions related to compartmental kinetics associated with drug disposition and elimination. Vaughan and Dennis' (1978) point-area method assumed a staircase input function for $\dot{f_r}$, defined as a finite set of rectangular pulses, the duration of which was not, in principle, constrained to be equal. Their analysis was applied to an *a priori* known simulated $C_p(t)$ dataset without the influence of noise which is known to influence the robustness and accuracy of numerical deconvolution methods (Gamel et al, 1973). Madden et al (1996) described the use of several numerical deconvolution methods applied to different sets of simulated noisy data. The methods studied were based on diverse mathematical principles such as Fourier transform, cubic splines, maximum entropy, and a genetic algorithm. It is beyond the scope of this chapter to analyze the various techniques in detail; however, it will be noted that the methods had differing levels of success. Thus, the term *numerical deconvolution* is a generic one representative of a collection of very diverse methods, and, as a result, caution is required when making qualifications in general about the performance of *numerical deconvolution*.

The focus in this subsection will be on a commonly utilized method of numerical deconvolution which involves the use of deconvolution-through convolution (Cutler, 1978; Veng-Pedersen and Modi, 1992) coupled with the use of smoothed "hat-type wavelets" as the basis function for the characterization of the drug input rate (Veng-Pedersen, 1997; Certara:Phoenix/WinNonlin, 2019). In the version of deconvolution-through-convolution implemented in Phoenix/WinNonlin, each subject UIR is fitted to a polyexponential function and convolved with an initially guessed subject input rate profile based on the hat-type wavelets [a schematic of the wavelets can be found in Kakhi et al (2017)]. Since the functions being convolved have closed-form expressions, an analytic solution is obtained which yields a predicted subject concentration-time profile. Central to this algorithm is a set of to-be-estimated parameters referred to as dose-scaling factors and within each observation time interval (from the measured data set), a dose-scaling factor is defined that constitutes the fraction of the dose applied in a given wavelet function. Numerical deconvolution converges toward a solution for the input rate function by iteratively updating the dose scaling factors in order to minimize the sum of squared residuals of the predicted and observed concentrations. The subject input rate of drug, thus generated, is then integrated over time to yield the subject cumulative fraction of drug released/absorbed. The dose scaling factors are not physiologically-based parameters; they are essentially ad-hoc parameters defined to ensure the best possible fit of the underlying observed concentration-time data when convolving the predicted input rate with the UIR. This observation is further reinforced by the fact that the calculated fraction input rate is de-coupled from the dose (ie, there is no boundedness criterion placed on the sum of all dose scaling factors) allowing for the cumulative sum of the *in vivo* fraction of drug release to exceed unity when the UIR is not derived from IV data (Kakhi et al, 2017).

The second stage of the two-stage approach to IVIVC development involves a regression analysis. In this step, a plot of $f_r$ against $f_d$ is used to explore the relationship between these two variables so that a suitable mathematical relationship can be postulated that might best fit the data spread. An alternative graph is known as the Levy plot which shows *in vivo* time against *in vitro* time required to achieve a given percent release. The Levy plot can provide quick feedback as to the need for time scaling in the IVIVC characterization to account for differences in the rate of *in vivo* and *in vitro* dissolution kinetics. A graphical workflow of the two-stage process is shown in Fig. 7-12.

**Level B Correlation** Level B correlation utilizes the principle of statistical moment in which the mean *in vitro* dissolution time is compared to either the mean residence time (MRT)[4] or the mean *in vivo* dissolution time (MDT). Level B correlation uses all of the *in vitro* and *in vivo* data, but is not a point-to-point correlation. Different profiles can give the same parameter values.

---

[4]MRT is the mean (average) time that the drug molecules stay in the body, whereas the MDT is the mean time for drug dissolution.

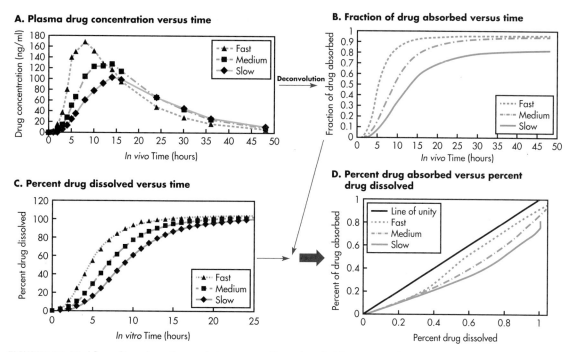

**A. Plasma drug concentration versus time**

**B. Fraction of drug absorbed versus time**

**C. Percent drug dissolved versus time**

**D. Percent drug absorbed versus percent drug dissolved**

*Deconvolution*

**FIGURE 7-12 •** Workflow of two-stage deconvolution process. (Reproduced with permission from Kakhi M, Marroum P, Chittenden J. Analysis of level A in vitro-in vivo correlations for an extended-release formulation with limited bioavailability, *Biopharm Drug Dispos.* 2013 Jul;34(5):262-277.)

The Level B correlation alone cannot justify formulation modification, manufacturing site change, excipient source change, batch-to-batch quality, etc.

**Level C Correlation**   A Level C correlation is not a point-to-point correlation. A Level C correlation establishes a single-point relationship between a dissolution parameter such as percent dissolved at a given time and a PK parameter of interest such as AUC and $C_{max}$. Level C correlation is useful for formulation selection and development but has limited regulatory application. *Multiple Level C correlation* relates one or several PK parameters of interest to the amount of drug dissolved at several time points of the dissolution profile. In general, if one is able to develop a multiple Level C correlation, then it may be feasible to develop a Level A correlation.

**Validation of IVIVCs**

Once an IVIVC has been developed using the techniques described above, it needs to be validated in order to determine its predictive accuracy. This is

essential if the IVIVC is to be applied with confidence in a situation where its use would be justified as a surrogate for *in vivo* BE trials. The data set comprising the *in vitro* and *in vivo* observations that were used to develop the IVIVC are referred to as the "internal data set". Essentially, the IVIVC has been calibrated with the internal data set. A validation of the IVIVC for this internal data set is called an internal validation, and this is the first line of investigation the modeler needs to perform to assess the accuracy of the IVIVC. Criteria for the assessment of internal predictability of an IVIVC are given in regulatory documents such as the FDA Guidance for Industry (1997b) and EMA guideline (2014). The FDA currently recommends that the criteria be based on how accurately the IVIVC-predicted PK parameters $C_{max}$ and AUC compare with the corresponding observations extracted from the averaged plasma concentration-time data, and not the average of the individual $C_{max}$ and AUC. As a side note, it is important to emphasize that the convolutions/deconvolutions used to develop the IVIVC should be based, where possible (eg, with suitable crossover data), on the individual PK data and not on averaged PK data. Depending on the outcome of the internal validation, it may be necessary to demonstrate the IVIVC's predictive robustness by predicting the PK of a formulation, which has not been used to develop the IVIVC. This is referred to as external validation. Another class of validation that serves to instill greater confidence in an IVIVC's predictability is the use of cross-validation, or the "leave one out" approach. For example, if three formulations are available to develop the IVIVC, one can re-perform the internal validation with just two of the formulations while excluding the third which can be used as an external validation (Kakhi et al, 2013). In the United States and in Europe, a BE study can be waived based on the established IVIVC if the predicted mean AUC and $C_{max}$ of the test and reference do not differ from each other by more than 20% (FDA Guidance for Industry, 1997b; EMA, 2014).

## Failure of Correlation of *In Vitro* Dissolution to *In Vivo* Absorption

A robust IVIVC should demonstrate its ability to predict the *in vivo* performance of a drug product from its *in vitro* dissolution characteristics over the range of *in vitro* release rates evaluated during the construction and validation (internal and external) of the correlation. Well-defined IVIVCs have been reported for ER drug products but have been more difficult to predict for IR drug products. The success for establishing a robust IVIVC depends on several factors including (1) the selection of a discriminating dissolution method that mimics the drug product's *in vivo* performance; (2) the number of formulations used in the construction of the correlation; (3) inclusion of formulations with significantly different release characteristics as demonstrated by dissolution similarity test; (4) design of the *in vivo* BA/BE study (eg, fast versus fed conditions); (5) modeling approach (physiologically-based/mechanistic versus non-mechanistic), etc. The following is a list of the most common reasons (besides not meeting the validation requirements) for a lack of successful IVIVCs (Suarez-Sharp et al, 2016):

1. Failing to meet the criteria for *in vitro* and *in vivo* experimentation in terms of the number of formulations used in the construction of the IVIVC.

2. *In vitro* release rates of formulations used in the construction of the IVIVC are similar.

3. Lack of a rank-order correlation.

4. Failure to develop the IVIVC in the fasted state unless the drug can only be tolerated in the fed state.

5. The use of averaged PK data to develop the IVIVC in place of individual data for both one- and two-stage approaches.

6. The IVIVC was over-parameterized.

7. Complex absorption processes (eg, gut wall metabolism, instability of drug in the GI tract) were not captured by the model.

8. The use of different scaling factors for the formulations when building/parameterizing the correlation function.

It should be noted that an IVIVC supersedes similarity (eg, $f_2$) testing in such a way that when an IVIVC is approved, the data that should be included to support the change (eg, post-approval changes, support of wider dissolution acceptance criteria) are the difference in predicted means for $C_{max}$ and AUC.

As noted above, the problem of poor correlation between systemic exposure and dissolution may be due to the complexity of drug absorption and the weakness of the dissolution method. The use of biorelevant dissolution methods can be used to understand the effects of formulation factors on release (dispersion, dissolution, drug precipitation, and stability), and the interactions between active pharmaceutical ingredients, dosage form, excipients, and the *in vivo* environment. These methods may increase the likelihood for the development of successful IVIVCs (Suarez-Sharp et al, 2018).

Biorelevant methods can range from using physiologically relevant dissolution media in standard dissolution apparatus as stated in the guidance for industry documents (FDA Guidance for Industry, 1997a) to more complicated media to mimic *in vivo* conditions such as food effects and alcohol dose dumping (Klein, 2010). Note, however, that successful IVIVCs have been possible when simple dissolution methods are used (Suarez-Sharp, 2012).

An excellent example of the importance of dissolution design is shown in Fig. 7-13. Dissolution tests using four different dissolution media were performed for two quinidine gluconate sustained-release

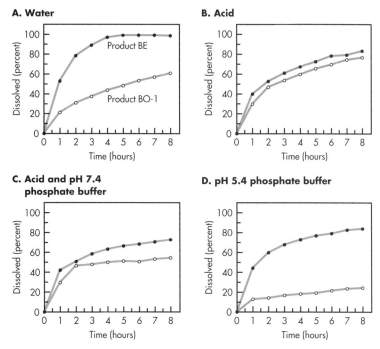

FIGURE 7-13 • Dissolution profile of two quinidine gluconate sustained-release products in different dissolution media. Each data point is the mean of 12 tablets. f(• = product BE, ° = product BO-1.) (Reproduced with permission from Prasad V, Shah V, Knight P, et al: Importance of media selection in establishment of in vitro–in vivo relationship for quinidine gluconate, 1982 *Int J Pharm* Dec;13(1):1–7.)

tablets (Prasad et al, 1983). Product "BE" was known to be bioavailable, whereas product BO-1 was known to be incompletely absorbed. It is interesting to see that using acid medium as well as acid followed by pH 7.4 buffer did not distinguish the two products well, whereas using water or pH 5.4 buffer as dissolution medium clearly distinguished the "good" product from the one that was not completely available. In this case, the use of an acid medium is consistent with the physiologic condition in the stomach, but this procedure would be misleading as a quality control tool. It is important that any new dissolution test be carefully researched before being adopted as a method for predicting drug absorption.

### Approaches to Establish Clinically Relevant Drug Product Specifications

Establishing the appropriate product specifications is critical in assuring that drug product quality is consistent throughout the product's life cycle. Product specifications are typically considered as those limits that define adequate quality and that support the *in vitro* determinations of identity, purity, potency, and strength of the drug product. On the other hand, clinically relevant specifications are those specifications that, in addition, take into consideration the clinical impact assuring a consistent safety and efficacy profile. In this case, the choice of acceptance criteria is no longer made based on the *in vitro* results but on predefined clinically acceptable outcomes. Understanding the relationship between the *in vitro* measures and the clinical outcomes may provide flexibility in setting specifications.

The ideal approach in setting drug product specifications would be to adopt a *quality by design* (QbD) approach in the drug development process. This approach should include an understanding of the *critical quality attributes* (CQAs), their respective interactions, and the impact that these may have on the quality target product profile (QTPP). Under the QbD paradigm, it is assumed that all the batches manufactured within the design space (DS) have the same *in vivo* performance[5]. The key question is: How

---

[5]Note that within the design space (DS) all batches are assumed BE, but that is only true if the DS is verified, for example, through the establishment of a safe space, as discussed further on.

do we achieve the goal of demonstrating that all the batches within the DS have the same *in vivo* performance? In answering this question, the use of biopharmaceutic tools such as dissolution and BA/BE studies becomes relevant because it would be rather impractical to determine the clinical relevance of movements within the DS through clinical efficacy and safety trials. As such, one ideal path toward establishing *clinically relevant drug product specifications* (CRDPS) may be to manufacture several product variants with different dissolution characteristics resulting in plasma concentration versus time profiles, which follow a rank order relationship. In so doing, one can also (a) assess the impact of changes in various product attributes or process parameters on *in vitro* dissolution and *in vivo* performance, (b) explore the relationship between *in vitro* dissolution and *in vivo* BA, and (c) determine relative BA or BE among product variants, using clinical trial material as a reference. Consequently, this approach not only facilitates the identification of the CMAs and CPPs but also facilitates establishing CRDPS. This understanding helps in defining and verifying the DS limits, which links the important *in vitro* performance of the drug product to the desired clinical performance.

Due to the critical role that dissolution plays in defining the BA of the drug, *in vitro* dissolution, if identified as a CQA, can serve as a relevant predictor of the *in vivo* performance of the drug product. In this case, clinically relevant dissolution methods and specifications will minimize the variability to the patient and therefore will optimize drug therapy.

There are several general approaches that can be used for establishing CRDPS, depending on whether *in vivo* data (ie, systemic exposure) are available (Suarez Sharp, 2011, 2012). These approaches enable dissolution testing to define the boundaries of a safe space, which is a region within which all product variants are bioequivalent. Equally, behavior falling outside of the safe space would imply bio-inequivalence and allow for justified rejection of these batches. The implementation of these approaches may or may not result in regulatory flexibility (Suarez Sharp et al, 2018). Some of the scenarios are examined below highlighting the impact of regulatory flexibility.

### Approach A: Data Linking In Vitro and In Vivo Performance are NOT Available

In this approach, although there is PK, efficacy, and safety data for the relevant phases of product development, no relationship has been established linking variations on the CMAs and CPPs and dissolution on clinical performance. Therefore, drug product specifications (ie, dissolution acceptance criterion) are established based on the mean dissolution values of batches tested in pivotal clinical trials. Any major changes implemented to a pivotal clinical trial formulation need to be supported by additional *in vivo* BA/BE studies since dissolution can only support the implementation of minor/moderate changes.

It is widely accepted that minor/moderate changes (refer to FDA Guidance for Industry, SUPAC IR,1995 and SUPAC MR, 1997c), with no or minimal expected effect on the BA, and consequently the safety and efficacy profile, can be evaluated by dissolution profile comparisons; however, there may be the case when certain minor/moderate apparent changes may have an *in vivo* impact, and the assessment of the impact on clinical performance depends on the discriminating ability of the method (ie, established using data from design of experiments studies). These limitations make this approach less desirable for drug product containing low solubility drug substances and it is likely to result in very tight drug product specifications.

### Approach B: Data Linking In Vitro and In Vivo Performance are Available

In this case, studies have been carried out to determine whether changes of the CMAs or CPPs has an effect on dissolution and systemic exposure. The *in vitro–in vivo* assessment process often involves the following steps:

(a) Prepare product variants using critical formulation and/or manufacturing variables to study their *in vitro* dissolution characteristics

(b) Develop a discriminating dissolution method

(c) Conduct *in vivo* PK study(ies) in appropriate groups of human subjects to test these product variants along with a reference standard (ie, the formulation used in pivotal Phase 3 clinical trials)

(d) Identify the products exhibiting the fastest and slowest dissolution characteristics

(e) Evaluate relative BA and/or BE of the product variants and determine whether a safe space can be established via either an IVIVR (eg, established by determining whether the drug product variants with extreme dissolution profiles are bioequivalent) or an IVIVC

Specifically, data analysis from these approaches will result in one of the following outcomes.

**Sub-Approach B1: An IVIVR Has Been Established.** In those cases where an IVIVC has been attempted but cannot be established, an IVIVR should be investigated as this would provide some leeway and support for further drug product formulation refinement. While an IVIVR can be considered a qualitative or semiquantitative approach, it can be an important tool in the QbD approach to formulation development and justification. For example, verification of the DS and the clinical relevance of the specifications for material attributes and process parameters can still be determined in the absence of an IVIVC; however, clinical relevance can only be assured for those changes whose dissolution profiles fall within the extremes of dissolution profiles for batches that were bioequivalent to the clinical trial formulation.

Figure 7-14 illustrates the advantage of this approach over approach A. This figure shows the relationship between drug substance particle size, dissolution, and BE. Under approach A with batch D failing similarity testing (ie, $f_2$ testing) and in the absence of BA/BE data, the appropriate specification was set at $Q = 80\%$ at 15 minutes in order to reject batch D. However, for this particular case there was a BE study showing that all the batches were BE to the clinical batch. Under these conditions, one can then set an acceptance criterion for dissolution that does not reject this batch, which in this case is $Q = 80\%$ at 20 minutes. Setting a wider dissolution acceptance criterion based on *in vivo* data allows for the setting of wider particle size specifications (referred to in this figure as lower and upper bounds of PSD). In the example of Fig. 7-14, the upper bound of PSD could be set based on the slowest releasing batch that is BE to the clinical batch.

A small variation to this approach, as described above, would be to use data from an *in vivo* BA/BE study where at least two formulation variants have been evaluated and determine whether the dissolution method and acceptance criterion are able to reject batches that are not bioequivalent. As explained above, when this happens the method and acceptance criteria are considered clinically relevant and the possibility exists of building a wider safe space.

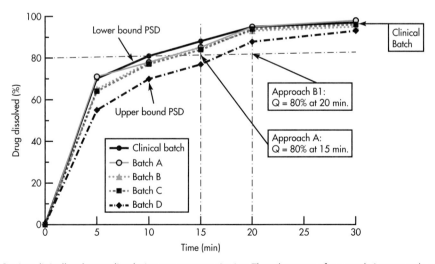

FIGURE 7-14 • Setting clinically relevant dissolution acceptance criterion. The advantage of approach A versus sub-approach B1 (Adapted with permission from Sharp SS: Establishing clinically relevant drug product specifications: FDA Perspective. AAPS Annual Meeting and Exposition. Chicago, IL: US Food and Drug Administration; 2012. http://www.fda.gov/downloads/AboutFDA /CentersOffices/OfficeofMedicalProductsandTobacco/CDER/UCM341185.pdf).

**Sub-Approach B2: An IVIVC Has Been Established.** This is the most desirable approach for setting CRDPS, including dissolution acceptance criteria. Since the mechanism for release of drug from IR dosage forms is simpler than that for MR dosage forms, one might expect that an IVIVC would be easier to develop with IR formulations. However, mainly Level C correlations for IR products have been successful in guiding drug product development, the identification of critical process parameters, and material attributes affecting product performance such as dissolution (Suarez-Sharp, 2018).

A validated IVIVC enhances drug product understanding and provides justification of manufacturing changes during a drug product's lifecycle. It enhances the significance of the *in vitro* testing leading to drug product specification settings (eg, dissolution acceptance criteria) based on targeted clinically relevant plasma concentrations. In addition, it allows for the prediction of the clinical impact of movements within the DS without the need for additional *in vivo* studies.

More recently, the scientific community is gaining confidence on the use of physiologically based modeling applied to support drug product quality; namely, physiologically based biopharmaceutics modeling (PBBM) (also more commonly referred to as PBAM, MAM, and PBPK) for the construction of mechanistic IVIVR or IVIVC (Heimbach et al, 2019; Pepin et al, 2021). Ultimately, with proper mechanistic absorption elements defined, PBBM would be able to predict the clinical impact of variations in the critical attributes measured in the chain of production, such as solid-state characteristics, particle size distributions or tablet tensile strength, porosity, and determinants for MR processes. Such an approach could, for example, be used in defining a safe space and in determining whether differences/variability in physiological conditions could affect product performance. This opens possibilities in multiple areas of regulatory applications from the level of supporting information, setting product specifications to full waivers of *in vivo* BA/BE studies. The regulatory impact of a proposed modeling study, in terms of the risk to product quality and the patient, should be assessed by the approach of the *in silico* model and the clarity of its communication with the regulatory agencies. Specifically, in order to achieve high confidence in the model's robustness,

the PBPM's ability to predict BE and non-BE should be demonstrated.

### Biopharmaceutic Drug Classification System

The BCS, discussed more fully in Chapter 8, is a scientific framework for classifying drug substances based on their aqueous solubility and intestinal permeability (FDA Guidance for Industry, December 2017). A BCS Class I drug product contains a highly soluble drug substance that is highly permeable and from which the drug rapidly dissolves from the drug product over the physiologic pH range of 1–6.8. Highly permeable drugs have an absolute BA greater than 85%. It is to be noted that the BCS only applies to oral IR formulations and cannot be applied to MR formulations or for buccally absorbed drug products (FDA Guidance for Industry, December 2017). Within the BCS framework, when certain criteria are met, the BCS can be used as a drug development tool to help sponsors/applicants justify requests for biowaivers (ie, for BCS Class 1 and 3).

### Drug Product Stability

The long-term stability of any drug product is a critical attribute of overall product quality, given that it defines the time period for which product quality, safety, and effectiveness are assured. Product stability is usually determined by testing a variety of stability indicating attributes such as drug potency, impurities, dissolution, and other relevant physicochemical measures of performance as necessary.

Stability studies are generally performed under well-controlled storage and testing conditions and provide evidence on how the quality of a drug product varies with time under the influence of a variety of environmental factors such as temperature, humidity, oxygen, and light. The time period during which a drug product is expected to remain within the established product quality specification under the labeled storage conditions is generally termed "*shelf-life*"; however, this term is often used interchangeably with expiration period, expiry date, or expiration date.

### Scale-Up and Postapproval Changes

Any change in a drug product after it has been approved for marketing by the FDA is known as a *postapproval change*. Postapproval changes may include formulation (component and composition), equipment, manufacturing process, site, and scale-up in a drug product after it has been approved for marketing by the FDA (FDA Guidance for Industry, April 2004). A major concern for industry and the FDA is whether these changes will affect the bioavailability, safety, and/ or efficacy of the approved drug product. In addition, any changes in raw material (ie, material used for preparing active pharmaceutical ingredient), excipients, or packaging (including container closure system) should also be shown not to affect the quality of the drug product. There are three levels of manufacturing changes.

Level 1 changes are defined as changes that are unlikely to have any detectable impact on formulation quality and performance and are usually reported in the annual report.

Level 2 changes could have a significant impact on formulation quality and performance and are usually reported in a change being affected supplement. Level 2 changes usually require dissolution profile comparisons in multiple media.

Level 3 changes are likely to have a significant impact on quality and performance and are usually reported in a prior approval supplement. Level 3 changes usually require the conduct of a bioequivalence study unless an IVIVC, or in general, a safe space has been established (Suarez-Sharp et al, 2018).

## CONSIDERATIONS IN THE DESIGN AND PERFORMANCE OF DRUG PRODUCTS

### Biopharmaceutic Considerations

As mentioned above, biopharmaceutics is the study of the manufacturing factors and physicochemical properties influencing the rate and extent of drug absorption from the site of administration of a drug and the use of this information to (1) anticipate potential clinical problems arising from poor absorption of a candidate drug and (2) optimize BA of newly developed compounds. Some of the major biopharmaceutic considerations in the design of a drug product are:

- Pharmacodynamics: Therapeutic objective, toxic effects, adverse reactions

- Drug substance: Physicochemical properties, PK, patents

- Drug product: BA, route of administration, desired dosage form

- Patient: Compliance and acceptability of drug product, cost

- Manufacturing: Cost, availability/stability of raw materials, quality controls, method of manufacturing, patents

The essential elements of the biopharmaceutical considerations in drug product design include (Kaplan, 1972) (1) studies done to decide the physicochemical nature of the drug to be used, for example, salt and particle size; (2) the timing of these studies in relation to the preclinical studies with the drug; (3) the determination of the solubility and dissolution characteristics; (4) the evaluation of drug absorption and physiological disposition studies; and (5) the design and evaluation of the final drug formulation.

The drug product must effectively deliver the active drug at an appropriate rate and amount to the target receptor site so that the intended therapeutic effect is achieved. It should not produce any additional side effects or discomfort due to the drug and/ or excipients. Ideally, all excipients in the drug product should be pharmacologically inactive ingredients alone or in combination in the final dosage form.

### Pharmacodynamic Considerations

*Pharmacodynamics* (PD) is the study of the effect of a drug in the body and its mechanism of action. Therapeutic considerations include the desired PD and pharmacologic properties of the drug, including the desired therapeutic response and the type and frequency of adverse reactions to the drug. The therapeutic objective influences the design of the drug product, route of drug administration, dose, dosage regimen, and manufacturing process. An oral drug used to treat an acute illness is generally formulated to release the drug rapidly, allowing for quick absorption and rapid onset. If more rapid drug absorption is desired (or if oral absorption is not feasible for chemical, metabolic, or tolerability reasons), then an injectable drug formulation might be formulated. In the case of nitroglycerin, which is highly metabolized if swallowed, a sublingual tablet formulation allows for rapid absorption of the drug from the buccal area of the mouth for the treatment of angina pectoris. Refer to additional notes in the section "Buccal and Sublingual Tablets."

In order to reduce unwanted systemic side effects, locally acting drugs such as inhaled drugs have been developed. The advantage of inhaled therapy for local action is that it is possible to deliver the drug directly into the lungs, reducing the amount needed to reach a therapeutic effect at the site of action and thereby reducing systemic side effects resulting in an improved benefit:risk ratio.

For the treatment of certain diseases, such as hypertension, chronic pain, etc, an ER dosage form is preferred. The ER dosage form releases the drug slowly, thereby controlling the rate of drug absorption and allowing for more constant plasma drug concentrations. In some cases, an immediate-drug-release component is included in the ER dosage form to allow for both rapid onset followed by a slower sustained release of the drug, for example, zolpidem tartrate ER tablets. MR dosage forms are discussed in Chapter 9.

## Pharmacokinetics of the Drug

Drug development is a laborious process that can be roughly grouped into the following five stages: (1) disease target identification, (2) target validation, (3) high-throughput identification of drug leads, (4) lead optimization, and (5) preclinical and clinical evaluation. Stages 3 to 5 mainly involve the characterization of the PK properties, namely absorption, distribution, metabolism, and excretion (ADME), of the molecules being investigated as potential drug candidates. The data obtained from these studies allow the development of a dose(s) and dosage regimen that are age appropriate, including avoidance of drug–drug interactions, food effect interactions, and achieving an appropriate drug release rate that will maintain a desired drug level in the body. Clinical failures of about 50% of the Investigational New Drug (IND) filings are attributed to their inadequate ADME attributes. It is, therefore, not surprising that the pharmaceutical industry is searching for ever more effective means to minimize this problem.

Building mathematical models (known as *in silico* screens) to reliably predict ADME attributes solely from molecular structure is at the heart of this effort in reducing costs as well as development cycle times (Gombar et al, 2003). Also, the integration of PK and PD allows for the characterization of the onset, intensity, and duration of the pharmacological effect of a drug and its interaction with the mechanism of action. In understanding the interrelationship of these two disciplines, light can be shed on situations where one or the other needs to be optimized in drug development. As such PK/PD modeling and simulation provides a quantitative assessment of dose/exposure-response relationships with extensive applications at the early and late-stage drug development as well as during decision making.

It is well known that there is a great degree of individual variation, called polymorphism, in the genes coding for drug-metabolizing enzymes. The degree of polymorphism can significantly affect the drug metabolism and, therefore, the PK and the clinical outcome of the drug. Thus, variations in oxidation of some drugs have been attributed to genetic differences in certain CYP enzymes. Genetic polymorphisms of CYP2D6 and CYP2C19 enzymes are well characterized, and human populations of "extensive metabolizers" and "poor metabolizers" have been identified. Applying pharmacogenomics (eg, genomic biomarkers) into the drug development and clinical trial evaluation allows for the selection of an optimal group of patients to be enrolled into trials and reduces the number of adverse events. This will lead to more successful clinical trials and decrease the time to market for compounds.

## Bioavailability of the Drug

Given that the pharmacologic response is generally related to the concentration of drug at its site of action, the BA of a drug from a dosage form is a critical element of a drug product's clinical efficacy. However, most BA studies involve the determination of drug concentration mainly in the plasma since it is rather difficult to measure the concentration at the site of action.

Numerous factors can affect how much of the absorbed drug reaches the intended site of action.

These include psychochemical properties of the drug, formulation and manufacturing variables, physiological factors, drug–drug interactions, and (for oral dosage forms) food effect interactions.

The stability of the drug in the GI tract, including the stomach and intestine, is another consideration. Some drugs, such as penicillin G, are unstable in the acidic medium of the stomach. The addition of buffering in the formulation or the use of an enteric coating on the dosage form will protect the drug from degradation at a low pH.

Some drugs have poor BA because of first-pass effects (presystemic elimination). If oral drug BA is poor due to metabolism by enzymes in the GI tract or in the liver, then a higher dose may be needed, as in the case of propranolol, or an alternative route of drug administration, as in the case of nitroglycerin. Incompletely absorbed drugs and drugs with highly variable BA have a risk that, under unusual conditions (eg, change in diet or disease condition, drug–drug interaction), excessive drug BA can occur leading to more intense PD activity and possible adverse events. If the drug is not absorbed after the oral route or a higher dose causes toxicity, then the drug must be given by an alternative route of administration, and a different dosage form such as a parenteral drug product might be needed.

## Dose Considerations

Some patients experience unique differences from the regular adult population in PK parameters due to differences in metabolic background, renal clearance, weight, volume of distribution, age, and disease stage (eg, liver impairment, renal impairment) and, consequently, require individualized dosing. Therefore, the drug product must usually be available in several dose strengths to allow for individualized dosing and possibly dose titration. Some tablets are also scored for breaking, to potentially allow (as supported by appropriate data) the administration of fractional tablet doses.

The absence of an available pediatric dosage form for some medications increases the potential for dosing errors and may produce serious complications in this patient population. Congress enacted the *Pediatric Research Equity Act* (PREA) and other laws requiring drug companies to study their products in children under certain circumstances. When pediatric studies are necessary, they must be conducted with the same drug and for the same use for which they were approved in adults. Thus, specific dosing guidelines and useful dosage forms for pediatric patients are being developed in order to optimize therapeutic efficacy and limit or prevent serious adverse side effects.

In the presence of renal or liver impairment, the drug metabolism or excretion process may be altered, requiring smaller dose. For example, in the case of renal insufficiency, phenobarbitone, which is mainly excreted by the kidneys, should be given in a smaller dose, and in patients with liver impairment, morphine should be given in smaller dose.

The size and the shape of a solid oral drug product are designed for easy swallowing. The total size of a drug product is determined by the dose of the drug and any additional excipients needed to manufacture the desired dosage form. For oral dosage forms, if the recommended dose is large (1 g or more), then the patient may have difficulty in swallowing the drug product. For example, many patients may find a capsule-shaped tablet (caplet) easier to swallow than a large round tablet. Large or oddly shaped tablets, which may become lodged in the esophageal sphincter during swallowing, are generally not manufactured. Some esophageal injuries due to irritating drug lodged in the esophagus have been reported with potassium chloride tablets and other drugs. Older patients may have more difficulty in swallowing large tablets and capsules. Most of these swallowing difficulties may be overcome by taking the product with a large amount of fluid.

## Dosing Frequency

The dose, the dosing frequency, and the total daily dose should be considered when developing a therapeutic dosage regimen for a patient. The dose is the amount of drug taken at any one time. This can be expressed as the mass of drug (eg, 100 mg), volume of drug solution (eg, 5 mL, 5 drops), or some other quantity (eg, 2 puffs). The dosage regimen is the frequency at which the drug doses are given. Examples include two puffs twice a day, one capsule two times a day, etc. The total daily dose is calculated from the dose and the number of times per day the dose is taken.

The dosing frequency is in part determined by the clearance of the drug and the target plasma drug concentration. When the dosing frequency or interval is less than the elimination half-life ($t_{1/2}$), greater accumulation occurs, that is, steady-state levels are higher and there is less fluctuation. If the dosing interval is much greater than the half-life of the drug, then minimum concentration, $C_{p\ min}$, approaches zero. Under these conditions, no accumulation will occur and the plasma concentration–time profile will approximate the result of administration of a series of single doses.

As such, if the drug has a short $t_{1/2}$ or rapid clearance from the body, the drug must be given more frequently or administered as an ER drug product. Simplifying the medication dosing frequency can improve compliance markedly (Jin et al, 2008). Thus, to minimize fluctuating plasma drug concentrations and improve patient compliance, an ER drug product may be preferred.

### Patient Considerations

The drug product and therapeutic regimen must be acceptable to the patient. Poor patient compliance may result from poor product attributes, such as difficulty in swallowing, disagreeable odor, bitter medicine taste, or too frequent and/or unusual dosage requirements.

In recent years, creative packaging has allowed the patient to remove one tablet each day from a specially designed package so that the daily doses are not missed. Orally disintegrating tablets and chewable tablets allow the patient to typically take the medication without water. These innovations improve compliance. Of course, PD factors, such as side effects of the drug or an allergic reaction, also influence patient compliance.

Transmucosal (nasal) administration of antiepileptic drugs may be more convenient, easier to use, just as safe, and an alternative to rectal administration.

### Route of Drug Administration

The route of drug administration affects the rate and extent (BA) of the drug, thereby affecting the onset, duration, and intensity of the pharmacologic effect (efficacy and safety).

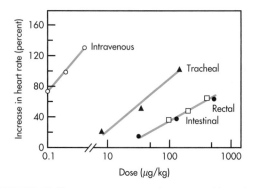

**FIGURE 7-15 •** Dose–response curve to isoproterenol by various routes in dogs. (Reproduced with permission from Gillette JR, Mitchell JR: Concepts in Biochemical Pharmacology. Berlin: Springer-Verlag; 1975.)

Although the PD activity of the drug at the receptor site is similar with different routes of administration, severe differences in the intensity of the PD response and the occurrence of adverse events may be observed. For example, isoproterenol has a thousandfold difference in activity when given orally or by IV injection. Figure 7-15 shows the change in heart rate due to isoproterenol with different routes of administration. Studies have shown that isoproterenol is metabolized in the gut and during passage through the liver (presystemic elimination or first-pass effects). The rate and types of metabolite formed are different depending on the routes of administration.

The use of novel drug delivery methods could enhance the efficacy and reduce the toxicity of antiepileptic drugs (AEDs). As such, slow-release oral forms of medication or depot drugs such as skin patches might improve compliance and, therefore, seizure control. In emergency situations, administration via rectal, nasal, or buccal mucosa can deliver the drug more quickly than can oral administration (Fisher and Ho, 2002).

## EXAMPLES RELATED TO THE DESIGN AND PERFOMANCE OF DRUG PRODUCTS

Pharmaceutical development companies are constantly looking at new approaches to deliver drugs safely and improve efficacy and patient compliance. Noninvasive systemic drug delivery such as oral, inhalation, intranasal, transdermal, etc are much more preferred compared to invasive drug delivery such as intramuscular, intravenous, and subcutaneous (Mathias and Hussain, 2010). Although the oral route of drug administration is preferred and is the most popular route of drug administration, alternate noninvasive systemic drug delivery is being considered for biotechnology-derived drugs (proteins), ease of self-administration (orally disintegrating tablets), or prolonged drug delivery (transdermal patch). The discussion below briefly describes some of the more popular drug products.

## Oral Drug Products

Oral administration of drug products is the most common, convenient, and economic route. The major advantages of oral drug products are the convenience of administration, safety, and the elimination of discomforts involved with injections. The hazard of rapid intravenous administration causing toxic high concentration of drug in the blood is avoided. The main disadvantages of oral drug products are the potential issues of reduced, erratic, or incomplete BA due to solubility, permeability, stability problems, and the presence of food that may alter the GI tract pH, gastric motility, and emptying time. Unabsorbed drug may also alter the contents and microbiologic flora of the GI tract. Some orally administered drugs may irritate the GI linings causing nausea or GI discomfort. BA may also be altered by any pathology of the GI tract such as ulcerative colitis (see Chapter 4).

Highly ionized drug molecules are not absorbed easily. The ganglion-blocking drugs hexamethonium, pentolinium, and bretylium are ionized at intestinal pH. Therefore, they are not sufficiently absorbed orally to be effective systemically. Drugs with large molecular weights may not be well absorbed when given orally. The antibiotics neomycin and vancomycin are large hydrophilic molecules that partition poorly across the GI mucosa. Consequently, they are not absorbed after oral administration and are used for local antibacterial effect in the GI tract. Some large molecules are absorbed when administered in solution with a surface-active agent. For example, cyclosporine has been given orally with good absorption when formulated with a surfactant in oil. A possible role of the oil is to stimulate the flow of lymph as well as to delay retention of the drug. Oily vehicles have been used to lengthen the GI transit time of oral preparations.

Delivering proteins and peptides by the oral route has been a big challenge, given the lack of stability due to enzymatic degradation in the digestive system prior to absorption. Considerable progress has been made over the past few years in developing innovative technologies for promoting absorption across the GI tract and the numbers of these approaches are demonstrating potential in clinical studies. In developing oral protein delivery systems with high BA, three practical approaches might be most helpful (Morishita and Peppas, 2006): (1) modification of the physicochemical properties of macromolecules; (2) addition of novel function to macromolecules; or (3) use of improved delivery carriers. Chemical modification and use of mucoadhesive polymeric systems for site-specific drug delivery seem to be promising candidates for protein and peptide drug delivery (Shaji and Patole, 2008). Also, nanoparticles with peptidic ligands are especially worthy of notice because they can be used for specific targeting in the GI tract.

## Absorption of Lipid-Soluble Drugs

Lipid solubility of drugs is a major factor affecting the extent of drug distribution, particularly to the brain, where the blood–brain barrier restricts the penetration of polar and ionized molecules. Inconsistently, drugs that are highly hydrophobic are also poorly absorbed, because they are poorly soluble in aqueous fluid and, therefore, cannot get to the surface of cells. For a drug to be readily absorbed, it must be mainly hydrophobic, but have some solubility in aqueous solutions. This is one reason why many successfully developed drugs are weak acids or weak bases to begin with.

The most significant issue to consider when formulating poorly water-soluble drugs is the risk of precipitation in the lumen of the GI tract. The *lipid formulation classification system* (LFCS) provides a simple framework that can be used, in combination with appropriate *in vitro* tests, to predict how the fate of a drug is likely to be affected by formulation, and to optimize the choice of lipid formulation for a particular drug (Puoton, 2006). Poorly water-soluble drug candidates present considerable formulation challenges. These drugs can be successfully formulated for oral administration. Some options available involve either reduction of particle size (of crystalline drug) or formulation of the drug in solution, as an amorphous system or lipid formulation (Puoton, 2006).

Lipophilic drugs are more soluble in lipids or oily vehicles. Lipid-soluble drugs given with fatty excipients mix with digested fatty acids, which are emulsified by bile in the small intestine. The emulsified drug is then absorbed through the GI mucosa or through the lymphatic system. A normal digestive function of the small intestine is the digestion and absorption of fats such as triglycerides. These fats are first hydrolyzed into monoglycerides and fatty acids by pancreatic lipase. The fatty acids then react with carrier lipoproteins to form chylomicrons, which are absorbed through the lymph. The chylomicrons eventually release the fatty acids, and any lipophilic drugs incorporated in the oil phase. Fat substances trigger receptors in the stomach to delay stomach emptying and reduce GI transit rates. Prolonged transit time allows more contact time for increased drug absorption.

When griseofulvin or phenytoin was given orally in corn oil suspensions, an increase in drug absorption was demonstrated (Bates and Equeira, 1975). The increase in absorption was attributed to the formation of mixed micelles with bile secretions, which aid drug dissolution. Hydrophobic drugs such as griseofulvin and metaxalone have greater BA when given with a high-fat meal. A meal high in lipids will delay stomach emptying depending on the volume and nature of the oil. For example, the BA of a water-insoluble antimalarial drug was increased in dogs when oleic acid was incorporated as part of a vehicle into a soft gelatin capsule (Stella et al, 1978). Calcium carbonate, a source of calcium for the body, was only about 30% available in a solid dosage form but was almost 60% bioavailable when dispersed in a special vehicle such as a soft gelatin capsule (Fordtran et al, 1986). Bleomycin (MW 1500), an anticancer drug, is poorly absorbed orally and therefore was formulated for absorption through the lymphatic system. The lymphotropic carrier was dextran sulfate. Bleomycin was linked by ionic bonds to the carrier to form a complex. The carrier dextran (MW 500,000) was too large to be absorbed through the membrane and pass into the lymphatic vessels (Yoshikawa et al, 1989).

## Gastrointestinal Side Effects

Many orally administered drugs such as aspirin are irritating to the stomach. These drugs may cause nausea or stomach pain due to local irritation when taken on an empty stomach. In some cases, food or antacids may be given together with the drug to reduce stomach irritation. Alternatively, the drug may be enteric coated to reduce gastric irritation. Buffered aspirin tablets, enteric-coated aspirin tablets, and rapidly dissolving effervescent tablets and granules are available to minimize local gastric irritation. However, enteric coating may sometimes delay or reduce the amount of drug absorbed. Furthermore, enteric coating may not abolish gastric irritation completely, because the drug may occasionally be regurgitated back to the stomach after the coating dissolves in the intestine. Enteric-coated tablets may be greatly affected by the presence of food in the stomach. The drug may not be released from the stomach for several hours when stomach emptying is delayed by food.

Buffering material or antacid ingredients have also been used with aspirin to reduce stomach irritation. When a large amount of antacid or buffering material is included in the formulation, dissolution of aspirin may occur quickly, leading to reduced irritation to the stomach.

It has been shown that acute aspirin-induced damage to the gastric mucosa can be reduced by chemically associating aspiring with the phospholipid, phosphatidylcholine and that the mechanism of mucosal protection provided by this compound is not related to any alteration in the ability of aspirin to inhibit mucosal COX activity (Bhupinderjit et al, 1999). Also, certain drugs have been formulated into soft gelatin capsules to improve drug BA and reduce GI side effects. If the drug is formulated in the soft gelatin capsule as a solution, the drug may disperse and dissolve more rapidly, leaving less residual drug in the gut and causing less irritation. This approach may be useful for a drug that causes local irritation but will be ineffective if the drug is inherently ulcerogenic. Indomethacin, for example, may cause ulceration in animals even when administered parenterally.

There are many options available to the formulator to improve the tolerance of the drug and minimize gastric irritation. The nature of excipients and the physical state of the drugs are important and must be carefully assessed before a drug product is formulated. Some excipients may improve the solubility of the drug and facilitate absorption, whereas others may physically adsorb the drug to reduce irritation. Often, a great number of formulations must be considered before an acceptable one is chosen.

## Immediate-Release and Modified-Release Drug Products

The USP differentiates between an IR drug product and an MR drug product. For the IR drug product, no deliberate effort has been made to modify the drug release rate. IR dosage forms release the active drug(s) within short time (eg, 80% of drug after 60 min). Applying particular formulation and process technologies, even faster drug release can be achieved. The basic approach used in development of tablets is the use of superdisintegrants like cross-linked crospovidone, sodium starch glycolate, carboxymethylcellulose, etc. These superdisintegrants provide instantaneous disintegration of tablets following oral administration.

For MR drug products, the pattern of drug release from the dosage form has been deliberately changed from that of a conventional (IR) form of the drug. Types of MR drug products include delayed release (eg, enteric coated) and ER. ER formulations are designed to reduce dosing frequency for drugs with a short elimination half-life and duration of effect. These forms reduce the fluctuation in plasma drug concentration, providing a more uniform therapeutic effect while minimizing adverse effects. Absorption rate is slowed by different methods including coating drug particles with wax or other water-insoluble material, by embedding the drug in a matrix that releases it slowly during transit through the GI tract, or by complexing the drug with ion-exchange resins.

An ER oral dosage form should meet the following characteristics: (1) The BA profile established for the drug product rules out the occurrence of any dose dumping; (2) the drug product's steady-state performance is comparable (eg, degree of fluctuation is similar or lower) to a currently marketed non-ER or ER drug product that contains the same active drug ingredient or therapeutic moiety and that is subject to an approved full New Drug Application; (3) the drug product's formulation provides consistent PK performance between individual dosage units; and (4) the drug product has a less frequent dosing interval compared to a currently marketed non-ER drug product.

### Buccal and Sublingual Tablets

A drug that diffuses and penetrates rapidly across mucosal membranes may be placed under the tongue and be rapidly absorbed. A tablet designed for release under the tongue is called a *sublingual tablet*. Nitroglycerin, isoproterenol, erythrityl tetranitrate, and isosorbide dinitrate are common examples. A tablet designed for release and absorption of the drug in the buccal (cheek) pouch is called a *buccal tablet*. The buccal cavity is the space between the mandibular arch and the oral mucosa, an area well supplied with blood vessels for efficient drug absorption.

Oral transmucosal absorption is generally rapid because of the rich vascular supply to the mucosa and the lack of a stratum corneum epidermis. This minimal barrier to drug transport results in a rapid rise in blood concentrations. Sublingual and buccal medications are compounded in the form of small, quick-dissolving tablets, sprays, lozenges, or liquid suspensions. A buccal tablet may be designed to release drug slowly for a prolonged effect. This form of drug product administration is very effective as it avoids first-pass metabolism by the liver before general distribution. Consequently, for a drug with significant first-pass effect, buccal/sublingual absorption may provide better BA than oral administration and rapid onset of action as it may be absorbed in the blood stream in minutes.

For example, Sorbitrate sublingual tablet, Sorbitrate chewable tablet, and Sorbitrate oral tablet (Zeneca) are three different dosage forms of isosorbide dinitrate for the relief and prevention of angina pectoris. The sublingual tablet is a lactose formulation that dissolves rapidly under the tongue and is then absorbed. The chewable tablet is chewed, and some drug is absorbed in the buccal cavity; the oral tablet is simply a conventional product for GI absorption. The chewable tablet contains flavor, confectioner's sugar, and mannitol, which are absent in both the oral and sublingual tablets. The sublingual tablet contains lactose and starch for rapid dissolution. The onset of sublingual nitroglycerin is rapid, much faster than when nitroglycerin is taken orally or absorbed through the skin. The duration of action, however, is shorter than with the other two routes. Some peptide drugs have been reported to be absorbed by the buccal route, which provides a route of administration without the drug being destroyed by enzymes in the GI tract.

A newer approach to drug absorption from the oral cavity has been the development of a translingual nitroglycerin spray (Nitrolingual Pumpspray). The spray, containing 0.4 mg per metered dose, is given by spraying one or two metered doses onto the oral mucosa at the onset of an acute angina attack.

Fentanyl citrate is a potent, lipid-soluble opioid agonist that crosses mucosal membranes rapidly. Fentanyl has been formulated as a transdermal drug product (Durapress˚) and as an oral lozenge on a handle (Actiq˚) containing fentanyl citrate for oral transmucosal delivery. According to the manufacturer, fentanyl BA from Actiq is about 50%, representing a combination of rapid absorption across the oral mucosa and slower absorption through swallowing and transport across the GI mucosa.

## Colonic Drug Delivery

Drugs that are destroyed following oral administration by the acidic environment of the stomach or metabolized by enzymes may only be slightly affected in the colon. Oral drug products for colonic drug delivery have been studied not only for the delivery of drugs for the treatment of local diseases associated with the lower bowel and colon (eg, Crohn's disease) but also for their potential for the delivery of proteins and therapeutic peptides (eg, insulin) for systemic absorption (Chourasia and Jain, 2003; Shareef et al, 2003). Targeting drug delivery to the colon has several therapeutic advantages. Crohn's disease or chronic inflammatory colitis may be more effectively treated by direct drug delivery to the colon. For example, mesalamine (5-aminosalicylic acid,

Asacol˚) is available in a delayed-release tablet coated with an acrylic-based resin that delays the release of the drug until it reaches the distal ileum and beyond. Other approaches include prodrugs (sulfasalazine and balsalazine) to deliver 5-aminosalicylic acid (5-ASA) for localized chemotherapy of inflammatory bowel disease (IBD). Drugs containing an azo bond (balsalazide) and azo cross-linked polymers used as a coating are degraded by anaerobic microbes in the lower bowel.

Protein drugs are generally unstable in the acidic environment of the stomach and are also degraded by proteolytic enzymes present in the stomach and small intestine. Researchers are investigating the oral delivery of protein and peptide drugs by protecting them against enzymatic degradation for later release in the colon.

Drug delivery to the colon is highly influenced by several factors including high bacterial level, the physiology of the colonic environment, level of fluid, and transit time. Thus availability of most drugs to the absorptive membrane is low because of the high water absorption capacity of the colon, the colonic contents are considerably viscous, and their mixing is not efficient. The human colon has over 500 distinct species of bacteria as resident flora. Within the cecum and colon, anaerobic species dominate and bacterial counts of $10^{12}$/mL have been reported. Among the reactions carried out by these gut flora are azoreduction and enzymatic cleavage, that is, glycosides. These metabolic processes may be responsible for the metabolism of many drugs and may also be applied to colon-targeted delivery of peptide-based macromolecules such as insulin by oral administration (Philip and Philip, 2010).

Drugs such as the beta-blockers, oxprenolol and metoprolol, and isosorbide-5-mononitrate, nonsteroidal anti-inflammatory drugs (NSAIDs), steroids, peptides, and vaccines are well absorbed in the colon, similar to absorption in the small intestine. Thus, these drugs are suitable candidates for colonic delivery. The NSAID naproxen has been formed into a prodrug naproxen–dextran that survives intestinal enzyme and intestinal absorption. The prodrug reaches the colon, where it is enzymatically decomposed into naproxen and dextran (Harboe et al, 1989).

## Rectal and Vaginal Drug Delivery

Products for rectal or vaginal drug delivery may be administered in either solid or liquid dosage forms. Rectal drug administration can be used for either local or systemic drug delivery. Rectal drug delivery for systemic absorption is preferred for drugs that cannot be tolerated orally (eg, when a drug causes nausea) or in situations where the drug cannot be given orally (eg, during an epileptic attack). Rectal route offers potential advantages for drug delivery such as rapid absorption of many low-molecular-weight drugs, partial avoidance of first-pass metabolism, potential for absorption into the lymphatic system, retention of large volumes, rate-controlled drug delivery, and absorption enhancement (Lakshmi et al, 2012). However, this route also has some disadvantages as many drugs are poorly or erratically absorbed across the rectal mucosa, dissolution problems, and drug metabolism in microorganisms among other factors. Thus to overcome these, various absorption-enhancing adjuvants, surfactants, mixed micelle, and cyclodextrins have been investigated.

The rate of absorption from this route can be affected by several factors including formulation, concentration of drug, pH of the rectal content, presence of stool, volume of fluid, etc. A sustained-release preparation may be prepared for rectal administration. The rate of release of the drug from this preparation is dependent on the nature of the base composition and on the solubility of the drug involved.

Release of drug from a suppository depends on the composition of the suppository base. A water-soluble base, such as polyethylene glycol and glycerin, generally dissolves and releases the drug; on the other hand, an oleaginous base with a low melting point may melt at body temperature and release the drug. Some suppositories contain an emulsifying agent that keeps the fatty oil emulsified and the drug dissolved in it.

Vaginal drug delivery offers a valuable route for drug delivery through the use of specifically designed carrier systems for both local and systemic applications. A range of drug delivery platforms suitable for intravaginal administration have been developed, such as intravaginal rings, vaginal tablets, creams, hydrogels, suppositories, and particulate systems.

For example, progesterone vaginal suppositories have been evaluated for the treatment of premenstrual symptoms of anxiety and irritability. Antifungal agents are often formulated into suppositories for treating vaginal infections. Fluconazole, a triazole antifungal agent, has been formulated to treat vulvovaginal candidiasis. The result of oral doses is comparable to that of a clotrimazole vaginal suppository. Many vaginal preparations are used for the delivery of antifungal agents.

The rate and extent of drug absorption after intravaginal administration may vary depending on formulation factors, age of the patient, vaginal physiology, and menstrual cycle. As such, exhaustive efforts have been made recently to evaluate the vagina as a potential route for the delivery of molecules, such as proteins, peptides, small interfering RNAs, oligonucleotides, antigens, vaccines, and hormones. However, successful delivery of drugs through the vagina remains a challenge, primarily due to the poor absorption across the vaginal epithelium, cultural sensitivity, hygiene, personal, gender specificity, local irritation, and other factors that need to be addressed during the design of a vaginal formulation (Ashok et al, 2012).

## Parenteral Drug Products

The parenteral route of administration refers to all forms of drugs administered via a syringe, needle, or catheter into body tissues or fluids such as intravenous (IV), intra-arterial, intraosseous, intramuscular, subcutaneous, and intrathecal routes.

In general, IV bolus administration of a drug provides the most rapid onset of drug action. After IV bolus injection, the drug is distributed via the circulation to all parts of the body within a few minutes. After intramuscular (IM) injection, drug is absorbed from the injection site into the bloodstream (Fig. 7-16). Plasma drug input after oral and IM administration involves an absorption phase in which the drug concentration rises to a peak and then declines according to the elimination half-life of the drug. (Note that the systemic elimination of all products is essentially similar; only the rate and extent of absorption may be modified by formulation.) The plasma drug level is at a maximum almost instantaneously after an IV bolus injection, so a peak is usually not visible. After 3 hours, however, the plasma level of the drug after IV administration has declined to a lower level than after the oral and IM administration. In this example (see Fig. 7-16), the areas under the plasma curves are all approximately equal, indicating that the oral and IM preparations are both well formulated and 100% available. Frequently, because of incomplete absorption or metabolism, oral preparations may have a lower area under the curve.

Drug absorption after an IM injection may be faster or slower than after oral drug administration. IM preparations are generally injected into a muscle mass such as in the buttocks (gluteus muscle) or in the deltoid muscle. Drug absorption occurs as the drug diffuses from the muscle into the surrounding tissue fluid and then into the blood. Different muscle tissues have different blood flow. For example, blood flow to the deltoid muscle is higher than blood flow to the gluteus muscle. IM injections may be formulated to have a faster or slower drug release by changing the vehicle of the injection preparation. Aqueous solutions release drug more rapidly, and the drug is more rapidly absorbed from the injection site,

whereas a viscous, oily, or suspension vehicle may result in a slow drug release and consequently slow and sustained drug absorption. Viscous vehicles generally slow down drug diffusion and distribution. A drug in an oily vehicle must partition into an aqueous phase before systemic absorption. A drug that is very soluble in oil and relatively insoluble in water may have a relatively long and sustained release from the absorption site because of slow partitioning.

MR parenteral dosage forms have been developed in which the drug is entrapped or encapsulated into inert polymeric or lipophilic matrices that slowly release the drug *in vivo* over a week or up to several years (Patil and Burgess, 2010). The polymers or lipophilic carriers used to deliver the drugs in MR parenterals are either biodegradable *in vivo* or are nonbiodegradable. Nonerodable, nonbiodegradable systems (eg, subcutaneous implants) are removed at the end of therapy. Drugs, including peptides and proteins, have also been formulated as emulsions, suspensions, liposomes, and nanoparticles for parenteral injection. A change in a parenteral drug product from a solution to an emulsion, liposome, etc will alter the drug's distribution and PK profile.

### Nasal Drug Products

The nasal route of administration has been used for the delivery of drug products for both topical and systemic actions. A variety of different drug products such as antihistamines, corticosteroids, anticholinergics, and vasoconstrictors are currently being marketed for the local treatment of congestion, rhinitis, sinusitis, and related allergic or chronic conditions. Recently, increasing investigations of the nasal route have focused especially on nasal application for systemic drug delivery. The intranasal delivery of drugs for systemic action is aimed at optimizing drug BA, given its large surface area, porous endothelial membrane, high total blood flow, and the avoidance of first-pass metabolism. Thus, peptides such as calcitonin and pituitary hormones have been successfully delivered through the nasal route. Intranasal delivery is also currently being marketed for treatments for migraine, smoking cessation, acute pain relief, osteoporosis, and vitamin $B_{12}$ deficiency. In addition, MedImmune Inc. and Wyeth marketed the first intranasal vaccine in the United States: FluMist®.

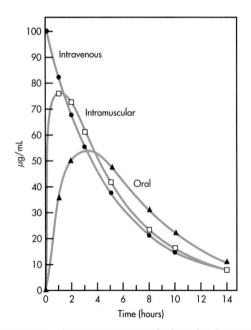

FIGURE 7-16 • Plasma concentration of a drug after the same dose is administered by three different routes.

Recently, the nasal route of administration has gained increasing consideration for obtaining systemic absorption and brain uptake of drugs. The delivery of drugs to the central nervous system (CNS) from the nasal route may occur via olfactory neuroepithelium. Drug delivery through nasal route into CNS has been reported for Alzheimer disease, brain tumors, epilepsy, pain, and sleep disorders (Pavan et al, 2008).

There are various factors that affect the systemic BA of drugs that are administered through the nasal route (Kumari et al, 2013). These factors can be classified as follows:

1. Physiochemical properties of the drugs: lipophilic–hydrophilic balance, chemical form, polymorphism, enzymatic degradation in nasal cavity, molecular size, solubility, and dissolution rate.

2. Delivery effect: formulation (concentration, pH, osmolarity), droplet/particle size distribution, viscosity.

3. Nasal effect: mucociliary clearance, diseased state (eg common cold), rhinitis, membrane permeability, environmental pH, anatomical and physiological considerations.

Nasal devices have progressively evolved from the pipettes and the droppers through to spraying devices such as squeeze bottles, toward, a nasal gel pump, pressurized metered dose inhalers (MDIs), and dry-powder inhalers (Djupesland, 2013). Drug development in the near future should not only rely on innovative new compounds and sophisticated formulations but also rely on the efficiency, safety, and comfort of the dispensing systems.

Certain studies should be performed to characterize the performance properties of the nasal drug product and to provide support in defining the optimal labeling statements regarding use. Delivery systems for nasal administration can vary in both design and mode of operation, and these characteristics may be unique to a particular drug product. Regardless of the design, the most crucial attributes are the reproducibility of the dose, the spray plume, and the particle/droplet size distribution, since these parameters can affect the delivery of the drug substance to the intended biological target. Studies to define these characteristics will help facilitate correct use and maintenance of the drug product and contribute to patient compliance. For the most part, these should be one-time studies, preferably performed on multiple batches (eg, two or three) of drug product representative of the product intended for distribution (FDA Guidance for Industry, 2002).

The concept of classical BE and BA may not be applicable for all nasal drug products specially those for local action. In addition, the doses administered are typically so small that blood or serum concentrations may not be detectable by routine analytical procedures. Therefore, for locally acting drug product, major manufacturing changes may require the need for safety and efficacy trials.

## Inhalation Drug Products

Localized drug delivery to the lungs is an important and effective therapeutic method for treating a variety of pulmonary disorders including asthma, bronchitis, and cystic fibrosis. The advantages of inhalation therapy for the treatment of lung disorders are the following: (1) Relatively small doses are needed for effective therapy, reducing exposure of drug to the systemic circulation, and potentially minimizes adverse effects; (2) wide surface area for absorption and relatively low metabolic activity of the lungs; (3) the lungs provide substantially greater BA for macromolecules than any other route of administration to the systemic circulation.

The therapeutic effect for locally acting inhaled drugs and the duration of this effect are determined mainly by the dose deposited at the site of action and its pulmonary clearance. In turn, drug distribution and deposition along the respiratory tract depend on several factors such as (1) characteristics of the inhaled formulation (particle size distribution, shape, electrical charge, density, and hygroscopicity) and (2) breathing patterns such as frequency, depth, and flow rate. It has been shown that increasing the drug substance lipophilicity (Derendorf et al, 2006) and optimization of particle size (MMAD <5 $\mu$m) (Gonda 1987; Labiris and Dolovich, 2003) and release rate (Gonda, 1987; Suarez et al, 1998), it is possible to increase the lung residence time of the drug. Labiris and Dolovich (2003) reported that there are more than 65 different inhaled products of more than 20 active ingredients marketed to treat respiratory diseases. Inhaled glucocorticoids (eg, fluticasone propionate, budesonide, triamcinolone acetonide, mometasone furoate, etc) are some drugs usually prescribed for the treatment of local pulmonary diseases.

Inhalation therapy for local action is generated by different devices that aim to deliver the drug to the lower airways. Inhalation devices can be classified into three different categories: MDIs, dry-powder inhalers (eg, Aerolizer˙, Diskus˙, Flexaler˙, Turbohaler˙, etc), and nebulizer inhalers. Some examples of inhalation and intranasal products are shown in Table 7-8. Dolovich (1999) reported that developments in inhalation devices made it possible to deliver larger drug doses (milligram compared with microgram dosing) to the airways and achieve greater deposition efficiency than the older devices (>50% lung deposition versus ≤20% with older devices).

The development of drugs for pulmonary drug delivery has focused mainly on the optimization of particle or device technologies to improve the aerosol generation and pulmonary deposition of inhaled drugs. Although substantial progress has been made in these areas, no significant advances have been made that would lead to pulmonary drug delivery beyond the treatment of some respiratory diseases. One main reason for this stagnation is the poor knowledge about (1) details on the fate of inhaled drug or carrier particles after deposition in the lungs; (2) the total amount of drug that reaches the lungs and validated method to demonstrate this; and (3) differential assessment on the region of drug deposition, for example, central portion vs. periphery lung deposition (O'Connor et al, 2011). Inhalation products are complex drug–device combination products, bearing quite distinctive performance characteristics and patient instructions for use and handling. BA/BE studies alone may not be sufficient for documentation of the locally acting drug products (FDA Guidance for Industry, 1989; FDA, 2019) following major manufacturing changes or for approval of generics, because for delivery to the target sites these drugs do not depend upon systemic circulation. Despite these arguments, it is believed that PK studies might be able to provide some key information (how much drug is deposited, where is it deposited, how long does it stay in the lung) needed for demonstration of BE of inhalation drugs for local action (Adams et al, 2010; O'Connor et al, 2011).

The role of aerosol therapy is emerging beyond the initial focus. This expansion has been driven by the Montreal protocol and the need to eliminate chlorofluorocarbons (CFCs) from traditional metered-dose inhalers, by the need for delivery devices and formulations that can efficiently and reproducibly target the systemic circulation for the delivery of proteins and peptides, and by developments in medicine that have made it possible to consider curing lung diseases with aerosolized gene therapy and preventing epidemics of influenza and measles with

## TABLE 7-8 • Examples of Inhalation and Intranasal Drug Products

|  | Drug Product | Generic Name | Indication |
|---|---|---|---|
| **Inhalation** | Proventil | Albuterol | Bronchodilator |
|  | Beconase | Beclomethasone diproprionate | Anti-inflammatory steroid |
|  | Foradil Aerolizer | Formoterol fumarate inhalation powder | Bronchodilator |
|  | Pulmicort Turbuhaler | Budesonide inhalation powder | Anti-inflammatory steroid |
|  | Virazole | Ribavirin for inhalation solution | Antiviral nucleoside |
|  | Mucomyst | Acetylcysteine | Mucolytic |
| **Intranasal** | Flonase | Fluticasone proprionate | Anti-inflammatory steroid |
|  | FluMist | Influenza virus intranasal vaccine | Live (attenuated) influenza virus |
|  | Nasalcrom | Cromolyn sodium | Mast cell stabilizer |
|  | Nasalcort | Triamcinolone actonide | Anti-inflammatory steroid |

aerosolized vaccines. The rate of absorption from the periphery of the lung has been shown to be twice as fast as that taking place from the central portions, owing to the variable thickness of the epithelial cells versus alveolar cells (Brown and Schanker, 1983). Therefore, to achieve maximum BA of drugs aimed for systemic delivery, attention should be paid on delivering the drug to the periphery of the lungs.

The continued expansion of the role of aerosol therapy will probably depend on factors such as the demonstration of the safety of this route of administration for drugs that have their targets outside the lung and are administered long term (eg, insulin aerosol) (Laube, 2005).

## Transdermal Drug Products

Transdermal drug products, sometimes referred to as transdermal delivery systems or "patches," are placed on the skin to deliver drug for both systemic and local activity. For example, Scopolamine˚ (Transderm Scop) delivers drug through the skin of the ear and is absorbed into the patient's systemic circulation for relief of motion sickness. Lidocaine patches are designed for local anesthetic activity due to pain from shingles, and diclofenac sodium patch is a topical NSAID.

Transdermal administration may release the drug over an extended period of several hours or days (eg, estrogen replacement therapy) without the discomforts of GI side effects or first-pass effects. Many transdermal products deliver drug at a constant rate to the body, similar to a zero-order infusion process. As a result, a stable, plateau level of the drug may be maintained. Many therapeutic categories of drugs are now available as transdermal products (Table 7-9).

Transdermal products vary in design (Gonzalez and Cleary, 2010). In general, the patch contains several parts: (1) a backing or support layer; (2) a drug layer (reservoir containing the dose); (3) a release-controlling layer (usually a semipermeable film), (4) a pressure-sensitive adhesive (PSA); and (5) a protective strip, which must be removed prior to application (see Chapter 9, Fig. 9-11). The release-controlling membrane may be a polymeric film such as ethylvinyl copolymer, which controls the release rate of the dose and its duration of action. The PSA layer is important for maintaining uninterrupted skin contact for drug

| TABLE 7-9 • Transdermal Products | | |
|---|---|---|
| **Drug** | **Product** | **Drug Class** |
| Estradiol | Vivelle | Estrogen |
| Fentanyl | Duragesic | Opiate agonist |
| Nicotine | Habitrol Tran | Smoking control |
| | Nicoderm | Smoking control |
| | Nicotrol | Smoking control |
| | Prostep patch | Smoking control |
| Naftifine HCl | Naftin | Antifungal |
| Nifedipine | Adalat | Calcium channel blocker |
| Nitroglycerin | Nitrodisc | Antiangina |
| | Nitro-Dur | Antiangina |
| Clonidine | Catopress | Antihypertensive |
| Ethinylestradiol and norelgestromin | Evra | Contraception |

diffusion through the skin. In some cases, the drug is blended directly into an adhesive, such as acrylate or silicone, performing the dual functions of release control and adhesion. This type of product is known as "drug in adhesive." In other products, the drug dose may be placed in a separate insoluble matrix layer, which helps control the release rate. This is generally known as a "matrix patch," and provides a little more control of the release rate as compared to the simple "reservoir" type of patch. Multilayers of drugs may be involved in other transdermal products using a "laminate" design. In many cases, drug permeation through the skin is the rate-limiting step in the transdermal delivery of drug into the body. See Chapter 9 for a discussion of MR drug products.

## Absorption Enhancers

A variety of excipients known as *absorption enhancers* or *permeation enhancers* have been incorporated into the drug product to promote systemic drug absorption from the application site. For oral drug products that contain poorly absorbed hydrophobic drugs, surfactants have been added to the formulation to help solubilize the drug by making the drug more miscible in water. The stratum corneum is the major barrier to systemic drug absorption from transdermal drug products. The addition of excipients or the use of physical approaches has been used to enhance drug permeation from transdermal products. For example, Estraderm˚, an estradiol transdermal system, contains ethanol, which promotes drug delivery through the stratum corneum of the skin. The use of ultrasound (phonophoresis or sonophoresis) has been used by physical therapists to enhance percutaneous absorption of hydrocortisone ointments and creams from intact skin. Iontophoresis is a technique using a small electric charge to deliver drug containing an ionic charge through the stratum corneum. Most of these absorption enhancement approaches attempt to disrupt the cellular barriers to drug transport and allow the drug to permeate better.

## CHAPTER SUMMARY

Biopharmaceutics is the study of the physicochemical properties of the drug and the drug product and links these properties to drug product quality and drug product performance. Biopharmaceutics has a crucial role in establishing a link between the *in vivo* product performance such as BA, onset of action, safety, and efficacy to the drug product CPPs and CMAs. Both *in vitro* (eg, dissolution) and *in vivo* methods (BA) are applied to evaluate drug product quality and drug product performance. Thus, the selection of a suitable salt form of the drug that has improved stability, aqueous solubility, and BA is based on the correct choice of the drug's physicochemical properties, the formulation excipients and the method of manufacture. Polymorphism refers to the arrangement of a drug substance in various crystalline forms. The selection of a suitable crystal, solvate, or hydrates may be crucial to improve the solubility and dissolution of a drug, and therefore its BA. The particle size distribution of the drug is an important property for insoluble, hydrophobic drugs. Decreasing the particle size for some low-solubility drugs may result in improved BA. Systemic drug absorption from a drug product consists of a succession of rate processes including (1) disintegration of the drug product and subsequent release of the drug, (2) dissolution of the drug in an aqueous environment, and (3) absorption of the drug across cell membranes into the systemic circulation. The slowest step in a series of kinetic processes is called the rate-limiting step. Dissolution is a dynamic process by which a solid drug substance becomes dissolved in a dissolution medium. Developing a discriminating dissolution method and setting the appropriate product specifications is critical in assuring that the manufacture of the dosage form is consistent and successful throughout the product's life cycle. Clinically relevant specifications are those specifications that, in addition, take into consideration the clinical impact assuring consistent safety and efficacy profile. In this case, clinically meaningful dissolution method and specifications will minimize the variability to the patient and, therefore, will optimize drug therapy. Due to the critical role that dissolution plays in defining the BA of the drug, *in vitro* dissolution, if identified as CQA, can serve as a relevant predictor of the *in vivo* performance of the drug product.

An *in vitro–in vivo* correlation (IVIVC) establishes a relationship between a biological property of the drug (such as PD effect or plasma drug concentration) and a physicochemical property of the drug product containing the drug substance, such as dissolution rate. A properly validated IVIVC enhances drug product understanding and provides justification of manufacturing changes during drug product development. It enhances the significance of the *in vitro* testing leading to drug product specifications' (eg, dissolution acceptance criteria) setting based on targeted clinically relevant plasma concentrations. In addition, it allows for the prediction of the clinical impact of movements within the design space without the need for additional *in vivo* studies.

The use of biopharmaceutic tools such as dissolution and BA/BE studies become very relevant in setting clinically relevant drug product specifications because it would be rather impractical to determine the clinical relevance of movements within the design space through clinical efficacy and safety trials.

# LEARNING QUESTIONS

1. What are the two rate-limiting steps possible in the oral absorption of a solid drug product? Which one would apply to a soluble drug? Which one could be altered by the pharmacist? Give examples.

2. What is the physiologic transport mechanism for the absorption of most drugs from the GI tract? What area of the GI tract is most favorable for the absorption of drugs? Why?

3. Explain why the absorption rate of a soluble drug tends to be greater than the elimination rate of the drug?

4. What type of oral dosage form generally yields the greatest amount of systemically available drug in the least amount of time? (Assume that the drug can be prepared in any form.) Why?

5. What effect does the oral administration of an anticholinergic drug, such as atropine sulfate, have on the BA of aspirin from an enteric-coated tablet? (*Hint:* Atropine sulfate decreases GI absorption.)

6. Drug formulations of erythromycin, including its esters and salts, have significant differences in BA. Erythromycin is unstable in an acidic medium. Suggest a method for preventing a potential BA problem for this drug.

# ANSWERS

## Frequently Asked Questions

*What physical or chemical properties of a drug substance are important in designing a drug for (a) oral administration or (b) parenteral administration?*

- For optimal drug absorption after oral administration, the drug should be water soluble and highly permeable so that it can be absorbed throughout the GI tract. Ideally, the drug should not change into a polymorphic form that could affect its solubility. The drug should be stable in both gastric and intestinal pH and preferably should not be hygroscopic.
- For parenteral administration, the drug should be water soluble and stable in solution, preferably at autoclave temperature. The drug should be non-hygroscopic and preferably should not change into another polymorphic form.

*For a lipid-soluble drug that has very poor aqueous solubility, what strategies could be used to make this drug more bioavailable after oral administration?*

- A lipid-soluble drug may be prepared in an oil-in-water (o/w) emulsion or dissolved in a nonaqueous solution in a soft gelatin capsule. A co-solvent may improve the solubility and dissolution of the drug.

*For a weak ester drug that is unstable in highly acidic or alkaline solutions, what strategies could be used to make this drug more bioavailable after oral administration?*

- The rate of hydrolysis (decomposition) of the ester drug may be reduced by formulating the drug in a co-solvent solution. A reduction in the percent of the aqueous vehicle will decrease the rate of hydrolysis. In addition, the drug should be formulated at the pH in which the drug is most stable.

## Learning Questions

1. The rate-limiting steps in the oral absorption of a solid drug product are the rate of drug dissolution within the GI tract and the rate of permeation of the drug molecules across the intestinal mucosal cells. Generally, disintegration of the drug product is rapid and not rate limiting. Water-soluble drugs dissolve rapidly in the aqueous environment of the GI tract, so the permeation of the intestinal mucosal cells may be the rate-limiting step. The drug absorption rate may be altered by a variety of methods, all of which depend on knowledge of the biopharmaceutic properties of the drug and the drug product and on the physiology of the GI tract. Drug examples are described in detail in this chapter.

2. Most drugs are absorbed by passive diffusion. The duodenum provides a large surface area and blood supply that maintains a large drug concentration gradient favorable for drug absorption from the duodenum into the systemic circulation.

3. If the initial drug absorption rate is smaller than the drug elimination rate, then therapeutic drug concentrations in the body would not be achieved. It should be noted that the rate of absorption is generally first order, ie rate of absorption is proportional to the amount of drug still available for absorption.

4. A drug product prepared as an oral aqueous solution is generally the most bioavailable compared to its solid oral counterpart. However, the same drug prepared as a well-designed IR tablet or capsule may have similar BA. In the case of an oral drug solution, there is no dissolution step; the drug molecules come into contact with the intestinal membrane, and the drug is subsequently absorbed. As a result of first-pass effects, a drug given in an oral drug solution may not be 100% bioavailable. If the drug solution is formulated with a high solute concentration—such as sorbitol solution, which yields a high osmotic pressure—gastric motility may be slowed, thus slowing the rate of drug absorption.

5. Anticholinergic drugs prolong gastric emptying, which will delay the absorption of an enteric-coated drug product.

6. Erythromycin may be formulated as enteric-coated granules to protect the drug from degradation at the stomach pH. Enteric-coated granules are less affected by gastric emptying and food (which delays gastric emptying) compared to enteric-coated tablets.

## REFERENCES

Achanta AS, Gray VA, Cecil TL, et al: Evaluation of the performance of prednisone and salicylic acid calibrators. *Drug Develop Ind Pharm* 21:1171–1182, 1995.

Adams W, et al: Demonstrating bioequivalence of locally acting orally inhaled drug products (OIPs): Workshop Summary Report. *J Aerol Med* 23(1):1–29, 2010.

Aguiar AJ, Krc J, Kinkel AW, Samyn JC: Effect of polymorphism on the absorption of chloramphenicol from chloramphenicol palmitate. *J Pharm Sci* 56:847–853, 1967.

Allen PV, Rahn PD, Sarapu AC, Vandewielen AJ: Physical characteristic of erythromycin anhydrate, monohydrate, and dihydrate crystalline solids. *J Pharm Sci* 67:1087–1093, 1978.

Armenante P, Muzzio F: Inherent Method Variability in Dissolution Testing: The Effect of Hydrodynamics in the USP II Apparatus. A Technical Report Submitted to the Food and Drug Administration, 2005.

Ashok V, Kumar MR, Murali D, Chatterjee A: A review of vaginal route as a systemic drug delivery. *Critical Rev in Pharm Sci* 1(1):1–19, 2012.

ASTM E2503-13: Standard Practice for Qualification of Basket and Paddle Dissolution Apparatus. *DOI: 10.1520/E2503-13E01*. West Conshohocken, PA, ASTM International, 2013.

Bai G, Armenante PM, Plank RV, Gentzler M, Ford K, Harmon P: Hydrodynamic investigation of USP dissolution test apparatus II. *J Pharm Sci* 96(9):2327–2349, 2007.

Bai G, Armenante PM: Hydrodynamic, mass transfer, and dissolution effects induced by tablet location during dissolution testing. *J Pharm Sci* 98(4):1511–1531, 2009.

Bates TR, Equeira JA: Bioavailability of micronized griseofulvin from corn oil in water emulsion, aqueous suspension and commercial dosage form in humans. *J Pharm Sci* 64:793–797, 1975.

Baxter JL, Kukura J, Muzzio FJ: Hydrodynamics-induced variability in the USP apparatus II dissolution test. *Int J Pharm* 292:17-28, 2005.

Beal SL, Sheiner LB: Estimating population kinetics. *Crit Rev Biomed Engineering* 8(3):195–222, 1982.

Beyer WF, Smith DL: Unexpected variable in the USP-NF rotating basket dissolution test. *J Pharm Sci* 60(3):496–497, 1971.

Bhupinderjit SA, et al: Phospholipid association reduces the gastric mucosal toxicity of aspirin in human subjects. *Am J Gastroent* 94(7):1817–1822, 1999.

Bocanegra LB, Morris GJ, Jurewicz JT, et al: Fluid and particle laser Doppler velocity measurements and mass transfer predictions for USP paddle method dissolution apparatus. *Drug Dev Ind Pharm* 16:1441–1462, 1990.

Boeckmann AJ, Sheiner LB, Beal SL: NONMEM Users Guide - Part V. Introductory Guide. NONMEM Project Group, University of California at San Francisco. ICON plc, Gaithersburg, Maryland, 2017.

Brown CK, Chokshi HP, Nickerson B, et al: Acceptable analytical practices for dissolution testing of poorly soluble compounds. *Pharm Tech* 28(12):56, 2004.

Brown CK, Buhse L, Friedel H-D, Keitel S et al: FIP Position paper on qualification of paddle and basket dissolution apparatus. *AAPS PharmSciTech* 10(3):924–927, 2009.

Brown CK, Friedel HD, Barker AR, Buhse LF et al: FIP/AAPS Joint Workshop Report: Dissolution/in vitro release testing of novel/special dosage forms. *Indian J Pharm Sci* 73(3):338–353, 2011.

Brown R, Schanker L: Absorption of aerosolized drugs from the rat lung. *Drug Metab Dispos* 11:355–360, 1983.

Buchwald P: Direct, differential-equation-based in-vitro–in-vivo correlation (IVIVC) method. *J Pharm Pharmacol* 55:495–504, 2003.

Certara: Phoenix/WinNonlin Version 8.1 User Manual. 2019. https://www.certara.com/.

Chang RK, Raw A, Lionberger R, Yu L: Generic development of topical dermatologic products: Formulation development, process development, and testing of topical dermatologic products. *AAPS J* **15**(1):41–52, 2013.

Chiou WL, Riegelman S: Pharmaceutical Applications of Solid Dispersion Systems. *J Pharm Sci* **60**(9):1281–1302, 1971.

Chourasia MK, Jain SK: Pharmaceutical approaches to colon targeted drug delivery systems. *J Pharm Pharm Sci* **6**(1):33–66, January–April 2003.

Code of Federal Regulations, Title 21, Volume 1, 21CFR3.2, Revised as of April 1, 2018. https://www.accessdata.fda.gov/scripts/cdrh/cfdocs/cfcfr/CFRSearch.cfm?fr=3.2 (last accessed September 2019).

Cohen JL, Hubert BB, Leeson LJ, Rhodes CT et al: The development of USP dissolution and drug release standards. *Pharm Res* **7**(10):983–987, 1990.

Commentaries in Dissolution Technologies 14(2), 2007.

Cox DC, Douglas CC, Furman WB, Kirchhoeffer RD, Myrick JW, Wells CE: Guidelines for dissolution testing. *Pharm Tech* **2**(40):41–53, 1978.

Cox DC, Furman WB: Systematic error associated with apparatus 2 of the USP dissolution test I: Effects of physical alignment of the dissolution apparatus. *J Pharm Sci* **71**(4):451–452, 1982.

Cox DC, Wells CE, Furman WB, Savage TS, King AC: Systematic error associated with apparatus 2 of the USP dissolution test II: Effects of deviations in vessel curvature from that of a sphere. *J Pharm Sci* **71**(4):395–399, 1982.

Cox DC, Furman WB, Thornton LK, Moore TW, Jefferson EH: Systematic error associated with apparatus 2 of the USP dissolution test III: Limitations of calibrators and the USP suitability test. *J Pharm Sci* **72**(8):910–913, 1983.

Cutler DJ: Linear systems analysis in pharmacokinetics. *J Pharmacokinet Biopharm* **6**(3):265–282, 1978.

D'Arcy DM, Corrigan OI, Healy AM: Evaluation of hydrodynamics in the basket dissolution apparatus using computational fluid dynamics—Dissolution rate implications. *Eur J Pharm Sci* **28**:259–267. 2006.

D'Arcy DM, Liu B, Bradley G, Healy AM, Corrigan OI: Hydrodynamic and species transfer simulations in the USP 4 dissolution apparatus: Considerations for dissolution in a low velocity pulsing flow. *Pharm Res* **27**(2):246–258, 2010.

Deng G, Ashley AJ, Brown WE, Eaton JW, et al: The USP performance verification test, Part I: USP Lot P prednisone tablets—quality attributes and experimental variables contributing to dissolution variance. *Pharm Res* **25**(5):1100–1109, 2008.

Derendorf H, Nave R, Drollmann A, et al: Relevance of pharmacokinetics and pharmacodynamics of inhaled corticosteroids to asthma. *ERJ* **28**(5):1042–1050, 2006.

DeStefano AJ, Hauck WW, Stippler ES, et al: Establishing new acceptance limits for dissolution performance verification of USPC apparatus 1 and 2 using uspc prednisone tablets reference standard. *Pharm Res* **28**:505–516, 2011.

Djupesland PG: Nasal drug delivery devices: Characteristics and performance in a clinical perspective—A review. *Drug Deliv Transl Res* **3**(1):42–62, 2013.

Dolovich M: New propellant-free technologies under investigation. *J Aerosol Med* **12**(1):s9–s17, 1999.

D'Souza S: A review of in vitro drug release test methods for nano-sized dosage forms advances in pharmaceutics, vol. 2014, Article ID 304757, 12 pages, 2014. https://doi.org/10.1155/2014/304757.

Ekstrom MP. A spectral characterization of the ill-conditioning in numerical deconvolution. *IEEE Trans Audio Electroacoust* **21**(4):344–348, 1973.

EMA Guideline on the pharmacokinetic and clinical evaluation of modified release dosage forms, November 2014.

Estudante M, Morais JG, Soveral G, Benet LZ: Intestinal drug transporters: An overview. *Advanced Drug Delivery Reviews* **65**:1340–1356, 2013.

FDA Guidance for Industry: In-vitro Bioequivalence Studies of Metaproterenol Sulfate and Albuterol Inhalation Aerosols (Metered Dose Inhalers). Division of Bioequivalence, Food and Drug Administration, Rockville, Maryland, 1989.

FDA Guidance for Industry: SUPAC-IR: Immediate Release Solid Oral Dosage Forms. November 1995.

FDA Guidance for Industry: Dissolution Testing of Immediate Release Solid Oral Dosage Forms. FDA, 1997a.

FDA Guidance for Industry: Extended Release Oral Dosage Forms: Development, Evaluation, and Application of In Vitro/In Vivo Correlations. FDA, 1997b.

FDA Guidance for Industry: SUPAC-MR: Modified Release Solid Oral Dosage Forms. FDA, 1997c.

FDA Guidance for Industry: Nasal Spray and Inhalation Solution, Suspension, and Spray Drug Products—Chemistry, Manufacturing, and Controls Documentation. 2002.

FDA Guidance for Industry: Changes to an Approved NDA or ANDA. April 2004.

FDA Guidance for Industry: The Use of Mechanical Calibration of Dissolution Apparatus 1 and 2: Current Good Manufacturing Practice (CGMP). January 2010.

FDA: Draft Guidance for Industry on Fluticasone Propionate; Salmeterol Xinafoate. May 2019.

FDA Guidance for Industry: Classification of Products as Drugs and Devices & Additional Product Classification Issues: Guidance for Industry and FDA Staff. September 2017.

FDA Guidance for Industry: Waiver of In Vivo Bioavailability and Bioequivalence Studies for Immediate-Release Solid Oral Dosage Forms Based on a Biopharmaceutics Classification System. December 2017.

FDA: Is The Product A Medical Device? March 2018.

Finkelstein L, Carson ER. *Mathematical Modelling of Dynamic Biological System*, 2nd ed. New York, Research Studies Press Ltd/John Wiley & Sons, 1985.

Fisher RS, Ho J: Potential new methods for antiepileptic drug delivery. *CNS Drugs* **16**(9):579–593, 2002.

FIP, Guidelines for dissolution testing of solid oral products. *Pharm Ind* **43**(4):334–343, 1981.

Fordtran J, Patrawala M, Chakrabarti S: Influence of vehicle composition on *in vivo* absorption of calcium from soft elastic gelatin capsule. *Pharm Res* **3**(suppl):645, 1986.

Foster T, Brown W: USP dissolution calibrators: Re-examination and appraisal. Dissolution Tech **12**(1), 2005.

Fujiwara K, Murashima K, Iwamoto K, et al: Influence of equipment vibration on dissolution rates. *JPF* **6**(1):46-48, 1997.

Fusari S, Grostic MF, Lewis AR, Poole J, Sarapu AC: Dissolution-test calibrators: PMA's collaborative study, 1978. *Pharm Tech* **5**(9) 135–143, September 1981.

Gamel J, Rousseau WF, Katholi CR, Mesel E: Pitfalls in digital computation of the impulse response of vascular beds from indicator-dilution curves. *Circ Res* **32**:516–523, 1973.

Gao Z, Moore TW, Doub WH, Westenberger BJ, Buhse LF: Effects of deaeration methods on dissolution testing in aqueous media: A study using a total dissolved gas pressure meter. *J Pharm Sci* **95**(7):1606–1613, 2006.

Gao Z, Moore TW, Smith AP, Doub W, Westenberger B, Buhse L: Gauge repeatability and reproducibility for accessing variability during dissolution testing: A technical note. *AAPS PharmSciTech* **8**(4):E1–E5, 2007a.

Gao Z, Moore TW, Smith AP, Doub WH, Westenberger BJ: Studies of variability in dissolution testing with USP apparatus 2. *J Pharm Sci* **96**(7):1794–1801, 2007b.

Gao Z, Moore TW, Buhse LF, Doub WH: The random vibration effects on dissolution testing with USP apparatus 2. *J Pharm Sci* **98**(1):297–306, 2009.

Gaynor C, Dunne A, Costello C, Davis J: A population approach to in vitro–in vivo correlation modelling for compounds with nonlinear kinetics. *J Pharmacokinet Pharmacodyn* **38**:317–332, 2011.

Gibaldi M, Feldman S: Establishment of sink conditions in dissolution rate determinations. Theoretical considerations and application to nondisintegrating dosage forms. *J Pharm Sci* **56**(10):1238–1242, 1967.

Gibaldi M, Perrier D: *Pharmacokinetics.* Boca Raton, FL, CRC Press; 2nd ed, September 15, 1982.

Gillespie, WR: Convolution based approaches for in-vivo in-vitro correlation modeling. *Adv Exper Med Biol* **423**:53–65, 1997.

Gillette JR, Mitchell JR: Routes of drug administration and response. In *Concepts in Biochemical Pharmacology.* Berlin, Springer-Verlag, 1975, Chap 6.

Glasgow M, Dressman S, Brown W, et al: The USP performance verification test, part II: collaborative study of USPs lot P prednisone tablets. *Pharm Res* **25**(5):1110–1115, 2008.

Gonda I: Drugs administered directly into the respiratory tract: Modeling of the duration of effective drug levels. *J Pharm Sci* **77**:340–346, 1987.

Gombar VK, Silver IS, Zhao Z: Role of ADME characteristics in drug discovery and their in silico evaluation: In silico screening of chemicals for their metabolic stability. *Curr Top Med Chem* **3**(11):1205–1225, 2003.

Gonzalez MA, Cleary GW: Transdermal dosage forms. In Shargel L, Kanfer I (eds). *Generic Drug Product Development–Specialty Dosage Forms.* New York, Informa Healthcare, 2010, Chap 8.

Gray VA, Hubert BB, Krasowski JA: Calibration of dissolution apparatuses 1 and 2. What to do when equipment fails. *Pharmacop Forum* **20**(6):8571–8573, 1994.

Gray VA, Foster TS: Utility of USP salicylic acid dissolution calibrator tablets. *Pharm Forum* **23**(6):5360–5363, 1997.

Gray VA, Brown CK, Dressman JB, Leeson J: A new general chapter on dissolution. *Pharm Forum* **27**:3432–3439, 2001.

Hamilton JF, Moore TW, Kerner CM: Reproducibility of dissolution test results. *Pharm Forum* **21**(5):1383–1386, 1995.

Hamlin WE, Nelson E, Ballard BE, Wagner JG. Loss of sensitivity in distinguishing real differences in dissolution rates due to increasing intensity of agitation. *J Pharm Sci* **51**(5):432–435, 1962.

Hanson R, Gray V: *Handbook of Dissolution Testing*, 3rd ed. Hockessin, DE, Dissolution Technologies, Inc., 2004, Chap 1.

Harboe E, Larsen C, Johansen A, Olesen HP: Macromolecular prodrugs. XV. Colon-targeted delivery–bioavailability of naproxen from orally administered dextran-naproxen ester prodrugs varying in molecular size in the pig. *Pharm Res* **6**(11):919–923, 1989.

Hauck WW, DeStefano AJ, Brown WE, Stippler ES et al.: Change in criteria for USP dissolution performance verification tests. *AAPS PharmSciTech* **10**(1):21–26, 2009.

Hauck WW, Li C, Stippler ES, Brown WE: Establishing acceptance limits for dissolution performance verification of USP apparatus 1 and 2 using USP prednisone tablets reference standard lot Q0H398. *Dissolution Tech* **20**(1):6–10, 2013.

Heimbach T, Suarez-Sharp S, Kakhi M, et al.: Dissolution and translational modeling strategies toward establishing an in vitro-in vivo link—a workshop summary report. *AAPS J* 21:29, 2019. https://doi.org/10.1208/s12248-019-0298-x.

ICH. Specifications: Test Procedures and Acceptance Criteria for New Drug Substances and New Drug Products: Chemical Substances. Q6A, October 1999.

Issa MG, Ferraz HG: Intrinsic dissolution as a tool for evaluating drug solubility in accordance with the biopharmaceutics classification system. *Dissolution Tech* **18**(3):6–13, 2011.

Jin J, Sklar, GE, Sen Oh VM, et al: Factors affecting therapeutic compliance: A review from the patient's perspective. *Ther Clin Risk Manag* **4**(1):269–286, 2008.

Kakhi M: Classification of the flow regimes in the flow-through cell. *Eur J Pharm Sci* **37**:531–544, 2009a.

Kakhi M: Mathematical modeling of the fluid dynamics in the flow-through cell. *Int J Pharm* **376**:22–40, 2009b.

Kakhi M, Marroum P, Chittenden J: Analysis of level A in vitro–in vivo correlations for an extended-release formulation with limited bioavailability. *Biopharm Drug Dispos* **34**:262–277, 2013.

Kakhi M, Chittenden J: Modeling of pharmacokinetic systems using stochastic deconvolution. *J Pharm Sci* **102**:4433–4443, 2013.

Kakhi M, Lukacova V: Metformin: Mechanistic absorption modeling and IVIVC development. *AAPS Annual Meeting and Exposition.* Orlando FL, October 25–29, 2015.

Kakhi M, Suarez-Sharp S, Shephard T, Chittenden J: Application of an NLME stochastic deconvolution approach to level A IVIVC modeling. *J Pharm Sci* **106**:1905–1916, 2017.

Kaniwa N, Katori N, Aoyagi N, et al: Collaborative study on the development of a standard for evaluation of vibration levels for dissolution apparatus. *Int J Pharm* **175**:119–129, 1998.

Kaplan SA: Biopharmaceutical considerations in drug formulation design and evaluation. *Drug Metab Rev* **1**:15–34, 1972.

Kesisoglou F, Mitra A: Application of absorption modeling in rational design of drug product under quality-by-design paradigm. *AAPS J* **17**(5):1224–1236, 2015.

Kesisoglou F, Xia B, Agrawal NGB: Comparison of deconvolution-based and absorption modeling IVIVC for extended release formulations of a BCS III drug development candidate. *AAPS J* **17**(6):1492–1500, 2015.

Klein S: The use of biorelevant dissolution media to forecast the *in vivo* performance of a drug. *AAPS J* **12**(3):397–406, 2010.

Kumari N, Kalyanwat R, Singh VK. Complete review on nasal drug delivery systems. *Int J Med Pharm Res* **1**(2):235–249, 2013.

Labiris NR, Dolovich MB: Pulmonary drug delivery. Part I: Physiological factors affecting therapeutic effectiveness of aerosolized medications. *Br J Clin Pharmacol* **56**(6):588–599, 2003.

Lakshmi PJ, Deepthi B, Rama RN: Rectal drug delivery: A promising route for enhancing drug absorption. *Asian J Res Pharm Sci* **2**(4):143–149, 2012.

Langenbucher F, Benz D, Kürth W, Möller H, Otz M: Standardized flow-cell method as an alternative to existing pharmacopeial dissolution testing. *Pharm Ind* **51**(11):1276–1281, 1989.

Laube B: The expanding role of aerosols in systemic drug delivery, therapy, and vaccination. *Resp Care* **50**(9):1161–1176, 2005.

Layloff T: Studies in the development of USP dissolution test method number 2. *Pharm Forum* **9**(6):3752–3757, 1983.

Lemmer HJR, Hamman JH: Paracellular drug absorption enhancement through tight junction modulation. *Exp Opin Drug Deliv* **10**(1):103–114, 2013.

Levy G: Effect of dosage form on drug absorption a frequent variable in clinical pharmacology. *Arch Int Pharmacodyn* **152**(1):59–68, 1964.

Liebenberg W, Engelbrecht E, Wessels A, Devarakonda B, Yang W, De Villiers MM: A comparative study of the release of active ingredients from semisolid cosmeceuticals measured with Franz, enhancer or flow-through cell diffusion apparatus. *J Food Drug Anal* **12**(1):19–28, 2004.

Loo JCK, Riegelman S: New method for calculating the intrinsic absorption rate of drugs. *J Pharm Sci* **57**(6):918–928, 1968.

Machado MB, Bittdorf KJ, Roussinova VT, Kresta SM: Transition from turbulent to transitional flow in the top half of a stirred tank. *Chem Eng Sci* **98**:218–230, 2013.

Madden FN, Godfrey KR, Chappell MJ, Hovorka R, Bates RA: A comparison of six deconvolution techniques. *J Pharmacokinet Biopharmaceut* **24**(3):283–299, 1996.

Mathias NR, Hussain MA: Non-invasive systemic drug delivery: Developability considerations for alternate routes of administration. *J Pharm Sci* **99**(1):1–20, 2010.

McCarthy LG, Bradley G, Sexton JC, Corrigan OI, Healy AM: Computational fluid dynamics modeling of the paddle dissolution apparatus: Agitation rate, mixing patterns, and fluid velocities. *AAPS PharmSciTech* **5**(2)e31, 2004

McCormick TJ: Industry Perspective on dissolution apparatus calibration. *Dissolution Tech* **2**(4):12–15, 1995.

Mistry B, Patel N, Jamei M, Rostami-Hodjegan A, Martinez MN: Examining the use of a mechanistic model to generate an in vivo/in vitro correlation: Journey through a thought process. *AAPS J*. **18**(5):1144–1158, 2016.

Mirza T: Mechanical versus chemical dissolution calibration. *Dissolution Tech* **7**(1):6–7, 2000.

Mirza T, Joshi Y, Liu Q, Vivilecchia R: Evaluation of dissolution hydrodynamics in the USP, Peak and flat-bottom vessels using different solubility drugs. *Dissolution Tech* **12**(1):11–16, 2005.

Moore TW, Hamilton JF, Kerner CM: Dissolution testing: Limitations of the USP prednisone and salicylic acid calibrator tablets. *Pharmacopeial Forum* **21**(5):1387–1396, 1995.

Moore JW, Flanner HH: Mathematical comparison of dissolution profiles. *Pharm Tech* **20**:64–74, 1996.

Moore TW, Shangraw RF, Habib Y: Dissolution calibrator tablets: A recommendation for new calibrator tablets to replace both current USP calibrator tablets. *Pharmacopeial Forum* **22**(3):2423–2428, 1996.

Moore TW, Cox DC, Demarest DA Jr: Dissolution calibrator tablets: A scaled-up lot of a new calibrator tablet recommended to replace both current USP calibrator tablets. *Pharmacopeial Forum* **23**(6):5352–5359, 1997.

Morishita M, Peppas N: Is the oral route possible for peptide and protein drug delivery? *Drug Discovery Today* **11**(19–20):905–910, 2006.

Noyes AA, Whitney WR: The rate of solution of solid substances in their own solutions. *J Am Chem Soc* **19**:930–934, 1897.

Oates M: Recent innovations in dissolution calibration. *Dissolution Tech* **6**(3):11,1999.

O'Connor D, et al: Role of pharmacokinetics in establishing bioequivalence for orally inhaled drug products: Workshop Summary Report. *J Aerol Med* **24**(3):119–135, 2011.

O'Hara T, Hayes S, Davis J, Devane J, Smart T, Dunne A: In vivo–in vitro correlation (IVIVC) modeling incorporating a convolution step. *J Pharmacokinet Pharmacodyn* **28**(3):277–298, 2001.

Parrott EL, Wurster DE, Higuchi T: Investigation of drug release from solids. I. Some factors influencing the dissolution rate. *J Am Pharm Assoc* **44**(5):269–273, 1955.

Patil SD, Burgess DJ: Pharmaceutical development of modified release parenteral dosage forms using bioequivalence (BE), quality by design (QBD) and in vitro-in vivo correlation (IVIVC) principles. In Shargel, L, Kanfer I (eds). *Generic Drug Product Development–Specialty Dosage Forms*. New York, Informa Healthcare, 2010, Chap 9.

Pavan B, Dalpiaz A, Ciliberti N, et al: Progress in drug delivery to the central nervous system by the prodrug approach. *Molecules* **13**:1035–1065, 2008.

Pepin XJH, Parrott N, Dressman J, Delvadia P, Mitra A, Zhang X, Babiskin A, Kolhatkar V, Suarez-Sharp S. Current State and Future Expectations of Translational Modeling Strategies to Support Drug Product Development, Manufacturing Changes and Controls: A Workshop Summary Report. *J Pharm Sci.* 2021 Feb;**110**(2):555-566. doi: 10.1016/j.xphs.2020.04.021. Epub 2020 May 4. PMID: 32380182.

PhRMA Subcommittee on Dissolution Calibration: Dissolution calibration: Recommendations for reduced chemical testing and enhanced mechanical calibration. *Pharmacopeial Forum* **26**(4):1149–1151, 2000.

Philip AK, Philip B: Colon targeted drug delivery systems: A review on primary and novel approaches. *OMJ* **25**:70–78, 2010.

Puoton CW: Formulation of poorly water-soluble drugs for oral administration: Physicochemical and physiological issues and the lipid formulation classification system. *Eur J Pharm Sci* **29**(3–4):27, 2006.

Prasad V, Shah V, Knight P, et al: Importance of media selection in establishment of *in vitro–in vivo* relationship for quinidine gluconate. *Int J Pharm* **13**:1–7, 1983.

Qiu Y, Samara EE, Cao G. In vitro-in vivo correlations in the development of solid oral controlled release dosage form. In Wise DL (ed). *Handbook of Pharmaceutical Controlled Release Technology*, Vol. 1. New York, Marcel Dekker, pp 527–549, 2000.

Qureshi SA, McGilveray IJ. A critical assessment of the USP dissolution apparatus suitability test criteria. *Drug Dev Ind Pharm* **21**(8):905–924, 1995.

Qureshi SA, McGilveray IJ. Typical variability in drug dissolution testing: Study with USP and FDA calibrator tablets and a marketed drug (Glibenclamide) product. *Eur J Pharm Sci* **7**:249, 1999.

Qureshi SA, Shabnam J: Cause of high variability in drug dissolution testing and its impact on setting tolerances. *Eur J Pharm Sci* **12**:271–276, 2001.

Röst M, Quist PO: Dissolution of USP prednisone calibrator tablets: Effects of stirring conditions and particle size distribution. *J Pharm Biomed Analysis* **31**:1129–1143, 2003.

Sarapu AC, Lewis AR, Grostic MF: Analysis of PMA collaborative studies of dissolution test calibrators. *Pharmacopeial Forum* **6**(2):172–176, 1980.

Schuirmann DJ: Analysis of a collaborative study of the USP prednisone dissolution calibrator. *Pharmacopeial Forum* **6**(1):75–89, 1980.

Shaji J, Patole V: Protein and peptide drug delivery: Oral approaches. *Indian J Pharm Sci* **70**(3):269–277, 2008.

Shareef MA, Ahuja A, Ahmad FJ, Raghava S: Colonic drug delivery: An updated review. *AAPS Pharm Sci* **54**:161–186, 2003.

Sheiner LB: The population approach to pharmacokinetic data analysis: Rationale and standard data analysis methods. *Drug Metab Rev* **15**(1&2):153–171, 1984.

Shen J, Lee K, Choi S, Qu W, Wang Ym, Burgess DJ: A reproducible accelerated in vitro release testing method for PLGA microspheres. *Int J Pharm* **498**:274–282, 2016.

Shiko G, Gladden LF, Sederman AJ, Connolly PC, Butler JM: MRI studies of the hydrodynamics in a USP 4 dissolution testing cell. *J Pharm Sci* **100**(3):976–991, 2011.

Siewart M, Dressman J, Brown CK, Shah VP: FIP/AAPS guidelines to dissolution/in vitro release testing of novel/special dosage forms. *AAPS Pharm Sci Tech* **4**(1):1–10, 2003.

Skoug JW: Calibration of dissolution rate apparatuses: A user's perspective. Dissolution Tech **1**(2):3–5, 1994.

Stella V, Haslam J, Yata N, et al: Enhancement of bioavailability of a hydrophobic amine antimalarial by formulation with oleic acid in a soft gelatin capsule. *J Pharm Sci* **67**:1375–1377, 1978.

Suarez S, et al. Effect of dose and release rate on pulmonary targeting of glucocorticoids using liposomes as a model dosage form. *Pharm Res* **15**:461–463, 1998.

Suarez Sharp S: Establishing clinically relevant drug product specifications: FDA Perspective. AAPS Annual Meeting and Exposition, Chicago, IL, 2011. http://www.fda.gov/downloads/AboutFDA/CentersOffices/OfficeofMedicalProductsandTobacco/CDER/UCM341185.pdf.

Suarez-Sharp S: FDA's Experience on IVIVC- New Drugs. PQRI Workshop on Application of IVIVC in Formulation Development. Bethesda, MD, 2012.

Suarez-Sharp S, Li M, Duan J, Shah H, Seo P: Regulatory experience with in vivo in vitro correlations (IVIVC) in new drug applications. *AAPS J* **18**(6):1379–1390, 2016.

Suarez-Sharp S, Cohen M, Kesisoglou F, et al. Applications of clinically relevant dissolution testing: Workshop summary report. AAPS J **20**(6), 2018.

Tatterson, GB. *Fluid Mixing and Gas Dispersion in Agitated Tanks.* McGraw-Hill, 1991.

Ueda CT, Shah VP, Derdzinski K, et al: Topical and transdermal drug products. *Pharmacopeial Forum* **35**(3):750–764, 2009.

United States Pharmacopeia 41/National Formulary 36 1S. 2018. General Chapter <701> Disintegration. Rockville, MD.

Vaughan DP, Dennis M: Mathematical basis of the point area deconvolution method for determining *in vivo* input functions. *J Pharm Sci* **67**(5):663–665, 1978.

Vangani S, Flick T, Tamayo G, Chiu R, Cauchon N: Vibration measurements on dissolution systems and effects on dissolution of prednisone tablets RS. *Dissolution Tech* **14**(1):6–14, 2007.

Veng-Pedersen, P: DRADAP Batch Version. Drug Release and Delivery Analysis Program V.1.0 User's Manual, 1997 (unpublished work).

Veng-Pedersen P, Modi NB: An algorithm for constrained deconvolution based on reparameterization. *J Pharm Sci* **81**(2):175–179, 1992.

Wagner JG, Nelson E: Per cent absorbed time plots derived from blood level and/or urinary excretion data. *J Pharm Sci* **52**(6):610–611, 1963.

Wood JH, Syarto JE, Letterman H: Improved holder for intrinsic dissolution rate studies. *J Pharm Sci* **54**(7):1068, 1965.

Yamaoka T, Nakamichi H, Miyata K: Studies on the characteristics of carbochromen hydrochloride crystals. II. Polymorphism and cracking in the tablets. *Chem Pharm Bull* **30**(10):3695–3700, 1982.

Yoshida H, Kuwana A, Shibata H, Izutsu K, Goda Y: Particle image velocimetry evaluation of fluid flow profiles in USP 4 flow-through dissolution cells. *Pharm Res* **32**:2950–2959, 2015.

Yoshikawa H, Nakao Y, Takada K, et al: Targeted and sustained delivery of aclarubicin to lymphatics by lactic acid oligomer microsphere in rat. *Chem Pharm Bull* **37**:802–804, 1989.

# BIBLIOGRAPHY

Aguiar AJ: Physical properties and pharmaceutical manipulations influencing drug absorption. In Forth IW, Rummel W (eds). *Pharmacology of Intestinal Absorption: Gastro-intestinal Absorption of Drugs,* Vol 1. New York, Pergamon, 1975, Chap 6.

Amidon GL, Lennernas H, Shah VP, Crison JR: A theoretical basis for a biopharmaceutic drug classification: The correlation of *in vitro* drug product dissolution and *in vivo* bioavailability. *Pharm Res* **12**:413–420, 1995.

Barr WH: The use of physical and animal models to assess bioavailability. *Pharmacology* **8**:88–101, 1972.

Berge S, Bighley L, Monkhouse D: Pharmaceutical salts. *J Pharm Sci* **66**:1–19, 1977.

Blanchard J: Gastrointestinal absorption, II. Formulation factors affecting bioavailability. *Am J Pharm* **150**:132–151, 1978.

Blanchard J, Sawchuk RJ, Brodie BB: *Principles and Perspectives in Drug Bioavailability.* New York, Karger, 1979.

Burks TF, Galligan JJ, Porreca F, Barber WD: Regulation of gastric emptying. *Fed Proc* **44**:2897–2901, 1985.

Cabana BE, O'Neil R: FDA's report on drug dissolution. *Pharm Forum* **6**:71–75, 1980.

Cadwalder DE: *Biopharmaceutics and Drug Interactions.* Nutley, NJ, Roche Laboratories, 1971.

Christensen J: The physiology of gastrointestinal transit. *Med Clin N Am* **58**:1165–1180, 1974.

Dakkuri A, Shah AC: Dissolution methodology: An overview. *Pharm Technol* **6**:28–32, 1982.

Dressman JB, Amidon GL, Reppas C, Shah VP: Dissolution testing as a prognostic tool for oral drug absorption: Immediate release dosage forms. *Pharm Res* **15**:11–22, 1998.

Eye IS: A review of the physiology of the gastrointestinal tract in relation to radiation doses from radioactive materials. *Health Phys* **12**:131–161, 1966.

Gilbaldi M: *Biopharmaceutics and Clinical Pharmacokinetics.* Philadelphia, Lea & Febiger, 1977.

Hansen WA: *Handbook of Dissolution Testing.* Springfield, OR, Pharmaceutical Technology Publications, 1982.

Hardwidge E, Sarapu A, Laughlin W: Comparison of operating characteristics of different dissolution test systems. *J Pharm Sci* **6**:1732–1735, 1978.

Houston JB, Wood SG: Gastrointestinal absorption of drugs and other xenobiotics. In Bridges JW, Chasseaud LF (eds). *Progress in Drug Metabolism,* Vol 4. London, Wiley, 1980, Chap 2.

Jollow DJ, Brodie BB: Mechanisms of drug absorption and drug solution. *Pharmacology* **8**:21–32, 1972.

LaDu BN, Mandel HG, Way EL: *Fundamentals of Drug Metabolism and Drug Disposition.* Baltimore, Williams & Wilkins, 1971.

Leesman GD, Sinko PJ, Amidon GL: Simulation of oral drug absorption: Gastric emptying and gastrointestinal motility. In Welling PW, Tse FLS (eds). *Pharmacokinetics: Regulatory, Industry, Academic Perspectives.* New York, Marcel Dekker, 1988, Chap 6.

Leeson LJ, Carstensen JT: Industrial pharmaceutical technology. In Leeson L, Carstensen JT (eds). *Dissolution Technology.* Washington, DC, Academy of Pharmaceutical Sciences, 1974.

Levine RR: Factors affecting gastrointestinal absorption of drugs. *Dig Dis* **15**:171–188, 1970.

McElnay JC: Buccal absorption of drugs. In Swarbrick J, Boylan JC (eds). *Encyclopedia of Pharmaceutical Technology,* Vol 2. New York, Marcel Dekker, 1990, pp 189–211.

Mojaverian P, Vlasses PH, Kellner PE, Rocci ML Jr: Effects of gender, posture and age on gastric residence of an indigestible solid: Pharmaceutical considerations. *Pharm Res* **5**:639–644, 1988.

Neinbert R: Ion pair transport across membranes. *Pharm Res* **6**:743–747, 1989.

Niazi S: *Textbook of Biopharmaceutics and Clinical Pharmacokinetics.* New York, Appleton, 1979.

Notari RE: *Biopharmaceutics and Pharmacokinetics: An Introduction.* New York, Marcel Dekker, 1975.

Palin K: Lipids and oral drug delivery. *Pharm Int* **11**:272–279, November 1985.

Palin K, Whalley D, Wilson C, et al: Determination of gastric-emptying profiles in the rat: Influence of oil structure and volume. *Int J Pharm* **12**:315–322, 1982.

Parrott EL: *Pharmaceutical Technology.* Minneapolis, Burgess, 1970.

Pernarowski M: Dissolution methodology. In Leeson L, Carstensen JT (eds). *Dissolution Technology.* Washington, DC, Academy of Pharmaceutical Sciences, 1975, p 58.

Pharmacopeial Forum: FDA report on drug dissolution. *Pharm Forum* **6**:71–75, 1980.

Prasad VK, Shah VP, Hunt J, et al: Evaluation of basket and paddle dissolution methods using different performance standards. *J Pharm Sci* **72**:42–44, 1983.

Robinson JR: *Sustained and Controlled Release Drug Delivery Systems.* New York, Marcel Dekker, 1978.

Robinson JR, Eriken SP: Theoretical formulation of sustained release dosage forms. *J Pharm Sci* **55**:1254, 1966.

Rubinstein A, Li VHK, Robinson JR: Gastrointestinal–physiological variables affecting performance of oral sustained release dosage forms. In Yacobi A, Halperin-Walega E (eds). *Oral Sustained Release Formulations: Design and Evaluation.* New York, Pergamon, 1988, Chap 6.

Schwarz-Mann WH, Bonn R: Principles of transdermal nitroglycerin administration. *Eur Heart J* **10**(suppl A):26–29, 1989.

Shaw JE, Chandrasekaran K: Controlled topical delivery of drugs for system in action. *Drug Metab Rev* **8**:223–233, 1978.

Siewart M, Dressman J, Brown CK, Shah VP: FIP/AAPS Guidelines to dissolution/in vitro release testing of novel/special dosase forms. *AAPS Pharm Sci Tech* **4**(1):1–10, 2003.

Swarbrick J: *In vitro* models of drug dissolution. In Swarbrick J (ed). *Current Concepts in the Pharmaceutical Sciences: Biopharmaceutics.* Philadelphia, Lea & Febiger, 1970.

Wagner JG: *Biopharmaceutics and Relevant Pharmacokinetics.* Hamilton, IL, Drug Intelligence Publications, 1971.

Welling PG: Dosage route, bioavailability and clinical efficacy. In Welling PW, Tse FLS (eds). *Pharmacokinetics: Regulatory, Industry, Academic Perspectives.* New York, Marcel Dekker, 1988, Chap 3.

Wurster DE, Taylor PW: Dissolution rates. *J Pharm Sci* **54**:169–175, 1965.

Yoshikawa H, Muranishi S, Sugihira N, Seaki H: Mechanism of transfer of bleomycin into lymphatics by bifunctional delivery system via lumen of small intestine. *Chem Pharm Bull* **31**:1726–1732, 1983.

York P: Solid state properties of powders in the formulation and processing of solid dosage form. *Int J Pharm* **14**:1–28, 1983.

Zaffaroni A: Therapeutic systems: The key to rational drug therapy. *Drug Metab Rev* **8**:191–222, 1978.

# 8

# Drug Product Performance, *In Vivo*: Bioavailability and Bioequivalence

Leon Shargel and Murray P. Ducharme

## CHAPTER OBJECTIVES

- Define bioavailability, bioequivalence, and drug product performance.

- Explain why certain drugs and drug products have low bioavailability.

- Distinguish between relative bioavailability and absolute bioavailability.

- Explain why first-pass effect as well as chemical instability of a drug can result in low relative bioavailability.

- Distinguish between bioavailability and bioequivalence.

- Explain why relative bioavailability may have values greater than 100%.

- Explain why bioequivalence may be considered as a measure of drug product performance.

- Describe various methods for measuring bioavailability and the advantages and disadvantages of each.

- Describe the statistical criteria for bioequivalence and 90% confidence intervals.

- Explain the conditions under which a generic drug product manufacturer may request a waiver (biowaiver) for performing an *in vivo* bioequivalence study.

- Define therapeutic equivalence and explain why bioequivalence is only one component of the regulatory requirements for therapeutic equivalence.

## DRUG PRODUCT PERFORMANCE

*Drug product performance,*[1] *in vivo*, may be defined as the release of the drug substance from the drug product leading to bioavailability of the drug substance. The assessment of drug product performance is important since bioavailability is related both to the pharmacodynamic response and to adverse events. Bioavailability studies are *in vivo* drug product performance studies that relate the physicochemical properties of the drug substance, the formulation of the drug and the manufacture process, to the expected clinical efficacy and safety of the drug product. Drug product performance studies are used in the development of both new and generic drug products.

Bioavailability studies are important to establish the *in vivo* performance of a new drug product. Bioequivalence studies are used to compare the performance of the original formulation that was used in clinical safety and efficacy studies to a to-be marketed drug product.[2] Bioequivalence studies are drug product performance tests that compare the bioavailability of the same active pharmaceutical ingredient from one drug product (test) to a second drug product (reference). Bioavailability and bioequivalence are measures of the drug product performance *in vivo*.

## PURPOSE OF BIOAVAILABILITY AND BIOEQUIVALENCE STUDIES

Bioavailability and bioequivalence studies are important in the process of approving pharmaceutical products for marketing. *Bioavailability* is defined as the rate and extent

---

[1]A glossary of terms appears at the end of this chapter.

[2]During new drug development, different dosage forms of the active drug may be formulated. The term "relative bioavailability" rather than "bioequivalence" may be used to compare the bioavailability of different dosage forms of the same drug.

to which the active ingredient or active moiety is absorbed from a drug product and becomes available at the site of action (US-FDA, CDER, 2014a). Bioavailability data provide an estimate of the fraction of drug absorbed from the formulation and provide information about the pharmacokinetics of the drug. *Relative bioavailability* studies compare two or more drug product formulations. A bioequivalence study is a relative bioavailability study. *Bioequivalence* is defined as the absence of a significant difference in the rate and extent to which the active ingredient or active moiety becomes available at the site of drug action when administered at the same molar dose under similar conditions in an appropriately designed study.

Bioavailability and bioequivalence study data are used in regulatory submissions for worldwide marketing approval of new and generic drugs. Each country's regulatory agency has its own guidelines for the conduct of acceptable bioavailability and bioequivalence studies. A recent survey of international bioequivalence guidelines showed that there are more similarities than differences among approaches used by various international jurisdictions (Davit et al, 2013). In this chapter, the relationship between bioavailability, bioequivalence, and drug approval requirements will focus on the regulatory perspective of the FDA.

## Bioequivalence Studies in New Drug Development

During new drug development, different dosage forms of the active drug may be formulated. The term *relative bioavailability* rather than *bioequivalence*

is often used to compare the bioavailability of different dosage forms of the same drug. Bioequivalence studies are used to compare (a) early and late clinical trial formulations; (b) formulations used in clinical trials and stability studies, if different; (c) clinical trial formulations and to-be-marketed drug products, if different; and (d) product strength equivalence, as appropriate. Bioequivalence studies are used to support new formulations of previously approved products, such as a new fixed-dose combination version of two products approved for coadministration, or modified-release (MR) versions of immediate-release products. After the drug has been approved for marketing, postapproval, *in vivo* bioequivalence studies may be needed to support regulatory approval of major changes in formulation, manufacturing, or site, in comparison to reference formulation (usually the prechange formulation) (Fig. 8-1).

During new drug development, the initial safety and clinical efficacy studies may use a simple formulation such as a hard gelatin capsule containing only the active ingredient diluted with lactose. If the new drug demonstrates appropriate human efficacy and safety, a to-be-marketed drug product (eg, compressed tablet) may be developed. Since the initial safety and efficacy studies were performed using a different formulation (ie, hard gelatin capsule), the pharmaceutical manufacturer must demonstrate that the to-be-marketed drug product (compressed tablet) demonstrates equivalent drug product performance to the original formulation (Fig. 8-1).

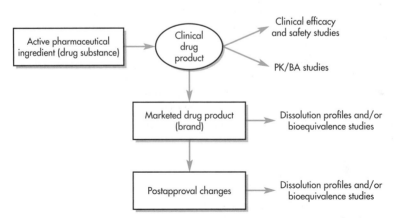

**FIGURE 8-1** • Drug product performance and new drug product development for NDAs. Drug product performance may be determined *in vivo* by bioequivalence studies or *in vitro* by comparative drug dissolution studies. BA = bioavailability.

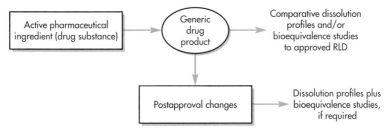

FIGURE 8-2 • Drug product performance and generic drug product development. Drug product performance may be determined *in vivo* by bioequivalence studies or *in vitro* by comparative drug/release dissolution studies.

### FREQUENTLY ASKED QUESTIONS

▶ Why are bioequivalence studies considered as drug product performance studies?

▶ What are the differences between a safety/efficacy study and an *in vivo* bioequivalence study? How do the study objectives differ?

▶ What is the difference between drug product performance and bioequivalence?

Equivalent drug product performance is generally demonstrated by an *in vivo* bioequivalence study in normal healthy volunteers. Under certain conditions, equivalent drug product performance may be demonstrated *in vitro* using comparative dissolution profiles (see Chapter 7).

The marketed drug product approved by the United States Food and Drug Administration (US FDA) may not be the same formulation that was used in the original safety and clinical efficacy studies. After the new drug product is approved by the FDA and marketed, the manufacturer may perform changes to the formulation. These changes to the marketed drug product are known as postapproval changes (see also Chapter 26). These postapproval changes, often termed SUPAC (scale-up and postapproval changes) are based on several FDA guidance documents and may include a change in the supplier of the active ingredient, a change in the formulation, a change in the manufacturing process, and/or a change in the manufacturing site. In each case, the manufacturer must demonstrate that drug product performance did not change and is the same for the drug product manufactured before and after the SUPAC change. As shown in Fig. 8-1, drug product performance may be determined by *in vivo*

bioequivalence studies or by *in vitro* comparative drug release or dissolution profiles.

### Bioequivalence Studies in Generic Drug Development (Abbreviated New Drug Applications)

Comparative drug product performance studies are important in the development of generic drug products (Fig. 8-2). A generic drug product is a multisource drug product[3] that has been approved by the FDA as a therapeutic equivalent to the reference listed drug (RLD) product[4] (usually the brand or innovator drug product) that has proven equivalent drug product performance. Since clinical safety and efficacy studies were performed on the brand drug product, these studies are not usually repeated for generic drug products. The formulation and method of manufacture of a generic drug product may be different from the brand drug product. Since these differences can affect the bioavailability and stability of the drug, the generic drug manufacturer must demonstrate that the generic drug product is pharmaceutically equivalent, bioequivalent, and therapeutically equivalent (ie, has the same drug product performance) to the comparator brand-name drug product. Drug product performance comparison for oral generic drug products is usually measured by *in vivo* bioequivalence

---

[3]Multisource drug products are drug products that contain the same active drug substance in the same dosage form and are marketed by more than one pharmaceutical manufacturer.

[4]Reference listed drugs corresponding to proposed generic versions are listed by the US-FDA in its publication Approved Drug Products with Therapeutic Equivalence Evaluations (Orange Book).

studies in normal healthy adult subjects under fasted and fed conditions. Drug product performance comparisons *in vitro* may also include comparative drug dissolution/release profiles. Similar to the brand-name drug product manufacturer, the generic drug manufacturer may make changes after FDA approval in the formulation, in the source of the active pharmaceutical ingredient, manufacturing process, or other changes. For any postapproval change, the manufacturer must demonstrate that the change did not alter the performance of the drug product.

## RELATIVE AND ABSOLUTE AVAILABILITY

Regulatory agencies such as the FDA require submission of bioavailability data in applications to market new and generic drug products. A drug product's bioavailability provides an estimate of the relative fraction of the administered dose that is absorbed into the systemic circulation. The determination of the fraction (*f*) of administered dose absorbed involves comparing the drug product's systemic drug exposure (represented by the concentration-versus-time or pharmacokinetic profile with that of a reference product. For systemically available

drug products, bioavailability is most often assessed by determining the area under the drug plasma concentration-versus-time profile (AUC). The AUC is considered the most reliable measure of a drug's bioavailability, as it is directly proportional to the total amount of unchanged drug that reaches the systemic circulation. Figure 8-3 shows how the drug concentration-versus-time profile is used to identify the pharmacokinetic parameters that form the basis of bioavailability and bioequivalence comparisons.

### Absolute Bioavailability

Absolute bioavailability compares the bioavailability of the active drug in the systemic circulation following extravascular (eg, oral) administration with the bioavailability of the same drug following intravenous administration (Fig. 8-4). Drug delivered by intravenous (IV) administration is considered 100% systemically absorbed. The route of extravascular administration can be by inhalation, intramuscular, oral, rectal, subcutaneous, sublingual, topical, transdermal, etc. The *absolute bioavailability* is the dose-corrected AUC of the extravascularly administered drug product divided by the AUC of the drug product given intravenously. The dose given by IV administration is generally smaller than the dose given by an extravascular route and therefore, the AUC is based on mg of dose given. For an oral

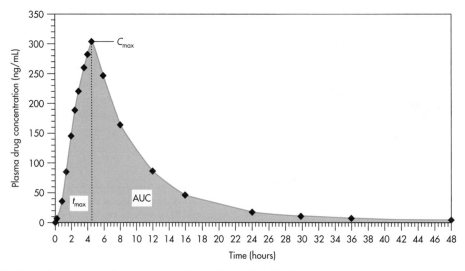

FIGURE 8-3 • Plasma drug concentration–time curve after oral drug administration.

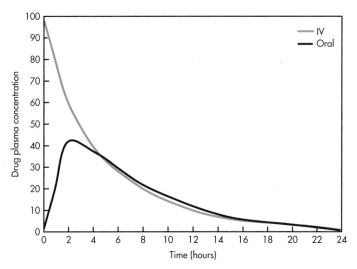

**FIGURE 8-4** • Relationship between plasma drug concentration-versus-time profiles for an intravenously administered formulation versus an orally administered formulation. In an absolute bioavailability study, the systemic exposure profile of a drug administered by the oral route (black curve) is compared with that of the drug administered by the intravenous route (green curve).

drug product, the absolute bioavailability is calculated as follows:

$$F_{abs} = \frac{[AUC]_{iv}/D_{iv}}{[AUC]_{po}/D_{po}}$$

where

$F_{abs}$ is the fraction of the dose absorbed, expressed as a percentage;

$AUC_{po}$ is the AUC following oral administration;

$D_{iv}$ is the dose administered intravenously;

$AUC_{iv}$ is the AUC following intravenous administration; and

$D_{po}$ is the dose administered orally.

Absolute availability, $F_{abs}$, may be expressed as a fraction or as a percent by multiplying $F_{abs} \times 100$. A drug given by the IV route will have an absolute bioavailability of 100% ($f = 1$). A drug given by an extravascular route may have an $F_{abs} = 0$ (no systemic absorption) and $F_{abs} = 1.0$ (100% systemic absorption).

$F_{ab}$ or F, fraction of drug absorbed, represents the relative fraction of the drug absorbed after oral drug administration.

### Relative Bioavailability

Another type of comparative bioavailability assessment is provided by a relative bioavailability study. In a relative bioavailability study, the systemic exposure of a drug in a test formulation is compared with that of the same drug administered in a reference formulation. In a relative bioavailability study, the AUCs of the two formulations are compared as follows:

$$F_{rel} = \frac{[AUC]_A/D_A}{[AUC]_B/D_B}$$

where

$F_{rel}$ is the relative bioavailability of treatment (formulation) A, expressed as a percentage;

$AUC_A$ is the AUC following administration of treatment (formulation) A; the value of $F_{rel}$ can be ±1 or ±100% since the test formulation may be more or less bioavailable compared to the reference formulation. A $F_{rel} = 1$ (100%) does not mean that the absolute bioavailability, $F_{rel}$ of the drug is 100%;

$D_A$ is the dose of formulation A;

$AUC_B$ is the AUC of formulation B; and

$D_B$ is the dose of formulation B.

Relative bioavailability studies are frequently included in regulatory submissions. For example, the FDA recommends that new drug developers routinely use an oral solution as the reference for a new oral formulation, for the purpose of assessing how formulation impacts bioavailability. Other types of relative bioavailability studies used in drug development include studies to characterize food effects and drug–drug interactions. In a *food-effect* bioavailability study, oral bioavailability of the drug product given with food (usually a high-fat, high-calorie meal) is compared to oral bioavailability of the drug product given under fasting conditions. The drug product given under fasting conditions is treated as the reference treatment. The goal of a *drug–drug interaction* study is to determine whether there is an increase, decrease, or no change in bioavailability in the presence of the interacting drug. As such, the general drug–drug interaction study design compares drug relative bioavailability with and without (reference treatment) the interacting drug. Relative bioavailability studies are used in developing new formulations of existing immediate-release drug products, such as new modified release, MR versions or new fixed-dose combination formulations. In the case of a new MR version, the reference product is the approved immediate-release product. In the case of a new fixed-dose combination, the reference product can be the single-entity drug products administered either separately (ie, three treatments for a fixed-dose combination doublet) or concurrently according to an approved combination regimen (ie, two treatments). Relative bioavailability study designs are also commonly used for bridging formulations during drug development, for example, to evaluate how drug systemic availability from a new premarket formulation compares with that from an existing premarket formulation.

## PRACTICE PROBLEM

The bioavailability of a new investigational drug was studied in 12 volunteers. Each volunteer received either a single oral tablet containing 200 mg of the drug, 5 mL of an aqueous solution containing 200 mg of the drug to be given orally, or a single IV bolus injection containing 50 mg of the drug. Plasma samples were obtained periodically up to 48 hours after the dose and assayed for drug concentration. The average AUC values (0–48 hours) are given in the table below. From these data, calculate (a) the relative bioavailability of the drug from the tablet compared to the oral solution and (b) the absolute bioavailability of the drug from the tablet.

| Drug Product | Dose (mg) | AUC (µg·h/mL) | Standard Deviation |
|---|---|---|---|
| Oral tablet | 200 | 89.5 | 19.7 |
| Oral solution | 200 | 86.1 | 18.1 |
| IV bolus injection | 50 | 37.8 | 5.7 |

### Solution

The relative bioavailability of the drug from the tablet compared to the oral solution is estimated by the equation below. No adjustment for the dose is necessary since the nominal doses are the same.

$$\text{Relative bioavailability} = \frac{89.5}{86.1} = 1.04 \quad \text{or} \quad 104\%$$

The relative bioavailability of the drug from the tablet is 1.04, or 104%, compared to the solution. In this study, the difference in drug bioavailability between tablet and solution would need to be analyzed statistically to determine whether the difference in drug bioavailability is statistically significant. It is possible for relative bioavailability to be greater than 100%. In this case, the tablet formulation may have some property or excipient that increases bioavailability.

The absolute drug bioavailability from the tablet is calculated and adjusted for the dose.

$$F = \text{absolute bioavailiability} = \frac{89.5 / 200}{37.5 / 50}$$

$$= 0.592 \quad \text{or} \quad 59.2\%$$

Because $F$, the fraction of dose absorbed from the tablet, is less than 1, the drug from the oral tablet is not completely absorbed systemically, as a result of either poor oral absorption of the drug itself, formulation effects that reduce oral bioavailability, or metabolism by first-pass effect (presystemic elimination). The relative bioavailability of the drug from the tablet is approximately 100% when compared to the oral solution.

The comparison between oral solution (little to no formulation effect) and IV administration gives information on the absorption of the drug itself when formulation effects are virtually nonexistent. With this knowledge, one can interpret the absolute bioavailability from the tablet and know if there is an effect of that formulation to change bioavailability or relative bioavailability is the same whether the tablet formulation was not even there.

Results from bioequivalence studies may show that the relative bioavailability of the test oral product is greater than, equal to, or less than 100% compared to the reference oral drug product. However, the results from these bioequivalence studies should not be misinterpreted to imply that the absolute bioavailability of the drug from the oral drug products is also 100% unless the oral formulation was compared to an intravenous injection (completely bioavailable) of the drug.

## METHODS FOR ASSESSING BIOAVAILABILITY AND BIOEQUIVALENCE

Direct and indirect methods may be used to assess drug bioavailability. The FDA's regulations (US-FDA, CDER, 2014a) list the following approaches to determining bioequivalence, in descending order of accuracy, sensitivity, and reproducibility:

- *In vivo* measurement of active moiety or moieties in biological fluid (ie, a pharmacokinetic study)
- *In vivo* pharmacodynamic (PD) comparison
- *In vivo* limited clinical comparison
- *In vitro* comparison
- Any other approach deemed acceptable (by the FDA)

For drug products that are not intended to be absorbed into the bloodstream, bioavailability may be assessed by measurements intended to reflect the rate and extent to which the active ingredient or active moiety becomes available at the site of action. The design of the bioavailability study depends on the objectives of the study, the ability to analyze the drug (and metabolites) in biological fluids, the pharmacodynamics of the drug substance, the route of drug administration, and the nature of the drug product. For all systemically active drugs, with a few exceptions, bioequivalence should be demonstrated by an *in vivo* study based on pharmacokinetic (PK) endpoints, as this is the most sensitive, accurate, and reproducible approach. The other approaches— pharmacodynamic, PD, clinical, or *in vitro*—may be more appropriate for locally acting drugs that are not systemically absorbed, such as those administered topically or those that act locally within the gastrointestinal (GI) tract. These latter bioequivalence approaches are considered on a case-by-case basis (Table 8-1). Detailed examples to illustrate when PD, clinical, or *in vitro* approaches are most suitable for establishing bioequivalence are presented below.

**TABLE 8-1 •** Methods for Assessing Bioavailability and Bioequivalence

*In vivo* **measurement of active moiety or moieties in biological fluids**

**Plasma drug concentration**
  Time for peak plasma (blood) concentration ($t_{max}$)
  Peak plasma drug concentration ($C_{max}$)
  Area under the plasma drug concentration–time curve (AUC)

**Urinary drug excretion**
  Cumulative amount of drug excreted in the urine ($D_u$)
  Rate of drug excretion in the urine ($dD_u/dt$)
  Time for maximum urinary excretion ($t$)

*In vivo* **pharmacodynamic (PD) comparison**
  Maximum pharmacodynamic effect ($E_{max}$)
  Time for maximum pharmacodynamic effect
  Area under the pharmacodynamic effect–time curve
  Onset time for pharmacodynamic effect

**Clinical endpoint study**
  Limited, comparative, parallel clinical study using predetermined clinical endpoint(s) and performed in patients

*In vitro* **studies**
  Comparative drug dissolution, $f_2$ similarity factor
  *In vitro* binding studies
  Examples: Cholestyramine resin—*In vitro* equilibrium and kinetic binding studies

**Any other approach deemed acceptable (by the FDA)**

## *IN VIVO* MEASUREMENT OF ACTIVE MOIETY OR MOIETIES IN BIOLOGICAL FLUIDS

### Plasma Drug Concentration

Measurement of drug concentrations in blood, plasma, or serum after drug administration is the most direct and objective way to determine systemic drug bioavailability. By appropriate blood sampling, an accurate description of the plasma drug concentration–time profile of the therapeutically active drug substance(s) can be obtained using a validated drug assay.

$t_{max}$: The *time of peak plasma concentration*, $t_{max}$, corresponds to the time required to reach maximum drug concentration after drug administration. At $t_{max}$, peak drug absorption occurs and the rate of drug absorption exactly equals the rate of drug elimination (Fig. 8-3). Drug absorption still continues after $t_{max}$ is reached, but at a slower rate. When comparing drug products, $t_{max}$ can be used as an approximate indication of drug absorption rate. The value for $t_{max}$ will become smaller (indicating less time required to reach peak plasma concentration) as the absorption rate for the drug becomes more rapid. Units for $t_{max}$ are units of time (eg, hours, minutes). For many systemically absorbed drugs, small differences in $t_{max}$ may have a little clinical effect on overall drug product performance. However, for some drugs, such as delayed action drug products, large differences in $t_{max}$ may have clinical impact.

$C_{max}$: The *peak plasma drug concentration*, $C_{max}$, represents the maximum plasma drug concentration obtained after oral administration of drug. For many drugs, a relationship is found between the pharmacodynamic drug effect and the plasma drug concentration. $C_{max}$ provides indications that the drug is sufficiently systemically absorbed to provide a therapeutic response. In addition, $C_{max}$ provides warning of possibly toxic levels of drug. The units of $C_{max}$ are concentration units (eg, mg/mL, ng/mL). Although not a unit for rate, $C_{max}$ is often used in bioequivalence studies as a surrogate measure for the rate of drug bioavailability. The expectation is that as the rate of drug absorption goes up, the peak or $C_{max}$ will also be larger. If the rate of drug absorption goes down, then the peak or $C_{max}$ is smaller.

**AUC:** The *area under the plasma level–time curve*, AUC, is a measurement of the *extent* of drug bioavailability (see Fig. 8-3). The AUC reflects the total amount of active drug that reaches the systemic circulation. The AUC is the area under the drug plasma level–time curve from $t = 0$ to $t = \infty$, and is equal to the amount of unchanged drug reaching the general circulation divided by the clearance.

$$[AUC]_0^\infty = \int_0^\infty C_p \, dt \tag{8.1}$$

$$[AUC]_0^\infty = \frac{FD_0}{\text{clearance}} = \frac{FD_0}{kV_D} \tag{8.2}$$

where $F$ = fraction of dose absorbed, $D_0$ = dose, $k$ = elimination rate constant, and $V_D$ = volume of distribution. The AUC is independent of the route of administration and processes of drug elimination as long as the elimination processes do not change. The AUC can be determined by a numerical integration procedure, such as the trapezoidal rule method. The units for AUC are concentration × time (eg, $\mu$g·h/mL).

For many drugs, the AUC is directly proportional to dose. For example, if a single dose of a drug is increased from 250 to 1000 mg, the AUC will also show a 4-fold increase (Figs. 8-5 and 8-6).

In some cases, the AUC is not directly proportional to the administered dose for all dosage levels. For example, as the dosage of drug is increased, one of the pathways for drug elimination may become

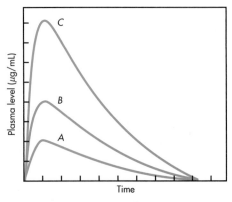

**FIGURE 8-5 •** Plasma level–time curve following administration of single doses of (*A*) 250 mg, (*B*) 500 mg, and (*C*) 1000 mg of drug.

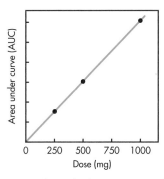

FIGURE 8-6 • Linear relationship between AUC and dose (data from Fig. 16-5).

saturated (Fig. 8-7). Drug elimination includes the processes of metabolism and excretion. Drug metabolism is an enzyme-dependent process. For drugs such as salicylate and phenytoin, continued increase of the dose causes saturation of one of the enzyme pathways for drug metabolism and consequent prolongation of the elimination half-life. The AUC thus increases disproportionally to the increase in dose, because a smaller amount of drug is being eliminated (ie, more drug is retained). When the AUC is not directly proportional to the dose, bioavailability of the drug is difficult to evaluate because drug kinetics may be dose dependent. Conversely, absorption may also become saturated resulting in lower-than-expected changes in AUC.

## Urinary Drug Excretion Data

Urinary drug excretion data is an indirect method for estimating bioavailability. The drug must be excreted in significant quantities as unchanged drug in the urine. In addition, timely urine samples must be collected and the total amount of urinary drug excretion must be obtained.

$D_u^\infty$: The *cumulative amount of drug excreted in the urine*, $D_u^\infty$, is related directly to the total amount of drug absorbed. Experimentally, urine samples are collected periodically after administration of a drug product. Each urine specimen is analyzed for free drug using a specific assay. A graph is constructed that relates the cumulative drug excreted to the collection-time interval (Fig. 8-8).

The relationship between the cumulative amount of drug excreted in the urine and the plasma level–time curve is shown in Fig. 8-8. When the drug is almost completely eliminated (point C), the plasma concentration approaches zero and the maximum amount of drug excreted in the urine, $D_u^\infty$, is obtained.

$dD_u/dt$: The *rate of drug excretion*. Because most drugs are eliminated by a first-order rate process, the rate of drug excretion is dependent on the first-order elimination rate constant, $k$, and the concentration of drug in the plasma, $C_p$. In Fig. 8-9, the *maximum rate of drug excretion*, $(dD_u/dt)_{max}$, is at point B, whereas the minimum rate of drug excretion is at points A and C. Thus, a graph comparing the rate of drug excretion with respect to time should be similar in shape to the plasma level–time curve for that drug (Fig. 8-10).

$t^\infty$: The *total time for the drug to be excreted*. In Figs. 8-9 and 8-10, the slope of the curve segment A–B is related to the rate of drug absorption, whereas point C is related to the total time required after

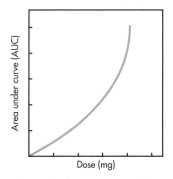

FIGURE 8-7 • Relationship between AUC and dose when metabolism (elimination) is saturable.

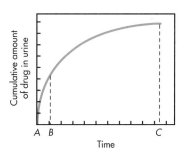

FIGURE 8-8 • Corresponding plots relating the plasma level–time curve and the cumulative urinary drug excretion.

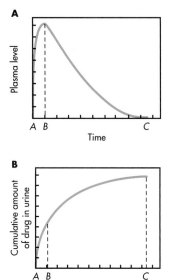

FIGURE 8-9 • Corresponding plots relating the plasma level–time curve and the cumulative urinary drug excretion.

## BIOEQUIVALENCE STUDIES BASED ON PHARMACODYNAMIC ENDPOINTS— *IN VIVO* PHARMACODYNAMIC COMPARISON

In some cases, the quantitative measurement of a drug in plasma is not available or *in vitro* approaches are not applicable. The following criteria for a PD endpoint study are important:

- A dose–response relationship is demonstrated.
- The PD effect of the selected dose should be at the rising phase of the dose–response curve, as shown in Fig. 8-11.
- Sufficient measurements should be taken to assure an appropriate PD response profile.
- All PD measurement assays should be validated for specificity, accuracy, sensitivity, and precision.

For locally acting, nonsystemically absorbed drug products, such as topical corticosteroids,

drug administration for the drug to be absorbed and completely excreted, $t = \infty$. The $t^\infty$ is a useful parameter in bioequivalence studies that compare several drug products.

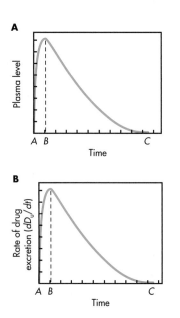

FIGURE 8-10 • Corresponding plots relating the plasma level–time curve and the rate of urinary drug excretion.

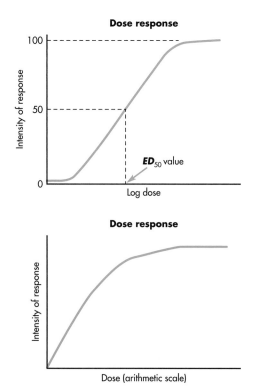

FIGURE 8-11 • Dose–response curves. Dose–response curves for dose versus response graphed on a log or arithmetic scale.

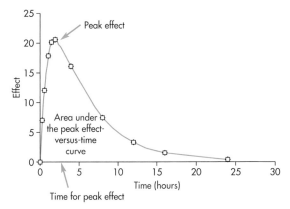

FIGURE 8-12 • Acute pharmacodynamic effect–time curve. It shows an acute pharmacologic effect that is measured periodically after a single oral dose. The effect curve is similar to Fig. 16-3.

plasma drug concentrations may not reflect the bioavailability of the drug at the site of action. An acute pharmacodynamic effect,[5] such as an effect on forced expiratory volume, $FEV_1$ (inhaled bronchodilators), or skin blanching (topical corticosteroids), can be used as an index of drug bioavailability. In this case, the acute pharmacodynamic effect is measured over a period of time after administration of the drug product. Measurements of the pharmacodynamic effect should be made with sufficient frequency to permit a reasonable estimate for a time period at least three times the half-life of the drug (Gardner, 1977). This approach may be particularly applicable to dosage forms that are not intended to deliver the active moiety to the bloodstream for systemic distribution (Zou and Yu, 2014).

The use of an acute pharmacodynamic effect to determine bioavailability generally requires demonstration of a dose–response curve (Fig. 8-11 and Chapter 22). Bioavailability is determined by characterization of the dose–response curve. For bioequivalence determination, pharmacodynamic parameters including the total area under the acute pharmacodynamic effect–time curve, peak pharmacodynamic effect, and time for peak pharmacodynamic effect are obtained from the pharmacodynamic effect–time curve (Fig. 8-12). The onset

time and duration of the pharmacokinetic effect may also be included in the analysis of the data. The use of pharmacodynamic endpoints for the determination of bioavailability and bioequivalence is much more variable than the measurement of plasma or urine drug concentrations. Some examples of drug products for which bioequivalence PD endpoints are recommended are listed in Table 8-2.

## BIOEQUIVALENCE STUDIES BASED ON CLINICAL ENDPOINTS—CLINICAL ENDPOINT STUDY

The clinical endpoint study is the most variable and least sensitive to bioavailability differences. A predetermined clinical endpoint is used to evaluate comparative clinical effect in a chosen patient population. Highly variable clinical responses require the use of a large number of patient study subjects, which increases study costs and requires a longer time to complete compared to the other approaches for determination of bioequivalence. A placebo arm is usually included to demonstrate that the study is sufficiently sensitive to identify the clinical effect in the patient population enrolled in the study. The FDA considers this approach only when analytical methods and pharmacodynamic methods are not available to permit use of one of the approaches described above. The clinical study is usually a limited, comparative, parallel clinical study using predetermined clinical endpoint(s).

Clinical endpoint bioequivalence studies are recommended for those products that have negligible systemic drug exposure, for which there is no identified PD measure, and for which the site of action is local. Comparative clinical studies have been used to establish bioequivalence for topical antifungal drug products (eg, ketoconazole) and for topical acne preparations. For dosage forms intended to deliver the active moiety to the bloodstream for systemic distribution, this approach may be considered acceptable only when analytical methods cannot be developed to permit use of one of the other approaches. Some examples of drug products where a clinical endpoint bioequivalence study is recommended (Davit and Conner, 2015) are listed in Table 8-3.

---

[5] A pharmacodynamic endpoint is an acute pharmacologic effect that is directly related to the drug's activity that can be measured quantitatively.

## TABLE 8-2 • Examples of Drug Products for Which FDA Recommends That Bioequivalence Studies Use Pharmacodynamic Endpoints

| Drug Product | Indication | Mechanism of Action | Endpoint |
|---|---|---|---|
| Acarbose tablet (if no Q1/Q2 sameness between test and reference) | Treatment of type 2 diabetes | Inhibition of intestinal $a$-glucosidase, thereby decreasing absorption of starch and oligosaccharides | Reduction in blood glucose concentrations |
| Lanthanum carbonate tablet | Reduction of serum phosphate levels in patients with end-stage renal disease | Inhibits phosphate absorption by forming highly insoluble lanthanum phosphate complexes in GI tract | Reduction in urinary phosphate excretion |
| Orlistat capsules | Treatment of obesity | Inhibition of intestinal lipase, thereby reducing absorption of free fatty acids and monoacylglycerols | Amount of fat excreted in feces over 24 hours at steady state |
| Fluticasone propionate cream | Relief of skin itching and inflammation | The application of corticosteroids causes blanching in the microvasculature of the skin (not the mechanism of action, but quantitatively measurable) | Skin chromameter measurements through at least 24 hours after application |
| Albuterol sulfate metered dose inhaler | Relaxes smooth muscle of airways, thus protecting against bronchoconstrictor challenges | A beta$_2$-adrenergic agonist | • Either a bronchoprovocation or bronchodilatation assay is suitable<br>• For bronchoprovocation, measure the concentration or dose of methacholine required to decrease $FEV_1$ by 20%<br>• For bronchodilatation, measure the $AUEC_{0-4h}$, $AUEC_{0-6h}$, and maximum $FEV_1$ through 6 hours post-dose |
| Fluticasone propionate/salmeterol xinafoate inhalation power | Treatment of asthma and chronic obstructive pulmonary disease (COPD) | • Fluticasone is an anti-inflammatory corticosteroid<br>• Salmeterol is a beta$_2$-adreneric agonist | Measure area under the $FEV_1$-time curve at designated intervals on first day and last day of 4-week daily treatment period |
| Low-molecular-weight heparins for IV administration | Anticoagulant | Inactivation of Factor Xa and Factor IIa in coagulation cascade | • To assure pharmaceutical equivalence of two formulations, measure anti-Xa and anti-IIa activities<br>• Demonstration of *in vivo* bioequivalence is waived because product is a true solution |

*Adapted with permission from LX Yu, Li BV: FDA Bioequivalence Standards. New York, NY: Springer; 2014.*

## TABLE 8-3 • Examples of Drug Products for Which FDA Recommends Bioequivalence Studies with Clinical Endpoints

| Product | Study Patients | Study Duration | Endpoint(s) |
|---|---|---|---|
| Calcipotriene cream | Plaque psoriasis | 56 days | Proportions of subjects in the PP population with treatment success on PGA and clinical success of PASI |
| Imiquimod cream | Actinic keratosis | 14 weeks | Proportion of subjects in the PP population with treatment success (100% clearance of all AK lesions) |
| Ketoconazole shampoo | Dandruff | 28 days | Proportion of subjects with treatment success or cure, defined as a score of 0 or 1 on the Global Evaluation Scale (erythema rating) |
| Miconazole nitrate vaginal cream | Vulvovaginal candidiasis | 21–30 days | Proportion of patients with therapeutic cure, defined as both mycological and clinical cure, at the test-of-cure visit |
| Nitazoxanide tablets | Diarrhea caused by Giardia lamblia | 10 days | Proportion of patients with a "well" clinical response, defined as either (1) no symptoms, no watery stool, and no more than 2 soft stools with no hematochezia within the past 24 hours or (2) no symptoms and no unformed stools within the past 48 hours |
| Sucralfate tablets | Active duodenal ulcer disease; patients must be *Helicobacter pylori* negative or continue to have the presence of an ulcer after appropriate *H. pylori* treatment | 8 weeks | Proportion of patients with ulcer healing at week 8 by endoscopic examination; if more than one ulcer is observed at enrollment, both must demonstrate healing at week 8 for success ("cure") |

## *IN VITRO* STUDIES

Comparative drug release/dissolution studies under certain conditions may give an indication of drug bioavailability and bioequivalence. Ideally, the *in vitro* drug dissolution rate should correlate with *in vivo* drug bioavailability (see Chapter 7 on *in vivo–in vitro* correlation, IVIVC). The test and reference products for which *in vitro* release rates form the basis of the bioequivalence usually demonstrate Q1/Q2 sameness (qualitatively same inactive ingredients in the quantitative same amounts). Comparative dissolution studies are often performed on several test formulations of the same drug during drug development. Comparative dissolution profiles may be considered similar if the similarity factor ($f_2$) is greater than 50 (see Chapter 7). For drugs whose dissolution rate is related to the rate of systemic absorption, the test formulation that demonstrates the most rapid rate of drug dissolution *in vitro* will generally have the most rapid rate of drug bioavailability *in vivo*. Under certain conditions, comparative dissolution profiles of higher and lower dose strengths of a solid oral drug product such as an immediate-release tablet are used to obtain a waiver of performing additional *in vivo* bioequivalence studies (see section on biowaivers).

## OTHER APPROACHES DEEMED ACCEPTABLE (BY THE FDA)

The FDA may also use *in vitro* approaches other than comparative dissolution for establishing bioequivalence. The use of *in vitro* biomarkers and *in vitro* binding studies has been proposed to establish bioequivalence. For example, cholestyramine resin is a basic quaternary ammonium anion-exchange resin that is hydrophilic, insoluble in water, and not absorbed in the GI tract. The bioequivalence of cholestyramine resin is performed by equilibrium and kinetic binding studies of the resin to bile acid salts. For calcium acetate tablets, which exert the therapeutic response by binding phosphate in the GI tract, the FDA recommends a relatively simple *in vitro* binding assay based on the test/reference binding ratio over a range of phosphate concentrations. Since this test is thought to be highly reproducible, the bioequivalence acceptance criterion is that the test/reference binding ratio should fall within limits of 0.9–1.1. The FDA accepts various other *in vitro* approaches for bioequivalence assessment of proposed generic locally-acting drug products. For the acyclovir topical ointment, recommended bioequivalence approaches consist of comparative *in vitro* release testing and physicochemical characterization.

## BIOEQUIVALENCE STUDIES BASED ON MULTIPLE ENDPOINTS

The FDA may recommend two or more bioequivalence studies, each based on a different approach, for some drug products with complex delivery systems or mechanisms of action. Some examples of drug products that the FDA requires multiple bioequivalence studies (Davit and Conner, 2015) are listed in Table 8-4.

## BIOEQUIVALENCE STUDIES

Differences in the predicted clinical response or an adverse event may be due to differences in the pharmacokinetic and/or pharmacodynamic behavior of the drug among individuals or to differences in the bioavailability of the drug from the drug product. Bioequivalent drug products that have the same systemic drug bioavailability will have the same predictable drug response. However, variable clinical responses among individuals that are unrelated to bioavailability may also be due to differences in the pharmacodynamics of the drug. Differences in pharmacodynamics may be due to individual differences in receptor sensitivity to the drug (see Chapter 21). Various factors affecting pharmacodynamic drug behavior may include age, drug tolerance, drug interactions, and unknown pathophysiologic factors.

### Bases for Determining Bioequivalence

Bioequivalence is established if the *in vivo* bioavailability of a test drug product (usually the generic product) does not differ significantly (ie, statistically not significant) from that of the *reference listed drug* (usually the brand-name product approved through the NDA route) in the product's rate and extent of drug absorption. Bioequivalence is determined by comparison of measured parameters (eg, concentration of the active drug ingredient in the blood, urinary excretion rates, or pharmacodynamic effects), when administered at the same molar dose of the active moiety under similar experimental conditions, either single dose or multiple doses.

In a few cases, a drug product that differs from the RLD in its rate of absorption, but not in its extent of absorption, may be considered bioequivalent if the difference in the rate of absorption is intentional and appropriately reflected in the labeling and/or the rate of absorption is not detrimental to the safety and effectiveness of the drug product.

## DESIGN AND EVALUATION OF BIOEQUIVALENCE STUDIES

### Objective

All scientific studies should have clearly stated objectives. The main objective for a bioequivalence study is that the drug bioavailability from test and reference products is not statistically different when administered to patients or subjects at the same molar dose from pharmaceutically equivalent drug products through the same route of administration under similar experimental conditions.

## TABLE 8-4 • Drug Products for Which FDA Recommends Multiple Bioequivalence Approaches

| Product | Indicated to Treat | Approach | Endpoint |
|---|---|---|---|
| Diclofenac gel | Osteoarthritis of the knee | Clinical | Pain score change from baseline |
| | | *In vivo* PK | AUC, $C_{max}$ |
| Nitazoxanide oral | Diarrhea caused by *Giardia lamblia* | Clinical | Proportion of patients with a "well" clinical response |
| | | *In vivo* PK | AUC, $C_{max}$ |
| Fluticasone propionate nasal suspension | Allergic rhinitis | Clinical | Total nasal symptom score (TNSS) change from baseline |
| | | *In vivo* PK | AUC, $C_{max}$ |
| | | *In vitro* | Comparison of device performance with regard to the amount of drug per actuation, droplet size distribution, and plume shape |
| Mesalamine DR and ER oral formulations | Ulcerative colitis | *In vivo* PK | AUC, pAUC, $C_{max}$ |
| | | *In vitro* | Comparison of dissolution profiles in several different media of varying pH values |
| Mesalamine rectal enema | Distal ulcerative colitis, proctitis, and proctosigmoiditis | *In vivo* PK | AUC, $C_{max}$ |
| | | *In vitro* | Dissolution profiles at pH 4.5, 6.8, 7.2 (Apparatus 2), 900 mL, 35, 50 rpm |
| Mesalamine suppository | Ulcerative proctitis | *In vivo* PK | AUC, $C_{max}$ |
| | | *In vitro* | Comparison of physicochemical properties |
| Risperidone long-acting injectable | Bipolar I disorder and schizophrenia | Steady-state PK in patients | $AUC_t$, $(C_{max})_{SS}$ |
| | | *In vitro* | Comparison of the time for 50% of drug to be released at two bracketing sampling times |
| Lansoprazole DR capsule | Gastroesophageal reflux disease | *In vivo* PK | AUC, $C_{max}$ |
| | | *In vitro* | Comparison of sedimentation volume, granule dispersion, recovery, and acid resistance, after dispersing into apple juice and dispensing into nasogastric tubes |
| Dexamethasone/ Tobramycin Ophthalmic Suspension | Prophylaxis against inflammation and infection during cataract surgery | *In vivo* PK | AUC, $C_{max}$, in aqueous humor of cataract surgery patients |
| | | *In vitro* | Microbial kill rates against specified microorganisms |

## Study Considerations

The basic design for a bioequivalence study is determined by (1) the scientific questions and objectives to be answered, (2) the nature of the reference material and the dosage form to be tested, (3) the availability of analytical methods, (4) the pharmacokinetics and pharmacodynamics of the drug substance, (5) the route of drug administration, and (6) benefit–risk and ethical considerations with regard to testing in humans.

Since bioequivalence studies are performed to compare the bioavailability of the test or generic drug product to the reference or brand-name product, the statistical techniques should be of sufficient sensitivity to detect differences in rate and extent of absorption that are not attributable to subject variability. Once bioequivalence is established, it is likely that both the generic and brand-name dosage forms will produce the same therapeutic effect. The FDA publishes guidances for bioequivalence studies. Sponsors may also request a meeting with the FDA to review the study design for a specific drug product. As discussed, pharmacokinetic parameters, pharmacodynamic parameters, clinical observations, and/or *in vitro* studies may be used to determine drug bioavailability from a drug product.

The design and evaluation of well-controlled bioequivalence studies require cooperative input from pharmacokineticists, statisticians, clinicians, bioanalytical chemists, and others. For some generic drugs, the FDA offers general guidelines for conducting these studies. For example, *Statistical Procedures for Bioequivalence Studies Using a Standard Two-Treatment Crossover Design* is available from the FDA (US-FDA, CDER, 2000a); the publication addresses three specific aspects, including (1) logarithmic transformation of pharmacokinetic data, (2) sequence effect, and (3) outlier consideration. However, even with the availability of such guidelines, the principal investigator should prepare a detailed protocol for the study. Some of the elements of a protocol for an *in vivo* bioavailability study are listed in Table 8-5.

For bioequivalence studies, the test and reference drug formulations must contain the same drug in the same dose strength and in similar dosage forms (eg, immediate release or controlled release), and must be given by the same route of administration. Before

## TABLE 8-5 • Elements of a Bioavailability Study Protocol

I. Title
  A. Principal investigator (study director)
  B. Project/protocol number and date
II. Study objective
III. Study design
  A. Design
  B. Drug products
    1. Test product(s)
    2. Reference product
  C. Dosage regimen
  D. Sample collection schedule
  E. Housing/confinement
  F. Fasting/meals schedule
  G. Analytical methods
IV. Study population
  A. Subjects
  B. Subject selection
    1. Medical history
    2. Physical examination
    3. Laboratory tests
  C. Inclusion/exclusion criteria
    1. Inclusion criteria
    2. Exclusion criteria
  D. Restrictions/prohibitions
V. Clinical procedures
  A. Dosage and drug administration
  B. Biological sampling schedule and handling procedures
  C. Activity of subjects
VI. Ethical considerations
  A. Basic principles
  B. Institutional review board
  C. Informed consent
  D. Indications for subject withdrawal
  E. Adverse reactions and emergency procedures
VII. Facilities
VIII. Data analysis
  A. Analytical validation procedure
  B. Statistical treatment of data
IX. Drug accountability
X. Appendix

beginning the study, the *Institutional Review Board* (IRB) of the clinical facility in which the study is to be performed must approve the study. The IRB is composed of both professional and laypersons with diverse backgrounds who have clinical experience and expertise as well as sensitivity to ethical issues and community attitudes. The IRB is responsible for all ethical issues including safeguarding the rights and welfare of human subjects.

The basic guiding principle in performing studies is *do not do unnecessary human research*. Generally, the study is performed in normal, healthy male and female volunteers who have given informed consent to be in the study. Critically ill patients are not included in an *in vivo* bioavailability study unless the attending physician determines that there is a potential benefit to the patient. The number of subjects in the study will depend on the expected intersubject and intrasubject variability. Patient selection is made according to certain established criteria for inclusion in, or exclusion from, the study. For example, the study might exclude any volunteers who have known allergies to the drug, are overweight, or have taken any medication within a specified period (often 1 week) prior to the study. Moderate smokers may be included in these studies. The subjects generally fast for 10–12 hours (overnight) prior to drug administration and may continue to fast for a 2- to 4-hour period after dosing.

### Reference Listed Drug

For bioequivalence studies of generic products, one formulation of the drug is chosen as a reference standard against which all other formulations of the drug are compared. The FDA designates a single RLD[6] as the standard drug product to which all generic versions must be shown to be bioequivalent. The FDA hopes to avoid possible significant variations among generic drugs and their brand-name counterparts. Such variations could result if generic drugs were compared to different RLDs.

The reference drug product should be administered by the same route as the comparison formulations unless an alternative route or additional route is needed to answer specific pharmacokinetic questions. For example, if an active drug is poorly bioavailable after oral administration, the drug may be compared to an oral solution or an intravenous injection. For bioequivalence studies on a proposed generic drug product, the reference standard is the RLD, which is listed in the FDA's *Approved Drug Products with Therapeutic Equivalence Evaluations*—the Orange Book (US-FDA, CDER, 2014d), and the proposed generic drug product is often referred to as the "test" drug product. The RLD is generally a formulation currently marketed with a fully approved NDA for which there are valid scientific safety and efficacy data. The RLD is usually the innovator's or original manufacturer's brand-name product and is administered according to the dosage recommendations in the labeling.

Before beginning an *in vivo* bioequivalence study, the total content of the active drug substance in the test product (generally the generic product) must be within 5% of that of the reference product. Moreover, *in vitro* comparative dissolution or drug-release studies under various specified conditions are usually performed for both test and reference products before performing the *in vivo* bioequivalence study.

### Regulatory Recommendations for Optimizing Bioavailability Study Design

The FDA lists a number of recommendations to consider in designing clinical relative bioavailability studies in drug development. These recommendations include the following:

- Use of a randomized crossover design whenever possible
- Enrolling both male and female subjects whenever possible
- Administering single doses rather than multiple doses, as single-dose studies are more sensitive to changes in bioavailability, although multiple-dose studies may be more suitable in some cases
- Conducting the studies under fasting and fed conditions[7]

---

[6]The reference listed drug (RLD) is listed in the Orange Book, Approved Drug Products with Therapeutic Equivalence Evaluations. http://www.accessdata.fda.gov/scripts/cder/ob/default.cfm.

[7]In a food-effect bioavailability study, the reference treatment is the oral formulation of the drug product given on an empty stomach, which is compared with the same oral formulation given with food, usually a high-fat, high-calorie meal.

- Measuring the parent drug rather than metabolites, unless the parent cannot be reliably measured. Presystemically formed metabolites (first pass effect) that contribute meaningfully to safety and efficacy should also be measured

In addition, the FDA recommends that $C_{max}$ and $t_{max}$ be measured to compare peak exposure and rate of absorption, and that $AUC_{0-t}$ (AUC to the last measurable drug concentration) and $AUC_{0-\infty}$ (AUC extrapolated to infinity) be measured to compare total exposure or extent of drug absorption. Drug exposure parameters should be log-transformed before statistical comparisons. Further detail about the statistical tests is discussed in Chapter 3 and is provided later in the discussion on bioequivalence study designs.

## Product-Specific Guidances for Generic Drug Development

FDA has published Product-Specific Guidances for Generic Drug Development to assist the generic pharmaceutical industry with identifying the most appropriate methodology for developing drugs and generating evidence needed to support Abbreviated New Drug Applications (ANDA) approval. FDA publishes product-specific guidances describing the Agency's current thinking and expectations on how to develop generic drug products therapeutically equivalent to specific RLDs (https://www.accessdata.fda.gov/scripts/cder/psg/index.cfm).

### FREQUENTLY ASKED QUESTIONS

▶ What are the study protocol considerations for conducting a bioequivalence study?

▶ What is the reference listed drug (RLD), and how is the RLD selected?

▶ How is a bioavailability study of a new molecular entity conducted?

▶ Why does the value for relative bioavailability sometimes exceed 1.0, whereas the value for absolute bioavailability cannot exceed 1.0[7]?

## Factors Influencing Bioavailability and Impact on Drug Development

Various factors influence bioavailability (Table 8-6). Some of these factors are listed below with implications for formulation development and optimization of dosing regimens.

*Physicochemical properties of the drug and formulation.* Formulations can be designed to improve the bioavailability of poorly soluble drugs, extend the absorption phase by slowing the rate of release of drugs (controlled-release formulations), or prevent dissolution in the gastric lumen for drugs that are destroyed by gastric acidity (enteric-coated formulations) (see also Chapter 7).

An example of how formulation design can improve bioavailability is shown by comparing the immunosuppressant drug cyclosporine systemic exposures provided by the Neoral® microemulsion formulation to the Sandimmune® formulation. The Neoral label states that, in a relative bioavailability study in renal transplant, rheumatoid arthritis, and psoriasis patients, the mean cyclosporine AUC was 20%–50% greater, and the mean cyclosporine $C_{max}$ was 40%–106% greater, compared to following administration with Sandimmune. In addition, the dose-normalized AUC in liver transplant patients administered Neoral for 28 days was 50% greater and $C_{max}$ was 90% greater than in those patients administered Sandimmune.

*Drug stability and pH effects.* Acid-labile drugs may have low oral bioavailability, due to acid-induced degradation in the low pH conditions of the stomach. To improve bioavailability, the drug may be formulated as a buffered product or enteric-coated products. Enteric-coated formulations protect acid-labile drugs in the stomach. Examples are didanosine (Damle et al, 2002), a purine nucleoside analog to treat HIV disease, and omeprazole and lansoprazole (Horn and Howden, 2005), which are proton pump inhibitors to treat acid reflux.

*Presystemic and first-pass metabolism.* The effects of presystemic metabolism on oral bioavailability is (Jagdale et al, 2009) illustrated by propranolol, a nonselective beta-adrenergic receptor blocking agent used as an antihypertensive, antianginal, and anti-arrhythmic, presystemic metabolism. Propranolol is almost completely absorbed after oral

---

[7]$F$ will appear to exceed 1.0, if the absolute bioavailability is near 100% and variability yields a result slightly higher than 1.0.

## TABLE 8-6 • Factors Influencing Bioavailability and Impacting Drug Development

- Physicochemical properties of the drug and formulation
  - The active drug ingredient has low solubility in water (eg, less than 5 mg/mL)
  - The dissolution rate of the product is slow (eg, <50% in 30 min when tested with a general method specified by the FDA)
  - The particle size and surface area of the active drug ingredient is critical in determining its bioavailability
  - Certain structural forms of the active drug ingredient (eg, polymorphic forms, solvates, complexes, and crystal modifications) dissolve poorly, thus affecting bioavailability
- Drug product
  - Drug products that have a high ratio of excipients to active ingredients (eg, >5:1)
  - Specific inactive ingredients (eg, hydrophilic or hydrophobic excipients and lubricants) either may be required for absorption of the active drug or may interfere with such absorption
- Drug stability
  - The drug (and drug product) has poor stability leading to short shelf life
  - The active drug ingredient or therapeutic moiety is unstable in specific portions of the GI tract and requires special coatings or formulations (eg, buffers, enteric coatings, etc) to ensure adequate absorption
- pH effects (eg, pH within the gastrointestinal lumen)
- Surface of dosage form and time available for absorption
- Presystemic metabolism, including hepatic first-pass effect
- Food effects, for orally administered formulations
- The active drug ingredient or its precursor is absorbed mostly in a particular segment of the GI tract or is absorbed from a localized site
- Drug–drug interactions
- Efflux transporters (such as P-glycoprotein)
- The drug product is subject to dose-dependent kinetics in or near the therapeutic range, and the rate and extent of absorption are important in establishing bioequivalence
- Age
- Disease state

administration, but due to extensive first-pass metabolism in the liver, only about 25% of the parent drug reaches the systemic circulation (see Chapter 21).

*A prodrug* is a chemically modified drug usually an inactive form to improve solubility, increase chemical stability, or increase bioavailability of the active drug by decreasing first-pass metabolism. After oral administration, the inactive prodrug is converted to the active drug generally by biotransformation or hydrolysis. For example, valacyclovir, a prodrug of the nucleoside analog antiviral compound acyclovir, undergoes rapid presystemic conversion to acyclovir. Both valacyclovir and acyclovir are effective in treating herpes infections. Acyclovir bioavailability is greatly enhanced when delivered as a prodrug valacyclovir, for treating herpes zoster, Valtrex˚ (valacyclovir) tablets are administered once

daily, compared to 5 times daily for Zovirax˚ (acyclovir) capsules.

*Food effects.* Food can either decrease drug bioavailability or increase bioavailability, or have no effect on bioavailability (Davit and Conner, 2008; Dehaven and Conner, 2014). Food can influence bioavailability in a number of ways, such as affecting GI pH, gastric emptying, intestinal transit, splanchnic blood flow, and first-pass metabolism. Food can also affect bioavailability by physical or chemical interactions that may affect the release mechanism of MR drug products. Most food effects on drug bioavailability are not clinically significant, and, consequentially, most drug products are labeled to be administered without regard to meals. If the food effects on drug bioavailability are clinically significant, then the drug product labeling will provide instructions about how to achieve the optimal dosing regimen—either to take the drug only on an empty stomach, or only with food, depending on the nature of the bioavailability effect and clinical consequences.

The bioavailability of didanosine is reduced by food, and this food effect is included in the approved labeling. Food prolongs gastric emptying, increasing the length of time that the acid-labile didanosine will be in contact with a low pH environment. The Videx® EC label states that food reduced the didanosine $C_{max}$ by 46% and its AUC by 19%. Consequently, the Videx EC label recommends that didanosine should be taken on an empty stomach in order to avoid the possibility of exposing a patient to subtherapeutic plasma levels if the product is taken with food.

Food-induced increase in drug bioavailability can be either desirable or undesirable. Food increases the bioavailability of isotretinoin (Accutane®) indicated to treat severe recalcitrant nodular acne. The Accutane label states that for isotretinoin capsules, both the $C_{max}$ and AUC were more than doubled when the drug product was taken with a meal compared with fasted conditions. Consequently, the label recommends that isotretinoin capsules should always be taken with food. By contrast, food-induced increases in oral bioavailability may be associated with safety concerns. This situation is illustrated by the drug efavirenz, a non-nucleoside reverse transcriptase inhibitor indicated to treat HIV disease. The Sustiva® label describes how coadministration of a high-fat, high-calorie meal increased the efavirenz AUC and $C_{max}$ by 22% and 39%, respectively, and coadministration of a lower-fat, lower-calorie meal increased the efavirenz AUC and $C_{max}$ by 17% and 51%, respectively. Due to concern that exposure to higher efavirenz systemic bioavailability could result in increased serious adverse events, the Sustiva label recommends that efavirenz capsules and tablets be taken on an empty stomach, preferably at bedtime.

*Effects of drug–drug interactions.* Changes in drug bioavailability due to drug–drug interactions can occur via a variety of mechanisms, such as inhibition of metabolizing enzymes, induction of metabolizing enzymes, inhibitor of transporters, and induction of transporters. The FDA recommends that interactions between an investigational new drug and other drugs be defined during drug development (US-FDA, CDER, 2012c). Two examples of drug–drug interactions, one of enzyme inhibition and the second of enzyme induction, will show how the ability of coadministered drugs to alter systemic bioavailability impacts both recommendations for optimal dosing regimens and development of new formulations to maximize bioavailability.

An example of a drug–drug interaction that increases bioavailability is provided by ritonavir (an HIV protease inhibitor indicated for treating HIV disease), which is a potent inhibitor of cytochrome P450 3A (CYP3A). As such, ritonavir coadministration increases systemic bioavailability of drugs that are metabolized by CYP3A. For drugs such as sedative hypnotics, antiarrhythmic, and ergot alkaloid preparations, large increases in systemic bioavailability caused by ritonavir coadministration can result in potentially serious and/or life-threatening adverse events; thus, ritonavir coadministration with these drugs is contraindicated. For other coadministered CYP3A substrate drugs for which ritonavir increases bioavailability, such as antidepressants, clarithromycin, immunomodulators, rifabutin, and trazodone, the Norvir® labeling recommends either dose adjustment or additional monitoring of the coadministered drug to maintain systemic bioavailability levels associated with safety and efficacy.

Because ritonavir can significantly increase the bioavailability of CYP3A substrates, it has been developed as a "booster" to improve systemic exposure of HIV therapies that are CYP3A substrates and that have low oral bioavailability due to extensive hepatic clearance (de Mendoza et al, 2006). Notably, ritonavir is formulated together with the HIV-1 protease inhibitor lopinavir in the fixed-dose combination product Kaletra®. Ritonavir in the Kaletra formulation inhibits the CYP3A-mediated metabolism of lopinavir, thereby increasing lopinavir systemic bioavailability to levels that achieve antiviral activity.

Enzyme inducers coadministered with drugs can potentially lower systemic bioavailability to subtherapeutic levels. An example is the antibacterial drug rifampin (used in treatment of tuberculosis), which is a potent inducer of cytochrome P-450 enzymes. Coadministration of rifampin with drugs metabolized by metabolic pathways induced by rifampin can result in lower bioavailability due to acceleration of metabolism. The Rifadin® label states that to maintain optimum therapeutic bioavailability, dosages of drugs metabolized by these enzymes may require dose adjustment when starting or stopping concomitantly administered rifampin. Some examples of these drugs for which rifampin lowers systemic bioavailability to the extent that dose adjustment is needed include anticonvulsants, antiarrhythmics, beta-blockers, calcium channel blockers, fluoroquinolones, oral hypoglycemic agents, transplant drugs, and tricyclic antidepressants. For some drugs, such as oral contraceptives, coadministration with rifampin is contraindicated due to concerns that rifampin coadministration can lower oral contraceptive systemic bioavailability to subtherapeutic levels.

*Efflux transporters.* The cardiac glycoside digoxin is a substrate for P-glycoprotein, at the level of intestinal absorption, renal tubular secretion, and biliary-intestinal secretion (Hughes and Crowe, 2010). Drugs that induce or inhibit P-glycoprotein have the potential to alter digoxin bioavailability. Examples of such drugs include amiodarone, propafenone, quinidine, and verapamil. As digoxin is a narrow therapeutic index drug, small changes in bioavailability can potentially result in serious adverse events due to loss of efficacy (bioavailability is lower than the therapeutic range) or life-threatening toxicity (bioavailability exceeds the therapeutic range). Digoxin oral solution USP labeling instructs the practitioner to measure serum digoxin concentrations before initiating concomitant drugs, reduce the digoxin dose once concomitant therapy is initiated, and continue to monitor digoxin serum concentrations.

*Age.* The systemic bioavailability of a drug is controlled by its absorption, distribution, metabolism, and elimination (ADME). In pediatric patients, growth and developmental changes in factors influencing ADME lead to drug bioavailability that can differ from that of adult patients (US-FDA, CDER, 2014e). The FDA recommends that sponsors developing pediatric formulations conduct pharmacokinetic studies in the pediatric population to determine how the dosing regimen should be adjusted to achieve the same systemic exposure that is safe and effective in adults (Chapter 24).

Systemic bioavailability of drugs can change with aging (Klotz, 2009). Impairments in the functional reserve of multiple organs can occur with advancing age, and such impairments might affect drug metabolism and pharmacokinetics. Advancing age is associated with changes such as decreases in liver mass and perfusion, changes in body composition, and decreases in renal function. Many of these changes result in increased drug bioavailability. As a result, it is recommended that clinicians carefully monitor dosing regimens and drug action in geriatric patients.

*Disease state.* The bioavailability of drugs eliminated primarily through renal excretory mechanisms is likely to increase in patients with impaired renal function (Chapter 25). The FDA recommends that, where appropriate, drug pharmacokinetics be characterized in patients with varying degrees of renal impairment. The results of such studies are used to determine how doses can be adjusted in patients with renal impairment in order to achieve the same systemic drug bioavailability as in patients with normal renal function (US-FDA CDER, 2020). Similarly, it may be advisable to conduct pharmacokinetic studies of drugs that are primarily cleared by the liver in patients with varying degrees of hepatic impairment (US-FDA, CDER, 2003a). The results of pharmacokinetic studies in hepatic-impaired patients can be useful in determining whether dose adjustments are required in such patients to achieve the same systemic drug bioavailability as in patients with normal liver function.

The systemic bioavailability of a drug in patients can differ from that in healthy normal subjects. Ordinarily, sponsors conduct single- and multiple-dose pharmacokinetic studies in both healthy normal subjects and the target patient population in early stage development, to characterize similarities and differences in drug systemic bioavailability.

### Analytical Methods

Analytical methods used for *in vivo* bioavailability, bioequivalence, or pharmacodynamic studies must be validated for accuracy and sufficient sensitivity (FDA Guidance for Industry, 2018).

The actual concentration of the active drug ingredient or therapeutic moiety, or its active metabolite(s), must be measured with appropriate precision in body fluids or excretory products. For bioavailability and bioequivalence studies, both the parent drug and its major active metabolites are generally measured. For bioequivalence studies, the parent drug or active moiety is measured rather than the metabolite. Measurement of the active moiety is more sensitive to changes in formulation performance than that of the metabolite, which is more reflective of metabolite formation, distribution, and elimination. Measurement of the active metabolite is important for very high-hepatic clearance (first-pass metabolism) drugs when the parent drug concentrations are too low to be reliable. The metabolite may be measured if it contributes to efficacy and/or safety.

The analytical method for measurement of the drug must be validated for accuracy, precision, sensitivity, specificity, and robustness. (US FDA-CDER 2018) The use of more than one analytical method during a bioequivalence study may not be valid, because different methods may yield different values. Data should be presented in both tabulated and graphic form for evaluation. The plasma drug concentration–time curve for each drug product and each subject should be available.

## STUDY DESIGNS

*In vivo* and/or *in vitro* methods can be used to establish bioequivalence. The studies in descending order of preference include pharmacokinetic, pharmacodynamic, clinical, and *in vitro* studies. For many drug products, the FDA provides specific guidance for the performance of *in vitro* dissolution and *in vivo* bioequivalence studies (US-FDA, CDER, 2010a). Generally, two bioequivalence studies are required for solid oral dosage forms, including (1) a fasting study and (2) a food intervention study. For extended-release capsules containing beads (pellets) that might be poured on a semisolid food such as applesauce, an additional "sprinkle" bioequivalence study is recommended. Other study designs such as parallel design, replicate design, and multiple-dose (steady-state) bioequivalence studies have been proposed by the FDA. Proper study design and statistical evaluation

are important considerations for the determination of bioequivalence.

### Pivotal and Pilot Bioequivalence Studies

A *pivotal* bioequivalence study is a large *in vivo* study that is properly designed with a sufficient number of subjects and appropriately timed blood samples that can well define the bioavailability of the active drug. Successful pivotal bioequivalence studies are submitted with the ANDA as part of the information required by the FDA for approval as a generic drug product.

Because a pivotal study is very costly, time consuming, and may not be successful to establish bioequivalence, a less expensive, smaller pilot study may be conducted prior to the large pivotal study. A *pilot study* is a relative bioavailability study in a small number of subjects. The pilot study is used to compare the bioavailability of various formulations of the proposed generic drug product against the RLD. Pilot bioavailability studies are often used for MR and complex drug products that are often more difficult to formulate compared to conventional, IR drug products. The pilot study is used to validate analytical methodology, assess intrasubject and intersubject variability, optimize sample collection time intervals, and provide other information. The results of the pilot study provide information as to the most appropriate design for the pivotal bioequivalence study.

Single-dose bioequivalence studies are preferred since single-dose BEs are generally more sensitive than steady-state studies in assessing differences in the release of the active drug from the drug product and its systemic bioavailability. The bioequivalence study compares the highest strength of the test and RLD products. A different strength may be used if there is a concern for safety.

### Fasting Study

Bioequivalence studies are usually evaluated by a single-dose, two-period, two-treatment, two-sequence, open-label, randomized crossover design comparing equal doses of the test and reference products in fasted, adult, healthy subjects. This study is requested for all IR and MR oral dosage forms. Both male and female subjects may be used in the study. Blood sampling is performed just before (zero time) the dose and at appropriate intervals after the dose to obtain an adequate description of the plasma drug concentration–time profile. The subjects should be in the fasting state (overnight fast of at least 10 hours) before drug administration and should continue to fast for up to 4 hours after dosing. No other medication is normally given to the subject for at least 1 week prior to the study. In some cases, a parallel design may be more appropriate for certain drug products, containing a drug with a very long elimination half-life. A replicate design may be used for a drug product containing a drug that has high intrasubject variability.

### Food Intervention Study

Coadministration of food with an oral drug product may affect the bioavailability of the drug. Food intervention or food effect studies are generally conducted using meal conditions that are expected to provide the greatest effects on GI physiology so that systemic drug availability is maximally affected. Food effects on bioavailability are generally greatest when the drug product is administered shortly after a meal is ingested. The nutrient and caloric contents of the meal, the meal volume, and the meal temperature can cause physiological changes in the GI tract in a way that affects drug product transit time, luminal dissolution, drug permeability, and systemic availability.

Meals that are high in total calories and fat content are more likely to affect the GI physiology and thereby result in a larger effect on the bioavailability of a drug substance or drug product (US-FDA, CDER, 2003b). In addition, the high fat meal can have a significant effect on certain MR drug products causing them to dose dump (ie, a large amount of the dose is prematurely released from the MR drug product). The test meal is a high-fat (approximately 50% of total caloric content of the meal) and high-calorie (approximately 800–1000 calories) meal. A typical test meal is two eggs fried in butter, two strips of bacon, two slices of toast with butter, 4 oz of brown potatoes, and 8 oz of milk. This test meal derives approximately 150, 250, and 500–600 calories from protein, carbohydrate, and fat, respectively (www.fda.gov/cder/guidance/4613dft.pdf).

For bioequivalence studies for generic drugs, drug bioavailability from both the test and reference products should be affected similarly by food. The usual study design uses a single-dose, randomized, two-treatment, two-period, crossover study comparing equal doses of the test and reference products. Following an overnight fast of at least 10 hours, subjects are given the recommended meal 30 minutes before dosing. The meal is consumed over 30 minutes, with administration of the drug product immediately after the meal. The drug product is given with 240 mL (8 fluid oz) of water. No food is allowed for at least 4 hours postdose. This study is requested for all MR dosage forms and may be requested for immediate-release dosage forms if the bioavailability of the active drug ingredient is known to be affected by food (eg, ibuprofen, naproxen).

*Sprinkle Bioequivalence Studies.* The labeling for certain extended-release capsules that contain coated beads indicates that the capsule contents can be sprinkled over soft foods such as applesauce. For the NDA, the contents of the capsule are sprinkled on applesauce, which is taken by the fasted subject, and the bioavailability of the drug is then measured. For generic drug products in ANDAs, the sprinkle study is performed as a bioequivalence study to demonstrate that both products, sprinkled on food, will have equivalent bioavailability. Bioavailability studies might also examine the effects of other foods and special vehicles such as apple juice.

## CROSSOVER STUDY DESIGNS

Subjects who meet the inclusion and exclusion study criteria and have given informed consent are selected at random. A complete crossover design is usually employed, in which each subject receives the test drug product and the reference product. Examples of *Latin-square crossover designs* for a bioequivalence study in human volunteers, comparing three different drug formulations (A, B, C) or four different drug formulations (A, B, C, D), are described in Tables 8-7 and 8-8. The Latin-square design plans the clinical trial so that each subject receives each drug product only once, with adequate time between medications for the elimination of the drug from the body. In this design, each subject is his own control,

**TABLE 8-7** • Latin-Square Crossover Design for a Bioequivalence Study of Three Drug Products in Six Human Volunteers

| Subject | Drug Product | | |
|---|---|---|---|
| | Study Period 1 | Study Period 2 | Study Period 3 |
| 1 | A | B | C |
| 2 | B | C | A |
| 3 | C | A | B |
| 4 | A | C | B |
| 5 | C | B | A |
| 6 | B | A | C |

**TABLE 8-8** • Latin-Square Crossover Design for a Bioequivalency Study of 4 Drug Products in 16 Human Volunteers

| Subject | Drug Product | | | |
|---|---|---|---|---|
| | Study Period 1 | Study Period 2 | Study Period 3 | Study Period 4 |
| 1 | A | B | C | D |
| 2 | B | C | D | A |
| 3 | C | D | A | B |
| 4 | D | A | B | C |
| 5 | A | B | D | C |
| 6 | B | D | C | A |
| 7 | D | C | A | B |
| 8 | C | A | B | D |
| 9 | A | C | B | D |
| 10 | C | B | D | A |
| 11 | B | D | A | C |
| 12 | D | A | C | B |
| 13 | A | C | D | B |
| 14 | C | D | B | A |
| 15 | D | B | A | C |
| 16 | B | A | C | D |

and subject-to-subject variation is reduced. Moreover, variations due to sequence, period, and treatment (formulation) are reduced, so that all patients do not receive the same drug product on the same day and in the same order. The order in which the drug treatments are given should not stay the same in order to prevent any bias in the data due to a residual effect from the previous treatment. Possible *carryover effects* from any particular drug product are minimized by changing the sequence or order in which the drug products are given to the subject. Thus, drug product B may be followed by drug product A, D, or C (Table 8-8). After each subject receives a drug product, blood samples are collected at appropriate time intervals so that a valid blood drug level–time curve is obtained. The time intervals should be spaced so that the peak blood concentration, the total area under the curve, and the absorption and elimination phases of the curve may be well described.

*Period* refers to the time period in which a study is performed. A two-period study is a study that is performed on two different days (time periods) separated by a *washout period* during which most of the drug is eliminated from the body—generally about 10 elimination half-lives. A *sequence* refers to the number of different orders in the treatment groups in a study. For example, a two-sequence, two-period study would be designed as follows:

| | Period 1 | Period 2 |
|---|---|---|
| Sequence 1 | T | R |
| Sequence 2 | R | T |

R = reference; T = treatment.

## Replicated Crossover Study Designs

The standard bioequivalence criterion using the two-way crossover design does not give an estimate of within-subject (intrasubject) variability. By giving the same drug product twice to the same subject, the replicate design provides a measure for within-subject variability. Replicate design studies may be used for highly variable drugs and for narrow therapeutic index drugs. In the case of highly variable drugs (%CV greater than 30), a large number of subjects (>80) would be needed to demonstrate bioequivalence using the standard two-way cross-over design. Drugs with high within-subject variability generally have a wide therapeutic window and despite high variability, these products have been demonstrated to be both safe and effective. Replicate designs for highly variable drugs/products require a smaller number of subjects and, therefore, do not unnecessarily expose a large number of healthy subjects to a drug when this large number of subjects is not needed for assurance of bioequivalence (Haidar et al, 2008).

Replicated crossover designs are used for the determination of individual bioequivalence, to estimate within-subject variance for both the test and reference drug products, and to provide an estimate of the subject-by-formulation interaction variance. A four-period, two-sequence, two-formulation design is shown below:

|            | Period 1 | Period 2 | Period 3 | Period 4 |
|------------|----------|----------|----------|----------|
| Sequence 1 | T        | R        | T        | R        |
| Sequence 2 | R        | T        | R        | T        |

*R = reference; T = treatment.*

In this design, the same reference and the same test are each given twice to the same subject. Other sequences are possible. In this design, reference-to-reference and test-to-test comparisons may also be made.

## Narrow Therapeutic Index Drugs

Narrow therapeutic index (NTI) drugs, also referred to as *critical dose drugs*, are drugs in which small changes in dose or concentration may lead to serious therapeutic failures or serious adverse drug reactions in patients. NTI drugs consistently display the following characteristics: (a) subtherapeutic concentrations may lead to serious therapeutic failure; (b) there is little separation between therapeutic and toxic doses (or the associated plasma concentrations); (c) they are subject to therapeutic monitoring based on pharmacokinetic or pharmacodynamic measures; (d) they possess low-to-moderate within-subject variability (<30%); and (e) in clinical practice, doses are generally adjusted in very small increments

(<20%). The FDA currently recommends that bioequivalence studies of NTI drugs should employ a four-way, fully replicated, crossover study design. The replicated study design permits comparison of both test and reference means and test and reference within-subject variability (Davit et al, 2013).

An additional test recommended in bioequivalence studies of generic NTI drugs is a test for within-subject variability. The test determines whether within-subject variability of the test narrow therapeutic index drug does not differ significantly from that of the reference by evaluating the test/reference ratio of the within-subject standard deviation. The FDA currently recommends that all bioequivalence studies on NTI drugs must pass both the reference-scaled approach and the unscaled average bioequivalence limits of 80.00%–125.00%.

## Reference Scaled Average Bioequivalence

Recently a three-sequence, three-period, two-treatment partially replicated crossover design for bioequivalence studies of highly variable drugs has been recommended by the FDA (Haidar et al, 2008). The partially replicated design allows the estimation of the within-subject variance and subject-by-formulation interaction for the reference product. The time for completion of this study is shorter than the fully replicated four-way cross-over design.

This design is usually used for highly variable drugs with within-subject variability ≥30%. Large numbers of subjects may be needed in bioequivalence studies of highly variable drugs; the FDA implemented the reference-scaled average bioequivalence approach to ease regulatory burden and reduce unnecessary human testing. Using this approach, the implied bioequivalence limits can widen to be larger than 80%–125% for drugs that are highly variable, provided that certain constraints are applied to this approach in order to maintain an acceptable type I error rate and satisfy any public health concerns (Davit et al, 2012).

|            | Period 1 | Period 2 | Period 3 |
|------------|----------|----------|----------|
| Sequence 1 | T        | R        | R        |
| Sequence 2 | R        | T        | R        |
| Sequence 3 | R        | R        | T        |

Under this design, if the test product has lower variability than the reference product, the study will need a smaller number of subjects to pass the bioequivalence criteria. Scaled average bioequivalence is evaluated for both AUC and $C_{max}$.

## Parallel Study Designs

A nonreplicate, parallel design is used for drug products that contain drugs that have a long elimination half-life or drug products such as depot injections in which the drug is slowly released over weeks or months. In this design, two separate groups of volunteers are used. One group will be given the test product and the other group will be given the reference product. It is important to balance the demographics of both groups of volunteers. Blood sample collection time should be adequate to ensure completion of GI transit (approximately 2–3 days) of the drug product and absorption of the drug substance. $C_{max}$ and a suitably truncated AUC, generally to 72 hours after dose administration, can be used to characterize peak and total drug exposure, respectively. For drugs that demonstrate low intrasubject variability in distribution and clearance, an AUC truncated at 72 hours ($AUC_0^{72}$ hours) can be used in place of $AUC_0^t$ or $AUC_0^\infty$. This design is not recommended for drugs that have high intrasubject variability in distribution and clearance.

## Multiple-Dose (Steady-State) Study Design

A bioequivalence study may be performed using a multiple-dose study design. Multiple doses of the same drug are given consecutively to reach steady-state plasma drug levels. The multiple-dose study is designed as a steady-state, randomized, two-treatment, two-way, crossover study comparing equal doses of the test and reference products in healthy adult subjects. Each subject receives either the test or the reference product separated by a "washout" period, which is the time needed for the drug to be completely eliminated from the body.

To ascertain that the subjects are at steady state, three consecutive trough concentrations ($C_{min}$) are determined. The last morning dose is given to the subject after an overnight fast, with continual fasting for at least 2 hours following dose administration. Blood sampling is then performed over one dosing interval. The area under the curve during a dosing interval at steady state should be the same as the area under the curve extrapolated to infinite time after a single dose.

Pharmacokinetic analyses for multiple-dose studies include calculation of the following parameters for each subject:

$AUC_{0\text{-tau}}$—Area under the curve during a dosing interval

$t_{max}$—Time to $C_{max}$ during a dosing interval

$C_{max}$—Maximum drug concentration during dosing interval

$C_{min}$—Drug concentration at the end of a dosing interval

$C_{av}$—The average drug concentration during a dosing interval

*Degree of fluctuation* $= (C_{max} - C_{min})/C_{max}$

*Swing* $= (C_{max} - C_{min})/C_{min}$

The data are analyzed statistically using analysis of variance (ANOVA) on the log-transformed AUC and $C_{max}$. To establish bioequivalence, both AUC and $C_{max}$ for the test (generic) product should be within 80%–125% of the reference product using a 90% confidence interval. Estimation of the absorption rate constant during multiple dosing is difficult, because the residual drug from the previous dose superimposes on the dose that follows. However, the data obtained in multiple doses are useful in calculating a steady-state plasma level.

The extent of bioavailability, measured by assuming the $[AUC]_0^\infty$, is dependent on clearance:

$$[AUC]_0^\infty = \frac{FD_0}{Cl_T}$$

Determination of bioavailability using multiple doses reveals changes that are normally not detected in a single-dose study. For example, nonlinear pharmacokinetics may occur after multiple drug doses due to the higher plasma drug concentrations saturating an enzyme system involved in absorption or elimination of the drug. Nonlinear pharmacokinetics after multiple-dose studies may be observed by rising $C_{min}$ drug concentrations and $AUC_t$ after each dosing interval. With some drugs, a drug-induced malabsorption syndrome can also alter the percentage of drug absorbed. In this case, drug bioavailability may decrease after repeated doses if the fraction of the dose absorbed ($F$) decreases or if the total body clearance ($kV_D$) increases. It should be noted that nonlinear PK can also be observed by high single doses of the drug.

There are several disadvantages of using the multiple-dose crossover method for the determination of bioequivalence. (1) The study takes more time to perform, because steady-state conditions must be reached. A longer time for completion of a study leads to greater clinical costs and the possibility of a subject dropping out and not completing the study. (2) More plasma samples must be obtained from the subject to ascertain that steady state has been reached and to describe the plasma level–time curve accurately. (3) Because $C_{av}^{\infty}$ depends primarily on the dose of the drug and the time interval between doses, the extent of drug systemically available is more important than the rate of drug availability. Small differences in the rate of drug absorption may not be observed with steady-state study comparisons

## Pharmacodynamic Endpoint Studies

Studies using pharmacodynamic endpoints are described in Chapter 22 and earlier in this chapter. In general, if the drug is intended to be absorbed from the drug product into the systemic circulation, then a PK approach is preferred to establish bioequivalence.

## Clinical Endpoint Bioequivalence Study

Study design for a clinical endpoint study generally consists of a randomized, double-blind, placebo-controlled, parallel-designed study comparing test product, reference product, and placebo product in patients. A placebo arm is usually included to demonstrate that the treatments are active (above the no-effect part of the effect versus dose curve, see Fig. 8-11) and the study is sufficiently sensitive to identify the clinical effect in the patient population enrolled in the study. In some cases, the use of a placebo may not be included for safety reasons. The primary analysis for bioequivalence is determined by evaluating the difference between the proportion of patients in the test and reference treatment groups who are considered a "therapeutic cure" at the end of

study. The superiority of the test and reference products against the placebo is also tested using the same dichotomous endpoint of "therapeutic cure."

## Determination of Bioequivalence of Drug Products in Patients Maintained on a Therapeutic Drug Regimen

A bioequivalence study may be performed in patients already maintained on the reference (brand-name) drug. Due to safety concerns, certain drugs such as clozapine, a dibenzodiazepine derivative with potent antipsychotic properties, should not be given to normal healthy subjects (US-FDA, CDER, 2011b). Instead, bioequivalence studies on clozapine should be performed in patients who have been stabilized on the highest strength (eg, 100 mg) using a multiple-dose bioequivalence study design. This study does not disrupt the patient's ongoing drug treatment. Patients on these or other drugs such as antipsychotics (US-FDA, CDER, 2013a) or cancer chemotherapeutic drugs (Kaur et al, 2013) would be at risk if a washout period is used between drug treatments. Therefore, the patient is maintained on his or her previous dose of medication or an equal dose of the test product, and blood sampling is performed during a dosage interval (Fig. 8-13, reference product A). Once blood sampling is accomplished, the patient takes equal oral doses of the other drug product (test or reference) and the previous drug product is discontinued. Drug dosing with each drug product continues until attainment of steady state. When steady state is reached, the plasma level–time curve for a dosage interval with the second drug product is described (Fig. 8-13, drug product B). Using the same plasma measures as before, the bioequivalence or lack of bioequivalence may be determined. The patient then continues with his or her therapy with the original drug product.

Products are given in random order: A then B, B then A. Failure to do this might lead to a sequence effect. The reference product that is tested is provided by the investigator from a known lot (not the patient's own prescription).

Since the patients are being treated with the reference (brand) product A, the drug concentrations are at steady state prior to the start of the study and the accumulation phase is not observed. The test

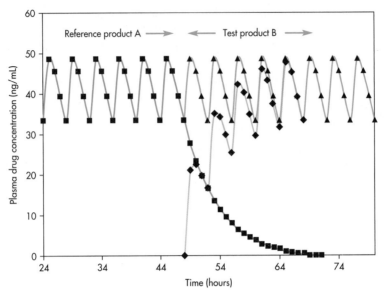

FIGURE 8-13 • Multiple-dose bioequivalence study in patients. Bioequivalence is determined by comparison of the steady-state plasma drug-versus-time profile after administration of the reference drug product A to the steady-state plasma drug–time profile after administration of the test drug product B.

drug product B is started and the reference drug product A is stopped. The total plasma drug concentrations are maintained. Bioequivalence is determined by comparison of the steady-state plasma drug-versus-time profile after administration of the reference drug product A to the steady-state plasma drug–time profile after administration of the test drug product B.

If the blood level–time curve of the second drug product is bioequivalent, as shown by $AUC_t$ and $C_{max}$, to that of the reference drug product, the second product is considered to be bioequivalent. If the second drug has less bioavailability (assuming that only the extent of drug absorption is less than that of the reference drug), the resulting $C_{av}^{\infty}$ will be smaller than that obtained with the first drug. $C_{av}^{\infty}$ is not used as a direct measurement. Usually, the drug manufacturer will perform dissolution and content uniformity tests before performing a bioequivalence study. These *in vitro* dissolution tests will help ensure that the $C_{av}^{\infty}$ obtained from each drug product *in vivo* will not be largely different from each other. In contrast, if the extent of drug availability is greater in the second drug product, the $C_{av}^{\infty}$ will be higher.

## CLINICAL EXAMPLE

### Levothyroxine Sodium Oral Tablets

A multiple dose relative bioavailability study[9] of two synthetic branded levothyroxine sodium oral tablets, product A and product B, were evaluated in 20 euthyroid patients. The investigation was designed as a two-way crossover study in which the patients who had been diagnosed as hypothyroid by their primary care physician were given a single 100-$\mu$g daily dose of either product A or product B levothyroxine sodium tablets for 50 days and then switched over immediately to the other treatment for 50 days. Predose blood samples were taken on days 1, 25, 48, 49, and 50 of each phase, and, on day 50, a complete blood sampling was performed. The serum from each blood sample was analyzed for total and free thyroxine (T4), total and free

[9]For the FDA-recommended bioequivalence study for levothyroxine sodium tablets, see FDA Guidance for Industry: Levothyroxine Sodium Tablets—In Vivo Pharmacokinetic and Bioavailability Studies, and In Vitro Dissolution Testing, December 2000.

triiodothyronine (T3), the major metabolite of T4, and thyrotropin (TSH).

a. Why were hypothyroid patients used in this study?

b. Why were the subjects dosed for 50 days with each thyroid product?

c. Why were blood samples obtained on days 48, 49, and 50?

d. Why was T3 measured?

e. Why was TSH measured?

### Solution

a. Normal healthy euthyroid subjects would be at risk if they were to take levothyroxine sodium for an extended period of time.

b. The long (50-day) daily dosing for each product was required to obtain steady-state drug levels because of the long elimination half-life of levothyroxine.

c. Serum from blood samples was taken on days 48, 49, and 50 to obtain three consecutive $C_{min}$ drug levels.

d. T3 is the active metabolite of T4.

e. The serum TSH concentration is inversely proportional to the free serum T4 concentrations and gives an indication of the pharmacodynamic activity of the active drug.

## CLINICAL EXAMPLE

### Mercaptopurine (Purinethol) Oral Tablets

Mercaptopurine (Purinethol) is a cytotoxic drug used to treat cancer and is available in a 50-mg oral tablet. The FDA recommends bioequivalence steady-state studies (US-FDA, CDER, 2011c) in patients receiving therapeutic oral doses (usually 100–200 mg/d in the average adult) or maintenance daily doses (usually 50–100 mg/d in the average adult).

Patients should be on a stable regimen using the same dosage unit (multiples of the same 50-mg strength). Plasma drug concentration–time profiles are obtained in these patients at steady state with the brand product. The proposed generic drug product is then given to these patients at the same dosage

regimen until steady state is reached. Plasma drug concentration–time profiles are obtained for the generic drug product; then the patients return to the original brand medication.

## SYSTEMIC DRUG EXPOSURE AND PHARMACOKINETIC EVALUATION OF THE DATA

The rate of drug absorption (peak exposure) is measured by the peak drug concentration, $C_{max}$ obtained without interpolation. When there is more than one $C_{max}$ that may be observed with certain MR drug products, then the first $C_{max}$ is used. The time to peak drug plasma concentrations, $t_{max}$, provides important information regarding the rate of drug absorption.

The extent of absorption (total drug exposure) is measured by the area under the plasma drug concentration versus time curve, AUC. For single-dose studies, $AUC_{0-t}$ is the area under the plasma drug concentration curve from zero time to time t which is the last time point for which there is a measureable drug concentration and $AUC_{0-inf}$ is the total AUC extrapolated to time infinity. For multiple-dose, steady-state studies, the $AUC_{0-tau}$ is the area under the plasma drug concentration curve where tau is the length of the dosing interval.

For single-dose studies, including a fasting study or a food intervention study, the pharmacokinetic analyses include calculation for each subject of the area under the curve to the last quantifiable concentration $(AUC_0^t)$ and to infinity $(AUC_0^\infty)$, $t_{max}$, and $C_{max}$.

Additionally, the elimination rate constant, $k$, the elimination half-life, $t_{1/2}$, and other parameters may be estimated. For multiple-dose studies, pharmacokinetic analysis includes calculation for each subject of the steady-state area under the curve, $(AUC_{\infty}^{t})$, $t_{max}$, $C_{min}$, $C_{max}$, and the percent fluctuation $[100 \times (C_{max} - C_{min})/C_{min}]$. Proper statistical evaluation should be performed on the estimated pharmacokinetic parameters.

## Statistical Evaluation of the Data

Bioequivalence is generally determined using a comparison of population averages of a bioequivalence metric, such as AUC and $C_{max}$. This approach, termed *average bioequivalence,* involves the calculation of a 90% confidence interval for the ratio of averages (population geometric means) of the bioequivalence metrics for the test and reference drug products (US-FDA, CDER, 2000a).

Many statistical approaches (parametric tests) assume that the data are distributed according to a normal distribution or "bell-shaped curve" (Chapter 3). The pharmacokinetic parameters such as $C_{max}$ and AUC may not be normally distributed, and the true distribution is difficult to ascertain because of the small number of subjects used in a bioequivalence study. The distribution of data that have been transformed to log values resembles more closely a normal distribution compared to the distribution of non-log-transformed data.

### Two One-Sided Tests Procedure

The two one-sided tests procedure is also referred to as the *confidence interval approach* (Schuirmann, 1987). This statistical method is used to demonstrate if the bioavailability of the drug from the test formulation is too low or high in comparison to that of the reference product. The objective of the approach is to determine if there are large differences (ie, greater than 20%) between the mean parameters.

The 90% confidence limits are estimated for the sample means. The interval estimate is based on Student's $t$ distribution of the data. In this test, presently required by the FDA, a 90% confidence interval about the ratio of means of the two drug products must be within ±20% for measurement of the rate and extent of drug bioavailability. For most drugs, up to a 20%

difference in AUC or $C_{max}$ between two formulations would have no clinical significance. The lower 90% confidence interval for the ratio of means cannot be less than 0.80, and the upper 90% confidence interval for the ratio of the means cannot be greater than 1.20. When log-transformed data are used, the 90% confidence interval is set at 80%–125%. These confidence limits have also been termed the *bioequivalence interval* (Midha et al, 1993). The 90% confidence interval is a function of sample size and study variability, including inter- and intra-subject variability.

For a single-dose, fasting or food intervention bioequivalence study, an ANOVA is usually performed on the log-transformed AUC and $C_{max}$ values. There should be no statistical differences between the mean AUC and $C_{max}$ parameters for the test (generic) and reference drug products. In addition, the 90% confidence intervals about the ratio of the means for AUC and $C_{max}$ values of the test drug product should not be less than 0.80 (80%) nor greater than 1.25 (125%) of that of the reference product based on log-transformed data. Table 8-9 summarizes the statistical analysis for average bioequivalence. Presently, the FDA

---

**TABLE 8-9 • Statistical Analysis for Average Bioequivalence**

- Based on log-transformed data
- Point estimates of the mean ratios
  Test/reference for AUC and $C_{max}$ are between 80% and 125%
- AUC and $C_{max}$
  90% confidence intervals (CI) must fit between 80% and 125%
- Bioequivalence criteria
  Two one-sided tests procedure
  - Test (T) is not significantly less than reference
  - Reference (R) is not significantly less than test
  - Significant difference is 20% ($a = 0.05$ significance level)
    T/R = 80/100 = 80%
    R/T = 80% (all data expressed as T/R, so this becomes 100/80 = 125%)
- The statistical model typically includes factors accounting for the following sources of variation: sequence, subjects nested in sequences, period, and treatment

*Data from US-FDA, CDER (2000).*

accepts only average bioequivalence estimates used to establish bioequivalence of generic drug products.

## Analysis of Variance

An analysis of variance (ANOVA) is a statistical procedure (see Chapter 3) used to test the data for differences within and between treatment and control groups. A bioequivalent product should produce no significant difference in all pharmacokinetic parameters tested. The parameters tested statistically usually include $AUC_\infty^t$, $AUC_0^\infty$, and $C_{max}$ obtained for each treatment or dosage form. Other metrics of bioavailability have also been used to compare the bioequivalence of two or more formulations. The ANOVA may evaluate variability in subjects, treatment groups, study period, formulation, and other variables, depending on the study design. If the variability in the data is large, the difference in means for each pharmacokinetic parameter, such as AUC, may be masked, and the investigator might erroneously conclude that the two drug products are bioequivalent.

A statistical difference between the pharmacokinetic parameters obtained from two or more drug products is considered statistically significant if there is a probability of less than 1 in 20 times or 0.05 probability ($p \leq .05$) that these results would have happened on the basis of chance alone. The probability, $p$, is used to indicate the level of statistical significance. If $p < .05$, the differences between the two drug products are not considered statistically significant.

To reduce the possibility of failing to detect small differences between the test products, a *power test* is performed to calculate the probability that the conclusion of the ANOVA is valid. The power of the test will depend on the sample size, variability of the data, and desired level of significance. Usually, the power is set at 0.80 with a $\beta = 0.2$ and a level of significance of 0.05. The higher the power, the test is more sensitive and the greater the probability that the conclusion of the ANOVA is valid.

## THE PARTIAL AUC IN BIOEQUIVALENCE ANALYSIS

Several drug delivery systems have a complex approach to drug release (eg, combinations of zero-order and first-order drug release) that produces an unusually shaped plasma drug concentration-versus-time profile. The shape of this plasma drug concentration-versus-time profile is related to the pharmacodynamics of the drug.

To evaluate a generic dosage form of these new drug delivery systems, the FDA recommends including the partial AUC (pAUC) as a pivotal bioequivalence metric. The pAUC is defined as the area under the plasma concentration-versus-time profile over two specified time points. The choice of sampling time points for calculating the pAUC is based on the pharmacokinetic/pharmacodynamic or efficacy/safety data for the drug under examination.

The FDA currently expects the pAUC to be analyzed statistically when determining bioequivalence of multiphasic MR formulations designed to achieve a rapid therapeutic response followed by a sustained response. Such products are generally formulated with both an immediate-release component and a delayed- or extended-release component. Figure 8-14 illustrates how a pAUC analysis, based on two partial AUCs, is applied. The two partial AUCs consist of an early pAUC measure $AUC_{0-T}$ to compare test and reference exposure responsible for early onset of response, and a late pAUC measure $AUC_{T-t}$ to compare test and reference exposure responsible for sustained response. The early $AUC_{0-T}$ is measured beginning at sampling time 0 to a truncation time $T$. The late $AUC_{T-t}$ is measured from the truncation time $T$ to the last sampling point with measurable drug concentration. These two metrics replace $AUC_{0-t}$ in bioequivalence evaluation. The bioequivalence determination is based on comparison of test and reference $C_{max}$, $AUC_{0-\infty}$, $AUC_{0-T}$, and $AUC_{T-t}$.

For some drug products, the shape of the plasma drug concentration versus time curve may be clinically relevant. FDA recommends the use of pAUC to compare the shapes of the plasma drug concentration curve. pAUC refers to the AUC between two specified, clinically relevant, time points on the drug plasma concentration-versus-time profile. The sampling time $T$ should be selected based on the pharmacokinetic and pharmacodynamic properties of the active ingredient.

## Examples of Partial AUC Analyses

pAUC analyses measure partial drug exposure for which the time to truncate the partial area should be related to a clinically relevant measurement.

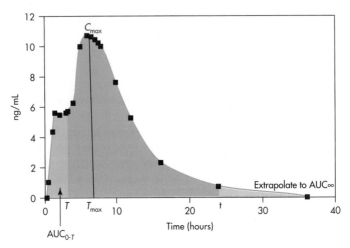

**FIGURE 8-14** • Partial AUC analysis in a bioequivalence study. The partial AUC (pAUC) refers to the AUC between two specified, clinically relevant, time points on the drug plasma concentration-versus-time profile. The sampling time $T$ should be selected based on the pharmacokinetic and pharmacodynamic properties of the active ingredient.

This approach has been applied to the zolpidem extended-release formulation. The reference for this product, Ambien CR, exhibits biphasic absorption characteristics which result in rapid initial absorption from the GI tract, similar to zolpidem tartrate immediate release, and then provide extended plasma concentrations beyond 3 hours of administration. As a result, patients receiving Ambien CR experience both rapid onset of sleep and maintenance of sleep. To ensure that a test zolpidem tartrate extended-release tablet provides the same pharmacodynamic response (timing of sleep onset and maintenance) when switched with the reference product, the FDA expects that, in a bioequivalence study comparing the two, the parameters $AUC_{0-1.5h}$, $AUC_{1.5h-t}$, $AUC_{0-\infty}$, and $C_{max}$ will all pass bioequivalence limits of 80.00%–125.00% (US-FDA, CDER, 2011d). The sampling time for the early and late pAUCs for the zolpidem extended-release tablet is selected based on zolpidem pharmacokinetic–pharmacodynamic relationships.

FDA recommends three pAUC metrics for bioequivalence studies of generic versions of the methylphenidate multiphasic MR tablet (US-FDA, CDER, 2014f). The RLD is Concerta, indicated for the treatment of attention deficit hyperactivity disorder. Concerta is labeled to be administered once in the morning, before the start of the school day, for pediatric patients. The three pAUC metrics are

proposed to ensure that when patients for whom Concerta treatment is indicated switch formulations, they will experience equivalent therapeutic responses over the course of the day. Thus, for an acceptable bioequivalence study, the 90% confidence intervals of the geometric mean test/reference ratios $C_{max}$, $AUC_{0-T1}$, $AUC_{T1-T2}$, $AUC_{T2-T3}$, and $AUC_{\infty}$ should fall within the limits of 80.00%–125.00%. The sampling time $T_1$ for the first pAUC ($AUC_{0-T1}$) is based on the time at which 90%–95% of subjects are likely to achieve an early onset of response. The middle pAUC ($AUC_{T1-T2}$) comparison is to ensure similar drug exposures during the remaining school hours (for pediatric patients) after early onset of exposure. The late pAUC comparison ($AUC_{T2-T3}$) is to ensure equivalent methylphenidate exposures during the latter part of the dosing interval, corresponding to the duration of the sustained response.

The pAUC is also used as a bioequivalence metric in studies comparing test and reference versions of mesalamine orally administered MR formulations (Table 8-10). Mesalamine is indicated to treat inflammatory diseases of the colon and rectum, and is thought to act locally rather than systemically. Table 8-10 summarizes the mesalamine RLD oral MR formulations, associated indications, and pAUC metrics used in bioequivalence studies against each of these RLDs. Mesalamine is well absorbed, most likely throughout the small and large intestines,

**TABLE 8-10** • Bioequivalence Metrics for *In Vivo* Studies of Mesalamine Modified-Release Oral Dosage Forms

| Formulation | Reference | Bioequivalence Metrics |
|---|---|---|
| Mesalamine delayed-release capsule | Delzicol[*] | For both fasting and fed studies: $C_{max}$, $AUC_{8-48\,h}$, $AUC_{0-t}$ |
| Mesalamine delayed-release tablet | Asacol[*] | |
| Mesalamine delayed-release tablet | Asacol HD[*] | |
| Mesalamine delayed-release tablet | Lialda[*] | |
| Mesalamine extended-release capsule | Pentasa[*] | For fasting study: $C_{max}$, $AUC_{0-3\,h}$, $AUC_{3\,h-t}$, $AUC_{0-t}$<br>For fed study: $C_{max}$ and $AUC_{0-t}$ are pivotal; $AUC_{0-3\,h}$ and $AUC_{0-t}$ are supportive |
| Mesalamine extended-release capsule | Apriso[*] | |

with the result that it is possible to measure plasma concentrations and determine PK profiles following oral administration (US-FDA, CDER, 2013b). Because the site of mesalamine action is the colon and rectum, the FDA concluded that comparisons of AUC and $C_{max}$ alone in bioequivalence studies would not distinguish between products with materially different mesalamine release profiles at the sites of drug action (US-FDA, CDER, 2010c). Thus, the pAUC is used to analyze systemic mesalamine concentrations over specified time intervals to determine whether mesalamine from test and reference products is available at the same rate and to

the same extent at the colon and rectum (Davit and Conner, 2015).

## BIOEQUIVALENCE EXAMPLES

A simulated example of the results for a single-dose, fasting study is shown in Table 8-11 and in Fig. 8-15. As shown by the ANOVA, no statistical differences for the pharmacokinetic parameters, $(AUC_0^t)$, $(AUC_0^\infty)$, and $C_{max}$, were observed between the test product and the brand-name product. The 90% confidence limits for the mean pharmacokinetic parameters of the test product were within 0.80–1.25

**TABLE 8-11** • Bioavailability Comparison of a Generic (Test) and Brand-Name (Reference) Drug Products (Log-Normal Transformed Data)

| Variable | Units | Geometric Mean | | % Ratio | 90% Confidence Interval (Lower Limit, Upper Limit) | *p* Values for Product Effects | Power of ANOVA | ANOVA %CV |
|---|---|---|---|---|---|---|---|---|
| | | Test | Reference | | | | | |
| $C_{max}$ | ng/mL | 344.79 | 356.81 | 96.6 | (89.5, 112) | 0.3586 | 0.8791 | 17.90% |
| $AUC_{0-t}$ | ng·h/mL | 2659.12 | 2674.92 | 99.4 | (95.1, 104) | 0.8172 | 1.0000 | 12.60% |
| $AUC_\infty$ | | 2708.63 | 2718.52 | 99.6 | (95.4, 103) | 0.8865 | 1.0000 | 12.20% |
| $t_{max}$ | h | 4.29 | 4.24 | 101 | | | | |
| $K_{elim}$ | 1/h | 0.0961 | 0.0980 | 98.1 | | | | |
| $t_{1/2}$ | h | 8.47 | 8.33 | 101.7 | | | | |

*The results were obtained from a two-way, crossover, single-dose study in 36 fasted, healthy, adult male and female volunteers. No statistical differences were observed for the mean values between test and reference products.*

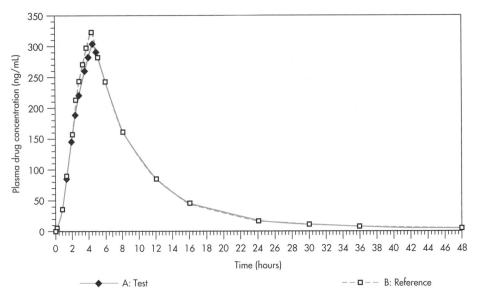

FIGURE 8-15 • Bioequivalence of test and reference drug products: mean plasma drug concentrations.

(80%–125%) of the reference product means based on log transformation of the data. The power test for the AUC measures was above 99%, showing good precision of the data. The power test for the $C_{max}$ values was 87.9%, showing that this parameter was more variable.

Table 8-12 shows the results for a hypothetical bioavailability study in which three different tablet formulations were compared to a solution of the drug given in the same dose. As shown in the table, the bioavailability from all three tablet formulations was greater than 80% of that of the solution. According to the ANOVA, the mean AUC values were not statistically different from one another, nor different from that of the solution. However, the 90% confidence interval for the AUC showed that for tablet A, the relative bioavailability was less than 80% (ie, 74%), compared to the solution at the low-range estimate, and would not be considered bioequivalent based on the AUC.

For illustrative purposes, consider a drug that has been prepared at the same dosage level in three formulations, A, B, and C. These formulations are given to a group of volunteers using a three-way, randomized crossover design. In this experimental design, all subjects receive each formulation once.

## TABLE 8-12 • Summary of the Results of a Bioavailability Study[*]

| Dosage Form | $C_{max}$ ($\mu$g/mL) | $t_{max}$ (h) | $AUC_{0-24}$ ($\mu$g h/mL) | $F^{\dagger}$ | 90% Confidence Interval for AUC |
|---|---|---|---|---|---|
| Solution | $16.1 \pm 2.5$ | $1.5 \pm 0.85$ | $1835 \pm 235$ | | |
| Tablet A | $10.5 \pm 3.2^{c}$ | $2.5 \pm 1.0^{\ddagger}$ | $1523 \pm 381$ | 81 | 74%–90% |
| Tablet B | $13.7 \pm 4.1$ | $2.1 \pm 0.98$ | $1707 \pm 317$ | 93 | 88%–98% |
| Tablet C | $14.8 \pm 3.6$ | $1.8 \pm 0.95$ | $1762 \pm 295$ | 96 | 91%–103% |

[*]The bioavailability of a drug from four different formulations was studied in 24 healthy, adult male subjects using a four-way Latin-square crossover design. The results represent the mean ± standard deviation.

[†]Oral bioavailability relative to the solution.

[‡]$p \le .05$.

**A**

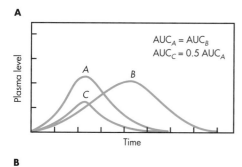

**B**

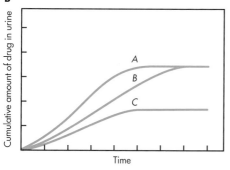

FIGURE 8-16 • Corresponding plots relating plasma concentration and urinary excretion data.

because the $t_{max}$ for formulation A is shorter. Because the AUC for formulation A is identical to the AUC for formulation B, the extent of bioavailability from both of these formulations is the same. Note, however, the $C_{max}$ for A is higher than that for B, because the rate of drug absorption is more rapid.

The $C_{max}$ is generally higher when the extent of drug bioavailability is greater. The rate of drug absorption from formulation C is the same as that from formulation A, but the extent of drug available is less. The $C_{max}$ for formulation C is less than that for formulation A. The decrease in $C_{max}$ for formulation C is proportional to the decrease in AUC in comparison to the drug plasma level data for formulation A. The corresponding urinary excretion data confirm these observations. These relationships are summarized in Table 8-13. The table illustrates how bioavailability parameters for plasma and urine change when only the extent and rate of bioavailability are changed, respectively. Formulation changes in a drug product may affect both the rate and extent of drug bioavailability.

From each subject, plasma drug level and urinary drug excretion data are obtained. With these data, we can observe the relationship between plasma and urinary excretion parameters and drug bioavailability (Fig. 8-16). The rate of drug absorption from formulation A is more rapid than that from formulation B,

## STUDY SUBMISSION AND DRUG REVIEW PROCESS

The contents of New Drug Applications (NDAs) and ANDAs are similar in terms of the quality of manufacture (Table 8-14). The submission for an

**TABLE 8-13 •** Relationship of Plasma Level and Urinary Excretion Parameters to Drug Bioavailability

| Extent of Drug Bioavailability Decreases | | Rate of Drug Bioavailability Decreases | |
|---|---|---|---|
| Parameter | Change | Parameter | Change |
| Plasma data | | | |
| $t_{max}$ | Same | $t_{max}$ | Increase |
| $C_{max}$ | Decrease | $C_{max}$ | Decrease |
| AUC | Decrease | AUC | Same |
| Urine data | | | |
| $t^{\infty}$ | Same | $t^{\infty}$ | Increase |
| $[dD_u/dt]_{max}$* | Decrease | $[dD_u/dt]_{max}$* | Decrease |
| $D_u^{\infty}$ | Decrease | $D_u^{\infty}$ | Same |

*Maximum rate of urinary drug excretion.

**TABLE 8-14 •** NDA Versus ANDA Review Process

| Brand-Name Drug NDA Requirements | Generic Drug ANDA Requirements |
|---|---|
| 1. Chemistry | 1. Chemistry |
| 2. Manufacturing | 2. Manufacturing |
| 3. Controls | 3. Controls |
| 4. Labeling | 4. Labeling |
| 5. Testing | 5. Testing |
| 6. Animal studies | 6. Bioequivalence |
| 7. Clinical studies | |
| 8. Bioavailability | |

*Reproduced with permission from Center for Drug Evaluation & Research, US Food & Drug Administration, http://www.fda.gov.*

NDA must contain safety and efficacy studies as provided by animal toxicology studies, clinical efficacy studies, and pharmacokinetic/bioavailability studies. For the generic drug manufacturer, the bioequivalence study is the pivotal study in the ANDA that replaces the animal, clinical, and pharmacokinetic studies.

An outline for the submission of a completed bioavailability to the FDA is shown in Table 8-15. The investigator should be sure that the study has been properly designed, the objectives are clearly defined, and the method of analysis has been validated (ie, shown to measure precisely and accurately the plasma drug concentration). The results are analyzed both statistically and pharmacokinetically. These results, along with case reports and various data supporting the validity of the analytical method, are included in the submission. The FDA reviews the study in detail according to the outline presented in Table 8-16. If necessary, an FDA investigator may inspect both the clinical and analytical facilities used in the study and audit the raw data used in support of the bioavailability study. For ANDA applications, the FDA Office of Generic Drugs reviews the entire ANDA as shown in Fig. 16-17. If the application is incomplete, the FDA will not review the submission and the sponsor will receive a *Refusal to File* letter.

**FREQUENTLY ASKED QUESTIONS**

▶ What is the most appropriate bioequivalence design for a solid oral drug product containing a drug for systemic absorption?

▶ What are some of the problems associated with clinical endpoint bioequivalence studies?

## BIOEQUIVALENCE FOR SPECIFIC DRUGS AND DRUG PRODUCTS

*Oral solutions.* For oral solutions including elixirs, syrups, tinctures, or other solubilized forms, an *in vivo* bioequivalence testing requirement may be waived for certain products on the grounds that *in vivo* bioequivalence is self-evident.

*Chewable tablets.* Chewable tablets should be given according to the directions on the label. If the label states that the tablet must be chewed before swallowing, the product should be chewed when administered in bioequivalence studies.

*Orally administered drugs intended for local action.* For oral drug products that produce their effects by local action in the GI tract, bioequivalence may be determined using PK endpoints. In other cases, bioequivalence may be determined using clinical endpoints, pharmacodynamic endpoints, and/or suitably designed and validated *in vitro* studies in addition to, or instead of, measuring drug plasma concentrations.

*Bioequivalence of topical drug products for local action.* Bioequivalence assessment of locally acting topical dosage forms is difficult. Bioequivalence is determined by various *in vitro* and *in vivo* approaches including the following: (a) Formulation sameness, in which the proposed formulation is both qualitative, Q1 and quantitatively, Q2 the same. The formulations have Q3 similarity in which the physical–chemical properties for the test and RLD formulations are similar. (b) *In vitro* drug release tests, which show that the test and RLD products have equivalent drug release. (c) *In vitro* permeation tests that show the rate and extent of drug permeation through excised human skin from the test and reference products are comparable (Dandamudi, 2017).

*Inhalation and nasal sprays for local drug action.* Bioequivalence of locally acting drugs from inhalation and nasal sprays is complicated by several

**TABLE 8-15** • Proposed Format and Contents of an *In Vivo* Bioequivalence Study Submission and Accompanying *In Vitro* Data

**Title page**
  Study title
  Name of sponsor
  Name and address of clinical laboratory
  Name of principal investigator(s)
  Name of clinical investigator
  Name of analytical laboratory
  Dates of clinical study (start, completion)
  Signature of principal investigator (and date)
  Signature of clinical investigator (and date)

**Table of contents**
  I. Study Résumé
    Product information
    Summary of bioequivalence study
    Summary of bioequivalence data
    Plasma
    Urinary excretion
    Figure of mean plasma concentration–time profile
    Figure of mean cumulative urinary excretion
    Figure of mean urinary excretion rates

  II. Protocol and Approvals
    Protocol
    Letter of acceptance of protocol from FDA
    Informed consent form
    Letter of approval of Institutional Review Board
    List of members of Institutional Review Board

  III. Clinical Study
    Summary of the study
    Details of the study
    Demographic characteristics of the subjects
    Subject assignment in the study
    Mean physical characteristics of subjects arranged by sequence
    Details of clinical activity
    Deviations from protocol
    Vital signs of subjects
    Adverse reactions report

  IV. Assay Methodology and Validation
    Assay method description
    Validation procedure
    Summary of validation
    Data on linearity of standard samples
    Data on interday precision and accuracy
    Data on intraday precision and accuracy
    Figure for standard curve(s) for low/high ranges
    Chromatograms of standard and quality control samples
    Sample calculation

  V. Pharmacokinetic Parameters and Tests
    Definition and calculations
    Statistical tests
    Drug levels at each sampling time and pharmacokinetic parameters
    Figure of mean plasma concentration–time profile
    Figures of individual subject plasma concentration–time profiles
    Figure of mean cumulative urinary excretion
    Figures of individual subject cumulative urinary excretion
    Figure of mean urinary excretion rates
    Fgures of individual subject urinary excretion rates
    Tables of individual subject data arranged by drug, drug/period, drug/sequence

  VI. Statistical Analyses
    Statistical considerations
    Summary of statistical significance
    Summary of statistical parameters
    Analysis of variance, least squares estimates, and least squares means
    Asessment of sequence, period, and treatment effects
    90% confidence intervals for the difference between test and reference products for the log-normal transformed parameters of $AUC_{0-t}$, $AUC_{0-\infty}$, and $C_{max}$ should be within 80% and 125%

  VII. Appendices
    Randomization schedule
    Sample identification codes
    Analytical raw data
    Chromatograms of at least 20% of subjects
    Medical record and clinical reports
    Clinical facilities description
    Analytical facilities description
    *Curricula* vitae of the investigators

  VIII. *In Vitro* Testing
    Dissolution testing
    Dissolution assay methodology
    Content uniformity testing
    Potency determination

  IX. Batch Size and Formulation
    Batch record
    Quantitative formulation

*Data from Dighe SV, Adams WP. Bioequivalence: A United States Regulatory Perspective. Pharmaceutical Bioequivalence. Volume 48 of Drugs and the Pharmaceutical Sciences. New York, NY: Mercel Dekker Inc; 1991.*

**TABLE 8-16 • General Elements of a Biopharmaceutics Review**

| Introduction | Summary and analysis of data |
|---|---|
| Study design | Comments |
| Study objective(s) | Deficiencies |
| Assay description and validation | Recommendation |

factors. For more details, the FDA's latest guidance for industry should be consulted. Various factors influence the bioavailability of the drug including release of the drug from the drug product including

droplet or drug particle sizes and distribution patterns within the nose (nasal spray) or trachea (inhalation product) that are dependent upon the drug substance, formulation, and device characteristics.

*Alcohol effects on MR drug products.* The consumption of alcoholic beverages can affect the release of a drug substance from an MR formulation. FDA recommends *in vitro* drug release studies to determine the potential for dose dumping in alcohol *in vivo. In vitro* assessments of the drug release from the drug product using media with various alcohol concentrations may be used.

*Endogenous substances.* Some drugs (eg, various hormones including estrogens, androgens, thyroxine, etc) are similar to endogenous substances

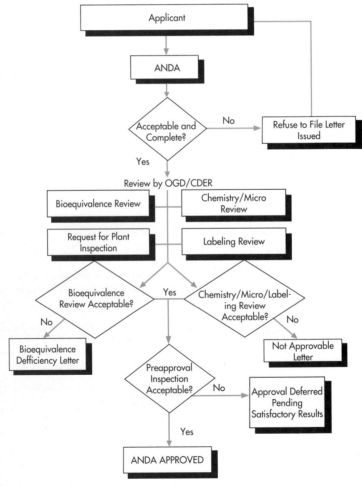

FIGURE 8-17 • Generic drug review process. (Reproduced with permission from Office of Generic Drugs, Center for Drug Evaluation & Research, US Food & Drug Administration.)

normally found in the body. FDA recommends that applicants measure and approximate the baseline endogenous levels in blood (plasma) and subtract these levels from the total concentrations measured from each subject after the drug product has been administered.

*Long-half-life drugs.* Adequate characterization of drugs with a long half-life (≥ 24 hours), should include blood sampling over a long period of time. For these drugs, an adequate washout period may be difficult. Therefore, a parallel design study may be used. $C_{max}$ and a truncated AUC can be used to characterize peak and total drug exposure, respectively. For drugs that demonstrate low intrasubject variability in distribution and clearance, a truncated AUC (eg, $AUC_{0-72}$ hr) can be used in place of $AUC_{0-t}$ or $AUC_{0-inf}$.

*Drug products with high intrasubject variability.* Highly variable drugs are drugs that have high intrasubject variability (≥30%). Various study designs may be considered for long-half-life drugs. One approach is an average BE study using replicate scaling. Another approach is the reference-scaled average bioequivalence approach which adjusts the bioequivalence limits of highly variable drugs by scaling to the within-subject variability of the reference product in the study. The FDA may be consulted for the most appropriate design of the bioequivalence study.

*Drug products with complex mixtures as the active ingredients.* Certain drug products may contain complex drug substances (ie, active moieties or active ingredients that are mixtures of multiple synthetic and/or natural source components). Some or all of the components of these complex drug substances may not be fully characterized with regard to chemical structure and/or biological activity. Quantification of all active or potentially active components in bioavailability and bioequivalence studies may not be possible. In such cases, FDA recommends that bioavailability and bioequivalence studies be based on a select number of components (FDA Guidance 2014).

## WAIVERS OF *IN VIVO* BIOEQUIVALENCE STUDIES (BIOWAIVERS)

*In vivo* bioequivalence studies may not be necessary for all drug products. In some cases, the FDA may waive the requirement for performing an *in vivo* bioequivalence study. For example, bioequivalence is self-evident based on certain characteristics of the drug product, such as a pure solution of the drug. However, the drug product will still need to meet certain *in vitro* comparison tests.

In some cases, bioequivalence studies *in vitro* dissolution testing may be used in lieu of *in vivo* bioequivalence studies. When the drug product is in the same dosage form but in different strengths and is proportionally similar in active and inactive ingredients, an *in vivo* bioequivalence study of one or more of the lower strengths can be waived based on the dissolution tests and an *in vivo* bioequivalence study on the highest strength. Ideally, if there is a strong correlation between dissolution of the drug and the bioavailability of the drug, then the comparative dissolution tests comparing the test product to the reference product should be sufficient to demonstrate bioequivalence. For most drug products, especially immediate-release tablets and capsules, no strong correlation exists, and the FDA requires an *in vivo* bioequivalence study. For oral solid dosage forms, an *in vivo* bioequivalence study may be required to support at least one dose strength of the product. Usually, an *in vivo* bioequivalence study is required for the highest dose strength. If the lower-dose-strength test product is substantially similar in active and inactive ingredients, then only a comparative *in vitro* dissolution between the test and brand-name formulations may be used.

For example, an immediate-release (IR) tablet is available in 200-mg, 100-mg, and 50-mg strengths. The 100- and 50-mg-strength tablets are made the same way as the highest-strength tablet. A human bioequivalence study is performed on the highest or 200-mg strength. Comparative *in vitro* dissolution studies are performed on the 100-mg and 50-mg dose strengths. If these drug products have no known bioavailability problems, are well absorbed systemically, are well correlated with *in vitro* dissolution, and have a large margin of safety, then arguments for not performing an *in vivo* bioavailability study may be valid. Methods for correlation of *in vitro* dissolution of the drug with *in vivo* drug bioavailability are discussed in Chapters 7 and 9. The manufacturer does not need to perform additional *in vivo* bioequivalence studies on the lower-strength products if the products meet all *in vitro* criteria.

## Regulatory Perspective for Biowaiver

The FDA permits the waiving of bioequivalence studies for products for which bioequivalence is self-evident. This includes solutions for parenteral, oral, or local use. There are generally additional criteria to be met before a biowaiver can be granted. Test and reference solutions intended for parenteral use should have the same active and inactive ingredients in the same amounts. The FDA generally refers to this as qualitative (Q1) and quantitative (Q2) sameness. Generic drug product solutions that are intended for oral or topical use can have different excipients than their corresponding RLD products but should not contain excipients that could potentially cause differences in drug substance absorption.

The FDA will consider granting biowaivers to non-biostudy strengths of a generic IR solid oral dosage form drug product line, provided that the following three criteria are met:

- An acceptable bioequivalence study is conducted on at least one strength.
- The strength(s) for which the biowaiver is sought should be proportionally similar to the strength on which bioequivalence was demonstrated.
- Acceptable *in vitro* dissolution should be demonstrated for the strength(s) for which the biowaiver is sought.

The FDA does not grant biowaivers for generic MR products, but may deem non-biostudy strength(s) bioequivalence to the corresponding biostudy strength(s) subject to certain criteria. This policy applies to all MR dosage forms, including but not limited to delayed-release tablets and capsules, extended-release tablets, transdermal products, and long-acting injectables (Davit et al, 2013).

## Dissolution Profile Comparisons

Comparative dissolution profiles are used as (1) the basis for formulation development of bioequivalent drug products and proceeding to the pivotal *in vivo* bioequivalence study (Chapter 15); (2) comparative dissolution profiles are used for demonstrating the equivalence of a change in the formulation of a drug product after the drug product has been approved for marketing (Chapters 26 and 27); and (3) the basis of a biowaiver of a lower-strength drug product that is dose proportional in active and inactive ingredients to the higher-strength drug product.

A model-independent mathematical method was developed by Moore and Flanner (1996) to compare dissolution profiles using two factors, $f_1$ and $f_2$. The factor $f_2$, known as the *similarity factor*, measures the closeness between the two profiles:

$$f_2 = 50 \times \log\left[\left(1 + \frac{1}{n}\sum_{t=1}^{n}(R_1 - T_1)^2\right)^{-0.5} \times 100\right]$$

where $n$ is the number of time points, $R_1$ is the dissolution value of the reference product at time $t$, and $T_1$ is the dissolution value of the test product batch at time $t$.

The reference may be the original drug product before a formulation change (prechange) and the test may be the drug product after the formulation was changed (postchange). Alternatively, the reference may be the higher-strength drug product and the test may be the lower-strength drug product. The $f_2$ comparison is the focus of several FDA guidances and is of regulatory interest in knowing the similarity of the two dissolution curves. When the two profiles are identical, $f_2 = 100$. An average difference of 10% at all measured time points results in an $f_2$ value of 50 (Shah et al, 1998). The FDA has set a public standard for $f_2$ value between 50 and 100 to indicate similarity between two dissolution profiles (US-FDA, CDER, 1997).

In some cases, two generic drug products may have dissimilar dissolution profiles and still be bioequivalent *in vivo*. For example, Polli et al (1997) have shown that slow-, medium-, and fast-dissolving formulations of metoprolol tartrate tablets were bioequivalent. Furthermore, bioequivalent MR drug products may have different drug release mechanisms and therefore different dissolution profiles. For example, for theophylline extended-release capsules, the *United States Pharmacopeia* (USP) lists 10 individual drug release tests for products labeled for dosing every 12 hours. However, only generic drug products that are FDA approved as bioequivalent drug products and listed in the current edition of the Orange Book may be substituted for each other.

**FREQUENTLY ASKED QUESTIONS**

▶ Why are preclinical animal toxicology studies and clinical efficacy drug studies in human subjects not required by the FDA to approve a generic drug product as a therapeutic equivalent to the brand-name drug product?

▶ Are bioequivalence studies needed for each dose strength of an oral drug product? For example, an oral drug product is commercially available in 200-mg, 100-mg, and 50-mg dose strengths.

## THE BIOPHARMACEUTICS CLASSIFICATION SYSTEM

The Biopharmaceutics Classification System (BCS) is a scientific framework for classifying drug substances based on their aqueous solubility and intestinal permeability. When combined with the dissolution of the drug product, the BCS takes into account three major factors that govern the rate and extent of drug absorption from IR solid oral dosage forms. These factors are dissolution, solubility, and intestinal permeability.

According to the BCS, drug substances are classified as follows:

- Class 1: high solubility–high permeability
- Class 2: low solubility–high permeability
- Class 3: high solubility–low permeability
- Class 4: low solubility–low permeability

A theoretical basis for correlating *in vitro* drug dissolution with *in vivo* bioavailability was developed by Amidon et al (1995). This approach is based on the aqueous solubility of the drug and the permeation of the drug through the GI tract. The classification system is based on Fick's first law applied to a membrane:

$$J_w = P_w C_w$$

where $J_w$ is the drug flux (mass/area/time) through the intestinal wall at any position and time, $P_w$ is the permeability of the membrane, and $C_w$ is the drug concentration at the intestinal membrane surface.

This approach assumes that no other components in the formulation affect the membrane permeability and/or intestinal transport. Using this approach, Amidon et al (1995) studied the solubility and permeability characteristics of various representative drugs and obtained a biopharmaceutic drug classification, BCS for predicting the *in vitro* drug dissolution of IR solid oral drug products with *in vivo* absorption.

The FDA may waive the requirement for performing an *in vivo* bioavailability or bioequivalence study for certain IR solid oral drug products that meet very specific criteria, namely, the permeability, solubility, and dissolution of the drug. These characteristics include the *in vitro* dissolution of the drug product in various media, drug permeability information, and assuming ideal behavior of the drug product, drug dissolution, and absorption in the GI tract. For regulatory purposes, drugs are classified according to the BCS in accordance with the solubility, permeability, and dissolution characteristics of the drug (US-FDA, CDER, 2000b).

### Solubility

An objective of the BCS approach is to determine the equilibrium solubility of a drug under approximate physiologic conditions. For this purpose, determination of pH–solubility profiles over a pH range of 1–8 is suggested. The solubility class is determined by calculating what volume of an aqueous medium is sufficient to dissolve the highest anticipated dose strength. A drug substance is considered highly soluble when the highest dose strength is soluble in 250 mL or less of aqueous medium over the pH range 1–8. The volume estimate of 250 mL is derived from typical bioequivalence study protocols that prescribe administration of a drug product to fasting human volunteers with a glass (8 oz) of water.

### Permeability

Studies of the extent of absorption in humans, or intestinal permeability methods, can be used to determine the permeability class membership of a drug. To be classified as highly permeable, a test drug should have an extent of absorption >90% in humans. Supportive information on permeability characteristics of the drug substance should also be derived from its physical–chemical properties (eg, octanol: water partition coefficient).

Some methods to determine the permeability of a drug from the GI tract include (1) *in vivo* intestinal perfusion studies in humans; (2) *in vivo* or *in situ* intestinal perfusion studies in animals; (3) *in vitro* permeation experiments using excised human or animal intestinal tissues; and (4) *in vitro* permeation experiments across a monolayer of cultured human intestinal cells. When using these methods, the experimental permeability data should correlate with the known extent-of-absorption data in humans.

After oral drug administration, *in vivo* permeability can be affected by the effects of efflux and absorptive transporters in the GI tract, by food, and possibly by the various excipients present in the formulation.

### Dissolution

The dissolution class is based on the *in vitro* dissolution rate of an IR drug product under specified test conditions and is intended to indicate rapid *in vivo* dissolution in relation to the average rate of gastric emptying in humans under fasting conditions. An IR drug product is considered rapidly dissolving when not less than 85% of the label amount of drug substance dissolves within 30 minutes using USP Apparatus I (Chapter 7) at 100 rpm or Apparatus II at 50 rpm in a volume of 900 mL or less in each of the following media: (1) acidic media such as 0.1 N HCl or simulated gastric fluid USP without enzymes, (2) a pH 4.5 buffer, and (3) a pH 6.8 buffer or simulated intestinal fluid USP without enzymes.

The FDA is in the process of revising the BCS guidance to permit biowaivers for generic formulations of Class 3 drugs (Mehta, 2014). Table 8-17 summarizes the recently proposed FDA criteria to be met for BCS biowaivers.

### Biopharmaceutics Drug Disposition Classification System

The major aspects of BCS are the consideration of solubility and permeation. According to BCS, permeability *in vivo* is considered high when the active drug is systemically absorbed ≥90%. Wu and Benet (2005) and Benet et al (2008) have proposed modification of the BCS system known as the *Biopharmaceutics Drug Disposition Classification System* (BDDCS), which takes into account drug metabolism (hepatic clearance) and transporters in the GI tract for drugs that are orally administered. For BCS 1 drugs (ie, high solubility and high permeability), transporter effects will be minimal. However, for BCS 2 drugs (low solubility and high permeability), transporter effects are more important. These investigators suggest that the BCS should be modified on the basis of the extent of

**TABLE 8-17** • Criteria Proposed by FDA for Consideration of BCS-Based Biowaivers of Immediate-Release Generic Drug Products

| BCS Class 1 | | | |
|---|---|---|---|
| **Highly Soluble** | **Oral Bioavailability** | **Dissolution** | **Criteria on Excipients** |
| Highest strength, over range of pH 1.0–6.8 | ≥85% | • ≥85% in 30 minutes at pH 1.0, 4.5, 6.8 ("rapidly dissolving")<br>• Volume = 500 mL<br>• Paddles at 50 rpm, or basket at 100 rpm | • Test and reference should be pharmaceutical equivalents<br>• Test and reference should not differ in amounts of excipients known to affect bioavailability |
| **BCS Class 3** | | | |
| **Highly Soluble** | **Oral Bioavailability** | **Dissolution** | **Criteria on Excipients** |
| Highest strength, over range of pH 1.0–6.8 | <85% | • ≥85% in 15 minutes at pH 1.0, 4.5, 6.8 ("very rapidly dissolving")<br>• Volume = 500 mL<br>• Paddles at 50 rpm, or basket at 100 rpm | • Test and reference should be pharmaceutical equivalents<br>• Test and reference formulations should be Q1 and Q2 the same |

drug metabolism, overall drug disposition, including routes of drug elimination and the effects of efflux, and absorptive transporters on oral drug absorption.

### Drug Products for Which Bioavailability or Bioequivalence May Be Self-Evident

The best measure of a drug product's performance is to determine the *in vivo* bioavailability of the drug. For some well-characterized drug products and for certain drug products in which bioavailability is self-evident (eg, sterile solutions for injection), *in vivo* bioavailability studies may be unnecessary or unimportant to the achievement of the product's intended purposes. The FDA will waive the requirement for submission of *in vivo* evidence demonstrating the bioavailability of the drug product if the product meets one of the following criteria (US-FDA, CDER, 2014a). However, there may be specific requirements for certain drug products, and the appropriate FDA division should be consulted.

1. The drug product (a) is a solution intended solely for IV administration and (b) contains an active drug ingredient or therapeutic moiety combined with the same solvent and in the same concentration as in an intravenous solution that is the subject of an approved, full NDA.

2. The drug product is a topically applied preparation (eg, a cream, ointment, or gel intended for local therapeutic effect). The FDA has released guidances for the performance of bioequivalence studies on topical corticosteroids and antifungal agents. The FDA is also considering performing dermatopharmacokinetic (DPK) studies on other topical drug products. In addition, *in vitro* drug release and diffusion studies may be required.

3. The drug product is in an oral dosage form that is not intended to be absorbed (eg, an antacid or a radiopaque medium). Specific *in vitro* bioequivalence studies may be required by the FDA. For example, the bioequivalence of cholestyramine resin is demonstrated *in vitro* by the binding of bile acids to the resin.

4. The drug product meets both of the following conditions:

    a. It is administered by inhalation as a gas or vapor (eg, as a medicinal or as an inhalation anesthetic).

    b. It contains an active drug ingredient or therapeutic moiety in the same dosage form as a drug product that is the subject of an approved, full NDA.

5. The drug product meets all of the following conditions:

    a. It is an oral solution, elixir, syrup, tincture, or similar other solubilized form.

    b. It contains an active drug ingredient or therapeutic moiety in the same concentration as a drug product that is the subject of an approved, full NDA.

    c. It contains no inactive ingredient that is known to significantly affect absorption of the active drug ingredient or therapeutic moiety.

## GENERIC BIOLOGICS (BIOSIMILAR DRUG PRODUCTS)

*Biologics*, or biotechnology-derived drugs, in contrast to drugs that are chemically synthesized, are derived from living sources such as humans, animals, or microorganisms. Many biologics are complex mixtures that are not easily identified or characterized and are manufactured using biotechnology or are purified from natural sources. Other biological drugs, such as insulin and growth hormone, are proteins derived by biotechnology and have been well characterized. Advances in analytical sciences (both physicochemical and biological) enable some protein products to be characterized extensively in terms of their physicochemical and biological properties. These analytical procedures have improved the ability to identify and characterize not only the desired product but also product-related substances and product- and process-related impurities. Advances in manufacturing science and production methods may enhance the likelihood that a product will be highly similar to another product by better targeting the original product's physiochemical and functional properties.

The assessment of biosimilarity between a proposed biosimilar product and its reference product involves the robust characterization of the proposed biosimilar product, including comparative physicochemical and functional studies. The FDA recommends the following factors that must be considered in assessing whether products are highly similar (US-FDA, CDER, 2014g).

- *Expression system*: Therapeutic protein products can be produced by microbial cells (prokaryotic, eukaryotic), cell lines of human or animal origin (eg, mammalian, avian, insect), or tissues derived from animals or plants. It is expected that the expression construct for a proposed biosimilar product will encode the same primary amino acid sequence as its reference product.

- *Manufacturing process*: A comprehensive understanding of all steps in the manufacturing process for the proposed biosimilar product should be established during product development.

- *Assessment of physicochemical properties*: Physicochemical assessment of the proposed biosimilar product and the reference product should consider all relevant characteristics of the protein product (eg, the primary, secondary, tertiary, and quaternary structure, post-translational modifications, and functional activity[ies]). The objective of this assessment is to maximize the potential for detecting differences in quality attributes between the proposed biosimilar product and the reference product.

- *Functional activities*: Functional assays serve multiple purposes in the characterization of protein products. These tests act to complement physicochemical analyses and are a quality measure of the function of the protein product.

- *Receptor binding and immunochemical properties*: When binding or immunochemical properties are part of the activity attributed to the protein product, analytical tests should be performed to characterize the product in terms of these specific properties.

- *Impurities*: The applicant should characterize, identify, and quantify impurities (product and process related) in the proposed biosimilar product and the reference product.

- *Reference product and reference standards*: A thorough physicochemical and biological assessment of the reference product should provide a base of information from which to develop the proposed biosimilar product and justify reliance on certain existing scientific knowledge about the reference product.

- *Finished drug product*: Product characterization studies should be performed on the most downstream intermediate best suited for the analytical procedures used.

- *Stability*: An appropriate physicochemical and functional comparison of the stability of the proposed biosimilar product with that of the reference product should be initiated including accelerated and stress stability studies, or forced degradation studies.

The foundation for an assessment of biosimilarity between a proposed biosimilar product and its reference product involves the robust characterization of the proposed biosimilar product, including comparative physicochemical and functional studies.

## Biosimilarity Versus Interchangeability

The Patient Protection and Affordable Care Act of 2010 contains provisions that establish an abbreviated regulatory approval pathway for generic versions of biological medicines (ie, biosimilars). The new legislation establishes two distinct categories of biosimilar products: (1) biological products that are "biosimilar" to a reference biological product, and (2) biological products that are "interchangeable" with the reference product.

*Biosimilar biological drug products* are biological products that are highly similar to the reference product notwithstanding minor differences in clinically inactive components. In addition, there are no clinically meaningful differences between the biological product and the reference product in terms of the safety, purity, and potency of the product.

*Interchangeable biological drug products* are biological products that are interchangeable with a reference biological product if (1) it meets the criteria for being biosimilar to the reference product, (2) it can be expected to produce the same clinical result as the reference product in any given patient, and (3) the risk in terms of safety or diminished efficacy in alternating or switching between use of the biological and reference product is not greater than the risk of using the reference product without such alteration or switch.

FDA determination of biosimilar drug products is based on the totality of the evidence provided by a sponsor to support a demonstration of biosimilarity. The FDA recommends that sponsors use a stepwise approach in their development of biosimilar products. FDA regulatory approval of a biosimilar drug product is based on a stepwise approach that includes a comparison of the proposed product and the reference product including:

- Analytical studies that demonstrate that the biological product is highly similar to the reference product notwithstanding minor differences in clinically inactive components
- Animal studies (including the assessment of toxicity)
- Clinical study or studies (including the assessment of immunogenicity and pharmacokinetics or pharmacodynamics) that are sufficient to demonstrate safety, purity, and potency

Biosimilars and interchangeable biotechnology-derived drugs will be considered on a case-by-case basis. After FDA approval, the manufacturer must provide robust postmarketing safety monitoring as an important component in ensuring the safety and effectiveness of biological products.

### FDA Guidance Documents

The legislation makes clear that the FDA will play a central role in defining the specific criteria needed to demonstrate biosimilarity for a given class of biological. In deference to the FDA's expertise in this area, the legislation specifically states that the FDA can issue guidance documents with respect to the approval of a biosimilar product. The guidance can be general or specific in nature, and the public must be provided with an opportunity to comment.

Advocates for the manufacture of generic biologics argue that bioequivalent biotechnology-derived drug products can be made on a case-by-case basis. Those opposed to the development of generic biologics or biosimilar drug products have claimed that generic manufacturers do not have the ability to fully characterize the active ingredient(s), that immunogenicity-related impurities may be present in the product, and that the manufacture of a biologic drug product is process dependent. Several biosimilar drug products have been approved in Europe. Currently, there are several applications for biosimilar drug products under review by the FDA. In the United States, FDA regulatory approval is based on a stepwise approach that includes a comparison of the proposed product and the reference product with respect to structure, function, animal toxicity, human PK and PD, clinical immunogenicity, and clinical safety and effectiveness.

### CLINICAL SIGNIFICANCE OF BIOEQUIVALENCE STUDIES

Bioequivalence of different formulations of the same drug substance involves equivalence with respect to the rate and extent of systemic drug absorption. Clinical interpretation is important in evaluating the results of a bioequivalence study. A small difference between drug products, even if statistically significant, may produce very little difference in therapeutic response. Generally, two formulations whose rate and extent of absorption differ by 20% or less are considered bioequivalent. The Report by the Bioequivalence Task Force (1988) considered that differences of less than 20% in AUC and $C_{max}$ between drug products are "unlikely to be clinically significant in patients." The Task Force further stated that "clinical studies of effectiveness have difficulty detecting differences in doses of even 50%–100%." Therefore, normal variation is observed in medical practice and plasma drug levels may vary among individuals greater than 20%.

According to Westlake (1973), a small, statistically significant difference in drug bioavailability from two or more dosage forms may be detected if the study is well controlled and the number of subjects is sufficiently large. When the therapeutic objectives of the drug are considered, an equivalent clinical response should be obtained from the comparison dosage forms if the plasma drug concentrations remain above the minimum effective concentration (MEC) for an appropriate interval and do not reach the minimum toxic concentration (MTC). Therefore, the investigator must consider whether any statistical difference in bioavailability would alter clinical efficiency.

Special populations, such as the elderly or patients on drug therapy, are generally not used for bioequivalence studies. Normal, healthy volunteers are preferred for bioequivalence studies, because these subjects are less at risk and may more easily endure the discomforts of the study, such as blood sampling. Furthermore, the objective of these studies is to evaluate the bioavailability of the drug from the dosage form, and use of healthy subjects should minimize both inter- and intrasubject variability. It is theoretically possible that the excipients in one of the dosage forms tested may pose a problem in a patient who uses the generic dosage form.

For the manufacture of a dosage form, specifications are set to provide uniformity of dosage forms. With proper specifications, quality control procedures should minimize product-to-product variability by different manufacturers and lot-to-lot variability with a single manufacturer (see Chapter 27).

## EXAMPLE ▷ ▷ ▷

### IMPACT OF EFFLUX TRANSPORTERS ON BIOEQUIVALENCE STUDY

Digoxin is a drug that may be absorbed differently in individuals that expressed the efflux gene MDR1.

### Questions
- What would be the impact of such an individual recruited into a bioavailability study?
- Would a protocol with the usual crossover design be able to adequately evaluate the bioequivalence of a generic digoxin product with a reference? Explain why or why not.

### Solution

Bioequivalence studies for generic drug products compare the bioavailability of the drug from the test (generic) product to the bioavailability of the drug from the reference (brand) product. The study design is a two-way, crossover design in which each subject takes each drug product. The study design usually includes males and females with different ethnic backgrounds. In addition, some studies include both smokers and non-smokers. Although there may be large intersubject variability due to gender, environmental, and genetic factors, the crossover design minimizes intrasubject variability by comparing the bioavailability of test and reference products in the same individual. Thus each individual subject should have similar drug absorption characteristics after taking the test or reference drug products.[10]

---

[10]For a few drug products, a high intrasubject variability (>30% CV) may be observed for which the bioavailability response changes for the same drug product each time the drug is dosed in the same subject.

## SPECIAL CONCERNS IN BIOAVAILABILITY AND BIOEQUIVALENCE STUDIES

The general bioequivalence study designs and evaluation, such as the comparison of AUC, $C_{max}$, and $t_{max}$, may be used for systemically absorbed drugs and conventional oral dosage forms. However, for certain drugs and dosage forms, systemic bioavailability and bioequivalence are difficult to ascertain (Table 8-18). Drugs and drug products (eg, cyclosporine, chlorpromazine, verapamil, isosorbide dinitrate, sulindac)

| TABLE 8-18 • Issues in Establishing in Bioavailability and Bioequivalence |
|---|
| Drugs with high intrasubject variability |
| Drugs with long elimination half-life |
| Biotransformation of drugs |
|    Stereoselective drug metabolism |
|    Drugs with active metabolites |
|    Drugs with polymorphic metabolism |
| Nonbioavailable drugs (drugs intended for local effect) |
|    Antacids |
|    Local anesthetics |
|    Anti-infectives |
|    Anti-inflammatory steroids |
| Dosage forms for nonoral administration |
|    Transdermal |
|    Inhalation |
|    Ophthalmic |
|    Intranasal |
| Bioavailable drugs that should not produce peak drug levels |
|    Potassium supplements |
| Endogenous drug levels |
|    Hormone replacement therapy |
| Biotechnology-derived drugs |
|    Erythropoietin interferon |
|    Protease inhibitors |
| Complex drug substances |
|    Conjugated estrogens |

are considered to be highly variable if the intrasubject variability in bioavailability parameters is greater than 30% by analysis of variance coefficient of variation (Shah et al, 1996). The number of subjects required to demonstrate bioequivalence for these drug products may be excessive, requiring more than 60 subjects to meet current FDA bioequivalence criteria. The intrasubject variability may be due to the drug itself or to the drug formulation or to both. The FDA has held public forums to determine whether the current bioequivalence guidelines need to be changed for these highly variable drugs (Davit et al, 2012).

For drugs with very long elimination half-lives or a complex elimination phase, a complete plasma drug concentration–time curve (ie, three elimination half-lives or an AUC representing 90% of the total AUC) may be difficult to obtain for a bioequivalence study using a crossover design. For these drugs, a truncated (shortened) plasma drug concentration–time curve (0–72 hours) may be more practical. The use of a truncated plasma drug concentration–time curve allows for the measurement of peak absorption and decreases the time and cost for performing the bioequivalence study.

Many drugs are stereoisomers, and each isomer may give a different pharmacodynamic response and may have a different rate of biotransformation. The bioavailability of the individual isomers may be difficult to measure because of problems in analysis. Some drugs have active metabolites, which should be quantitated as well as the parent drug. Drugs such as thioridazine and selegiline have two active metabolites. The question for such drugs is whether bioequivalence should be proven by matching the bioavailability of both metabolites and the parent drug. Assuming both biotransformation pathways

follow first-order reaction kinetics, then the metabolites should be in constant ratio to the parent drug. Genetic variation in metabolism may present a bioequivalence problem. For example, the acetylation of procainamide to *N*-acetylprocainamide demonstrates genetic polymorphism, with two groups of subjects consisting of rapid acetylators and slow acetylators. To decrease intersubject variability, a bioequivalence study may be performed on only one phenotype, such as the rapid acetylators.

Some drugs (eg, benzocaine, hydrocortisone, anti-infectives, antacids) are intended for local effect and formulated as topical ointments, oral suspensions, or rectal suppositories. These drugs should not have significant systemic bioavailability from the site of administration. The bioequivalence determination for drugs that are not absorbed systemically from the site of application can be difficult to assess. For these nonsystemic-absorbable drugs, a "surrogate" marker is needed for bioequivalence determination (Table 8-19). For example, the acid-neutralizing capacity of an oral antacid and the binding of bile acids to cholestyramine resin have been used as surrogate markers in lieu of *in vivo* bioequivalence studies.

Various drug delivery systems and newer dosage forms are designed to deliver the drug by a nonoral route, which may produce only partial systemic bioavailability. For the treatment of asthma, inhalation of the drug (eg, albuterol, beclomethasone dipropionate) has been used to maximize drug in the respiratory passages and to decrease systemic side effects. Drugs such as nitroglycerin given transdermally may differ in release rates, in the amount of drug in the transdermal delivery system, and in the surface area of the skin to which the transdermal

## TABLE 8-19 • Possible Surrogate Markers for Bioequivalence Studies

| Drug Product | Drug | Possible Surrogate Marker for Bioequivalence |
|---|---|---|
| Metered-dose inhaler | Albuterol | Forced expiratory volume ($FEV_1$) |
| Topical steroid | Hydrocortisone | Skin blanching |
| Anion-exchange resin | Cholestyramine | Binding to bile acids |
| Antacid | Magnesium and aluminum hydroxide gel | Neutralization of acid |
| Topical antifungal | Ketoconazole | Drug uptake into stratum corneum |

delivery system is applied. Thus, the determination of bioequivalence among different manufacturers of transdermal delivery systems for the same active drug is difficult. Dermatopharmacokinetic studies investigate drug uptake into skin layers after topical drug administration. The drug is applied topically, the skin is peeled at various time periods after the dose, using transparent tape, and the drug concentrations in the skin are measured.

Drugs such as potassium supplements are given orally and may not produce the usual bioavailability parameters of AUC, $C_{max}$, and $t_{max}$. For these drugs, more indirect methods must be used to ascertain bioequivalence. For example, urinary potassium excretion parameters are more appropriate for the measurement of bioavailability of potassium supplements. However, for certain hormonal replacement drugs (eg, levothyroxine), the steady-state hormone concentration in hypothyroid individuals, the thyroidal-stimulating hormone level, and pharmacodynamic endpoints may also be appropriate to measure.

## GENERIC SUBSTITUTION

Drug product selection and generic drug product substitution are major responsibilities for physicians, pharmacists, and others who prescribe, dispense, or purchase drugs. To facilitate such decisions, the FDA publishes annually, in print and on the Internet, *Approved Drug Products with Therapeutic Equivalence Evaluations*, also known as the Orange Book (www.fda.gov/cder/ob/default.htm). The Orange Book identifies drug products approved on the basis of safety and effectiveness by the FDA and contains therapeutic equivalence evaluations for approved multisource prescription drug products. These evaluations serve as public information and advice to state health agencies, prescribers, and pharmacists to promote public education in the area of drug product selection and to foster containment of healthcare costs.

To contain drug costs, most states have adopted generic substitution laws to allow pharmacists to dispense a generic drug product for a brand-name drug product that has been prescribed. Some states have adopted a *positive formulary*, which lists therapeutically equivalent or interchangeable drug products that pharmacists may dispense. Other states use

a *negative formulary*, which lists drug products that are not therapeutically equivalent, and/or the interchange of which is prohibited. If the drug is not in the negative formulary, the unlisted generic drug products are assumed to be therapeutically equivalent and may be interchanged.

### Approved Drug Products with Therapeutic Equivalence Evaluations (Orange Book)

The Orange Book contains therapeutic equivalence evaluations for approved drug products made by various manufacturers. These marketed drug products are evaluated according to specific criteria. The evaluation codes used for these drugs are listed in Table 8-20. The drug products are divided into two major categories: "A" codes apply to drug products considered to be therapeutically equivalent to other pharmaceutically equivalent products, and "B" codes apply to drug products that the FDA, at this time, does not consider to be therapeutically equivalent to other pharmaceutically equivalent products. A list of therapeutic-equivalence-related terms and their definitions are also given in the monograph. FDA evaluations provide public information and do not mandate drugs to be prescribed. The FDA evaluation of the drug products should be used as a guide only, with the practitioner exercising professional care and judgment.

The concept of therapeutic equivalence as used to develop the Orange Book applies only to drug products containing the same active ingredient(s) and does not encompass a comparison of different therapeutic agents used for the same condition (eg, amoxicillin versus ampicillin for the treatment of an infection). Any drug product in the Orange Book that is repackaged and/or distributed by other than the application holder is considered to be therapeutically equivalent to the application holder's drug product even if the application holder's drug product is single source or coded as nonequivalent (eg, BN). Also, distributors or repackagers of an application holder's drug product are considered to have the same code as the application holder. Therapeutic equivalence determinations are not made for unapproved, off-label indications. With this limitation, however, the FDA believes that products classified as therapeutically equivalent can be substituted with

## TABLE 8-20 • Therapeutic Equivalence Evaluation Codes

### A Codes

Drug products considered to be therapeutically equivalent to other pharmaceutically equivalent products

| | |
|---|---|
| AA | Products in conventional dosage forms not presenting bioequivalence problems |
| AB | Products meeting bioequivalence requirements |
| AN | Solutions and powders for aerosolization |
| AO | Injectable oil solutions |
| AP | Injectable aqueous solutions |
| AT | Topical products |

### B Codes

Drug products that the FDA does not consider to be therapeutically equivalent to other pharmaceutically equivalent products

| | |
|---|---|
| B* | Drug products requiring further FDA investigation and review to determine therapeutic equivalence |
| BC | Extended-release tablets, extended-release capsules, and extended-release injectables |
| BD | Active ingredients and dosage forms with documented bioequivalence problems |
| BE | Delayed-release oral dosage forms |
| BN | Products in aerosol–nebulizer drug delivery systems |
| BP | Active ingredients and dosage forms with potential bioequivalence problems |
| BR | Suppositories or enemas for systemic use |
| BS | Products having drug standard deficiencies |
| BT | Topical products with bioequivalence issues |
| BX | Insufficient data |

*Adapted with permission from Approved Drug Products with Therapeutic Equivalence Evaluations (Orange Book), 2003.*

the full expectation that the substituted product will produce the same clinical effect and safety profile as the prescribed product (www.fda.gov/cder/ob/default.htm).

Professional care and judgment should be exercised in using the Orange Book. Evaluations of therapeutic equivalence for prescription drugs are based on scientific and medical evaluations by the FDA. Products evaluated as therapeutically equivalent can be expected, in the judgment of the FDA, to have equivalent clinical effect and no difference in their potential for adverse effects when used under the conditions of their labeling. However, these products may differ in other characteristics such as shape, scoring configuration, release mechanisms, packaging, excipients (including colors, flavors, preservatives), expiration date/time, and, in some instances, labeling. If products with such differences are substituted for each other, there is a potential for patient confusion due to differences in color or shape of tablets, inability to provide a given dose using a partial tablet if the proper scoring configuration is not available, or decreased patient acceptance of certain products because of flavor. There may also be better stability of one product over another under adverse storage conditions or allergic reactions in rare cases due to a coloring or a preservative ingredient, as well as differences in cost to the patient.

FDA evaluation of therapeutic equivalence in no way relieves practitioners of their professional responsibilities in prescribing and dispensing such products with due care and with appropriate information to individual patients. In those circumstances where the characteristics of a specific product, other

**TABLE 8-21** • Nifedipine Extended-Release Oral Tablet

| TE Code | RLD | Active Ingredient | Dosage Form; Route | Strength | Proprietary Name | Applicant |
|---------|-----|-------------------|---------------------|----------|------------------|-----------|
| AB1 | Yes | Nifedipine tablet | Extended release; oral | 90 mg | **Adalat CC** | Bayer Healthcare |
| AB1 | No | Nifedipine tablet | Extended release; oral | 90 mg | Nifedipine | Actavis |
| AB1 | No | Nifedipine tablet | Extended release; oral | 90 mg | Nifedipine | Valeant Intl |
| AB2 | Yes | Nifedipine tablet | Extended release; oral | 90 mg | **Procardia XL** | Pfizer |
| AB2 | No | Nifedipine tablet | Extended release; oral | 90 mg | Nifedipine | Mylan |
| AB2 | No | Nifedipine tablet | Extended release; oral | 90 mg | Nifedipine | Osmotica Pharm |

TE = therapeutic equivalent.
Adapted with permission from Approved Drug Products with Therapeutic Equivalence Evaluations (Orange Book), 2003.

than its active ingredient, are important in the therapy of a particular patient, the physician's specification of that product is appropriate. Pharmacists must also be familiar with the expiration dates/times and labeling directions for storage of the different products, particularly for reconstituted products, to assure that patients are properly advised when one product is substituted for another.

## EXAMPLE ▷ ▷ ▷

### INTERPRETATION OF THERAPEUTIC EVALUATION CODE FOR NIFEDIPINE EXTENDED-RELEASE TABLETS

The FDA has approved a few drug products containing the same active drug from different pharmaceutical manufacturers, each of which has provided a separate New Drug Application (NDA) for its own product. Since no information is available to demonstrate whether the two NDA-approved drug products are bioequivalent, each branded drug product becomes a separate RLD (Table 8-21). Generic drug manufacturers must demonstrate to which RLD product is bioequivalent.

In Table 8-21, AB1 products are bioequivalent to each other and can be substituted. AB2 products are bioequivalent to each other and can be substituted. However, an AB1 product cannot be substituted for an AB2 product.

### GLOSSARY[11]

**Abbreviated New Drug Application (ANDA):** Drug manufacturers must file an ANDA for approval to market a generic drug product. The generic manufacturer is not required to perform clinical efficacy studies or nonclinical toxicology studies for the ANDA.

**Bioavailability:** Bioavailability means the rate and extent to which the active ingredient or active moiety is absorbed from a drug product and becomes available at the site of action. For drug products that are not intended to be absorbed into the bloodstream, bioavailability may be assessed by measurements intended to

---

[11]The definitions are from *Approved Drug Products with Therapeutic Equivalence Evaluations* (*Orange Book*). [www.fda.gov/Drugs/InformationOnDrugs/ucm129662.htm], Code of Federal Regulations, 21 CFR 320, and other sources.

reflect the rate and extent to which the active ingredient or active moiety becomes available at the site of action.

**Bioequivalence requirement:** A requirement imposed by the FDA for *in vitro* and/or *in vivo* testing of specified drug products, which must be satisfied as a condition for marketing.

**Bioequivalent drug products:** This term describes pharmaceutical equivalent or pharmaceutical alternative products that display comparable bioavailability when studied under similar experimental conditions. For systemically absorbed drugs, the test (generic) and RLD (brand name) shall be considered bioequivalent if (1) the rate and extent of absorption of the test drug do not show a significant difference from the rate and extent of absorption of the reference drug when administered at the same molar dose of the therapeutic ingredient under similar experimental conditions in either a single dose or multiple doses or (2) the extent of absorption of the test drug does not show a significant difference from the extent of absorption of the reference drug when administered at the same molar dose of the therapeutic ingredient under similar experimental conditions in either a single dose or multiple doses and the difference from the reference drug in the rate of absorption of the drug is intentional, is reflected in its proposed labeling, is not essential to the attainment of effective body drug concentrations on chronic use, and is considered medically insignificant for the drug.

When the above methods are not applicable (eg, for drug products that are not intended to be absorbed into the bloodstream), other *in vivo* or *in vitro* test methods to demonstrate bioequivalence may be appropriate. Bioequivalence may sometimes be demonstrated using an *in vitro* bioequivalence standard, especially when such an *in vitro* test has been correlated with human *in vivo* bioavailability data. In other situations, bioequivalence may sometimes be demonstrated through comparative clinical trials or pharmacodynamic studies.

Bioequivalent drug products may contain different inactive ingredients, provided the manufacturer identifies the differences and provides information that the differences do not affect the safety or efficacy of the product.

**Biosimilar or biosimilarity:** The biological product is highly similar to the reference product notwithstanding minor differences in clinically inactive components, and there are no clinically meaningful differences between the biological product and the reference product in terms of the safety, purity, and potency of the product.

**Brand name:** The trade name of the drug. This name is privately owned by the manufacturer or distributor and is used to distinguish the specific drug product from competitor's products (eg, Tylenol, McNeil Laboratories).

**Chemical name:** The name used by organic chemists to indicate the chemical structure of the drug (eg, *N*-acetyl-*p*-aminophenol).

**Drug product:** The finished dosage form (eg, tablet, capsule, or solution) that contains the active drug ingredient, generally, but not necessarily, in association with inactive ingredients.

**Drug product performance:** Drug product performance, *in vivo*, may be defined as the release of the drug substance from the drug product, leading to bioavailability of the drug substance and leading to a pharmacodynamic response. Bioequivalence studies are drug product performance tests.

**Drug product selection:** The process of choosing or selecting the drug product in a specified dosage form.

**Drug substance:** A drug substance is the active pharmaceutical ingredient (API) or component in the drug product that furnishes the pharmacodynamic activity.

**Equivalence:** Relationship in terms of bioavailability, therapeutic response, or a set of established standards of one drug product to another.

**Generic name:** The established, nonproprietary, or common name of the active drug in a drug product (eg, acetaminophen).

**Generic substitution:** The process of dispensing a different brand or an unbranded drug product in place of the prescribed drug product. The substituted drug product contains the same active ingredient or therapeutic moiety as the same salt or ester in the same dosage form but is made by a different manufacturer. For example, a prescription for Motrin brand of ibuprofen might be dispensed by the pharmacist as Advil brand of ibuprofen or as a nonbranded generic ibuprofen if generic substitution is permitted and desired by the physician.

**Pharmaceutical alternatives:** Drug products that contain the same therapeutic moiety but as different salts, esters, or complexes. For example, tetracycline phosphate and tetracycline hydrochloride equivalent to 250-mg tetracycline base are considered pharmaceutical alternatives. Different dosage forms and strengths within a product line by a single manufacturer are pharmaceutical alternatives (eg, an extended-release dosage form and a standard immediate-release dosage form of the same active ingredient). The FDA currently considers a tablet and capsule containing the same active ingredient in the same dosage strength as pharmaceutical alternatives.

**Pharmaceutical equivalents:** Drug products in identical dosage forms that contain the same active ingredient(s), that is, the same salt or ester, are of the same dosage form, use the same route of administration, and are identical in strength or concentration (eg, chlordiazepoxide hydrochloride, 5-mg capsules). Pharmaceutically equivalent drug products are formulated to contain the same amount of active ingredient in the same dosage form and to meet the same or compendial or other applicable standards (ie, strength, quality, purity, and identity), but they may differ in characteristics such as shape, scoring configuration, release mechanisms, packaging, excipients (including colors, flavors, preservatives), expiration time, and, within certain limits, labeling. When applicable, pharmaceutical equivalents must meet the same content uniformity, disintegration times, and/or dissolution rates. Modified-release dosage forms that require a reservoir or overage or certain dosage forms such as prefilled syringes in which residual volume may vary must deliver identical amounts of active drug ingredient over an identical dosing period.

**Pharmaceutical substitution:** The process of dispensing a pharmaceutical alternative for the prescribed drug product. For example, ampicillin suspension is dispensed in place of ampicillin capsules, or tetracycline hydrochloride is dispensed in place of tetracycline phosphate. Pharmaceutical substitution generally requires the physician's approval.

**Reference listed drug:** The reference listed drug (RLD) is identified by the FDA as the drug product on which an applicant relies when seeking approval of an ANDA. The RLD is generally the brand-name drug that has a full NDA. The FDA designates a single RLD as the standard to which all generic versions must be shown to be bioequivalent. The FDA hopes to avoid possible significant variations among generic drugs and their brand-name counterparts. Such variations could result if generic drugs were compared to different RLDs.

**Therapeutic alternatives:** Drug products containing different active ingredients that are indicated for the same therapeutic or clinical objectives. Active ingredients in therapeutic alternatives are from the same pharmacologic class and are expected to have the same therapeutic effect when administered to patients for such condition of use. For example, ibuprofen is given instead of aspirin; cimetidine may be given instead of ranitidine.

**Therapeutic equivalents:** Drug products are considered to be therapeutic equivalents only if they are pharmaceutical equivalents and if they can be expected to have the same clinical effect and safety profile when administered to patients under the conditions specified in the labeling. The FDA classifies as therapeutically equivalent those products that meet the following general criteria: (1) they are approved as safe and effective; (2) they are pharmaceutical equivalents in that they (a) contain identical amounts of the same active drug ingredient in the same dosage form and route of administration, and (b) meet compendial or other applicable standards of strength, quality, purity, and identity; (3) they are bioequivalent in that (a) they do not present a known or potential bioequivalence problem, and they meet an acceptable *in vitro* standard, or (b) if they do present such a known or potential problem, they are shown to meet an appropriate bioequivalence standard; (4) they are adequately labeled; and (5) they are manufactured in compliance with Current Good Manufacturing Practice regulations. The FDA believes that products classified as therapeutically equivalent can be substituted with the full expectation that the substituted product will produce the same clinical effect and safety profile as the prescribed product.

**Therapeutic substitution:** The process of dispensing a therapeutic alternative in place of the prescribed drug product. For example, amoxicillin is dispensed instead of ampicillin or ibuprofen is dispensed instead of naproxen. Therapeutic substitution can also occur when one NDA-approved drug is substituted for the same drug that has been approved by a different NDA, for example, the substitution of Nicoderm (nicotine transdermal system) for Nicotrol (nicotine transdermal system).

---

**FREQUENTLY ASKED QUESTIONS**

▶ Can pharmaceutic equivalent drug products that are not bioequivalent have similar clinical efficacy?

▶ What is the difference between generic substitution and therapeutic substitution?

---

## CHAPTER SUMMARY

Drug product performance may be defined as the release of the drug substance from the drug product leading to bioavailability of the drug substance. Bioequivalence is a relative bioavailability study and is a measure of comparative drug product performance *in vivo*. Bioavailability studies relate the quality of a drug product to clinical safety and efficacy. The absolute availability of drug is the systemic availability of a drug estimated by comparing the extravascular administration (eg, oral, rectal, transdermal, subcutaneous) compared to IV dosing. Relative bioavailability compares the bioavailability of a drug from two or more drug products. The most direct method to assess drug bioavailability is to determine the rate and extent of systemic drug absorption by measurement of the active drug concentrations in plasma. The main pharmacokinetic parameters, $C_{max}$ and AUC, are used to determine bioequivalence. However, other pharmacokinetic parameters such as $t_{max}$ and elimination $t_{1/2}$ should also be assessed. The most common statistical design for bioequivalence studies is the two-way, crossover design in normal healthy volunteers. Bioequivalence is generally determined if the 90% confidence intervals for $C_{max}$ and AUC fall within 80%–125% of the reference listed drug based on log transformation of the data. Food intervention or food effect studies are generally conducted using meal conditions that are expected to provide the greatest effects on GI physiology so that systemic drug availability is maximally affected. The Biopharmaceutics Classification System (BCS) is based on the solubility, permeability, and dissolution characteristics of the drug. However, systemic drug bioavailability may also be affected by transporters in the GI tract, hepatic clearance, GI transit and motility, and the contents of the GI tract.

Drug product selection and generic substitution are important responsibilities of the pharmacist. A listing of approved drug products of generic drug products that may be safely substituted is available in *Approved Drug Products with Therapeutic Equivalence Evaluations* (Orange Book).

## LEARNING QUESTIONS

1. An antibiotic was formulated into two different oral dosage forms, A and B. Biopharmaceutic studies revealed different antibiotic blood level curves for each drug product (Fig. 8-18). Each drug product was given in the same dose as the other. Explain how the various possible formulation factors could have caused the differences in blood levels. Give examples where possible.

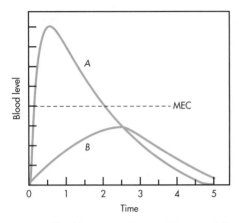

**FIGURE 8-18** ∙ Blood level curves for two different oral dosage forms of a hypothetical antibiotic.

How would the corresponding urinary drug excretion curves relate to the plasma level–time curves?

2. Assume that you have just made a new formulation of acetaminophen. Design a protocol to compare your drug product against the acetaminophen drug products on the market. What criteria would you use for proof of bioequivalence for your new formulation? How would you determine if the acetaminophen was completely (100%) systemically absorbed?

3. The data in Table 8-22 represent the average findings in antibiotic plasma samples taken from 10 humans (average weight 70 kg), tabulated in a 4-way crossover design.

   **a.** Which of the four drug products in Table 8-22 would be preferred as a reference standard for the determination of relative bioavailability? Why?

   **b.** From which oral drug product is the drug absorbed more rapidly?

   **c.** What is the absolute bioavailability of the drug from the oral solution?

   **d.** What is the relative bioavailability of the drug from the oral tablet compared to the reference standard?

   **e.** From the data in Table 8-15, determine:

      **(i)** Apparent $V_D$

      **(ii)** Elimination $t_{1/2}$

**TABLE 8-22** ∙ Comparison of Plasma Concentrations of Antibiotic, as Related to Dosage Form and Time

| | Plasma Concentration ($\mu$g/mL) | | | |
| --- | --- | --- | --- | --- |
| Time after Dose (h) | IV Solution (2 mg/kg) | Oral Solution (10 mg/kg) | Oral Tablet (10 mg/kg) | Oral Capsule (10 mg/kg) |
| 0.5 | 5.94 | 23.4 | 13.2 | 18.7 |
| 1.0 | 5.30 | 26.6 | 18.0 | 21.3 |
| 1.5 | 4.72 | 25.2 | 19.0 | 20.1 |
| 2.0 | 4.21 | 22.8 | 18.3 | 18.2 |
| 3.0 | 3.34 | 18.2 | 15.4 | 14.6 |
| 4.0 | 2.66 | 14.5 | 12.5 | 11.6 |
| 6.0 | 1.68 | 9.14 | 7.92 | 7.31 |
| 8.0 | 1.06 | 5.77 | 5.00 | 4.61 |
| 10.0 | 0.67 | 3.64 | 3.16 | 2.91 |
| 12.0 | 0.42 | 2.30 | 1.99 | 1.83 |
| AUC $\left(\dfrac{\text{mg}}{\text{mL}} \times \text{h}\right)$ | 29.0 | 145.0 | 116.0 | 116.0 |

(iii) First-order elimination rate constant $k$

(iv) Total body clearance

f. From the data above, graph the cumulative urinary excretion curves that would correspond to the plasma concentration–time curves.

4. Aphrodisia is a new drug manufactured by the Venus Drug Company. When tested in humans, the pharmacokinetics of the drug assumes a one-compartment open model with first-order absorption and first-order elimination:

$$D_{GI} \xrightarrow{k_a} D_B V_D \xrightarrow{k}$$

The drug was given in a single oral dose of 250 mg to a group of college students 21–29 years of age. Mean body weight was 60 kg. Samples of blood were obtained at various time intervals after the administration of the drug, and the plasma fractions were analyzed for active drug. The data are summarized in Table 8-23.

a. The minimum effective concentration of Aphrodisia in plasma is 2.3 $\mu$g/mL. What is the onset time of this drug?

b. The minimum effective concentration of Aphrodisia in plasma is 2.3 $\mu$g/mL. What is the duration of activity of this drug?

c. What is the elimination half-life of Aphrodisia in college students?

d. What is the time for peak drug concentration $(t_{max})$ of Aphrodisia?

e. What is the peak drug concentration $(C_{max})$?

f. Assuming that the drug is 100% systemically available (ie, fraction of drug absorbed equals unity), what is the AUC for Aphrodisia?

5. You wish to do a bioequivalence study on three different formulations of the same active drug. Lay out a Latin-square design for the proper sequencing of these drug products in six normal, healthy volunteers. What is the main reason for using a crossover design in a bioequivalence study? What is meant by a "random" population?

6. Four different drug products containing the same antibiotic were given to 12 volunteer adult males (age 19–28 years, average weight 73 kg) in a 4-way crossover design. The volunteers fasted for 12 hours prior to taking the drug product. Urine samples were collected up to 72 hours after the administration of the drug to obtain the maximum urinary drug excretion, $D_u^\infty$. The data are presented in Table 8-24.

a. What is the absolute bioavailability of the drug from the tablet?

b. What is the relative bioavailability of the capsule compared to the oral solution?

7. According to the prescribing information for cimetidine (Tagamet$^*$), following IV or IM administration, 75% of the drug is recovered from the urine after 24 hours as the parent compound. Following a single oral dose, 48% of the drug is recovered from the urine after 24 hours as the parent compound. From this information, determine what fraction of the drug is absorbed systemically from an oral dose after 24 hours.

**TABLE 8-23 • Data Summary of Active Drug Concentration in Plasma Fractions**

| Time (h) | $C_p$ ($\mu$g/mL) | Time (h) | $C_p$ ($\mu$g/mL) |
|---|---|---|---|
| 0 | 0 | 12 | 3.02 |
| 1 | 1.88 | 18 | 1.86 |
| 2 | 3.05 | 24 | 1.12 |
| 3 | 3.74 | 36 | 0.40 |
| 5 | 4.21 | 48 | 0.14 |
| 7 | 4.08 | 60 | 0.05 |
| 9 | 3.70 | 72 | 0.02 |

**TABLE 8-24 • Urinary Drug Excretion Data Summary**

| Drug Product | Dose (mg/kg) | Cumulative Urinary Drug Excretion 0–72 h |
|---|---|---|
| IV solution | 0.2 | 20 |
| Oral solution | 4 | 380 |
| Oral tablet | 4 | 340 |
| Oral capsule | 4 | 360 |

8. Define *bioequivalence requirement*. Why does the FDA require a bioequivalence requirement for the manufacture of a generic drug product?

9. Why can we use the time for peak drug concentration ($t_{max}$) in a bioequivalence study for an estimate of the rate of drug absorption, rather than calculating the $k_a$?

10. Ten male volunteers (18–26 years of age) weighing an average of 73 kg were given either 4 tablets each containing 250 mg of drug (drug product A) or 1 tablet containing 1000 mg of drug (drug product B). Blood levels of the drug were obtained and the data are summarized in Table 8-25.

    a. State a possible reason for the difference in the time for peak drug concentration ($t_{max,A}$) after drug product A compared to the $t_{max,B}$ after drug product B. (Assume that all the tablets were made from the same formulation—ie, the drug is in the same particle size, same salt form, same excipients, and same ratio of excipients to active drug.)

    b. Draw a graph relating the cumulative amount of drug excreted in urine of patients given drug product A compared to the cumulative drug excreted in urine after drug product B. Label axes.

    c. In a second study using the same 10 male volunteers, a 125-mg dose of the drug was given by IV bolus and the AUC was computed as 20 $\mu g \cdot h/mL$. Calculate the fraction of drug systemically absorbed from drug product B (1 × 1000-mg) tablet using the data in Table 8-25.

11. After performing a bioequivalence test comparing a generic drug product to a brand-name drug product, it was observed that the generic drug product had greater bioavailability than the brand-name drug product.

    a. Would you approve marketing the generic drug product, claiming it was superior to the brand-name drug product?

    b. Would you expect identical pharmacodynamic responses to both drug products?

    c. What therapeutic problem might arise in using the generic drug product that might not occur when using the brand-name drug product?

12. The following study is from Welling et al (1982):

    *Tolazamide Formulations*: Four tolazamide tablet formulations were selected for this study. The tablet formulations were labeled A, B, C, and D. Disintegration and dissolution tests were performed by standard USP-23 procedures.

    *Subjects*: Twenty healthy adult male volunteers between the ages of 18 and 38 years (mean, 26 years) and weighing between 61.4 and 95.5 kg (mean, 74.5 kg) were selected for the study. The subjects were randomly assigned to four groups

## TABLE 8-25 • Blood Level Data Summary for Two Drug Products

| Kinetic Variable | Unit | Drug Product | | Statistic |
| --- | --- | --- | --- | --- |
| | | A, 4 × 250-mg Tablet | B, 1000-mg Tablet | |
| Time for peak drug concentration (range) | h | 1.3 (0.7–1.5) | 1.8 (1.5–2.2) | $p < .05$ |
| Peak concentration (range) | $\mu g/mL$ | 53 (46–58) | 47 (42–51) | $p < .05$ |
| AUC (range) | $\mu g \cdot h/mL$ | 118 (98–125) | 103 (90–120) | NS |
| $t_{1/2}$ | h | 3.2 (2.5–3.8) | 3.8 (2.9–4.3) | NS |

of five each. The 4 treatments were administered according to 4 × 4 Latin-square design. Each treatment was separated by 1-week intervals. All subjects fasted overnight before receiving the tolazamide tablet the following morning. The tablet was given with 180 mL of water. Food intake was allowed at 5 hours postdose. Blood samples (10 mL) were taken just before the dose and periodically after dosing. The serum fraction was separated from the blood and analyzed for tolazamide by high-pressure liquid chromatography.

*Data Analysis*: Serum data were analyzed by a digital computer program using a regression analysis and by the percent of drug unabsorbed by the method of Wagner and Nelson (1963). AUC was determined by the trapezoidal rule and an analysis of variance was determined by Tukey's method.

a. Why was a Latin-square crossover design used in this study?

b. Why were the subjects fasted before being given the tolazamide tablets?

c. Why did the authors use the Wagner–Nelson method rather than the Loo–Riegelman method for measuring the amount of drug absorbed?

d. From the data in Table 8-26 only, from which tablet formulation would you expect the highest bioavailability? Why?

e. From the data in Table 8-26, did the disintegration times correlate with the dissolution times? Why?

f. Do the data in Table 8-27 appear to correlate with the data in Table 8-26? Why?

g. Draw the expected cumulative urinary excretion–time curve for formulations A and B. Label axes and identify each curve.

h. Assuming formulation A is the reference formulation, what is the relative bioavailability of formulation D?

i. Using the data in Table 8-27 for formulation A, calculate the elimination half-life ($t_{1/2}$) for tolazamide.

13. If *in vitro* drug dissolution and/or release studies for an oral solid dosage form (eg, tablet) does not correlate with the bioavailability of the drug *in vivo*, why should the pharmaceutical manufacturer continue to perform *in vitro* release studies for each production batch of the solid dosage form?

14. Is it possible for two pharmaceutically equivalent solid dosage forms containing different inactive ingredients (ie, excipients) to demonstrate bioequivalence *in vivo* even though these drug products demonstrate differences in drug dissolution tests *in vitro*?

15. For bioequivalence studies, $t_{max}$, $C_{max}$, and AUC, along with an appropriate statistical analysis, are the parameters generally used to demonstrate the bioequivalence of two similar drug products containing the same active drug.

a. Why are the parameters $t_{max}$, $C_{max}$, and AUC acceptable for proving that two drug products are bioequivalent?

b. Are pharmacokinetic models needed in the evaluation of bioequivalence?

c. Is it necessary to use a pharmacokinetic model to completely describe the plasma drug concentration–time curve for the determination of $t_{max}$, $C_{max}$, and AUC?

d. Why are log-transformed data used for the statistical evaluation of bioequivalence?

e. What is an add-on study?

## TABLE 8-26 • Disintegration Times and Dissolution Rates of Tolazamide Tablets*

| Tablet | Mean Disintegration Time[†] min (Range) | Percent Dissolved in 30 min[‡] (Range) |
|---|---|---|
| A | 3.8 (3.0–4.0) | 103.9 (100.5–106.3) |
| B | 2.2 (1.8–2.5) | 10.9 (9.3–13.5) |
| C | 2.3 (2.0–2.5) | 31.6 (26.4–37.2) |
| D | 26.5 (22.5–30.5) | 29.7 (20.8–38.4) |

*N = 6.
[†]By the method of USP-23.
[‡]Dissolution rates in pH 7.6 buffer.
Reproduced with permission from Welling PG, Patel RB, Patel UR, et al: Bioavailability of tolazamide from tablets: comparison of in vitro and in vivo results, J Pharm Sci. 1982 Nov;71(11):1259–1263.

## TABLE 8-27 • Mean Tolazamide Concentrations* in Serum

| Time (h) | Treatment (µg/mL) A | B | C | D | Statistic[†] |
|---|---|---|---|---|---|
| 0 | $10.8 \pm 7.4$ | $1.3 \pm 1.4$ | $1.8 \pm 1.9$ | $3.5 \pm 2.6$ | $\overline{ADCB}$ |
| 1 | $20.5 \pm 7.3$ | $2.8 \pm 2.8$ | $5.4 \pm 4.8$ | $13.5 \pm 6.6$ | $\overline{ADCB}$ |
| 3 | $23.9 \pm 5.3$ | $4.4 \pm 4.3$ | $9.8 \pm 5.6$ | $20.0 \pm 6.4$ | $\overline{ADCB}$ |
| 4 | $25.4 \pm 5.2$ | $5.7 \pm 4.1$ | $13.6 \pm 5.3$ | $22.0 \pm 5.4$ | $\overline{ADCB}$ |
| 5 | $24.1 \pm 6.3$ | $6.6 \pm 4.0$ | $15.1 \pm 4.7$ | $22.6 \pm 5.0$ | $\overline{ADCB}$ |
| 6 | $19.9 \pm 5.9$ | $6.8 \pm 3.4$ | $14.3 \pm 3.9$ | $19.7 \pm 4.7$ | $\overline{ADCB}$ |
| 8 | $15.2 \pm 5.5$ | $6.6 \pm 3.2$ | $12.8 \pm 4.1$ | $14.6 \pm 4.2$ | $\overline{ADCB}$ |
| 12 | $8.8 \pm 4.8$ | $5.5 \pm 3.2$ | $9.1 \pm 4.0$ | $8.5 \pm 4.1$ | $\overline{CADB}$ |
| 16 | $5.6 \pm 3.8$ | $4.6 \pm 3.3$ | $6.4 \pm 3.9$ | $5.4 \pm 3.1$ | $\overline{CADB}$ |
| 24 | $2.7 \pm 2.4$ | $3.1 \pm 2.6$ | $3.1 \pm 3.3$ | $2.4 \pm 1.8$ | $\overline{CBAD}$ |
| $C_{max}$, µg/mL[‡] | $27.8 \pm 5.3$ | $7.7 \pm 4.1$ | $16.4 \pm 4.4$ | $24.0 \pm 4.5$ | $\overline{ADCB}$ |
| $t_{max}$, h[§] | $3.3 \pm 0.9$ | $.7.0 \pm 2.2$ | $5.4 \pm 2.0$ | $4.0 \pm 0.9$ | $\overline{BCDA}$ |
| $AUC_{0-24}$, µg h/mL[‖] | $260 \pm 81$ | $112 \pm 63$ | $193 \pm 70$ | $231 \pm 67$ | $\overline{ADCB}$ |

*Concentrations ± 1 SD, n = 20.
[†]For explanation see text.
[‡]Maximum concentration of tolazamide in serum.
[§]Time of maximum concentration.
[‖]Area under the 0–24-h serum tolazamide concentration curve calculated by trapezoidal rule.
Reproduced with permission from Welling PG, Patel RB, Patel UR, et al: Bioavailability of tolazamide from tablets: comparison of in vitro and in vivo results, J Pharm Sci. 1982 Nov;71(11):1259–1263.

## ANSWERS

### Frequently Asked Questions

*Why are preclinical animal toxicology studies and clinical efficacy drug studies in human subjects not required by the FDA to approve a generic drug product as a therapeutic equivalent to the brand-name drug product?*

- Preclinical animal toxicology and clinical efficacy studies were performed on the marketed *brand* drug product as part of the NDA prior to FDA approval. These studies do not have to be repeated for the *generic* bioequivalent drug product. The manufacturer of the generic drug product must submit an ANDA to the FDA, demonstrating that the generic drug product is a therapeutic equivalent (see definitions in Chapter 15) to the brand drug product.

*What do sequence, washout period, and period mean in a crossover bioavailability study?*

- The *sequence* is the order in which the drug products (ie, treatments) are given (eg, brand product followed by generic product or vice versa). Sequence is important to prevent any bias due to the order of the treatments in the study. The term *washout* refers to the time for total elimination of the dose. The time for washout is determined by the elimination half-life of the drug. *Period* refers to the drug-dosing day on which the drug is given to the subjects. For example, for Period 1, half the subjects receive treatment A, brand product, and the other half of the subjects receive treatment B, generic product.

*Why does the FDA require a food intervention (food-effect) study for generic drug products before granting approval?*

■ Manufacturers are required to perform a food-intervention bioavailability study on all drugs whose bioavailability is known to be affected by food. In addition, a food-intervention bioavailability study is required on all MR products since (1) the MR formulation (eg, enteric coating, sustained-release coating) may be affected by the presence of food and (2) MR products have a greater potential to be affected by food due to their longer residence time in the GI tract and changes in GI motility.

*What type of bioequivalence studies are required for drugs that are not systemically absorbed or for those drugs in which the $C_{max}$ and AUC cannot be measured in the plasma?*

■ If the drug is not absorbed systemically from the drug product, a surrogate marker must be used as a measure of bioequivalence. This surrogate marker may be a pharmacodynamic effect or, as in the case of cholestyramine resin, the binding capacity for bile acids *in vitro*.

## Learning Questions

3. **a.** Oral solution: The drug is in the most bioavailable form.

   **b.** Oral solution: Same reason as above.

   **c.** Absolute bioavailability

   $$= \frac{[AUC]_{soln}/dose_{soln}}{[AUC]_{IV}/dose_{IV}}$$

   $$= \frac{145/10}{29/2} = 1.0$$

**d.** Relative bioavailability

$$= \frac{[AUC]_{tab}/dose_{tab}}{[AUC]_{soln}/dose_{soln}}$$

$$= \frac{116/10}{145/10} = 0.80$$

**e. (1)** $C_p^0 = 6.67\ \mu g/mL$

(by extrapolation of IV curve)

$$V_D = \frac{2000\ \mu g/kg}{6.67\ \mu g/mL} = 300\ mL/kg$$

**(2)** $t_{1/2} = 3.01\ h$

**(3)** $k = 0.23\ h^{-1}$

**(4)** $Cl_T = kV_D = 69\ m/kg \cdot h$

4. Plot the data on both rectangular and semi-log graph paper. The following answers were obtained from estimates from the plotted plasma level–time curves. More exact answers may be obtained mathematically by substitution into the proper formulas.

   **a.** 1.37 hours

   **b.** 13.6 hours

   **c.** 8.75 hours

   **d.** 5 hours

   **e.** 4.21 $\mu g/mL$

   **f.** 77.98 $\mu g\ h/mL$

5. **Drug Product**

| Subject | Period 1 | Period 2 | Week 3 |
|---------|----------|----------|--------|
| 1 | A | B | C |
| 2 | B | C | A |
| 3 | C | A | B |
| 4 | A | C | B |
| 5 | C | B | A |
| 6 | B | A | C |

6. **a.** Absolute bioavailability

$$= \frac{D_{u,PO}^{\infty}/dose_{PO}}{D_{u,IV}^{\infty}/dose_{IV}} = \frac{340/4}{20/0.2}$$

$$= 0.85\ or\ 85\%$$

**b.** Relative bioavailability

$$= \frac{D_{ucap}^{\infty} / dose_{cap}}{D_{usoln}^{\infty} / dose_{sol}} = \frac{360 / 4}{380 / 4}$$

$$= 0.947 \text{ or } 94.7\%$$

Fraction of drug absorbed

$$= \frac{\% \text{ of dose excreted after PO}}{\% \text{ of dose excreted after IV}}$$

$$= \frac{48\%}{75\%} = 0.64$$

7. The fraction of drug absorbed systemically is the absolute bioavailability.

## REFERENCES

Amidon, GL, Lennernas H, Shah VP, Crison JR: A theoretical basis for a biopharmaceutic drug classification: The correlation of *in vitro* drug product dissolution and *in vivo* bioavailability. *Pharm Res* **12**:413, 1995.

Benet LZ, Amidon, GL, Barends DM, et al: The use of BDDCS in classifying the permeability of marketed drugs. *Pharm Res* **52**:483, 2008.

Damle BD, Kaul S, Behr D, Knupp C: Bioequivalence of two formulations of didanosine, encapsulated enteric-coated beads and buffered tablets, in healthy volunteers and HIV-infected subjects. *J Clin Pharmacol* **42**:791, 2002.

Davit B, Braddy A, Conner D, Yu X: International guidelines for bioequivalence of systemically-available orally-administered generic drug products: a survey of similarities and differences. *AAPSJ* **15**:974, 2013.

Davit BM, Chen ML, Conner DP, et al: Implementation of a reference-scaled average bioequivalence approach for highly variable generic drug products by the US Food and Drug Administration. *AAPSJ* **14**:915, 2012.

Davit BM, Conner DP: Food effects on drug bioavailability: implications for new and generic drug development. In Yu L, Krishna R (eds). *Biopharmaceutics Applications in Drug Development*. New York, Springer, 2008, p 317.

Davit BM, Conner DP: United States of America. In Kanfer I, Shargel L (eds). *Generic Drug Product Development—International Regulatory Requirements for Bioequivalence*. Boca Raton, CRC Press, 2015, in press (with permission).

de Mendoza C, Valer L, Ribera E, et al: Performance of six different ritonavir-boosted protease inhibitor-based regimens in heavily antiretroviral-experienced HIV-infected patients. *HIV Clin Trials* **7**:163, 2006.

Dehaven WI, Conner DP: The effects of food on drug bioavailability and bioequivalence. In Li BV, Yu LX (eds). *FDA Bioequivalence Standards*. New York, Springer, 2014, p 95.

Dandamudi S: In Vitro Bioequivalence Data for a Topical Product: Bioequivalence Review Perspective. FDA Public Workshop. Topical Dermatological Generic Drug Products: Overcoming Barriers to Development and Improving Patient Access, October 20, 2017.

FDA: Abbreviated New Drug Application (ANDA) Forms and Submission Requirements https://www.fda.gov/drugs/abbreviated-new-drug-application-anda/abbreviated-new-drug-application-anda-forms-and-submission-requirements, Accessed August 11, 2021

FDA: Filing Review of Abbreviated New Drug Applications, Manual of Policies and Procedures, Center for Drug Evaluation And Research, Office of Generic Drugs, 09/01/2017, https://www.fda.gov/media/107325/download, Accessed August 11, 2021

Gardner S: Bioequivalence requirements and *in vivo* bioavailability procedures. *Fed Reg* **42**:1651, 1977.

Haidar SH, Davit BM, Chen ML, et al: Bioequivalence approaches for highly variable drugs and drug products. *Pharm Res* **25**:237, 2008.

Horn JR, Howden CW: Review article: Similarities and differences among delayed-release proton pump inhibitor formulations. *Aliment Pharmacol Ther* **22**(S3):20, 2005.

Hughes J, Crowe A: Inhibition of P-glycoprotein-mediated efflux of digoxin and its metabolites by macrolide antibiotics. *J Pharmacol Sci* **113**:315, 2010.

Jagdale SC, Agavekar AJ, Pandya SV, Kuchekar BS, Chabukswar AR: Formulation and evaluation of a gastroretentative drug delivery system of propranolol hydrochloride. *AAPS PharmSciTech* **10**:1071, 2009.

Kaur P, Chaurasia CS, Davit BM, Conner DP: Bioequivalence study designs for generic solid oral anticancer drug products: Scientific and regulatory considerations. *J Clin Pharmacol* **53**:1252, 2013.

Klotz U: Pharmacokinetics and drug metabolism in the elderly. *Drug Metab Rev* **41**:67, 2009.

Mehta M: The criteria for BCS-based biowaiver and the regulatory experience gathered in the US. Open Forum presentation, American Association of Pharmaceutical Sciences Annual Meeting, San Diego, CA, 2014.

Midha KA, Ormsby ED, Hubbard JW, et al: Logarithmic transformation in bioequivalence: Application with two formulations of perphenazine. *J Pharm Sci* **82**:138, 1993.

Moore JW, Flanner HH: Mathematical comparison of curves with an emphasis on *in vitro* dissolution profiles. *Pharm Tech* **20**:64, 1996.

Polli JE, Rekhi GS, Augsburger LL, Shah VP: Methods to compare dissolution profiles and a rationale for wide dissolution specifications for metoprolol tartrate tablets. *J Pharm Sci* **86**:690, 1997.

Report by the Bioequivalence Task Force 1988 on Recommendations from the Bioequivalence Hearings Conducted by the Food and Drug Administration, Sept 29–Oct 1, 1986. Rockville, MD, 1988.

Shah VP, Tsong Y, Sathe P: In vitro dissolution profile comparison—Statistics and analysis of the similarity factor, $f_2$. *Pharm Res* **15**:896, 1998.

Shah PV, Yacobi A, Barr WH, et al: Evaluation of orally administered highly variable drugs and drug formulations. *Pharm Res* **13**:1590, 1996.

Schuirmann DJ: A comparison of the two one-sided tests procedure and the power approach for assessing the equivalence of average bioavailability. *J Pharmacokinet Biopharm* **15**:657, 1987.

US-FDA, CDER: Guidance for Industry: Bioanalytical Method Validation, May 2018.

US-FDA, CDER: Guidance for Industry: Bioavailability and Bioequivalence Studies Submitted in NDAs or INDs —General Considerations, Draft Guidance, March 2014.

US-FDA, CDER: Guidance for Industry, Dissolution Testing of Immediate-Release Solid Oral Dosage Forms. http://www.fda.gov/downloads/Drugs/GuidanceComplianceRegulatory Information/Guidances/UCM070237.pdf. Silver Spring, MD, 1997.

US-FDA, CDER: Guidance for Industry, Statistical Approaches to Establishing Bioequivalence. http://www.fda.gov/downloads/GuidanceComlianceRegulatoryInformation/Guidances/UCM070244.pdf. Silver Spring, MD, 2000a.

US-FDA, CDER: Guidance for Industry, Waiver of In Vivo Bioavailability and Bioequivalence Studies for Immediate-Release Solid Oral Dosage Forms Based on A Biopharmaceutics Classification System. http://www.fda.gov/downloads/Drugs/GuidanceComplianceRegulatoryInfomration/Guidances/UCM070246.pdf. Silver Spring, MD, 2000b.

US-FDA, CDER: Guidance for Industry, Pharmacokinetics in Patients with Impaired Hepatic Function: Study Design, Data Analysis, and Impact on Dosing and Labeling. http://www.fda.gov/downloads/Drugs/GuidanceComplianceRegulatory-Information/Guidances/UCM072123.pdf. Silver Spring, MD, 2003a.

US-FDA, CDER: Guidance for Industry, Food-Effect Bioavailability Studies and Fed Bioequivalence Studies. http://www.fda.gov/downloads/Drugs/GuidanceComplianceRegulatory-Information/Guidances/UCM070241.pdf. Silver Spring, MD, 2003b.

US-FDA, CDER: Guidance for Industry, Bioequivalence Recommendations for Specific Products. http://www.fda.gov/downloads/GuidanceComplianceRegulatoryInformatoin/Guidances/UCM072872.pdf Silver Spring, MD, 2010a.

US-FDA, CDER: Guidance for Industry Pharmacokinetics in Patients with Impaired Renal Function—Study Design, Data Analysis, and Impact on Dosing and Labelling.

http://www.fda.gov/downloads/Drugs/GuidanceCompliance RegulatoryInformation/Guidances/UCM204959.pdf. Silver Spring, MD, 2014.

US-FDA, CDER: Response to Warner Chilcott Company LLC petition part approval and denial. http://www.regulations.Gov/#!documentDetail;D=FDA-2010-P-0111-0011. Silver Spring, MD, 2010c.

US-FDA, CDER: Draft Bioequivalence Recommendations for Cholestyramine Oral Powder. US-FDA, CDER: Draft Bioequivalence Recommendations for Calcium Acetate Tablets. http://www.fda.gov/downloads/GuidanceComplianceRegulatoryInformation/Guidances/UCM148185.pdf. Silver Spring, MD, 2011a.

US-FDA, CDER: Draft Bioequivalence Recommendations for Clozapine Tablets. http://www.fda.gov/downloads/Drugs/GuidanceComplianceRegulatoryInformation/Guidances/UCM249219.pdf. Silver Spring, MD, 2011b.

US-FDA, CDER: Draft Bioequivalence Recommendations for Mercaptopurine Tablets. http://www.fda.gov/downloads/Drugs/GuidanceComplianceRegulatoryInformation/Guidances/ucm088658.pdf. Silver Spring, MD, 2011c.

US-FDA, CDER: Bioequivalence Recommendations for Zolpidem Extended-ReleaseTablets.http://www.fda.gov/downloads/Drugs/GuidanceComplianceRegulatoryInformation/Guidances/UCM175029.pdf. Silver Spring, MD, 2011d.

http://www.fda.gov/downloads/Drugs/ComplianceGuidance-RegulatoryInformation/Guidances/UCM273910.pdf. Silver Spring, MD, 2012a.

US-FDA, CDER: Draft Bioequivalence Recommendations for Acyclovir Topical Ointment. http://www.fda.gov/downloads/GuidanceComplianceRegulatoryInformation/Guidances/UCM296733.pdf. Silver Spring, MD, 2012b.

US-FDA, CDER: Guidance for Industry Drug-Drug Interaction Studies—Study Design, Data Analysis, Implications for Dosing, and Labeling Recommendations. http://www.fda.gov/downloads/Drugs/GuidanceComplianceRegulatoryInformation/Guidances/UCM292362.pdf. Silver Spring, MD, 2012c.

US-FDA, CDER: Draft Bioequivalence Recommendations for Risperidone Intramuscular Injection. http://www.fda.gov/downloads/Drugs/GuidanceComplianceRegulatory Information/Guidances/UCM201272.pdf. Silver Spring, MD 2013a.

US-FDA, CDER: Drugs@FDA, Delzicol˚ Approval Summary. http://www.accessdata.fda.gov/drugsatfda_docs/nda/2013/204412_delzicol_toc.cfm. Silver Spring, MD, 2013b.

US-FDA, CDER: CFR Code of Federal Regulations Title 21 Part 320 Bioavailability Bioequivalence Requirements. http://www.accessdata.fda.gov/scripts/cdrh/cfdocs/cfcfr/CFRSearch.cfm?CFRPart=320&showFR=1&subpartNode=21:5.0.1.1.8.1. Silver Spring, MD 2014a.

US-FDA, CDER: CFR Code of Federal Regulations Title 21 Part 314 Applications for FDA Approval to Market a New Drug. http://www.accessdata.fda.gov/scripts/cdrh/cfdocs/cfcfr/cfrsearch.cfm?cfrpart=314. Silver Spring, MD, 2014b.

US-FDA, CDER: Draft Guidance for Industry Bioavailability and Bioequivalence Studies Submitted in NDAs or INDs—General Considerations.http://www.fda.gov/downloads/Drugs/GuidanceComplianceRegulatoryInformation/Guidances/UCM389370.pdf. Silver Spring, MD, 2014c.

US-FDA, CDER: Orange Book: *Approved Drug Products with Therapeutic Equivalence Evaluations*. http://www.accessdata.fda.gov/scripts/cder/ob/default.cfm. Silver Spring, MD, 2014d.

US-FDA, CDER: Guidance for Industry General Considerations for Pediatric Pharmacokinetic Studies for Drugs and Biological Products. U.S. Food and Drug Administration Drugs Guidance. http://www.fda.gov/downloads/Drugs/GuidanceComplianceRegulatoryInformation/Guidances/UCM425885.pdf. Silver Spring, MD, 2014e.

US-FDA, CDER: Draft Bioequivalence Recommendations for Methylphenidate Extended-Release Tablets. http://www.fda.gov/downloads/Drugs/GuidanceComplianceRegulatoryInformation/Guidances/UCM320007.pdf. Silver Spring, MD, 2014f.

US-FDA, CDER. Guidance for Industry, Clinical Pharmacology Data to Support a Finding of Biosimilarity to a Reference Product.

http://www.fda.gov/downloads/drugs/guidancecomplianceregulatoryinformation/guidances/ucm397017.pdf. Silver Spring, MD, 2014g.

US-FDA CDER Guidance for Industry, Pharmacokinetics in Patients with Impaired Renal Function – Study Design, Data Analysis, and Impact on Dosing, Draft Guidance, September 2020

Wagner JG, Nelson E: Per cent absorbed time plots derived from blood level and/or urinary excretion data. *J Pharm Sci* **52**:610, 1963.

Welling PG, Patel RB, Patel UR, et al: Bioavailability of tolazamide from tablets: Comparison of *in vitro* and *in vivo* results. *J Pharm Sci* **71**:1259, 1982.

Westlake WJ: Use of statistical methods in evaluation of *in vivo* performance of dosage forms. *J Pharm Sci* **61**:1340, 1973.

Wu CY, Benet LZ: Predicting drug disposition via application of BCS: Transport/absorption/elimination interplay and development of a biopharmaceutics drug disposition classification system. *Pharm Res* **22**:11, 2005.

Zou P, Yu LX: Pharmacodynamic endpoint bioequivalence studies. In LX Yu, Li BV (eds). *FDA Bioequivalence Standards*. New York, Springer, 2014, p 217.

# 9

# Modified-Release Drug Products and Drug Devices

## Hong Ding

## CHAPTER OBJECTIVES

- Define modified-release drug products.
- Differentiate between conventional, immediate-release, extended-release, delayed-release, and targeted drug products.
- Explain the advantages and disadvantages of extended-release drug products.
- Describe the kinetics of extended-release drug products compared to immediate-release drug products.
- Explain when an extended-release drug product should contain an immediate-release drug dose.
- Explain why extended-release beads in capsule formulation may have a different bioavailability profile compared to an extended-release tablet formulation of the same drug.
- Describe several approaches for the formulation of an oral extended-release drug product.
- Explain why a transdermal drug product (patch) may be considered an extended-release drug product.
- Describe the components of a transdermal drug delivery system.
- Explain why an extended-release formulation of a drug may have a different efficacy profile compared to the same dose of drug given in as a conventional,

immediate-release, oral dosage form in multiple doses.

- List the studies that might be required for the development of an extended-release drug product.
- List the several advantages of drug devices based on modified-release drug design.

## MODIFIED-RELEASE DRUG PRODUCTS AND CONVENTIONAL (IMMEDIATE-RELEASE) DRUG PRODUCTS

Most conventional (also called immediate release [IR]) oral drug products, such as tablets, capsules, and solutions, are formulated to release the active pharmaceutical ingredient (API) immediately after oral administration. In the formulation of conventional drug products, no deliberate effort is made to modify the drug release rate. IR products generally provide relatively rapid drug absorption and onset of accompanying pharmacodynamic (PD) effects, but not always. In the case of conventional oral products containing prodrugs, the PD activity may be altered due to the time for conversion from prodrugs to the active drug by hepatic or intestinal metabolism or by chemical hydrolysis. Alternatively, in the case of conventional oral products containing poorly soluble (lipophilic drugs), drug absorption may be gradual due to slow dissolution in or selective absorption across the GI tract, also resulting in a delayed onset time.

To achieve a desired therapeutic objective and/or better patient compliance, the pattern of drug release from modified-release (MR) dosage forms is deliberately changed from that of a conventional (also called immediate-release, IR) dosage formulation. MR drug products are often a more effective therapeutic alternative to conventional or IR dosage forms. The objective of MR drug products for oral administration is to prolong the therapeutic effect of the active drug by controlling the rate of drug absorption from the gastrointestinal (GI) tract. MR formulations release a drug in a controlled manner during the absorption period, so they have advantages over IR formulas such as fewer pills to be taken and less peak–trough fluctuations of drug concentration in serum which may be associated with decreased adverse effects. Types of MR drug products include but are not limited to extended-release (ER), delayed-release (eg, enteric coated), targeted-release, and orally disintegrating tablets (ODT).

The term *modified-release (MR) drug product* is used to describe products that are formulated to alter the timing and/or rate of release of the drug. An MR dosage form is a formulation in which the drug-release characteristics of the time course and/or location are chosen to accomplish therapeutic or convenience objectives, which is not offered by conventional dosage forms. Several types of MR oral drug products are as follows.

1. *Extended-release (ER) drug products.* A dosage form that allows at least a 2-fold reduction in dosage frequency as compared to that drug presented as an IR (conventional) dosage form. ER drug products are formulated so that the active drug is available over an extended period of time following administration. ER products can be used for reducing fluctuations in plasma concentrations. Several terms have been used to describe ER formulations. Examples of ER dosage forms include controlled-release (CR), sustained-release (SR), prolonged-release, long-acting (LA), and time-release drug products.

2. *Delayed-release (DR) drug products.* A dosage form that releases a discrete portion/portions of drugs at a time later than immediately after administration (USP-NF). An initial portion may be released promptly after administration. The delayed release may be time sensitive or dependent on the environment (eg, GI pH). *Enteric-coated* dosage forms are common DR products (eg, enteric-coated aspirin and other NSAID products) that do not dissolve in the acid conditions in the stomach but release the drug in the higher pH of the duodenum.

3. *Targeted-release (TR) drug products.* A dosage form that releases drug at or near the intended physiologic site of action (see Chapter 10). TR dosage forms may have either immediate- or extended-release characteristics.

4. *Orally disintegrating tablets* (ODTs). ODTs disintegrate rapidly in the saliva after oral administration. ODTs may be used without the addition of water. The drug is dispersed in saliva and swallowed with little or no water.

The term *controlled-release drug product* was previously used to describe various types of oral extended-release-rate dosage forms including SR, sustained-action, prolonged-action, long-action, slow-release, and programmed drug delivery. Other terms, such as ER (extended-release), SR (sustained-release), XL & XR (other acronyms for extended-release), and CR (controlled-release), are also used to indicate the mechanism of the extended-release drug product. Retarded release is an older term for a slow-release drug product. Many of these terms for MR drug products were introduced by drug companies to reflect either a special design for an ER drug product or for use in marketing.

MR drug products are designed for different routes of administration based on the physicochemical, PD, and pharmacokinetic (PK) properties of the drug and on the properties of the materials used in the dosage form (Table 9-1). Several different terms are now defined to describe the available types of MR drug products based on the drug release characteristics of the products.

## Other Examples of Modified-Release Oral Dosage Forms

The pharmaceutical industry uses various terms to describe MR drug products. New and novel drug delivery systems are being developed by the pharmaceutical industry to alter the drug release profile, which in turn results in a unique plasma drug concentration versus time profile and PD effect. In many cases, the industry will patent their novel drug delivery systems. Due to the proliferation of these MR dosage forms, the following terms are general descriptions and should not be considered definitive.

**TABLE 9-1 •** Modified Drug Delivery Products

| Route of Administration | Drug Product | Examples | Comments |
|---|---|---|---|
| Oral drug products | Extended release | Diltiazem HCl extended release | Once-a-day dosing. |
| | Delayed release | Diclofenac sodium delayed release | Enteric-coated tablet for drug delivery into small intestine. |
| | Delayed (targeted) drug release | Mesalamine delayed release | Coated for drug release in terminal ileum. |
| | Oral mucosal drug delivery | Oral transmucosal fentanyl citrate | Fentanyl citrate is in the form of a flavored sugar lozenge that dissolves slowly in the mouth. |
| | Oral soluble film | Ondansetron | The film is placed top of the tongue. Film will dissolve in 4 to 20 seconds. |
| | Orally disintegrating tablets (ODT) | Aripiprazole | ODT is placed on the tongue. Tablet disintegration occurs rapidly in saliva. |
| Transdermal drug delivery systems | Transdermal therapeutic system (TTS) | Clonidine transdermal therapeutic system | Clonidine TTS is applied every 7 days to intact skin on the upper arm or chest. |
| | Iontophoretic drug delivery | | Small electric current moves charged molecules across the skin. |
| Ophthalmic drug delivery | Insert | Controlled-release pilocarpine | Elliptically shaped insert designed for continuous release of pilocarpine following placement in the cul-de-sac of the eye. |
| Intravaginal drug delivery | Insert | Dinoprostone vaginal insert | Hydrogel pouch containing prostaglandin within a polyester retrieval system. |
| Parenteral drug delivery | Intramuscular drug products | Depot injections | Lyophilized microspheres containing leuprolide acetate for depot suspension. |
| | | Water-immiscible injections (eg, oil) | Medroxyprogesterone acetate (Depo-Provera). |
| | Subcutaneous drug products | Controlled-release insulin | Basulin is a controlled-release, recombinant human insulin delivered by nanoparticulate technology. |
| Targeted delivery systems | IV injection | Daunorubicin citrate liposome injection | Liposomal preparation to maximize the selectivity of daunorubicin for solid tumors *in situ*. |

*(Continued)*

| Route of Administration | Drug Product | Examples | Comments |
|---|---|---|---|
| Implants | Brain tumor | Polifeprosan 20 with carmustine implant (Gliadel wafer) | Implant designed to deliver carmustine directly into the surgical cavity when a brain tumor is resected. |
| | Intravitreal implant | Fluocinolone acetonide intravitreal implant | Sterile implant designed to release fluocinolone acetonide locally to the posterior segment of the eye. |

**TABLE 9-1** • Modified Drug Delivery Products (*Continued*)

An *enteric-coated* tablet is one kind of DR type within the MR dosage family designed to release drug in the small intestine. Different from the film coating on tablets or capsules to prevent bitter taste from medicine or protect tablets from microbial growth as well as color alteration, usually the enteric coating materials are polymer-based barriers applied on oral medicine. This enteric coating may delay release of the medicine until after it leaves the stomach, either for the purpose of drug protection under harsh pH circumstances or alleviation of irritation on cell membrane in the stomach from the drug itself. For example, aspirin irritates the gastric mucosal cells of the stomach, and the enteric coating on the aspirin tablet may prevent the tablet from disintegrating promptly and releasing its contents at the low pH in the stomach. The coating and the tablet later dissolve and release the drug in the relatively mild pH of the duodenum, where the drug is rapidly absorbed with less irritation to the mucosal cells. Mesalamine (5-aminosalicylic acid) tablets (Asacol, Proctor & Gamble) is also a DR tablet coated with acrylic-based resin that delays the release of mesalamine until it reaches the terminal ileum and colon. Mesalamine tablets can also be considered *targeted-release*.

Some manufacturers have combined a delayed-release drug product with an ER component. Esomeprazole magnesium (Nexium* 24) capsules contain enteric-coated beads with an ER core. Esomeprazole is not stable in acid. The enteric coating prevents the release of esomeprazole in the stomach. In the duodenum, the enteric coating dissolves and the bead's inner core slowly releases esomerprazole in an extended period.

*Extended-release* (ER) drug products are MR formulations whose activity continues for a longer time than conventional, IR drug products. As mentioned, the pharmaceutical industry has developed many types of MR drug products. Therefore, it is difficult for the pharmacist and patient to distinguish among the many names and purported ER properties that the name conveys. For example, bupropion hydrochloride (Wellbutrin) tablets, 100 mg are conventional, IR tablets given three times a day (TID). Bupropion hydrochloride SR (Wellbutrin SR) tablets, 150 mg is an ER tablet given twice a day (BID), whereas bupropion hydrochloride extended-release (Wellbutrin XL) tablets, 300 mg, are given once a day. In each case, the patient receives a daily bupropion hydrochloride dose of 300 mg.

A *repeat-action tablet* is a type of MR drug product that is designed to release one dose of drug initially, followed by a second or more doses of drug at a later time. It provides the required dosage initially and then maintains or repeats it at desired intervals. *Repeat-action tablets*, along with various formulations such as prolonged, sustained, delayed, and timed-release dosage forms, may generally be considered as having the property of prolonged action. It purports to describe just when and how much of a drug is released, and simplified curves of blood levels or clinical response claim to depict how the preparation will act *in vivo*.

An extended-release drug product may contain an IR component. This ER drug product delivers an initial therapeutic dose, followed by a slower and constant release. The IR component acts as a loading dose is to provide immediate or fast drug release to quickly provide therapeutic drug concentrations in the plasma. The rate of release of the maintenance dose is designed so that the amount of drug loss from the body by elimination is constantly replaced.

Extended-release drug products often imply that drug release is at a constant or zero-order drug release rate. Fig. 9-1 shows the dissolution rate of three SR products without loading dose. The plasma concentrations resulting from the SR products are shown in Fig. 9-2.

Although some ER drug products release the drug at a zero-order rate, *in vitro*, drug absorption from the GI tract may not be zero order. Some MR drug products are formulated with materials that are more soluble at a specific pH, and the product may release the drug depending on the pH of a particular region of the GI tract. Ideally, an extended-release drug product should release the drug at a constant rate, independent of the pH, the ionic content, and other contents within the entire segment of the GI tract.

An extended-release dosage form with zero- or first-order drug absorption is compared to drug absorption from a conventional dosage form given in multiple doses in Figs. 9-3 and 9-4, respectively.

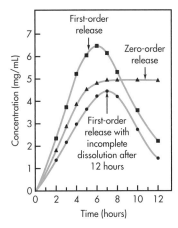

FIGURE 9-2 • Simulated plasma–drug concentrations resulting from three different sustained-release products in Fig. 9-1.

Drug absorption from conventional (IR) dosage forms generally follows first-order drug absorption.

**FREQUENTLY ASKED QUESTIONS**

▶ What is the difference between extended release, delayed release, sustained release, modified release, and controlled release?

▶ Why does the drug bioavailability from some conventional, IR drug products resemble an extended-release drug product?

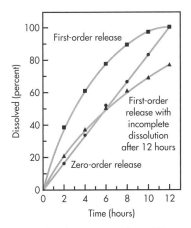

FIGURE 9-1 • Drug dissolution rates of three different extended-release products *in vitro*.

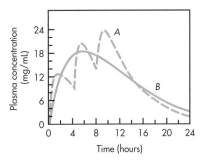

FIGURE 9-3 • Plasma level of a drug from a conventional tablet containing 50 mg of drug given at 0, 4, and 8 hours (*A*) compared to a single 150-mg drug dose given in an extended-release dosage form (*B*). The drug absorption rate constant from each drug product is first order. The drug is 100% bioavailable and the elimination half-life is constant.

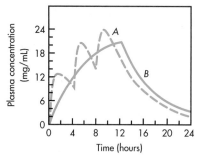

FIGURE 9-4 • Bioavailability of a drug from an immediate-release tablet containing 50 mg of drug given at 0, 4, and 8 hours compared to a single 150-mg drug dose given in an extended-release dosage form. The drug absorption rate constant from the immediate-release drug product is first order, whereas the drug absorption rate constant from the extended-release drug product is zero order. The drug is 100% bioavailable and the elimination half-life is constant.

## BIOPHARMACEUTIC FACTORS

Some drugs are well-established medicine in the treatment of specific diseases because of their effectiveness and good tolerance. However, the relatively short plasma half-life of their active drug may require frequent dosing, which is associated with a poor compliance. In the case of DR drug products, the enteric coating minimizes gastric irritation of the drug in the stomach. The major objective of ER drug products is to achieve a prolonged therapeutic effect while minimizing unwanted side effects due to fluctuating plasma drug concentrations.

An ideal ER drug product should demonstrate complete bioavailability versus its IR or reference formulation counterpart, minimal fluctuations in drug concentration at steady state, reproducibility of release characteristics independent of food, and minimal diurnal variation. Hence, an ER drug product should release the drug at a constant or zero-order rate. As the drug is released from the drug product, the drug is rapidly absorbed, and the drug absorption rate should follow zero-order kinetics similar to an intravenous drug infusion. The drug product is designed so that the rate of systemic drug absorption is limited by the rate of drug release from the drug delivery system. Unfortunately, most ER drug products that release a drug by zero-order kinetics *in vitro* do not demonstrate zero-order drug absorption

*in vivo*. The lack of zero-order drug absorption from these ER drug products after oral administration may be due to a number of unpredictable events occurring in the GI tract during drug absorption.

The ER oral drug products remain in the GI tract longer than conventional, IR drug products. Thus, drug release from an ER drug product is more subject to be affected by the anatomy and physiology of the GI tract, GI transit, pH, and its contents, such as food, compared to an IR oral drug product. The physiologic characteristics of the GI tract, including variations in pH, blood flow, GI motility, presence of food, enzymes and bacteria, etc, affects the local action of the ER drug product within the GI tract and may affect the drug release rate from the product in addition to transporters and metabolizing enzymes located in the gut wall. In some cases, there may be a specific absorption site or location within the GI tract in which the ER drug product should release the drug. This specific drug absorption site or location within the GI tract is referred to as an *absorption window*. The absorption window is the optimum site for drug absorption. If drug is not released and available for absorption within the absorption window, the ER tablet moves further distally in the GI tract and incomplete drug absorption may occur and may give rise to unsatisfactory drug absorption *in vivo* despite excellent *in vitro* release characteristics.

### Stomach

The stomach is a muscular, hollow, dilated part of the digestive system located on the left side of the upper abdomen. The stomach receives food or liquids from the esophagus. In this "mixing and secreting" organ, the stomach secretes protein-digesting enzymes called proteases and strong acids to aid in food digestion, through smooth muscular contortions before sending partially digested food (chyme) periodically to the small intestines. However, the movement of food or drug product in the stomach and small intestine varies greatly depending on the physiologic state. In the presence of food, the stomach is in the *digestive phase*; in the absence of food, the stomach is in the *interdigestive phase* (Chapter 4). During the digestive phase, food particles or solids larger than 2 mm are retained in the stomach, whereas smaller particles are emptied through the pyloric sphincter at a first-order rate depending on the content and size of the meals. During the interdigestive phase, the stomach rests for a period of up to 30 to 40 minutes, coordinated with an equal resting period in the small intestine. Peristaltic contractions then occur, which end with strong *housekeeper contractions* that move everything in the stomach through to the small intestine. Similarly, large particles in the small intestine are moved along only in the housekeeper contraction period.

A drug may remain for several hours in the stomach if it is administered during the digestive phase. Fatty material, nutrients, and osmolality may further extend the time the drug stays in the stomach. When the drug is administered during the interdigestive phase, the drug may be swept along rapidly into the small intestine. The drug release rates from some ER drug products are affected by mechanism of drug release (Sujja-areevath et al, 1998; Basu et al, 2019), viscosity (Rahman et al, 2011; Ghayas et al, 2019), pH and ionic strength (Asare-Addo et al, 2011; Zhu et al, 2018), and food (Abrahamsson et al, 2004; Ikeuchi et al, 2018). Dissolution of drugs in the stomach may also be affected by the presence or absence of food. When food and nutrients are present, the stomach pH may change from 1 to 2 by stomach acid (usually HCl) secretion to about 3 to 5 because of the food and nutrient neutralization.

In one example, drug release from Nifedipine ER formulations could be influenced (either increased or decreased) by concomitant intake of food compared to fasting conditions (Jonkman, 1989; Gao et al, 2019). Food can alter drug exposure in several ways, including by delaying gastric emptying, stimulating bile flow, altering GI pH, increasing splanchnic blood flow, or physically and/or chemically interacting with the drug. Food intake can influence the rate of drug release from the dosage form, the rate of drug absorption, the amount of drug absorbed, or all of these parameters simultaneously. The rate of drug release of various ER formulations can be affected by the composition of the coadministered meal. This effect may result in both "positive" and "negative." Positive food effects usually come with drug release speeding up from ER formulation, which may cause a high risk for patients in extreme cases by tablets coating erosion (Petrides et al, 2018). The solubilization effect by bile micelles in the presence of food may have a positive effect on drug absorption (Kawai et al, 2011). Negative food effects may take effect in an opposite direction by increasing the viscosity in the upper GI tract, delaying the absorption rate, and prolonging the passage time of the ER drug product in the GI tract (Marasanapalle et al, 2009; Margolesky and Singer, 2017). A longer retention time in the stomach may expose the drug to stronger agitation in the acid environment. The stomach has been described as having "jet mixing" action, which sends mixture at up to 50 mm Hg pressure toward the pyloric sphincter, causing it to open and periodically release chyme to the small intestine.

### Small Intestine and Transit Time

The small intestine is about 10 to 14 ft in length. The duodenum is sterile, while the terminal part of the small intestine that connects the cecum contains some bacteria. The proximal part of the small intestine has a pH of about 6, because of neutralization of acid by bicarbonates secreted into the lumen by the duodenal mucosa and the pancreas. The small intestine provides an enormous surface area for drug absorption because of the presence of microvilli. The small intestine transit time of a solid preparation has been concluded to be about 3 hours or less in 95% of the population (Hofmann et al, 1983). As Table 9-2 summarizes, the small intestinal transit time is more reproducible around 3 to 4 hours. The transit time from mouth to cecum ranges from 3 to 7 hours. Colonic transit time has the highest variation which is typically from 10 to 20 hours (Shareef et al, 2003; WA, 1991; Yu et al, 1996). Various investigators have used the lactulose hydrogen test, which measures the appearance of hydrogen in a patient's breath, to estimate transit time. Lactulose is metabolized rapidly by bacteria in the large intestine, yielding hydrogen that is exhaled. Hydrogen is normally absent in a person's breath. These results and the use of gamma-scintigraphy studies confirm a relatively short GI transit time from mouth to cecum of 4 to 6 hours (Shareef et al, 2003), and this technique has been applied in exploring extended oro-cecal transit time in the intestine (Eisenmann et al, 2008; Razavi et al, 2015).

**TABLE 9-2 • pH Values against Transit Time at Different Segments of GI Tract**

| Anatomical Location | Fasting Condition | | Food Condition | |
|---|---|---|---|---|
| | pH | Transition Time (h) | pH | Transition Time (h) |
| Stomach | 1–3 | 0.5–0.7 | 4.3–5.4 | 1 |
| Duodenum | ~6 | <0.5 | 5.4 | <0.5 |
| Jejunum | 6–7 | 1.7 | 5.4–5.6 | 1.7 |
| Ileum | 6.6–7.4 | 1.3 | 6.6–7.4 | 1.3 |
| Cecum | 6.4 | 4.5 | 6.4 | 4.5 |
| Colon | 6.8 | 13.5 | 6.8 | 13.5 |

This transit time interval was concluded to be too short for ER dosage forms that last up to 12 hours, unless the drug is to be absorbed in the colon. The colon has little fluid, and the abundance of bacteria may make drug absorption erratic and incomplete.

In one Phase I study of 12 healthy males, at a controlled rate, new gastro-resistant, ER tablets with multi-matrix structure (ie, MMX® tablets containing 9 mg budesonide) have been developed. The noninvasive technique of gamma-scintigraphy was employed to monitor the GI transit of orally ingested dosage forms for the purpose of identification of the exact time and region of disintegration and to follow the release of the active ingredient from the ER formulation. The effect of food was tested by comparing plasma PKs after intake of a high fat and high calorie breakfast with fasting controls. The results showed that 153 Sm-labelled MMX-budesonide ER tablets reached the colonic region after a mean of 9.8 h. Initial tablet disintegration was observed in the ileum in 42% of subjects, whereas in 33% the main site of disintegration was either the ascending or transverse colon. The budesonide plasma concentrations were first detected after 6.8 ± 3.2 h (Brunner et al, 2006).

### Large Intestine

The large intestine is about 4 to 5 ft long. It consists of the cecum, the ascending and descending colons, and eventually ends at the rectum. Little fluid is in the colon, and drug transit is slow. Not much is known about drug absorption in this area, although unabsorbed drug that reaches this region may be metabolized by bacteria. Incompletely absorbed antibiotics may affect the normal flora of the bacteria. The rectum has a pH of about 6.8 to 7.0 and contains more fluid compared to the colon. Drugs are absorbed rapidly when administered as rectal preparations. However, the transit rate through the rectum is affected by the rate of defecation. Presumably, drugs formulated for 24-hour duration must remain in this region to be absorbed.

Several ER and DR drug products, such as mesalamine DR tablets (Asacol), are formulated to take advantage of the physiological conditions of the GI tract (Shareef et al, 2003). This kind of efficient site-specific delivery can also be used for treatment of inflammatory bowel disorder (IBD) (Sharma et al, 2018). Enteric-coated beads have been found to release drug over 8 hours when taken with food because of the gradual emptying of the beads into the small intestine. Specially formulated "floating tablets" that remain in the top of the stomach have been used to extend the residence time of the product in the stomach. None of these methods, however, are consistent enough to predict reliably what would happen for potent medications. More experimental research is needed in this area.

In 2016, Jin et al reported an oral pH-enzyme double dependent mesalamine colon–specific delivery system. This chitosan-coated particle-based system produced sustained target release after oral administration with low toxicity potential for other organs, and was efficient in delivering mesalamine to its target tissue of colon. Their conclusion was that using this type of ER drug system can maintain the concentration of mesalamine in the target range for a long time; reduce the influence caused by fluctuations in drug concentrations, reducing adverse events; ensure the efficiency of treatment and reduce the frequency of administration; and improve patient compliance (Jin et al, 2016).

## DOSAGE FORM SELECTION

The properties of the drug and required dosage are important in formulating an ER product since the selection of appropriate dissolution media, apparatus, and test parameters reflect *in vivo* drug release. For example, a drug with low aqueous solubility generally should not be formulated into a non-disintegrating tablet, because the risk of incomplete drug dissolution is high. Instead, a drug with low solubility at neutral pH should be formulated to an erodible tablet, so that most of the drug is released before it reaches the colon, since the lack of fluid in the colon may make complete dissolution difficult. Erodible tablets are more reliable for these drugs because the entire tablet eventually dissolves.

A drug that is highly water soluble in the acid pH in the stomach but very insoluble at intestinal pH may be difficult to formulate into an ER drug product. An ER drug product with too much coating protection may result in low drug bioavailability, while too little coating protection may result in rapid drug release or dose dumping in the stomach. A moderate extension of duration with enteric-coated beads may be possible. However, the risk of erratic performance is higher than with a conventional dosage form. The osmotic type of controlled drug release system may be more suitable for this type of drug.

With most single-unit dosage forms, there is a risk of erratic performance due to variable stomach emptying and GI transit time. The size and shape of the single-unit dosage form will also influence GI transit time. Selection of a pellet or bead dosage form may minimize the risk of erratic stomach emptying, because pellets are usually scattered soon after ingestion. Disintegrating tablets have the same advantages because they break up into small particles soon after ingestion. The goal of the dissolution test is to predict the *in vivo* performance of products from *in vitro* test by a proper *in vitro/in vivo* correlation (IVIVC) (Chapter 7). These tests may not be pharmacopeia standard. However, dissolution tests should be sensitive, reliable, and discriminatory about the *in vitro* drug release characteristics. This technique is applied in IR ER drug products (Honório et al, 2013; Cheng et al, 2014; Meulenaar et al, 2014; Grimm et al, 2019).

## ADVANTAGES AND DISADVANTAGES OF EXTENDED-RELEASE PRODUCTS

To maintain a long therapeutic effect, frequent administration of conventional formulations of many drugs with short half-life is necessary. Otherwise, concentration under the therapeutic window occurs frequently in the course of treatment, which may induce drug resistance. ER dosage forms may solve these issues by having a number of advantages in safety and efficacy over IR drug products in that the frequency of dosing can be reduced, drug efficacy can be prolonged, and the incidence and/or intensity of adverse effects can be decreased.

### Advantages

1. **Sustained therapeutic blood levels of the drug.** ER drug products offer several important advantages over conventional dosage forms of the same drug by optimizing biopharmaceutics, PK, and PD properties of drugs. ER allows for sustained therapeutic blood levels of the drug. Sustained blood levels provide for a prolonged and consistent clinical response in the patient. Moreover, if the drug input rate is constant, the blood levels should not fluctuate much between a maximum and minimum compared to a multiple-dose regimen with an IR drug product. Highly fluctuating blood concentrations of drug may produce unwanted side effects in the patient if the drug level is too high or may fail to exert the proper therapeutic effect if the drug level is too low. In such a way, ER drug products may maintain a constant plasma drug concentration within the therapeutic window for a prolonged period. ER dosage forms maximize the therapeutic effect of drugs while minimizing possible resistance.

2. **Improved patient compliance.** An advantage of the ER formulation is improved patient compliance. Dosing frequency of one tablet twice daily (eg, morning and night) or one tablet once

daily is easier for patients to comply with compared to taking an IR tablet three or four times a day. Some ER drug products reduce dosing frequency to once-daily dosing for therapeutic management through a more uniform plasma exposure over time providing longer PD activity with a reduction in the associated systemic side effects. For example, if the patient needs to take the medication only once daily, they will not have to remember to take additional doses at specified times during the day. Furthermore, because the dosage interval is longer, the patient's sleep may not be interrupted to take another drug dose. With longer therapeutic drug concentrations, the patient awakens without having subtherapeutic drug levels.

3. **Reduction in adverse side effects and improvement in tolerability.** Drug plasma levels are maintained within a narrow window with no sharp peaks and with AUC of plasma concentration versus time curve equivalent to the AUC from multiple dosing with IR dosage form. Because of the controlled drug concentration in the therapeutic and safe window, the possible side effects can be significantly decreased due to the absence of drug plasma levels higher than toxic level or lower, trough plasma levels that might be subtherapeutic.

4. **Reduction in healthcare cost.** The patient may also derive an economic benefit in using an ER drug product. For patients under nursing care, the cost of nursing time required to administer medication is decreased if only one drug dose is given to the patient each day.

For some drugs with long elimination half-lives, such as chlorpheniramine, the inherent duration of pharmacologic activity is long. Minimal fluctuations in blood concentrations of these drugs are observed after multiple doses are administered. Therefore, there is no rationale for ER formulations of these drugs. However, such drug products are marketed with the justification that ER products minimize toxicity, decrease adverse reactions, and provide patients with more convenience and thus better compliance. In contrast, drugs with very short half-lives need to be given at frequent dosing intervals to maintain therapeutic efficacy. For drugs with very short elimination half-lives, an ER drug product maintains the efficacy over a longer duration.

### Disadvantages

There are also some disadvantages with using ER medications.

1. **Dose dumping.** *Dose dumping* is defined either as the release of more than the intended fraction of drug or the release of drug at a greater rate than the customary amount of drug per dosage interval, such that potentially adverse plasma levels may be reached. Dose dumping is a phenomenon whereby a relatively large quantity of drug in a controlled release formulation is rapidly released, introducing a potentially toxic quantity of the drug into systemic circulation. Dose dumping can lead to severe conditions for patients, especially for a drug with a narrow therapeutic index. Usually, dose dumping is a result of poor formulation design.

2. **Less flexibility in accurate dose adjustment.** If the patient suffers from an adverse drug reaction or accidentally becomes intoxicated, removal of drug from the system is more difficult with an ER drug product. In conventional dosage forms, dose adjustments are much simpler, eg, tablet can be divided into two fractions.

3. **Less possibility for high dosage.** Orally administered ER drug products may yield erratic or variable drug absorption as a result of various drug interactions with the contents of the GI tract and changes in GI motility. The formulation of ER drug products may not be practical for drugs that are usually given in large doses (eg, 500 mg) in conventional dosage forms (eg, amoxicillin). Because the ER drug product may contain two or more times the dose given at more frequent intervals, the size of the ER drug product may have to be quite large—too large for the patient to swallow easily.

In addition to the above-mentioned disadvantages, other issues including increased potential for first-pass clearance and poor IVIVC correlation, etc, are also challenges. For example, with delayed release or enteric drug products, two possible problems may occur if the enteric coating is poorly formulated. First, the enteric coating may become degraded in the stomach, allowing for early release of the drug,

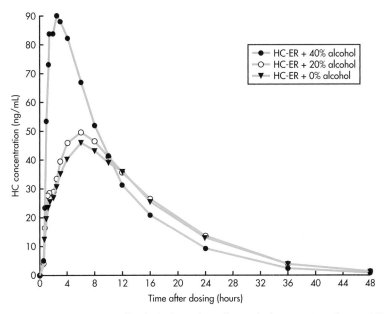

FIGURE 9-5 • Plasma concentration by time profiles for hydrocodone after oral administration of 50 mg HC-ER with or without alcohol.

possibly causing irritation to the gastric mucosal lining. Second, the enteric coating may fail to dissolve at the proper site, and therefore the tablet may be lost from the body prior to drug release, resulting in incomplete absorption (Nagaraju et al, 2010; Wilson et al, 2013). Enteric-coated drug products may unintentionally release drug in the stomach in patients with achlorhydria or in patients who have taken certain medications (eg, proton pump inhibitors such as omeprazole) that block acid secretion and increases the pH of the content in the stomach.

The side effects may remain longer after the administration, and an omitted dose of an ER drug product may lead to a reduced plasma concentration. Also, ER drug products have less flexibility in the dosing regimen and may cost more than IR formulations (Brandt and May, 2018).

### Effect of Alcohol Ingestion on ER Formulation of Hydrocodone

There have been several reported failures of ER formulations of opiates in patients who have consumed alcohol along with their medication. Figure 9-5 shows the plasma drug concentrations of an ER formulation in healthy volunteers who have also ingested 40%, 20%, or no (0%) alcohol.

In this study, subjects ingested 240 mL of 40% alcohol in the orange group; the equivalent of 5-6 shots (220–264 mL or 44 mL per shot of 80-proof vodka (Farr et al, 2015). The higher dose of alcohol dramatically raised the plasma hydrocodone levels.

### KINETICS OF EXTENDED-RELEASE DOSAGE FORMS

The amount of drug required in an ER dosage form to provide a sustained drug level in the body is determined by the PKs of the drug, the desired therapeutic level of the drug, and the intended duration of action. In general, the total dose required ($D_{tot}$) is the sum of the maintenance dose ($D_m$) and the initial dose ($D_I$) released immediately to provide a therapeutic blood level.

$$D_{tot} = D_I + D_m \tag{9.1}$$

In practice, $D_m$ (mg) is released over a period of time and is equal to the product of $t_d$ (the duration of drug release) and the zero-order rate $k_r^0$ (mg/h). Therefore, Equation 9.1 can be expressed as

$$D_{tot} = D_I + K_r^0 t_d \tag{9.2}$$

Ideally, the maintenance dose ($D_m$) is released after $D_I$ has produced a blood level equal to the therapeutic drug level ($C_p$). However, due to the limits of formulations, $D_m$ actually starts to release at $t = 0$. Therefore, $D_I$ may be reduced from the calculated amount to avoid *topping*.[1]

$$D_{tot} = D_I - K_r^0 t_p + K_r^0 t_d \quad (9.3)$$

Equation 9.3 describes the total dose of drug needed, with $t_p$ representing the time needed to reach peak drug concentration after the initial dose.

For any drug, the rate of elimination ($R$) needed to maintain the drug at a therapeutic level ($C_p$) is dependent on the drug's clearance (CL/F) and the desired stable concentration:

$$R = C_p.CL/F \quad (9.4)$$

where $k_r^0$ must be equal to $R$ in order to provide a stable blood level of the drug. Equation 9.4 provides an estimation of the release rate ($k_r^0$) required in the formulation. Equation 9.4 may also be written as 9.5 if we assume that the PK of the drug product will be described by a one-compartment model, where $CL/F = k.V_D/F$:

$$R = C_p.k.V_D/F \quad (9.5)$$

In designing an ER product, $D_I$ would be the loading dose that would raise the drug concentration in the body to $C_p$, and the total dose needed to maintain therapeutic concentration in the body would be simply

$$D_{tot} = D_I + C_p CL_T \tau \quad (9.6)$$

For many SR drug products, there is no built-in loading dose (ie, $D_I = 0$). The dose needed to maintain a therapeutic concentration for $\tau$ hours is

$$D_0 = (C_p \tau CL_T)/F \quad (9.7)$$

where $\tau$ is the dosing interval and F is the drug product's bioavailability.

---

[1]Topping is a spiking peak following subsequent doses due to the addition of the IR component releasing drug and the ER component releasing drug.

## EXAMPLE ▷ ▷ ▷

Which dose is needed to maintain a therapeutic concentration of 10 $\mu$g/mL for 12 hours in a SR product? (**a**) Assume that the clearance of the drug is 2 L/h with a bioavailability of 100%, or assuming a 1-cpt model that the elimination $t_{1/2}$ for the drug is 3.46 hours and its $V_D$ is 10 L. (**b**) Assume a change in elimination $t_{1/2}$ of the drug to 1.73 hours and the $V_D$ to 5 L.

a. $$k = \frac{0.693}{3.46} = 0.2 \text{ L/h}$$

$$CL_T = kV_D = 0.2 \times 10 = 2 \text{ L/h}$$

From Equation 9.7,

$$D_0 = (10 \ \mu\text{g/mL})(1000 \text{ mL/L})(12 \text{ h})(2 \text{ L/h})/1$$
$$= 240,000 \ \mu\text{g or } 240 \text{ mg}$$

b. $$k = \frac{0.693}{1.73} = 0.4 \text{ h}$$

$$CL_T = 0.4 \times 10 = 2 \text{ L/h}$$

From Equation 9.7,

$$D_0 = 10 \times 2 \times 1000 \times 12 / 1 = 240,000 \ \mu\text{g or } 240 \text{ mg}$$

The amount of drug needed in a SR product to maintain therapeutic drug concentration is dependent on the clearance In part **b** of the example, the clearance changes because the elimination half-life is shorter and the volume of distribution smaller.

---

The desired concentrations are as we have indicated dependent on the drug product's clearance. When clearance changes are resulting in the exact same changes in $t_{1/2}$ without a corresponding effect on volumes of distribution, the desired concentrations can be shown to change according to the half-life. Table 9-3 shows the influence of $t_{1/2}$ on the amount of drug needed for an ER drug product. Table 9-3 was constructed by assuming that the drug has a desired serum concentration of 5 $\mu$g/mL and an apparent volume of distribution of 20,000 mL. The release rate needed to achieve the desired concentration, $R$, decreases as the elimination half-life

**TABLE 9-3 •** Release Rates for Extended-Release Drug Products as a Function of Elimination Half-Life*

| $t_{1/2}$ (h) | $k$ (h⁻¹) | $R$ (mg/h) | Total (mg) to Achieve Duration | | | |
|---|---|---|---|---|---|---|
| | | | 6 h | 8 h | 12 h | 24 h |
| 1 | 0.693 | 69.3 | 415.8 | 554.4 | 831.6 | 1663 |
| 2 | 0.347 | 34.7 | 208.2 | 277.6 | 416.4 | 832.8 |
| 4 | 0.173 | 17.3 | 103.8 | 138.4 | 207.6 | 415.2 |
| 6 | 0.116 | 11.6 | 69.6 | 92.8 | 139.2 | 278.4 |
| 8 | 0.0866 | 8.66 | 52.0 | 69.3 | 103.9 | 207.8 |
| 10 | 0.0693 | 6.93 | 41.6 | 55.4 | 83.2 | 166.3 |
| 12 | 0.0577 | 5.77 | 34.6 | 46.2 | 69.2 | 138.5 |

*Assume $C_{desired}$ is 5 µg/mL and the $V_D$ is 20,000 mL; $R = kV_DC_p$; no immediate-release dose.

increases. Because elimination is slower for a drug with a long half-life, the input rate should be slower. The total amount of drug needed in the ER drug product is dependent on both the release rate $R$ and the desired duration of activity for the drug. For a drug with an elimination half-life of 4 hours and a release rate of 17.3 mg/h, the extended-release product must contain 207.6 mg to provide a duration of activity of 12 hours. The bulk weight of the extended-release product will be greater than this amount, due to the presence of excipients needed in the formulation. The values in Table 9-3 show that, to achieve a long duration of activity (≥12 hours) for a drug with a very short half-life (1–2 hours), the high drug doses cause the ER drug product to become quite large and impractical for most patients to swallow.

## PHARMACOKINETIC SIMULATION OF EXTENDED-RELEASE PRODUCTS

The plasma drug concentration profiles of many ER products can be described appropriately using a simple oral one-compartment model assuming first-order absorption and elimination. Compared to an IR product, the ER product typically shows a smaller absorption rate constant because of the slower absorption of the ER product. The time for peak concentration ($t_{max}$) is usually longer (Fig. 9-6), and the peak drug concentration ($C_{max}$) is reduced.

If the drug product is properly formulated so if the relative bioavailability of the ER formulation to the IR is 1, then the area under the plasma drug concentration curve will be the same. Parameters such as $C_{max}$, $t_{max}$, and AUC conveniently show how successfully the ER product performs *in vivo*. For example, a product with an excessively high $C_{max}$ and short $t_{max}$ may be a sign of dose dumping due to inadequate formulation. The PK analysis of single- and multiple-dose plasma data has been used by regulatory agencies to evaluate many SR products. The analysis is practical because many products can be fitted to this model even though the drug is not released in a first-order manner. The limitation of this type of prediction is that the absorption rate constant may not relate to the rate of drug dissolution *in vivo*. If the

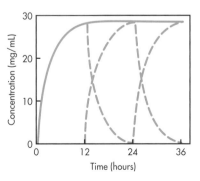

FIGURE 9-6 • Simulated plasma drug level of an extended-release product administered every 12 hours. The plasma level shows a smooth rise to steady-state level with no fluctuations.

drug strictly follows zero-order release and absorption, more complex models will be needed.

Various other models have been used to simulate plasma drug levels of ER products (Welling, 1983). The plasma drug levels from a zero-order, ER drug product may be simulated with Equation 9.8 assuming a one compartment model.

$$C_p = \frac{R.F}{k.V_D}(1 - e^{-kt})$$ (9.8)

where $R$ = rate of drug release (mg/min), $F$ = expected drug product's bioavailability, $C_p$ = plasma drug concentration, $k$ = elimination rate constant, and $V_D$ = volume of distribution. In the absence of a loading dose, the drug level in the body rises slowly to a plateau with minimum fluctuations (Fig. 9-7). This simulation assumes that (1) rapid drug release occurs without delay, (2) perfect zero-order release and absorption of the drug takes place, and (3) the drug is given exactly every 12 hours. In practice, the above assumptions are not precise, and fluctuations in drug level do occur.

When an SR drug product with a loading dose (rapid release) and a zero-order maintenance dose is given, assuming a one-compartment model, the resulting plasma drug concentrations may be estimated by

$$C_p = \frac{D_i F k_a}{V_D(k_a - k)}(e^{-kt} - e^{-k_a t}) + \frac{D_s F}{kV_D}(1 - e^{-kt})$$ (9.9)

where $D_i$ = IR (loading dose) dose and $D_s$ = maintenance dose (zero-order). This expression is the sum of the oral absorption equation due to the loading dose (first part) and the zero-order equation describing the constant release (second part).

## Extended-Release Drug Product with Immediate-Release Component

ER drug products may be formulated with or without an IR loading dose. ER drug products that are given to patients in daily multiple doses to maintain steady-state therapeutic drug concentrations do not need a built-in loading dose when given subsequent doses. PK models have been proposed for ER drug products that have a rapid first-order drug release component and a slow zero-order release maintenance dose component. Some models assume a long elimination $t_{1/2}$ in which drug accumulation occurs until steady state is attained. The models would predict spiking peaks due to the loading dose component when the ER drug product is given continuously in multiple doses. In these models, a rapid-release loading dose along with the ER drug dose given in a daily multiple dose regimen introduces more drug into the body than is necessary. This is observed by a "topping" effect. As shown in the example, amoxicillin ER tablets (Moxatag) are designed to consist of three components, one IR and two DR parts, each containing amoxicillin. The three components are combined in a specific ratio to prolong the release of amoxicillin from Moxatag compared to IR amoxicillin.

When a loading dose is necessary, a RR or IR drug product may be given separately as a loading dose to initially bring the patient's plasma drug level to the desired therapeutic level. In certain clinical situations, an ER drug product with an IR component along with a CR core can provide a specific PK profile that provides rapid onset and prolonged plasma drug concentrations that relates to the time course for the desired PD activity. For these ER drug products with initial IR components, the active drug must have a relatively short elimination $t_{1/2}$ so that the drug does not accumulate between dosing.

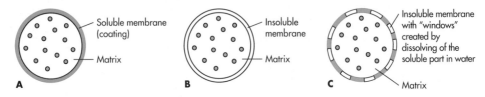

**FIGURE 9-7 •** Examples of three different types of modified matrix-release mechanisms.

# CLINICAL EXAMPLES

## Methylphenidate HCl Extended-Release Tablets (Concerta®)

Methylphenidate HCl is a central nervous system (CNS) stimulant indicated for the treatment of attention deficit-hyperactivity disorder (ADHD) and is often used in children 6 years of age and older. Methylphenidate is readily absorbed after oral administration and has an elimination $t_{1/2}$ of about 3.5 hours. Methylphenidate HCl ER tablets (Concerta) have an osmotically active controlled release core with an IR drug overcoat. Concerta uses osmotic pressure to deliver methylphenidate HCl at a controlled rate. The system, which resembles a conventional tablet in appearance, comprises an osmotically active trilayer core surrounded by a semipermeable membrane with an IR drug overcoat. The trilayer core is composed of two drug layers containing the drug and excipients, and a push layer containing osmotically active components. Each ER tablet for once-a-day oral administration contains 18, 27, 36, or 54 mg of methylphenidate HCl USP and is designed to have 12-hour duration of effect. After oral administration of Concerta, the plasma methylphenidate concentration increases rapidly, reaching an initial maximum at about 1 hour, followed by gradual ascending concentrations over the next 5 to 9 hours, after which a gradual decrease begins. Mean $t_{max}$ occurs between 6 to 10 hours. When the patient takes this product in the morning, the patient receives an initial loading dose followed by a maintenance dose that is mostly eliminated by the evening when the patient wants to go to sleep. Due to the short

elimination $t_{1/2}$, the drug does not accumulate significantly even when administered daily.

By measuring the mean methylphenidate plasma concentrations, Concerta 18 mg once daily was found to minimize the fluctuations between peak and trough concentrations associated with immediate-release methylphenidate three times daily administrated every four hours (see Figure 9-8). The relative bioavailability of Concerta once daily and methylphenidate three times daily in adults is comparable (Concerta [methylphenidate HCl] Extended-Release Tablets, FDA approved label, December 2013)

## Oxymorphone Extended-Release Tablets (Opana ER)

Oxymorphone ER tablets (Opana ER) are approved for the management of chronic pain. The PK profile of oxymorphone ER is predictable, linear, and dose proportional. Opana ER may maintain steady plasma levels over a 12-hour period with $t_{1/2}$ of about 9 to 11 hours. It has a low fluctuation index of less than 1 after achieving steady state, as do its two metabolites. Oxymorphone is metabolized primarily via hepatic glucuronidation to one active metabolite (6-OH-oxymorphone) and to one inactive metabolite (oxymorphone-3-glucuronide). It is neither metabolized by CYP enzymes nor inhibited or induced by CYP substrates. Since oxymorphone ER has minimal potential for PK interactions, its use with sedatives, tranquilizers, hypnotics, phenothiazines, and other CNS depressants can produce additive effects. Hence, as with other opioids, vigilance is required in preventing PD interactions during therapy with oxymorphone ER (Craig, 2010).

## Zolpidem Tartrate Extended-Release Tablets (Ambien CR)

Zolpidem tartrate ER tablets are indicated for the treatment of insomnia characterized by difficulties with sleep onset and/or sleep maintenance. Zolpidem has a mean elimination $t_{1/2}$ of 2.5 hours. Zolpidem tartrate ER tablets exhibit biphasic absorption characteristics, which results in rapid initial absorption from the GI tract similar to zolpidem tartrate IR, then provides extended plasma concentrations beyond 3 hours after administration.[2] Patients who use this product

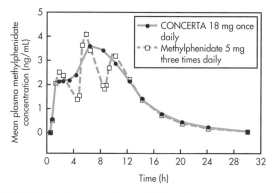

FIGURE 9-8 • The relative bioavailability of Concerta® once daily and methylphenidate three times daily.

---

[2]Approved label for Ambien CR, April 2010.

have a more rapid onset of sleep due to the initial dose and are able to maintain sleep due to the maintenance dose. Due to the short elimination $t_{1/2}$, the drug does not accumulate. In adult and elderly patients treated with zolpidem tartrate ER tablets, there was no evidence of accumulation after repeated once-daily dosing for up to 2 weeks. A food-effect study compared the PKs of zolpidem tartrate ER tablets 12.5 mg when administered while fasting or within 30 minutes after a meal. Results demonstrated that with food, mean AUC and $C_{max}$ were decreased by 23% and 30%, respectively, while median $t_{max}$ was increased from 2 hours to 4 hours. The half-life was not changed. These results suggest that, for faster sleep onset, zolpidem tartrate ER tablets should not be administered with or immediately after a meal.

### Divalproex Sodium Extended-Release Tablets (Depakote ER)

Divalproex sodium is used to treat seizure disorders, mental/mood conditions (such as manic phase of bipolar disorder), and to prevent migraine headaches. It works by restoring the balance of certain natural substances (neurotransmitters) in the brain. The mechanisms by which valproate exerts its therapeutic effects have not been established. It has been suggested that its activity in epilepsy is related to increased brain concentrations of gamma-aminobutyric acid (GABA). The absolute bioavailability of divalproex sodium ER tablets administered as a single dose after a meal was approximately 90% relative to intravenous infusion. The median time to maximum plasma valproate concentrations ($C_{max}$) after divalproex sodium ER tablet administration ranged from 4 to 17 hours. Mean terminal $t_{1/2}$ for valproate monotherapy ranged from 9 to 16 hours depending on the dosage applied.

## TYPES OF EXTENDED-RELEASE PRODUCTS

The pharmaceutical industry has been developing newer MR drug products at a very rapid pace. Many of these MR drug products have patented drug delivery systems. This chapter provides an overview of some of the more widely used methods for the manufacture of modified drug products.

The ER drug product is designed to contain a drug dose, which will release drug at a desired rate over a specified period of time. As discussed previously, the ER drug product may also contain an IR component. The general approaches to manufacturing an ER drug product include the use of a matrix structure in which the drug is suspended or dissolved, the use of a rate-controlling membrane through which the drug diffuses, or a combination of both. None of the ER drug products works by a single drug-release mechanism. Most ER products release drug by a combination of processes involving drug dissolution, permeation, erosion, and diffusion. The single most important factor is water permeation into the drug product, without which none of the product release mechanisms would operate. Controlling the rate of water influx into the product generally dictates the rate at which the drug dissolves in the GI tract. Once the drug is dissolved, the rate of drug diffusion may be further controlled to a desirable rate. Table 9-4 describes some common MR product examples and the mechanisms for controlling drug release. Table 9-5 lists the composition for some drugs.

### Drug Release from Matrix

A *matrix* is an inert solid vehicle in which a drug is uniformly suspended. A variety of excipients based on wax, lipid, as well as natural and synthetic polymers have been used as carrier material in the preparation of such matrix-type of drug delivery systems. The drug release from such matrix systems is mainly controlled by the diffusion process, concomitant swelling, and/or erosion processes. A matrix may be formed by compressing or fusing the drug and the matrix material together. When an erodible or swellable polymer matrix is involved, the drug release kinetics are further complicated by the presence of a second moving boundary, namely the swelling or eroding front which moves either opposite to or in the same direction as the diffusion front. Generally, the drug is present in a small percentage, so that the matrix protects the drug from rapid dissolution and the drug slowly diffuses out over time. Most matrix materials are water insoluble, although some matrix materials may swell slowly in water. Drug release using a matrix dosage form may be achieved using tablets or small beads, depending

## TABLE 9-4 • Examples of Oral Modified-Release Drug Products

| | Type | Trade Name | Rationale |
|---|---|---|---|
| Extended-release drug products | Erosion tablet | Constant-T | Theophylline |
| | | Tenuate Dospan | Diethylpropion HCl dispersed in hydrophilic matrix |
| | | Tedral SA | Combination product with a slow-erosion component (theophylline, ephedrine HCl) and an initial-release component theophylline, ephedrine HCl, phenobarbital |
| | Waxy matrix tablet | Kaon *Cl* | Slow release of potassium chloride to reduce GI irritation |
| | Coated pellets in capsule | Ornade spansule | Combination phenylpropanolamine HCl and chlorpheniramine with initial- and extended-release component |
| | Pellets in tablet Leaching | Theo-Dur | Theophylline |
| | | Ferro-Gradumet (Abbott) | Ferrous sulfate in a porous plastic matrix that is excreted in the stool; slow release of iron decreases GI irritation |
| | | Desoxyn gradumet tablet (Abbott) | Methamphetamine methylacrylate methylmethacrylate copolymer, povidone, magnesium stearate; the plastic matrix is porous |
| | Coated ion exchange | Tussionex | Cation ion-exchange resin complex of hydrocodone and phenyltoloxamine |
| | Flotation–diffusion | Valrelease | Diazepam |
| | Osmotic delivery | Acutrim | Phenylpropanolamine HCl (Oros delivery system) |
| | | Procardia-XL | GITS—Gastrointestinal therapeutic system with NaCl-driven (osmotic pressure) delivery system for nifedipine |
| | Microencapsulation | Bayer timed-release | Aspirin |
| | | Nitrospan | Microencapsulated nitroglycerin |
| | | Micro-K Extencaps | Potassium chloride microencapsulated particles |
| Delayed-release drug products | | Diclofenac sodium enteric-coated tablets mesalamine) delayed-release tablets | Enteric coating dissolves at pH >5 for release of drug in duodenum |
| | | | Delayed-release tablets are coated with acrylic-based resin, Eudragit S (methacrylic acid copolymer B, NF), which dissolves at pH 7 or greater, releasing mesalamine in the terminal ileum and beyond for topical anti-inflammatory action in the colon |
| Orally disintegrating tables | | | |

**TABLE 9-5 •** Composition and Examples of Some Modified-Release Products

| | |
|---|---|
| K-Tab (Abbott) | 750 mg or 10 mEq of potassium chloride in a film-coated matrix tablet. The matrix may be excreted intact, but the active ingredient is released slowly without upsetting the GI tract.<br>Inert ingredients: Cellulosic polymers, castor oil, colloidal silicon dioxide, polyvinyl acetate, paraffin. The product is listed as a waxy/polymer matrix tablet for release over 8–10 h. |
| Toprol-XL tablets (Astra) | Contains metoprolol succinate for sustained release in pellets, providing stable beta-blockade over 24 h with one daily dose. Exercise tachycardia was less pronounced compared to immediate-release preparation. Each pellet separately releases the intended amount of medication.<br>Inert ingredients: Paraffin, PEG, povidone, acetyltributyl citrate, starch, silicon dioxide, and magnesium stearate. |
| Quinglute Dura tablets (Berlex) | Contains 320 mg quinidine gluconate in a prolonged-action matrix tablet lasting 8–12 h and provides PVC protection.<br>Inert ingredients: Starch, confectioner's sugar and magnesium stearate. |
| Brontil Slow-Release capsules (Carnrick) Slow Fe tablets (Ciba) | Phendimetrazine tartrate 105 mg sustained pellet in capsule.<br>Slow-release iron preparation (OTC medication) with 160 mg ferrous sulfate for iron deficiency.<br>Inert ingredients: HPMC, PEG shellac, and cetostearyl alcohol. |
| Tegretol-XR tablets (Ciba Geneva) | Carbamazepine extended-release tablet.<br>Inert ingredients: Zein, cetostearyl alcohol, PEG, starch, talc, gum tragacanth, and mineral oil. |
| Sinemed CR tablets (Dupont pharma) | Contains a combination of carbidopa and levodopa for sustained-release delivery. This is a special erosion polymeric tablet for Parkinson's disease treatment. |
| Pentasa capsules (Hoechst Marion/Roussel) | Contains mesalamine for ulcerative colitis in a sustained-release mesalamine coated with ethylcellulose. For local effect mostly, about 20% absorbed versus 80% otherwise. |
| Isoptin SR (Knoll) | Verapamil HCI sustained-release tablet.<br>Inert ingredients: PEG, starch, PVP, alginate, talc, HPMC, methylcellulose, and microcrystalline cellulose. |
| Pancrease capsules (McNeil) | Enteric-coated microspheres of pancrelipase. Protects the amylase, lipase, and protease from the action of acid in the stomach.<br>Inert ingredients: CAP, diethyl phthalate, sodium starch glycolate, starch, sugar, gelatin, and talc. |
| Cotazym-S (Organon) | Enteric-coated microspheres of pancrelipase. |
| Eryc (erythromycin delayed-release capsules) (Warner-Chilcott) | Erythromycin enteric-coated tablet that protects the drug from instability and irritation. |
| Dilantin Kapseals (Parke-Davis) | Extended-release phenytoin capsule which contains beads of sodium phenytoin, gelatin, sodium lauryl sulfate, glyceryl monooleate, PEG 200, silicon dioxide, and talc. |
| Micro-K Extencaps (Robbins) | Ethylcellulose forms semipermeable film surrounding granules by microencapsulation for release over 8–10 h without local irritation.<br>Inert ingredients: Gelatin and sodium lauryl sulfate. |
| Quinidex Extentabs (Robbins) | 300-mg dose, 100-mg release immediately in the stomach and is absorbed in the small intestine. The rest is absorbed later over 10–12 h in a slow-dissolving core as it moves down the GI tract.<br>Inert ingredients: White wax, carnauba wax, acacia, acetylated monoglyceride, guar gum, edible ink, calcium sulfate, corn derivative, and shellac. |
| Compazine Spansules (GSK) | Initial dose of prochlorperazine release first, then release slowly over several hours.<br>Inert ingredients: Glycerylmonostearate, wax, gelatin, sodium lauryl sulfate. |
| Slo-bid Gyrocaps (Rhone-Poulenc Rorer) | A controlled-release 12–24-h theophylline product. |
| Theo-24 capsules (UCB Pharma) | A 24-h sustained-release theophylline product.<br>Inert ingredients: Ethylcellulose, edible ink, talc, starch, sucrose, gelatin, silicon dioxide, and dyes. |
| Sorbitrate SA (Zeneca) | The tablet contains isosorbide dinitrate 10 mg in the outer coat and 30 mg in the inner coat.<br>Inert ingredients: Carbomer 934P, ethylcellulose, lactose magnesium stearate, and Yellow No. 10. |

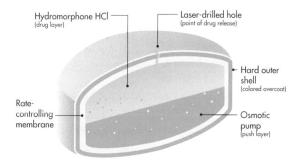

FIGURE 9-9A • Cross section of the extended-release hydromorphone tablet. (Adapted with permission from Gupta S, Sathyan G. Providing constant analgesia with OROS® hydromorphone, *J Pain Symptom Manage* 2007 Feb;33(2 suppl): S19–S24.)

on the formulation composition and therapeutic objective (Lee, 2011). Figure 9-9 shows three common approaches by which matrix mechanisms are employed. In Fig. 9-9A, the drug is coated with a soluble coating, so drug release relies solely on the regulation of drug release by the matrix material. If the matrix is porous, water penetration will be rapid and the drug will diffuse out rapidly. A less porous matrix may give a longer duration of release. Unfortunately, drug release from a simple matrix tablet is not zero order. Takeru Higuchi was the first one in the pharmaceutical field to tackle this moving boundary mathematical problem for drug release from matrix systems (Siepmann and Peppas, 2011). The Higuchi equation was originally derived to describe the drug release from an ointment layer containing suspended drug at an initial concentration (or amount

of drug loading per unit volume), which is substantially greater than the solubility of the drug per unit volume in the vehicle matrix. The *Higuchi equation* describes the release rate of a matrix tablet:

$$Q = DS\left(\frac{P}{\lambda}\right)(A - 0.5SP)1/2\sqrt{t} \qquad (9.10)$$

where $Q$ = amount of drug release per cm² of surface at time $t$, $S$ = solubility of drug in g/cm³ in the dissolution medium, $A$ = content of drug in insoluble matrix, $P$ = porosity of matrix, $D$ = diffusion coefficient of drug, and $\lambda$ = tortuosity factor.

Figure 9-9B represents a matrix enclosed by an insoluble membrane, so the drug release rate is regulated by the permeability of the membrane as well as the matrix. Figure 9-9A represents a matrix tablet

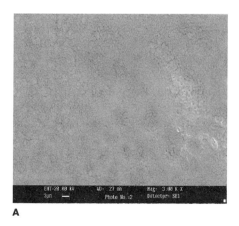

**A**

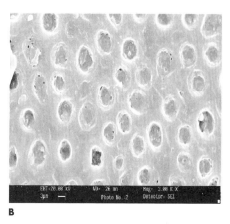

**B**

FIGURE 9-9B • SEM micrograph of the membrane of controlled porosity osmotic pump (CPOP) tablet containing diltiazem hydrochloride (A) before and (B) after dissolution studies.

enclosed with a combined film. The film becomes porous after dissolution of the soluble part of the film. An example of this is the combined film formed by ethylcellulose and methylcellulose. Close to zero-order release has been obtained with this type of release mechanism.

## Classification of Matrix Tablets

Based on the retarded materials used, matrix tablets can be divided into five types: (1) hydrophobic matrix (plastic matrix), (2) lipid matrix, (3) hydrophilic matrix, (4) biodegradable matrix, and (5) mineral matrix. Matrix systems can also be classified according to their porosity situation, including macroporous, microporous, and nonporous systems. By the usage frequency, matrix tablets can also be categorized as follows.

### Gum-Type Matrix Tablets

Some excipients have a remarkable ability to swell in the presence of water and form a substance with a gel-like consistency. When this happens, the gel provides a natural barrier to drug diffusion from the tablet. Natural gum polysaccharides consisting of multiple sugar units link together to create large molecules. Natural gums are biodegradable and nontoxic, which hydrate and swell on contact with aqueous media, and these have been used for the preparation of dosage form. They are used in pharmaceuticals for their diverse properties and applications. They can receive modification for the purpose of hydration rate control, pH-dependent solubility adjustment, thickness alteration and viscosity change, etc (Rana et al, 2011; Pachuau and Mazumder, 2012; Nur et al, 2016).

Because the gel-like material is quite viscous and may not disperse for hours, this approach provides a means for maintaining the drug for hours until all the drug has been completely dissolved and diffused into the intestinal fluid. Gelatin is a common gelling material. However, gelatin dissolves rapidly after the gel is formed. Drug excipients such as methylcellulose, gum tragacanth, Veegum, and alginic acid form a viscous mass and provide a useful matrix for controlling drug release and dissolution. Drug formulations with these excipients provide extended drug release for hours.

### Polymeric Matrix Tablets

Various polymeric materials have been used to prolong the rate of drug release. The most important characteristic of this type of preparation is that the prolonged release may last for days or weeks rather than for a shorter duration (as with other techniques). An early example of an oral polymeric matrix tablet was Gradumet (Abbott Laboratories), which was marketed as an iron preparation. The non-biodegradable plastic matrix provides a rigid geometric surface for drug diffusion, so that a relatively constant rate of drug release is obtained. In the case of the iron preparation, the matrix reduces the exposure of the irritating drug to the GI mucosal tissues. The matrix is usually expelled unchanged in the feces after all the drug has leached out.

Polymeric matrix tablets for oral use can be regarded as release-controlling excipients which can be divided into water-soluble (or hydrophilic) and insoluble (or hydrophobic) carriers (Grund et al, 2014; Barmpalexis et al, 2018). Considering the application in formulation, they should be quite safe. However, for certain patients with reduced GI motility caused by disease, polymeric matrix tablets should be avoided, because accumulation or obstruction of the GI tract by matrix tablets has been reported (Franek et al, 2014). As an oral SR product, the matrix tablet has not been popular. In contrast, the use of the matrix tablet in implantation has been more popular.

The use of biodegradable polymeric material for ER has been the focus of more recent research. Chitosan–carrageenan matrix tablets were characterized and used for the controlled release of highly soluble drug of trimetazidine hydrochloride (Li et al, 2013). One such example is poly(lactic acid-co-glycolic acid) copolymer, which degrades to lactic/gaalatic acid and eliminates the problem of retrieval after implantation (Clark et al, 2014; Sequeira et al, 2018), and the associated mathematical modeling is used for advanced analysis of the release/delivery process of polymeric-based matrix tablets, including porous, microporous, and nonporous matrix. With generating more and more complex models or a parametric fitting process, these modeling efforts can help the practitioner to achieve a better formulation design and understanding (Peppas and Narasimhan, 2014; Ong et al, 2018).

Other polymers for drug formulations include polyacrylate, methacrylate, polyester, ethylene-vinyl acetate copolymer (EVA), polyglycolide, polylactide, and silicone. Of these, the hydrophilic polymers, such as polylactic acid and polyglycolic acid, erode in water and release the drug gradually over time (Clark et al, 2014). Polymer properties may affect the integrity and drug release from insoluble matrices. Typical examples of insoluble carriers are Kollidon° SR (co-processed polyvinyl acetate and polyvinyl pyrrolidone, ratio 8:2), Eudragit° RS (ammonium methacrylate copolymer), and ethyl cellulose. A hydrophobic and also a non-degradable polymer such as EVA releases the drug over a longer duration of weeks or months. The rate of release may be controlled by blending two polymers and increasing the proportion of the more hydrophilic polymer, thus increasing the rate of drug release. The addition of a low-molecular-weight polylactide to a polylactide polymer formulation increased the release rate of the drug and enabled the preparation of an ER system (Krivoguz et al, 2013; Kleiner et al, 2014). The type of plasticizer and the degree of cross-linking provide additional means for modifying the release rate of the drug. Many drugs are incorporated into the polymer as the polymer is formed chemically from its monomer. Light, heat, and other agents may affect the polymer chain length, degree of cross-linking, and other properties. This may provide a way to modify the release rate of the polymer matrices prepared. Drugs incorporated into polymers may have release rates that last over days, weeks, or even months. These vehicles have been often recommended for protein and peptide drug administration. For example, EVA is biocompatible and was shown to prolong insulin release in rats.

Hydrophobic polymers with water-labile linkages are prepared so that partial breakdown of the polymers allows for desired drug release without deforming the matrix during erosion. Hydrophilic polymer such as Hypromellose (hydroxypropyl methylcellulose (HPMC) may be integrated with hydrophobic block, eg, polyacrylate polymers, Eudragit RL100 and Eudragit RS100, with or without incorporating ethyl cellulose on a matrix-controlled Metformin hydrochloride drug delivery system (Viridén et al, 2009; Jain et al, 2014). For oral drug delivery, the problem of incomplete drug release from the matrix is a major hurdle that must be overcome with the polymeric matrix dosage form. Another problem is that drug release rates may be affected by the amount of drug loaded. For implantation and other uses, the environment is more stable compared to oral routes,

so a stable drug release from the polymer matrix may be attained for days or weeks.

## Slow-Release Pellets, Beads, or Granules

Pellets or beads are small spherical particles that can be formulated to provide a variety of modified drug release properties. These beads can be very small (microencapsulation) for injections or larger for oral drug delivery. Several approaches have been used to manufacture beaded formulations including pan coating, spray drying, fluid bed drying, and extrusion-spheronization.

An early approach to the manufacture of ER drug products was the use of encapsulated drugs in a beaded or pellet formulation. In general, the beads are prepared by coating the powdered drug onto preformed cores known as *nonpareil seeds*. The nonpareil seeds are made from slurry of starch, sucrose, and lactose. The drug-coated beads are then coated by a variety of materials that act as barriers to drug release. The beads may have a blend of different thicknesses to provide the desired drug release. The beads may be placed in a capsule (eg, amphetamine ER capsules, Adderall XR) or with the addition of other excipients compressed into tablets (eg, metoprolol succinate ER tablets, Toprol XL).

*Pan coating* is a modified method adopted from candy manufacturing. Cores or nonpareil seeds of a given mesh size are slowly added to known amount of fine drug powder and coating solution and rounded for hours to become coated drug beads. The drug-coated beads are then coated with a polymeric layer which regulates drug release rate by changing either the thickness of the film or the composition of the polymeric material. Coatings may be aqueous or nonaqueous. Aqueous coatings are generally preferred. Nonaqueous coatings may leave residual solvents in the product, and the removal of solvents during manufacture presents danger to workers and the environment. Cores are coated by either sprayed pan coating or by air-suspension coating. Once the drug beads are prepared, they may be further coated with a protective coating to allow a sustained or prolonged release of the drug. *Spray dry coating*, or *fluid-bed coating*, is a more recent approach and has several advantages over pan coating. Drug may be dissolved in a solution that is sprayed or dispersed in small droplets in a chamber. A stream of hot air evaporates the solvent, and the drug becomes a dry powder. The powdered material, which is aerated, may be coated with a variety of excipients to achieve the desired drug release. Several experimental process variables for fluid-bed coating include inlet air temperature, spray rate (g/min), atomizing air pressure, solid content, and curing time. Pelletization may also be obtained by *extrusion-spheronization* in which the powdered drug and excipients are mixed in a mixer/granulator. The moist mixture is then fed through an extruder at a specified rate and becomes spheronized on exit though small diameter dies. A wide range of extrusion screen sizes and configurations are available for optimization of pellet diameter.

The use of various amounts of coating solution can provide beads with various coating protection. A careful blending of beads is used to achieve a desired drug release profile. The finished drug product (eg, beads in capsule or beads in tablet) may contain a blend of beads coated with materials of different solubility rates to provide a means of controlling drug release and dissolution.

The orally administered ER drug products may display in single or multiple-unit dosage forms. In single-unit formulations, they contain the active ingredient within the single tablet or capsule, whereas multiple-unit dosage forms are comprised of number of discrete particles that are combined into one dosage unit. Both may exist as pellets, granules, sugar seeds (nonpareil), minitablets, ion-exchange resin particles, powders, and crystals, with drugs being entrapped in or layered around cores. In this way, multiple-unit dosage forms offer several advantages over single-unit systems such as nondisintegrating tablets or capsules, although the drug release profiles are similar. Once multiple-unit systems are taken orally, the subunits of multiple-unit preparations distribute readily over a large surface area in the GI tract, and because of the small particles (<2 mm), multiple-unit preparations can enable them to be well distributed along the GI tract, which could improve the bioavailability (Rosiaux et al, 2014; Tyagi and Subramony, 2018). Some products take advantage of bead blending to provide two doses of drug in one formulation. For example, a blend of rapid-release beads with some pH-sensitive enteric-coated material may provide a second dose of drug release when the drug reaches the intestine.

The pellet dosage form can be prepared as a capsule or tablet. When pellets are prepared as tablets, the beads must be compressed lightly so that they do not break. This process is called compaction of pellets, which is also a challenging area. Only a few multiple-unit-containing tablet products are available, such as Beloc° ZOK, Antra° MUPS, and Prevacid° SoluTab™. Compaction of multiparticulates into tablets could either result in a disintegrating tablet providing a multiparticulate system during GI transit or intact tablets due to the fusion of the multiparticulates in a larger compact. Usually, a disintegrant is included in the tablet, causing the beads to be released rapidly after administration. Formulation of a drug into pellet form may reduce gastric irritation because the drug is released slowly over a period of time, therefore avoiding high drug concentration in the stomach (Abdul et al, 2010). Figure 9-10 shows the two types of multiple unit pellets in tablets, coated by polymer (reservoir-type)

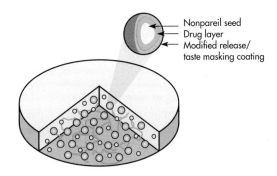

Nonpareil seed
Drug layer
Modified release/ taste masking coating

**A** MUPS containing polymer coated pellets

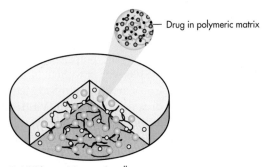

Drug in polymeric matrix

**B** MUPS containing matrix pellets

FIGURE 9-10 • Schematic representation of types of multiple unit pellet system (MUPS) in tablets — (a) comprised of coated pellets, and (b) uncoated/matrix pellets.

(a) compaction of matrix and/or uncoated drug pellets (b). The drug release from both pellets shows significant extended characterization, regardless of the polymer coating or matrix dispersion. For the reservoir-type coated-pellet dosage forms, the polymeric coating must be able to withstand the compaction force. It may deform but should not rupture since any crack on the coating layer may cause unexpected drug release. The type and amount of coating agent, the size of subunits, selection of external additives, and the rate and magnitude of pressure applied must be considered carefully to maintain the desired drug release properties.

Dextroamphetamine sulfate formulated as timed-release pellets in capsules (Dexedrine spansule) is an early example of a beaded dosage form. Another older product is a pellet-type ER product of theophylline (Gyrocap). Table 9-6 shows the frequency of adverse reactions after theophylline is administered as a solution or as pellets. If theophylline is administered as a solution, a high drug concentration is reached in the body due to rapid drug absorption. Some side effects may be attributed to the high concentration of theophylline. Pellet dosage form allows drug to be absorbed gradually, therefore reducing the incidence of side effects by preventing a high $C_{max}$.

Bitolterol mesylate (Tornalate) is a $\beta_2$-adrenergic receptor agonist used as a bronchodilator in asthma. A study in dogs indicated that the incidence of tachycardia was reduced using an ER bead preparation, whereas the bronchodilation effect was not reduced. Administering the drug as ER pellets apparently reduced excessively high drug concentration in the body and avoided stimulating an increase in heart rate. Studies also reported reduced GI side effects of the drug potassium chloride in pellet or microparticulate form. Potassium chloride is irritating to the GI tract. Formulation of potassium chloride in pellet form reduces the chance of exposing high concentrations of potassium chloride to the mucosal cells in the GI tract.

Many ER cold products also employ the bead formulation approach. A major advantage of pellet dosage forms is that the pellets are less affected by stomach emptying. Because numerous pellets are within a capsule, some pellets will gradually reach the small intestine each time the stomach empties, whereas a single ER tablet may be delayed in the stomach for a long time because of erratic stomach emptying. Stomach emptying time is particularly important in the formulation and *in vivo* behavior of enteric-coated products. Enteric-coated tablets may be delayed for hours by the presence of food in the stomach, whereas enteric-coated pellets are relatively unaffected by the presence of food.

## TABLE 9-6 • Incidence of Adverse Effects of Sustained-Release Theophylline Pellet Versus Theophylline Solution*

| | Volunteers Showing Side Effects | |
| Side Effects | Using Solution | Using Sustained-Release Pellets |
| --- | --- | --- |
| Nausea | 10 | 0 |
| Headache | 4 | 0 |
| Diarrhea | 3 | 0 |
| Gastritis | 2 | 0 |
| Vertigo | 5 | 0 |
| Nervousness | 3 | 1 |

* After 5-day dosing at 600 mg theophylline/24 h, adverse reaction points on fifth day: solution, 135; pellets, 18.
Data from Breimer DD, Dauhof M: Towards Better Safety of Drugs and Pharmaceutical Products. Amsterdam: Elsevier/North-Holland; 1980.

### Prolonged-Action Tablets

An alternate approach to prolong the action of a drug is to reduce the aqueous solubility of the drug so that the drug dissolves slowly over a period of several hours. The solubility of a drug is dependent on the salt form used. An examination of the solubility of the various salt forms of the drug is performed in early drug development. In general, the nonionized base or acid form of the drug is usually much less soluble than the corresponding salt. For example, sodium phenobarbital is more water soluble than phenobarbital, the acid form of the drug. Diphenhydramine hydrochloride is more soluble than the base form, diphenhydramine.

In cases where it is inconvenient to prepare a less soluble form of the drug, the drug may be granulated with an excipient to slow dissolution of the drug.

Often, fatty or waxy lipophilic materials are employed in formulations. Stearic acid, castor wax, high-molecular-weight polyethylene glycol (Carbowax), glyceryl monostearate, white wax, and spermaceti oil are useful ingredients in providing an oily barrier to slow water penetration and the dissolution of the tablet. Many of the lubricants used in tableting may also be used as lipophilic agents to slow dissolution. For example, magnesium stearate and hydrogenated vegetable oil (Sterotex) are actually used in high percentages to cause sustained drug release in a preparation. The major disadvantage of this type of preparation is the difficulty in maintaining a reproducible drug release from patient to patient because oily materials may be subjected to digestion, temperature, and mechanical stress, which may affect the release rate of the drug.

Another application of prolonged-action tablets is also called as pulsatile drug delivery system. This chronopharmaceutical formulation is usually used in the treatment of circadian rhythms dysfunction diseases. This effort may improve the therapeutic efficacy of oral drug administration for some specific chrono treatment. In one study, drug was compressed into regular tablets with ingredients of starch, lactose, magnesium stearate, etc. Then the tablet was put at a lower position into the capsule with another erodible plug composed of hydroxypropyl methylcellulose (HMPC):lactose, whose erodible process was controlled by osmotic extent from outer water. After a determined time point, the drug containing tablet was ejected from this pulsincap capsule by the mechanism of osmotic control (Wu et al, 2006; Ranjan et al, 2013; Lopez-Agullo et al, 2018). Time-controlled devices are also prepared by tablet surface coating with different compositions in order to defer the onset of release. Depending to the coating agent(s) employed, various type mechanisms can be involved, such as in erodible, permeable, or diffusive reservoir systems (Gefter (Federovich) et al, 2018).

## Ion-Exchange Products

The ion-exchange technique has been popularly applied in water purification and chemical extraction. Ion-exchange preparations usually involve an insoluble resin capable of reacting with either an anionic or cationic drug. An anionic resin is negatively charged so a positively charged cationic drug may attach the resin to form an insoluble nonabsorbable resin–drug complex. Upon exposure in the GI tract, cations in the gut, such as potassium and sodium, may displace the drug from the resin, releasing the drug, which is absorbed freely. Researchers have already applied the combination technique of iontophoresis and cation-exchange fibers as drug matrices for the controlled transdermal delivery of the antiparkinsonian drug apomorphine (Malinovskaja et al, 2013; Janićijević and Radovanović, 2018). The main disadvantage of ion-exchange preparations is that the amount of cation–anion in the GI tract is not easily controllable and varies among individuals, making it difficult to provide a consistent mechanism or rate of drug release. A further disadvantage is that resins may provide a potential means of interaction with nutrients and other drugs.

Ion exchange may be used in ER liquid preparations. An added advantage is that the technique provides some protection for very bitter or irritating drugs. Ion exchange has been combined with a coating to obtain a more effective SR product. Examples include dextromethorphan polistirex (Delsym®), an oral suspension formulated as an ion-exchange complex to mask the bitter taste and to prolong the duration of drug action, and Tussionex Pennkinetic®, an oral suspension containing chlorpheniramine polistirex and hydrocodone polistirex.

A general mechanism for the formulation of cationic drugs is

$$H^+ + resin - SO_3^- drug \rightleftharpoons resin - SO_3^- H^+ + drug^+$$
$$\text{Insoluble drug complex} \qquad \text{Soluble drug}$$

For anionic drugs, the corresponding mechanism is

$$Cl^- + resin - N^+(CH_3)_3\, drug^- \rightleftharpoons resin - N^+(CH_3)_3\, Cl^- + drug^-$$
$$\text{Insoluble drug complex} \qquad \text{Soluble drug}$$

The insoluble drug complex containing the resin and drug dissociates in the GI tract in the presence of the appropriate counter ions. The released drug dissolves in the fluids of the GI tract and is rapidly absorbed.

## Core Tablets

A core tablet is a tablet within a tablet. The inner core is usually used for the slow-drug-release component, and the outside shell contains a rapid-release dose of drug. Formulation of a core tablet requires two granulations. The core granulation is usually compressed lightly to form a loose core and then transferred to a second die cavity, where a second granulation containing additional ingredients is compressed further to form the final tablet.

The core material may be surrounded by hydrophobic excipients so that the drug leaches out over a prolonged period of time. This type of preparation is sometimes called a *slow-erosion core tablet* because the core generally contains either no disintegrant or insufficient disintegrant to fragment the tablet. The composition of the core may range from wax to gum or polymeric material. Numerous slow-erosion tablets have been patented and are sold commercially under various trade names.

The success of core tablets depends on the nature of the drug and the excipients used. As a general rule, this preparation is very hardness dependent in its release rate. Critical control of hardness and processing variables are important in producing a tablet with a consistent release rate. OSDrC°OptiDose" is a new commercial core tablet whose manufacture is conducted in a solvent-free, dry compression, single-process operation. Its single- or multi-cored tablets, with a range of dose forms including fixed-dose combination tablets, offer differentiated controlled-release functionality. This product is produced by Catalent, partnering with Sanwa Kagaku Kenkyusho Co., Ltd.

Core tablets are occasionally used to avoid incompatibility in preparations containing two physically incompatible ingredients. For example, in an oral enteric coated tablet of Adenovirus*, the final vaccine drug delivery system composed of two tablets (one tablet of Adenovirus Type 4 and one tablet of Adenovirus Type 7) is designed to pass intact through the stomach and release the live virus in the intestine for active immunization for the prevention of febrile acute respiratory disease.

### Microencapsulation

Microencapsulation is a process of encapsulating microscopic drug particles with a special coating material, therefore providing more desirable physical and chemical characteristics to the drug products. A common drug that has been encapsulated is aspirin. Aspirin has been microencapsulated with ethylcellulose, making the drug superior in its flow characteristics; when compressed into a tablet, the drug releases more gradually compared to a simple compressed tablet (Garekani et al, 2018). Usually, biodegradable polymers, such as dextran, collagen, chitosan, poly(lactide), ethyl cellulose, casein, etc, are natural materials applied in microencapsulation. After forming the encapsulation material as flowing powder, it is suitable for formulation as compressed tablets, hard gelatin capsules, suspensions, and other dosage forms (Baracatet al, 2012; Zhou et al, 2019).

Many techniques are used in microencapsulating a drug. One process used in microencapsulating acetaminophen involves suspending the drug in an aqueous solution while stirring. The coating material, ethylcellulose, is dissolved in cyclohexane, and the two liquids are added together with stirring and heating. As the cyclohexane is evaporated by heat, the ethylcellulose coats the microparticles of the acetaminophen. The microencapsulated particles have a slower dissolution rate because the ethylcellulose is not water soluble and provides a barrier for diffusion of drug. The amount of coating material deposited on the acetaminophen determines the rate of drug dissolution. The coating also serves as a means of reducing the bitter taste of the drug. In practice, microencapsulation is not consistent enough to produce a reproducible batch of product, and it may be necessary to blend the microencapsulated material in order to obtain a desired release rate.

### Osmotic Drug Delivery Systems

Osmotic drug delivery systems have been developed for both oral ER products known as GI therapeutic systems (GITS) and for parenteral drug delivery as an implantable drug delivery (eg, osmotic minipump). Drug delivery is controlled by the use of an osmotically controlled device in which a constant amount of water flows into the system causing the dissolving and releasing of a constant amount of drug per unit time. Drug is released via a single laser-drilled hole in the tablet.

Figure 9-9A describes an osmotic drug delivery system in the form of a tablet, which contains an outside semipermeable membrane and an inner core filled with a mixture of drug and osmotic agent (salt solution). When the tablet is placed in water, osmotic pressure is generated by the osmotic agent within the core. Water moves into the device, forcing the dissolved drug to exit the tablet through an orifice. The rate of drug delivery is relatively constant and unaffected by the pH of the environment. Figure 9-9B provides the surface electronic micrograph (SEM) images of the membrane of controlled porosity osmotic pump (CPOP) tablet containing diltiazem hydrochloride (A) before and (B) after dissolution studies, which can clearly find the drug release mechanism under microscopic domain (Adibkia et al, 2014).

Newer osmotic drug delivery systems are considered "push-pull" systems. Nifedipine (Procardia XL) ER tablets have the appearance of a conventional tablet. Procardia XL ER tablets have a semipermeable membrane surrounding an osmotically active drug core. The core itself is divided into two layers: an "active" layer containing the drug and a "push" layer containing pharmacologically inert (but osmotically active) components. As water from the GI tract enters the tablet, pressure increases in the osmotic layer and "pushes" against the drug layer, releasing drug through a laser-drilled tablet orifice in the active layer. Drug delivery is essentially constant (zero order) as long as the osmotic gradient remains constant, and then gradually falls to zero. Upon swallowing, the biologically inert components of the tablet remain intact during GI transit and are eliminated in the feces as an insoluble shell.

Methylphenidate HCl (Concerta) ER tablets use osmotic pressure to deliver methylphenidate HCl at a controlled rate. The system, which resembles a conventional tablet in appearance, comprises an osmotically active trilayer core surrounded by a semipermeable membrane with an IR drug overcoat. The trilayer core is composed of two drug layers containing the drug and excipients, and a push layer containing osmotically active components. A laser-drilled orifice on the drug-layer end of the tablet allows for exit of the drug. This product is similar to the GI therapeutic systems discussed earlier. The biologically inert components of the tablet remain intact during GI transit and are eliminated in the stool as an insoluble tablet shell.

The frequency of side effects experienced by patients using GI therapeutic systems was considerably less than that with conventional tablets. When the therapeutic system was compared to the regular 250-mg tablet given twice daily, ocular pressure was effectively controlled by the osmotic system. The blood level of acetazolamide using GI therapeutic systems, however, was considerably below that from the tablet. In fact, the therapeutic index of the drug was measurably increased by using the therapeutic system. The use of ER drug products, which release drug consistently, may provide promise for administering many drugs that previously had frequent adverse side effects because of the drug's narrow therapeutic index. The osmotic drug delivery system has become a popular drug vehicle for many products that require an extended period of drug delivery for 12 to 24 hours (Table 9-7).

A newer osmotic delivery system is the L-Oros Softcap (Alza), which claims to enhance bioavailability of poorly soluble drug by formulating the drug in a soft gelatin core and then providing extended drug delivery through an orifice drilled into an osmotic driven shell (Fig. 9-11). The soft gelatin capsule is surrounded by the barrier layer, the expanding osmotic layer, and the release-rate-controlling membrane. A delivery orifice is formed through the three outer layers but not through the gelatin shell. When the system is administered, water permeates through the rate-controlling membrane and activates the osmotic engine. As the engine expands, hydrostatic pressure inside the system builds up, thereby forcing the liquid formulation to break through the hydrated gelatin capsule shell at the delivery orifice and be pumped out of the system. At the end of the operation, liquid drug fill is squeezed out, and the gelatin capsule shell becomes flattened. The osmotic layer, located between the inner layer and the rate-controlling membrane, is the driving force for pumping the liquid formulation out of the system. This layer can gel when it hydrates. In addition, the high osmotic pressure can be sustained to achieve a constant release. This layer should comprise, therefore, a high-molecular-weight hydrophilic polymer and an osmotic agent. It is a challenge to develop a coating solution for a high-molecular-weight hydrophilic polymer. A mixed solvent of water and ethanol was used for this coating composition.

## TABLE 9-7 • OROS Osmotic Therapeutic Systems*

| Trade Name | Manufacturer | Generic Name | Description |
|---|---|---|---|
| Acutrim | Ciba | Phenylpropanolamine | Once-daily, over-the-counter appetite suppressant |
| Covera-HS | Searle | Verapamil | Controlled-Onset Extended-Release (COER-24) system for hypertension and angina pectoris |
| DynaCirc CR | Sandoz Pharmaceuticals | Isradipine | Treatment of hypertension |
| Efidac 24 | Ciba Self-Medication | | Over-the-counter, 24-h extended-release tablets providing relief of allergy and cold symptoms, containing either chlorpheniramine maleate, pseudoephedrine hydrochloride, or a combination of pseudoephedrine hydrochloride/brompheniramine maleate |
| Glucotrol XL | Pfizer | Glipizide | Extended-release tablets indicated as an adjunct to diet for the control of hyperglycemia in patients with non-insulin-dependent diabetes |
| Minipress XL | Pfizer | Prazosin | Extended-release tablets for treatment of hypertension |
| Procardia XL | Pfizer | Nifedipine | Extended-release tablets for treatment of angina and hypertension |
| Adalat CR | Bayer AG | Nifedipine | An Alza-based OROS system of nifedipine introduced internationally |
| Volmax | Glaxo-Wellcome | Albuterol | Extended-release tablets for the relief of bronchospasm in patients with reversible obstructive airway disease |

*Alza's OROS Osmotic Therapeutic Systems use osmosis to deliver drug continuously at controlled rates for up to 24 h.

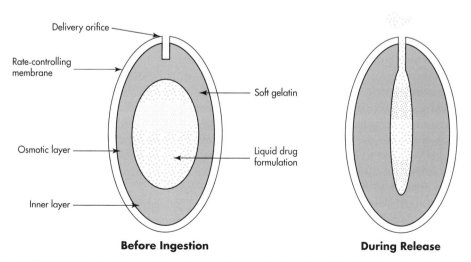

**Before Ingestion**      **During Release**

FIGURE 9-11 • Configuration of L-Oros Softcap. (Reproduced with permission from Dong L, Shafi K, Wong P, et al: L-OROS˚ SOFTCAP™ for controlled release of non-aqueous liquid formulation. *Drug Deliv Technol* 2002 2(1):52–55.)

## Gastroretentive System

The ER drug product should release the drug completely within the region in the GI tract in which the drug is optimally absorbed. Due to GI transit, the ER drug product continuously moves distally down the GI tract. In some cases, the ER drug product containing residual drug may exit from the body. Pharmaceutical formulation developers have used various approaches to retain the dosage form in the desired area of the GI tract. One such approach is a *gastroretentive system* that can remain in the gastric region for several hours and prolong the gastric residence time of drugs. Usually, the gastroretentive systems can be classified into several types based on the mechanism applied such as: (i) high density systems; (ii) floating systems; (iii) expandable systems; (iv) superporous hydrogels; (v) mucoadhesive or bioadhesive systems; (vi) magnetic systems; and (vii) dual working systems (Tripathi et al, 2019).

One of the most commonly used gastroretentive systems is the *floating* drug delivery system (FDDS). For example, diazepam (Valium) was formulated using methylcellulose to provide sustained release (Valrelease). The manufacturer of Valrelease claimed that the hydrocolloid (gel) floated in the stomach to give sustained release diazepam. In other studies, however, materials of various densities were emptied from the stomach without any difference as to whether the drug product was floating on top or sitting at the bottom of the stomach (Eberle et al, 2014). Another gastroretentive system is mucoadhesive or bioadhesive drug delivery system. These systems permit a given drug delivery system to be incorporated with the bio/mucoadhesive agents, enabling the device to adhere to the stomach (or other GI) walls, thus resisting gastric emptying. Sometimes bio/mucoadhesive substance is a natural or synthetic polymer capable of adhering to biological membrane (bioadhesive polymer) or the mucus lining of the GIT (mucoadhesive polymer) (Ways et al, 2018).

The most important consideration in this type of formulation appears to be the gelling strength of the gum material and the concentration of gummy material. Modification of the release rates of the product may further be achieved with various amounts of talc or other lipophilic lubricant. However, the gastroretentive system is not feasible for drugs having solubility or stability problems in gastric fluid or having irritation on gastric mucosa. Drugs such as nifedipine, which is well absorbed along the entire GIT and which undergoes significant first-pass metabolism, may not be desirable candidates for FDDS since the slow gastric emptying may lead to reduced systemic bioavailability.

## Transdermal Drug Delivery Systems

Skin represents the largest and most easily accessible organ of the body. A transdermal drug delivery system (patch) is a dosage form intended for delivering drug across the skin for systemic drug absorption (see Chapters 6, 21). Transdermal drug absorption also avoids presystemic metabolism or "first-pass" effects. Transdermal drug delivery systems deliver the drug through the skin in a controlled rate over an extended period of time. Examples of transdermal drug delivery systems are shown in Tables 9-8 and 9-9. Transdermal delivery drug products vary in patch design (Fig. 9-12). Generally, the transdermal patch consists of (i) a backing or support layer that protects the patch, (ii) a drug layer that might be in the form of a solid gel reservoir or in a matrix, (iii) a pressure-sensitive adhesive layer, and (iv) a release liner or protective strip that is removed before placing the patch on the skin. In some cases, the adhesive layer may also contain the active drug (Gonzalez and Cleary, 2010).

The skin is a natural barrier to prevent the influx of foreign chemicals (including water) into the body and loss of water from the body. To be a suitable candidate for transdermal drug delivery, the drug must possess the right physicochemical properties. The drug must be highly potent so that only a small systemic drug dose is needed, and the size of the patch (dose is also related to surface area) need not be exceptionally large, not greater than 50 cm$^2$. Physicochemical properties of the drug include a small molecular weight (<500 Da), and high lipid solubility. The elimination half-life should not be too short, to avoid having to apply the patch more frequently than once a day.

In general, drugs given at a dose of over 100 mg would require too large a patch to be used practically. The increase of skin penetration of drug from patch maybe a design direction. The first generation of transdermal drug delivery systems focused

## TABLE 9-8 • Examples of Transdermal Delivery Systems

| Type | Trade Name | Rationale |
|------|-----------|-----------|
| Membrane-controlled system | Transderm-Nitro (Novartis) | Drug in reservoir, drug release through a rate-controlling polymeric membrane |
| Adhesive diffusion-controlled system | Deponit system (Pharma-Schwartz) | Drug dispersed in an adhesive polymer and in a reservoir |
| Matrix-dispersion system | Nitro-Dur (Key) | Drug dispersed into a rate-controlling hydrophilic or hydrophobic matrix molded into a transdermal system |
| Microreservoir system | Nitro-Disc (Searle) | Combination reservoir and matrix-dispersion system |

on chemical drugs tailoring of the physicochemical properties; second-generation research focused on improving the skin permeability of drugs using chemical enhancers and stimulators through external driving force, such as heat, electricity, and ultrasound; third-generation works pay more attention to the microscopic destruction of epidermis to facilitate the delivery of drugs, such as radiofrequency ablation, laser, and microneedle. Due to the size of the microneedles leaving the dermal and hypodermal layers untouched, the microneedle is considered painless and minimally invasive (Lee et al, 2018).

Microneedles were first reported to deliver calcein by permeation improvement in 1998 (Henry et al, 1998). It can painlessly disrupt the skin barrier and create pores inside the skin to increase drug penetration. In recent years, microneedles have been extensively investigated for the delivery of compounds like diclofenac, desmopressin, and even as vectors for gene therapy (Badran et al, 2009). The possible problems such as low dosage, accurate dose administration, and patient compliance can be solved by introducing development of dissolvable/degradable and hollow microneedles to deliver drugs at a higher dose and to engineer drug release.

## TABLE 9-9 • Transdermal Delivery Systems

| Trade Name | Manufacturer | Generic Name | Description |
|------------|-------------|--------------|-------------|
| Catapres-TTS | Boehringer Ingelheim | Clonidine | Once-weekly product for the treatment of hypertension |
| Duragesic | Janssen Pharmaceutical | Fentanyl | Management of chronic pain in patients who require continuous opioid analgesia for pain that cannot be managed by lesser means |
| Estraderm | Ciba-Geigy | Estradiol | Twice-weekly product for treating certain postmenopausal symptoms and preventing osteoporosis |
| Nicoderm CQ | Hoechst Marion | Nicotine | An aid to smoking cessation for the relief of nicotine-withdrawal symptoms |
| Testoderm | Alza | Testosterone | Replacement therapy in males for conditions associated with a deficiency or absence of endogenous testosterone |
| Transderm-Nitro | Novartis | Nitroglycerin | Once-daily product for the prevention of angina pectoris due to coronary artery disease; contains nitroglycerin in a proprietary, transdermal therapeutic system |
| Transderm Scop | | Scopolamine | Prevention of nausea and vomiting associated with motion sickness |

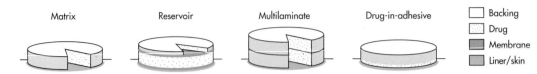

FIGURE 9-12 • The four basic configurations for transdermal drug delivery systems.

In addition to steel, microneedles may be fabricated from a microelectromechanical system employing silicon, metals, polymers, or polysaccharides. Solid-coated microneedles can be used to pierce the superficial skin layer, followed by delivery of the drug. Microneedles can be used to deliver macromolecules such as insulin, growth hormones, immunobiologicals, proteins, and peptides (Lee et al, 2018).

The transdermal drug delivery system has been extensively studied for 40 years. Currently, only about 40 drug products are commercial for 20 drug substances, due to the drug diffusion problem, since all approaches to drug delivery need to overcome the barrier function of skin. Drug diffusion may be controlled by a semipermeable membrane next to the reservoir layer. In other cases, drug diffusion is controlled by passage through the epidermal layer of the skin. The transdermal delivery system generally contains large drug concentrations to produce the ideal drug delivery with a zero-order rate. The patch may contain residual drug when it is removed from the application site.

Nitroglycerin is commonly administered by transdermal delivery (eg, Nitro-Dur, Transderm-Nitro*). Transdermal delivery systems of nitroglycerin may provide hours of protection against angina, whereas the duration of nitroglycerin given in a sublingual tablet (Nitrostat*) or sublingual spray (Nitrolingual) may be only a few minutes. The nitroglycerin patch is placed over the chest area and provides up to 12 hours of angina protection. In a study comparing these three dosage forms in patients, no substantial difference was observed among the three preparations. In all cases, the skin was found to be the rate-limiting step in nitroglycerin absorption. There were fewer variations among products than of the same product among different patients.

After the application of a transdermal patch, there is generally a lag time before the onset of the drug action because of the drug's slow diffusion into the dermal layers of the skin. When the patch is removed, diffusion of the drug from the dermal layer to the systemic circulation may continue for some time until the drug is depleted from the site of application. The solubility of drug in the skin rather than the concentration of drug in the patch layer is the most important factor controlling the rate of drug absorption through the skin. Humidity, temperature, and other factors have been shown to affect the rate of drug absorption through the skin. With most drugs, transdermal delivery provides a more stable blood level of the drug than oral dosing. However, with nitroglycerin, the sustained blood level of the drug provided by transdermal delivery is not desirable, due to induced tolerance to the drug not seen with sublingual tablets.

Transdermal therapeutic systems (TTS) consist of a thin, flexible composite of membranes, resembling a small adhesive bandage, which is applied to the skin and delivers drug through intact skin into the bloodstream. Other examples of products delivered using this system are shown in Table 9-8. Transdermal Nitro consists of several layers: (1) an aluminized plastic backing that protects nitroglycerin from loss through vaporization; (2) a drug reservoir containing nitroglycerin adsorbed onto lactose, colloidal silicon dioxide, and silicone medical fluid; (3) a diffusion-controlling membrane consisting of ethylene–vinyl acetate copolymer; (4) a layer of silicone adhesive; and (5) a protective strip.

Other transdermal delivery manufacturers have made transdermal systems in which the adhesive functions both as a pressure-sensitive adhesive and as a controlling matrix. Dermaflex (Elan) is a uniquely passive transdermal patch system that employs a hydrogel matrix into which the drug is incorporated. Dermaflex regulates both the availability and absorption of the drug in a manner that allows for controlled and efficient systemic delivery of many drugs.

An important limitation of transdermal preparation is the amount of drug that is needed in the transdermal patch to be absorbed systemically to provide the optimum therapeutic response. The amount of drug absorbed is related to the amount of drug in the patch, the size of the patch, and the method of manufacture. A dose–response relationship is obtained by applying a proportionally larger transdermal patch that differs only in surface area. For example, a 5-cm² transdermal patch will generally provide twice as much drug absorbed systemically as a 2.5-cm² transdermal patch.

Among these efforts, new advances in pharmaceutic solvents may provide a mechanism for an increased amount of drug to be absorbed transdermally. Ideally, the increase in permeation enhancement should not cause skin irritation or any other kind of damage to the skin. To achieve this goal, the localization of the enhancer's effect only to the stratum corneum is necessary, though it is very difficult. Azone, one of chemical permeation enhancers, is a solvent that increases the absorption of many drugs through the skin. Azone is usually composed of organic solvents such as dimethylformamide, dimethylacetamide, etc (Chen et al, 2014). These solvents can only be regarded as relatively nontoxic.

Among physical transdermal permeation enhancers, for ionic drugs, absorption may be enhanced by *iontophoresis*, a method in which an electric field is maintained across the epidermal layer with special mini electric current (0.1–1.0 mA/cm²). Some drugs, such as lidocaine, verapamil, insulin, and peptides, have been absorbed through the skin by iontophoresis. A number of transdermal iontophoretic products have received approval, including LidoSite® Topical System (lidocaine for local anesthesia: Vyteris Inc., Fairlawn, NJ), Ionsys® (fentanyl iontophoretic transdermal system for patient-controlled analgesia; developed by Alza Corporation then acquired in sequence by Johnson & Johnson, Incline Therapeutics, and The Medicines Company), and Zecuity® (6.5 mg sumatriptan delivered over 4 h for migraine: NuPathe Inc./Teva).

A process in which transdermal drug delivery is aided by high-frequency acoustic sound is called *sonophoresis*. Sonophoresis has been used with hydrocortisone cream applied to the skin to enhance penetration for treating "tennis elbow" and other mild inflammatory muscular problems. Characteristic drug delivery enhancements in drug transport induced by therapeutic ultrasound have been approximately 10-fold compared to passive drug delivery. Many such novel systems are being developed by drug delivery companies (Benson et al, 2019). A sonophoresis-based device is Sonoprep® (approved in 2004 and withdrawn in 2007). Prelude® skin prep system, prepared by Echo Therapeutics, is now looking for commercial applications.

Panoderm XL patch technology (Elan) is a new system that delivers a drug through a concealed miniature probe which penetrates the stratum corneum. Panoderm XL is fully disposable and may be programmed to deliver drugs as a preset bolus, in continuous or pulsed regimen. The complexity of the device is hidden from the patient and is simple to use. Panoderm (Elan) is an electrotransdermal drug delivery system that overcomes the skin diffusion barriers through the use of low-level electric current to transport the drug through the skin. Several transdermal products, such as fentanyl, hydromorphone, calcitonin, and luteinizing hormone–releasing hormone (LHRH), are in clinical trials. More improvements in transdermal delivery of larger molecules and the use of absorption enhancers will be available in future transdermal delivery systems.

Several additional studies that are unique to the development of a transdermal drug delivery system include (1) wear and adhesiveness of the patch, (2) skin irritation, (3) skin sensitization, and (4) residual drug in the patch after removal. The FDA is asking drug companies to consider minimizing the amount of residual drug left in transdermal patches. Marketed products that use transdermal and transmucosal drug delivery systems can contain between 10% and 95% of the initial active drug even after use, according to the FDA's Guidance published in August, 2011 (FDA Guidance, https://www.fda.gov/media/79401/download). Adverse events have been reported after patients have failed to remove a patch, resulting in increased or prolonged effects of the drug (eg, fentanyl patch).

## Combination Products

Combination products are defined in 21 CFR 3.2(e).[3] The term *combination product* includes the following.

1. A product comprised of two or more regulated components, ie, drug/device, biologic/device, drug/biologic, or drug/device/biologic, that are physically, chemically, or otherwise combined or mixed and produced as a single entity

2. Two or more separate products packaged together in a single package or as a unit and comprised of drug and device products, device and biological products, or biological and drug products

3. A drug, device, or biological product packaged separately that according to its investigational plan or proposed labeling is intended for use only with an approved individually specified drug, device, or biological product where both are required to achieve the intended use, indication, or effect and where upon approval of the proposed product the labeling of the approved product would need to be changed, eg, to reflect a change in intended use, dosage form, strength, route of administration, or significant change in dose

4. Any investigational drug, device, or biological product packaged separately that according to its proposed labeling is for use only with another individually specified investigational drug, device, or biological product where both are required to achieve the intended use, indication, or effect

Examples of combination products where the components are physically, chemically, or otherwise combined:

- Monoclonal antibody combined with a therapeutic drug
- Device coated or impregnated with a drug or biologic
- Drug-eluting stent; pacing lead with steroid-coated tip; catheter with antimicrobial coating; condom with spermicide
- Skin substitutes with cellular components; orthopedic implant with growth factors
- Prefilled syringes, insulin injector pens, metered dose inhalers, transdermal patches
- Drug or biological product packaged with a delivery device
- Surgical tray with surgical instruments, drapes, and lidocaine or alcohol swabs
- Photosensitizing drug and activating laser/light source
- Iontophoretic drug delivery patch and controller

In summary, combination products consist of the drug in combination with a device that is physically, chemically, or otherwise combined or mixed and produced as a single entity. The device and/or biologic is intended for use with the approved drug and influences the route of administration and PKs of the drug.

One example of combination product presented in USP 9,872,859 descripted a long-term nanoformulated drug product (US Patent 9,872,859, 2018). In this patent, nanoformulation is encapsulated into an enteric-coated capsule for in vivo drug delivery targeted to gut-associated lymphoid tissue (GALT). The nanocarrier inside the enteric-coated capsule is associated with an agent for targeting microfold cells (M-cells), for treating retrovirus infections, including, for example, HIV, and the drug can be selected as Efavirenz (EFV).

An *enteric-coated* tablet is one kind of DR type within the MR dosage family designed to release drug in the small intestine. The nanocarrier encapsulated in the enteric capsule is a carboxylated Pluronic® block copolymer abbreviated F127COOH, loading the HIV treatment drug of EFV in the hydrophobic core of polymeric nanoparticles. After lyophilization, the nanoformulation is encapsulated into the enteric-coated capsule for *in vivo* drug delivery targeted to GALT in the intestine. Advantageously, the capsule will sustain stomach digestion to escape intervention from enzymatic digestion and acid in stomach due to the enteric-coated layer on the capsule surface after oral administration. The loaded drug can then release in the gut under intestine pH circumstances from the erupted capsule and bind to M-cells and incorporate to GALT, where it will facilitate sustained

---

[3]http://www.fda.gov/CombinationProducts/AboutCombination Products/ucm118332.htm.

release of the incorporated drug. Applying this nano-formulated combination drug product can synergize the advantages of conventional therapeutic systems and achieve the goals of drug targeting with diminished side effects, and this concept of combination of conventional formulation with nanocarrier can be applied to several therapy fields.

## Modified-Release Parenteral Dosage Forms

MR parenteral dosage forms are parenteral dosage forms that maintain plasma drug concentrations through rate-controlled drug release from the formulation over a prolonged period of time (Patil and Burgess, 2010; Lau et al, 2018). Some examples of MR parenteral dosage forms include microspheres, liposomes, drug implants, inserts, drug-eluting stents, and nanoparticles. These formulations are designed by entrapment or microencapsulation of the drug into inert polymeric or lipophilic matrices that slowly release the drug, *in vivo*, for a duration of several days up to several years. MR parenteral dosage forms may be biodegradable or nonbiodegradable. Nonbiodegradable implants need to be surgically removed at the end of therapy.

## Implants and Inserts

Even though the oral route should be considered highly desirable by patients, it still represents a huge challenge, such as low bioavailability for peptides or proteins after oral administration. Alternative routes of administration (pulmonary, nasal, buccal, transdermal, ocular, and rectal) have also shown drawbacks such as enzymatic degradation or low/variable absorption. As a result, there is a renewed interest in parenteral administration because of the increased innovation on new inactive ingredient development, especially as there have been many improvements in pain reduction. Among these approaches, biodegradable polymer-based implants and inserts display excellent drug delivery characteristics and very good compatibility.

*In situ* forming implants based on phase separation by solvent exchange is a conventional preformed implant and microparticles for parenteral applications. After administration, the polymeric solutions may precipitate at the site of injection, thus forming a drug-eluting depot. Drug release may then initiate

in three phases: (i) burst during precipitation of the depot, (ii) diffusion of drug through the polymeric matrix, and finally (iii) drug release by implant degradation. They are easier to manufacture, and their administration does not require surgery, therefore improving patient compliance. The drawbacks of this drug delivery system are lack of reproducibility in depot shape, burst during solidification, and potential toxicity (Parent et al, 2013).

*In situ* gelling mucoadhesive formulations are applied as simple eyedrops, forming a semisolid gel as soon as they meet the ocular surface. The gel forms a homogeneous layer on the corneal surface, exhibiting pseudoplastic behavior during blinking to avoid patient discomfort and blurred vision while facilitating drug diffusion (Yadav et al, 2019).

Polymeric drug implants can deliver and sustain drug levels in the body for an extended period. Both biodegradable and nonbiodegradable polymers can be impregnated with drugs in a controlled drug delivery system. For example, levonorgestrel implants (Norplant system, Wyeth-Ayerst) are sets of six flexible closed capsules made of silastic (dimethylsiloxane/methylvinylsiloxane copolymer), each containing 36 $\mu$g of the progestin levonorgestrel. The capsules are sealed with silastic adhesive and sterilized. The Norplant system is available in an insertion kit to facilitate subdermal insertion of all six capsules in the mid-portion of the upper arm. The dose of levonorgestrel is about 85 $\mu$g/day, followed by a decline to about 50 $\mu$g/day by 9 months and to about 35 $\mu$g/day by 18 months, declining further to about 30 $\mu$g/day. The levonorgestrel implants are effective for up to 5 years for contraception and then must be replaced. An intrauterine progesterone contraceptive system (Progestasert, Alza) is a T-shaped unit that contains a reservoir of 38 $\mu$g of progesterone. Contraceptive effectiveness for Progestasert is enhanced by continuous release of progesterone into the uterine cavity at an average rate of 65 $\mu$g/day for 1 year.

A dental insert available for the treatment of periodontitis is the doxycycline hyclate delivery system (Atrigel). This is a subgingival CR product consisting of two syringe mixing systems that, when combined, form a bioabsorbable, flowable polymeric formulation. After administration under the gum, the liquid solidifies and then allows for controlled release of doxycycline for a period of 7 days.

## Nanotechnology-Derived Drugs

*Nanotechnology* is the manufacture of materials in the nanometer size range, usually less than 100–200 nm. Nanotechnology has been applied to drug development, food, electronics, biomaterials, and other applications. Nanoscale materials have chemical, physical, or biological properties that are totally different in comparison to those of their larger counterparts. Such differences may include altered surface area, magnetic properties, altered electrical or optical activity, increased structural integrity, or altered chemical or biological activity (FDA guidance, https://www.fda.gov/media/88423/download, June 2014). Because of these properties, nanoscale materials have great potential for use in a variety of therapeutic agents. Because of some of their special properties, nanoscale materials may pose different safety and efficacy issues compared to their larger or smaller (ie, molecular) counterparts.

According to the material composition, nanoparticles can be categorized into two main aspects: organic and inorganic. Organic-based nanoparticles may be composed of biodegradable materials, such as polylactide (PLA), polyglycolide (PGA), poly(lactide-co-glycolide) (PLGA), polyethylene glycol (PEG), etc, and some biocompatible materials, eg, poly(propylene oxide)(PPO), polyvinylpyrrolidone (PVP), etc. Inorganic-based nanoparticles can be formed from gold, iron oxide, etc. All of these show a bright future in the area of controlled drug delivery (Ding et al, 2007, 2011).

In addition to the large surface area of nanoparticles, surface modification of the nanoparticles such as binding different chemical groups to the surface with surfactants or biocompatible polymers (eg, PEG) changes the PKs, toxicity, and surface reactivity of the nanoparticles *in vivo*. Therefore, nanoparticles can have a wide variety of properties that are markedly different from the same materials in larger particle forms (Couvreur and Vauthier, 2006) (see also Chapter 28).

## Liposomes

Liposomes are vesicles composed of a bilayer (unilamellar) and/or a concentric series of multiple bilayers (multilamellar) separated by aqueous compartments formed by amphipathic molecules such as phospholipids that enclose a central aqueous compartment In the current FDA Guidance, the particle size of liposome is not specified; it is preferably defined on the basis of volume or mass if particle density is known. Typically, water-soluble drugs are contained in the aqueous compartment(s) and hydrophobic drugs are contained in the lipid bilayer(s) of the liposomes. Release of drugs from liposome formulations, among other characteristics such as liposomal clearance and circulation half-life, can be modified by the presence of polyethylene glycol and/or cholesterol or other potential additives in the liposome (FDA Guidance, https://www.fda.gov/media/70837/download, April 2018).

Daunorubicin has been used for the treatment of ovarian cancer, AIDS-related Kaposi sarcoma, and multiple myeloma. Two different liposomal formulations of daunorubicin are currently marketed. DaunoXome® contains an aqueous solution of the citrate salt of daunorubicin encapsulated within lipid vesicles (liposomes) composed of a lipid bilayer of distearoylphosphatidylcholine and cholesterol, whereas Doxil® is doxorubicin HCl encapsulated in liposomes that are formulated with surface-bound methoxypolyethylene glycol (MPEG). The use of MPEG is a process often referred to as pegylation, to protect liposomes from detection by the mononuclear phagocyte system (MPS) and to increase blood circulation time. Each of these products has different PKs, and they are not interchangeable.

Another application of liposome is to change the PK profile and optimize the immunogenicity of loaded protein drugs. In one study, PEGylated phosphatidylinositol (PI) containing liposome was designed to load recombinant FVIII by reducing immunogenicity and prolonging the circulating half-life. Reduced activity *in vitro* and improved retention of activity in the presence of antibodies suggested strong shielding of FVIII by the particle; thus, *in vivo* studies were conducted in hemophilia A mice showing that the apparent terminal half-life was improved versus both free FVIII and FVIII–PI, but exposure determined by AUC was reduced. The formation of inhibitory antibodies after subcutaneous immunization with FVIII–PI/PEG was lower than free FVIII but resulted in a significant increase in inhibitors following intravenous administration (Peng et al, 2012).

Liposomes were first described in 1965 and soon proposed as drug delivery systems. With numerous important chemical structure improvements such as remote drug loading, size homogeneity, long-circulating (PEGylated) modification, triggered release, combination drug loading, etc. Liposomes have been used in numerous clinical trials in such diverse areas as the delivery of anticancer, antifungal, and antibiotic drugs; the delivery of gene medicines; and the delivery of anesthetics and anti-inflammatory drugs. Some liposome products are on the market, and many more are in the pipeline. These lipidic nanoparticles are the first nanomedicine delivery system to make the transition from concept to clinical application, and they are now an established technology platform with considerable clinical acceptance (Allen and Cullis, 2013). Table 9-10 lists the liposomal or lipid-based drug products in the market or still in the clinical trials. From this table, not only the chemical drugs but also the antibodies, vaccine, nucleic acids, and gene medicine can be loaded into liposomes for treatment of infections and for cancer treatment, for lung disease, and for skin conditions. When the long-circulating liposomes are bioconjugated with additional targeting molecules on their surface, the common "passive" liposomal drug delivery system may be evolved to an "active" system.

Over the last several years, the concept of continuous manufacturing has evolved from bulk APIs and solid oral dosages into the more complex realm of biologics. If proper procedures and equipment are selected, the possibility of continuous manufacturing

## TABLE 9-10 • Marketed and in Clinic Trial Liposomal and Lipid-Based Drug Products

| Trade Name | Manufacturer | Generic Name | Description |
|---|---|---|---|
| **Marketed** | | | |
| Doxil/Caelyx | Johnson & Johnson | Doxorubicin | Kaposi sarcoma, ovarian cancer, breast cancer, multiple myeloma + velcade |
| Myocet | Cephalon | Doxorubicin | Breast cancer + cyclophosphamide |
| DaunoXome | Galen | Daunorubicin | Kaposi sarcoma |
| Amphotec | Intermune | Amphotericin B | Invasive aspergillosis |
| DepoDur | Pacira | Morphine sulfate | Pain following surgery |
| DepoCyt | Pacira | Cytosine + Arabinoside | Lymphomatous, meningitis, neoplastic |
| Diprivan | AstraZeneca | Propofol | Anesthesia |
| Estrasorb | King | Estrogen | Menopausal therapy |
| Marqibo | Talon | Vincristine | Acute lymphoblastic leukemia |
| **Clinic Trials** | | | |
| SPI-077 | Alza | Cisplatin | Solid tumors (Phase II) |
| CPX-351 | Celator | Cytarabine: daunorubicin | Acute myeloid leukemia (Phase II) |
| MM-398 | Merrimack | CPT-11 | Gastric and pancreatic cancer (Phase II) |
| Lipoplatin | Regulon | Cisplatin | Non-small cell lung cancer (Phase III) |
| ThermoDox | Celsion | Thermosensitive doxorubicin | Primary hepatocellular, carcinoma, refractory chest wall breast cancer, colorectal liver metastases (Phase III) |
| Stimuvax | Oncothyreon/ Merck | Anti-MUC1 cancer vaccine | Non-small cell lung cancer (Phase III) |
| Exparel | Pacira | Bupivacaine | Nerve block (Phase II) |

for liposomal formulation turns to be a reality. The challenge may come from formulation improvement, lipid/API selection, and the microbial control (Worsham et al, 2019).

## Polymer-Based Nano Drug Delivery System

The term "polymer therapeutics" was coined to describe the therapeutics associated with polymers, including polymeric drugs, polymer conjugates of proteins, drugs, and aptamers, together with those block copolymer micelles and multicomponent non-viral vectors. These nonviral vectors may display as micelles, implants, inserts, or nanoparticles.

PLGA, PLA, and PGA are perhaps the most commonly studied polymers due to their versatility in tuning biodegradation time and high biocompatibility arising from their natural by-products, lactic acid and glycolic acid. Now polylactide is commonly used in surgery, while polyglycolide or its drug conjugates is being increasingly used as a drug carrier. Their molecular weight can be tailored to the expected extent upon the requirements. Because of the unique property of biodegradability and integration of quality by design (QbD) approach concept during development, this polymer therapeutics can be applied to preclinical structure optimization and manufacturing process control.

Lupron Depot˚ (LD) is the first US Food and Drug Administration (FDA)-approved microparticle-based depot drug delivery system, developed by Takeda-Abbott Products. LD consists of leuprolide encapsulated in PLGA microspheres. LD is a long-term product (1–6 months, depending on the API loaded in particle), which slowly releases encapsulated leuprolide acetate for at least 1 month, to reduce injection frequency relative to daily injections of soluble peptide for treatment of hormone-sensitive prostate cancer, breast cancer, endometriosis, and uterine fibroids.

LD has been commercially successful from the beginning of marketing (Anselmo and Mitragotri, 2014). LD can be intramuscularly injected, having dosage schedule as 7.5 mg 1×/month, 22.5 mg 1× for every 3 months or 30 mg 1× for every 4 months. The peptide drug is released from these depot formulations at a functionally constant daily rate for 1, 3, or 4 months, depending on the polymer type

(PLGA for a 1-month depot and PLA) for depot of >2 months), with doses ranging between 3.75 and 30 mg. Mean peak plasma leuprorelin concentrations ($C_{max}$) of 13.1, 20.8 to 21.8, 47.4, 54.5, and 53 µg/L occur within 1 to 3 hours of depot subcutaneous administration of 3.75, 7.5, 11.25, 15, and 30 mg, respectively, compared with 32 to 35 µg/L at 36 to 60 min after a subcutaneous injection of 1 mg of a non-depot formulation. Sustained drug release from the PLGA microspheres maintains plasma concentrations between 0.4 and 1.4 µg/L over 28 days after single 3.75, 7.5, or 15 mg depot injections. Mean AUCs are similar for subcutaneous or intravenous injection of short-acting leuprorelin. A 3-month depot PLA formulation of leuprorelin acetate 11.25 mg ensures a $C_{max}$ of around 20 µg/L at 3 hours after subcutaneous injection and continuous drug concentrations of 0.43 to 0.19 µg/L from day 7 until before the next injection (Dreicer et al, 2011; Zhou et al, 2018).

In polymer therapeutics, polymeric drugs, polymeric sequestrants, and PEG conjugates (both protein conjugates and the PEG-aptamer conjugate) have progressed to market or under clinic trials. Table 9-11 shows the marketed and clinical trial polymeric therapeutics. Success stories include Copaxone as a treatment for multiple sclerosis (a complex random copolymer of three amino acids), PEGylated interferons (Pegasys; Peg-Intron), and PEGylated rhG-CSF (Neulasta) as a more convenient once-per-cycle adjunct to cancer chemotherapy (Duncan and Vicent, 2013).

## 3D Printed Formulation

3D printing technology is one of the most revolutionary and powerful tools for precise manufacturing of individual dosage forms, combined with tissue engineering and disease modeling (Kotta et al, 2018). The conventional manufacturing procedure of granulation for tablets and capsules is designed for large-scale production, whereas the 3D printing technique presents potential for small batches of personalized medicines. Its reproducible character can be used to prepare complex drug-release dosages (Verstraete et al, 2018). With 3D printed technology, the building formulation can be achieved by unique digitally coded layering without compression or traditional molding techniques. In this 3D printing

**TABLE 9-11 •** Marketed and Clinical Trials Polymeric Therapeutics

| Trade Name | Subclass | Composition | Market/Clinic Trial |
|---|---|---|---|
| Copaxone | | Glu, Ala, Tyr copolymer | Market |
| Vivagel | Polymeric drugs | Lysine-based dendrimer | Phase III |
| Hyaluronic acid | | Hyalgal, Synvisc | Market |
| Zinostatin Stimaler | Polymer–protein conjugates | Styrene maleic anhydride-neocarzinostatin (SMANCS) | Market (Japan) |
| Cimzia | | PEG-anti-TNF Fab | Market |
| Peg-intron | PEGylated proteins | PEG-Interferon alpha 2b | Market |
| Neulasta | | PEG-hrGCSF | Market |
| Macugen | PEGylated-aptamer | PEG-aptamer (apatanib) | Market |
| CT-2103; Xyotax | Polymer–drug conjugate | Poly-glutamic acid (PGA)-paclitaxel | Phase II/III |
| NKTR-118 | | PEG-naloxone | Phase III |
| IT-101 | Self-assembled polymer conjugate nanoparticles | Polymer conjugated-cyclodextrin nanoparticle-camptothecin | Phase II |
| NK-6004 | Block copolymer micelles | Cisplatin block copolymer micelle | Phase II |

technology, the manufacturing of 3D solid objects can be achieved by repeatedly spreading thin layers of powdered medication on the top of one another and fusing successive layers of material until the desired object is generated.

The concept of 3D printing evolved in the 1970s; 3D technology was created at the Massachusetts Institute of Technology in the 1980s as a rapid prototyping technique. The application has been in existence since 2012. Based on the first commercial technology of stereolithography (SLA), fused deposition modeling (FDM) is one of the most commonly used low-cost techniques in the field of 3D printing. Over 40 years' development, the three predominant 3D printing methods are (1) power solidification (drop on solid deposition, selective laser sintering, or melting); (2) liquid solidification (drop on drop deposition, stereolithography), and (3) extrusion (fused deposition modeling, pressure assistant syringe) (Jamróz et al, 2018). The main benefit of 3D construction in the pharmaceutical field is delivering patient-centered and on-demand medications to avoid variable effects and adverse reactions during drug therapy.

In 2015, the FDA approved the first 3D printed prescription drug, Spritam (Levetiracetam), to treat partial-onset seizures, myoclonic seizures, and primary generalized tonic-clonic seizures. In 3D printed Spritam manufacturing, materials are assembled layer by layer without compression or traditional molding. Thin layers of powdered medication are repeatedly spread on top of one another, as patterns of liquid droplets are printed onto selected regions of each powder layer. Interactions between the powder and liquid bond the materials together at a microscopic level. The tablet allows the pill to disintegrate in the mouth with just a little bit of water. This also provides an option for patients who struggle to swallow a pill (Kite-Powerll, 2016). In December 2017, the FDA published a guidance to provide specific recommendation on 3D printing drug technology R&D: Technical Considerations for Additive Manufactured Devices. (FDA Guidance, https://www.fda .gov/media/97633/download, 2017).

### Imaging-Guided Drug Delivery System

In addition to the common stimuli-responsive drug delivery systems such as pH, enzyme, temperature, magnetic field, and light, imaging-guided drug delivery system (IGDDS) has been applied in bio-medicine and in clinics due to its noninvasive features, including magnetic resonance imaging (MRI), x-ray computed tomography (CT), positron emission tomography (PET), single-photon emission computed tomography (SPECT), electron microscopy, autoradiography, optical imaging, and ultrasound (US). Among these imaging modalities, PET and optical imaging are regarded as quantitative or semi-quantitative, especially the near-infrared (NIR) range light on image-assisted biodistribution of the labeled drugs due to the characteristics of deep tissue penetration and high sensitivity of NIR light (Centelles et al, 2018). CT and MRI are normally used for anatomical imaging purposes (Yang et al, 2018); for example, the imaging of the brain. This noninvasive technique, used for combination purposes, has been called *theranostics* (therapy + diagnostic).

The ability to quantitatively image the biodistribution of therapeutics or drug delivery systems in a noninvasive manner can aid in the development of new theranostics, dose optimization, and treatment monitoring. However, development of an endogenous system with both contrast and quantitative delivery capabilities is still a challenge for imaging-guided drug delivery systems and clinical applications.

### FREQUENTLY ASKED QUESTIONS

▶ How do patient-specific variables influence performance of MR dosage forms?

▶ What is the difference between the different types of MR dosage forms?

## CONSIDERATIONS IN THE EVALUATION OF MODIFIED-RELEASE PRODUCTS

The development of an MR formulation has to be based on a well-defined clinical need and integration of physiological, PD, and PK considerations. The two important requirements in the development of ER products are (1) demonstration of safety and efficacy and (2) demonstration of controlled drug release.

Safety and efficacy data are available for many drugs given in a conventional or IR dosage form. Bioavailability data of the drug from the ER drug product should demonstrate sustained plasma drug concentrations and bioavailability equivalent to giving the conventional dosage in the same total daily dose in two or more doses. The bioavailability data requirements are specified in the Code of Federal Regulations, 21 CFR 320.25(f). The important points are as follows.

1. The product should demonstrate sustained release, as claimed, without *dose dumping* (abrupt release of a large amount of the drug in an uncontrolled manner).

2. The drug should show steady-state levels comparable to those reached using a conventional dosage form given in multiple doses, and which was demonstrated to be effective.

3. The drug product should show consistent PK performance between individual dosage units.

4. The product should allow for the maximum amount of drug to be absorbed while maintaining minimum patient-to-patient variation.

5. The demonstration of steady-state drug levels after the recommended doses are given should be within the effective plasma drug levels for the drug.

6. An *in vitro* method and data that demonstrate the reproducible ER nature of the product should be developed. The *in vitro* method usually consists of a suitable dissolution procedure that provides a meaningful *in vitro–in vivo* correlation.

7. *In vivo* PK data consist of single and multiple dosing comparing the ER product to a reference standard (usually an approved nonsustained-release or a solution product).

The PK data usually consist of plasma drug data and/or drug excreted into the urine. PK analyses are performed to determine such parameters as $t_{1/2}$, $V_D$, $t_{max}$, AUC, and $k$.

### Pharmacodynamic and Safety Considerations

Pharmacodynamic and safety issues must be considered in the development and evaluation of an MR dosage form. The most critical issue is to consider whether the MR dosage form truly offers an advantage over the same drug in an IR (conventional) form. This advantage may be related to better efficacy, reduced toxicity, or better patient compliance. However, because the cost of manufacture of an MR dosage form is generally higher than the cost for a conventional dosage form, economy or cost savings for patients also may be an important consideration.

Ideally, the ER dosage form should provide a more prolonged PD effect compared to the same drug given in the IR form. However, an ER dosage form of a drug may have a different PD activity profile compared to the same drug given in an acute, intermittent, rapid-release dosage form. For example, transdermal patches of nitroglycerin, which produce prolonged delivery of the drug, may produce functional tolerance to vasodilation that is not observed when nitroglycerin is given sublingually for acute angina attacks. Certain bactericidal antibiotics such as penicillin may be more effective when given in intermittent (pulsed) doses compared to continuous dosing. The continuous blood level of a hormone such as a corticosteroid might suppress adrenocorticotropic hormone (ACTH) release from the pituitary gland, resulting in atrophy of the adrenal gland. Furthermore, drugs that act indirectly or cause irreversible toxicity may be less efficacious when given in an ER rather than in conventional dosage form.

Several manufacturers are developing MR drug products based on their PK and PD relationship. Concerta (methylphenidate HCl) ER tablets approved for the treatment of ADHD, and Ambien CR (zolpidem tartrate ER tablets) approved for the treatment of adults with trouble falling asleep and/or waking up often during the night were developed in consideration of the therapeutic objectives and PKs of the active drug.

Because the MR dosage form may be in contact with the body for a prolonged period, the recurrence of sensitivity reactions or local tissue reactions due to the drug or constituents of the dosage form is possible. For oral MR dosage forms, prolonged residence time in the GI tract may lead to a variety of interactions with GI tract contents, and the efficiency of absorption may be compromised as the drug moves distally from the duodenum to the large intestine.

Moreover, dosage form failure due to either dose dumping or to the lack of drug release may have important clinical implications. Another possible unforeseen problem with MR dosage forms is an alteration in the metabolic fate of the drug, such as nonlinear biotransformation or site-specific disposition.

Design and selection of ER products are often aided by dissolution tests carried out at different pH units for various time periods to simulate conditions in the GI tract. This in *vitro-in vivo* correlation (IVIVC) for oral ER drug product (discussed later in this chapter). The supporting documents have been involved in the FDA submission of new drug application (NDA), abbreviated new drug application (ANDA), or antibiotic drug application (AADA). Topographical plots of the dissolution data may be used to graph the percent of drug dissolved versus two variables (time, pH) that may affect dissolution simultaneously. For example, Skelley and Barr have shown that ER preparations of theophylline have a more rapid dissolution rate at a higher pH of 8.4, whereas Theo-Dur is less affected by pH (Fig. 9-13) (Skelly and Barr, 1987; Li et al, 2018; Lozoya-Agullo et al, 2018). These dissolution tests *in vitro* may help predict the *in vivo* bioavailability performance of the dosage form (see Chapter 7).

### FREQUENTLY ASKED QUESTION

▶ Does the ER drug product have the same safety and efficacy compared to a conventional dosage form of the same drug?

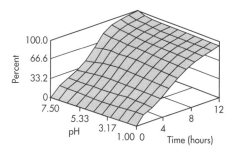

FIGURE 9-13 • Topographical dissolution characterization of theophylline extended release. Topographical dissolution characterization (as a function of time and pH) of Theo-Dur, a theophylline controlled-release preparation, the bioavailability of which was essentially the same whether administered with food or under fasted conditions.

# EVALUATION OF MODIFIED-RELEASE PRODUCTS

## Dissolution Studies

Dissolution requirements for each of the three types of MR dosage form are published in the USP-NF. Some of the key elements for the *in vitro* dissolution/drug release studies are listed in Table 9-12. Dissolution studies may be used together with bioavailability studies to predict IVIVC of the drug release rate of the dosage forms.

### In Vitro–In Vivo Correlations

A general discussion of correlating in vitro drug product performance (eg, dissolution rate) to an *in*

---

**TABLE 9-12 •** Suggested Dissolution/Drug Release Studies for Modified-Release Dosage Forms

**Dissolution Studies**

1. Reproducibility of the method.
2. Proper choice of medium.
3. Maintenance of sink conditions.
4. Control of solution hydrodynamics.
5. Dissolution rate as a function of pH, ranging from pH 1 to pH 8 and including several intermediate values.
6. Selection of the most discriminating variables (medium, pH, rotation speed, etc) as the basis for the dissolution test and specification.

**Dissolution Procedures**

1. Lack of dose dumping, as indicated by a narrow limit on the 1-h dissolution specification.
2. Controlled-release characteristics obtained by employing additional sampling windows over time. Narrow limits with an appropriate Q value system will control the degree of first-order release.
3. Complete drug release of the drug from the dosage form. A minimum of 75%–80% of the drug should be released from the dosage form at the last sampling interval.
4. The pH dependence/independence of the dosage form as indicated by percent dissolution in water, appropriate buffer, simulated gastric juice, or simulated intestinal fluid.

*Data from Robinson JR, Lee VHL: Controlled Drug Delivery: Fundamentals and Applications, 2nd ed. New York, NY: Marcel Dekker; 1987.*

---

*vivo* biologic response (eg, blood-level versus time profile) is discussed in Chapter 7. Ideally, the *in vitro* drug release of the ER drug product should relate to the bioavailability of the drug *in vivo*, so that changes in drug dissolution rates will correlate directly to changes in drug bioavailability.

Per the European Medicines Agency and the FDA on the quality control of oral modified release drug products, the *in vitro* profile for drug products has relationship with PK, PD, and clinical efficacy/safety. *In vitro* dissolution testing is not only important as a necessary quality assurance for batch-to-batch consistency but also to indicate consistency within a batch (ie, that individual dosage units will have the desired *in vivo* performance). By establishing a meaningful correlation between *in vitro* release characteristics and *in vivo* bioavailability parameters, the *in vitro* dissolution test can serve as a surrogate marker for *in vivo* behavior and thereby confirm consistent therapeutic performance of batches from routine production. The variability of the data should be reported and discussed when establishing a correlation. In general, the higher the variability in the data used to generate the IVIVC, the less confidence can be placed on the predictive power of the correlation (FDA Guidance, https://www.fda.gov/media/70939/download).

For MR dosage forms, IVIVC is highly desirable in that it provides a critical linkage between product quality and clinical performance. With an established IVIVC, an *in vitro* test, such as dissolution test, can serve as a critical tool for product and process understanding; aid product/process development, manufacturing, and control; provide significantly increased assurance for consistent product performance; and predict *in vivo* performance throughout the life cycle of an MR product (Cardot et al, 2018) (Chapter 7).

## Pharmacokinetic Studies

In many cases, the active drug is first formulated in an IR drug product. After market experience with the IR drug product, a manufacturer may design an MR or an ER drug product based on the PK profile of the IR drug product, as discussed earlier in this chapter. Various types of PK studies may be required by the FDA for marketing approval of the MR drug product, depending on knowledge about the drug, its clinical PKs and PD, and its biopharmaceutic properties[4] (Skelley et al, 1990). Usually, a complete PK data package is required for a new chemical entity developed as MR formulation. Additional documentation specific to the MR dosage form includes studies evaluating factors affecting the biopharmaceutic performance of the MR formulation. Moreover, the ER dosage form should be available in several dosage strengths to allow flexibility for the clinician to adjust the dose for the individual patient.

Single-dose ranging studies and multiple-dose steady-state crossover studies using the highest strength of the dosage form may be performed. In addition, a food intervention bioavailability study is also performed, since food interactions may be related to the drug substance itself and/or the formulation, the latter being most important in the case of MR products. The reference dosage form may be a solution of the drug or the full NDA-approved conventional, IR dosage form given in an equal daily dose as the ER dosage form. If the dosage strengths differ from each other only in the amount of the drug–excipient blend, but the concentration of the drug–excipient blend is the same in each dosage form, then the FDA may approve the NDA or ANDA on the basis of single- and multiple-dose studies of the highest dosage strength, whereas the other lower-strength dosage forms may be approved on the basis of comparative *in vitro* dissolution studies. The latest FDA Guidance for Industry should be consulted for regulatory requirements (https://www.fda.gov/regulatory-information/search-fda-guidance-documents/). Researchers have described several types of such PK studies (Daousani and Karalis, 2015; Blume, 2019).

## Clinical Considerations of Modified-Release Drug Products

Clinical efficacy and safety may be altered when drug therapy is changed from a conventional, IR drug product given several times a day to a modified, ER drug product given once or twice a day. Usually, the original marketed drug is a conventional, IR drug product.

After experience with the IR drug product, a pharmaceutical manufacturer (sponsor) may develop an ER product containing the same drug. In this case, the sponsor needs to demonstrate that the PK profile of the ER drug product has sustained plasma drug concentrations compared to the conventional drug product. In addition, the sponsor may perform a clinical safety and efficacy study comparing both drug products.

Bupropion hydrochloride (Wellbutrin), an antidepressant drug, is available as an IR drug product given three times a day, an SR[5] drug product given twice a day, and an ER (XL) drug product given once a day. Jefferson et al reviewed the PKs of these three products. These investigators reported that although the PKs profiles are different for each drug product, the clinical efficacy for each drug product is similar if bupropion hydrochloride is given in equal daily doses. According to the approved label information for Wellbutrin XL, patients who are currently being treated with Wellbutrin tablets at 300 mg/day (for example, 100 mg three times a day) may be switched to Wellbutrin XL 300 mg once daily. Patients who are currently being treated with Wellbutrin SR tablets at 300 mg/day (for example, 150 mg twice daily) may be switched to Wellbutrin XL 300 mg once daily. Thus, for bupropion HCl, the fluctuations in plasma drug concentration versus time profiles do not affect clinical efficacy as long as the patient is given the same daily dose of drug (Jefferson et al, 2005).

## Generic Substitution of Modified-Release Drug Products

Generic ER drug products may have different drug release mechanisms compared to the brand-drug product. The different drug release mechanisms may lead to slightly different PK profiles. Generic ER drug products are approved by FDA and are bioequivalent based on AUC and $C_{max}$ criteria and therapeutic equivalence to the brand name equivalent. For some drugs, several different MR products containing exactly the same active ingredient are commercially available. These MR drug products have different pharmacokinetic profiles and may have different clinical efficacy

---

[4]The FDA has specific regulatory requirements for an approved drug that a manufactured wants to develop as a different dosage form. Both bioavailability studies and clinical efficacy studies may be required for market approval. (FDA Draft Guidance for Industry: Determining Whether to Submit an ANDA or a 505(b)(2), October 2017.)

[5]A sustained-release drug product may also be called an extended-release drug product.

compared to the conventional form of the drug given in the same daily dose and compared to other ER products containing the same active drug. Since the pharmacokinetic profiles may differ, the practitioner needs to consult the FDA publication, Approved Drug Products with Therapeutic Equivalence Evaluations (Orange Book),[6] to determine which of these drug products may be substituted.

## EXAMPLE ▷ ▷ ▷

### METHYLPHENIDATE DRUG PRODUCTS

Methylphenidate hydrochloride is a central nervous system (CNS) stimulant indicated for the treatment of attention deficit hyperactivity disorder (ADHD). Numerous conventional and MR drug products containing methylphenidate hydrochloride are available (Table 9-13). Although each of these methylphenidate hydrochloride drug products has the same indication, the prescriber needs to understand which product would be most appropriate for the patient.

**TABLE 9-13** • Various Methylphenidate Hydrochloride Drug Products

| Drug Product | Formulation | Comments |
|---|---|---|
| Ritalin | Immediate release | Conventional drug product |
| Ritalin SR | Extended release | ER drug product with no initial dose |
| Ritalin LA | Extended release with an initial IR dose | Produces a bi-modal plasma concentration-time profile when given orally; not interchangeable with Concerta |
| Concerta | Extended release with an initial IR dose | Not interchangeable for Ritalin LA |
| Daytrana | Film, extended release; transdermal | Provides extended release via transdermal drug absorption |
| Methylin | Solution; oral | Immediate release drug product |
| Methylin | Tablet, chewable; oral | Immediate release drug product |

6 www.fda.gov/Drugs/InformationOnDrugs/ucm129662.htm.

## EVALUATION OF *IN VIVO* BIOAVAILABILITY DATA

The data from a properly designed *in vivo* bioavailability study are evaluated using both pharmacokinetic and statistical analysis methods. The evaluation may include a PK profile, steady-state plasma drug concentrations, rate of drug absorption, occupancy time, and statistical evaluation of the computed PK parameters.

### Pharmacokinetic Profile

The plasma drug concentration–time curve should adequately define the bioavailability of the drug from the dosage form. The bioavailability data should include a profile of the fraction of drug absorbed (Wagner–Nelson) and should rule out dose dumping or lack of a significant food effect. The bioavailability data should also demonstrate the ER characteristics of the dosage form compared to the reference or IR drug product.

### Steady-State Plasma Drug Concentration

The fluctuation between the $C_{max}^{\infty}$ (peak) and $C_{min}^{\infty}$ (trough) concentrations should be calculated:

$$\text{Fluctuation} = \frac{C_{max}^{\infty} - C_{min}^{\infty}}{C_{av}^{\infty}} \qquad (9.11)$$

where $C_{av}^{\infty}$ is equal to $[\text{AUC}]/\tau$

An ideal ER dosage form should have minimum fluctuation between $C_{max}$ and $C_{min}$. A true zero-order release will have no fluctuation. In practice, the fluctuation in plasma drug levels after the ER dosage form should be less than the fluctuation after the same drug given in an IR dosage form.

### Rate of Drug Absorption

For the ER drug product to claim zero-order absorption, an appropriately calculated input function such as used in the Wagner–Nelson approach should substantiate this claim. The difference between first-order and zero-order absorption of a drug is shown in Fig. 9-14. The rate of drug absorption from the conventional or IR dosage form is generally first order, as shown by Fig. 9-14. Drug absorption after an ER dosage form may be zero order (Fig. 9-14, curve B), first order

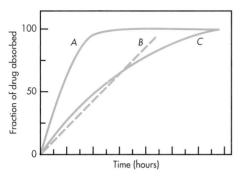

FIGURE 9-14 • The fraction of drug absorbed using the Wagner–Nelson method may be used to distinguish between the first-order drug absorption rate of a conventional (immediate-release) dosage form (A) and an extended-release dosage form (C). Curve B represents an extended-release dosage form with zero-order absorption rate.

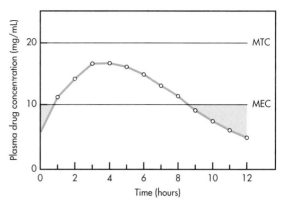

FIGURE 9-15 • Occupancy time.

(see Fig. 9-14, curve A), or an indeterminate order (Fig. 9-14, curve C). For many ER dosage forms, the rate of drug absorption is first order, with an absorption rate constant $k_a$ smaller than the elimination rate constant $k$. The PK model when $k_a > k$ is termed *flip-flop pharmacokinetics* and is discussed in Chapter 7.

## Occupancy Time

In drugs for which the therapeutic window is known, the plasma drug concentrations should be maintained above the minimum effective drug concentration (MEC) and below the minimum toxic drug concentration (MTC). The time required to obtain plasma drug levels within the therapeutic window is known as *occupancy time* (Fig. 9-15).

## Bioequivalence Studies

Bioequivalence studies for ER drug products are discussed in detail in Chapter 7. Bioequivalence studies may include (1) a fasting study, (2) a food-intervention study, and (3) a multiple-dose study. The FDA's Center for Drug Evaluation and Research (CDER) maintains

a website (www.fda.gov/cder) that lists regulatory guidances to provide the public with the FDA's latest submission requirements for NDAs and ANDAs.

## Statistical Evaluation

Variables subject to statistical analysis generally include plasma drug concentrations at each collection time, AUC (from zero to last sampling time), AUC (from zero to time infinity), $C_{max}$, $t_{max}$, and elimination half-life $t_{1/2}$. Statistical testing may include an analysis of variance (ANOVA), computation of 90% and 95% confidence intervals on the difference in formulation means, and the power of ANOVA to detect a 20% difference from the reference mean.

### FREQUENTLY ASKED QUESTIONS

▶ Are ER drug products always more efficacious than IR drug products containing the same drug?

▶ Why do some ER formulations of a drug have a different efficacy profile compared to a conventional dosage form, given in multiple doses?

▶ What are the advantages and disadvantages of a zero-order rate design for drug absorption?

## CHAPTER SUMMARY

The term *modified-release (MR) drug product* is used to describe drug products that are formulated to alter the timing and/or rate of release of the drug. A MR dosage form is a formulation in which the

drug-release characteristics of time course and/or location are chosen to accomplish therapeutic or convenience objectives, which is not offered by conventional dosage forms. Delayed-release and ER drug products are common types of MR dosage forms. The goal of ER drug products is to prolong the duration of drug activity by prolonging effective plasma drug concentrations. ER formulations reduce the peak-to-trough fluctuations of drug concentrations, which may reduce adverse events. Patient compliance often improves due to less frequent dosing.

The timing and rate of drug release can be adjusted according to the therapeutic objective along with efficacy and safety considerations, which cannot be achieved by conventional dosage forms. Oral MR drug products are easily affected by the anatomy and physiology of the GI tract, GI transit, pH, and its contents compared to conventional oral drug products. MR drug products may also have a different PD and safety profile compared to IR drug products containing the same drug. Various approaches have been used to manufacture modified- and extended-release drug products including matrix tablets, coated beads, osmotic release, ion-exchange, liposome, polymeric therapeutics, 3D printed formulation, imaging-guided drug delivery systems, etc. The physical–chemical properties of the drug, the drug dose, the therapeutic objective, and the route of administration are all considerations in designing a MR drug product. Although the route of administration and PK parameters may be different, the bioequivalence should be equal or improved between IR formulations with MR drug products. More and more pharmacometrics have been applied to predict the *in vivo* and clinic performance, including single-dose studies, steady-state studies, partial AUC calculation, IVIVC, assay, etc. Overall, MR products may have different clinical efficacy compared to other ER products containing the same active drug.

## LEARNING QUESTIONS

1. The design for most ER or SR oral drug products allows for the slow release of the drug from the dosage form and subsequent slow absorption of the drug from the GI tract.

   a. Why does the slow release of a drug from an ER drug product produce a longer-acting PD response compared to the same drug prepared in a conventional, oral, IR drug product?

   b. Why do manufacturers of SR drug products attempt to design this dosage form to have a zero-order rate of systemic drug absorption?

2. The dissolution profiles of three drug products are illustrated in Fig. 9-14.

   a. Which of the drug products in Fig. 9-14 releases drug at a zero-order rate of about 8.3% every hour?

   b. Which of the drug products does not release drug at a zero-order rate?

   c. Which of the drug products has an almost zero rate of drug release during certain hours of the dissolution process?

   d. Suggest a common cause of slowing drug dissolution rate of many rapid-release drug products toward the end of dissolution.

   e. Suggest a common cause of slowing drug dissolution of a SR product toward the end of a dissolution test.

3. A drug is normally given at 10 mg four times a day. Suggest an approach for designing a 12-hour, zero-order release product.

   a. Calculate the desired zero-order release rate.

   b. Calculate the concentration of the drug in an osmotic pump type of oral dosage form that delivers 0.5 mL/h of fluid.

4. An industrial pharmacist would like to design a SR drug product to be given every 12 hours. The active drug ingredient has an apparent volume of distribution of 10 L, an elimination half-life of 3.5 hours, and a desired therapeutic plasma drug concentration of 20 $\mu$g/mL. Calculate the zero-order release rate of the SR drug product and the total amount of drug needed, assuming no loading dose is required.

# ANSWERS

## Frequently Asked Questions

*What is the difference between extended release, delayed release, sustained release, modified release, and controlled release?*

■ The several types of modified-release (MR) drug products can be recognized as the following subtypes such as extended release, delayed release, sustained release, and controlled release, based on the drug release characteristics of the products for the purpose of timing and/or rate and/or location control. The above terms are frequently used interchangeably, but individual products may differ in design, performance, and therapeutic purpose.

*Why does the drug bioavailability from some conventional IR drug products resemble an extended-release drug product?*

■ IR products generally provide relatively rapid drug absorption and onset of accompanying pharmacodynamic (PD) effects, but not always, especially for lipophilic drugs. The extended-release drug product can control the drug release during an extended period, at a predetermined rate, duration, and location after administration. An extended-release dosage form with zero or first-order drug absorption may have comparable drug bioavailability to drug absorption from a conventional dosage form given in multiple doses and the elimination half-life is constant.

*How do patient-specific variables influence performance of MR dosage forms?*

■ MR dosage forms have complex formulations that can offer an advantage over conventional release medication for some specific patients. By improving the features of patience compliance, less administration frequency, delivering poorly soluble active pharmaceutical ingredients (APIs), product differentiation, and longer life cycle, MR dosage has the patient-specific benefits such as improved efficacy and reduced adverse events.

*What is the difference between the different types of MR dosage forms?*

■ The USP recognizes several types of MR dosage forms such as extended release, delayed release, sustained release, and controlled release or targeted release. MR dosage forms can be designed to deliver drugs in a controlled and predictable manner or at a target location by expressing the features of prolonged, controlled, pulsatile, combination, targeted delivery, etc. The above terms are frequently used interchangeably, depending on the purpose of design, performance, and therapeutics.

*Does the ER drug product have the same safety and efficacy compared to a conventional dosage form of the same drug?*

■ The safety and efficacy are two critical issues for ER drug product development. In comparison to conventional dosage form of the same drug, besides better efficacy, reduced toxicity, or better patient compliance, ER drug products should provide a prolonged pharmacodynamic (PD) effect.

*Are ER drug products always more efficacious than IR drug products containing the same drug?*

■ The safety and efficacy are two critical issues for ER drug product development. In comparison to conventional dosage form of the same drug, besides better efficacy, reduced toxicity, or better patient compliance, ER drug product should provide a prolonged pharmacodynamic effect. However, an ER dosage form of a drug may have a different pharmacodynamic (PD) activity profile in comparison to the same drug given in an acute, intermittent, rapid-release dosage form. ER formulation may not be able always to provide more efficacious than IR drug products, eg, the functional tolerance effect in ER transdermal patches and certain bactericidal antibiotics issues in ER pulsed doses. Furthermore, drugs that act indirectly or have irreversible toxicity may be less efficacious when given in an ER rather than in conventional dosage form.

*Why do some ER formulations of a drug have a different efficacy profile compared to a conventional dosage form, given in multiple doses?*

■ There is no rationale for ER formulations development for the conventional dosage form with minimal fluctuations in blood concentrations after multiple doses are administered. In contrast, drugs with very short half-lives need to be given at frequent dosing intervals to maintain therapeutic efficacy. For drugs with very short elimination half-lives, an ER drug product maintains the efficacy over a longer duration. Under this situation, ER formulations of a drug have a different efficacy profile compared to a conventional dosage form and ER drug products should show steady-state levels comparable to those reached using a conventional dosage form given in multiple doses.

*What are the advantages and disadvantages of a zero-order rate design for drug absorption?*

■ Zero-order kinetic (such as drug absorption and elimination) from the dosing site into/out of the plasma usually occurs by a saturable process with constant amount (eg, milligrams) per unit time. Alcohol, aspirin, phenytoin, etc. can be regarded as zero-order drugs. Zero-order rate drug formulation leads to the best control of plasma concentration and offers the following advantages: 1) sustained therapeutic blood levels of the drug; 2) improved patient compliance; and 3) reduction in adverse side effects. The disadvantages are: 1) dose dumping; 2) less flexibility in accurate dose adjustment; and 3) less possibility for high dosage.

## REFERENCES

Abdul S, Chandewar AV, Jaiswal SB: A flexible technology for modified-release drugs: Multiple-unit pellet system (MUPS). *JCR* **147**(1):2–16, 2010. doi: http://dx.doi.org/10.1016/j.jconrel.2010.05.014

Abrahamsson B, Albery T, Eriksson A, Gustafsson I, Sjöberg M: Food effects on tablet disintegration. *Eur J Pharm Sci* **22**(2–3):165–172, 2004. doi: http://dx.doi.org/10.1016/j.ejps.2004.03.004

Adibkia K, Ghanbarzadeh S, Shokri MH, Arami Z, Arash Z, Shokri J: Micro-porous surfaces in controlled drug delivery systems: Design and evaluation of diltiazem hydrochloride controlled porosity osmotic pump using non-ionic surfactants as pore-former. *Pharm Dev Technol* **19**(4):507–512, 2014. doi: 10.3109/10837450.2013.805774

Allen TM, Cullis PR: Liposomal drug delivery systems: From concept to clinical applications. *Adv Drug Deliv Rev* **65**(1):36–48, 2013. doi: http://dx.doi.org/10.1016/j.addr.2012.09.037

Anselmo AC, Mitragotri S: An overview of clinical and commercial impact of drug delivery systems. *J Control Release* **190**(0):15–28, 2014. doi: http://dx.doi.org/10.1016/j.jconrel.2014.03.053

Asare-Addo K, Levina M, Rajabi-Siahboomi AR, Nokhodchi A: Effect of ionic strength and pH of dissolution media on theophylline release from hypromellose matrix tablets—Apparatus USP III, simulated fasted and fed conditions. *Carbohydr Polymer* **86**(1):85–93, 2011. doi: http://dx.doi.org/10.1016/j.carbpol.2011.04.014

Badran MM, Kuntsche J, Fahr A: Skin penetration enhancement by a microneedle device (Dermaroller®) in vitro: Dependency on needle size and applied formulation. *Eur J Pharm Sci* 36(4–5),511-523, 2009. doi: http://dx.doi.org/10.1016/j.ejps.2008.12.008

Baracat, M, Nakagawa A, Casagrande R, Georgetti S, Verri, W Jr, de Freitas O: Preparation and characterization of microcapsules based on biodegradable polymers: Pectin/casein complex for controlled drug release systems. *AAPS PharmSciTech* **13**(2):364–372, 2012. doi: 10.1208/s12249-012-9752-0

Barmpalexis P, Kachrimanis K, Malamataris S: Statistical moments in modelling of swelling, erosion and drug release of hydrophilic matrix-tablets. *Int J Pharm* **540**(1-2):1–10, 2018. https://doi.org/10.1016/j.ijpharm.2018.01.052

Basu S, Yang H, Fang L, et al: Physiologically based pharmacokinetic modeling to evaluate formulation factors influencing bioequivalence of metoprolol extended-release products. *J Clin Pharmacol* **59**(9):1252–1263, 2019. https://doi.org/10.1002/jcph.1017

Benson HAE, et al: Topical and transdermal drug delivery: From simple potions to smart technologies. *Curr Drug Deliv* **16**(5):444–460, 2019. Doi: 10.2174/1567201816666190201143457

Blume HH: Bioequivalence. In: Hock F, Gralinski M. (eds). *Drug Discovery and Evaluation: Methods in Clinical Pharmacology.* Springer, Cham, 2019, pp 1–16. doi: https://doi.org/10.1007/978-3-319-56637-5_17-1

Brandt C, May TW: Extended-release drug formulations for the treatment of epilepsy. *Exp Opin Pharmacother* **19**(8):843–850, 2018. DOI: https://doi.org/10.1080/14656566.2018.1465561

Brunner M, Ziegler S, Di Stefano AFD, et al: Gastrointestinal transit, release and plasma pharmacokinetics of a new oral budesonide formulation. *British J Clin Pharmacol* **61**(1):31–38, 2006. doi: 10.1111/j.1365-2125.2005.02517.x

Cardot JM, Luckas JC, Muniz P: Time scaling for in vitro-in vivo correlation: The inverse release function (IRF) approach. *AAPS J* **20**:95, 2018. https://doi.org/10.1208/s12248-018-0250-5

Centelles MN, et al: Image-guided thermosensitive liposomes for focused ultrasound drug delivery: Using NIRF-labelled lipids and topotecan to visualise the effects of hyperthermia in tumors. *J Control Release* 280:87–98, 2018. https://doi.org/10.1016/j.jconrel.2018.04.047

Chen Y, Cun D, Quan P, et al: Saturated long-chain esters of isopulegol as novel permeation enhancers for transdermal drug delivery. *Pharm Res* 31(8):1907–1918, 2014. doi: 10.1007/s11095-013-1292-0

Cheng C, Wu P-C, Lee H-Y, Hsu K-Y: Development and validation of an in vitro–in vivo correlation (IVIVC) model for propranolol hydrochloride extended-release matrix formulations. *J Food Drug Anal* 22(2):257–263, 2014. doi: http://dx.doi.org/10.1016/j.jfda.2013.09.016

Clark A, Milbrandt TA, Hilt JZ, Puleo DA: Mechanical properties and dual drug delivery application of poly(lactic-co-glycolic acid) scaffolds fabricated with a poly(β-amino ester) porogen. *Acta Biomaterialia* 10(5):2125–2132, 2014. doi: http://dx.doi.org/10.1016/j.actbio.2013.12.061

Couvreur P, Vauthier C: Nanotechnology: Intelligent design to treat complex disease. *Pharm Res* 23(7):1417–1450, 2006. doi: 10.1007/s11095-006-0284-8

Craig D: Oxymorphone extended-release tablets (Opana ER) for the management of chronic pain. *PharmTherapeut* 35(6):324–329, 2010.

Daousani C, Karalis V: Bioequivalence studies in Europe before and after 2010. *Clin Res Reg Affairs* 32(1): 9–21, 2015. https://doi.org/10.3109/10601333.2014.976229

Ding H, Wu F, Nair MP: Image-guided drug delivery to the brain using nanotechnology. *Drug Discov Today* 18(21–22): 1074–1080, 2013. doi: http://dx.doi.org/10.1016/j.drudis.2013.06.010

Ding H, Yong K, Roy I, et al: Gold nanorods coated with multilayer polyelectrolyte as contrast agents for multimodal imaging. *J Phys Chem C* 111(34):12552–12557, 2007. doi: 10.1021/jp0733419

Ding H, Yong KT, Roy I, et al: Bioconjugated PLGA-4-arm-PEG branched polymeric nanoparticles as novel tumor targeting carriers. [Research Support, N.I.H., Extramural]. *Nanotechnology* 22(16):165101, 2011. doi: 10.1088/0957-4484/22/16/165101

Dreicer R, Bajorin DF, McLeod DG, Petrylakemail DP, Moul JW; New data, new paradigms for treating prostate cancer patients—VI: Novel hormonal therapy approaches. *Urology* 78(5):S494–S498, 2011.

Duncan R, Vicent MJ: Polymer therapeutics-prospects for 21st century: The end of the beginning. *Adv Drug Deliv Rev* 65(1):60–70, 2013. doi: http://dx.doi.org/10.1016/j.addr.2012.08.012

Eberle VA, Schoelkopf J, Gane PAC, Alles R, Huwyler J, Puchkov M: Floating gastroretentive drug delivery systems: Comparison of experimental and simulated dissolution profiles and floatation behavior. *Eur J Pharm Sci* 58(0):34–43, 2014. doi: http://dx.doi.org/10.1016/j.ejps.2014.03.001

Eisenmann A, Amann A, Said M., Datta B, Ledochowski M: Implementation and interpretation of hydrogen breath tests. *J Breath Res* 2:046002, 2008. (046009pp).

Farr SJ, Robinson CY, Rubino CM: Effects of food and alcohol on the pharmacokinetics of an oral, extended-release formulation of hydrocodone in healthy volunteers. *Clin Pharmacol* 7:1–9, 2015.

FDA: Guidance for Industry. Extended-Release oral dosage Forms: Development, evaluation, and application of in vitro/in vivo correlations. Food and Drug Administration (FDA). Guideline on quality of oral modified release products. European Medicines Agency, 2012.

Franek F, Holm P, Larsen F, Steffansen B: Interaction between fed gastric media (Ensure Plus') and different hypromellose based caffeine-controlled release tablets: Comparison and mechanistic study of caffeine release in fed and fasted media versus water using the USP dissolution apparatus 3. *Int J Pharm* 461(1–2):419–426, 2014. doi: http://dx.doi.org/10.1016/j.ijpharm.2013.12.003

Gao Z, Ngo C, Ye W, et al: Effects of dissolution medium pH and simulated gastrointestinal contraction on drug release from Nifedipine extended-release tablets. *J Pharm Sci* 108(3): 1189–1194, 2019. https://doi.org/10.1016/j.xphs.2018.10.014

Garekani HA, et al: Peculiar effect of polyethylene glycol in comparison with triethyl citrate or diethyl phthalate on properties of ethyl cellulose microcapsules containing propranolol hydrochloride in process of emulsion-solvent evaporation. *Drug Devel Indust Pharm* 44(3):421–431, 2018. https://doi.org/10.1080/03639045.2017.1395460

Gefter (Shenderovich) J, et al: Chlorhexidine sustained-release varnishes for catheter coating – Dissolution kinetics and anti-biofilm properties. *Eur J Pharm Sci* 112:1–7, 2018. https://doi.org/10.1016/j.ejps.2017.10.041

Ghayas S, Shoaib MH, Qazi F, et al: Influence of different viscosity grade cellulose-based polymers on the development of valsartan controlled release tablets. *Polymer Bulletin* published online: 06 May 2019. https://doi.org/10.1007/s00289-019-02802-2

Gonzalez MA, Cleary GW: Transdermal dosage forms. In Shargel L, Kanfer I (eds). *Generic Drug Product Development–Specialty Dosage Forms*. New York. Informa Healthcare, 2010, Chapter 8.

Grimm M, Ball K, Scholz E, et al: Characterization of the gastrointestinal transit and disintegration behavior of floating and sinking acid-resistant capsules using a novel MRI labeling technique. *Eur J Pharm Sci* 129:163–172, 2019. https://doi.org/10.1016/j.ejps.2019.01.012

Grund J, Koerber M, Walther M, Bodmeier R: The effect of polymer properties on direct compression and drug release from water-insoluble controlled release matrix tablets. *Int J Pharm* 469(1):94–101, 2014. doi: http://dx.doi.org/10.1016/j.ijpharm.2014.04.033

Henry S, McAllister DV, Allen MG, Prausnitz MR: Microfabricated microneedles: A novel approach to transdermal drug delivery. [In Vitro Research Support, Non-U.S. Gov't Research Support, U.S. Gov't, Non-P.H.S.]. *J Pharm Sci* 87(8):922–925, 1998. doi: 10.1021/js980042+

Hofmann AF, Pressman JH, Code CF, Witztum KF: Controlled entry of orally administered drugs: Physiological considerations. *Drug Devel Indust Pharm* 9(7):1077–1109, 1983. doi: 10.3109/03639048309046314

Honório TD, Pinto E, Rocha H, at al: In vitro–in vivo correlation of Efavirenz tablets using GastroPlus'. *AAPS PharmSciTech* **14**(3):1244–1254, 2013. doi: 10.1208/s12249-013-0016-4

Ikeuchi SY, Kambayashi A, Kojima H, Naoto Oku N, Asai T: Prediction of the oral pharmacokinetics and food effects of Gabapentin Enacarbil extended-release tablets using biorelevant dissolution tests. *Biol Pharm Bull* **41**(11):1708–1715, 2018. https://doi.org/10.1248/bpb.b18-00456

Jain AK, Söderlind E, Viridén, A, et al: The influence of hydroxypropyl methylcellulose (HPMC) molecular weight, concentration and effect of food on in vivo erosion behavior of HPMC matrix tablets. *J Control Release* **187**(0):50–58, 2014. doi: http://dx.doi.org/10.1016/j.jconrel.2014.04.058

Jefferson JW, Pradko JF, Muir KT: Bupropion for major depressive disorder: Pharmacokinetic and formulation considerations. [Review]. *Clin Ther* **27**(11):1685–1695, 2005. doi: 10.1016/j.clinthera.2005.11.011

Jamróz W, et al: 3D Printing in pharmaceutical and medical applications – recent achievements and challenges. *Pharm Res* **35**(9):176, 2018. doi: 10.1007/s11095-018-2454-x

Janićijević Ž, Radovanović F: Polyethersulfone/poly(acrylic acid) composite hydrogel membrane reservoirs for controlled delivery of cationic drug formulations. *Polymer* **147**:56–66, 2018. https://doi.org/10.1016/j.polymer.2018.05.065

Jin L, Ding Y-C, Zhang Y, Xu X-Q, Cao Q: A novel pH–enzyme-dependent mesalamine colon-specific delivery system. *Drug Des Devel Ther* **10**:2021–2028, 2016. doi: 10.2147/DDDT.S10728

Jonkman JHG: Food interactions with sustained-release theophylline preparations. *Clin Pharmacokinet* **16**(3):162–179, 1989. doi: 10.2165/00003088-198916030-00003

Kawai Y, Fuji Y, Tabata F, et al: Profiling and trend analysis of food effects on oral drug absorption considering micelle interaction and solubilization by bile micelles. *Drug Metab Pharmacokinet* **26**(2):180–191, 2011. doi: 10.2133/dmpk.DMPK-10-RG-098

Kite-Powell J: FDA approved 3D printed drug available in the US. Forbes, 2016. link: https://www.forbes.com/sites/jenniferhicks/2016/03/22/fda-approved-3d-printed-drug-available-in-the-us/#2da2f5ba666b

Kotta S, Nair A, Alsabeelah N: 3D printing technology in drug delivery: Recent progress and application. *Curr Pharm Des* **24**(42):5039–5048, 2018. doi: 10.2174/1381612825666181206123828

Kleiner LW, Wright JC, Wang Y: Evolution of implantable and insertable drug delivery systems. *J Control Rel* **181**(0):1–10, 2014. doi: http://dx.doi.org/10.1016/j.jconrel.2014.02.006

Krivoguz YM, Guliyev AM, Pesetskii SS: Free-radical grafting of trans-ethylene-1,2-dicarboxylic acid onto molten ethylene-vinyl acetate copolymer. *J Applied Polymer Sci* **127**(4):3104–3113, 2013. doi: 10.1002/app.37703

Lau ETL, et al: Dosage form modification and oral drug delivery in older people. *Adv Drug Deliv Rev* **135**:75–84, 2018. https://doi.org/10.1016/j.addr.2018.04.012

Lee H, et al: Device-assisted transdermal drug delivery. *Adv Drug Deliv Rev* **127**:35–45, 2018. https://doi.org/10.1016/j.addr.2017.08.009

Lee PI: Modeling of drug release from matrix systems involving moving boundaries: Approximate analytical solutions. *Int J Pharm* **418**(1):18–27, 2011. doi: http://dx.doi.org/10.1016/j.ijpharm.2011.01.019

Li L, Wang L, Shao Y, et al: Elucidation of release characteristics of highly soluble drug trimetazidine hydrochloride from chitosan–carrageenan matrix tablets. *J Pharm Sci* **102**(8):2644–2654, 2013. doi: 10.1002/jps.23632

Li Z, et al: In vitro-in vivo predictive dissolution-permeation-absorption dynamics of highly permeable drug extended-release tablets via drug dissolution/absorption simulating system and pH alteration. *AAPS PharmSciTech* **19**(4):1882–1893, 2018. https://doi.org/10.1208/s12249-018-0996-1

Lozoya-Agullo I, et al: Preclinical models for colonic absorption, application to controlled release formulation development. *Eur J Pharmaceut Biopharmaceut* **130**:247–259, 2018. https://doi.org/10.1016/j.ejpb.2018.07.008

Malinovskaja K, Laaksonen., Kontturi K, Hirvonen J: Ion-exchange and iontophoresis-controlled delivery of apomorphine. *Eur J Pharmaceut Biopharmaceut* **83**(3):477–484, 2013. doi: http://dx.doi.org/10.1016/j.ejpb.2012.11.014

Marasanapalle VP, Crison JR, Ma J, Li X, Jasti BR: Investigation of some factors contributing to negative food effects. *Biopharmaceut Drug Disp* **30**(2):71–80, 2009. doi: 10.1002/bdd.647

Margolesky J, Singer C. Extended-release oral capsule of carbidopa–levodopa in Parkinson disease. *TAND* **11**:1–12, 2017. https://doi.org/10.1177/1756285617737728

Meulenaar J, Keizer RJ, Beijnen JH, Schellens JHM, Huitema ADR, Nuijen B: Development of an extended-release formulation of capecitabine making use of in vitro–in vivo correlation modelling. *J Pharm Sci* **103**(2):478–484, 2014. doi: 10.1002/jps.23779

Nagaraju R, Swapna Y, Baby RH, Kaza R: Design and evaluation of delayed and extended release tablets of mesalamine. *J Pharm Technol* **2**(1):103–110, 2010.

Ong YXJ, et al: Production of drug-releasing biodegradable microporous scaffold using a two-step micro-encapsulation/supercritical foaming process. *J Supercrit Fluids* **133**(1):263–269, 2018. https://doi.org/10.1016/j.supflu.2017.10.018

Pachuau L, Mazumder B: Albizia procera gum as an excipient for oral controlled release matrix tablet. *Carbohydr Polymer* **90**(1):289–295, 2012. doi: http://dx.doi.org/10.1016/j.carbpol.2012.05.038

Parent M, Nouvel C, Koerber M, Sapin A, Maincent P, Boudier A: PLGA in situ implants formed by phase inversion: Critical physicochemical parameters to modulate drug release. *J Control Release* **172**(1):292–304, 2013. doi: http://dx.doi.org/10.1016/j.jconrel.2013.08.024

Patil SD, Burgess DJ: Pharmaceutical development of modified release parenteral dosage forms using bioequivalence (BE), quality by design (QBD) and in vitro in vivo correlation (IVIVC) principles. In Shargel I, Kanfer I (eds). *Generic Drug Product Development–Specialty Dosage Forms*. New York, Informa Healthcare, 2010, Chapter 9.

Peng A, Kosloski M, Nakamura G, Ding H, Balu-Iyer S: PEGylation of a factor VIII–phosphatidylinositol complex: Pharmacokinetics and immunogenicity in hemophilia A mice. *AAPS J* **14**(1):35–42, 2012. doi: 10.1208/s12248-011-9309-2

Peppas NA, Narasimhan B: Mathematical models in drug delivery: How modeling has shaped the way we design new drug delivery systems. *J Control Release* **190**(0):75–81, 2014. doi: http://dx.doi.org/10.1016/j.jconrel.2014.06.041

Petrides PE, Schoergenhofer C, Widmann R, Bernd JB, Klade CS: Pharmacokinetics of a novel anagrelide extended-release formulation in healthy subjects: Food intake and comparison with a reference product. *Clin Pharmacol Drug Dev* **7**(2):123–131, 2018. doi: 10.1002/cpdd.340

Rahman M, Roy S, Das SC, Jha MK, Begum T, Ahsan Q: Evaluation of various grades of hydroxypropyl methylcellulose matrix systems as oral sustained release drug delivery systems. *J Pharm Sci Res* **3**(1):390–398, 2011.

Rana V, Rai P, Tiwary AK, Singh RS, Kennedy JF, Knill CJ: Modified gums: Approaches and applications in drug delivery. *Carbohydr Polymer* **83**(3):1031–1047, 2011. doi: http://dx.doi.org/10.1016/j.carbpol.2010.09.010

Ranjan OP, Nayak UY, Reddy MS, Dengale SJ, Musmade PB, Udupa N: Osmotically controlled pulsatile release capsule of montelukast sodium for chronotherapy: Statistical optimization, in vitro and in vivo evaluation. *Drug Deliv* **0**(0):1–10, 2013. doi: 10.3109/10717544.2013.853209

Razavi M, Karimian H, Yeong CH, et al: Gamma scintigraphic study of the hydrodynamically balanced matrix tablets of metformin HCl in rabbits. *Drug Des Devel Ther* **9**:3125–3139, 2015. doi: 10.2147/DDDT.S82935

Ritschel WA: Targeting in the gastrointestinal tract: new approaches, method and find. Exp Clin Pharmacol **13**(5):313–336, 1991.

Rosiaux Y, Velghe C, Muschert S, et al: Mechanisms controlling theophylline release from ethanol-resistant coated pellets. *Pharm Res* **31**(3):731–741, 2014. doi: 10.1007/s11095-013-1194-1

Sequeira JAD, et al: Poly(lactic-co-glycolic acid) (PLGA) matrix implants. *Nanostructures for the Engineering of Cells, Tissues and Organs, From Design to Applications.* William Andrew 2018, pp 375–402, Chapter 10. https://doi.org/10.1016/B978-0-12-813665-2.00010-7

Shareef MA, Khar RK, Ahuja A, Ahmad FJ, S, R: Colonic drug delivery: An updated review. *AAPS PharmSci* **5**(2):E17, 2003.

Sharma S, Sinha VR: Current pharmaceutical strategies for efficient site specific delivery in inflamed distal intestinal mucosa. *J Control Release* **272**:97–106, 2018. https://doi.org/10.1016/j.jconrel.2018.01.003

Siepmann J, Peppas NA: Higuchi equation: Derivation, applications, use and misuse. *Int J Pharm* **418**:6–12, 2011. Doi: https://doi.org/10.1016/j.ijpharm.2011.03.051

Skelley JP, Amidon GL, Barr WH, et al: Report of the workshop on in vitro and in vivo testing and correlation for oral controlled/modified-release dosage forms. *J Pharm Sci* **79**(9):849–854, 1990. doi: 10.1002/jps.2600790923

Skelly JP, Barr WH: Regulatory assessment. In Robinson JR, Lee VHL (eds). Controlled Drug Delivery: Fundamentals and applications, 2nd ed. New York, Marcel Dekker, 1987.

Sujja-areevath J, Munday DL, Cox PJ, Khan KA: Relationship between swelling, erosion and drug release in hydrophilic natural gum mini-matrix formulations. *Eur J Pharm Sci* **6**(3):207–217, 1998. doi: http://dx.doi.org/10.1016/S0928-0987(97)00072-9

Tripathi J, et al: Current state and future perspectives on gastroretentive drug delivery systems. *Pharmaceutics* **11**(4):193, 2019. https://doi.org/10.3390/pharmaceutics11040193

Tyagi P, Subramony A: Nanotherapeutics in oral and parenteral drug delivery: Key learnings and future outlooks as we think small. *J Control Release* **272**:159–168, 2018. https://doi.org/10.1016/j.jconrel.2018.01.009

US Patent 9,872,859, issued on Jan 23, 2018.

Verstraete G, et al: 3D printing of high drug loaded dosage forms using thermoplastic polyurethanes. *Int J Pharm* **536**(1):318–25, 2018. https://doi.org/10.1016/j.ijpharm.2017.12.002

Viridén A, Wittgren B, Larsson A: Investigation of critical polymer properties for polymer release and swelling of HPMC matrix tablets. *Eur J Pharm Sci* **36**(2–3):297–309, 2009. doi: http://dx.doi.org/10.1016/j.ejps.2008.10.021

Ways TM, Lau MM, Khutoryanskiy VV: Chitosan and its derivatives for application in mucoadhesive drug delivery systems. *Polymer* **10**(3):267, 2018. https://doi.org/10.3390/polym10030267

Welling PG: Oral controlled drug administration, pharmacokinetic considerations. *Drug Devel Indust Pharm* **9**(7):1185–1225, 1983. doi:10.3109/03639048309046316

Wilson B, Babubhai PP, Sajeev MS, Jenita JL, SRB P: Sustained release enteric coated tablets of pantoprazole: Formulation, in vitro and in vivo evaluation. *Acta Pharmaceutica* **63**(1):131–140, 2013.

Worsham RD, Thomas V, Farid SS: Potential of continuous manufacturing for liposomal drug products. *Biotechnol J* **14**:1700740, 2019. https://doi.org/10.1002/biot.201700740|

Wu F, Ding H, Zhang ZR: Investigation of the in vivo desintegration and transit behavior of tetramethylpyrazine phosphate pulsincap capsule in the GI tract of dogs by gamma scintigraphy. *J Biomed Eng* **23**(4):790–794, 2006.

Yadav M, et al: Bimatoprost loaded nanovesicular long-acting sub-conjunctival in-situ gelling implant: In vitro and in vivo evaluation. *Mater Sci Eng C* **103**:109730, 2019. https://doi.org/10.1016/j.msec.2019.05.015

Yang K, et al: Cooperative assembly of magneto-nanovesicles with tunable wall thickness and permeability for MRI-guided drug delivery. *J Am Chem Soc* **140**(13):4666–4677, 2018. https://doi.org/10.1021/jacs.8b00884

Yu, LX, Crison JR, Amidon GL: (1996). Compartmental transit and dispersion model analysis of small intestinal transit flow in humans. Int J Pharm **140**(1):111–118, 1996. doi: http://dx.doi.org/10.1016/0378-5173(96)04592-9

Zhou J, et al: Reverse engineering the 1-month Lupron Depot. *AAPS J* **10**:105, 2018. https://doi.org/10.1208/s12248-018-0253-2

Zhou Y, et al: Concomitant drugs-loaded microcapsules of roxithromycin and theophylline with pH-sensitive controlled-releasing properties. *Int J Polymer Mat Polymer Biomat.* Published online: 12 Apr 2019. https://doi.org/10.1080/00914037.2019.1596917

Zhu Q, Wei Y, Li C, Mao S: Inner layer-embedded contact lenses for ion-triggered controlled drug delivery. *Mat Sci Eng C* **93**:36–48, 2018. https://doi.org/10.1016/j.msec.2018.07.065.

## BIBLIOGRAPHY

Akala EO, Collett JH: Influence of drug loading and gel structure on in-vitro release kinetics from photopolymerized gels. *Ind Pharm* **13**:1779–1798, 1987.

Arnon R: In Gregoriadis G, Senior J, Trouet A (eds): *Targeting of Drugs*. New York, Plenum Press, 1982, pp 31–54.

Arnon R, Hurwitz E: In Goldberg EP (ed): *Targeted Drugs*. New York, Wiley, 1983, pp 23–55.

Bayley H, Gasparro F, Edelson R: Photoactive drugs. *TIPS* **8**: 138–144, 1987.

Boxenbaum HG: Physiological and pharmacokinetic factors affecting performance of sustained release dosage forms. *Drug Dev Ind Pharm* **8**:1–25, 1982.

Brodsky FM: Monoclonal antibodies as magic bullets. *Pharm Res* **5**:1–9, 1988.

Bruck S (ed): *Controlled Drug Delivery*. Boca Raton, FL, CRC Press, 1983.

Cabana BE: Bioavailability regulations and biopharmaceutic standard for controlled release drug delivery. *Proceedings of 1982 Research and Scientific Development Conference*. Washington, DC, The Proprietary Association, 1983, pp 56–69.

Chien YW: *Novel Drug Delivery Systems*. New York, Marcel Dekker, 1982.

Chien YW: Oral controlled drug administration. *Drug Dev Ind Pharm* **9**: 1983.

Chien YW, Siddiqui O, Shi WM, et al: Direct current iontophoretic transdermal delivery of peptide and protein drugs. *J Pharm Sci* **78**:376–383, 1989.

Chu BCF, Whiteley JM: High molecular weight derivatives of methotrexate as chemotherapeutic agents. *Mol Pharmacol* **13**:80, 1980.

Fiume L, Busi C, Mattioli A: Targeting of antiviral drugs by coupling with protein carriers. *FEBS Lett* **153**:6, 1983.

Fiume L, Busi C, Mattioli A, et al: Hepatocyte targeting of antiviral drugs coupled to galactosyl-terminating glycoproteins. In Gregoriadis G, Senior J, Trouet A (eds). *Targeting of Drugs*. New York, Plenum, 1982, pp 1–18.

Friend DR, Pangburn S: Site-specific drug delivery. *Medicinal Res Rev* **7**:53–106, 1987.

Gros L, Ringsdorf H, Schupp H: Polymeric antitumor agents on a molecular & cellular level. *Angew Chem Int Ed Engl* **20**:312, 1981.

Heller J: Controlled drug release from monolithic bioerodible polymer devices. *Pharm Int* **7**:316–318, 1986.

Hunter E, Fell JT, Sharma H: The gastric emptying of pellets contained in hard gelatin capsules. *Drug Dev Ind Pharm* **8**: 151–157, 1982.

Joshi HN: Recent advances in drug delivery systems: Polymeric prodrugs. *Pharm Technol* **12**:118–125, 1988.

Langer R: New methods of drug delivery. *Science* **249**:1527–1533, 1990.

Levy G: Targeted drug delivery: Some pharmacokinetic considerations. *Pharm Res* **4**:3–4, 1987.

Malinowski HJ: Biopharmaceutic aspects of the regulatory review of oral controlled release drug products. *Drug Dev Ind Pharm* **9**:1255–1279, 1983.

Miyazaki S, Ishii K, Nadai T: Controlled release of prednisolone from ethylene-vinyl acetate copolymer matrix. *Chem Pharm Bull* **29**:2714–2717, 1981.

Mueller-Lissner SA, Blum AL: The effect of specific gravity and eating on gastric emptying of slow-release capsules. *N Engl J Med* **304**:1365–1366, 1981.

Okabe K, Yamoguchi H, Kawai Y: New ionotophoretic transdermal administration of the beta-blocker metoprolol. *J Control Release* **4**:79–85, 1987.

Park H, Robinson JR: Mechanisms of mucoadhesion of poly(acrylic acid) hydrogels. *Pharm Res* **4**:457–464, 1987.

Pozansky MJ, Juliano RL: Biological approaches to the controlled delivery of drugs: A critical review. *Pharmacol Rev* **36**: 277–336, 1984.

Robinson JR: *Sustained and Controlled Release Drug Delivery Systems*. New York, Marcel Dekker, 1978.

Robinson JR: Oral drug delivery systems. *Proceedings of 1982 Research and Scientific Development Conference*. Washington, DC, The Proprietary Association, 1983, pp 54–69.

Robinson JR, Eriksen SP: Theoretical formulation of sustained release dosage forms. *J Pharm Sci* **53**:1254–1263, 1966.

Robinson JR, Lee VHL (eds): *Controlled Drug Delivery: Fundamentals and Applications*, 2nd ed. New York, Marcel Dekker, 1987.

Rosement TJ, Mansdorf SZ: *Controlled Release Delivery Systems*. New York, Marcel Dekker, 1983.

Schechter B, Wilchek M, Arnon R: Increased therapeutic efficacy of cis-platinum complexes of poly L-glutamic acid against a murine carcinoma. *Int J Cancer* **39**:409–413, 1987.

Urquhart J: *Controlled-Release Pharmaceuticals*. Washington, DC, American Pharmaceutical Association, 1981.

United States Pharmacopeial Convention, Inc., "In Vitro-In Vivo Correlation for Extended Release Oral Dosage Forms," Pharmacopeial Forum Stimuli Article, July 1988, 4160-4161

# 10

# Targeted Drug Delivery Systems and Biotechnology Products

Dhaval K. Shah, Zhe Li, and Donald E. Mager

## CHAPTER OBJECTIVES

- Describe basic classification categories of protein therapeutics and discuss example drugs in each group.

- Compare and contrast the general pharmacokinetic characteristics of small-molecule and biological drugs.

- Describe the unique targeting mechanisms of monoclonal antibodies and novel antibody-based constructs along with general determinants of their disposition and effects.

- Identify the need and rationale for drug carriers and formulations for biologics along with the major components of targeted drug delivery systems.

- Recognize integrating and non-integrating delivery vectors that address disposition challenges and enable effective gene therapies.

- Describe the major processes governing the pharmacokinetic properties of biopharmaceuticals.

## INTRODUCTION

Early clinical applications of protein therapeutics focused on the replacement of deficient or abnormal protein concentrations, such as insulin in type 1 diabetes mellitus, and relied on the purification of proteins from animal origins. Breakthroughs in molecular biology, recombinant DNA technology, protein engineering, and drug formulations and delivery systems have fueled a revolution in protein-based therapeutics and innovative targeted drug delivery systems. Biological drugs are now a major sector of the pharmaceutical industry, with biologics making up 29% of new drug approvals by the Food and Drug Administration (FDA) in 2018. There are several advantages of biopharmaceuticals over small-molecule drugs, including highly specific mechanisms of action and better tolerability profiles with a decreased potential for adverse drug effects. Small-molecule drugs often cannot mimic the full range of pharmacological effects of protein-based therapeutics, are typically associated with off-target toxicities, and safety and efficacy remain the primary reasons for the attrition of new chemical entities during drug development. In contrast, biotechnological products have tremendous potential for treating disease and can also be incorporated into targeted delivery systems to improve the therapeutic index of potent small-molecule drugs.

The molecular properties and physiological processes that govern the pharmacokinetics of biological drugs are unique from those of small-molecule drugs, and incomplete understanding of the determinants of drug absorption and disposition is a major challenge to the development and utilization of these innovative agents. There is substantial variability in the pharmacokinetic properties of biological drugs. Monoclonal antibody and antibody-based drugs tend to exhibit long circulating half-lives as compared to cytokines, peptides, and relatively small proteins owing to an endogenous recycling pathway. Another important factor is target-mediated drug disposition (TMDD), in which interactions of protein-based therapeutics with cell-surface receptors influence the pharmacokinetic characteristics of the drug. Numerous drug-specific physicochemical properties also influence the disposition of biologics, including molecular size, charge heterogeneity, hydrophobicity, and other engineered modifications. In contrast to small-molecule drugs, immunogenic reactions to protein therapeutics can also alter their pharmacokinetics and/or pharmacodynamics. This chapter will introduce a diverse array of biotechnology products and targeted delivery systems, highlight the advantages and challenges associated with biological drugs, and review their salient pharmacokinetic properties.

## BIOTECHNOLOGY

### Protein Drugs

The discovery of recombinant DNA technology in the 1970s revolutionized the development of biopharmaceuticals by enabling the production of human proteins from host bacterial or mammalian cells, such as *Escherichia coli* and Chinese hamster ovary (CHO) cells. In 1982, recombinant insulin became the first approved recombinant protein drug by the FDA for the treatment of diabetes mellitus. Protein therapeutics no longer need to be extracted and purified from animal sources, and recombinant proteins from human genes improve specific activity and can reduce the likelihood of mounting an immunogenic response to foreign proteins. Today, the biopharmaceutical industry can mass-produce large quantities of naturally occurring and engineered proteins to treat diseases across the therapeutic areas. Protein drugs can be classified into three groups based on their pharmacological action (Leader et al, 2008), including proteins that: (1) replace deficient or abnormal protein concentrations, (2) augment activity through an existing pathway, and (3) provide a novel function or activity. Selected examples of FDA-approved recombinant protein drugs from these three categories are listed in Table 10-1.

Protein drugs within the first group in Table 10-1 are prescribed to supplement or replace missing endogenous proteins. Classical examples include insulin for patients with diabetes mellitus, Factor VIII for hemophiliacs, and β-glucocerebrosidase for treating Gaucher disease. Such disorders are characterized by a deficiency in critical proteins that would be normally present, and patients suffer from the pathophysiological sequelae that result from an absence of the biological functions associated with the missing or abnormal concentrations of proteins. A major challenge for this group is that most endogenous proteins may exhibit irregular temporal profiles owing to circadian rhythms, their transient release in response to perturbations (such as insulin release in response to elevated glucose intake from meals), or other complexities associated with disease processes, comorbidities, and/or environmental factors. Thus, attempting to mimic typical endogenous profiles is often impractical, especially with the relatively short half-lives of most systemically circulating proteins. Engineered modifications to proteins, such as point mutations and polymeric conjugation, or innovative delivery systems, including nanoparticulate formulations and antibody conjugation, can improve the pharmacokinetic properties of proteins, and specific examples are covered in subsequent sections of this chapter.

The next group of therapeutic proteins (Table 10-1) seek to leverage and enhance the biological activities of these molecules by increased exposure. The interferons (IFNs) are a good example and represent a family of endogenous proteins that exhibit antiviral, antiproliferative, and immunomodulatory effects. These type II cytokines are classified as IFN-α (leukocyte IFN), IFN-β (fibroblast IFN), or IFN-γ. IFN-α and IFN-β are referred to as type I interferons, and share a common receptor, whereas IFN-γ is classified as a type II interferon. The biological effects of IFNs include antiviral activity, changes in cell distribution, activation of cytotoxic activities of lymphocytes, macrophages, and natural killer (NK) cells, regulation of cytokine and cytokine receptor gene expression, induction of class I major histocompatibility complex (MHC) molecules, stimulation of Fc receptor expression, *in vivo* induction of NK-cell and memory T-cell proliferation, and an increase in expression of some tumor-associated antigens (Pestka et al, 1987). Although specific pathways have been described to explain the activity

# TABLE 10-1 • Sample of Approved Recombinant Drugs

| Therapeutic | Trade Name | Function | Examples of Clinical Use |
|---|---|---|---|
| **Group 1: Proteins replacing deficient or abnormal protein concentrations** | | | |
| Insulin | Humulin, Novolin | Regulates blood glucose, shifts potassium into cells | Diabetes mellitus, diabetic ketoacidosis, hyperkalemia |
| Insulin zinc extended | Lente, Ultralente | Insulin zinc hexameric complex with slower onset of action and longer duration of action | Diabetes mellitus |
| Growth hormone (GH), somatotropin | Genotropin, Humatrope, Norditropin, NorlVitropin, Nutropin, Omnitrope, Protropin, Siazen, Serostim, Valtropin | Anabolic and anticatabolic effector | Growth failure due to GH deficiency or chronic renal insufficiency, Prader-Willi syndrome, Turner syndrome, AIDs wasting or cachexia with antiviral therapy |
| Factor VIII | Bioclate, Helixate, Kogenate, Recombinate, ReFacto | Coagulation factor | Hemophilia A |
| Factor IX | Benefix | Coagulation factor | Hemophilia B |
| β-Gluco-cerebrosidase | Cerezyme | Hydrolyzes glucocerebroside to glucose and ceramide | Gaucher disease |
| Alglucosidase-α | Myozyme | Degrades glycogen by catalyzing the hydrolysis of α-1,4 and α-1,6 glycosidic linkages of lysosomal glycogen | Pompe disease (glycogen storage disease type II) |
| Agalsidase-β (human α-galactosidase A) | Fabrazyme | Enzyme that hydrolyzes globotriaosylceramide (GL3) and other glycosphingolipids, reducing deposition of these lipids in capillary endothelium of the kidney and certain other cell types | Fabry disease; prevents accumulation of lipids that could lead to renal and cardiovascular complications |
| ‡α-1-Proteinase inhibitor | Aralast, Prolastin | Inhibits elastase-mediated destruction of pulmonary tissue; purified from pooled human plasma | Congenital α-1-antitrypsin deficiency |
| ‡Adenosine deaminase (pegademase bovine, PEG-ADA) | Adagen | Metabolizes adenosine, prevents accumulation of adenosine; purified from cows | Severe combined immunodeficiency disease due to adenosine deaminase deficiency |
| **Group 2: Proteins augmenting on existing pathways** | | | |
| Erythropoietin, Epoetin-α | Epogen, Procrit | Stimulates erythropoiesis | Anemia of chronic disease, myelodysplasia, anemia due to renal failure or chemotherapy, preoperative preparation |
| Darbepoetin-α | Aranesp | Modified erythropoietin with longer half-life; stimulates red blood cell production in the bone marrow | Treatment of anemia in patients with chronic renal insufficiency and chronic renal failure (+/− dialysis) |
| Filgrastim (granulocyte colony stimulating factor; G-CSF) | Neupogen | Stimulates neutrophil proliferation, differentiation, and migration | Neutropenia in AIDs or post-chemotherapy or bone marrow transplantation, severe chronic neutropenia |
| Pegfilgrastim (Peg-G-CSF) | Neulasta | Stimulates neutrophil proliferation, differentiation, and migration | Neutropenia in AIDs or post-chemotherapy or bone marrow transplantation, severe chronic neutropenia |
| Interferon-α2a (IFNα2a) | Roferon-A | Mechanism unknown; immunoregulator | Hairy cell leukemia, chronic myelogenous leukemia, Kaposi sarcoma, chronic hepatitis C infection |

*(Continued)*

## TABLE 10-1 • Sample of Approved Recombinant Drugs (*Continued*)

| Therapeutic | Trade Name | Function | Examples of Clinical Use |
|---|---|---|---|
| Peginterferon-α2a | Pegasys | Recombinant interferon-α2a conjugated to polyethylene glycol (PEG) to increase half-life | Adults with chronic hepatitis C who have compensated liver disease and who have not been previously treated with IFNα; used alone or in combination with ribavirin |
| Interferon-β1a (rIFN-β) | Avonex, Rebif | Mechanism unknown; antiviral and immunoregulator | Multiple sclerosis |
| Alteplase (tissue plasminogen activator; tPA) | Activase | Promotes fibrinolysis by binding fibrin and converting plasminogen to plasmin | Pulmonary embolism, myocardial infarction, acute ischemic stroke, occlusion of central venous access devices |
| Teriparatide (human parathyroid hormone residues) | Forteo | Markedly enhances bone formation; administered as a once-daily injection | Severe osteoporosis |
| Exenatide | Byetta | Incretin mimetic with actions similar to glucagon-like peptide 1 (GLP1); increases glucose-dependent insulin secretion, suppresses glucagon secretion, slows gastric emptying, decreases appetite (first identified in saliva of the Gila monster *Heloderma suspectum*) | Type 2 diabetes resistant to treatment with metformin and a sulphonylurea |
| **Group 3: Proteins providing a novel function or activity** | | | |
| Human deoxyribonuclease I, dornase-α | Pulmozyme | Degrades DNA in purulent pulmonary secretions | Cystic fibrosis; decreases respiratory tract infections in selected patients with FVC greater than 40% of predicted |
| Hyaluronidase (recombinant human) | Hylenex | Catalyzes the hydrolysis of hyaluronic acid to increase tissue permeability and allow faster drug absorption | Used as an adjuvant to increase the absorption and dispersion of injected drugs, particularly anesthetics in ophthalmic surgery and certain imaging agents |
| ‡L-Asparaginase | ELSPAR | Provides exogenous asparaginase activity, removing available asparagine from serum; purified from *Escherichia coli* | Acute lymphocytic leukemia, which requires exogenous asparagine for proliferation |
| ‡Peg-asparaginase | Oncaspar | Provides exogenous asparaginase activity, removing available asparagine from serum; purified from *E. coli* | Acute lymphocytic leukemia, which requires exogenous asparagine for proliferation |
| ‡Streptokinase | Streptase | Converts plasminogen to plasmin; produced by group C β-hemolytic streptococci | Acute evolving transmural myocardial infarction, pulmonary embolism, deep vein thrombosis, arterial thrombosis or embolism, occlusion of arteriovenous cannula |
| ‡Anistreplase[241,242] (anisoylated plasminogen streptokinase activator complex; APSAC) | Eminase | Converts plasminogen to plasmin; *p*-anisoyl group protects the catalytic center of the plasminogen–streptokinase complex and prevents premature deactivation, thereby providing longer duration of action than streptokinase | Thrombolysis in patients with unstable angina |

‡Non-recombinant

Data from Leader B, Baca QJ, Golan DE: Protein therapeutics: a summary and pharmacological classification, Nat Rev Drug Discov 2008 Jan;7(1):21–39.

of IFNs (van Boxel-Dezaire et al, 2006), the mechanisms by which they exert all of their biological effects are still being elucidated. Based on their pharmacological properties, IFNs have been approved for the treatment of certain viral infections, malignancies, and multiple sclerosis. Another example in this group is erythropoietin (EPO), which is an endogenous cytokine primarily released by the kidney in response to hypoxia to stimulate the survival, proliferation, and differentiation of erythroid progenitor cells in the bone marrow resulting in an increase in circulating reticulocytes and red blood cells (Elliott et al, 2008). Recombinant human EPO is indicated for the treatment of anemia resulting from chronic kidney disease, AIDS, and chemotherapy-induced anemia. Both IFN-β 1a and recombinant human EPO have shown nonlinear pharmacokinetic behavior in humans (Veng-Pedersen et al, 1995; Buchwalder et al, 2000) in which net drug exposure is not directly proportional to dose (see Chapter 18), and this has been attributed to high-affinity, capacity-limited interactions with their respective receptors or TMDD (Chapel et al, 2001; Mager and Jusko, 2002; Woo et al, 2007; Abraham et al, 2010). Engineered modifications have also been used to alter the pharmacokinetic and/or pharmacodynamic properties of these protein drugs, and both TMDD and protein structural changes will be described later in this chapter.

The last group of compounds (Table 10-1) include endogenous and foreign proteins that introduce novel therapeutic uses. As an example, hyaluronidases represent a family of enzymes that degrade hyaluronic acid, a glycosaminoglycan that supports the extracellular matrix of connective and epithelial tissues. The extracellular matrix in the subcutaneous (SC) space limits the amount of fluid that can be injected at sites of administration and can represent a major barrier to the effective delivery of subcutaneously administered biotherapeutics (Richter and Jacobsen, 2014). Recombinant human hyaluronidase was developed to be co-administered with subcutaneously injected protein therapeutics to degrade hyaluronic acid at the injection site, which transiently reduces the resistance to fluid flow, allows for greater injection volumes with limited discomfort, and enhances drug absorption (Frost, 2007). This excipient was added to a formulation of rituximab,

a monoclonal antibody used to treat hematological malignancies and arthritis (introduced in the next section), and enabled the conversion of rituximab from an hours long intravenous (IV) infusion (anywhere from 1.5 to 6 hrs) to a 5- to 7-min SC injection, thereby improving patient access to the drug, decreasing clinical resource requirements for treatment, and potentially improving patient compliance and convenience (Davies et al, 2017).

In contrast to small-molecule drugs, therapeutic proteins are complex macromolecules, with a range of molecular weights from relatively small peptides (1–10 kDa) to larger peptidic molecules (10–50 kDa) that are characterized by their hierarchical structural features: primary (amino acid sequence and connectivity), secondary (short-term ordered structures such as alpha helices and beta sheets), tertiary (3-dimensional structural confirmation/folding), and quaternary (spatial arrangement of subunits) structures. Accurate and reproducible manufacturing, drug storage, and the route of administration of proteins are major challenges owing to the numerous pathways by which these compounds are susceptible to chemical and physical instability. Changes in manufacturing can result in subtle to large changes in hierarchical structures of proteins, which could alter their stability, immunogenic potential, and pharmacokinetic and/or pharmacodynamic properties. Cold storage conditions are required to achieve a desirable shelf-life for protein drugs and to improve their stability. Whereas most small-molecule drugs are taken orally, the enzymatic degradation of proteins limits their administration to parenteral routes (mainly IV, SC, and intramuscular [IM]). These challenges contribute to the limited global reach of biologics, and innovative formulation and drug delivery systems (described later in this chapter) are needed to reduce the costs associated with manufacturing protein drugs and to realize the potential of these molecules for improving global health.

### Monoclonal Antibodies

Monoclonal antibodies (mAbs) are another class of protein therapeutics, which are inspired by immunoglobin (Ig) molecules in the immune system that can recognize and neutralize specific targets in the body. The discovery of these molecules dates back to 1890, when Emil von Behring received the first Nobel Prize in physiology/medicine for demonstrating that one can acquire immunity against diphtheria by injecting the blood serum from an infected individual. However, until the late 1970s, when Georges Kohler and Cesar Milstein discovered how to make mAbs from hybridomas, these molecules were not widely used for therapeutic purposes. Since then, protein engineering methods have evolved tremendously, and it has become much easier to produce these molecules in research and manufacturing laboratories.

mAbs are "Y"-shaped proteoglycans with ~150 kDa molecular weight (Fig. 10-1). They have two antigen-binding domains (Fab) that provide specific binding capabilities to the molecule, and one Fc domain that can interact with Fc receptors in the body. Whereas most of the early therapeutic mAbs were of murine origin, mAbs gradually became more humanized primarily owing to issues related to immunogenicity. As such, mAbs can originate from animal or human genes, and depending on the species of origin, the nomenclature of these molecules varies. Completely murine mAbs end with the suffix –momab, chimeric mAbs with murine variable regions and human constant regions end with –ximab, humanized mAbs with murine complementarity-determining regions (CDRs) end with –zumab, and completely human mAbs end with –mumab. Completely human mAbs are typically produced using display libraries (eg, phage-display) or transgenic mice bearing a human immune system.

Since mAbs can recognize a specific targeted moiety, they have been tremendously useful for *in vitro* and *in vivo* diagnostic applications. Because of their selectivity and high affinity, these molecules can detect very small amounts of target antigens in diverse biological matrices. A popular example for *in vitro* diagnostic application of mAbs is pregnancy tests. These lateral-flow immunoassay strips contain mAbs directed against human chorionic gonadotropin (hCG) and can detect low levels of this pregnancy hormone in urine or serum samples as early as a few weeks after onset of pregnancy (Hamad et al, 2018). In addition, mAbs are also widely used in companion diagnostics, which are *in vitro* tests that guide safe and effective use of drug products (Scheerens et al, 2017). An example *in vivo* diagnostic application of mAbs is Oncoscint Cr/Ov (Satumomab pendetide), which is the first FDA-approved antibody for tumor imaging. This mAb is labeled with indium ([111]In) and binds to tumor-associated glycoprotein 72 (TAG-72) for detecting colorectal and ovarian cancer cells in the body (Abdel-Nabi et al, 1990).

The ability of mAbs to hone into specific targets in the body also makes them highly attractive molecules for developing targeted therapeutics. mAbs can act via binding to a specific ligand or receptor in the body to neutralize these molecules and prevent any pharmacology resulting from the natural ligand–receptor interaction. mAbs can also bind to cell surface receptors and act as an agonist or antagonist to modulate intracellular signaling. mAbs can eliminate targeted cells in the body via an antibody-dependent cell-mediated cytotoxic (ADCC) effect. During this process, mAb molecules bind on the surface of targeted cells via the Fab domain, and recruit immune-effector cells expressing Fc-gamma receptors via the Fc domain. The immune-effector cells get activated via the formation of a trimeric complex which leads to the killing of the targeted cells. mAbs can also eliminate targeted cells via a complement-dependent cytotoxic (CDC) effect, in which antibody-coated target cells recruit and activate the complement cascade, which leads to the formation of a membrane-attack complex (MAC) on the cell surface and eventual cell lysis. Since mAbs have two binding sites, they can demonstrate very high affinity for cell surface targets via the avidity effect, which helps them exhibit the above-mentioned pharmacological effects with

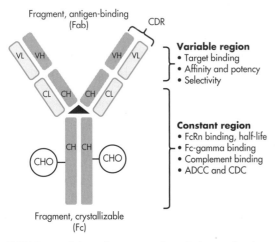

**FIGURE 10-1** • Schematic structure of a typical monoclonal antibody molecule.

great efficiency. In addition, since the interaction with FcRn receptors bestows an unusually long half-life (~21 days) to mAbs, they can provide therapeutic benefits for prolonged periods of time following a single administration.

Since the approval of first therapeutic mAb by the FDA in 1986, at least 570 therapeutic mAbs have been tested in the clinic so far, and 79 therapeutic mAbs have been approved by the FDA. mAbs are now considered the best-selling drugs on the market, and eight of the top ten bestselling drugs worldwide in 2018 were biologics. It is expected that the global therapeutic mAb market will generate revenue of ~$300 billion by 2025 (Lu et al, 2020). mAbs have been used to treat a wide array of disorders, such as asthma, arthritis, cancer, Crohn's disease, headaches/migraine, infectious diseases, macular degeneration, psoriasis, and transplant rejection. Some notable examples include (i) adalimumab, an anti-TNF alpha antibody that is used to treat arthritis and many other inflammatory disorders; (ii) omalizumab, an anti-IgE antibody that is used to treat asthma; (iii) nivolumab, an anti-PD-1 antibody that is used to activate the suppressed immune system to treat various cancers; (iv) ustekinumab, an anti-IL12 and IL23 antibody that is used to treat psoriasis and other inflammatory disease; (v) eculizumab, an anti-complement component 5 antibody that is used to treat hemoglobinuria and other complement-mediated disorders; (vi) trastuzumab, an anti-HER2 antibody that is used to treat breast and gastric cancer; (vii) bevacizumab, an anti-VEGF-A antiangiogenic antibody that is used to treat several cancers and macular degeneration; (viii) palivizumab, an antiviral protein F antibody that used for the prevention of respiratory syncytial virus (RSV) infections; and (ix) rituximab, an anti-CD20 antibody that is used to treat blood tumors, arthritis, and even multiple sclerosis (off-label use).

Apart from being pharmacologically active by themselves, mAbs can also be conjugated to various other moieties to achieve their targeted delivery within the body. This area of targeted drug delivery is discussed later in this chapter.

## Antibody Fragments and Novel Constructs

Despite the therapeutic and commercial success of mAbs, there are certain limitations to these molecules. These include (i) large size and steric hindrance

that restricts tissue penetration into solid tumors and poorly vascularized tissues, (ii) planar binding interfaces that make the binding to certain grooves and the catalytic sites difficult, (iii) physical and chemical instability, (iv) requirement for large doses, (v) potential immunogenicity, (vi) cost of goods, and (vii) intellectual property issues (Wurch et al, 2012; Shah, 2015; Skrlec et al, 2015). To overcome these issues, protein engineering is employed to develop the next generation of protein therapeutics, which are either derived from mAbs or generated using novel scaffolds.

The modular nature of mAbs provides a unique opportunity to remove or alter components of mAbs to alter their functionality. Antibody fragments are one such class of protein therapeutics, which are either generated via enzymatic digestion of mAbs (ie, Fab and $F(ab)_2$) or genetic fusion of mAb variable domains (ie, scFv). These molecules lack the Fc domain and hence exhibit very short half-lives and lack ADCC and CDC effects. In addition, since scFv (25 kDa) and Fab (50 kDa) can easily succumb to glomerular filtration, they have even shorter half-lives (ie, a few hours). Because of the smaller size of mAb fragments, they also demonstrate larger volumes of distribution and can permeate deeper into tissues and cross blood vessels more efficiently. These properties make antibody fragments excellent candidates for toxin neutralization and imaging purposes. For example, DigiFab™ is an FDA-approved anti-digoxin Fab fragment that is used for life-threatening toxicity or overdose of digoxin. CroFab° and Alacramyn° are polyvalent Fab fragments that are used as antivenom to treat snake and scorpion poisons. Anascorp° is a $F(ab)_2$ fragment that is used to treat scorpion poison. For imaging applications, Verluma° and CEA-Scan® are Technetium ($^{99}$mTc)-labeled Fab fragments, and Licartin° is $^{131}$I-labeled $F(ab)_2$ fragment, which are used for diagnosing various cancers. Fab fragments have also been used for the treatment of various disorders. For example, abciximab is an anti-GP IIb/IIIa Fab fragment that is used to inhibit platelet aggregation. Ranibizumab is an anti-VEGF-A Fab fragment that is used as an anti-angiogenic agent to treat macular degeneration. Certolizumab pegol is an anti-TNF alpha Fab fragment that is used to treat Crohn's disease, rheumatoid arthritis, psoriatic arthritis, and ankylosing spondylitis.

mAbs can also be engineered to enhance or abrogate their pharmacological function and pharmacokinetic properties. The Fc domain can be altered to enhance mAb binding to the FcγIIIa receptor for enhancing the effector function (eg, 3M mutation - S239D/A330L/I332E). The Fc domain can also be altered to reduce the affinity of mAb for Fcγ receptors and C1q for abrogating the effector function (eg, TM mutation - L234F/L235E/P331S). The half-life of mAbs can be increased by altering the Fc domain to increase the binding to the FcRn receptor (eg, YTE mutation - M252Y/S254T/T256E). Glycosylation site/pattern of mAbs can also be altered to change their pharmacology. For example, mogamulizumab is an afucosylated mAb targeting CCR4, which demonstrates a superior ADCC effect as compared to a fucosylated mAb and efficiently treats T-cell leukemia/lymphoma (Ishii et al, 2010).

The structure of antibodies has also been further modified to develop bi/multi-specific protein therapeutics, which are designed to bind to two or more antigens/epitopes simultaneously to achieve improved binding, tissue selectivity, and efficacy (Labrijn et al, 2019). Some of these molecules are simple IgG-like molecules with each arm binding to a different antigen. Catumaxomab is one such molecule whose one arm binds to EpCAM and the other arm binds to the T-cell receptor CD3. There are also symmetric IgG-like molecules in which each arm can bind to more than one antigen. Many bi/multi-specific proteins are also designed by fusion of multiple variable of Fc domains of mAbs (eg, Bis-Fab, Fab-Fv, BiTE, and DART). Blinatumomab is a clinically approved drug and an example of one such protein that is created by fusion of two different ScFv domains that bind to CD19 and CD3. This molecule brings CD19 expressing cancerous B-cells and CD3 expressing T-cells together to trigger the killing of cancer cells (Nagorsen et al, 2009).

Another innovative and fastest growing class of protein therapeutics is novel scaffolds that do not bear any resemblance to mAbs (Wurch et al, 2012). These proteins are highly engineered to obtain more attractive physical and chemical properties, and can possess greater affinity per unit mass of the molecule (Caravella and Lugovskoy, 2010). They are typically single polypeptidic chains with less than 200 amino acids and contain a highly structured core with variable portions that have high conformational tolerance.

This allows for insertions, deletions, or other substitutions without affecting the stability of the protein. There are more than 50 such scaffolds discovered so far, such as AdNectin, Anticalin, Avimer, and DARPin. Ecallantide is an example of an FDA-approved novel scaffold, which is developed by modifying the Kunitz domain. It is a 60 amino-acid protein discovered through phage display, which inhibits the kallikrein protein and provides the treatment for hereditary angioedema (Schneider et al, 2007).

Natural ligands and receptors have also been engineered to develop novel therapeutics with improved safety and efficacy (Kariolis et al, 2013). They provide an efficient way to overcome ligand multiplicity of a receptor, where a receptor has multiple ligands that complicate the design of an effective protein therapeutic. For example, the ErbB family consists of four receptors with eleven distinct ligands that bind to and activate these receptors. This diversity and ligand multiplicity present an important challenge for drug development, which has been overcome by developing a "ligand trap" approach such as TRAP-Fc (Lindzen et al, 2012). This molecule comprises of ligand-binding domains of EGFR and ErbB-4 fused to the Fc domain of IgG, and can antagonize all ligand family members targeting ErbB receptors. Similarly, a "receptor decoy" strategy has been developed to block multiple ligand–receptor interactions, which drive separate pathways leading to synergistic effects within a single biological signal. Eylea˙ and Zaltrap˙ are different formulations of aflibercept, an example of such clinically approved molecules, which are designed to neutralize multiple ligands that drive the angiogenic pathway independently (Al-Halafi, 2014).

## Gene Therapy

Gene therapy refers to the effective delivery of recombinant genetic material to cells for the ameliorative or curative treatment of inherited or acquired diseases. The primary goal is to restore or enhance the expression and function of a target gene (ie, transgene) in a safe and effective manner. Early applications of gene therapy failed owing to a lack of therapeutic effect and/or unanticipated toxicities; however, following decades of basic and translational research into addressing these major challenges, several gene therapies have been approved by regulatory agencies (Table 10-2), with hundreds more in clinical

## TABLE 10-2 • Regulatory Milestones in Gene Therapy*

| Year | Milestone | Regulatory Authority | Indication | Vector† | Route of Administration |
|------|-----------|----------------------|------------|---------|--------------------------|
| 2003 | Approval of recombinant human p53 adenovirus for injection (Gendicine, Sibiono GeneTech) | NMPA | Head and neck squamous-cell carcinoma | Ad–p53 | Intratumoral injection; intracavity or intravascular injection |
| 2012 | Approval of alipogene tiparvovec (Glybera, uniQure) | EMA‡ | Lipoprotein lipase deficiency | AAV1–LPL | Intramuscular injection |
| 2015 | Approval of talimogene laherparepvec (Imlygic, Amgen) | EMA and FDA | Melanoma | HSV–GM-CSF | Intratumoral injection |
| 2016 | Approval of autologous CD34+ cells encoding adenosine deaminase cDNA sequence (Strimvelis, Orchard Therapeutics) | EMA | Adenosine deaminase-deficient SCID | RV–ADA | Transplantation of autologous gene-modified CD34+ cells |
| 2017 | Approval of tisagenlecleucel (Kymriah, Novartis) | FDA | Patients younger than 25 y of age with relapsed or refractory ALL | LV–CD19 | Intravenous infusion of autologous gene-modified T cells |
|  | Approval of axicabtagene ciloleucel (Yescarta, Kite Pharma) | FDA | Certain types of non-Hodgkin lymphoma | RV–CD19 | Intravenous infusion of autologous gene-modified T cells |
|  | Approval of voretigene neparvovec-rzyl (Luxturna, Spark Therapeutics) | FDA | Biallelic *RPE65*-associated retinal dystrophy | AAV2–RPE65 | Subretinal injection |
| 2018 | Approval of tisagenlecleucel (Kymriah) | EMA | Patients younger than 25 y of age with relapsed or refractory ALL | LV–CD19 | Intravenous infusion of autologous gene-modified T cells |
|  | Approval of axicabtagene ciloleucel (Yescarta) | EMA | Certain types of non-Hodgkin lymphoma | RV–CD19 | Intravenous infusion of autologous gene-modified T cells |
|  | Review of gene-therapy IND applications in United States streamlined to single reviewing agency, the FDA | FDA and NIH | — | — | — |
|  | Approval of voretigene neparvovec (Luxturna) | EMA | Biallelic RPE65-associated retinal dystrophy | AAV2–RPE65 | Subretinal injection |
| 2019 | Conditional approval of autologous CD34+ cells encoding $\beta^{A-T87Q}$-globin gene (Zynteglo, Bluebird Bio) | EMA | Patients older than 12 y of age with transfusion-dependent β-thalassemia without $\beta^0/\beta^0$ genotype | LV–β-globin | Transplantation of autologous gene-modified CD34+ cells |
|  | Approval of onasemnogene abeparvovec-xioi (Zolgensma, AveXis) | FDA | Patients younger than 2 y of age with spinal muscular atrophy | AAV9–SMN1 | Intravenous infusion |

ALL, acute lymphoblastic leukemia; cDNA, complementary DNA; EMA, European Medicines Agency; FDA, U.S. Food and Drug Administration; IND, investigational new drug; NIH, National Institutes of Health; NMPA, National Medicine Products Administration (China).
†Vector designations indicate the type of vector (adeno-associated viral [AAV], adenoviral (Ad), herpes simplex viral [HSV], lentiviral [LV], or retroviral [RV]) and the gene transduced.
‡Regulatory approval was allowed to lapse by the sponsor in 2017.
Reproduced with permission from High KA, Roncarolo MG. Gene Therapy, N Engl J Med. 2019 Aug 1;381(5):455–464.

development (Dunbar et al, 2018; Anguela and High, 2019; High and Roncarolo, 2019).

Gene therapy can be broadly categorized into *integrating* and *non-integrating* delivery vectors (vehicles for transferring genes into cells). Integrating vectors introduce a target gene that gets incorporated into the DNA of precursor or stem cells, such that the functional target gene is passed on following cellular division. Gene transduction in stem cells is generally performed under *ex vivo* conditions in a manner similar to hematopoietic stem cell transplantation (HSCT), in which specific patient cells are isolated from harvested peripheral blood or bone marrow, a transgene is integrated into the DNA of patient HSCs using a viral (retroviral or lentiviral) or non-viral vector, and the cells modified to express the transgene are re-infused to the patient after a myeloablative conditioning regimen. In contrast, non-integrating vectors deliver the target gene outside of chromosomes (ie, episomal DNA) in mature, terminally differentiated cells no longer undergoing mitosis. In order to target these cells in specific tissue(s), the non-integrating vector is administered *in vivo* directly, and the transgene must be stable in episomes to ensure the adequate expression of the encoded therapeutic peptide or protein.

Genetically modified cell–based therapies have resulted in breakthrough treatments for inherited immunodeficiency and hematological disorders as well as acquired hematological malignancies. In 2016, the European Medicines Agency (EMA) approved the first *ex vivo* HSC gene therapy, Strimvelis®, autologous CD34+ cells encoding adenosine deaminase cDNA sequence, for the treatment of severe combined immunodeficiency due to adenosine deaminase deficiency (ADA-SCID), which is a rare disease resulting from an inherited mutation in the ADA gene. Patients with ADA deficiency exhibit severe lymphocytopenia, and the absence of sufficient B and T cell lymphocytes and NK cells increases the risk for fatal infections, certain cancers, and organ damage. First-line therapy for ADA-SCID is HSCT from an HLA-identical sibling; however, this is often not an available option for most patients. Gene therapy has been shown to provide a durable reconstitution of the immune system in ADA-SCID patients (Aiuti et al, 2009) and may be a more desirable and effective alternative to enzyme replacement

therapy. Engineered T cells for the treatment of hematological cancers is another example of successful *ex vivo* gene therapy, and in 2017, the FDA approved tisagenlecleucel (trade name Kymriah) and axicabtagene ciloleucel (trade name Yescarta); two chimeric antigen receptor T cell (CAR-T) therapies that enhance tumor killing by targeting T cells to the CD19 antigen expressed on malignant B cells. Both of these autologous T cell immunotherapies are indicated for patients with relapsed or refractory large B cell lymphoma after two or more lines of systemic therapy, and tisagenlecleucel is also indicated for the treatment of patients less than 25 years of age with refractory B-cell precursor acute lymphoblastic leukemia in second or later relapse. The initial response rates in select leukemias and lymphomas are greater than 50%, with long-term durable responses in about 30–40% of patients (June and Sadelain, 2018). Although there are therapeutic challenges associated with *ex vivo* gene therapy (discussed later in this section), other genetically modified HSC therapies are under clinical development to extend this treatment modality to other blood (Dhakal et al, 2020) and solid (Patterson et al, 2020) tumors, as well as allogeneic or "off-the-shelf" cell-based therapies to eliminate the need for harvesting patient-specific HSCs (Mohanty et al, 2019).

In contrast to cell-based gene therapies that utilize *ex vivo* gene transduction in HSCs, long-term expression of the transgene in postmitotic cells can be achieved with direct *in vivo* injection, often to the site of action or using organ/tissue targeting modalities. Whereas retroviral and lentiviral vectors, which can integrate up to 8 kb of DNA, are typically used for *ex vivo* gene transduction in HSCs, the adeno-associated virus (AAV), which is limited to transgenes less than 5 kb, appears to be the leading platform for *in vivo* gene delivery (Wang et al, 2019). The first approved AAV gene therapy in the United States was voretigene neparvovec-rzyl (trade name Luxterna) and is indicated for the treatment of biallelic RPE65-associated retinal dystrophy. RPE65 is critical isomerase usually expressed in retinal pigment epithelium that converts all-trans-retinyl esters to 11-cis-retinol, thereby supporting the visual cycle. This rare inherited deficiency in RPE65 results in early-onset blindness unless treated. Voretigene neparvovec-rzyl is injected directly into the subretinal space in an outpatient surgical procedure, and the AAV-transgene vector remains stable in episomes, expresses RPE65 protein, and improves functional vision in this otherwise untreatable disorder (Russell et al, 2017). Although the long-term durability of voretigene neparvovec-rzyl is still being evaluated (Jacobson et al, 2015), the initial positive response has inspired the field of gene therapy, and interdisciplinary research is ongoing to address challenges and engineer improved gene delivery platforms for a variety of genetic and acquired human diseases (Wang et al, 2019).

Despite the recent approvals of gene therapies (Table 10-2), there are many challenges associated with their design, development, and therapeutic use to ensure that sufficient extent and duration of gene expression is achieved safely. Some safety concerns are general, whereas others may be drug specific. For example, the risk of insertional mutagenesis of integrating retroviral vectors leading to off-target genotoxicity, and adverse immune responses raised against the viral vector or transgene administered *in vivo*, were early major safety concerns for gene therapy. Although these risks are still general concerns, they have been reduced (but not eliminated) with vector design modifications, such as moving from retroviral to lentiviral vectors that exhibit a safer integration profile, and immune responses can be prevented or treated with immunomodulatory drugs. For non-integrating vectors used for *ex vivo* gene transduction (eg, AAV), improved myeloablative conditioning, through dose individualization or alternative antibody-based regimens, might minimize the toxicities associated with these pre-transplant therapies and enhance the engraftment of modified HSCs. Interestingly, some patients have pre-existing anti-AAV neutralizing antibodies, which could mount an immunogenic reaction to the viral vector and render it inactive.

Some safety concerns may be drug-specific and manifest from the pharmacodynamic effects of gene-based drugs. For example, CAR-T therapy can be associated with severe adverse drug reactions, such as cytokine release syndrome (CRS), which is characterized by high concentrations of harmful circulating proinflammatory cytokines in response to activated T cell proliferation (Fitzgerald et al, 2017). In addition, more than 50% of patients receiving CAR-T cells show signs of neurological symptoms, and grade 3−4 neurotoxicity is associated with decreased overall survival (Karschnia et al, 2019). Corticosteroids are currently used to help control inflammation and CRS, but long-term use of steroids (greater than 10 days) is itself a negative prognostic factor for overall survival (Karschnia et al, 2019). Tocilizumab, an anti-interleukin-6 monoclonal antibody, is approved to treat CRS; however, the rate of severe neurotoxicity was increased when tocilizumab was given prophylactically to patients with refractory, aggressive non-Hodgkin lymphoma treated with axi-cel, an autologous anti-CD19 CAR-T therapy (Locke et al, 2017). Gene therapies are clearly complex drug products, and the positive results of approved gene therapies and those in development suggest great promise for disorders with few or no treatment options. Further research is needed to improve the design and clinical use of gene therapies to expand the list of indications, establish clinically significant and long-lasting transgene expression, and minimize treatment-related adverse effects.

## Oligonucleotide Drugs

Oligonucleotides are short, single- or double-stranded DNA or RNA sequences that have been developed primarily to block the transcription of genes or RNA translation to protein(s) (albeit new functions are being developed including modulating splice variants and gene activation) that are implicated in a variety of diseases. These nucleic acid drugs bind to their target via simple complementary base pairing and are therefore designed based on detailed knowledge of the target DNA or RNA sequence. Oligonucleotides can be classified into two main groups, namely antisense oligonucleotides (ASOs), which are single-stranded DNA molecules that bind complementary to target mRNA, and oligonucleotides that act by RNA interference (RNAi), which are comprised of single-stranded (miRNAs) or double-stranded (siRNAs) RNAi molecules. A list of FDA-approved oligonucleotides are shown in Table 10-3 (Roberts et al, 2020). ASOs can be further distinguished based on their mechanisms of target engagement and subsequent processing (Bennett et al, 2017). Fomivirsen, mipomersen, and inotersen are three ASOs that bind to their target mRNA, which then undergoes degradation catalyzed by the RNase H

**TABLE 10-3 •** FDA-Approved Oligonucleotide Therapeutics

| Name (Market Name), Company | Target (Indication) | Organ (ROA) | FDA Approval | Comments |
|---|---|---|---|---|
| Fomivirsen (Vitravene), Ionis Pharma Novartis | CMV UL123 (cytomegalovirus retinitis) | Eye (IVI) | August 1998 | First approved nucleic acid drug Local delivery Withdrawn from use owing to reduced clinical need |
| Pegaptanib (Macugen), NeXstar Pharma Eyetech Pharma | VEGF-165 (neovascular age-related macular degeneration) | Eye (IVI) | December 2004 | First approved aptamer drug Local delivery Limited commercial success due to competition |
| Mipomersen (Kynamro), Ionis Pharma Genzyme Kastle Tx | *APOB* (homozygous familial hypercholesterolemia) | Liver (SC) | January 2013 | Rejected by EMA owing to safety Limited commercial success due to competition |
| Defibrotide (Defitelio), Jazz Pharma | *NA* (hepatic veno-occlusive disease) | Liver (IV) | March 2016 | Unique sequence-independent mechanism of action |
| Eteplirsen (Exondys 51), Sarepta Tx | *DMD* exon 51 (Duchenne muscular dystrophy) | Skeletal muscle (IV) | September 2016 | Systemic delivery to non-hepatic tissue Low efficacy |
| Nusinersen (Spinraza), Ionis Pharma Biogen | *SMN2* exon 7 (spinal muscular atrophy) | Spinal cord (IT) | December 2016 | Local delivery |
| Patisiran (Onpattro), Alnylam Pharma | *TTR* (hereditary transthyretin amyloidosis, polyneuropathy) | Liver (IV) | August 2018 | First approved RNAi drug Nanoparticle delivery system Requires co-treatment with steroids and antihistamines |
| Inotersen (Tegsedi), Ionis Pharma Akcea Pharam | *TTR* (hereditary transthyretin amyloidosis, polyneuropathy) | Liver (SC) | October 2018 | Same gapmer ASO platform as mipomersen |
| Givosiran (Givlaari), Alnylam Pharma | *ALAS1* (acute hepatic porphyria) | Liver (SC) | November 2019 | Enhanced stability chemistry Hepatocyte-targeting bioconjugate |
| Golodirsen (Vyondys 53), Sarepta Tx | *DMD* exon 53 (Duchenne muscular dystrophy) | Skeletal muscle (IV) | December 2019 | Same PMO chemistry platform as eteplirsen |

ASO, antisense oligonucleotide; IT, intrathecal; IV, intravenous; IVI, intravitreal injection; NA, not applicable; PMO, phosphorodiamidate morpholino oligonucleotide; ROA, route of administration; SC, subcutaneous
Reproduced with permission from Roberts TC, Langer R, Wood MJA. Advances in oligonucleotide drug delivery, Nat Rev Drug Discov 2020 Oct;19(10):673–694.

enzyme RNASEH1 that cleaves such RNA-DNA heteroduplexes and thereby silences gene translation. Other post-binding mechanisms, including RNA splice modulation/switching, inhibiting, or enhancing translation, and blocking miRNA function, can result in modulation of gene function without inducing target degradation. Eteplirsen, golodirsen, and nusinersen are FDA-approved splice-switching ASOs. Similar to ASOs, siRNAs interact with their target through complementary binding; however, these potent RNAi agents insert into Argonaute 2 protein (AGO2) to form an RNA-induced silencing complex (RISCA) with target transcripts. High homology in target–base pairing is required and results in AGO2-cleavage and effective gene silencing. Two siRNAs have been approved by the FDA: patisiran is indicated for the treatment of polyneuropathy in patients with hereditary transthyretin-mediated amyloidosis, and givosiran targets 5-aminolevulinic acid synthase for treating patients with acute hepatic porphyria.

The most challenging issue for the translation of oligonucleotide technology to their use as clinical drugs is their successful *in vivo* delivery. Some ASOs can be delivered directly to an anatomical site that enables their effective biodistribution. For example, nusinersen is administered as a direct intrathecal (IT) injection into the cerebrospinal fluid for the treatment of spinal muscular atrophy (SMA) (Table 10-3). In a safety, tolerability, and pharmacokinetic study in 28 patients with childhood SMA, the IT injection of nusinersen resulted in prolonged exposure in the CSF, with drug concentrations still measurable at the 9- to 14-month evaluation, despite plasma concentrations decreasing below the limit of detection of the assay 8 days after dosing (Chiriboga et al, 2016). In the absence of direct injection, many oligonucleotides are targeted toward the liver owing to its highly perfused and porous sinusoidal membrane. However, macrophages in the liver are part of the reticuloendothelial system (RES), which is a primary site for the catabolism and elimination of therapeutic proteins. Therefore, chemical modification and delivery systems are needed to improve the *in vivo* delivery of oligonucleotides. One of the most common chemical modifications to stabilize ASOs involves substituting one of the non-bridging oxygen atoms in the phosphate backbone with sulfur.

Many other chemical modification techniques are utilized, and care must be taken to balance the improvement in drug stability with the potential of chemical modifications to interfere with ASO-target-binding affinity (Roberts et al, 2020). Some strategies for improving the delivery of oligonucleotides (and proteins in general) are covered in the next section of this chapter.

## DRUG CARRIERS AND TARGETING

### Formulation and Delivery of Protein Drugs

The biotechnology revolution has ushered in a remarkable era of protein-based drugs and major therapeutic breakthroughs for a staggering number of previously untreatable or poorly managed disorders. The specificity and improved adverse effect profiles are often superior to small molecule approaches. Nevertheless, the relatively large size and fragility of these complex therapeutic proteins, along with their immunogenicity risk potential, represent major challenges in their development. Strategic drug delivery systems are now commonplace for improving the design and development of new proteins as well as enhancing the properties of existing agents. Proven methods include, among others, engineered protein structure modifications (eg, covalent polymers), albumin fusion proteins, formulation systems, such as liposomal encapsulation, and antibody conjugation (Pisal et al, 2010; Roberts et al, 2020). This section provides an overview of several techniques that improve the pharmacokinetic, efficacy, and safety properties of protein therapeutics.

One strategy to modify the pharmacokinetic properties of protein drugs is via pegylation, which involves the covalent modification of proteins by polyethylene glycol (PEG) moieties (Harris et al, 2001). PEG is a hydrophilic, biocompatible polymer, and pegylation can increase the half-life of proteins, reduce renal elimination, alter distribution, and reduce the likelihood of developing an immune reaction toward the protein drug (Harris and Chess, 2003; Ekladious et al, 2019). The process of pegylation involves its chemical activation and the covalent attachment of PEG, moieties at site-specific protein residues. The increase in the molecular size of the protein provides a hydrophilic shield that protects against proteolysis, renal filtration, and some non-specific interactions that might elicit an immunogenic response. One limiting factor is that this protective shield can also reduce drug-target binding affinity and decrease the potency of the drug. Care must be taken to ensure that any reduction in target binding is sufficiently offset by significant improvements in circulating half-life, enhanced safety, and potentially reduced immunogenicity. Pegylation of interferon-α–2b (PEGINTRON') increases its molecular weight from 19 to 31 kDa and increases its half-life from 3 to 8 hours to 65 hours. The antiviral activity of pegylated interferon-α–2b is also 12- to 136-fold greater than its unpegylated form, and the net result is a substantial decrease in the frequency of administration, which can improve patient adherence and clinical outcomes. There are approximately 15 polymer–drug conjugates currently approved in the United States, with many more in clinical development (Ekladious et al, 2019). This technique has also been extended to liposomal technology (described in this section) to enhance the half-life and biodistribution pattern of these nanoparticulate delivery systems.

Human serum albumin is a large protein (67 kDa) that has a circulating half-life of approximately 3 weeks. Similar to antibodies, albumin also binds to FcRn, which is responsible for the extended half-life of albumin. Based on its favorable half-life, many small-molecule drugs have been conjugated to albumin to improve their pharmacokinetic properties. For example, albumin-bound paclitaxel (Abraxane') is a microparticulate suspension that has a greater maximum tolerated dose than the traditional cremophor-based formulation and is also associated with a greater clinical response rate (Gradishar et al, 2005). This approach has been extended to therapeutic proteins as well (Strohl, 2015), and the first approved albumin fusion protein product was albiglutide (Tanzeum'), which is a GLP-1 receptor agonist conjugated to human albumin. The drug was approved by the FDA in 2014 and is indicated in the treatment of adults with type 2 diabetes mellitus. The GLP-1 incretin hormone has a very short half-life, on the order of 1 to 2 min, and the conjugation to albumin results in a circulating half-life of about 5 days, which supports its once-weekly dosing regimen. In 2016, the FDA approved a recombinant Factor IX albumin fusion protein (Idelvion') for the treatment of hemophilia B. A long-term safety and efficacy study suggested extended dosing intervals of 14 or 21 days demonstrated comparable efficacy to once weekly regimens providing added dosing flexibility for reducing treatment burden and individualizing dosing regimens (Mancuso et al, 2020). Albumin fusion proteins constitute a promising class of protein therapeutics with improved stability and pharmacokinetic characteristics.

Liposomes are microscopic lipid vesicles with an aqueous internal space enclosed by one or more synthetic phospholipid bilayer membranes. There has been a sustained effort to develop liposomal delivery systems, particularly for small-molecule cytotoxic anticancer agents, to improve their biodistribution by enhancing their deposition in tumors, prolonging circulating half-life, and reducing drug exposure to healthy tissue sites associated with adverse drug effects (Ait-Oudhia et al, 2014). A schematic of the most common types of liposomal carriers is shown in Fig. 10-2. Chemotherapy drugs can be incorporated in either the aqueous core or within the membrane of the liposome, depending on their hydrophobicity or effective partition coefficient. The structure of the liposome can be modified to alter drug release and the pharmacokinetic properties of the liposome. For unmodified conventional liposomes, its charge reflects the molar ratio of neutral or negatively charged phospholipids. The external

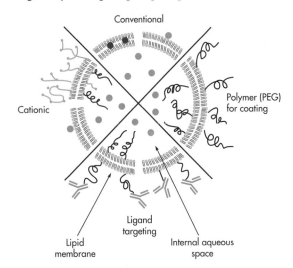

FIGURE 10-2 • Schematic representation of four types of drug-loaded liposomes. (Adapted with permission from Storm G, Crommelin DJA: Liposomes: Quo vadis? *Pharm Sci Technol Today* 1998 April 1;1(1):19–31.)

surface of the lipid bilayer can be modified to include (i) polymers, such as PEG, to prolong the plasma circulation half-life; (ii) antibodies or antibody fragments to target antigens or receptors specifically expressed on tumors and thereby improve selectivity; or (iii) positive charge (cationic liposomes). The overall size of the liposome can also be engineered for a specific range to exploit the extended permeability and retention of nanoparticulates in tumor interstitial spaces. Renal filtration is usually negligible for typical sized liposomes (>30 nm), and the main mechanism for the clearance of liposomes is through certain cells within the tissues of the RES, such as macrophages in the liver and spleen. Pegylated liposomal doxorubicin (Doxil') is an example of an approved liposome formulation, indicated for AIDS-related Kaposi sarcoma, metastatic ovarian and breast cancer, and multiple myeloma, which shows reduced cardiotoxicity as compared to the non-liposomal form. CPX-351 (Vyxeos') is a liposomal co-formulation of two anticancer drugs, cytarabine and daunorubicin, which was approved in 2017 for the treatment of adults with newly-diagnosed therapy-related acute myeloid leukemia (t-AML) or AML with myelodysplasia-related changes (AML-MRC). The liposomal formulation showed an improvement in overall survival, with a median overall survival of 9.6 months compared to the 5.9 months observed with the control arm featuring the standard regimen of the non-liposomal drugs (Krauss et al, 2019). Safety was comparable between the arms; however, neutropenia and thrombocytopenia were extended with the liposomal formulation. The engineering of liposomal drug properties has come a long way, and there are now many liposomal anticancer drugs in clinical development. Although no liposomal formulations of protein drugs have been approved, there is considerable interest in developing lipidic nanoparticle formulations of proteins to stabilize and enhance their circulating half-lives and reduce the potential for immunogenic reactions (Pisal et al, 2010).

## Antibody–Drug Conjugates

Antibody–drug conjugates (ADCs) provide an efficient way to accomplish targeted delivery of drug molecules inside the desired cells. While these molecules have been under investigation for decades, their clinical potential has been realized only recently.

Advances in protein engineering and linker-chemistry have allowed rapid optimization and efficient production of these molecules. ADCs are made by chemically conjugating mAbs with one or more very potent small molecules (ie, payloads) using specifically designed linkers. The average number of drug molecules attached to an antibody is known as the drug:antibody ratio (DAR). Depending on the nature of the linker, the ADC can deliver the drug molecules at different intracellular locations (ie, endosome, lysosome, etc.). Initially, the drug molecules were randomly conjugated to lysine or cysteine amino acids of mAbs to produce a heterogeneous formulation with different DAR, but lately, specifically engineered mAbs are being used to enable site-specific conjugation of drug molecules to yield a more homogenous product.

So far, the clinical development of ADCs has been focused on cancer. The ability of mAbs to specifically bind to cancer antigens provides a unique opportunity to deliver cytotoxic drug molecules only inside the cancer cells while sparing the normal cells, resulting in a better therapeutic index for anticancer drug molecules. The eight FDA-approved ADCs are (i) Gemtuzumab ozogamicin, for treating relapsed AML; (ii) Brentuximab vedotin, for treating relapsed HL and relapsed sALCL; (iii) Trastuzumab emtansine, for treating HER2-positive metastatic breast cancer; (iv) Inotuzumab ozogamicin, for treating CD22-positive B-cell lymphoblastic leukemia; (v) Polatuzumab vedotin-piiq, for treating relapsed or refractory diffuse large B-cell lymphoma; (vi) Enfortumab vedotin, for treating urothelial cancer; (vii) Trastuzumab deruxtecan, for treating HER2-positive breast cancer; and (viii) Sacituzumab govitecan, for treating metastatic triple-negative breast cancer. In addition, there are currently more than 200 ADCs at different stages of clinical and preclinical drug development.

The application of ADCs to treat the diseases beyond oncology is also emerging (Yu et al, 2018). These applications have been mainly confined to the field of immunology and infectious disease. Some notable examples include conjugation of anti-CD163 or anti-CD11a antibodies with dexamethasone, LXR agonist, or PDE4 inhibitor, to deliver immunosuppressive drug molecules to macrophages. Anti-CD70 antibody has been conjugated with budesonide to target the immunosuppressive therapy to immune cells. Anti-CXCR4 antibody has been conjugated to dasatinib to deliver the immunosuppressive tyrosine kinase inhibitor to T-cells. Scientists from Genentech have reported an interesting application of ADC to develop antibody-antibiotic conjugates (AAC) (Lehar et al, 2015). This ADC comprises of anti-*Staphylococcus aureus* antibody conjugated to a highly efficacious antibiotic, which is activated upon its release in the proteolytic environment of the phagolysosome. As such, this ADC is uniquely capable of effectively killing the intracellular *S. aureus* reservoirs, which comprise of virulent bacteria that can establish the infection even in the presence of vancomycin.

mAbs have also been conjugated with radiolabeled molecules to develop radioimmunoconjugates (RICs), which can specifically deliver radioisotopes at the site of action. Two clinically approved RICs include [131]I-tositumomab and 90Y-ibritumomab tiuxetan. Both of these RICs target CD20 antigen and provide treatment for non-Hodgkin lymphoma. In addition, more than a dozen RICs have been evaluated in the clinic (Dash et al, 2013). With the advent of new beta emitters with better physical properties (eg, lutetium 177), new alpha emitters that can eradicate microscopic clusters of tumor cells (eg, bismuth 213 and astatine 211), and personalized treatments based on positron emission tomography (PET), the next generation of RICs is also under development (Kraeber-Bodere et al, 2014).

Immunotoxins also represent a similar class of immunoconjugates, where antibody-based targeting domains are fused to bacterial/plant toxins for targeted cell killing. When the immunotoxin binds to the targeted cell, it is taken through endocytosis, and the toxin kills the cell. The application of these molecules has been limited to cancer and a few viral infections. Moxetumomab pasudotox is an example of one such molecule that is approved by FDA for the treatment of relapsed or refractory hairy cell leukemia (Lin and Dinner, 2019). This molecule consists of anti-CD22 antibody fragment that is fused to a Pseudomonas exotoxin PE38. Once the molecule binds to CD22 expressing cancer cells, it internalizes into the cell and releases the toxin, which inhibits protein translation process and kills the cancer cell. However, clinical success of immunotoxins

has been limited due to immunogenicity problems (Kim et al, 2020).

## TARGETED DRUG DELIVERY

Once drug molecules reach systemic circulation, their distribution and elimination (ie, disposition) in the body is governed by their inherent physicochemical properties and anatomical and physiological characteristics of the patient. In general, the drug molecules distribute throughout the body, and in addition to acting on the diseased cells, they can also act on various other cell types to elicit desired or undesired pharmacological effects. This leads to a relatively small margin between the concentrations that induce efficacy and toxicity, resulting in a narrow therapeutic index (TI), which may necessitate tight regulation of drug dosing and therapeutic drug monitoring (TDM). To overcome this issue, targeted drug delivery systems have been developed, which can provide targeted, localized, prolonged, and protected exposure of drug molecules at the site of action, resulting in a wider TI (Fig. 10-3). These systems are often compared with the "magic bullet" concept presented by Paul Ehrlich in 1900, where he hypothesized that a compound could be made so that it can selectively target an organism that is causing the disease without affecting normal host cells (Bosch and Rosich, 2008).

Targeted drug delivery can be obtained using several different strategies, which are classified into passive targeting or active targeting (Takakura and Hashida, 1996). In passive targeting, unique

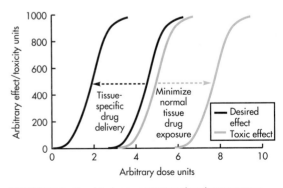

FIGURE 10-3 • Graphical representation that demonstrates how a targeted drug delivery system can be used to achieve a wider therapeutic index.

physicochemical properties and natural disposition profile of a drug carrier (eg, nanoparticle) is exploited to accomplish targeted delivery of drug molecules at the site of action. This process also depends on specific anatomical and physiological characteristics of the target tissue. In active targeting, either the drug is conjugated to a targeted carrier (eg, mAb) or natural disposition of a drug carrier is altered to direct it to specific cells, tissues, or organs. Most active targeting strategies either exploit cognate ligand–receptor interactions or employ mAbs that are targeted against antigens preferentially expressed at the site of action.

Targeted drug delivery systems can also be classified into three other categories depending on the site of drug delivery within a tissue (Friend and Pangburn, 1987): first-order systems, which deliver drug molecules to the capillary bed of target site, organ, or tissue; second-order systems, which deliver drug molecules to specific cell types (eg, tumor cells) while sparing the other cells; and third-order systems, which deliver drug molecules to specific intracellular location within the targeted cells. In general, the first-order targeting is determined by the shape, size, and other materialistic properties of the drug carrier, whereas the second- and third-order targeting depends on specific interactions between the drug/carrier and target cells. Some examples of first-order targeting include specific targeting of lymphatics, peritoneal/pleural cavity, joints, eyes, and cerebral space. An example of second-order targeting is the FDA-approved drug Givlaari™. This drug is designed by conjugating a therapeutic siRNA with GalNAc residues, which help with targeting the drug to the liver cells via hepatocyte-specific asialoglycoprotein receptors (ASGPR) (Springer and Dowdy, 2018). Examples of the third-order targeting include ADCs, RICs, and immunotoxins, which are discussed in detail earlier in this chapter.

## General Considerations in Targeted Drug Delivery

Targeted drug delivery is similar to the development of a precision-guided missile containing warheads. In order to successfully accomplish it, one needs to meticulously plan and comprehensively understand the properties of target location, targeted vehicle, and the payload. Thus, it is important to consider anatomical and physiological characteristics of the target tissue before devising a targeted drug delivery system. It is equally important to consider physical and chemical characteristics of the drug carrier, along with its PK properties and targeting abilities, before choosing a modality as an optimal system for carrying the drug. Inherent physicochemical properties of the drug molecule, its stability in different biological milieu, and its PK characteristics should also be considered, to get maximum selectivity in drug exposure at the site of action. A few of these considerations are discussed in detail below.

## Target Site

While all tissues in the body are connected via blood and lymph circulation, they each possess unique anatomical and physiological characteristics that make targeted drug delivery easier or more challenging. For example, to achieve targeted delivery of drug molecules in the eye, one can simply inject the drug in the eye to obtain a passively targeted drug delivery. However, for tissues like brain, which is highly impermeable to drug molecules, such local delivery strategy would be difficult to accomplish. While one can administer the drug into the spinal region via intrathecal administration, this route is marred with the possibility of nerve damage and lifelong pain, and drugs administered in the CSF may not efficiently penetrate brain parenchyma. Nonetheless, one can employ an active targeting strategy in the form of receptor-mediated transcytosis to cross the blood–brain barrier and accomplish active targeting of drug molecules in the brain (Pulgar, 2018). Certain tissues like solid tumors possess unique vasculature, which makes them amenable to passive targeting. Owing to the hypervascularization, aberrant vascular architecture, extensive production of vascular permeability factors, and lack of lymphatic drainage, particulate drug delivery systems like nanoparticles are able to accomplish passive targeting and preferential accumulation into the solid tumor via the enhanced permeability and retention effect. It has also been observed that certain tissues like spleen, bone marrow, and liver contain the RES made from phagocytic cells, which is able to rapidly take up particulate drug delivery systems like nanoparticles and liposomes.

## Site-Specific Properties

An efficient targeted drug delivery system should be able to hone into specific cell types within a tissue and efficiently release drug molecules at the site of action. To accomplish these goals, it is important to identify unique properties of the target site that makes it different from other organs or tissue systems within the body. One popular way to accomplish this is to use omics-based approaches to identify specific proteins/antigens that are only or preferentially expressed at the site of action. These molecules can then serve as a target for developing mAbs or other scaffolds that can specifically carry the drug molecules at the site of action. Most therapeutic mAbs, ADCs, and coated particulate systems (eg, nanoparticles, liposomes, etc) use this strategy to accomplish active targeting of drug molecules. One can also exploit naturally occurring ligand–receptor combinations to accomplish active targeting of drug molecules in a similar manner. Tissues can also differ in their chemical compositions, which can be leveraged to obtain targeted drug delivery. For example, it is known that tumor interstitial space can be hypoxic, acidic, and enriched with proteases and chemicals like ATP. Consequently, one can make drug delivery systems (eg, nanoparticles, liposomes, ADCs, etc) that trigger the release of drug molecules only in the presence of these environmental conditions. In order to develop an efficient third-order drug delivery system, it is also possible to identify certain intracellular properties that allow preferential delivery of drug molecules inside the cells. For example, it is well-known that intracellular glutathione concentrations are 1 to 3 orders of magnitude higher than extracellular values (Montero et al, 2013). Therefore, glutathione responsive nanoparticles (Ling et al, 2019) and ADCs (Lu et al, 2016) have been developed that can specifically release the drug molecule inside the cells in the presence of this antioxidant.

## Drug Characteristics

The goal of developing a targeted drug delivery system is either to protect the drug from a degradation-prone environment before it reaches the site of action, or to deliver a very potent drug with narrow TI specifically to the site of action. As such, it is important to bear in mind physicochemical properties, inherent stability, and disposition characteristics of the drug molecule that one intends to deliver. These properties also play an important role in deciding the final formulation and manufacturing process for the delivery system. If the drug molecule is unstable in the systemic circulation and possesses a very short half-life, it is typically delivered as an encapsulated formulation that can circulate in the system for long time and provide sustained release of the drug. In this manner, one changes the PK of the drug and makes it formation-rate limited. If the drug is very hydrophobic, it can nonspecifically distribute throughout the body, and it may help to make a delivery system that can preferentially accumulate and release the drug at the site of action. If the drug is very hydrophilic, it may not be able to cross the cell membrane and reach the target inside the cell. For this kind of drug, it may be helpful to make a delivery system that can penetrate the cell membrane and efficiently deliver the drug molecules inside the cell. For very potent or toxic drug molecules that have narrow TI, similar targeted intracellular delivery strategy may need to be employed.

## Targeting Modality

While advances in material science, chemistry, and protein engineering have created numerous options to develop a targeted drug delivery system, they need to be applied properly to accomplish the goals. An ideal drug delivery system should be nontoxic, biocompatible, non-immunogenic, biodegradable, and stealthy (ie, able to avoid recognition by the host's immune system). Most targeting modalities can be classified into particulate drug delivery systems or some form of conjugation/fusion of drug molecules with targeted peptides or proteins. While the latter modalities provide more selectivity, they have limitations in terms of their ability to deliver numbers of drug molecules per molecule of the carrier. As such, the total amount of active drug molecules that can be delivered at clinically acceptable dose levels is very limited, and only very potent drug molecules can be delivered using these modalities. On the contrary, while targeted or nontargeted particulate drug carriers can deliver a larger amount of drug molecules in a dose-efficient manner, they possess dominant PK characteristics, and it is hard to achieve efficient active targeting using these modalities.

## PHARMACOKINETICS OF BIOPHARMACEUTICALS

The pharmacokinetics of macromolecules is distinct from the physiological processes controlling the absorption, distribution, metabolism, and elimination of small-molecule drugs, and major differences are listed in Table 10-4 (Mahmood and Green, 2007). Whereas many routes of administration are available for small-molecule drugs, the relatively larger size and molecular instability of protein drugs necessitates a parenteral route. Traditional protein binding concepts for small-molecule drugs, in which the free fraction of the drug unbound to plasma proteins is important for distribution and clearance mechanisms, tend to be of little consequence due to the nonspecific binding of macromolecules. The steady-state volume of distribution of small-molecule drugs is determined according to drug- and tissue-specific properties, with many weak bases exhibiting extensive tissue distribution owing to moderate plasma protein binding and extensive binding to tissue

proteins. In contrast, the distribution of protein drugs is limited by their larger molecular size to primarily blood volume. The half-life of small-molecule drugs is often measured in hours, and although smaller peptide and protein drugs can have very short half-lives, larger antibodies and antibody-based constructs may have half-lives on the order of 3 weeks or longer. In contrast to the biotransformation (hepatic and extrahepatic metabolism) and excretion (eg, renal and biliary) pathways for small-molecule drugs, the elimination of biotechnology products is regulated by cellular processes, such as proteolysis, pinocytosis, and receptor-mediated endocytosis. Renal filtration is size-dependent and is operable for smaller peptides and proteins. Finally, immunogenic reactions to protein drugs can result in adverse reactions, rapid clearance of the drug, and diminished bioactivity, which is not relevant for small-molecule drugs. This section presents the main physiological processes controlling the pharmacokinetics of therapeutic proteins.

### Absorption

Biologics are usually administered parenterally such as IV, SC, or IM routes of administration. Compared to IV, SC administration offers several potential advantages, such as ease of administration and

**TABLE 10-4 • Differences Between Macromolecules and Small-Molecule Drugs**

|  | Protein Drugs | Small-Molecule Drugs |
|---|---|---|
| Molecular weight | >1000 Dalton | <1000 Dalton |
| Route of administration | Parenteral (IV, SC, IM) | All routes |
| Drug substance | Micro heterogeneous mixture | Single entity; high chemical purity |
| Impurities | Difficult to standardize | Purity standards well established |
| Plasma protein binding | Of negligible importance | May be important |
| Volume of distribution | Mainly limited to blood volume | Dictated by hydrophobicity and plasma and tissue protein binding |
| Half-life | Long (in days and weeks) | Short (in hours) |
| Cell-surface receptor interactions | Plays a significant role | May be important in some cases |
| Elimination | Phagocytosis, endocytosis, proteolysis, and renal | Biotransformation (oxidation and conjugation), renal |
| Immunogenicity | May play a significant role | Not important |

Reproduced with permission from Mahmood I, Green MD. Drug interaction studies of therapeutic proteins or monoclonal antibodies, J Clin Pharmacol. 2007 Dec;47(12):1540–1554.

improved patient compliance. However, compared to injecting drugs directly into the systemic circulation as with IV dosing, SC administration injects drugs to the extracellular space of the SC tissue. From there, the protein molecule needs to reach the lymphatic vessels or blood capillaries prior to reaching the blood circulation.

The injection site of SC administration is the skin hypodermis. In general, the hypodermis consists of adipose tissues that are separated by areolar connective tissues. The main cellular compartments in the hypodermis are adipose cells, and to a minor extent, fibroblasts and macrophages. Fibroblasts produce components of the extracellular matrix such as collagen and glycosaminoglycans (Richter and Jacobsen, 2014). Once in the interstitium, protein molecules can transport through both convection and diffusion. Convective transportation is driven by the lymphatic flow, which is from the capillaries to the lymphatic vessels. In contrast, diffusive transportation is driven by solute concentration gradient, which is from the injection site to neighboring space with lower drug concentration. The rate of drug transportation in the interstitial space of the SC injection site could be dependent on molecular size and charge. The convection of different-sized dextrans (3 to 71 kDa) in the interstitial space of mouse tail dermis showed molecular size dependency, where molecules with larger Stokes-Einstein radii are transported faster (Reddy et al, 2006). The net negatively charged interstitial matrix leads to faster transportation of negatively charged molecules. This result does not necessarily indicate that larger proteins absorb more quickly, because smaller proteins can diffuse faster and eventually reach the capillaries earlier. In a study of the SC absorption of four different-sized proteins, a positive correlation between absorption half-life ($t_{1/2}$) and protein size was demonstrated, suggesting that smaller proteins exhibit greater absorption rates (Richter et al, 2012).

The lymphatic system represents a major absorption site for mAbs and protein therapeutics (Supersaxo et al, 1990; Richter et al, 2012), and the percentage of lymphatic absorption is correlated to protein size. In one of the first studies examining the relationship between protein size and lymphatic recovery, it was shown that with increasing protein size, the percentage of drug absorbed through the lymphatic system increased in sheep (Supersaxo et al, 1990). In another study measuring the axillary lymph node recovery of four different-sized proteins in mice showed that the total lymphatic exposure was proportional to the molecular weight of the proteins (Wu et al, 2012), and although the trend was similar, the absolute values of lymphatic protein recovery differ substantially across species. For example, a 48-kDa pegylated peptide showed 73 and 27% recovery in the thoracic duct of cannulated dogs and rats (Zou et al, 2013); however, the observed value reported in sheep for the same sized protein was greater than 80%. The role of lymphatic recovery is not well studied in humans, but there is consensus that lymphatic drainage plays a major role in the delivery of therapeutic proteins following SC injection. Smaller proteins can get absorbed directly into blood capillaries, whereas the lymphatics play an increasing role in delivering protein drugs to the systemic circulation as molecular size increases. For smaller proteins, the dual update by the blood and lymphatics can give rise to "flip-flop" kinetics, a phenomenon in which the terminal elimination phase of the drug after SC administration is slower than after IV administration owing to the slower delayed delivery of the drug via the lymphatics. In contrast, although absorption is still delayed, mAbs typically do not show flip-flop kinetics after SC injection owing to their relatively longer half-lives as compared to small protein drugs.

The bioavailability of protein therapeutics (ie, net amount of drug dose making it to the systemic circulation) following SC administration is usually incomplete. Although the exact mechanisms that determine the bioavailability of therapeutic proteins after SC administration is incomplete, several important factors have been reported, such as differences across species, anatomic injection sites, blood and lymphatic flow at the site of administration, molecular size, TMDD at the local administration site, FcRn binding affinity, and co-administered formulation excipients (Deng et al, 2012; Zheng et al, 2012; Kagan and Mager, 2013; Richter and Jacobsen, 2014). Another major source of incomplete absorption is protein degradation at the site of administration, but the role of molecular drug and formulation properties that influence this process is still unclear. In humans, the bioavailability for mAbs is usually high (50% to 100%), with even greater variability for smaller protein therapeutics, which can range from 20% to 100% (Wang et al, 2008; Diao and Meibohm, 2013). It is hypothesized that the greater bioavailability of antibodies may be owing to the FcRn-mediated recycling pathway. The effect of molecular size on the bioavailability of protein therapeutics following SC administration is also unclear, and most studies show no relationship between bioavailability and protein size (Richter and Jacobsen, 2014). It is likely that the relationships between molecular drug properties and bioavailability are multifactorial, and more studies are needed to better predict and understand the incomplete bioavailability of protein therapeutics.

## Distribution

The tissue distribution of protein therapeutics is usually limited owing to the greater molecular size of proteins relative to small-molecule drugs, which tend to have greater tissue penetration. The typical volume of distribution of protein therapeutics tends to be approximately 1 to 2 times blood volume (about 15 L in a 70-kg human). Once in the systemic circulation, biologics can enter the interstitial space of peripheral tissues via three different pathways—convection, diffusion, and transcytosis. Convection is thought to be the predominant tissue extravasation pathway for antibodies, and greater than 98% of antibodies are estimated to enter tissue interstitium via convection (Baxter et al, 1994). However, for smaller proteins, this may not be the case.

The convective transportation pathway is driven by the blood–tissue hydrostatic pressure gradient. Because the pressure at the arterial end of capillaries is greater than the pressure of surrounding tissues, blood fluid will leave the capillary and enter the tissue interstitial space through the paracellular pores on the vascular endothelial cell layer. The efficiency of this pathway is determined by the relative size between protein molecules and pores, as well as the flow rate. Different tissues have different types of capillaries with varying sizes of pores. Tissues with continuous capillaries, such as muscle, CNS, and skin show the smallest pore sizes (about 3.5 to 4 nm) (Lin, 2009). Other tissues with fenestrated capillaries, such as the glomerulus, have circular openings of about 40 to 60 nm in diameter. In the liver, spleen,

and bone marrow, where discontinuous capillaries are found, the sinusoidal width can be up to 5 μm. Therefore, different tissues have different accessibility to convectively transported proteins. In addition, the extent of extravasation into the same tissue will also be different for different-size proteins.

The diffusive transportation pathway is a passive process, which is driven by the concentration gradient between the vascular and interstitial spaces. The rate of diffusion is governed by the permeability surface area product ($PS$), which can be defined by the following equation: $PS = \dfrac{D_s}{\Delta x} A$. In this equation, $D_s$ is the diffusion coefficient of the molecule, $\Delta x$ is the diffusion distance across the endothelial cell layer, and $A$ is the apparent pore area available for diffusion. $D_s$ is inversely related to protein size. As a result, large proteins, such as antibodies, cannot diffuse efficiently. Furthermore, $PS$ across certain types of pores is inversely related to $r^2$, in which $r$ refers to the pore radius (Rippe and Haraldsson, 1994). Therefore, from theoretical calculations, it is expected that proteins with small molecular size will show faster diffusive transportation rates, and tissues with larger pores on the endothelial cell layer will allow faster diffusion of proteins. As a result, for small proteins, diffusive transportation may be a significant pathway in tissue distribution.

Transcytosis transportation starts from the entry of the protein drug into the vascular endothelial cell via one of three mechanisms: receptor-mediated endocytosis, phagocytosis, and fluid-phase pinocytosis. Receptor-mediated endocytosis requires antigen–protein binding on the cell surface, and given that most tissue endothelial cells do not express drug targets, this pathway is often considered insignificant for therapeutic proteins. Phagocytosis takes place primarily in specialized cells such as macrophages, monocytes, and neutrophils. Therefore, this pathway does not play an important role in the transcytosis of therapeutic proteins. Fluid-phase pinocytosis is a nonspecific pathway driven by the concentration of drug at the extracellular side and is thought to be an important pathway for therapeutic proteins to enter endothelial cells. Once in the endothelial cells, depending on the presence of a functional Fc domain (eg, antibodies and Fc-fusion proteins), the protein molecule may bind to FcRn in the endosome. The bound protein will then undergo transcytosis and get released to the tissue interstitium or be recycled back to the vascular side of the cell and get released to the vascular space. The quantitative significance of FcRn in transcytosis of therapeutic proteins is not clear. It is hypothesized that FcRn binding can facilitate tissue extravasation of IgG antibodies; however, experimental evidence in other tissues is not conclusive.

### Metabolism and Elimination

The clearance of protein therapeutics from the body is mainly through three pathways: (i) non-metabolic elimination pathways like renal clearance, (ii) non-specific metabolic pathways like proteolysis in the extracellular environment or inside cells following pinocytosis, and (iii) specific metabolic pathways, such as TMDD.

Protein therapeutics can be excreted in the kidney by glomerular filtration, which is solute-size dependent (Haraldsson et al, 2008) and well supported by numerous studies in both preclinical species and humans using a variety of indicators (Ohlson et al, 2000; Lund et al, 2003). Antibodies are generally thought to be minimally excreted in the kidney owing to their larger molecular size. Molecules with an effective radius of less than 1.8 nm (or <12 kDa) are freely filtered, and molecules greater than 4.2 nm (or <70 kDa) are filtered to a limited extent (Vegt et al, 2010). Pharmacokinetic studies show that for smaller proteins, such as IL-10, total drug clearance is positively correlated with renal function as measured by creatinine clearance (Meibohm and Zhou, 2012). In contrast, renal filtration is insignificant for antibodies and antibody-based constructs (Wang et al, 2008). Molecular charge is another important factor that influences glomerular filtration of small protein therapeutics. In a study in which glomerular sieving coefficient ($\theta$) values were measured for solutes with four different charges (highly negative, negative, neutral, and positive) across a wide molecular weight range, solutes with the same charge showed an inverse relationship between $\theta$ and molecular weight (Haraldsson et al, 2008). For solutes with the same size, more positively charged molecules were associated with greater $\theta$ values. These results are consistent with an experimental study showing that antibodies that were chemically modified to have more basic (higher) isoelectric point (pI) values

showed increased systemic clearance in rodents (Boswell et al, 2010).

Protein therapeutics are also catabolized in the body via proteolysis. Whereas proteolysis occurs widely throughout the body, its kinetics and mechanistic details are poorly understood (Vugmeyster et al, 2012). Proteins with an Fc domain may bind to the Fc$\gamma$ receptor on the surface of macrophages and monocytes, followed by internalization and proteolysis in the lysosome (Raghavan and Bjorkman, 1996). Alternatively, these proteins can be protected from proteolysis by binding to FcRn in endothelial cells. The FcRn receptor is a widely-expressed 52-kDa membrane-bound heterodimeric glycoprotein, which is located in the endosomes of endothelial cells, and binds to the Fc domain of antibodies in a pH-dependent manner. It binds tightly to the Fc domain at acidic pH (6.0 to 6.5), but binds weakly or not at all at physiological pH (7.0 to 7.5). Therefore, Fc-containing proteins in the endothelial cells can escape subsequent proteolysis in the lysosome by binding to the FcRn in the endosome, followed by their release to either side of the cell.

TMDD is an important mechanism that can result in dose-dependent changes in both the distribution and elimination of therapeutic proteins. As discussed earlier in this chapter, TMDD is a phenomenon in which drug binding to its pharmacological target influences the pharmacokinetic properties of the drug. Levy was the first to coin the term TMDD in 1994, which was originally intended to describe the unique properties of a few small-molecule drugs that showed nonlinear or saturable tissue binding that was reflected in the time-course of drug exposure (Levy, 1994). However, the biotechnology revolution resulted in the plethora of protein-based therapeutics introduced in this chapter, and many proteins and antibodies exhibit TMDD (Wang et al, 2008; Diao and Meibohm, 2013). Essentially, drug binding to the pharmacological target may result in receptor-mediated endocytosis and subsequent lysosomal catabolism of the drug–target complex. As drug concentrations approach and exceed target concentrations, this process becomes saturated and can manifest as dose-dependent distribution and/or elimination properties. Lower dose levels of the drug often show very steep distributive phases but with extended terminal elimination, half-lives owing to drug–target binding. At high dose levels, these processes can become saturated, and the drug may follow linear kinetics until concentrations begin to decrease toward nonsaturating concentrations. Complex nonlinear behavior, such as TMDD, can complicate the analysis of pharmacokinetics and the evaluation of subsequent exposure-response relationships (Mager, 2006).

## Immunogenicity

The unwanted development of anti-therapeutic antibodies (ATAs), or immunogenic reactions, toward a protein drug can significantly alter the bioactivity and the pharmacokinetics of this important class of compounds (Chirmule et al, 2012). Such humoral responses to therapeutic proteins can result in ATAs that are either just binding or binding and neutralizing (ie, interfere with the activity of the drug). The hierarchical structure of the protein, its aggregation state, and the drug formulation can contribute to the risk of developing ATA. Factors related to the dosing regimen such as dose, frequency, and route of administration are also important determinants. The SC route is thought to be more associated with ATA

formation than IV dosing; however, studies may be confounded by the role of drug product–specific, disease-related, and individual-specific variables, which are still poorly understood. For some proteins, the development of ATA to endogenous proteins can cause serious adverse events, eg, red cell aplastic anemia with anti-erythropoietin antibodies. Immunogenic reactions can take time to develop and are often associated with the rapid clearance of the protein drug, which can have an impact on drug efficacy. For example, recombinant human interferon-β-1a is a first-line treatment for multiple sclerosis. The proportion of patients developing neutralizing antibodies can range from 2% to 25% depending on the frequency and route of administration (Panitch et al, 2002), and disease activity in ATA-positive patients can be similar to that of placebo-treated patients (1996). Further research is needed to better predict (1) the factors associated with a high likelihood of ATA formation, (2) whether an ATA response will alter the pharmacokinetics and/or pharmacodynamics of a therapeutic protein, and (3) optimum manufacturing and formulation strategies to mitigate immunogenic responses.

## CHAPTER SUMMARY

The pharmacokinetic properties of biotechnology products are distinct from those of small-molecule drugs, and although much is known about the processes controlling the *in vivo* fate of these compounds, research continues to identify the drug- and system-specific factors that influence the time-course of protein drug exposure. The relative size and instability of biotechnology products require robust and targeted drug delivery strategies to ensure the therapeutic protein achieves sufficient concentrations at the site of action with minimal adverse drug effects. Whereas great strides have been made in

understanding the pharmacokinetic properties of proteins, antibodies, and antibody-based constructs, research into the pharmacokinetic behavior of novel biotechnology products, such as the emerging cell-based therapies, is in its infancy. In addition, despite the emerging availability of lower cost biosimilars, healthcare systems will continue to struggle with the high costs associated with these complex medicines. There is promise of technological advances and innovations in clinical drug development and utilization practices to improve access to safe and effective biotechnology drugs.

## REFERENCES

Abdel-Nabi H, Doerr RJ, Chan HW, Balu D, Schmelter RF, Maguire RT: In-111-labeled monoclonal antibody immunoscintigraphy in colorectal carcinoma: Safety, sensitivity, and preliminary clinical results. *Radiology* 175:163–171, 1990.

Abraham AK, Kagan L, Kumar S, Mager DE: Type I interferon receptor is a primary regulator of target-mediated drug disposition of interferon-beta in mice. *J Pharmacol Exp Ther* 334:327–332, 2010.

Ait-Oudhia S, Mager DE, Straubinger RM: Application of pharmacokinetic and pharmacodynamic analysis to the development of liposomal formulations for oncology. *Pharmaceutics* 6:137–174, 2014.

Aiuti A, Cattaneo F, Galimberti S, et al: Gene therapy for immunodeficiency due to adenosine deaminase deficiency. *N Engl J Med* 360:447–458, 2009.

Al-Halafi AM: Vascular endothelial growth factor trap-eye and trap technology: Aflibercept from bench to bedside. *Oman J Ophthalmol* 7:112–115, 2014.

Anguela XM, High KA: Entering the Modern Era of Gene Therapy. *Annu Rev Med* 70:273–288, 2019.

Baxter LT, Zhu H, Mackensen DG, Jain RK: Physiologically based pharmacokinetic model for specific and nonspecific monoclonal antibodies and fragments in normal tissues and human tumor xenografts in nude mice. *Cancer Res* 54:1517–1528, 1994.

Bennett CF, Baker BF, Pham N, Swayze E, Geary RS: Pharmacology of antisense drugs. *Annu Rev Pharmacol Toxicol* 57:81–105, 2017.

Bosch F, Rosich L: The contributions of Paul Ehrlich to pharmacology: A tribute on the occasion of the centenary of his Nobel Prize. *Pharmacology* 82:171–179, 2008.

Boswell CA, Tesar DB, Mukhyala K, Theil FP, Fielder PJ, Khawli LA: Effects of charge on antibody tissue distribution and pharmacokinetics. *Bioconjug Chem* 21:2153–2163, 2010.

Buchwalder PA, Buclin T, Trinchard I, Munafo A, Biollaz J: Pharmacokinetics and pharmacodynamics of IFN-beta 1a in healthy volunteers. *J Interferon Cytokine Res* 20:857–866, 2000.

Caravella J, Lugovskoy A: Design of next-generation protein therapeutics. *Curr Opin Chem Biol* 14:520–528, 2010.

Chapel S, Veng-Pedersen P, Hohl RJ, Schmidt RL, McGuire EM, Widness JA: Changes in erythropoietin pharmacokinetics following busulfan-induced bone marrow ablation in sheep: Evidence for bone marrow as a major erythropoietin elimination pathway. *J Pharmacol Exp Ther* 298:820–824, 2001.

Chiriboga CA, Swoboda KJ, Darras BT, et al: Results from a phase 1 study of nusinersen (ISIS-SMN(Rx)) in children with spinal muscular atrophy. *Neurology* 86:890–897, 2016.

Chirmule N, Jawa V, Meibohm B: Immunogenicity to therapeutic proteins: Impact on PK/PD and efficacy. *AAPS J* 14:296–302, 2012.

Dash A, Knapp FF, Pillai MR: Targeted radionuclide therapy--an overview. *Curr Radiopharm* 6:152–180, 2013.

Davies A, Berge C, Boehnke A, et al: Subcutaneous rituximab for the treatment of B-cell hematologic malignancies: A review of the scientific rationale and clinical development. *Adv Ther* 34:2210–2231, 2017.

Deng R, Meng YG, Hoyte K, et al: Subcutaneous bioavailability of therapeutic antibodies as a function of FcRn binding affinity in mice. *MAbs* 4:101–109, 2012.

Dhakal B, Hari PN, Usmani SZ, Hamadani M: Chimeric antigen receptor T cell therapy in multiple myeloma: Promise and challenges. *Bone Marrow Transplant* 56:1038, 2020.

Diao L, Meibohm B: Pharmacokinetics and pharmacokinetic-pharmacodynamic correlations of therapeutic peptides. *Clin Pharmacokinet* 52:855–868, 2013.

Dunbar CE, High KA, Joung JK, Kohn DB, Ozawa K, Sadelain M: Gene therapy comes of age. *Science* 359:eaan4672, 2018.

Ekladious I, Colson YL, Grinstaff MW: Polymer-drug conjugate therapeutics: Advances, insights and prospects. *Nat Rev Drug Discov* 18:273–294, 2019.

Elliott S, Pham E, Macdougall IC: Erythropoietins: A common mechanism of action. *Exp Hematol* 36:1573–1584, 2008.

Fitzgerald JC, Weiss SL, Maude SL, et al: Cytokine release syndrome after chimeric antigen receptor t cell therapy for acute lymphoblastic leukemia. *Crit Care Med* 45:e124–e131, 2017.

Friend DR, Pangburn S: Site-specific drug delivery. *Med Res Rev* 7:53–106, 1987.

Frost GI: Recombinant human hyaluronidase (rHuPH20): An enabling platform for subcutaneous drug and fluid administration. *Expert Opin Drug Deliv* 4:427–440, 2007.

Gradishar WJ, Tjulandin S, Davidson N, et al: Phase III trial of nanoparticle albumin-bound paclitaxel compared with polyethylated castor oil-based paclitaxel in women with breast cancer. *J Clin Oncol* 23:7794–7803, 2005.

Hamad EM, Hawamdeh G, Jarrad NA, Yasin O, Al-Gharabli SI, Shadfan R: Detection of human chorionic gonadotropin (hCG) hormone using digital lateral flow immunoassay. *Conf Proc IEEE Eng Med Biol Soc* 2018:3845–3848, 2018.

Haraldsson B, Nystrom J, Deen WM: Properties of the glomerular barrier and mechanisms of proteinuria. *Physiol Rev* 88:451–487, 2008.

Harris JM, Chess RB: Effect of pegylation on pharmaceuticals. *Nat Rev Drug Discov* 2:214–221, 2003.

Harris JM, Martin NE, Modi M: Pegylation: A novel process for modifying pharmacokinetics. *Clin Pharmacokinet* 40:539–551, 2001.

High KA, Roncarolo MG: Gene therapy. *N Engl J Med* 381:455–464, 2019.

Ishii T, Ishida T, Utsunomiya A, et al: Defucosylated humanized anti-CCR4 monoclonal antibody KW-0761 as a novel immunotherapeutic agent for adult T-cell leukemia/lymphoma. *Clin Cancer Res* 16:1520–1531, 2010.

Jacobson SG, Cideciyan AV, Roman AJ, et al: Improvement and decline in vision with gene therapy in childhood blindness. *N Engl J Med* 372:1920–1926, 2015.

June CH, Sadelain M: Chimeric antigen receptor therapy. *N Engl J Med* 379:64–73, 2018.

Kagan L, Mager DE: Mechanisms of subcutaneous absorption of rituximab in rats. *Drug Metab Dispos* 41:248–255, 2013.

Kariolis MS, Kapur S, Cochran JR: Beyond antibodies: Using biological principles to guide the development of next-generation protein therapeutics. *Curr Opin Biotechnol* 24:1072–1077, 2013.

Karschnia P, Jordan JT, Forst DA, et al: Clinical presentation, management, and biomarkers of neurotoxicity after adoptive immunotherapy with CAR T cells. *Blood* 133:2212–2221, 2019.

Kim JS, Jun SY, Kim YS: Critical issues in the development of immunotoxins for anticancer therapy. *J Pharm Sci* 109:104–115, 2020.

Kraeber-Bodere F, Bodet-Milin C, Rousseau C, et al: Radioimmunoconjugates for the treatment of cancer. *Semin Oncol* 41:613–622, 2014.

Krauss AC, Gao X, Li L, et al: FDA Approval Summary: (Daunorubicin and Cytarabine) Liposome for injection for the treatment of adults with high-risk acute myeloid leukemia. *Clin Cancer Res* 25:2685–2690, 2019.

Labrijn AF, Janmaat ML, Reichert JM, Parren P: Bispecific antibodies: A mechanistic review of the pipeline. *Nat Rev Drug Discov* 18:585–608, 2019.

Leader B, Baca QJ, Golan DE: Protein therapeutics: A summary and pharmacological classification. *Nat Rev Drug Discov* 7:21–39, 2008.

Lehar SM, Pillow T, Xu M, et al: Novel antibody-antibiotic conjugate eliminates intracellular *S. aureus*. *Nature* 527:323–328, 2015.

Levy G: Pharmacologic target-mediated drug disposition. *Clin Pharmacol Ther* 56:248–252, 1994.

Lin AY, Dinner SN: Moxetumomab pasudotox for hairy cell leukemia: Preclinical development to FDA approval. *Blood Adv* 3:2905–2910, 2019.

Lin JH: Pharmacokinetics of biotech drugs: Peptides, proteins and monoclonal antibodies. *Curr Drug Metab* 10:661–691, 2009.

Lindzen M, Carvalho S, Starr A, et al: A recombinant decoy comprising EGFR and ErbB-4 inhibits tumor growth and metastasis. *Oncogene* 31:3505–3515, 2012.

Ling X, Tu J, Wang J, et al: Glutathione-responsive prodrug nanoparticles for effective drug delivery and cancer therapy. *ACS Nano* 13:357–370, 2019.

Locke FL, Neelapu SS, Bartlett NL, et al: Preliminary results of prophylactic tocilizumab after axicabtagenecilolleucel (axi-cel; KTEC19) treatment for patients with refractory, aggressive non-Hodgkin lymphoma (NHL). *Blood* 130:Abstract 1547, 2017.

Lu J, Jiang F, Lu A, Zhang G: Linkers having a crucial role in antibody-drug conjugates. *Int J Mol Sci* 17:561, 2016.

Lu RM, Hwang YC, Liu IJ, et al: Development of therapeutic antibodies for the treatment of diseases. *J Biomed Sci* 27:1, 2020.

Lund U, Rippe A, Venturoli D, Tenstad O, Grubb A, Rippe B: Glomerular filtration rate dependence of sieving of albumin and some neutral proteins in rat kidneys. *Am J Physiol Renal Physiol* 284:F1226–1234, 2003.

Mager DE: Target-mediated drug disposition and dynamics. *Biochem Pharmacol* 72:1–10, 2006.

Mager DE, Jusko WJ: Receptor-mediated pharmacokinetic/pharmacodynamic model of interferon-beta 1a in humans. *Pharm Res* 19:1537–1543, 2002.

Mahmood I, Green MD: Drug interaction studies of therapeutic proteins or monoclonal antibodies. *J Clin Pharmacol* 47:1540–1554, 2007.

Mancuso ME, Lubetsky A, Pan-Petesch B, et al: Long-term safety and efficacy of rIX-FP prophylaxis with extended dosing intervals up to 21 days in adults/adolescents with hemophilia B. *J Thromb Haemost* 18:1065–1074, 2020.

Meibohm B, Zhou H: Characterizing the impact of renal impairment on the clinical pharmacology of biologics. *J Clin Pharmacol* 52:54S–62S, 2012.)

Mohanty R, Chowdhury CR, Arega S, Sen P, Ganguly P, Ganguly N: CAR T cell therapy: A new era for cancer treatment (Review). *Oncol Rep* 42:2183–2195, 2019.

Montero D, Tachibana C, Rahr Winther J, Appenzeller-Herzog C: Intracellular glutathione pools are heterogeneously concentrated. *Redox Biol* 1:508–513, 2013.

Nagorsen D, Bargou R, Ruttinger D, Kufer P, Baeuerle PA, Zugmaier G: Immunotherapy of lymphoma and leukemia with T-cell engaging BiTE antibody blinatumomab. *Leuk Lymphoma* 50:886–891, 2009.

Neutralizing antibodies during treatment of multiple sclerosis with interferon beta-1b: Experience during the first three years. The IFNB Multiple Sclerosis Study Group and the University of British Columbia MS/MRI Analysis Group. *Neurology* 47:889–894, 1996.

Ohlson M, Sorensson J, Haraldsson B: Glomerular size and charge selectivity in the rat as revealed by FITC-ficoll and albumin. *Am J Physiol Renal Physiol* 279:F84–91, 2000.

Panitch H, Goodin DS, Francis G, et al: Efficacy ESGEoID-rENAC and University of British Columbia MSMRIRG Randomized, comparative study of interferon beta-1a treatment regimens in MS: The EVIDENCE Trial. *Neurology* 59:1496–1506, 2002.

Patterson JD, Henson JC, Breese RO, Bielamowicz KJ, Rodriguez A: CAR T cell therapy for pediatric brain tumors. *Front Oncol* 10:1582, 2020.

Pestka S, Langer JA, Zoon KC, Samuel CE: Interferons and their actions. *Annu Rev Biochem* 56:727–777, 1987.

Pisal DS, Kosloski MP, Balu-Iyer SV: Delivery of therapeutic proteins. *J Pharm Sci* 99:2557–2575, 2010.

Pulgar VM: Transcytosis to cross the blood brain barrier: New advancements and challenges. *Front Neurosci* 12:1019, 2018.

Raghavan M, Bjorkman PJ: Fc receptors and their interactions with immunoglobulins. *Annu Rev Cell Dev Biol* 12:181–220, 1996.

Reddy ST, Berk DA, Jain RK, Swartz MA: A sensitive in vivo model for quantifying interstitial convective transport of injected macromolecules and nanoparticles. *J Appl Physiol (1985)* 101:1162–1169, 2006.

Richter WF, Bhansali SG, Morris ME: Mechanistic determinants of biotherapeutics absorption following SC administration. *AAPS J* 14:559–570, 2012.

Richter WF, Jacobsen B: Subcutaneous absorption of biotherapeutics: Knowns and unknowns. *Drug Metab Dispos* 42:1881–1889, 2014.

Rippe B, Haraldsson B: Transport of macromolecules across microvascular walls: The two-pore theory. *Physiol Rev* 74:163–219, 1994.

Roberts TC, Langer R, Wood MJA: Advances in oligonucleotide drug delivery. *Nat Rev Drug Discov*, 2020.

Russell S, Bennett J, Wellman JA, et al: Efficacy and safety of voretigene neparvovec (AAV2-hRPE65v2) in patients with RPE65-mediated inherited retinal dystrophy: A randomised, controlled, open-label, phase 3 trial. *Lancet* 390:849–860, 2017.

Scheerens H, Malong A, Bassett K, et al: Current status of companion and complementary diagnostics: Strategic considerations for development and launch. *Clin Transl Sci* 10:84–92, 2017.

Schneider L, Lumry W, Vegh A, Williams AH, Schmalbach T: Critical role of kallikrein in hereditary angioedema pathogenesis: A clinical trial of ecallantide, a novel kallikrein inhibitor. *J Allergy Clin Immunol* 120:416–422, 2007.

Shah DK: Pharmacokinetic and pharmacodynamic considerations for the next generation protein therapeutics. *J Pharmacokinet Pharmacodyn* **42**:553–571, 2015.

Skrlec K, Strukelj B, Berlec A: Non-immunoglobulin scaffolds: A focus on their targets. *Trends Biotechnol* **33**:408–418, 2015.

Springer AD, Dowdy SF: GalNAc-siRNA conjugates: Leading the way for delivery of RNAi therapeutics. *Nucleic Acid Ther* **28**:109–118, 2018.

Strohl WR: Fusion proteins for half-life extension of biologics as a strategy to make biobetters. *BioDrugs* **29**:215–239, 2015.

Supersaxo A, Hein WR, Steffen H: Effect of molecular weight on the lymphatic absorption of water-soluble compounds following subcutaneous administration. *Pharm Res* **7**:167–169, 1990.

Takakura Y, Hashida M: Macromolecular carrier systems for targeted drug delivery: Pharmacokinetic considerations on biodistribution. *Pharm Res* **13**:820–831, 1996.

van Boxel-Dezaire AH, Rani MR, Stark GR: Complex modulation of cell type-specific signaling in response to type I interferons. *Immunity* **25**:361–372, 2006.

Vegt E, de Jong M, Wetzels JF, et al: Renal toxicity of radiolabeled peptides and antibody fragments: Mechanisms, impact on radionuclide therapy, and strategies for prevention. *J Nucl Med* **51**:1049-1058, 2010.

Veng-Pedersen P, Widness JA, Pereira LM, Peters C, Schmidt RL, Lowe LS: Kinetic evaluation of nonlinear drug elimination by a disposition decomposition analysis. Application to the analysis of the nonlinear elimination kinetics of erythropoietin in adult humans. *J Pharm Sci* **84**:760–767, 1995.

Vugmeyster Y, Xu X, Theil FP, Khawli LA, Leach MW: Pharmacokinetics and toxicology of therapeutic proteins: Advances and challenges. *World J Biol Chem* **3**:73–92, 2012.

Wang D, Tai PWL, Gao G: Adeno-associated virus vector as a platform for gene therapy delivery. *Nat Rev Drug Discov* **18**: 358–378, 2019.

Wang W, Wang EQ, Balthasar JP: Monoclonal antibody pharmacokinetics and pharmacodynamics. *Clin Pharmacol Ther* **84**:548–558, 2008.

Woo S, Krzyzanski W, Jusko WJ: Target-mediated pharmacokinetic and pharmacodynamic model of recombinant human erythropoietin (rHuEPO). *J Pharmacokinet Pharmacodyn* **34**:849–868, 2007.

Wu F, Bhansali SG, Law WC, Bergey EJ, Prasad PN, Morris ME: Fluorescence imaging of the lymph node uptake of proteins in mice after subcutaneous injection: Molecular weight dependence. *Pharm Res* **29**:1843–1853, 2012.

Wurch T, Pierre A, Depil S: Novel protein scaffolds as emerging therapeutic proteins: From discovery to clinical proof-of-concept. *Trends Biotechnol* **30**:575–582, 2012.

Yu S, Lim A, Tremblay MS: Next horizons: ADCs beyond oncology. In Damelin M (ed). *Innovations for Next-Generation Antibody-Drug Conjugates*. Cham, Springer International Publishing, pp 321–347, 2018.

Zheng Y, Tesar DB, Benincosa L, et al: Minipig as a potential translatable model for monoclonal antibody pharmacokinetics after intravenous and subcutaneous administration. *MAbs* **4**:243–255, 2012.

Zou Y, Bateman TJ, Adreani C, et al: Lymphatic absorption, metabolism, and excretion of a therapeutic peptide in dogs and rats. *Drug Metab Dispos* **41**:2206–2214, 2013.

# PART III

# Pharmacokinetic Principles

# Introduction to Pharmacokinetic and Pharmacodynamic Models and Analyses

Murray P. Ducharme and Luciano Gama Braga

## CHAPTER OBJECTIVES

- Define what a pharmacokinetic model is.
- Explain how pharmacokinetics (PK) relate to the pharmacodynamics (PD) of a drug.
- Explain the relationship between the "old" and the "current" compartmental PK approaches.
- Explain the differences between using differential and integrated equations in pharmacokinetics.
- Explain the term "residual variability."
- List the assumptions, advantages, and disadvantages of the noncompartment model.
- Discuss the differences between the compartmental, noncompartmental, and physiological-based PK approaches.

## INTRODUCTION

Pharmacokinetics (PK) describes the dynamics of drug absorption, distribution, and elimination and relates these processes to the pharmacodynamics (PD) of a drug, its efficacy, and its safety. Pharmacokinetic and pharmacodynamic (PK/PD) processes are complex, since drug events occur simultaneously and are time dependent. Drug exposure calculations and simulations in the systemic circulation and in other body fluids and tissues (eg, urine, cerebrospinal fluid, tumor cells) can be estimated using PK methods, while PK/PD will enable the same for efficacy and safety markers.

Mathematical models use simplified assumptions to reduce the complexity of these processes. A mathematical model is used to better understand the relationship of drug concentrations in the body with the observed and/or desired response. It allows the prediction of optimal dosing regimens and time courses of drug action. The validity of the model is based on the choice of the underlying assumptions. It is important that the model reliably fits the observed experimental data.

The availability of different mathematical and statistical techniques to characterize the PK/PD of drugs can be confusing. The objective of this chapter is to introduce the reader to the use of models and analyses in PK/PD, to show how methods are related to one another, and to explain when to use a particular model or analysis. This chapter will briefly describe various types of pharmacokinetic models that are currently used, their assumptions, as well as the experimental data needed for their development. These pharmacokinetic models and analyses will be discussed in more detail in the subsequent chapters.

## THE DIFFERENT METHODS FOR CALCULATING PK/PD

The science of pharmacokinetics was born before the widespread availability of computers. It relied for a long time mostly on "curve stripping" techniques and the use of semi-log graphical papers. The notions that "exponentials" could describe appropriately the rise (absorption), distribution (historically, "alpha"), and elimination (historically, "beta") of concentrations versus time curves are attributed to that period (Teorell, 1937; Wagner, 1975; Gibaldi et al, 1982). These notions are used to this day, but instead of discussing "individual" PK curves we now focus more on "populations" of individuals. In addition, instead of presenting PK parameters that are difficult to relate to from a clinical point of view (eg, Intercepts A, B, and C, and exponentials alpha, beta, and gamma), we now utilize noncompartmental and compartmental models that use clinically relevant parameters such as clearances and volumes.

One drawback of the "compartmental" approach has always been that the obtained calculations depend on the scientist or clinician conducting them. This is due to the possibility of using different steps and assumptions within data fitting, and to its overall complexity. The introduction of the noncompartmental method to PK in the late 1970s solved this issue. Now we had a method that could be described as an "observational" one, in that the maximum concentrations ($C_{max}$) and systemic exposure ($AUC_{0-t}$) could be "observed" (or easily computed in the case of $AUC_{0-t}$) instead of being fitted and predicted. This method soon became the norm for regulatory submissions of "Phase I" studies, in which healthy volunteers are typically administered single or multiple doses of a drug and where a large number of concentration time points can be collected after each dose.

Although this is largely misunderstood, the use of either method will lead to the same results if the parameters can be computed robustly. It is also appropriate to "mix" formulas from both methods for the same problem. For example, clearance could be fitted by the compartmental method, and then the $AUC_{0-inf}$ could be obtained by the noncompartmental method by simply dividing the administered dose with the clearance, or vice versa.

## COMPARTMENT MODELS

Compartment models are the ones the most widely used in PK/PD. The compartmental method groups "tissues" and "organs" where the drug distributes into one or more compartments, in which drugs move into and from the central compartment in a relatively homogenous manner. The central compartment includes the volume where the concentrations are sampled from (plasma, serum, or whole blood) as well as all the organs and tissues that are perfused in a similar manner by cardiac blood flow (eg, kidney, liver). The additional compartments are commonly called "peripheral," and represent organs and tissues that are not as well perfused by cardiac blood flow as the central, but which are perfused in a similar manner between them. The compartmental approach does not normally consider the physiologic processes between and within individual organs or tissues in the body, otherwise, it would be considered to be a physiologically-based PK (PBPK) approach, another method that will be introduced at the end of this chapter. Simply speaking, a drug that is polar and only eliminated unchanged in the urine will usually be very well described by a one-compartment model, while a drug that distributes extensively in many organs and tissues that are perfused in a slower manner by cardiac blood flow will be described by a two- or three-compartment model. There are no theoretical limits to the number of compartments that may be needed to appropriately describe the PK of a drug, but it is relatively rare to have to use a model with more than three compartments. Each peripheral compartment will include organs and tissues that are perfused in a similar manner by cardiac blood flow. Knowing exactly which organs and which tissues comprise each compartment is normally not needed with this method, but some hypotheses can often be formulated, especially when the PK of a drug is fitted with its PD.

The most commonly used compartmental model is the mammillary model. The *mammillary model* consists of the central compartment with peripheral compartments connecting to it. There are no direct interconnections between the peripheral compartments. The mammillary model is a strongly connected system in which the amount of drug in any compartment of the system may be estimated after drug is introduced into a given compartment. In these compartment models, drug can be both directly added to (IV administration) and eliminated from the central compartment. Elimination of drug occurs from the central compartment because the organs involved in drug elimination, primarily kidney and liver, are extremely well perfused by cardiac blood flow, and in an analogous manner. Because of this, clearances are considered between these organs to be additive, in that the total clearance will be equal to the sum of the renal, hepatic, and non-renal non-hepatic clearances. Examples of mammillary compartment models are shown in Fig. 11-1. Mammillary models make sense physiologically and pharmacologically, because the heart and the cardiac blood flow perfusing the different organs and tissues originates from the central compartment.

MODEL 1. One-compartment open model

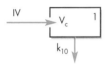

MODEL 2. Two-compartment open model

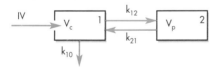

MODEL 3. Three-compartment open model

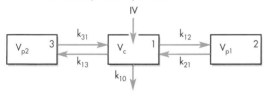

FIGURE 11-1 • Examples of mammillary PK compartmental models. Compartment 1 is the central compartment. Compartments 2 and 3 are peripheral compartments. $k_{12}$, $k_{21}$, $k_{13}$, and $k_{31}$ are first-order rate transfer constants. $K_{10}$ is the first order elimination rate constant from the central compartment. IV represents a dose administered intravenously by either a bolus or a constant infusion.

## Model Fitting versus Curve Stripping/Fitting

The fundamentals of PK/PD were developed before computers became widely available. Computers with high processing power are ubiquitous today, from within watches to smartphones. Before their wide availability, PK parameters had to be estimated using curve stripping on semi-log papers, and/or using scientific calculators. One-compartment models display mono-exponential declines of concentration-versus-time profiles on semi-log graphs, and so the terminal rate constant (terminal slope) can be estimated with ordinary or weighted least square regressions. We rarely or never do this anymore. We instead fit the data to a computer model, using better least squares techniques such as maximum likelihood or Bayesian analyses (Sheiner et al, 1979), use more accurate weighting approaches (eg, 1 over the variance) (Draper and Smith, 1998), and link important clinical covariates such as the actual body weight or the body surface area of our patients to our estimations of clearances and volumes of distribution. All of this can now easily be done using our personal smartphones that we carry with us all the time. In this section of the book, you will learn the "old" (curve stripping) and the "current" (model fitting) approaches to PK and PK/PD calculations, and how these methods are related to one another.

## Example of One-Compartment Model after Bolus IV Administration

The initial development of any model must be based on the observable data. In many cases, the observable data are plasma drug concentrations obtained from blood samples that were taken from a subject at various time intervals after the administration of a drug. Let us consider the example of a single bolus drug intravenous dose given to a subject, with plasma samples taken at various times after the dose. A plasma drug concentration-versus-time profile is thereby obtained, and is shown in Fig. 11-2.

We can observe that the data in Fig. 11-2 are very well described by a one-compartment model or mono-exponential decline (Panel B) using the semi-log scale, meaning that only one exponential is necessary to adequately characterize the concentration-versus-time profile. A PK model made of

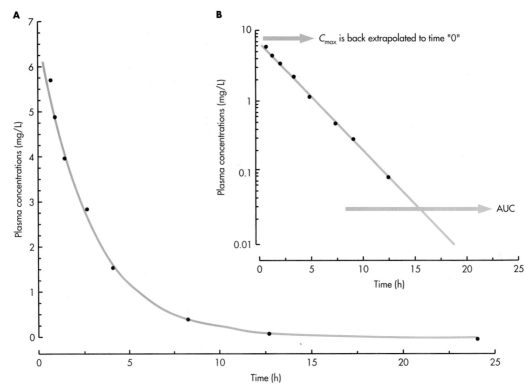

**FIGURE 11-2** • Plasma drug concentrations versus time profile after a single bolus IV administration (Panel A) linear scale, and (Panel B) semi-log scale.

only one compartment describes very well the pharmacokinetics of drugs that are polar in nature (eg, they distribute within the extracellular fluid volume, which is 0.3 L/kg) and that are readily excreted by the kidneys. A typical example is that of the aminoglycoside antibiotics (gentamicin, tobramycin, amikacin) (Sawchuk et al, 1977) that are polar and are

almost completely eliminated unchanged in the urine. The one-compartment model with intravenous bolus administration will be discussed extensively in Chapter 12.

The approach to calculate the PK of this data is presented in Fig. 11-3. Historically, we would have plotted the data on a semi-log paper and would have

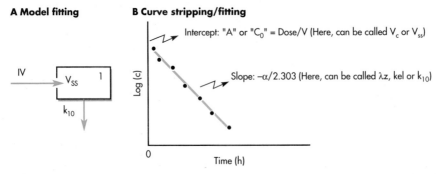

**FIGURE 11-3** • Representation of a one-compartment PK model and an example of an intravenous administration of a drug with its associated concentrations over time that would be well fitted by a mono-exponential decline.

estimated the slope by linear regression, so that the elimination rate constant could be calculated. We would then have "back-extrapolated" the concentration to time zero in order to get the predicted $C_{max}$ and the volume of distribution. The clearance would then have been obtained by multiplying the volume of distribution with the elimination rate constant. This is presented on Panel B of Fig. 11-3. Panel A represents the compartmental model that one would use nowadays to fit and characterize these concentration time data.

### Example of a Two-Compartment Model after IV Administration

Drugs that are less polar will distribute in a greater volume than the extracellular fluid, and their PK will then have to be characterized by adding one or more additional compartments to the central. Vancomycin, for example, is an antibiotic that is best described by a two-compartment model in adults (Lamarre et al, 2000). The central compartment is similar to the one that we have seen with a one-compartment model. It includes the plasma volume (when concentrations are measured in plasma), and it includes all the organs and tissues that are extremely well perfused by cardiac blood flow such as the kidney and the liver. The peripheral compartment includes all the organs and tissues that are not as well perfused by cardiac blood flow, but in a similar manner between them. Figure 11-4 illustrates the curve that we would observe on a semi-log paper (Panel B). This curve is

actually composed of two different exponentials, $\lambda_1$ and $\lambda_z$ (ie, historically they were called a and b)). The slope associated with $\lambda_1$ or a is representative of the "distribution" process, while the terminal slope $\lambda_z$ or b is representative of the terminal elimination of the drug. Panel A represents the compartmental model that one would use nowadays to fit and characterize these concentration time data.

### Relationship Between the "Old" Semi-Log Paper Stripping Method and the "Current" Modeling Approach

While a few decades ago we would have estimated the PK of the drug using semi-log paper and doing curve "stripping," we now simply use a computer where we define the compartment model as is shown in Panel A of Fig. 11-4. Instead of estimating the slope and intercept of each exponential, the computer is fitting the data to a two-compartment model represented by a central ($V_c$) and a peripheral ($V_p$) compartment. Importantly, though, all parameters fitted from Panel A can be used to find parameters describing the exponentials from Panel B, and vice versa, as shown in Table 11-1.

### Programs or Tools Used for PK/PD Modeling

The first computer programs available in PK were "stripping" programs. They executed processes that we were doing manually, but in a quicker and automatic fashion. Some of the programs available early on were CStrip\*, NonLin\*, and Topfit\*. These programs

**A Model fitting**

MODEL 2. Two-compartment open model

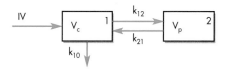

**B Curve stripping/fitting**

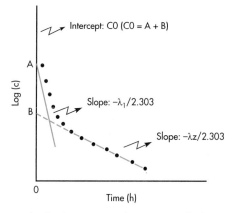

FIGURE 11-4 • Representation of a two-compartment PK model and an example of an intravenous administration of a drug with its associated concentrations on a semi-log paper that would be well fitted by a bi-exponential decline

**TABLE 11-1** • Relationships between the "Curve Stripping" Old Method of Finding PK Parameters and the Current Compartmental Approach

| | Parameters Obtained by "Stripping" ("Old Approach") | Parameters Obtained by Fitting A Compartment Model ("Current Approach") | Relationships between the "Old" and the "Current" Approaches |
|---|---|---|---|
| Parameters directly obtained | A and $\lambda_1$: First intercept and exponential representatives of "distribution process"<br><br>B and $\lambda_z$: Second intercept and exponential representatives of the "elimination process" | $V_c$: Central volume of distribution<br><br>$K_{10}$: Elimination rate constant from the central compartment<br><br>$K_{12}$: Transfer rate constant from the central to the peripheral compartments<br><br>$K_{21}$: Transfer rate constant from the peripheral to the central compartments | $V_c = $ Dose IV/(A + B)<br><br>$K_{21} = (A \times \lambda_z + B \times \lambda_1)/(A + B)$<br><br>$K_{10} = \lambda_1 \times \lambda_z / K_{21}$<br><br>$K_{12} = \lambda_1 + \lambda_z - K_{10} - K_{21}$<br><br>$\lambda_1 = K_{10} + K_{12} + K_{21} + $ SQRT $[(K_{10} + K_{12} + K_{21})^2 - 4 \times K_{10} \times K_{21}]/2$<br><br>$\lambda_z = K_{10} + K_{12} + K_{21} - $ SQRT $[(K_{10} + K_{12} + K_{21})^2 - 4 \times K_{10 \times} K_{21}]/2$ |
| Parameters that can be calculated in a second step | $C_0 = A + B$<br><br>$AUC_{0\text{-inf}} = A/\lambda_1 + B/\lambda_z$<br><br>$T_{1/2}$(distribution) $= 0.693/\lambda_1$<br><br>$T_{1/2}$(elimination) $= 0.693/\lambda_z$ | $Vp = V_c \times K_{12}/K_{21}$<br><br>$CL = K_{10} \times Vc$<br><br>$CLd = K_{12} \times Vc$<br><br>$Vss = V_c + Vp$ | |

could fit one, two, or three exponentials to a curve, an equivalent fit of a one-, two-, or three-compartment model.

Two programs that revolutionized PK/PD modeling were NONMEM® (Sheiner and Beal, 1981) and ADAPT-II® (D'Argenio and Schumitzky, 1979). They were made available for personal computers in the early 1980s and allowed PK models to be specified not only in terms of integrated equations (such as the exponential equations), but also in terms of matrix equations, and more importantly, *differential equations*. PK models are very easily specified in terms of differential equations, and models can become so complex that a solution to these equations can only be approximated by a computerized differential equation solver. These programs allowed these mathematical problems to be solved in addition to providing essential statistical algorithms for fitting such as maximum likelihood (ML) and maximum *a posteriori* probability (MAP, a Bayesian method). These two programs are still available today. NONMEM is currently in version 7.4 from ICON LLC, and ADAPT5®, version 61, from David D'Argenio

at the Biomedical Simulations Resource of the University of Southern California. They have been and are still arguably the gold standards in terms of PK and PK/PD modeling tools. They allow scientists to determine the PK/PD of drugs from both individual and population points of view. The latter permits the creation of a population PK model, that typically includes clinical covariates such as body weight, age, gender, serum creatinine, and other parameters such that simulations and predictions can be done. Once a population PK/PD model has been created and published, pharmacists can simply use the reported parameters within these programs to do therapeutic drug monitoring of their patients using a Bayesian methodology (MAP). With the miniaturization of computers, and with the advent of smartphones, technology now enables pharmacists and medical doctors to use these powerful tools everywhere they go. Currently available tools and programs for PK/PD are discussed in Chapter 20, and an example of a tool that can easily be created on an Excel spreadsheet on a smartphone to optimize aminoglycoside dosing in clinical practice can be found there.

## Concepts Behind Modeling

The modeling of a system, in this case the kinetics of a drug or biological in the body, can be translated as the reduction or a simplification of a problem to its core components. To achieve this, models are generally expressed as boxes with arrows indicating the movement of the analyte(s) in the body. The boxes often represent a *compartment*, which is a defined hypothetical region where the analyte transits through or accumulates. Since modeling is a simplification of a problem, the results obtained are not completely identical to the observed data, and the residual error that will not be explained by the model in the data is called *residual variability*. Despite their shortcomings, models can be accurate enough to predict the behavior of a drug in the body and to optimize drug therapy.

In the example presented in Fig. 11-5, the box reflects the one compartment model, and the compartment is called "1." The first arrow indicates the drug coming into the compartment (for example here an IV bolus) and the second arrow, the drug leaving the compartment. As the arrow is leaving the compartment 1, then by default, the rate constant (k) leaving the compartment "1" is called "$k_{10}$" for "K one-zero" or "K one-out."

### Number of "Boxes" versus "Compartments" in a PK Model

PK models do not always use the same number of *boxes* and *compartments*. A PK model describing the oral absorption of a modified release product may need several boxes to describe what is happening mathematically just regarding its absorption process, but if the drug is well described by a mono-exponential decline once it appears systemically, and therefore a one-compartment, it will then still be called a "one-compartment" model even though many "boxes" may be needed. An example is presented

in Fig. 11-6 for a PK model that could describe the behavior of the modified release product Concerta˚, a long-acting formulation of methylphenidate, after oral administration. There are three boxes in this model, because mathematically we have to define differential equations for what is happening in these three separate boxes, but it is still a one-compartment model (from a systemic point of view) despite the three boxes. PK models are therefore specified in terms of compartments that are associated with IV administration, because once the drug will be absorbed in Fig. 11-6 by either the immediate-release first-order rate constant ($ka_{IR}$) or by the extended-release first-order rate constant ($ka_{ER}$), then the concentration-time profile will be described by a mono-exponential decline and therefore a one-compartment model.

### Modeling with Differential and/or Integrated Equations

In modeling, terms like "coming into" and "leaving from" a compartment are translated as mass flow. In other words, the arrows represent the rate by which

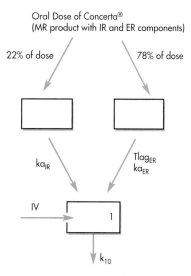

FIGURE 11-6 • The number of "boxes" in compartmental modeling is not always equal to the number of "compartments." Here is a representation of a one-compartment PK model for Concerta˚, but using three boxes mathematically, due to the two different absorption processes related to this specific drug product formulation. The Concerta product includes 22% and 78% of its labeled dose as IR and ER components, respectively.

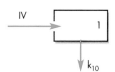

FIGURE 11-5 • Representation of a mathematical PK model using a box and two arrows.

the drug moves into and out of a compartment. By default, rates will have two suffixes after them to indicate where the flow is coming out of and where it is going to. For example, in a two-compartment model, the rate constants going between the central and peripheral compartments will be called $k_{12}$ ("k one-two," to indicate flow from the central to the peripheral compartment) and $k_{21}$ ("k two-one," to indicate flow from the peripheral to the central compartment). Similarly to velocity calculations in physics, where movement is expressed in space per time (as in miles per hour), in pharmacokinetics movement is expressed as the rate of mass units or amount of drug per time. This flow can be mathematically expressed using derivatives as:

$$\frac{dX}{dt} \qquad (11.1)$$

where $X$ is the amount of drug and $t$ is time.

In order to write a model, an equation is written to describe the quantity of drug in the compartment of interest. Therefore, a minimum of one equation has to be written for each "box" whether there are one or more boxes describing a compartment mathematically. For instance, in the example in Fig. 11-3, there is one arrow going into the compartment and one arrow leaving the compartment. The arrow coming into the compartment is written as a positive flow, while the arrow leaving the compartment is a negative one. What is happening to the amount of drug in that one compartment (Fig. 11-3) can then be described as:

$$\frac{dx1}{dt} = +IV - k_{10} \cdot x1 \qquad (11.2)$$

where $x1$ is the amount of drug in compartment 1, $IV$ represents the dose arriving per unit of time in the compartment intravenously, and $k_{10}$ is the elimination rate constant out of that same compartment.

Integration of the previous equation provides the predicted amount of drug in that compartment for any given time. By also considering the volume of distribution, the equation can be modified to provide concentration values of the drug. Systemic concentrations are more useful in pharmacokinetics than systemic amounts, because the effect of a drug (both from a safety and efficacy point of view) are related to concentrations, not to amounts. Once integrated and expressed in concentration units, Equation 11.2 becomes:

$$C_t = + \text{Dose}/V \times \exp(-k_{10} \times t) \qquad (11.3)$$

where $C_t$ is the predicted concentration for any given time $t$, Dose is the intravenous amount administered, V is the volume of distribution of that one-compartment model, and $k_{10}$ is the elimination rate constant from the compartment. Equation 11.3 is called "integrated," as it will provide only one solution for any given time t. The main advantage of an *integrated equation* is that it is already solved mathematically, so it can be used directly in Excel or any other type of computer spreadsheet to easily predict or fit concentration-versus-time profiles. Their disadvantage in PK is that many models, because of their complexity, cannot be solved in terms of integrated equations because they are not associated with a unique solution. They can, however, easily be described using *differential equations*. This explains why in PK and PK/PD we often work with differential equations, and therefore have to use differential equations solver to approximate what may be a solution. As mentioned previously, NONMEM and ADAPT5 are two of the main software or tools that pharmacokinetic scientists use when describing and using models in terms of differential equations.

## Fitting Data with a Model

Notice that the solved equation above (11.3) is populated with constants. The values of these constants are obtained through the process of model fitting. To fit, a model requires experimental observations. In pharmacokinetics, a subject's drug concentrations measured over time are used as observational data. The fitting of the model by the computer algorithm starts by assigning each constant in the model the value that is prespecified *a priori* by the modeler. These are called *initial estimates* or *priors*. The model uses these initial estimates and determines how close the calculated obtained concentrations are similar to the observed data. In each subsequent step, called *iterations*, the algorithm chooses new sets of estimates so that the calculated obtained concentrations are closer and closer to the observed data, until final results or *convergence* is obtained based on predefined criteria.

When fitting, the experimental measurements are associated with uncertainty or errors. These will arise because of inter-occasion and inter-individual variability, human error, pharmaceutical variability, bioanalytical uncertainty, and experimental errors such as sampling times or volumes. All these contribute to the overall error, which in PK is called the *residual variability*. The residual variability is the total variability in the data that is left unexplained by the model. This number also gives an indication of the quality of the fit, if one can suspect or can hypothesize what this overall error would ideally be, before model misspecifications are introduced. Say for example that we are fitting Phase-1 data and expecting that the experimental errors such as sampling times, administered drug potency, and bioanalytical variability are kept to a minimum, then one may expect that if we were to have a "perfect" fit where the model does not contribute anything to the overall error, then this residual variability may be within 5 to 15%. But if the residual variability is instead 30%, we may therefore conclude that the model may be contributing to this extra 15% error, because it is not yet the most appropriate one to use (eg, a one-compartment model instead of a two, a linear model instead of a nonlinear one).

Despite our best efforts, if the observed data used for modeling has too much error, the model will invariably not predict well the pharmacokinetics of a drug in the body. This is known in computer science as *garbage in, garbage out*, where noisy input used to create a model will result in a noisy and uncertain output. Here noise will be associated with error. In sum, the quality of the observed data used to generate the model is essential to its performing accurate calculations, predictions, and simulations. Different modeling approaches are further elaborated in Chapter 19, while the tools used to solve modeling problems are described in Chapter 20.

## Selecting the Most Appropriate PK Model

Selecting the most appropriate PK model is an essential step of conducting compartmental PK analyses. By definition, *models* are an approximation of the truth and are therefore always "wrong" to a certain degree. A model will, however, be judged to be appropriate if the following conditions are all met:

1. The model enables one to correctly characterize all observational data available.
2. The model is appropriately validated for its desired purposes.
3. The model makes physiological and pharmacological sense.
4. The model is the simplest that one can use while still being "optimal" in its associated quality of fit (ie, if both two- and one-compartment models are associated with the same overall quality of fit, then the one-compartment model has to be selected). This follows the *Law of parsimony*, in that increasing the complexity of the model is only justified when it significantly increases its accuracy.

The exercise of comparing models to one another for the purpose of selecting the most appropriate one is called *model discrimination*. To help us decide which models to use, scientists usually compare the model "-2 log likelihood" number, also called the *objective function* (OF) or the *minimum value of the objective function* (MOF). A model will be better than another one if the OF or MOF is statistically better while considering the increase in complexity. This can be done "automatically" by just comparing the *Akaike information criterion test* (AIC) obtained from two different models (Akaike, 1974), because that number is essentially the OF plus a penalty of 2 times the number of parameters. It therefore means that a model including two additional parameters will have to display an OF that is lower than 4 ($2 \times 2$) in order to be considered significantly better. Alternatively, OF or MOF can be compared assuming a chi-square distribution. For example, a model with one additional parameter will need to display an OF that is inferior by more than 3.84 ($p < 0.05$) to be considered significantly better.

## Linear versus Nonlinear PK Processes

Most processes in pharmacokinetics can be explained by linear-type relationships. The oral absorption of a drug from the gastrointestinal tract can often be characterized using a first-order rate constant (ka), while the transfer rate constants between compartments (eg, $k_{12}$ and $k_{21}$) or going outside of them (eg, $k_{10}$) are also often best described using first-order rate constants, all expressed in h$^{-1}$. An absorption rate constant, ka, or an elimination rate constant, $k_{10}$, of 0.4 h$^{-1}$ means that 40% of drug left to be absorbed or eliminated actually do so per hour. The majority of the subsequent chapters focus on PK behavior and characterization that are based on these linear concepts, simply because the vast majority of drugs marketed and used in clinical practice exhibit linear PK behavior. The absorption, distribution, and/or elimination processes of certain drugs can be saturable, and in those cases, the PK behavior will need to be characterized with nonlinear equations. Examples are the absorption of amoxicillin or of Levodopa that are saturable and best expressed by zero-order absorption rate constants (denoted "$k_0$" in amount units per time, for example, mg/h). An example of saturable distribution includes Paclitaxel distribution between red blood cells and plasma for intravenous formulations containing cremophor (Sparreboom et al, 1999), while a classical example of saturable elimination is that of phenytoin (Mawer et al, 1974). Nonlinear relationships and equations are presented in Chapter 18.

## Mathematical Introduction of a Drug into a Compartment

The introduction of a drug into the circulatory system can occur via various methods. If the drug is administered intravenously, it may be administered by intravenous push over a few seconds or minutes, if it is safe to do so, and will then be best described mathematically as a *bolus*, which is an instantaneous change in a system (Chapters 12 and 13). Nowadays, most intravenously administered drugs are administered more slowly, either by syringe-pumps over a period of 15 to 30 minutes, or by continuous infusion from a bag over 1 to 2 hours. Mathematically these infusions will be described as *rates*, where the change in a system or compartment will be in amounts per hour (eg, mg/h) and will be turned on and off in the dataset that will be read by the model. Chapter 14 describes the PK of drugs administered via intravenous infusions.

## Building Multicompartment Models

Mathematical models containing more than one compartment are built using the same principles seen previously, where each arrow or flow into and out of a compartment is added to the equation describing the mass of drug in that compartment. Compartments are mathematical tools used to fit the data and are not necessarily correlated to a chemical or biological event in the body. Multicompartmental models are presented in Chapter 13.

The differential equation describing the central compartment for a one (11.4), two (11.5), or three (11.6) compartment models are shown below for an administered IV bolus, as represented in Fig. 11-1.

$$\frac{dC_1}{dt} = -k_{10}C_1 \tag{11.4}$$

$$\frac{dC_1}{dt} = -k_{10}C_1 - k_{12}C_1 + k_{21}C_2 \tag{11.5}$$

$$\frac{dC_1}{dt} = -k_{10}C_1 - k_{12}C_1 + k_{21}C_2 - k_{13}C_{1-} + k_{31}C_3 \tag{11.6}$$

After a model is built, its solution, or the integration of the differential equation, will be another equation relating time to mass, what we have described earlier as an integrated equation. Normally in pharmacokinetics, the mass is divided by a volume, yielding the concentration. Hence, the solution of a pharmacokinetic model results in an equation relating time and concentrations. The solutions, or integrations, of models comprised of one to three compartments are given below in equations 11.7 to 11.9 for the central compartment for a drug administered via an instantaneous (bolus) intravenous administration:

$$C_1 = Ae^{-\alpha t} \tag{11.7}$$

$$C_1 = Ae^{-\alpha t} + Be^{-\beta t} \tag{11.8}$$

$$C_1 = Ae^{-\alpha t} + Be^{-\beta t} + Ce^{-\gamma t} \tag{11.9}$$

where α, β, and γ are the first, second, and third exponentials that are needed to characterize concentration-time profiles up to a three-compartment model, and A, B, and C are the intercepts associated with each of these exponentials.

For non-intravenous administrations, the equations must account for the rate by which the drug will enter the systemic circulation. Chapter 16 discusses the PK of drug absorption. Multiple-dosage regimens are discussed in Chapter 17.

# NONCOMPARTMENTAL MODEL

In contrast to compartmental modeling, *noncompartmental analysis* was developed to facilitate the calculation of essential pharmacokinetic parameters without the need for generating, solving, and optimizing complex models. The noncompartment model or approach is based on *statistical moment theory* (Yamaoka et al, 1978), providing scientists with an easy method that uses the least amount of fitting possible. The main assumptions of this model are that the PK behavior of the drug has to be linear (in terms of both time and dose), the drug product has to be eliminated from where the sampling occurs, and finally, the terminal phase of the concentration-time profile has to be monoexponential. Because of these assumptions, this method should not be called "model independent," as some call it, hence the more appropriate *noncompartmental* name. Some pharmacokinetic parameters are obtained directly from the concentration-time profile data and are thus considered to be "observed," such as the $C_{max}$, $T_{max}$, and $AUC_{0-t}$ (Fig. 11-7). The terminal first-order rate constant ($\lambda_z$ or $k_{el}$) is, however, calculated using the slope of the linear regression of the terminal ln-linear phase, and the extrapolated AUC (ie, $AUC_{t-inf}$) obtained by dividing the last detectable concentration time point (t) by the terminal rate constant. The clearance (CL) or apparent clearance (CL/F, when the dose has been administered via extravascular administration) is calculated as the ratio of dose divided by the $AUC_{0-inf}$. Both mean residence time (MRT, defined as the average time molecules of the drug spend in the body) and the total volume of distribution ($V_{ss}$) can be calculated after intravenous single-dose administration using statistical moment theory (see Chapter 23).

The first drawback of this method is that it is relying on a lot of observations in order to be robust. AUCs are usually considered accurate, for example, when at least 12 concentration samples are obtained to characterize a single-dose administration. The $C_{max}$ can only be "obtained" if multiple samples are taken before and after that concentration ("no first point $C_{max}$"). The second main drawback is that the method will not allow the computing of MRT and therefore $V_{ss}$ if the PK is assessed at steady state, and/or if the drug was administered extravascularly. Because of these two main limitations, the noncompartmental approach is really appropriate for Phase 1 studies where a drug's pharmacokinetic profile is characterized in healthy volunteers mostly in terms of maximum and extent of exposure (ie, $C_{max}$ and $AUC_{0-t}$), but not for studies conducted in patients or in clinical practice when very few observations are collected, rarely just after a single dose, and where additional predictions and extensive simulations are typically needed.

A comparison of the compartmental and of the noncompartmental approaches is shown in Table 11-2.

# PHYSIOLOGICALLY-BASED PHARMACOKINETIC MODEL

The physiologically-based pharmacokinetic (PBPK) method can be considered an extension of the compartmental approach. It is based on the same mathematical principles (they are models based on different compartments), but instead of having compartments that include several organs that are perfused in the same manner within them, a PBPK model will separate each of them into their individual organ units. For example, the central compartment in compartmental PK may be broken into the blood volume, extracellular volume, heart, kidney, liver, and so on for a PBPK model. While it is appealing to have more organ details within a PBPK model, the caveat is that most of these individual organs or compartments are actually not identifiable, so many parameters have to be assumed or fixed to sometimes arbitrarily chosen values. Nevertheless, years of

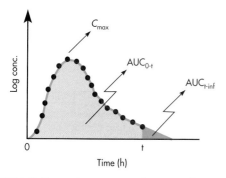

**FIGURE 11-7** • Plasma drug concentration versus time curve showing PK parameters obtained by the noncompartmental approach.

**TABLE 11-2 •** Comparison of the Compartmental and Noncompartmental Approaches in PK

| Attributes | Compartmental Model | Noncompartmental Model |
|---|---|---|
| Assumptions | • Distribution within each compartment normally assumed to be instantaneous. | • PK linearity.<br>• Terminal phase is mono-exponential.<br>• Drug product eventually eliminated. |
| Advantages | • Can be used to calculate any PK parameters and for all types of drug administration.<br>• Can be used for simulations and predictions. | • Simple and rapid calculations. |
| Disadvantages | • Can be very complicated and time consuming.<br>• Results can be "scientist-dependent." | • Limited utility in clinical practice or in patient studies with few observations.<br>• Can be used to calculate any PK parameters and for all types of drug administration. |
| Ideal for | • Patient studies or in clinical practice where a limited number of observations can be taken.<br>• Simulations and predictions. | • Phase-1 PK studies conducted in healthy volunteers.<br>• IV, single dose administrations, and steady state conditions (only for calculating $C_{avg(ss)}$, $AUC_{tau(ss)}$, $C_{min(ss)}$, and CL). |

PBPK modeling research have been beneficial in that these models can now predict drug–drug interactions, bioavailability, and clearance of drugs much better than they were able to just a few decades ago. A theoretical representation of a PBPK model is presented in Fig. 11-8.

In contrast to an estimated and/or fitted overall volume of distribution using the compartmental model, each desired tissue and organ volume has to be estimated and/or specified in a PBPK model. Because there are many tissues and organs in the body, each of them and their associated drug concentrations would have to be obtained for the PBPK model to be completely validated, an unrealistic and unfeasible feat at this point in time. PBPK models are therefore best viewed as a work in progress, becoming more accurate and useful as time goes by. PBPK models are not useful for data fitting, as they include too many parameters that are associated with severe identifiability issues and therefore cannot replace compartmental models. Their appeal and utility are in predicting mean PK concentration-time profiles without any PK data for any drug product when basic information about the drug is known, something that a simple compartmental model cannot provide.

Hence, the major advance brought by the PBPK approach in the last 20 years has been the prediction

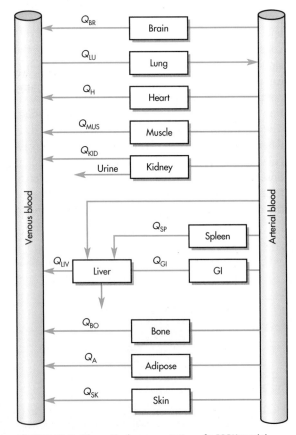

FIGURE 11-8 • Theoretical representation of a PBPK model.

of human PK for investigational drugs using only data obtained from drug discovery experiments. With minimal inputs to the model, such as a drug's physicochemical characteristics, protein binding, molecular weight, metabolic fate, and partition coefficient, for example, current PBPK models available from Gastroplus® or SimCYP® are able to predict mean human PK profiles with a much higher degree of precision than just a few decades ago. Early PBPK models developed in the 1970s and 1980s focused mostly on "physiological" alternatives to the well-stirred liver clearance model (see Chapter 6). These early PBPK "hepatic" models were complex, like the sinusoidal parallel tube or the dispersion models, and although they appeared at first glance to "look" much more "physiologic" than the simpler well-stirred model, they were found to be much worse at predicting drug–drug interaction study results. The explosion in the power capabilities of the personal computers in the 1990s led to a resurgence in the interest of full-scale PBPK models, but using the well-stirred model for organ clearances. The human genome project and all its associated research (Sachidanandam et al, 2001) brought major advances to our knowledge of enzymes and transporters that are responsible for drug absorption and metabolism. Current PBPK models have incorporated this new knowledge and are now much better at predicting oral bioavailability of drugs and drug–drug interactions.

## PHARMACOKINETIC/ PHARMACODYNAMIC (PK/PD) MODEL

A major objective of pharmacokinetics is to relate the plasma drug concentration–time profiles to the effect or pharmacodynamics of the drug (efficacy and/or safety). These can be very complex and difficult to simplify in a PK/PD model (see Chapter 22). In order to develop a PK/PD model, there needs to be a thorough evaluation of the drug concentration versus response (effect) so that the relationship is best understood and best described in a model. Models to be tested and compared will have to make physiological and pharmacological sense, otherwise they should not be pursued.

For most drugs, the systemic exposure (represented by AUCs or partial AUCs) will relate best with safety and efficacy, with a relationship often described

with an $E_{max}$ type model. Maximum exposure most often relates best with the occurrence of certain side effects (eg, high blood pressure with cyclosporine), but may also relate to efficacy when concentrations are within a range during which the efficacy increases (eg, antibiotics that have concentration-dependent killing activity such as aminoglycosides or fluoroquinolones). The relationship between most drugs and efficacy can therefore be characterized with the $E_{max}$-type response illustrated in Fig. 11-9. Efficacy starts when concentrations rise above a "threshold" value, indicated on the graph as the minimum effective concentration (MEC). For antibiotics and antiviral agents, this parameter will be related to the *in vitro* minimum inhibitory concentration (MIC) once protein binding has been taken into account. Figure 11-9 illustrates an $E_{max}$ type relationship, where the effect starts to plateau past a concentration called plateau in effective concentrations (PEC). For antibiotics, the PEC is typically seen when free concentrations become higher than 10 to 20 times the MIC for drugs associated with what is called *concentration-dependent killing activity*, such as aminoglycosides and fluoroquinolones, and with free concentrations that are higher than 4 to 6 times the MIC for drugs displaying what is commonly called *concentration-independent killing activity* (Ducharme et al, 2008). For both types of antibiotics, once concentrations are above the PEC, the killing activity is at the $E_{max}$, and the killing activity then becomes *time dependent*.

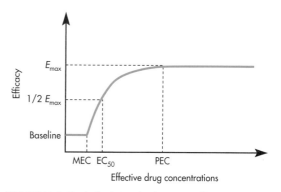

**FIGURE 11-9** • Typical relationship between Effective drug concentrations (ie, at the site of action or in equilibrium with the site of action) and the efficacy. Abbreviations: $E_{max}$, maximum theoretical effect of the drug; MEC, minimum effective concentration; EC50, concentration associated with ½ of the $E_{max}$; PEC: plateau in effective concentrations.

PK/PD models are typically constructed in a sequential fashion. The PK model is first determined and validated. The PD component is then added and validated to the fixed PK component of the model, because for most drugs, the PD marker that is being evaluated will not affect the PK. A PK/PD model is presented in Fig. 11-10 for a drug that would be well characterized by a one-compartment PK model, and where the effect of the drug would be directly related to its systemic concentrations, for example, an aminoglycoside treating a systemic bacterial infection.

PK/PD models are crucial in order to better understand the relationship between exposure, efficacy, and safety. In drug development, PK/PD models help better define the optimal dosing regimen of a drug for an intended indication and population

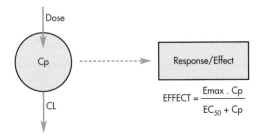

FIGURE 11-10 • Scheme for a simple PKPD model. Abbreviations: $E_{max}$, maximum effect of the drug; EC50, plasma drug concentration that is associated with 50% of the maximum drug effect; Cp, systemic drug concentration.

(see Chapter 30), while in clinical practice they will help optimize an individual patient's drug therapy.

## CHAPTER SUMMARY

Pharmacokinetics describes the variation of the drug concentration in the body versus time using mathematical models and different theoretical assumptions. Originally, pharmacokinetic parameters were calculated manually or with calculators, with the help of semi-log graphical papers and "stripping" methods. For many decades now, computers have been the main tools used for these calculations. Briefly, there are three main different approaches to pharmacokinetic calculations: the compartmental based, the non-compartmental based, and the physiologically based pharmacokinetic models. The compartmental model analysis assumes that the drug will distribute into one or more groups of "tissues" and "organs" in the body, that are perfused in a similar manner by cardiac blood flow. The drug concentration profiles in these compartments can be described using integrated equations when the models are simple, and differential equations when the models are complex. The noncompartmental approach to pharmacokinetics does not depend on complex equations, and

is a method that can be qualified as "observed," with minimal fitting. On the downside, it necessitates the taking of many observations (eg, concentration time points) for the PK to be robustly characterized. Finally, the physiologically-based pharmacokinetic model tries to take into account separately all the individual organs in the body where the drug may distribute and may be eliminated. These models are very complex, as they involve hundreds of compartments and parameters, but they have recently been shown to be useful in drug discovery and development for predicting and simulating mean PK profiles based on physicochemical characteristics of a drug product, and for predicting drug–drug interactions. Ultimately the understanding of the pharmacokinetic behavior of a drug is important in order to create a relationship between drug concentration and drug effect in the body, or pharmacodynamics, in order to optimize drug therapy in a given patient or population of patients.

## REFERENCES

Akaike H: A new look at the statistical model identification. *IEEE Trans Automat Control* 19:716–723, 1974.

D'Argenio DZ, Schumitzky A: A program package for simulation and parameter estimation in pharmacokinetic systems. *Comput Programs Biomed* 9(2):115–134, 1979.

Draper NR, Smith H: *Applied Regression Analysis*, 3rd ed. John Wiley and Sons, 1998.

Ducharme MP: Principes d'utilisation des antibiotiques. In Elsevier Masson (ed). *Pharmacie clinique et thérapeutique*. 3rd ed. Paris, Masson, 2008, pp 935–958.

Gibaldi M, Perrier D: *Pharmacokinetics*. 2nd ed. New York, NY, Marcel Dekker, 1982.

Lamarre P, Lebel D, Ducharme MP: A population pharmacokinetic model for vancomycin in pediatric patients and its predictive value in a naive population. *Antimicrob Agents Chemother* **44**(2):278–282, 2000.

Mawer GE, Mullen PW, Rodgers M, Robins AJ, Lucas SB: Phenytoin dose adjustment in epileptic patients. *BJCP* **1**(2): 163–168, 1974. https://doi.org/10.1111/j.1365-2125.1974 .tb00226.x.

Sachidanandam R, Weissman D, Schmidt SC, et al: A map of human genome sequence variation containing 1.42 million single nucleotide polymorphisms. *Nature* **409**(6822):928–934, 2001.

Sawchuk RJ, Zaske DE, Cipolle RJ, Wargin WA, Strate RG: Kinetic model for gentamicin dosing with the use of individual patient parameters. *Clin Pharmacol Ther* **21**(3):362–369, 1977.

Sheiner LB, Beal SL: Evaluation of methods for estimating population pharmacokinetic parameters II. Biexponential model and experimental pharmacokinetic data. *J Pharmacokinet Biopharmaceut* **9**(5):635–651, 1981.

Sheiner LB, Beal S, Rosenberg B, Marathe V, et al. Forecasting individual pharmacokinetics. *Clinical Pharmacology and Therapeutics* 1979;31:294–305.

Sparreboom A, van Zuylen L, Brouwer E, et al: Cremophor EL-mediated alteration of paclitaxel distribution in human blood: Clinical pharmacokinetic implications. *Cancer Res* **59**(7):1454–1457, 1999.

Teorell T: II. The intravascular modes of administration. *Arch internationales pharmacodynamie therapie* **57**:226, 1937.

Wagner JG: *Fundamentals of Clinical Pharmacokinetics*. Hamilton, IL, Drug Intelligence Publications Inc., 1975.

Yamaoka K, Nakagawa T, Uno T: Statistical moments in pharmacokinetics. *J Pharmacokinet Biopharm* **6**(6):547–558, 1978.

# 12

# One-Compartment Open Model: Intravenous Bolus Administration

Kayleigh Wight, Philippe Colucci, and Murray P. Ducharme

## CHAPTER OBJECTIVES

- Discuss the clinical relevance of IV bolus injection and introduce concepts of the one-compartment linear model with this route of administration.

- Define volume of distribution, elimination rate constant, and clearance, and explain how to calculate these parameters in a one-compartment linear model with IV bolus injection.

- Explain the clinical utility of the one-compartment model

## INTRODUCTION

### Intravenous Bolus Administration

Intravenous (IV) bolus injection is a method of parenteral drug administration. The term *parenteral* is derived from the Greek words *para* (ie, beside or near) and *enteron* (ie, the intestine). In medicine, *parenteral* refers to the administration of a drug through a route that does not involve gastrointestinal absorption. IV bolus injection is the administration of an entire dose of medicine into the veins over a short period of time (less than 1 minute). Intravenous administration is the most direct route of drug administration because absorption processes are bypassed when a drug is deposited directly into the bloodstream (ie, systemic circulation). Furthermore, bolus injection is the fastest method of IV drug administration, compared to IV infusion (see Chapter 14). This quality of complete and instantaneous absorption has its advantages and disadvantages.

A therapeutic effect may be seen almost immediately with IV bolus injection because the entire dose of medication enters the bloodstream directly, skipping absorption processes, and is thereby distributed throughout the body via the systemic circulation. For this reason, IV bolus injection is preferred in emergency situations where it is critical to reach therapeutic levels quickly (eg, heart attack, stroke, or narcotic overdose). Another benefit to IV bolus injection is that it can be used when a drug is not able to be absorbed by the gastrointestinal tract or when a patient cannot receive oral medication (eg, unable to swallow or unconscious). Alternatively, an IV bolus preparation would be selected if a clinician does not have the appropriate equipment to administer an IV infusion and it is safe to administer the drug quickly.

The rapid onset of effects following IV bolus injection can be harmful if the patient has an adverse reaction, and it is too late to stop the injection and impossible to

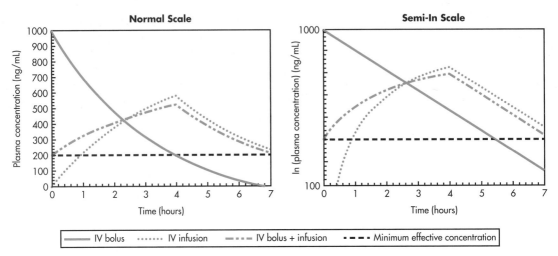

FIGURE 12-1 • Graph of a theoretical drug after IV bolus injection and IV infusion.

retrieve the medication once it has been administered. Higher concentrations of drug in systemic circulation (higher $C_{max}$ and early AUC exposure) are achieved following IV bolus injection compared to other routes of administration, because the entire dose is deposited directly into the bloodstream rapidly. This can result in unnecessary exposure to a drug because a large portion of the dose contributes to systemic concentrations that are higher than what is needed for a therapeutic effect, and if the drug is eliminated rapidly, then the duration of the therapeutic effect will be shorter after IV bolus injection compared to IV infusion (Fig. 12-1). These higher concentrations increase the risk of negative side effects without improving efficacy. Increasingly, IV bolus administration is used in combination with IV infusion, where the bolus dose is given at the start of infusion, in order to immediately achieve and then to maintain desirable drug levels (see Chapter 14).

The disadvantages of IV bolus administration often outweigh the advantages, thus this route is only used when necessary. Although other routes of administration are used more often, IV bolus injection is the easiest to understand in compartmental pharmacokinetics (PK) because absorption does not occur, and the entire dose is immediately distributed throughout the central compartment from a mathematical point of view. Not only is IV bolus injection a good example for introducing concepts of compartmental PK, but clinicians can use these methods to make rough estimates for drugs that are not given by IV bolus injection because calculations are so simple that they can be done "at the bedside."

## One-Compartment Open Model

As its name implies, the *one-compartment open model* represents the body as a single uniform compartment (ie, one compartment) where drugs can enter and leave (ie, open model). The one-compartment model can be characterized by two PK parameters, one for drug distribution and one for drug elimination (which may include metabolism). Distribution is only parameterized by the volume of distribution, whereas elimination may be parameterized by one of multiple PK parameters that describe elimination (eg, elimination rate constant or clearance). For simplicity, this chapter will only discuss the one-compartment model in relation to IV bolus administration and linear (first-order) elimination (Fig. 12-2).

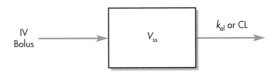

FIGURE 12-2 • One-compartment linear model with IV bolus administration. IV = intravenous; $V_{ss}$ = apparent volume of distribution; $k_{el}$ = elimination rate constant, CL = clearance.

The volume of distribution in a one-compartment model is often referred to as the central volume of distribution ($V_c$) because the volume mainly consists of extracellular fluid. The central compartment represents blood (systemic circulation) plus the organs and tissues that are highly perfused by the blood such as the heart, brain, lungs, liver, and kidney. As such, drugs that follow a one-compartment model are usually polar, distribute rapidly within the body, and are readily eliminated in the urine. Since there is only one compartment, the total volume of distribution ($V_{ss}$) is equal to $V_c$. Thus, the volume of distribution can be denoted as either $V_c$ or $V_{ss}$ because this model contains only one compartment (Fig. 12-2). Similarly, the elimination rate constant ($k_{el}$) can also be denoted as $k_{10}$ because there is only one compartment (compartment = 1) and the drug is eliminated from that compartment; note that this would not be true for a multicompartment model.

The model above illustrates a drug entering the body through an IV bolus injection, being mathematically instantaneously distributed throughout the one compartment, and leaving this compartment at a given rate. Note that drug distribution is not truly instantaneous after an IV bolus injection, as it takes a few minutes for blood to actually circulate throughout the body and throughout this compartment due to cardiac blood flow being approximately 5 to 6 L/min in a typical adult. This explains why we made the distinction between this distribution being instantaneous mathematically (assumed by the PK model), but in clinical practice it is not, and it takes a few minutes. This one-compartment model is a simplistic representation of complex biological processes, yet it is useful in describing and predicting the PK of many drugs.

## CALCULATIONS OF PHARMACOKINETIC PARAMETERS

### Volume of Distribution

The *volume of distribution* ($V_{ss}$) is a mathematical representation of the space (ie, volume) in which a given drug appears to distribute based on the relationship between the dose administered and the concentrations achieved. The one-compartment model considers the body to have a constant volume of distribution over time if the PK is linear, and therefore,

$V_{ss}$ for any given drug in any given patient will be constant. The reader is referred to Chapter 5 for more detail on the physiological aspects of the volume of distribution and how it will distribute in the body, with the assumption that this volume is proportional to the concentration of drug measured in a biological fluid. As we have seen in previous chapters, this is not an actual physiological volume but a theoretical volume in which the drug uniformly distributes after being injected into the body.

The $V_{ss}$ is derived from drug concentrations in the body measured over specified intervals of time. This means that there is a direct relationship between the amount of drug in the body, drug concentrations collected periodically, and the $V_{ss}$, where a measured concentration is simply the amount of drug in the body at the time of collection divided by the volume of distribution. Thus, the $V_{ss}$ relates the concentration of drug in plasma ($C_p$) and the amount of drug in the body ($D_B$) as represented by the following equation:

$$D_B = V_{ss} \cdot C_p \qquad (12.1)$$

The easiest way to estimate the volume of distribution is by characterizing the relationship between the dose (ie, amount of drug administered) and the concentration of drug in the systemic circulation at a theoretical time 0 (ie, immediately after the drug is administered), referred to as $C_p^0$. After time 0, the amount of drug in the body at any given time would not represent the amount administered, because drug is also being eliminated. Thus, the $V_{ss}$ in a one-compartment IV bolus model can be calculated with the following equation:

$$V_{ss} = \frac{D_B^0}{C_p^0} = \frac{\text{Dose}}{C_p^0} \qquad (12.2)$$

where $C_p^0$ represents the instantaneous drug concentration after drug equilibration in the body at $t = 0$. As instantaneous distribution is assumed, the dose of drug given by IV bolus is equivalent to $D_B^0$ (ie, the amount of drug in the body at $t = 0$).

In practice, it is not possible to collect a sample and measure the concentration at Time 0. Therefore, $C_p^0$ must be estimated through back-extrapolation of the slope (m) of concentrations measured after drug administration (ie, post-dose). Since the semi-ln graph of a one-compartment linear IV bolus model

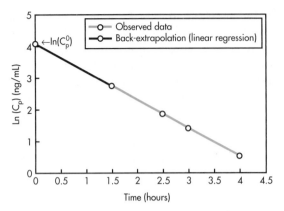

FIGURE 12-3 • Semi-ln graph of the estimation of $C_p^0$ in a one-compartment linear model. Ln($C_p$) = log-normal transformed plasma concentration; ln ($C_p^0$) = log-normal transformed plasma concentration at time 0.

is a straight line (Fig. 12-3), a linear regression can be used to find $C_p^0$.

Ln($C_p$) = log-normal transformed plasma concentration; ln ($C_p^0$) = log-normal transformed plasma concentration at time 0.

Due to the relationship between drug amount, concentration, and volume (see Equation 12.2), and because $V_{ss}$ remains constant over time, concentrations of drug in plasma can be estimated at any time after IV bolus administration when the drug's pharmacokinetic parameters are known. The standard equation for a one-compartment model (IV bolus administration, linear elimination), can be written as:

$$C_p = C_p^0 \cdot e^{-k_{el} \cdot t} \qquad (12.3)$$

where $C_p$ = concentration of drug in plasma at time t and $C_p^0$ = concentration of drug in plasma at $t = 0$.

This formula is also valid for any concentration to be determined at time $t$ based on a concentration measured before time t (Equation 12.4).

$$C_p^{t_2} = C_p^{t_1} \cdot e^{-k_{el} \cdot t_{(2-1)}} \qquad (12.4)$$

where $C_p^{t_2}$ = concentration estimated at time $t_2$, $C_p^{t_1}$ = concentration observed before time $t_2$, and $t_{2-1}$ = the difference between $t_2$ and $t_1$.

## Clearance

Clearance (CL) considers the entire body (or compartment, in the case of a one-compartment model)

as a drug-eliminating system (see Chapters 6 and 15). In other words, clearance is the measure of the capacity of one or more organs to eliminate a drug and it is unaffected by the $V_{ss}$ of a drug *per se*, although in certain circumstances, a clinical situation affecting one may affect the other, for example, a change in a patient body weight will affect both $V_{ss}$ and CL because both PK parameters vary with "body size." CL is a useful parameter clinically, because the overall exposure (AUC$_{\tau(ss)}$ or AUC$_{0-inf}$) relates directly with it and the dose administered as per Equation 12.5, and the overall exposure is the parameter that most correlates with efficacy and safety of drugs.

$$CL = \frac{Dose}{AUC_{0-inf} \text{ or } AUC_{\tau(ss)}} \qquad (12.5)$$

For this reason, pharmacokineticists often prefer to express drug elimination in terms of clearance rather than rate constants. Alternatively, CL can be calculated as:

$$CL = \frac{k_{el} \cdot C_p \cdot V_{ss}}{C_p} = k_{el} \cdot V_{ss} \qquad (12.6)$$

This equation can be rearranged to obtain the $k_{el}$ when CL and $V_{ss}$ are known, or to find the $V_{ss}$ when CL and $k_{el}$ are known. All these parameters are related to one another. There is no such thing as some parameters being really "independent" from the others as is often stipulated. If there is a clinical change resulting in one parameter changing, then one or two of the others may consequently change. For example, and as previously mentioned, a change in body weight in a patient will result in a change in CL and $V_{ss}$ with none or very little change in $k_{el}$. A change in the liver ability to metabolize drugs, such as cirrhosis, will affect $k_{el}$ and CL with no or little effect in $V_{ss}$ if protein binding is unaffected. A change in protein binding will affect both $V_{ss}$ and CL, while not affecting $k_{el}$ if the organ(s) ability at eliminating the drug is (are) unchanged.

To estimate the concentration of drug in plasma at a given time ($C_p$), Equation 12.3 can be re-written in terms of CL and $V_{ss}$:

$$C_p = \frac{Dose}{V_{ss}} \cdot e^{-(CL/V_{ss}) \cdot t} \qquad (12.7)$$

where $C_p$ is the estimated plasma concentration and t is the time associated with the estimated $C_p$.

When only one sample is available ($C_p$) at one sample time point ($t$) after a given dose, Equation 12.7 cannot be solved unambiguously because two unknown parameters must be found (ie, CL and $V_{ss}$). However, CL and $V_{ss}$ can be estimated using known population values (eg, from the literature) if it is not possible to obtain two samples for a given patient. A Bayesian approach can then be used to obtain the patient's $V_{ss}$ and CL based on what is known from the population and the one concentration collected for that patient. Bayesian analyses rely on known population PK parameter values to estimate values for an individual that will best explain data from the one sample that was collected. Clinical pharmacists have applied many variations of this approach to therapeutic drug monitoring and drug dosage adjustments in patients. Special software packages are available to calculate these parameters in a clinical setting (see Chapter 20).

## Elimination Rate Constant

The elimination for most drugs from an organ, tissue, or from the body as a whole is described with first-order processes. The first-order elimination rate constant ($k_{el}$) describes the removal of drug from the body in units of time (eg, $h^{-1}$ or $1/h$) (see Chapters 6 and 13 for information on elimination). The fact that $k_{el}$ is constant over time for a drug displaying linear PK makes it convenient to summarize drug elimination from the body independently of time from the last dose administered or the amount of drug in the body that remains to be eliminated.

The slope of concentrations plotted over time on a semi-ln graph represents the elimination rate constant. In a one-compartment model where two concentrations are obtained (C1 and C2), $k_{el}$ can therefore be calculated using the following equation:

$$k_{el} = \frac{\ln C_1 - \ln C_2}{t_2 - t_1} \tag{12.8}$$

Also, $k_{el}$ can be calculated by rearrangement of Equation 12.6 (Equation 12.9) when $V_{ss}$ and CL are known:

$$k_{el} = \frac{CL}{V_{ss}} \tag{12.9}$$

When data from blood samples are used, the elimination rate constant ($k_{el}$) can be obtained from Equation 12.8. The $k_{el}$ does not identify a route of elimination, but it can be further divided by organs if more information is collected. For example, if urinary excretion data is collected, then the renal elimination rate constant can be calculated, and the overall $k_{el}$ will be the sum of renal ($k_R$) and nonrenal ($k_{NR}$) elimination rate constants as per the following equation.

$$k_{el} = k_R + k_{NR} \tag{12.10}$$

### Renal Elimination Rate Constant

When a drug is eliminated renally, a renal first-order elimination rate constant ($k_R$) can be calculated from urinary excretion data. There are practical considerations to remember when collecting urine for drug analysis. Urine is produced at an approximate rate of 1 mL/min and accumulates in the bladder until voided for sample collection, thus it cannot be collected at specific timepoints like blood samples. Therefore, it is common practice to collect and combine ("pool") urine samples over specified time intervals, and to analyze the urine collected over each interval as one specimen.

Since the urinary excretion rate ($k_R$) of a drug cannot be determined at a specific moment in time, an average urinary excretion rate is calculated for that collection period. The average rate of urinary drug excretion ($D_u/t$) is obtained from dividing the amount of drug measured in urine ($D_u$) by the time associated with end of the collection period ($t$). A straight line is obtained when plotting $D_u/t$ over the midpoint of the collection period ($t_{mid}$) on the semi-ln scale (Fig. 12-4).

Given both $k_{el}$ and $k_R$, the nonrenal rate constant ($k_{NR}$) for any route of elimination other than renal excretion can be determined by as follows:

$$k_{NR} = k_{el} - k_R \tag{12.11}$$

### Elimination Half-Life

The elimination half-life ($t_{1/2}$) represents the amount of time that is required for drug concentrations in the body to be reduced by 50%, as shown in Table 12-1.

When a drug follows first-order elimination, $t_{1/2}$ is independent of the drug concentrations in the body.

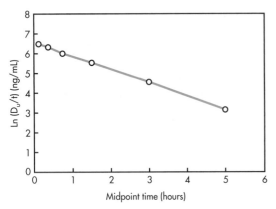

FIGURE 12-4 • Semi-ln graph of renal elimination in a one-compartment linear model with IV bolus administration. Ln(D$_u$/t) = log-normal transformed amount of drug in urine over time.

It is a clinically important parameter, as we will soon see, that can easily be derived from $k_{el}$ or CL and $V_{ss}$:

$$t_{1/2} = \frac{\ln(2)}{k_{el}} \qquad (12.12)$$

$$t_{1/2} = \frac{\ln(2) \cdot V_{ss}}{CL} \qquad (12.13)$$

It is important to consider both the drug dose and the drug's elimination half-life to ensure safe

and effective drug administration. Clinicians can use $t_{1/2}$ to determine an appropriate dosing regimen for an individual patient because this parameter can predict how long it will take for concentrations in the body to fall below a level that would necessitate additional doses. For instance, rearrangement of Equation 12.12 gives Equation 12.14, which leads to Equation 12.15, an expression of the percentage of the drug to be eliminated that remains in the body.

$$0.5 = e^{-k_{el} \cdot t_{1/2}} \qquad (12.14)$$

$$\%\text{Dose remaining} = 0.5^n \cdot 100 \qquad (12.15)$$

where $n$ is the number of half-lives that have elapsed since time of administration. Note that because $t_{1/2}$ is derived from $k_{el}$ or $V_{ss}$ and CL, it considers the impact that changes in these parameters will have on the dosing regimen of a patient.

As demonstrated in Table 12-1, it can be calculated that less than 5% and 1% of drug remains to be eliminated after 5 and 7 half-lives, respectively. Therefore, it is generally assumed that the administered dose is virtually eliminated after either 5 or 7 half-lives. The same is said for the amount of time needed to reach steady state. Steady state is attained within 5 to 7 half-lives, independent of the interval (dosing frequency) at which IV bolus doses are administered. The dosing interval will only affect the concentration levels reached at steady state; short dosing intervals will lead to higher steady-state concentrations than longer intervals.

The $t_{1/2}$ is important in clinical practice because it is used in determining the appropriate dosing interval for a given patient. As discussed in the following sections, the dosing interval can be decided based on (1) whether you want an immediately effective AUC or you want the AUC to be built up over time with accumulation, or (2) the desired $C_{min}$.

### Dosing Interval Based on Accumulation Ratio

The accumulation ratio (AR) is the relationship between dosing interval (τ) and rate of drug elimination ($k_{el}$, $t_{1/2}$) from single dose to steady state (see Chapter 13 for more detail). Accumulation is lower when the τ is long compared to the $t_{1/2}$, and

**TABLE 12-1 • Percentage of Drug Remaining to be Eliminated According to the Half-Life**

| Number of Half-Lives | Drug Eliminated (%) | Drug Remaining (%) |
|---|---|---|
| 1 | 50.00 | 50.00 |
| 2 | 75.00 | 25.00 |
| 3 | 87.50 | 12.50 |
| 4 | 93.75 | 6.250 |
| 5 | 96.88 | 3.125 |
| 6 | 98.44 | 1.563 |
| 7 | 99.22 | 0.781 |
| 8 | 99.61 | 0.391 |
| 9 | 99.80 | 0.195 |
| 10 | 99.90 | 0.098 |

accumulation is higher when the $\tau$ is short compared to the $t_{1/2}$. The AR is calculated as:

$$AR = \frac{AUC_{\tau(SS)}}{AUC_{\tau(SD)}} \qquad (12.16)$$

where $AUC_{\tau(SS)}$ is the AUC over a dosing interval at steady state, and $AUC_{\tau(SD)}$ is the AUC over the first dosing interval (ie, after a single dose).

The AR may be estimated after a single dose with the following equation:

$$AR = \frac{1}{1 - e^{-k_{el} \cdot \tau}} \qquad (12.17)$$

The AR is important in determining dosing regimens because it can be used when one wants the effective AUC to be built up over time. For instance, antipsychotic medications are often associated with adverse side effects that are better tolerated with time. In such cases, one would want a higher accumulation ratio and would therefore want the $\tau$ to be equal to or shorter than the $t_{1/2}$. Another example of using AR in the determination of a patient dosing regimen is when there are limitations to the amount/volume of drug that can be administered. For instance, a maximum volume of 1.5 mL can be administered subcutaneously (SC) and a maximum of 5 mL can be given intramuscularly (IM) due to the discomfort experienced by patients when larger volumes are given. Therefore, for biologics that need to be administered SC or IM only, it may be necessary to slowly build up to an effective AUC through shorter dosing intervals. The AR can also be useful in situations where one is not limited by factors such as adverse side effects or amount of drug that can be administered. For example, drugs with a short elimination half-life, such as antibiotics or beta blockers, can be given in larger doses so that they do not have to be administered as often. The AR would be used to ensure that the drug would not accumulate to toxic levels while allowing for less frequent dosing.

### Dosing Interval Based on $C_{min}$

The trough concentration ($C_{min}$) is the concentration of drug in the target biological fluid (eg, plasma) at steady state and is the lowest concentration before a subsequent dose. When the minimum effective concentration (MEC) of a drug is known or can be determined, $C_{min}$ and MEC can be used to determine an appropriate dosing regimen for a patient. In this situation, there would be a goal $C_{max}$ (ie, concentration below the known level of toxicity and/or concentration that is known to be effective) and a goal $C_{min}$ (ie, the MEC), therefore one would know exactly how many elimination half-lives the dosing interval would need to be.

## CLINICAL UTILITY OF THE ONE-COMPARTMENT MODEL

In clinical practice, compartmental PK can be used to determine appropriate dosing regimens for individual patients. The one-compartment linear model with IV bolus administration is associated with the simplest PK equations. The advantage of using this model is that calculations can be done without the assistance of specialized computer software.

The one-compartment model can be used to determine dosing regimens for drugs that are best characterized by multicompartment models, or when the pharmacokinetic model of a drug is unknown. When doing so, one must consider the potential errors that are being made. By visualizing the concentration-time curves of one-compartment versus two-compartment IV bolus drugs (Fig. 12-5), one can see that relatively little error would be made when predicting $C_{min}$ and $C_{max}$. Therefore the one compartment model can be used to predict $C_{max}$ and $C_{min}$ for drugs that are characterized by multicompartments, if the dosing interval stays unchanged.

The one-compartment model with IV bolus injection can also be used to determine dosing regimens for drugs given by IV infusion (Fig. 12-6). To do so, one must assume that the distribution phase is not important and can be ignored. To avoid the distribution phase, peak concentrations must be measured 1 to 3 hours after the end of infusion.

A prime example of the utility of the one-compartment model to determine dosing regimens for IV infusion drugs is the method described by Sawchuk and Zaske in 1976 (Sawchuk and Zaske, 1976). The Sawchuk–Zaske method can be used for aminoglycosides, such as gentamycin and vancomycin (Sawchuk and Zaske, 1976; Rodvold et al, 1995; Miller et al, 2018). The following section details the use of this method for vancomycin.

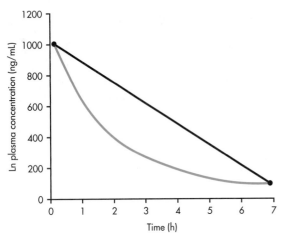

FIGURE 12-5 • PK profiles of hypothetical one-compartment and two-compartment model drugs.

### Example: Sawchuk–Zaske Method for Vancomycin

The Sawchuk–Zaske method uses a one-compartment model to determine parameters and dosing regimens. Therefore, it is assumed that concentrations during the distribution phase can be ignored. To avoid the distribution phase, peak vancomycin concentrations are obtained 1 to 3 hours after the end of infusion. The Sawchuk–Zaske method is commonly used for individualizing dosing regimens for vancomycin based on serum concentration–time data (Rodvold et al, 1995).

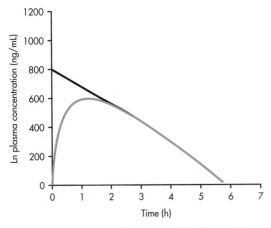

FIGURE 12-6 • PK profiles of hypothetical IV bolus and IV infusion drugs.

The Sawchuk–Zaske method involves using two or more concentration measurements, calculating the $K_{el}$ and $V_D$, and then using the calculated $K_{el}$ and $V_D$ to determine the new dose. Typically, the two concentrations used are a peak ($C_{max}$) and a trough ($C_{min}$) concentration. The first step is to estimate the elimination half-life (Equation 12.18) and apparent volume of distribution (Equation 12.19):

$$t_{1/2} = \frac{0.693}{\ln(C_1/C_2)/(t_2 - t_1)} \tag{12.18}$$

$$V_D = (1.44 \cdot R_0 \cdot t_{1/2}) \cdot \frac{1 - e^{-(0.693/t_{1/2}) \cdot \tau}}{C_{max} - (C_{min} \cdot e^{-(0.693/t_{1/2}) \cdot t'})} \tag{12.19}$$

where $R_0$ is the infusion rate, $\tau$ is the dosing interval, and $t' \rightarrow$ is the length of the infusion period.

Then one must select the desired peak ($C_{max}$) and trough ($C_{min}$) serum vancomycin concentrations and determine the dosing interval:

$$\tau = (1.44 \cdot t_{1/2} \cdot \log \frac{C_{max}}{C_{min}}) + t' \tag{12.20}$$

Next, determine the infusion rate of vancomycin required to obtain the desired $C_{max}$ and $C_{min}$:

$$R_0 = (0.693/t_{1/2}) \cdot V_D \cdot C_{max} \cdot \frac{1 - e^{-(0.693/t_{1/2}) \cdot \tau}}{1 - e^{-(0.693/t_{1/2}) \cdot t'}} \tag{12.21}$$

Finally, estimate the $C_{max}$ (Equation 12.22) after the end of infusion and the $C_{min}$ (Equation 12.23) that would result from the new dosage regimen:

$$C_{max} = \frac{R_0 \cdot t_{1/2} \cdot 1.44}{V_D} \cdot \frac{1 - e^{-(0.693/t_{1/2}) \cdot t'}}{1 - e^{-(0.693/t_{1/2}) \cdot \tau}} \tag{12.22}$$

$$C_{min} = C_{max} \cdot e^{-(0.693/t_{1/2}) \cdot [\tau - (t' + t)]} \tag{12.23}$$

It should be noted that although this method can be used to determine dosing regimens for aminoglycosides, the calculated PK parameter values may not be accurate. Furthermore, up to four concentration measurements may be required to accurately estimate the $K_{el}$ and $V_D$ (Sawchuk and Zaske, 1976; Rodvold et al, 1995).

## CHAPTER SUMMARY

The one-compartment model assumes that a drug is uniformly distributed within a single hypothetical compartment from which the drug concentration can be easily sampled and assayed. The one-compartment model can be parameterized by a volume of distribution and either an elimination rate constant or a clearance. The volume of distribution ($V_{ss}$) is a mathematical representation of the space in which a given drug will distribute in the body, and the magnitude of the $V_{ss}$ relates to the amount of drug outside the sampling compartment (eg, extravascular tissues). Clearance (CL) is a measure of the body's ability to eliminate a drug, and it is expressed as a volume per unit of time (eg, L/h or mL/min). The first-order elimination rate constant ($k_{el}$) represents the fraction of drug that is removed from the body per unit of time, and it is expressed in units of time

(eg, h$^{-1}$ or 1/h). The decision of which parameter to use is largely based on the clinician's preferences. Another important parameter related to elimination is the elimination half-life ($t_{1/2}$), which describes the amount of time required for drug concentrations in the body to be reduced by 50%. These elimination parameters can be calculated using measurements of drug concentration in whole blood, plasma, serum, or urine when the drug is eliminated renally.

Ultimately, the one-compartment model with IV bolus administration is useful in clinical practice, as the calculations are so simple that they can be done without the assistance of a computer. Therefore, clinicians can use this model to make predictions for drugs that either fit multiple compartment models or that are given by IV infusion.

## LEARNING QUESTIONS

1. A 50-kg woman was given a single IV dose of an antibacterial drug at a dose level of 6 mg/kg. The following plasma concentration data were obtained:

| t (hours) | $C_p$ (µg/mL) |
|-----------|---------------|
| 0.25 | 8.21 |
| 0.50 | 7.87 |
| 1.00 | 7.23 |
| 3.00 | 5.15 |
| 6.00 | 3.09 |
| 12.0 | 1.11 |
| 18.0 | 0.40 |

   a. What are the values for $V_{ss}$, $k_{el}$, and $t_{1/2}$ for this drug?

   b. How long would it take for 99.9% of this drug to be eliminated?

2. A drug has an elimination $t_{1/2}$ of 6 hours and follows first-order kinetics. If a single 200-mg dose is given to an adult male patient (68 kg) by IV bolus injection, what percent of the dose is lost in 24 hours?

3. A single IV bolus injection containing 140 mg of gentamicin is given to an adult female patient

(63 years, 55 kg, 5 foot 1) for a sepsis due to E.coli which has been tested to be sensitive to gentamicin (MIC = 0.5 mg/L). The apparent volume of distribution is 0.3 L/kg and the patient has a normal renal function as evidenced by her serum creatinine (Screat) of 0.9 mg/dL. Assuming the drug is well described by first-order kinetics and may be described by a one-compartment model, calculate the following:

   a. The expected Kel of gentamicin in this patient using the following gentamicin nomogram (Ducharme MP et al, Pharmacie clinique et Therapeutique, 3rd ed)

   $k_{el} = 0.01 + 0.003 \times ((140\text{-Age}) \times 0.85)/\text{Screat}$

   b. The $C_p^0$

   c. The concentration of drug in the body 4 hours after the dose is given

   d. The time for the drug to decline to the minimum inhibitory concentration

4. A drug has an elimination half-life of 8 hours and follows first-order elimination kinetics. If a single 600-mg dose is given to an adult female patient (62 kg) by rapid IV injection, what percent of the dose is eliminated (lost) in 24 hours

assuming the apparent $V_{ss}$ is 400 mL/kg? What is the expected plasma drug concentration ($C_p$) at 24 hours postdose?

**5.** For drugs that follow the kinetics of a one-compartment open model, must the tissues and plasma have the same drug concentration? Why?

## ANSWERS

**1.** Dose (IV bolus) = 6 mg/kg × 50 kg = 300 mg

**a.** First, the concentration at time zero (Cp0) must be extrapolated. To find it, the slope describing the disappearance of the concentrations over time must be calculated. This slope will be equal to the kel.

In excel, using linear regression, we find a kel of 0.17028 h$^{-1}$

- The half life is therefore 0.693/0.17028 = 4.07 h
- We now need to back extrapolate the concentration at time zero from the measure concentration at time 0.25 h:

$$C_t = C_0 \times \exp(-k_{el} \times t),$$

therefore $C_0 = C0.25/\exp(-k_{el} \times 0.25)$ = 8.21/exp (−0.17028 × 0.25) = 8.57 mg/L

- The $V_{ss}$ can now be calculated:

$$V_{ss} = \frac{dose}{C_p^0} == \frac{300 \text{ mg}}{8.57 \text{ mg/L}} = 35 \text{ L}$$

**b.** Time required for 99.9% of the drug to be eliminated:

Approximately 10 $t_{1/2}$

$t = 10 \times 4.07 = 40.7$ h

**2.** For first-order elimination kinetics, one-half of the initial quantity is lost each $t_{1/2}$. The following table may be developed:

| Time (hours) | Number of $t_{1/2}$ | Amount of Drug in Body (mg) | Percent of Drug in Body | Percent of Drug Lost |
|---|---|---|---|---|
| 0 | 0 | 200 | 100 | 0 |
| 6 | 1 | 100 | 50 | 50 |
| 12 | 2 | 50 | 25 | 75 |
| 12 | 2 | 50 | 25 | 75 |
| 18 | 3 | 25 | 12.5 | 87.5 |
| 24 | 4 | 12.5 | 6.25 | 93.75 |

From the above table the percent of drug remaining in the body after each $t_{1/2}$ is equal to 100% times (1/2) $n$, where $n$ is the number of half-lives, as shown below:

| Number of $t_{1/2}$ | Percent of Drug in Body | Percent of Drug Remaining in Body after $n\, t_{1/2}$ |
|---|---|---|
| 0 | 100 | |
| 1 | 50 | 100 × 1/2 |
| 2 | 25 | 100 × 1/2 × 1/2 |
| 3 | 12.5 | 100 × 1/2 × 1/2 × 1/2 |
| N | | 100 × (1/2)$^n$ |

Percent of drug remaining $\frac{100}{2^n}$, where $n$ = number of $t_{1/2}$

Percent of drug lost = $100 - \frac{100}{2^n}$

At 24 hours, $n = 4$, since $t_{1/2} = 6$ hours.

Percent of drug lost = $100 - \frac{100}{16} = 93.75\%$

**3. a.** The kel in this patient can be predicted via a nomogram first. Then later on concentrations could be taken, and the $K_{el}$ calculated in the patients. From the nomogram, the kel can be predicted to be:

$k_{el} = 0.01 + 0.003 \times (140 - \text{AGE}) \times 0.85/\text{Screat}$
$= 0.01 + 0.003 \times 77 \times 0.85/0.9 = 0.228$ h$^{-1}$

The $T_{1/2}$ is therefore predicted to be: $T_{1/2}$ = 0.693/0.228 = 3 h

**b.** $C_p^0 = \frac{dose}{V_{ss}} = \frac{140 \text{ mg}}{0.3 \text{ vL/kg·55 kg}} = 8.48$ mg/L

**c.** $C_t = C_0 \times \exp(-k_{el} \times t)$
$C_4 = C_0 \times \exp(-k_{el} \times 4) = 8.48 \times \exp(-0.228 \times 4)$
$= 3.4$ mg/L

**c.** $C_t = C_0 \times \exp(-k_{el} \times t)$ therefore, $C_t/C_0 = \exp(-k_{el} \times t)$, $\mathrm{Ln}(c_t/C_0) = -k_{el} \times t$

and finally $t = \mathrm{Ln}(c_t/C_0)/k_{el}$

Therefore, for this patient the time to reach the MIC concentration of 0.5 mg/L is

$t = \ln(0.5/8.48)/-0.228 = 12.4$ hours

**4. a.** $\log D_B = \dfrac{-k_{el} \cdot t}{2.3} + \log D_B^0$

$= \dfrac{(-0.693/8)(24)}{2.3} + \log 600$

$D_B = 74.9$ mg

Percent drug lost $= \dfrac{600 - 74.9}{600} \cdot 100 = 87.5\%$

$C_p$ at $t = 24$ hours:

$C_p = \dfrac{74.9 \text{ mg}}{(0.4 \text{ L/kg})(62 \text{ kg})} = 3.02 \text{ mg/L}$

**5.** If a drug is well described by a one-compartment model after IV administration, then the concentrations in the plasma will eventually also reach different tissues from the systemic circulation, such that drug concentrations in tissues will never be as high as those in the plasma (penetration in the bone may only be 40%, for example), but because the elimination of the drug only occurs from the systemic circulation (liver and kidney), the minimum concentration achieved in the different tissues will never be lower than the one achieved in the systemic circulation. The drug concentrations in the tissues may also differ from those achieved systemically because of differences in drug-protein binding between tissues and plasma, partitioning of drug into fat, differences in pH in different regions of the body causing a different degree of ionization for a weakly dissociated electrolyte drug, active tissue uptake process, etc.

## REFERENCES

Ducharme MP. Principes d'utilisation des antibiotiques. Pharmacie clinique et thérapeutique. 3e ed. Paris: Masson. 2008:935–958

Miller C, Winans A, Veillette J, Forland S: Use of individual pharmacokinetics to improve time to therapeutic vancomycin trough in pediatric oncology patients. *J Pediatr Pharmacol Ther* 23(2):92–99, 2018.

Rodvold KA, Erdman SM, Pryka RD: Vancomycin. *Therapeutic Drug Monitoring*. Schumacher GE (ed). East Norwalk, Appleton & Lange, 1995. Chapter 19.

Sawchuk R, Zaske D: Pharmacokinetics of dosing regimens which utilize multiple intravenous infusions: Gentamicin in burn patients. *J Pharmacokinet Biopharm* 4(2):183–195, 1976.

## BIBLIOGRAPHY

Doyle GR, and McCutcheon JA: *Clinical Procedures for Safer Patient Care.* BC Campus, 2015.

Gibaldi M, Nagashima R, Levy G: Relationship between drug concentration in plasma or serum and amount of drug in the body. *J Pharm Sci* 58:193–197, 1969.

Riegelman S, Loo JCK, Rowland M: Shortcomings in pharmacokinetic analysis by conceiving the body to exhibit properties of a single compartment. *J Pharm Sci* 57:117–123, 1968.

Riegelman S, Loo J, Rowland M: Concepts of volume of distribution and possible errors in evaluation of this parameter. *Science* 57:128–133, 1968.

Wagner JG, Northam JI: Estimation of volume of distribution and half-life of a compound after rapid intravenous injection. *J Pharm Sci* 58:529–531, 1975.

# 13

# Multicompartment Models: Intravenous Bolus Administration

Shabnam N. Sani and Rodney C. Siwale

## CHAPTER OBJECTIVES

- Define the pharmacokinetic terms used in a two- and three-compartment model.

- Explain using examples why drugs follow one-compartment, two-compartment, or three-compartment kinetics.

- Use equations and graph to simulate plasma drug concentration at various time periods after an IV bolus injection of a drug that follows the pharmacokinetics of a two- and three-compartment model drug.

- Relate the relevance of the magnitude of the volume of distribution and clearance of various drugs to underlying processes in the body.

- Explain the consequences of using $V_c$, $V_{area}$ (or $V_\beta$), versus $V_{ss}$ to calculate a loading dose

- Estimate two-compartment model parameters by using the method of residuals.

- Calculate clearance and alpha and beta half-lives of a two-compartment model drug.

- Explain how drug metabolic enzymes, transporters, and binding proteins in the body may modify the distribution and/or elimination phase of a drug after IV bolus.

Pharmacokinetic models are used to simplify all the complex processes that occur during drug administration, including drug distribution and elimination in the body. The model simplification is necessary because of the inability to measure quantitatively all the rate processes in the body, including the lack of access to biological samples from the interior of the body. As described in Chapter 1, pharmacokinetic models are used to simulate drug disposition under different conditions/time points so that optimal dosing regimens for individuals or groups of patients can be designed.

Compartmental models are classic pharmacokinetic models that simulate the kinetic processes of drug absorption, distribution, and elimination with minimal physiologic details. In contrast, the more sophisticated physiologic models are discussed in Chapter 19. In compartmental models, drug concentrations are assumed to be uniform and instantly distributed within each given hypothetical compartments. Hence, all muscle mass and connective tissues may be lumped into one hypothetical tissue compartment that equilibrates with drug from the central (composed of blood, extracellular fluid, and highly perfused organs/tissues such as heart, liver, and kidneys) compartment. Conventionally, since no data are collected on the tissue mass, the theoretical tissue concentration cannot be confirmed and used to forecast actual tissue drug levels. Only a theoretical, $C_t$, concentration of drug in the tissue compartment (or more commonly referred to as the peripheral compartment as $C_p$) can be calculated. Obviously, in contrast to compartment models, the drug concentrations in a particular tissue mass may not be homogeneously distributed. In reality, the body is more complex than depicted in the simple one- and multicompartment models, and the eliminating organs, such as the liver and kidneys, are much more complex than being simple extractors. Multicompartment models are helpful to gain a better appreciation regarding how drugs are handled in the body. Contrary to the mono-exponential decay observed with the simple one-compartment model, most drugs given by IV bolus dose decline in a biphasic fashion; that is, plasma drug concentrations rapidly decline soon after IV bolus injection, and then decline moderately as some of the drug distributes (equilibrates) into the tissue and moves back into the plasma. The early decline phase is commonly called the *distribution phase* (because distribution into tissues primarily determines the early rapid decline in plasma concentration) and the latter phase is called the terminal *elimination phase*. During the distribution phase, changes in the concentration of drug in plasma primarily reflect the movement of drug within the body, rather than elimination. However, with time, distribution equilibrium is established in more and more tissues between the tissue and plasma, and eventually changes in plasma concentration reflect proportional changes in the concentrations of drug in all other tissues (assuming drug follows first-order rate of elimination). During this proportionality phase, the body kinetically acts as a single compartment and because decline of the plasma concentration is now associated solely with elimination of drug from the body, this phase is often called the elimination phase.

Concentration of the drug in the tissue compartment ($C_t$), may not necessarily be a useful parameter due to the nonhomogenous tissue distribution of drugs, although relationships have been found between the predicted peripheral ("tissue") concentrations of digoxin and its pharmacological effect on the heart. The amount of the drug in the tissue compartment ($X_t$ or $X_p$) is also a predicted indicator of how much drug accumulates extravascularly in the body at any given time. The two-compartment model provides a simple way to keep track of the mass balance of the drug in the body.

Multicompartment models provide answers to such questions as: (1) How much of a dose is eliminated? (2) How much drug remains in the plasma compartment at any given time?, and (3) How much drug accumulates in the tissue compartment? The latter information is particularly useful for drug safety since the amount of drug in a deep tissue compartment may accumulate and be harder to eliminate by renal excretion or by dialysis after drug overdose.

Multicompartment models explain the observation that, after a rapid IV bolus drug injection, the plasma level–time curve does not decline in a mono-exponential decline, implying that the drug does not equilibrate rapidly in the body, as observed for a single first-order rate process in a one-compartment model. Instead, a biphasic or triphasic drug concentration decline is often observed. The initial decline phase represents the drug leaving the plasma compartment and entering one or more tissue compartments as well as being eliminated. Later, after drug distribution to the tissues is completed, the plasma drug concentrations decline more gradually when eventually plasma drug equilibrium with peripheral tissues occurs. Classically, in a two-compartment model, the two phases observed were called α and β, representing the distribution and elimination phases, respectively. The issue with this terminology was that the terminal phase would be associated with a different term depending on the number of exponentials or compartments needed in the PK model. For example, the only terminal phase for a one-compartment model could be called a, while for two and three compartment models it would be called b and d. It is therefore less confusing to call the different phases λ, with the terminal phase always specified as $\lambda_z$, and the previous phases denoted by λ with successive numbers (1, 2, 3, etc). Thereby, the exponentials would be $\lambda_z$ for a monoexponential decline (a one-compartment model), $\lambda_1$ and $\lambda_z$ for a bi-exponential decline (a two-compartment model), $\lambda_1$ $\lambda_2$, and $\lambda_z$ for a tri-exponential decline (a three-compartment model), and so on. Figure 13-1 illustrates

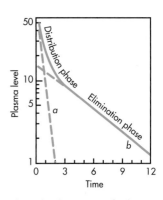

FIGURE 13-1 • Plasma level–time curve for the two-compartment open model (single IV dose) described in Fig. 13-2 (model A).

the elimination phase that can be obtained from the terminal slope of the plasma level–time curve using a semilogarithmic plot (Fig. 13-1).

Nonlinear plasma drug level–time decline occurs because some drugs distribute at various rates into different tissue groups. Multicompartment models were developed to explain and predict plasma and tissue concentrations for those types of drugs. In these models, each compartment represents organs that are perfused in a similar manner by cardiac blood flow. In a one-compartment model, these will include the blood, the extracellular fluid volume, and all organs that are extremely well perfused by the heart such as the kidney and the liver. When drugs distribute in other organs that are not as well perfused by cardiac blood flow but in a similar manner, additional compartments are added. In a two- and a three-compartment model, for example, one would find organs that are not well perfused by the heart and even less well perfused, respectively. The extent of drug distribution in tissues and organs is partially determined by the physical-chemical properties of the drug. For instance, aminoglycosides are polar, water-soluble molecules, and their distribution is primarily limited to extracellular water. Their pharmacokinetics is thereby well described by a one-compartment model. Lipophilic drugs with more extensive distribution into tissues such as the benzodiazepines or those with extensive intracellular uptake are better described by more complex models. For both one- and multicompartment models, the drug in those tissues that have the highest blood perfusion equilibrates rapidly with the drug in the plasma. These highly perfused tissues and blood make up the *central compartment* (often called the *plasma compartment*). While this initial drug distribution is taking place, multicompartment drugs are delivered concurrently to one or more *peripheral compartments* (often considered as the *tissue compartment that includes fat, muscle, and cerebrospinal fluid*) composed of groups of tissues with lower blood perfusion and different affinity for the drug. A drug will concentrate in a tissue in accordance with the *affinity* of the drug for that particular tissue. For example, lipid-soluble drugs tend to accumulate in adipose tissues. Drugs that bind plasma proteins may be more concentrated in the plasma, because only free (from protein binding) drugs diffuse easily into the tissues. Drugs may also bind with tissue proteins and other macromolecules, such as DNA and melanin.

Tissue sampling is invasive, and the drug concentration in the tissue sample may not represent the drug concentration in the entire organ due to the nonhomogenous tissue distribution. In recent years, the development of novel experimental methods such as magnetic resonance spectroscopy (MRS), single-photon emission computed tomography (SPECT), and tissue microdialysis have enabled the study of the drug distribution in the target tissues of animals and humans (Eichler and Müller, 1998; Müller, 2009). These innovative technologies have enabled us to follow the path of the drug from the plasma compartment into anatomically defined regions or tissues. More importantly, for some classes of drugs, the concentration in the interstitial fluid space of the target tissue can be measured. This also affords a means to quantify, for the first time, the inter- or intra-individual variability associated with the *in vivo* distribution process. Although these novel techniques are promising, measurement of drug or active metabolite concentrations in target tissues and the subsequent development of associated pharmacokinetic models is not a routine practice in standard drug development and is not mandated by regulatory requirements. Occasionally, tissue samples may be collected after a drug overdose episode. For example, the two-compartment model has been used to describe the distribution of colchicine, even though the drug's toxic tissue levels after fatal overdoses have only been recently described (Rochdi et al, 1992). Colchicine distribution is now known to be affected by P-gp (also known as ABCB1 or MDR1, a common transport protein of the ABC [ATP-binding cassette] transporter subfamily found in the body). Drug transporters are now known to influence the curvature in the log plasma drug concentration–time graph of drugs. The drug isotretinoin has a long half-life because of substantial distribution into lipid tissues.

Kinetic analysis of a multicompartment model initially assumes that all transfer rate processes for the passage of drug into or out of individual compartments are first-order processes. On the basis of this assumption, the plasma level–time curve for a drug that follows a multicompartment model is best

## TABLE 13-1 • Blood Flow to Human Tissues

| Tissue | Percent Body Weight | Percent Cardiac Output | Blood Flow (mL/100 g tissue per min) |
|---|---|---|---|
| Adrenals | 0.02 | 1 | 550 |
| Kidneys | 0.4 | 24 | 450 |
| Thyroid | 0.04 | 2 | 400 |
| Liver | | | |
|   Hepatic | 2.0 | 5 | 20 |
|   Portal | | 20 | 75 |
| Portal-drained viscera | 2.0 | 20 | 75 |
| Heart (basal) | 0.4 | 4 | 70 |
| Brain | 2.0 | 15 | 55 |
| Skin | 7.0 | 5 | 5 |
| Muscle (basal) | 40.0 | 15 | 3 |
| Connective tissue | 7.0 | 1 | 1 |
| Fat | 15.0 | 2 | 1 |

Data from Spector WS: Handbook of Biological Data. Philadelphia, PA: Saunders; 1956; Glaser O: Medical Physics, Vol II. Chicago, IL: Year Book Publishers; 1950; Butler TC: Proc First International Pharmacological Meeting, vol 6. Philadelphia, PA: Pergamon Press; 1962.

described by the summation of a series of exponential terms, each corresponding to first-order rate processes associated with a given compartment. Most multicompartment models used in pharmacokinetics are *mamillary models*. Mamillary models are well connected and dynamically exchange drug concentration between compartments making them very suitable for modeling drug distribution.

Because of numerous distribution factors, drugs will generally concentrate unevenly in the tissues, and different groups of tissues will accumulate the drug at very different rates. A summary of the approximate blood flow to major human tissues is presented in Table 13-1. Many different tissues and

rate processes are involved in the distribution of drugs. However, limited physiologic significance has been assigned to a few groups of tissues (Table 13-2).

The nonlinear profile of plasma drug concentration–time is the result of many factors interacting together, including blood flow to the tissues, the permeability of the drug into the tissues (fat solubility), partitioning, the capacity of the tissues to accumulate drug, and the effect of disease factors on these processes (see Chapter 5). Impaired cardiac function may produce a change in blood flow, and these affect the drug distributive phase, whereas impairment of the kidney or the liver may decrease drug elimination, as shown by a prolonged elimination half-life

## TABLE 13-2 • General Grouping of Tissues According to Blood Supply*

| Blood Supply | Tissue Group | Percent Body Weight |
|---|---|---|
| Highly perfused | Heart, brain, hepatic-portal system, kidney, and endocrine glands | 9 |
| | Skin and muscle | 50 |
| | Adipose (fat) tissue and marrow | 19 |
| Slowly perfused | Bone, ligaments, tendons, cartilage, teeth, and hair | 22 |

*Tissue uptake will also depend on such factors as fat solubility, degree of ionization, partitioning, and protein binding of the drug.
Adapted with permission from Papper EM, Kitz JR: Uptake and Distribution of Anesthetic Agents. New York, NY: McGraw Hill; 1963.

and corresponding reduction in the slope of the terminal elimination phase of the curve. Frequently, multiple factors can complicate the distribution profile in such a way that the profile can only be described clearly with the assistance of a computer simulation model.

## TWO-COMPARTMENT OPEN MODEL

Many drugs given in a single intravenous bolus dose demonstrate a plasma level–time curve that does not decline as a single exponential (first-order) process. The plasma level–time curve for a drug that follows a two-compartment model (Fig. 13-1) shows that the plasma drug concentration declines *biexponentially* as the sum of two first-order processes—distribution and elimination. A drug that follows the pharmacokinetics of a two-compartment model does not equilibrate rapidly throughout the body, as is assumed for a one-compartment model. In this model, the drug distributes into two compartments, the central compartment and the tissue, or peripheral, compartment. The drug distributes rapidly and uniformly in the central compartment. A second compartment, known as the *tissue* or *peripheral compartment,* contains tissues in which the drug equilibrates more slowly. Drug transfer between the two compartments is assumed to take place by first-order processes.

There are several possible two-compartment models (Fig. 13-2). Model A is used most often and describes the plasma level–time curve observed in Fig. 13-1. By convention, compartment 1 is the central compartment and compartment 2 is the tissue or peripheral compartment. The rate constants $k_{12}$ and $k_{21}$ represent the first-order rate transfer constants for the movement of drug from compartment 1 to compartment 2 ($k_{12}$) and from compartment 2 to compartment 1 ($k_{21}$). The transfer constants are sometimes termed *microconstants*, and their values cannot be estimated directly on a semi-log graph. Most two-compartment models assume that elimination occurs from the central compartment model, as shown in Fig. 13-2 (model A), unless other information about the drug is known. Drug elimination is presumed to occur from the central compartment, because the major sites of drug elimination (renal excretion and hepatic drug metabolism) occur in organs such as the kidney and liver, which are highly perfused with blood.

The plasma level–time curve for a drug that follows a two-compartment model may be divided into two parts, (a) a distribution phase and (b) an elimination phase. After an IV bolus injection, the relatively rapid cardiac blood flow (5 to 6 liters per minute in a typical adult) will ensure that drug equilibrates rapidly within the central compartment. It is important to note that compartment models assumed mathematically that the distribution within each compartment is instantaneous. This is obviously not the case, as cardiac blood flow is not infinite, but for most drugs, the PK behavior will be well characterized (in rare cases where the metabolism is faster than the cardiac blood flow, for example adenosine, different compartmental models will need to be specified to take this into account). The *distribution phase* of the curve represents the initial, more rapid decline of drug from the central compartment into the peripheral compartment (Fig. 13-1, line *a*). Although drug elimination and distribution occur *concurrently* during the distribution phase, there is a net transfer of drug from the central compartment to the peripheral compartment because the rate of distribution is faster than the rate of elimination. The fraction of drug in the peripheral compartment during the distribution phase increases up to a maximum in a given tissue, whose value may be greater or less than the plasma drug concentration. At maximum peripheral concentrations, the rate of drug entry into the peripheral compartment equals the rate of drug exit from

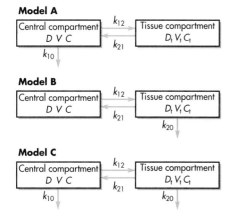

• Two-compartment open models, intravenous injection.

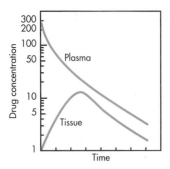

**FIGURE 13-3** • Relationship between tissue and plasma drug concentrations for a two-compartment open model. The maximum tissue drug concentration may be greater or less than the plasma drug concentration.

the peripheral compartment. The fraction of drug in the peripheral compartment is now in equilibrium (*distribution equilibrium*) with the fraction of drug in the central compartment (Fig. 13-3), and the

drug concentrations in both the central and peripheral compartments decline in parallel and more slowly compared to the distribution phase. This decline is a first-order process and is called the *elimination phase* or the *β* or *λ_z* *phase* (Fig. 13-1, line *b*). Since plasma and tissue concentrations decline in parallel, plasma drug concentrations provide some indication of the concentration of drug in the peripheral compartment. At this point, drug kinetics appears to follow a one-compartment model in which drug elimination is a first-order process described by *β* or *λ_z*. A typical tissue drug level curve after a single intravenous dose is shown in Fig. 13-3.

The processes that contribute to drug disposition after IV bolus administration in a two-compartment system are illustrated schematically in Fig. 13-4.

Peripheral drug concentrations in the pharmacokinetic model are theoretical only. The drug level in the theoretical peripheral compartment can

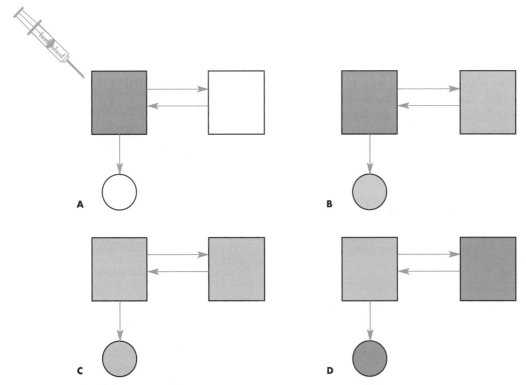

**FIGURE 13-4** • (A) Drug equilibrates instantly within the central compartment upon administration and the hypothetical concentration in the peripheral compartment is zero. (B) Drug is distributed into both the peripheral compartment and being systemically eliminated. (C) unbound drug in the central and peripheral compartments exists in a state of distributional equilibrium. (D) Drug elimination from the central compartment shifts the concentration gradient and drug moves back from the peripheral to the central compartment.

be calculated once the parameters for the model are estimated. However, the drug concentration in the peripheral compartment represents the *average* predicted drug concentration in a group of tissues rather than any real anatomic tissue drug concentration. In reality, drug concentrations may vary among different tissues and possibly within an individual tissue. These varying tissue drug concentrations are due to differences in the partitioning of drug into the tissues, as discussed in Chapter 5. Thus, tissue drug concentration may be higher or lower than the plasma drug concentrations, depending on the properties of the individual tissue and the binding properties of the drug in the tissues. Moreover, the transfer rate of drug from the tissue compartment is unlikely to be the same as the elimination rate directly from the central compartment. For example, if $k_{12} \cdot C_p$ is greater than $k_{21} \cdot C_t$ (rate into tissue > rate out of tissue), tissue drug concentrations will increase and plasma drug concentrations will decrease. Compartment models can also be modified to include actual tissue drug concentrations, such as synovial fluid or cancer cells for example, and can therefore explain not just concentrations in plasma, but concentrations that can be collected at different sites of action.

Despite the hypothetical nature of the peripheral compartment, the theoretical tissue level is still valuable information for clinicians. The theoretical tissue concentration, together with the blood concentration, gives an accurate method of calculating the total amount of drug remaining in the body at any given time (see digoxin example in Table 13-5). This information would not be available without pharmacokinetic models.

In practice, a blood sample is removed periodically from the central compartment and the plasma is analyzed for the presence of drug. The drug plasma level–time curve represents a phase of initial rapid equilibration with the central compartment (the distribution phase), followed by an elimination phase after the peripheral compartment has also equilibrated with drug. The distribution phase may take minutes or hours and may be missed entirely if the blood is sampled too late or at wide intervals after drug administration.

In the model depicted above, $k_{12}$ and $k_{21}$ are first-order rate constants that govern the rate of drug distribution into and out of the peripheral and plasma:

$$\frac{dC_p}{dt} = k_{12}C - k_{21}C_p \qquad (13.1)$$

$$\frac{dC}{dt} = k_{21}C_p - k_{12}C - k_{10}C \qquad (13.2)$$

The relationship between the amount of drug in each compartment and the concentration of drug in that compartment is shown by Equations 13.3 and 13.4:

$$C = \frac{X_c}{V_c} \qquad (13.3)$$

$$C_p = \frac{X_p}{V_p} \qquad (13.4)$$

where $X_c$ = amount of drug in the central compartment, $X_p$ = amount of drug in the peripheral compartment, $V_c$ = volume of drug in the central compartment, and $V_p$ = volume of drug in the peripheral compartment.

$$\frac{dX_c}{dt} = -k_{10}X_c - k_{12}X_c + k_{21}X_p \qquad (13.5)$$

$$\frac{dX_p}{dt} = k_{12}X_c - k_{21}X_p \qquad (13.6)$$

Solving Equations 13.5 and 13.6 using Laplace transforms and matrix algebra will give Equations 13.7 and 13.8, which describe the change in drug concentration in the blood and in the tissue with respect to time:

$$C = \frac{X_c^0}{V_c}\left(\frac{k_{21}-\alpha}{\beta-\alpha}e^{-\alpha t} + \frac{k_{21}-\beta}{\alpha-\beta}e^{-\beta t}\right) \qquad (13.7)$$

$$C_p = \frac{k_{21}-X_c^0}{V_p(\alpha-\beta)}(e^{-\beta t} - e^{-\alpha t}) \qquad (13.8)$$

$$X = X_c^0\left(\frac{k_{21}-\alpha}{\beta-\alpha}e^{-\alpha t} + \frac{k_{21}-\beta}{\alpha-\beta}e^{-\beta t}\right) \qquad (13.9)$$

$$X_p = \frac{k_{21}-X_c^0}{(\alpha-\beta)}(e^{-\beta t} - e^{-\alpha t}) \qquad (13.10)$$

where $X_c^0$ is dose given intravenously, $t$ is time after administration of dose, and $\alpha$ and $\beta$ are constants that depend solely on $k_{12}$, $k_{21}$, and $k_{10}$. The amount of drug remaining in the plasma and tissue compartments at any time may be described realistically by Equations 13.9 and 13.10.

The rate constants for the transfer of drug between compartments are referred to as *microconstants* or *transfer constants*. They relate the amount of drug being transferred per unit of time from one compartment to the other. The values for these microconstants cannot be determined by direct measurement, but they can be estimated by a graphical method.

$$\alpha + \beta = k_{12} + k_{21} + k_{10} \qquad (13.11)$$

$$\alpha\beta = k_{21} k_{10} \qquad (13.12)$$

The constants $\alpha$ and $\beta$ are hybrid first-order rate constants for the distribution phase and elimination phase, respectively. The mathematical relationships of $\alpha$ and $\beta$ to the rate constants are given by Equations 13.11 and 13.12, which are derived after integration of Equations 13.5 and 13.6. Equation 13.7 can be transformed into the following expression:

$$C = Ae^{-\alpha t} + Be^{-\beta t} \qquad (13.13)$$

The constants $\alpha$ and $\beta$ are rate constants for the distribution phase and elimination phase, respectively. The constants $A$ and $B$ are intercepts on the $y$ axis for each exponential segment of the curve in Equation 13.13. These values may be obtained graphically by the method of residuals or by computer. Intercepts $A$ and $B$ are actually hybrid constants, as shown in Equations 13.14 and 13.15, and do not have actual physiologic significance.

$$A = \frac{X_0(\alpha - k_{21})}{V_c(\alpha - \beta)} \qquad (13.14)$$

$$B = \frac{X_0(k_{21} - \beta)}{V_c(\alpha - \beta)} \qquad (13.15)$$

Note that the values of $A$ and $B$ are empirical constants directly proportional to the dose administered. All the rate constants involved in two-compartment model will have units consistent with the first-order process (Jambhekar and Breen, 2009).

## Method of Residuals

The *method of residuals* (also known as *feathering*, *peeling*, or *curve stripping*) is a commonly employed technique for resolving a curve into various exponential terms. This method allows the separation of the monoexponential constituents of a biexponential plot of plasma concentration against time, and therefore it is a useful procedure for fitting a curve to the experimental data of a drug when the drug does not clearly follow a one-compartment model. For example, 100 mg of a drug was administered by rapid IV injection to a healthy 70-kg adult male. Blood samples were taken periodically after the administration of drug, and the plasma drug concentration of each sample was assayed. The following data were obtained:

| Time (hour) | Plasma Drug Concentration ($\mu$g/mL) |
|---|---|
| 0.25 | 43.00 |
| 0.5 | 32.00 |
| 1.0 | 20.00 |
| 1.5 | 14.00 |
| 2.0 | 11.00 |
| 4.0 | 6.50 |
| 8.0 | 2.80 |
| 12.0 | 1.20 |
| 16.0 | 0.52 |

When these data are plotted on semilogarithmic graph paper, a curved line is observed (Fig. 13-5). The curved-line relationship between the logarithm of the plasma concentration and time indicates that the drug is distributed in more than one compartment. From these data, a biexponential equation, Equation 1.13, may be derived, either by computer or by the method of residuals.

As shown in the biexponential curve in Fig. 13-5, the decline in the initial distribution phase is more rapid than the elimination phase. The rapid distribution phase is confirmed with the constant $\alpha$ being larger than the rate constant $\beta$. Therefore, at some later time (generally at a time following the attainment of distribution equilibrium), the term $Ae^{-\alpha t}$ will approach 0, while $Be^{-\beta t}$ will still have a

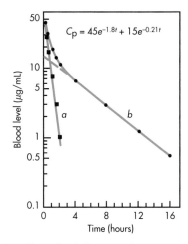

FIGURE 13-5 • Plasma level–time curve for a two-compartment open model. The rate constants and intercepts were calculated by the method of residuals.

finite value. At this later time, Equation 13.13 will reduce to:

$$C = Be^{-\beta t} \tag{13.16}$$

which, in common logarithms, is:

$$\log C = \log B - \frac{\beta t}{2.3} \tag{13.17}$$

From Equation 13.17, the rate constant can be obtained from the slope $(-\beta/2.3)$ of a straight line representing the terminal exponential phase (Fig. 13-5).

The $t_{1/2}$ for the elimination phase (beta half-life) can be derived from the following relationship:

$$t_{1/2\beta} = \frac{0.693}{\beta} \tag{13.18}$$

In the sample case considered here, $\beta$ was found to be 0.21 h$^{-1}$. From this information the regression line for the terminal exponential or $\beta$ phase is extrapolated to the $y$ axis; the $y$ intercept is equal to $B$, or 15 $\mu$g/mL. Values from the extrapolated line are then subtracted from the original experimental data points (Table 13-3) and a straight line is obtained. This line represents the rapidly distributed $\alpha$ phase (Fig. 13-5).

The new line obtained by graphing the logarithm of the residual plasma concentration $(C - C')$ against time represents the $\alpha$ phase. The value for $\alpha$ is 1.8 h$^{-1}$, and the $y$ intercept is 45 $\mu$g/mL. The elimination $t_{1/2\beta}$ is computed from $\beta$ by the use of Equation 13.18 and has the value of 3.3 hours.

A number of pharmacokinetic parameters may be derived by proper substitution of rate constants $\alpha$ and $\beta$ and $y$ intercepts $A$ and $B$ into the following equations:

$$k_{10} = \frac{\alpha\beta(A+B)}{A\beta + B\alpha} \tag{13.19}$$

$$k_{12} = \frac{AB(\beta-\alpha)^2}{(A+B)(A\beta + B\alpha)} \tag{13.20}$$

$$k_{21} = \frac{(A\beta + B\alpha)}{A+B} \tag{13.21}$$

## TABLE 13-3 • Application of the Method of Residuals

| Time (hour) | $C_p$ Observed Plasma Level | $C_p'$ Extrapolated Plasma Concentration | $C_p - C_p'$ Residual Plasma Concentration |
|---|---|---|---|
| 0.25 | 43.0 | 14.5 | 28.5 |
| 0.5 | 32.0 | 13.5 | 18.5 |
| 1.0 | 20.0 | 12.3 | 7.7 |
| 1.5 | 14.0 | 11.0 | 3.0 |
| 2.0 | 11.0 | 10.0 | 1.0 |
| 4.0 | 6.5 | | |
| 8.0 | 2.8 | | |
| 12.0 | 1.2 | | |
| 16.0 | 0.52 | | |

When an administered drug exhibits the characteristics of a two-compartment model, the difference between the distribution rate constant $\alpha$ and the slow post-distribution/elimination rate constant $\beta$ plays a critical role. The greater the difference between $\alpha$ and $\beta$, the greater is the need to apply two-compartment model. Failure to do so will result in false clinical predictions (Jambhekar and Breen, 2009). On the other hand, if this difference is small, it will not cause any significant difference in the clinical predictions, regardless of the model chosen to describe the pharmacokinetics of a drug. Then it may be prudent to follow the principle of *parsimony* when selecting the compartment model by choosing the simpler of the two available models (eg, one-compartment versus two) (Jambhekar and Breen, 2009).

## CLINICAL APPLICATION

### Digoxin in a Normal Patient and in a Renal-Failure Patient—Simulation of Plasma and Tissue Level of a Two-Compartment Model Drug

Once the pharmacokinetic parameters are determined for an individual, the amount of drug remaining in the plasma and tissue compartments may be calculated using Equations 13.9 and 13.10. The pharmacokinetic data for digoxin were calculated in a normal and in a renal-impaired, 70-kg subject using the parameters in Table 13-4 as reported in the literature. The amount of digoxin remaining in the plasma and tissue compartments is tabulated in Table 13-5

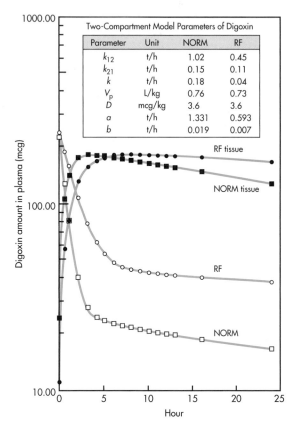

| Two-Compartment Model Parameters of Digoxin | | | |
|---|---|---|---|
| Parameter | Unit | NORM | RF |
| $k_{12}$ | t/h | 1.02 | 0.45 |
| $k_{21}$ | t/h | 0.15 | 0.11 |
| $k$ | t/h | 0.18 | 0.04 |
| $V_p$ | L/kg | 0.76 | 0.73 |
| $D$ | mcg/kg | 3.6 | 3.6 |
| $a$ | t/h | 1.331 | 0.593 |
| $b$ | t/h | 0.019 | 0.007 |

**FIGURE 13-6** • Amount of digoxin (simulated) in the plasma and tissue compartment after an IV dose to a normal and a renal-failure (RF) patient.

and plotted in Fig. 13-6. It can be seen that digoxin stored in the plasma declines rapidly during the initial distributive phase, while drug amount in the tissue compartment takes 3 to 4 hours to accumulate for a normal subject. It is interesting that clinicians have recommended that digoxin plasma samples be taken at least several hours after IV bolus dosing (3–4+ hours) (Reuning et al, 1973; Jelliffe, 2014) for a normal subject, since the equilibrated level is more representative of myocardium digoxin level. In the simulation below, the amount of the drug in the plasma compartment at any time divided by $V_c$ (54.6 L for the normal subject) will yield the plasma digoxin level. At 4 hours after an IV dose of 0.25 mg, $C = X_c/V_c = 24.43\ \mu g/54.6\ L = 0.45\ ng/mL$, corresponding to $3 \times 0.45\ ng/mL = 1.35\ ng/mL$ if a full loading dose of 0.75 mg is given in a single dose.

**TABLE 13-4** • Two-Compartment Model Pharmacokinetic Parameters of Digoxin

| Parameters | Unit | Normal | Renal Impaired |
|---|---|---|---|
| $k_{12}$ | h⁻¹ | 1.02 | 0.45 |
| $k_{21}$ | h⁻¹ | 0.15 | 0.11 |
| $k$ | h⁻¹ | 0.18 | 0.04 |
| $V_p$ | L/kg | 0.78 | 0.73 |
| $D$ | μg/kg | 3.6 | 3.6 |
| $a$ | 1/h | 1.331 | 0.593 |
| $b$ | 1/h | 0.019 | 0.007 |

## TABLE 13-5 • Amount of Digoxin in Plasma and Tissue Compartment after an IV Dose of 0.252 mg in a Normal and a Renal-Failure Patient Weighing 70 kg*

| | Digoxin Amount | | | |
| | Normal Renal Function | | Renal Failure | |
| Time (hour) | $D_p$ (µg) | $D_t$ (µg) | $D_p$ (µg) | $D_t$ (µg) |
|---|---|---|---|---|
| 0.00 | 252.00 | 0.00 | 252.00 | 0.00 |
| 0.10 | 223.68 | 24.04 | 240.01 | 11.01 |
| 0.60 | 126.94 | 105.54 | 189.63 | 57.12 |
| 1.00 | 84.62 | 140.46 | 158.78 | 85.22 |
| 2.00 | 40.06 | 174.93 | 107.12 | 131.72 |
| 3.00 | 27.95 | 181.45 | 78.44 | 156.83 |
| 4.00 | 24.43 | 180.62 | 62.45 | 170.12 |
| 5.00 | 23.17 | 177.91 | 53.48 | 176.88 |
| 6.00 | 22.53 | 174.74 | 48.39 | 180.04 |
| 7.00 | 22.05 | 171.50 | 45.45 | 181.21 |
| 8.00 | 21.62 | 168.28 | 43.69 | 181.29 |
| 9.00 | 21.21 | 165.12 | 42.59 | 180.77 |
| 10.00 | 20.81 | 162.01 | 41.85 | 179.92 |
| 11.00 | 20.42 | 158.96 | 41.32 | 178.89 |
| 12.00 | 20.03 | 155.97 | 40.89 | 177.77 |
| 13.00 | 19.65 | 153.04 | 40.53 | 176.60 |
| 16.00 | 18.57 | 144.56 | 39.62 | 173.00 |
| 24.00 | 15.95 | 124.17 | 37.44 | 163.59 |

*$D_p$, drug in plasma compartment; $D_t$, drug in tissue compartment.
Data from Harron DWG: Digoxin pharmacokinetic modelling—10 years later, Int J Pharm 1989 Aug 1;53(3):181–188.

Although the initial plasma drug levels were much higher than after equilibration, the digoxin plasma concentrations are generally regarded as not toxic, since drug distribution is occurring rapidly.

The tissue drug levels were not calculated. The tissue drug concentration represents the hypothetical tissue pool, which may not represent actual drug concentrations in the myocardium. In contrast, the amount of drug remaining in the tissue pool is real, since the amount of drug is calculated using mass balance. The rate of drug entry into the tissue in micrograms per hour at any time is $k_{12}X_c$, while the rate of drug leaving the tissue is $k_{21}X_p$ in the same units. Both of these rates may be calculated from Table 13-5 using $k_{12}$ and $k_{21}$ values listed in Table 13-4.

Although some clinicians for practical purposes assume that tissue and plasma concentrations are equal when at equilibration (in reality, full equilibration only occurs with constant infusion administration. otherwise, the concentrations constantly change and full equilibration is not achievable), tissue and plasma drug ratios are determined by the partition coefficient (a drug-specific physical ratio that measures the lipid/water affinity of a drug) and the extent of protein binding of the drug. Figure 13-6 shows that the time for the RF (renal-failure or renal-impaired) patient to reach stable tissue drug levels is longer than the time for the normal subject due to changes in the elimination and transfer rate constants. As expected, a significantly higher amount of digoxin remains in both the plasma and tissue compartments in the renally impaired subject compared to the normal subject.

## PRACTICE PROBLEM

From Figure 13-6 or Table 13-4, how many hours does it take for maximum tissue concentration to be reached in the normal and the renal-impaired patient?

### Solution

At maximum tissue concentration, the rate of drug entering the tissue compartment is equal to the rate of leaving (ie, at the peak of the tissue curve, where the slope = 0 or not changing). This occurs at about 3 to 4 hours for the normal patient and at 7 to 8 hours for the renal-impaired patient. This may be verified by examining at what time $X_c k_{12} = X_p k_{21}$ using the data from Tables 13-4 and 13-5. Before maximum $C_p$ is reached, there is a net flux of drug into the tissue, that is, $X_c k_{12} > X_p k_{21}$, and beyond this point, there is a net flux of drug out of the tissue compartment, that is, $X_p k_{12} > X_c k_{12}$.

## PRACTICAL FOCUS

The distribution half-life of digoxin is about 31 minutes ($t_{1/2}\alpha = 0.694/\alpha = 0.694/1.331 = 31$ min) based on Table 13-4. Both clinical experience and simulated tissue amount in Table 13-4 recommend "several hours" for equilibration, longer than $5t_{1/2}\alpha$ or $5 \times 32$ minutes. (1) Is digoxin elimination in tissue adequately modeled in this example? (2) Digoxin was not known to be a P-gp substrate when the data were analyzed; can the presence of a transporter at the target site change tissue drug concentration, necessitating a longer equilibration time?

Generally, the ability to obtain a blood sample and get accurate data in the alpha (distribution) phase is difficult for most drugs because of its short duration. Moreover, the alpha phase may not be very reproducible because it is affected by short-term physiologic changes. For example, stress may result in short-term change of the hematocrit or plasma volume and possibly other hemodynamic factors.

### Apparent Volumes of Distribution

Volumes of distributions are useful parameters to relate concentrations to an amount within a specific compartment. For drugs with large extravascular distribution which are characterized by multicompartment models, the apparent total volume of distribution ($V_{ss}$) will be generally large and will be the sum of the individual compartment volumes (eg, in a two-compartment model, $V_{ss} = V_c + V_p$). Conversely, for polar drugs with low lipid solubility that are well described by a one-compartment model, the apparent $V_{ss}$ will be generally small ($V_{ss}$ will be equal to $V_c$) and will approximate extracellular fluid volume when protein binding is not too prevalent (see Chapter 5). One major confusing factor is the tendency in the literature and in the official product label of drugs to not specify exactly what $V$ are described, with the non-informative term volume of distribution or ($V_d$). Sometimes $V_d$ is used for $V_{ss}$, sometimes for $V_c$, and sometimes for hybrid parameters such as the $V_\beta$ or $V_z$. Volumes of distribution generally reflect the extent of drug distribution in the body on a relative basis, and the calculations depend on the availability of data. In general, it is important to refer to the same volume parameter when comparing kinetic changes in disease states. Unfortunately, and as mentioned, values of apparent volumes of distribution of drugs from tables in the clinical literature are often listed without specifying the underlying kinetic processes, model parameters, or methods of calculation.

### Volume of the Central Compartment

*Volume of the central compartment ($V_c$) is a proportionality constant that relates the amount or mass of drug and its systemic concentration. On a semi-log* graph paper and when the drug product is given via a bolus IV injection, the $V_c$ can be estimated by extrapolating the systemic concentrations at time zero. The volume of the central compartment is useful for determining the drug concentration directly after an IV injection into the body. Obviously in a multi-compartment model situation, the $V_c$ will be smaller than the total volume of distribution ($V_{ss}$). The magnitude difference of volume of distributions is important in terms of designing an appropriate bolus-loading dose for a drug whose PK is well described by a two-compartment model.

$$V_c = \frac{X_0}{C_0} \qquad (13.22)$$

At zero time ($t = 0$), the entire drug in the body is in the central compartment. $C_0$ can be shown to be equal to $A + B$ by the following equation:

$$C = Ae^{-\alpha t} + Be^{-\beta t} \qquad (13.23)$$

at $t = 0$, $e^0 = 1$. Therefore,

$$C_0 = A + B \qquad (13.24)$$

$V_c$ is determined from Equation 13.25 by measuring $A$ and $B$ after feathering the curve, as discussed previously:

$$V_c = \frac{X_0}{A + B} \qquad (13.25)$$

Alternatively, the volume of the central compartment may be calculated from the $[AUC]_0^\infty$ in a manner similar to the calculation for the apparent $V_D$ in the one-compartment model. For a one-compartment model

$$[AUC]_0^\infty = \frac{X_0}{kV_D} \qquad (13.26)$$

In contrast, $[AUC]_0^\infty$ for the two-compartment model is:

$$[AUC]_0^\infty = \frac{X_0}{kV_c} \qquad (13.27)$$

Rearrangement of this equation yields:

$$V_c = \frac{X_0}{k[AUC]_0^\infty} \qquad (13.28)$$

### Apparent total Volume of Distribution

Apparent total volume of distribution (previously referred to as volume of distribution at steady state, $V_{ss}$) is a proportionality constant that relates the plasma concentration and the amount of drug remaining in the body at a time, following the attainment of practical steady state (which is reached at a time greater by at least four elimination half-lives of the drug). At the exact steady-state conditions, the rate of drug entry into the tissue compartment from the central compartment is equal to the rate of drug exit from the tissue compartment into the central compartment. These rates of drug transfer are described by the following expressions:

$$X_p k_{21} = X_c k_{12} \qquad (13.29)$$

| Group | A µg/mL | B µg/mL | α h⁻¹ | β h⁻¹ | k h⁻¹ |
|---|---|---|---|---|---|
| 1 | $138.9 \pm 114.9$ | $157.8 \pm 87.1$ | $6.8 \pm 4.5$ | $0.20 \pm 0.12$ | $0.38 \pm 0.26$ |
| 2 | $115.4 \pm 65.9$ | $115.0 \pm 40.8$ | $5.3 \pm 3.5$ | $0.27 \pm 0.08$ | $0.50 \pm 0.17$ |
| 3 | $102.9 \pm 39.4$ | $89.0 \pm 36.7$ | $5.6 \pm 3.8$ | $0.37 \pm 0.09$ | $0.71 \pm 0.16$ |
| Group | Cl mL/min | $V_p$ L/kg | $V_t$ L/kg | $(V_D)_{ss}$ L/kg | $(V_D)_\beta$ L/kg |
| 1 | $40.5 \pm 14.5$ | $0.12 \pm 0.05$ | $0.08 \pm 0.04$ | $0.20 \pm 0.09$ | $0.21 \pm 0.09$ |
| 2 | $73.7 \pm 13.1$ | $0.14 \pm 0.06$ | $0.09 \pm 0.04$ | $0.23 \pm 0.10$ | $0.24 \pm 0.12$ |
| 3 | $125.9 \pm 28.0$ | $0.15 \pm 0.05$ | $0.10 \pm 0.05$ | $0.25 \pm 0.08$ | $0.29 \pm 0.09$ |

**TABLE 13-6 •** Pharmacokinetic Parameters (mean ± SD) of Moxalactam in Three Groups of Patients

$$D_p = \frac{k_{12}X_c}{k_{21}} \qquad (13.30)$$

Because the amount of drug in the central compartment, $D_p$, is equal to $V_pC_p$, by substitution in the above equation,

$$D_p = \frac{k_{12}C\,V_c}{k_{21}} \qquad (13.31)$$

The total amount of drug in the body at steady state is equal to the sum of the amount of drug in the peripheral compartment, $X_p$, and the amount of drug in the central compartment, $X_c$. At steady state for a constant infusion, the apparent volume of drug at steady state $V_{ss}$ may be calculated by dividing the total amount of drug in the body by the concentration of drug in the central compartment at steady state:

$$(V_D)_{ss} = \frac{X_c + X_p}{C} \qquad (13.32)$$

Substituting Equation 13.31 into Equation 13.32, and expressing $X_c$ as $V_cC$, the equation for the calculation of $(V_D)_{ss}$ is obtained:

$$(V_D)_{ss} = \frac{C\,V_c + k_{12}V_cC\,/k_{21}}{C} \qquad (13.33)$$

which reduces to

$$(V_D)_{ss} = V_c + \frac{k_{12}}{k_{21}}\,V_c$$

### Volume of Distribution by Area

Another volume term sometimes used and reported is the $V_\beta$, $V_z$, or $V_{area}$. Although these terms are slightly different, they all represent the same volume but the terminology explains how they are calculated. $V_\beta$ or $V_z$ is the volume of distribution calculated using the clearance divided by the terminal rate constant (either denoted as $\beta$ or $\lambda_z$). $V_{area}$ is simply the same volume but calculated as $Dose/AUC_{inf}$.

$$V_\beta = CL/\beta \qquad (13.35)$$

$$V_z = CL/\lambda_z \qquad (13.36)$$

$$V_{area} = Dose/(AUC_{inf} \times \lambda_z) \qquad (13.37)$$

The $V_\beta$, $V_z$, $V_{area}$ will be equal to the total volume of distribution only if the drug is well described by a one-compartment model. For drugs that are distributed in two compartments, the $V_\beta$, $V_z$, $V_{area}$ will be a hybrid volume, one that will not be equal to the $V_c$ nor the $V_{ss}$, but will be between the two. Some refer to this volume as the "volume during the terminal phase," as it is calculated as the ratio of CL by the terminal rate.

## PRACTICE PROBLEM

Simulated plasma drug concentrations after an IV bolus dose (100 mg) of an antibiotic in two patients, Patient 1 with a normal $k$, and Patient 2 with a reduced $k$, are shown in Fig. 13-7. The data in the two patients were simulated with parameters using the two-compartment model equation. The parameters used are as follows:

Normal subject, $k_{10} = 0.3\ h^{-1}$, $V_c = 10\ L$, $CL = 3\ L/h$

$$k_{12} = 5\ h^{-1}, k_{21} = 0.2\ h^{-1}$$

Subject with moderate renal impairment, $k_{10} = 0.1\ h^{-1}$, $V_c = 10\ L$, $CL = 1\ L/h$

$$k_{12} = 2\ h^{-1}, k_{21} = 0.25\ h^{-1}$$

### Questions

1.  Is a reduction in drug clearance generally accompanied by an increase in plasma drug concentration, regardless of which compartment model the drug follows?

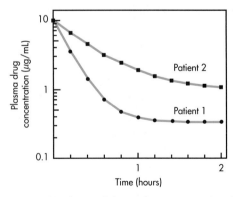

**FIGURE 13-7** • Simulation of plasma drug concentration after an IV bolus dose (100 mg) of an antibiotic in two patients, one with a normal $k$ (Patient 1) and the other with reduced $k$ (Patient 2).

2. Many antibiotics follow multiexponential plasma drug concentration profiles indicating drug distribution into tissue compartments. In clinical pharmacokinetics, the terminal half-life is often determined with limited early data. Which patient has a greater terminal half-life based on the simulated data?

### Solutions

1. A reduction in drug clearance results in less drug being removed from the body per unit time. *CL* is the same regardless of the number of compartments Therefore, the plasma drug concentration should be higher in subjects with decreased drug clearance compared to subjects with normal drug clearance, regardless of which compartment model is used (see Fig. 13-7).

2. Both patients have the same $\beta$ value ($\beta = 0.011$ h$^{-1}$); the terminal slopes are identical. Ignoring early points by only taking terminal data would lead to an erroneous conclusion that the renal elimination process is the same in both patients, while the volume of distribution of the renally impaired patient is smaller. In this case, the renally impaired patient has a clearance of 1 L/h compared with 3 L/h for the normal subject, and yet the terminal slopes are the same. The rapid distribution of drug into the tissue in the normal subject causes a longer and steeper distribution phase. Later, redistribution of drug out of tissues masks the effect of rapid drug elimination through the kidney. In the renally impaired patient, distribution to tissue is reduced; as a result, little drug is redistributed out from the tissue in the $\beta$ phase. Hence, it appears that the beta phases are identical in the two patients.

---

#### FREQUENTLY ASKED QUESTIONS

▶ What is the significance of the apparent volume of distribution?

▶ Why are there different volumes of distribution in the multiple-compartment models?

---

#### Drug in the Tissue Compartment

The apparent volume of the tissue or peripheral compartment ($V_p$) is a conceptual volume only and does not represent true anatomic volumes. The $V_p$ may be calculated from knowledge of the transfer rate constants and $V_c$:

$$V_p = \frac{V_c k_{12}}{k_{21}} \qquad (13.38)$$

The calculation of the amount of drug in the tissue compartment does not entail the use of $V_p$. Calculation of the amount of drug in the tissue compartment provides an estimate for drug accumulation in the tissues of the body. This information is vital in estimating chronic toxicity and relating the duration of pharmacologic activity to dose. Tissue compartment drug concentration is an average estimate of the tissue pool and does not mean that all tissues have the same concentration. The drug concentration in a tissue biopsy will provide an estimate for drug in that tissue sample. Due to differences in blood flow and drug partitioning into the tissue, and tissue heterogenicity, biopsies from the different locations in the same tissue may have different drug concentrations. Together with $V_c$ and $C$, used to calculate the amount of drug in the plasma, the compartment model provides mass balance information. Moreover, the pharmacodynamic activity may correlate better with the tissue drug concentration–time curve. To calculate the amount of drug in the tissue compartment $X_p$, the following expression is used:

$$X_p = \frac{k_{12}X_c}{\alpha - \beta}(e^{-\beta t} - e^{-\alpha t}) \qquad (13.39)$$

#### PRACTICAL FOCUS

The therapeutic plasma concentration of digoxin is between 1 and 2 ng/mL, Because digoxin has a long elimination half-life, it takes a long time to reach a stable, constant (steady-state) level in the body. A loading dose is usually given with the initiation of digoxin therapy. Consider the implications of the loading dose of 1 mg suggested for a 70-kg subject. The clinical source cited an apparent volume of distribution of 7.3 L/kg for digoxin in determining the loading dose. Use the pharmacokinetic parameters for digoxin in Table 13-4.

## Solution

Although digoxin is well described by a two-compartmental model, the loading dose was calculated by considering the body as one compartment during steady state, at which time the drug well penetrates the tissue compartment. The loading dose is calculated to load the $V_c$ only as the drug has not yet have time to distribute enough into the $V_p$. The volume of distribution $(V_D)_\beta$ of digoxin is much larger than $V_c$ or the volume of the central compartment.

Using Equation 13.35,

$$V\beta = k\, V_c/\beta$$

where $D_L = (V_D)_\beta \cdot (C)_{ss}$. The desired steady plasma concentration, $(C)_{ss}$, was selected by choosing a value in the middle of the therapeutic range. The loading dose is generally divided into two or three doses or is administered as 50% in the first dose with the remaining drug given in two divided doses 6 to 8 hours apart to minimize potential side effects from overdigitization. If the entire loading dose were administered intravenously, the plasma level would be about 4 to 5 ng/mL after 1 hour, while the level would drop to about 1.5 ng/mL at about 4 hours. The exact level after a given IV dose may be calculated using Equation 13.7 at any time desired. The pharmacokinetic parameters for digoxin are available in Table 13-4.

In addition to metabolism, digoxin distribution is affected by a number of processes besides blood flow. Digoxin and many other drugs are P-gp (P-glycoprotein) substrates, a transporter that is often located in cell membranes that efflux drug in and out of cells, and can theoretically affect cell uptake and cell efflux. Some transporters such as P-gp or ABC transporters exhibit genetic variability and therefore can contribute to pharmacokinetic variability between patients. For example, if drug transporters avidly carry drug to metabolic sites, then metabolism would increase, and plasma levels AUC would decrease. The converse is also true; examples of drugs that are known to increase digoxin level include amiodarone, quinidine, and verapamil. Verapamil is a potent P-gp inhibitor and a common agent used to test if an unknown substrate can be blocked by a P-gp inhibitor.

Many anticancer drugs such as taxol, vincristine, and vinblastine are P-gp substrates. P-gp can be located in GI, kidney, liver, and entry to blood brain barrier (BBB) (see Chapter 5 for distribution and Chapter 21 for genetically expressed transporters). There are other organic anion and cation transporters in the body that contribute to efflux of drug into and out of cells. Efflux and translocation of a drug can cause a drug to lose efficacy (MDR resistance) in many anticancer drugs. It may not always be possible to distinguish a specific drug transporter in a specific organ or tissue *in vivo* due to ongoing perfusion and the potential for multiple transporter/carriers involved. These factors—drug binding to proteins in blood, cell, and cell membranes—and diffusion-limiting processes contribute to "multiexponential" drug distribution kinetically for many drugs. Much of *in vivo* kinetics information can be learned by examining the kinetics of the IV bolus time–concentration profile when a suitable substrate probe is administered.

### Drug Clearance

The definition of clearance of a drug that follows a two-compartment model is similar to that of the one-compartment model. *Clearance* is the volume of plasma that is removed from the drug per unit of time. Clearance may be calculated without consideration of the compartment model. Thus, clearance may be viewed as a physiologic concept for drug removal.

Clearance is one parameter that is easily calculated using noncompartmental approaches, as in Equation 13.37, in which the bolus IV dose is divided by the area under the plasma concentration–time curve from zero to infinity, $[AUC]_0^\infty$. In evaluating the $[AUC]_0^\infty$ early time points must be collected frequently to observe the rapid decline in drug concentrations (distribution phase) for drugs with multicompartment pharmacokinetics. In the calculation of clearance using the noncompartmental approach, underestimating the area can inflate the calculated value of clearance.

$$CL = \frac{X_0}{[AUC]_0^\infty} \qquad (13.42)$$

Equation 13.42 may be rearranged to Equation 13.43 to show that *CL* in the two-compartment model is the product of $V_c$ and $k_{10}$

$$CL = V_c k_{10} \qquad (13.43)$$

## Elimination Rate Constant

In the two-compartment model (IV administration), the transfer rate constant, $k_{10}$, represents the elimination of drug from the central compartment, whereas $\beta$ or $\lambda_z$ represents the elimination rate constant. Because of redistribution of drug out of the tissue compartment, the plasma drug level curve declines more slowly in the $\beta$ phase. $\beta$ is smaller than $k_{10}$. $k_{10}$ is the transfer rate constant from the central compartment, whereas $\beta$ is the overall elimination rate constant that is influenced by the rate of transfer of drug into and out of the tissue compartment. When it is impractical to determine $k_{10}$, $\beta$ is calculated from the $\beta$ slope.

## THREE-COMPARTMENT OPEN MODEL

The three-compartment model is an extension of the two-compartment model, with an additional deep tissue compartment. A drug that demonstrates the necessity of a three-compartment open model is distributed most rapidly to a highly perfused central compartment, less rapidly to the second or tissue compartment, and very slowly to the third or deep tissue compartment, containing such poorly perfused tissue as bone and fat. The deep tissue compartment may also represent tightly bound drug in the tissues. The three-compartment open model is shown in Fig. 13-8.

A solution of the differential equation describing the rates of flow of drug into and out of the central compartment gives the following equation:

$$C_p = Ae^{-\alpha t} + Be^{-\beta t} + Ce^{-\gamma t} \qquad (13.44)$$

where $A$, $B$, and $C$ are the $y$ intercepts of extrapolated lines for the central, tissue, and deep tissue

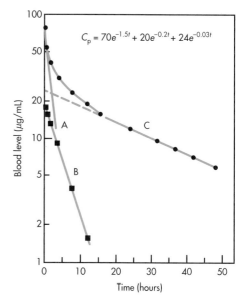

FIGURE 13-9 • Plasma level–time curve for a three-compartment open model. The rate constants and intercepts were calculated by the method of residuals.

compartments, respectively, and $\alpha$, $\beta$, and $\gamma$ are first-order rate constants for the central, tissue, and deep tissue compartments, respectively. Using lambdas, the equation becomes:

$$C_p = Ae^{-\lambda_1 t} + Be^{-\lambda_2 t} + Ce^{-\lambda_3 t} \qquad (13.44a)$$

Instead of $\alpha$, $\beta$, $\gamma$, etc, $\lambda_1$, $\lambda_2$, $\lambda_z$ are substituted to express the triexponential feature of the equation. Similarly, the $n$-compartment model may be expressed with $\lambda_1$, $\lambda_2$, . . . , $\lambda_n$. The preexponential terms are sometimes expressed as $C_1$, $C_2$, and $C_3$.

The parameters in Equation 13.44 may be solved graphically by the method of residuals (Fig. 13-9) or by computer. The calculations for the elimination rate constant from the central compartment

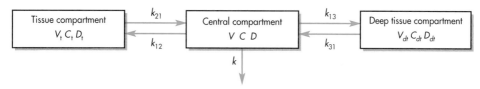

FIGURE 13-8 • Three-compartment open model. This model, as with the previous two-compartment models, assumes that all drug elimination occurs via the central compartment.

*k10*, volume of the central compartment, and overall exposure (AUCinf) are shown in the following equations:

$$k = \frac{(A+B+C)\alpha\beta\delta}{A\beta\delta + B\alpha\delta + C\alpha\beta} \quad (13.45)$$

$$V_c = \frac{X_0}{A+B+C} \quad (13.46)$$

$$[AUC] = \frac{A}{\alpha} + \frac{B}{\beta} + \frac{C}{\delta} \quad (13.47)$$

## CLINICAL APPLICATION

### Hydromorphone (Dilaudid)

Three independent studies on the pharmacokinetics of hydromorphone after a bolus intravenous injection reported that hydromorphone followed the pharmacokinetics of a one-compartment model (Vallner et al, 1981), a two-compartment model (Parab et al, 1988), or a three-compartment model (Hill et al, 1991), respectively. A comparison of these studies is listed in Table 13-7.

### Comments

The adequacy of the pharmacokinetic model will depend on the sampling intervals and the drug assay. The first two studies showed a similar elimination half-life. However, both Vallner et al (1981) and Parab et al (1988) did not observe a three-compartment pharmacokinetic model due to lack of appropriate description of the early distribution phases for hydromorphone. After an IV bolus injection, hydromorphone is very rapidly distributed into the tissues. Hill et al (1991) obtained a triexponential function

by closely sampling early time periods after the dose. Average distributions half-lives were 1.27 and 14.7 minutes, and the average terminal elimination was 184 minutes ($t_{1/2\beta}$). The average value for systemic clearance (*CL*) was 1.66 L/min; the initial dilution volume was 24.4 L. If distribution is rapid, the drug becomes distributed during the absorption phase. Thus, hydromorphone pharmacokinetics follows a one-compartment model after a single oral dose.

Hydromorphone is administered to relieve acute pain in cancer or postoperative patients. Rapid pain relief is obtained by IV injection. Although the drug is effective orally, about 50% to 60% of the drug is cleared by the liver through first-pass effects. The pharmacokinetics of hydromorphone after IV injection suggests a multicompartment model. The site of action is probably within the central nervous system, as part of the tissue compartment. The initial volume or initial dilution volume, $V_c$, is the volume into which IV injections are injected and diluted. Hydromorphone follows linear kinetics, that is, drug concentration is proportional to dose. Hydromorphone systemic clearance is much larger than the glomerular filtration rate (GFR) of 120 mL/min (see Chapter 15), hence the drug is probably metabolized significantly by the hepatic route. A clearance of 1.66 L/min is faster than the blood flow of 1.2–1.5 L/min to the liver. The drug must be rapidly extracted or, in addition, must have extrahepatic elimination. When the distribution phase is short, the distribution phase may be disregarded provided that the targeted plasma concentration is sufficiently low and the terminal elimination phase is relatively long. If the drug has a sufficiently high target plasma drug

| **TABLE 13-7** • Comparison of Hydromorphone Pharmacokinetics | | |
|---|---|---|
| **Study** | **Timing of Blood Samples** | **Pharmacokinetic Parameters** |
| 6 Males, 25–29 years; mean weight, 76.8 kg Dose, 2-mg IV bolus (Vallner et al, 1981) | 0, 15, 30, 45 minutes 1, 1.5, 2, 3, 4, 6, 8, 10, 12 hours | One-compartment model Terminal $t_{1/2} = 2.64 \, (\pm 0.88)$ hours |
| 8 Males, 20–30 years; weight, 50–86 kg Dose, 2-mg IV bolus (Parab et al, 1988) | 0, 3, 7, 15, 30, 45 minutes 1, 1.5, 2, 3, 4, 6, 8, 10, 12 hours | Two-compartment model Terminal $t_{1/2} = 2.36 \, (\pm 0.58)$ hours |
| 10 Males, 21–38 years; mean weight, 72.7 kg Dose, 10, 20, and 40 µg/kg IV bolus (Hill et al, 1991) | 1, 2, 3, 4, 5, 7, 10, 15, 20, 30, 45 minutes 1, 1.5, 2, 2.5, 3, 4, 5 hours | Three-compartment model Terminal $t_{1/2} = 3.07 \, (\pm 0.25)$ hours |

concentration and the elimination half-life is short, the distributive phase must not be ignored. For example, lidocaine's effective target concentration often lies close to the distributive phase, since its beta elimination half-life is very short, and ignoring the alpha phase will result in a large error in dosing projection.

## CLINICAL APPLICATION

Loperamide (Imodium®) is an opioid antidiarrheal agent that is useful for illustrating the importance of understanding drug distribution. Loperamide has little central opiate effect. Loperamide is a P-gp (an efflux transporter) substrate. The presence of P-gp transporter at the blood–brain barrier allows the drug to be pumped out of the cell at the cell membrane surface without the substrate (loperamide) entering into the interior of the cell. Mice that have had the gene for P-gp removed experimentally show profound central opioid effects when administered loperamide. Hypothesizing the presence of a tissue compartment coupled with a suitable molecular probe can provide a powerful approach toward elucidating the mechanism of drug distribution and improving drug safety.

## DETERMINATION OF COMPARTMENT MODELS

Models based on compartmental analysis should always use the fewest number of compartments necessary to describe the experimental data adequately. Once an empirical equation is derived from the experimental observations, it becomes necessary to examine how well the theoretical values that are calculated from the derived equation fit the experimental data.

The observed number of compartments or exponential phases will depend on (1) the route of drug administration, (2) the rate of drug absorption, (3) the total time for blood sampling, (4) the number of samples taken within the collection period, and (5) the assay sensitivity. If drug distribution is rapid, then after oral administration the drug will become distributed during the absorption phase and the distribution phase will not be observed. For example, theophylline follows the kinetics of a

one-compartment model after oral absorption, but after IV bolus (given as aminophylline), theophylline follows the kinetics of a two-compartment model. Furthermore, if theophylline is given by a slow intravenous infusion rather than by intravenous bolus, the distribution phase will not be observed. Hydromorphone (Dilaudid), which follows a three-compartment model, also follows a one-compartment model after oral administration, since the first two distribution phases are rapid.

Depending on the sampling intervals, a compartment may be missed because samples may be taken too late after administration of the dose to observe a possible distributive phase. For example, the data plotted in Fig. 13-10 could easily be mistaken for those of a one-compartment model, because the distributive phase has been missed and extrapolation of the data to $C_0$ will give a lower value than was actually the case. Slower drug elimination compartments may also be missed if sampling is not performed at later sampling times, when the dose or the assay for the drug cannot measure very low plasma drug concentrations.

The total time for collection of blood samples is usually estimated from the terminal elimination half-life of the drug. However, lower drug concentrations may not be measured if the sensitivity of the assay is not adequate. As the assay for the drug becomes more sensitive in its ability to measure lower drug concentrations, then another compartment with a smaller first-order rate constant may be observed.

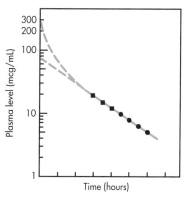

FIGURE 13-10 • The samples from which data were obtained for this graph were taken too late to show the distributive phase; therefore, the value of $C_0$ obtained by extrapolation (straight broken line) is deceptively low.

Compartment models having more than three compartments rarely need to be used. In certain cases, it is possible to "lump" a few compartments together to get a smaller number of compartments, which, together, will describe the data adequately.

An adequate description of several tissue compartments can be difficult. When the addition of a compartment to the model seems necessary, it is important to realize that the drug may be retained or slowly concentrated in a deep tissue compartment.

## PRACTICAL FOCUS

### Two-Compartment Model: Relation Between Distribution and Apparent (Beta) Half-Life

The distribution half-life of a drug is dependent on the type of tissues the drug penetrates as well as blood supply to those tissues. In addition, the capacity of the tissue to store drug is also a factor. Distribution half-life is generally short for many drugs because of the ample blood supply to and rapid drug equilibration in the tissue compartment. However, there is some supporting evidence that a drug with a long elimination half-life is often associated with a longer distribution phase. It is conceivable that a tissue with little blood supply and affinity for the drug may not attain a sufficiently high drug concentration to exert its impact on the overall plasma drug concentration profile during rapid elimination. In contrast, drugs such as digoxin have a long elimination half-life, and drug is eliminated slowly to allow more time for distribution to tissues. Human follicle-stimulating hormone (hFSH) injected intravenously has a very long elimination half-life, and its distribution half-life is also quite long. Drugs such as lidocaine, theophylline, and milrinone have short elimination half-lives and generally relatively short distributional half-lives.

In order to examine the effect of changing $k_{10}$ (from 0.6 to 0.2 $h^{-1}$) on the distributional (alpha phase) and elimination (beta phase) half-lives of various drugs, four simulations based on a two-compartment model were generated (Table 13-8). The simulations show that a drug with a smaller $k_{10}$ has a longer beta elimination half-life. Keeping all other parameters ($k_{12}$, $k_{21}$, $V_c$) constant, a smaller $k_{10}$ will result in a smaller $\alpha$, or a slower distributional phase. Examples of drugs with various distribution and elimination half-lives are shown in Table 13-8.

## TABLE 13-8 • Comparison of Beta Half-Life and Distributional Half-Life of Selected Drugs

| Drug | Beta Half-Life | Distributional Half-Life |
|------|---------------|--------------------------|
| Lidocaine | 1.8 hours | 8 minutes |
| Cocaine | 1 hours | 18 minutes |
| Theophylline | 4.33 hours | 7.2 minutes |
| Ergometrine | 2 hours | 11 minutes |
| Hydromorphone | 3 hours | 14.7 minutes |
| Milrinone | 3.6 hours | 4.6 minutes |
| Procainamide | 2.5–4.7 hours | 6 minutes |
| Quinidine | 6–8 hours | 7 minutes |
| Lithium | 21.39 hours | 5 hours |
| Digoxin | 1.6 days | 35 minutes |
| Human FSH | 1 day | 60 minutes |
| IgG1 kappa MAB | 9.6 days (monkey) | 6.7 hours |
| Simulation 1 | 13.26 hours | 36.24 minutes |
| Simulation 2 | 16.60 hours | 43.38 minutes |
| Simulation 3 | 26.83 hours | 53.70 minutes |
| Simulation 4 | 213.7 hours | 1.12 hours |

Simulation was performed using $V_p$ of 10 L; dose = 100 mg; $k_{12} = 0.5\ h^{-1}$; $k_{21} = 0.1\ h^{-1}$; $k = 0.6, 0.4, 0.2,$ and 0.02 hour for simulations 1–4, respectively (using Equations 5.11 and 5.12).
Data from Schumacher GE: Therapeutic Drug Monitoring. Norwalk, CT: Appleton & Lange; 1995.

## CLINICAL APPLICATION

### Moxalactam Disodium—Effect of Changing Renal Function in Patients with Sepsis

The pharmacokinetics of moxalactam disodium, a recently discontinued antibiotic (see Table 13-6), was examined in 40 patients with abdominal sepsis (Swanson et al, 1983). The patients were grouped according to creatinine clearances into three groups:

Group 1: Average creatinine clearance = 35.5 mL/min/1.73 m²

Group 2: Average creatinine clearance = 67.1 ± 6.7 mL/min/1.73 m²

Group 3: Average creatinine clearance = 117.2 ± 29.9 mL/min/1.73 m²

After intravenous bolus administration, the serum drug concentrations followed a biexponential

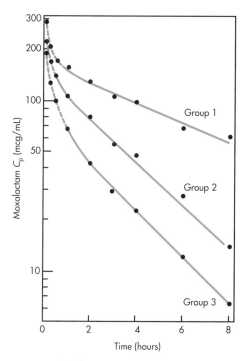

FIGURE 13-11 • Moxalactam serum concentration in three groups of patients: group 1, average creatinine concentration = 35.5 mL/min/1.73 m²; group 2, average creatinine concentration = 67.1 ± 6.7 mL/min/1.73 m²; group 3, average creatinine concentration = 117.2 ± 29.9 mL/min/1.73 m².

decline (Fig. 13-11). The pharmacokinetics at steady state (2 g every 8 hours) was also examined in these patients. Mean steady-state serum concentrations ranged from 27.0 to 211.0 $\mu g$/mL and correlated inversely with creatinine clearance ($r = 0.91, p < 0.0001$). The terminal half-life ranged from 1.27 to 8.27 hours and reflected the varying renal function of the patients. Moxalactam total body clearance ($CL$) had excellent correlation with creatinine clearance ($r^2 = 0.92$). $CL$ determined by noncompartmental data analysis was in agreement with $CL$ determined by nonlinear least squares regression ($r = 0.99, p < 0.0001$). Moxalactam total body clearance was best predicted from creatinine clearance corrected for body surface area.

## Questions (Refer to Table 13-6)

1. Calculate the beta half-life of moxalactam in the most renally impaired group.

2. What indicator is used to predict moxalactam clearance in the body?

3. What is the beta volume of distribution of patients in group 3 with normal renal function?

4. What is the initial volume ($V_i$) of moxalactam?

## Solutions

1. Mean beta half-life is 0.693/0.20 = 3.47 hours in the most renally impaired group.

2. Creatinine is mainly filtered through the kidney, and creatinine clearance is used as an indicator of renal glomerular filtration rate. Group 3 has normal renal function (average creatinine clearance = 117.2 mL/min/1.73 m²) (see Chapter 15).

3. Beta volume of distribution: Moxalactam clearance in group 3 subjects is 125.9 mL/min. From Equation 13.38,

$$(V_D)_\beta = \frac{Cl}{\beta}$$

$$= \frac{125.9 \text{ mL/min} \times 60 \text{ min/h}}{0.37 \text{ h}^{-1}}$$

$$= 20,416 \text{ mL or } 20.4 \text{ L}$$

4. The volume of the central compartment, $V_c$, is sometimes referred to as the initial volume. $V_c$ ranges from 0.12 to 0.15 L/kg among the three groups and is considerably smaller than the steady-state volume of distribution.

## CLINICAL EXAMPLE

### Azithromycin Pharmacokinetics

Following oral administration, azithromycin (Zithromax®) is an antibiotic that is rapidly absorbed and widely distributed throughout the body. Azithromycin is rapidly distributed into tissues, with high drug concentrations within cells, resulting in significantly higher azithromycin concentrations in tissue than in plasma. The high values for plasma clearance (630 mL/min) suggest that the prolonged half-life is due to extensive uptake and subsequent release of drug from tissues.

Plasma concentrations of azithromycin decline in a polyphasic pattern, resulting in an average terminal half-life of 68 hours. With this regimen, $C_{min}$ and $C_{max}$ remained essentially unchanged from day

2 through day 5 of therapy. However, without a loading dose, azithromycin $C_{min}$ levels required 5 to 7 days to reach desirable plasma levels.

The pharmacokinetic parameters of azithromycin in healthy elderly male subjects (65 to 85 years) were similar to those in young adults. Although higher peak drug concentrations (increased by 30% to 50%) were observed in elderly women, no significant accumulation occurred.

## Questions

1. Do you agree with the following statements for a drug that is described by a two-compartment pharmacokinetic model? At peak $C_p$, the drug is well equilibrated between the plasma and the tissue compartment, $C = C_p$, and the rates of drug diffusion into and from the plasma compartment are equal.

2. What happens after peak $C_p$?

3. Why is a loading dose used?

4. What is $V_i$? How is this volume related to $V_c$?

5. What population factors could affect the concentration of azithromycin?

## Solutions

1. For a drug that follows a multicompartment model, the rates of drug diffusion into the tissues from the plasma and from the tissues into the plasma are equal at peak tissue concentrations. However, the tissue drug concentration is generally not equal to the plasma drug concentration.

2. After peak $C_p$, the rate out of the tissue exceeds the rate into the tissue, and $C_t$ falls. The decline of $C_p$ parallels that of $C$, and occurs because distribution equilibrium has occurred.

3. When drugs are given in a multiple-dose regimen, a loading dose may be given to achieve desired therapeutic drug concentrations more rapidly (see Chapter 17).

4. The volume of the central compartment, $V_c$, is sometimes referred to as the initial volume.

5. Age and gender may affect the $C_{max}$ level of the drug.

## PRACTICAL PROBLEM

### Clinical Example—Etoposide Pharmacokinetics

Etoposide is a drug used for the treatment of lung cancer. Understanding the distribution of etoposide in normal and metastatic tissues is important to avoid drug toxicity. Etoposide follows a two-compartment model. The $(V_D)_\beta$ is 0.28 L/kg, and the beta elimination half-life is 12.9 hours. Total body clearance is 0.25 mL/min/kg.

### Questions

1. What is the $(V_D)_\beta$ in a 70-kg subject?

2. How is the $(V_D)_\beta$ different than the volume of the plasma fluid, $V_c$?

3. Why is the $(V_D)_\beta$ useful if it does not represent a real tissue volume?

4. How is $(V_D)_\beta$ calculated from plasma time–concentration profile data for etoposide? Is $(V_D)_\beta$ related to total body clearance?

5. Etoposide was recently shown to be a P-gp substrate. How may this affect drug tolerance in different patients?

### Solutions

1. $(V_D)_\beta$ of etoposide in a 70-kg subject is 0.28 L/kg × 70 kg = 19.6 L.

2. The plasma fluid volume is about 3 L in a 70-kg subject and is much smaller than $(V_D)_\beta$. The apparent volume of distribution, $(V_D)_\beta$, is also considerably larger than the volume of the plasma compartment (also referred to as the initial volume by some clinicians), which includes some extracellular fluid.

3. Etoposide is a drug that follows a two-compartment model with a beta elimination phase. Within the first few minutes after an intravenous bolus dose, most of the drug is distributed in the plasma fluid. Subsequently, the drug will diffuse into tissues and drug uptake may occur. Eventually, plasma drug levels will decline due to elimination, and some redistribution as etoposide in tissue diffuses back into the plasma fluid.

The real tissue drug level will differ from the plasma drug concentration, depending on the partitioning of drug in tissues and plasma. This allows the AUC, the volume distribution $(V_D)_\beta$, to be calculated, an area that has been related to toxicities associated with many cancer chemotherapy agents.

The two-compartment model allows continuous monitoring of the amount of the drug present in and out of the vascular system, including the amount of drug eliminated. This information is important in pharmacotherapy.

4. $(V_D)_\beta$ may be determined from the total drug clearance and beta:

$$CL = \beta \times (V_D)_\beta$$

$(V_D)_\beta$ is also calculated from Equation 13.37 where

$$(V_D)_\beta = (V_D)_{area} = \frac{X_0}{\beta[AUC]_0^\infty}$$

This method for $(V_D)_\beta$ determination using $[AUC]_0^\infty$ is popular because $[AUC]_0^\infty$ is easily calculated using the trapezoidal rule. Many values for apparent volumes of distribution reported in the clinical literature are obtained using the area equation. In general, both volume terms reflect extravascular drug distribution. $(V_D)_\beta$ appears to be affected by the dynamics of drug disposition in the beta phase. In clinical practice, many potent drugs are not injected by bolus dose. Instead, these drugs are infused over a short interval, making it difficult to obtain accurate information on the distributive phase. As a result, many drugs that

follow a two-compartment model are approximated using a single compartment. It should be cautioned that there are substantial deviations in some cases. When in doubt, the full equation with all parameters should be applied for comparison. A small bolus (test) dose may be injected to obtain the necessary data if a therapeutic dose injected rapidly causes side effects or discomfort to the subject.

---

## FREQUENTLY ASKED QUESTIONS

▶ What is the error assumed in a one-compartment model compared to a two-compartment or multicompartment model?

▶ What kind of improvement in terms of patient care or drug therapy is made using the compartment model?

---

## CLINICAL APPLICATION

### Dosing of Drugs with Different Biexponential Profiles

Drugs are usually dosed according to clearance principles with an objective of achieving a steady-state therapeutic level after multiple dosing (see Chapter 17). Overall dose is calculated using the CL as Dose = CL/AUC$_{inf}$. The distributive phase is not a major issue if the distribution phase has a short duration (Fig. 13-12) relative to the beta phase

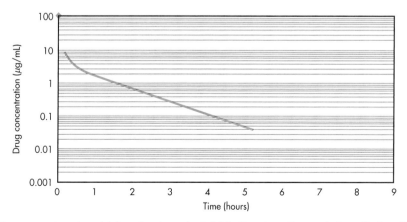

**FIGURE 13-12** • A two-compartment model drug showing a short distributive phase. The graph shows the log of the drug concentrations ($\mu$g/mL) versus time (hours). Drug mass rapidly distributes within the general circulation and highly vascular organs (central compartment) and is gradually distributed into other tissues or bound to cellular transporters or proteins.

for chronic dosing. However, from the adverse reaction perspective, injury may occur even with short exposure to sensitive organs or enzyme sites. The observation of where the therapeutically effective levels are relative to the time-concentration profile presents an interesting case below.

## PRACTICAL APPLICATION

Drugs *A*, *B*, and *C* are investigated for the treatment of arrhythmia (Fig. 13-13). Drug *A* has a very short distributive phase. The short distributive phase does not distort the overall kinetics when drug *A* is modeled by the one-compartment model. Simple one-compartment model assumptions are often made in practice and published in the literature for simplicity.

Drugs *B* and *C* have different distributive profiles. Drug *B* has a gradual distributive phase followed by a slower elimination (beta phase). The pharmacokinetic profile for drug *C* shows a longer and steeper distributive phase. Both drugs are well described by the two-compartment model.

Assuming drugs *A* and *B* both have the same effective level of 0.1 $\mu$g/mL, which drug would you prefer for dosing your patient based on the above plasma profiles provided and assuming that both drugs have the same toxic endpoint (as measured by plasma drug level)?

At what time would you recommend giving a second dose for each drug? Please state your supportive reasons. Hints: Draw a line at 0.1 $\mu$g/mL and see how it intersects the plasma curve for drugs *B* and *C*.

If you ignore the distributive phase and dose a drug based only on clearance or the terminal half-life, how would this dose affect the duration above minimum effective drug concentration of 0.1 $\mu$g/mL for each drug after an IV bolus dose?

Drug *A* represents a drug that has limited tissue distribution with mostly a linear profile and is dosed by the one-compartment model. Can you recognize when the terminal phase starts for drugs *B* and *C*?

Drug *A*—short distribution, drug *B*—intermediate distribution, drug *C*—long distribution phase due to transporter or efflux.

- Which drug is acceptable to be modeled by a simple one-compartment model?
- When re-dosed (ie, at 0.1 $\mu$g/mL), which drug was equilibrated with the tissue compartment?

### Significance of Distribution Phase

With many drugs, the initial phase or transient concentration is not considered as important as the steady-state "trough" level during long-term drug dosing. However, for a drug with the therapeutic endpoint (eg, target plasma drug concentration) that lies within the steep initial distributive phase, it is much harder to

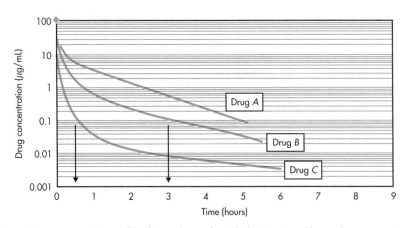

FIGURE 13-13 • Plasma drug concentration profile of three drugs after IV bolus injection. Plasma drug concentration (*C*$_p$)–time profiles of three drugs (*A, B, C*) with different distributive (*a*) phase after single IV bolus injection are plotted on a semilogarithmic scale. Plasma concentrations are in $\mu$g/mL (*x* axis) and time in hours (*y* axis). Drugs *A, B*, and *C* are each given at a dose of 10 mg/kg to subjects by IV bolus injection, and each drug has minimum effective concentration of 0.1 $\mu$g/mL.

dose accurately and not overshoot the target endpoint. This scenario is particularly true for some drugs used in critical care where rapid responses are needed and IV bolus routes are used more often. Many new biotechnological drugs are administered intravenously because of instability by oral route. The choice of a proper dose and rate of infusion relative to the half-life of the drug is an important consideration for safe drug administration. Individual patients may behave very differently with regard to drug metabolism, drug transport, and drug efflux in target cell sites. Drug receptors can be genetically expressed differently making some people more prone to allergic reactions and side effects. Simple kinetic half-life determination coupled with a careful review of the patient's chart by a pharmacist can greatly improve drug safety.

## CLINICAL APPLICATION

Lidocaine is a drug with low toxicity and a long history of use for anesthetization and for treating ventricular arrhythmias. The drug has a steep distributive phase and is biphasic. The risk of adverse effects is dose related and increases at intravenous infusion rates of above 3 mg/min. Dosage and dose rate are important for proper use (Greenspon et al, 1989). A case of inappropriate drug use was reported (Avery, 1998).

An overdose of lidocaine was given to a patient by an inexperienced hospital personnel to anesthetize the airway due to bronchoscopy. The patient was then left unobserved and subsequently developed convulsions

and cardiopulmonary arrest. He survived with severe cerebral damage. His lidocaine concentration was 24 $\mu$g/mL about 1 hour after initial administration (a blood concentration over 6 $\mu$g/mL is considered to be toxic). What is the therapeutic plasma concentration range? Is the drug highly protein bound? Is $V_D$ sufficiently large to show extravascular distribution?

A second case of adverse drug reaction based on inappropriate use of this drug due to rapid absorption was reported by Pantuck et al (1997). A 40-year-old woman developed seizures after lidocaine gel 40 mL was injected into the ureter. Vascular absorption can apparently be very rapid depending on the site of application even if the route is not directly intravenous. It is important to note that for a drug with a steeply declining elimination plasma profile, it is harder to maintain a stable target level with dosing because a small change on the time scale ($x$ axis) can greatly alter the drug concentration ($y$ axis). Some drugs that have a steep distributive phase may easily cause a side effect in a susceptible subject.

### FREQUENTLY ASKED QUESTIONS

▸ A new experimental drug can be modeled by a two-compartment model. What potential adverse event could occur for this drug if given by single IV bolus injection?

▸ A new experimental drug can be modeled by a three-compartment model. What potential adverse event could occur for this drug if given by multiple IV bolus injections?

## CHAPTER SUMMARY

*Compartment* is a term used in pharmacokinetic models to describe a theoreticized region within the body in which the drug concentrations are presumed to be uniformly distributed.

- A two-compartment model typically shows a biexponential plasma drug concentration–time curve with an initial distributive phase and a later terminal phase.
- One or more tissue compartments may be present in the model depending on the shape of the polyexponential curve representing log plasma drug concentration versus time.

- The central compartment refers to the volume of the plasma and body regions that are in rapid equilibrium with the plasma.
- The amount of drug within each compartment after a given dose at a given time can be calculated once the model is developed and model parameters are obtained by data fitting.
- A pharmacokinetic model is a quantitative description of how drug concentrations change over time. Pharmacokinetic parameters are numerical values of model descriptors derived from data that are fitted to a model. These parameters

are initially estimated and later refined using computing curve-fitting techniques such as least squares.

- Mamillary models are pharmacokinetic models that are well connected or dynamically exchange drug concentration between compartments. The two- and three-compartment models are examples.

- Compartment models are useful for estimating the mass balance of the drug in the body. As more physiological and genetic information is known, the model may be refined. Efflux and

special transporters are now known to influence drug distribution and plasma profile. The well-known ABC transporters (eg, P-gp) are genetically expressed and vary among individuals. During curve fitting, simplifying the two-compartment model after an IV bolus dose and ignoring the presence of the distributive phase may cause serious errors unless the beta phase is very long relative to the distributive phase.

- An important consideration is whether the effective concentration lies near the distributive phase after the IV bolus dose is given.

## LEARNING QUESTIONS

1. A drug was administered by rapid IV injection into a 70-kg adult male. Blood samples were withdrawn over a 7-hour period and assayed for intact drug. The results are tabulated below. Using the method of residuals, calculate the values for intercepts $A$ and $B$ and slopes $\alpha$, $\beta$, $k$, $k_{12}$, and $k_{21}$.

| Time (hours) | C (µg/mL) | Time (hours) | C (µg/mL) |
|---|---|---|---|
| 0.00 | 70.0 | 2.5 | 14.3 |
| 0.25 | 53.8 | 3.0 | 12.6 |
| 0.50 | 43.3 | 4.0 | 10.5 |
| 0.75 | 35.0 | 5.0 | 9.0 |
| 1.00 | 29.1 | 6.0 | 8.0 |
| 1.50 | 21.2 | 7.0 | 7.0 |
| 2.00 | 17.0 | | |

2. A 70-kg male subject was given 150 mg of a drug by IV injection. Blood samples were removed and assayed for intact drug. Calculate the slopes and intercepts of the three phases of the plasma level–time plot from the results tabulated below. Give the equation for the curve.

| Time (hours) | C (µg/mL) | Time (hours) | C (µg/mL) |
|---|---|---|---|
| 0.17 | 36.2 | 3.0 | 13.9 |
| 0.33 | 34.0 | 4.0 | 12.0 |
| 0.50 | 27.0 | 6.0 | 8.7 |
| 0.67 | 23.0 | 7.0 | 7.7 |
| 1.00 | 20.8 | 18.0 | 3.2 |
| 1.50 | 17.8 | 23.0 | 2.4 |
| 2.00 | 16.5 | | |

3. Mitenko and Ogilvie (1973) demonstrated that theophylline followed a two-compartment pharmacokinetic model in human subjects. After administering a single intravenous dose (5.6 mg/kg) in nine normal volunteers, these investigators demonstrated that the equation best describing theophylline kinetics in humans was as follows:

$$C = 12e^{-.58t} + 18e^{-0.16t}$$

What is the plasma level of the drug 3 hours after the IV dose?

4. A drug has a distribution that can be described by a two-compartment open model. If the drug is given by IV bolus, what is the cause of the initial or rapid decline in blood levels ($\alpha$ phase)? What is the cause of the slower decline in blood levels ($\beta$ phase)?

5. What does it mean when a drug demonstrates a plasma level–time curve that indicates a three-compartment open model? Can this curve be described by a two-compartment model?

6. A drug that follows a multicompartment pharmacokinetic model is given to a patient by rapid IV injection. Would the drug concentration in each tissue be the same after the drug equilibrates with the plasma and all the tissues in the body? Explain.

7. Park and associates (1983) studied the pharmacokinetics of amrinone after a single IV bolus injection (75 mg) in 14 healthy adult male volunteers. The pharmacokinetics of this drug

followed a two-compartment open model and fit the following equation:

$$C = Ae^{-\alpha t} + Be^{-\beta t}$$

where

$A = 4.62 \pm 12.0\ \mu g/mL$

$B = 0.64 \pm 0.17\ \mu g/mL$

$\alpha = 8.94 \pm 13\ h^{-1}$

$\beta = 0.19 \pm 0.06\ h^{-1}$

From these data, calculate:

a. The volume of the central compartment
b. The volume of the tissue compartment
c. The transfer constants $k_{12}$ and $k_{21}$
d. The elimination rate constant from the central compartment
e. The elimination half-life of amrinone after the drug has equilibrated with the tissue compartment

8. A drug may be described by a three-compartment model involving a central compartment and two peripheral tissue compartments. If you could sample the tissue compartments (organs), in which organs would you expect to find a drug level corresponding to the two theoretical peripheral tissue compartments?

9. A drug was administered to a patient at 20 mg by IV bolus dose and the time–plasma drug concentration is listed below. Use a suitable compartment model to describe the data and list the fitted equation and parameters. What are the statistical criteria used to describe your fit?

| Hour | mg/L |
|------|------|
| 0.20 | 3.42 |
| 0.40 | 2.25 |
| 0.60 | 1.92 |
| 0.80 | 1.80 |
| 1.00 | 1.73 |
| 2.00 | 1.48 |
| 3.00 | 1.28 |
| 4.00 | 1.10 |
| 6.00 | 0.81 |
| 8.00 | 0.60 |
| 10.00 | 0.45 |
| 12.00 | 0.33 |

| Hour | mg/L |
|------|------|
| 14.00 | 0.24 |
| 18.00 | 0.13 |
| 20.00 | 0.10 |

10. The toxicokinetics of colchicine in seven cases of acute human poisoning was studied by Rochdi et al (1992). In three further cases, postmortem tissue concentrations of colchicine were measured. Colchicine follows the two-compartment model with wide distribution in various tissues. Depending on the time of patient admission, two disposition processes were observed. The first, in three patients, admitted early, showed a biexponential plasma colchicine decrease, with distribution half-lives of 30, 45, and 90 minutes. The second, in four patients, admitted late, showed a monoexponential decrease. Plasma terminal half-lives ranged from 10.6 to 31.7 hours for both groups.

11. Postmortem tissue analysis of colchicine showed that colchicine accumulated at high concentrations in the bone marrow (more than 600 ng/g), testicle (400 ng/g), spleen (250 ng/g), kidney (200 ng/g), lung (200 ng/g), heart (95 ng/g), and brain (125 ng/g). The pharmacokinetic parameters of colchicine are:

Fraction of unchanged colchicine in urine = 30%

Renal clearance = 13 L/h

Total body clearance = 39 L/h

Apparent volume of distribution = 21 L/kg

a. Why is colchicine described by a monoexponential profile in some subjects and a biexponential in others?

b. What is the range of distribution of half-life of colchicine in the subjects?

c. Which parameter is useful in estimating tissue drug level at any time?

d. Some clinical pharmacists assumed that, at steady state when equilibration is reached between the plasma and the tissue, the tissue drug concentration would be the same as the plasma. Do you agree?

e. Which tissues may be predicted by the tissue compartment?

## ANSWERS

### Frequently Asked Questions

*Are "hypothetical" or "mathematical" compartment models useful in designing dosage regimens in the clinical setting? Does "hypothetical" mean "not real"?*

- *Mathematical* and *hypothetical* are used to simplify observed physiologic processes in the body. Mathematical equations can be used to calculate how much drug is in the vascular fluid and outside the vascular fluid (ie, extravascular or in the tissue pool). *Hypothetical* refers to an unproven model. The assumptions in the compartmental models imply that the model simulates the mass transfer of drug between the circulatory system and the tissue pool. Mass balance describes drug moving into and out of the plasma fluid. The tissue pool represents the virtual tissue mass that receives drug from the blood. While the model is a less-than-perfect representation, we can interpret the model knowing its limitations. All pharmacokinetic models need validation that the model fits the observed data. The model also needs interpretation. As long as we know the model limitations (ie, that the tissue compartment is not the brain or the muscle!) and stay within the bounds of the model, we can extract useful information from it. For example, we may determine the amount of drug that is stored outside the plasma compartment at any desired time point. After an IV bolus drug injection, the drug distributes rapidly throughout the plasma fluid and more slowly into the fluid-filled tissue spaces. Drug distribution is initially rapid and confined to a fixed fluid volume known as the $V_c$ or the initial volume. As drug distribution expands into other tissue regions, the volume of the penetrated spaces increases, until a critical point (steady state) is obtained when all penetrable tissue regions are equilibrated with the drug. Knowing that there is heterogeneous drug distribution within and between tissues, the tissues are grouped into compartments to determine the amount of drugs in them. Mass balance, including drug inside and outside the vascular pool, accounts for all body drug storage ($X_B = X_p + Xc$).

At steady state, the tissue drug concentration is in equilibrium[1] with the plasma drug concentration, $(C)_{ss}$, and size of the tissue volume using $X_p/C_{ss}$ may be determined. This volume is really a "numerical factor" that is used to describe the relationship of the tissue storage drug relative to the drug in the blood pool. The sum of the two volumes is the steady-state volume of distribution. The product of the steady-state concentration, $C_{ss}$, and the $(V_D)_{ss}$ yields the amount of drug in the body at steady state. The amount of drug in the body at steady state is considered vital information in dosing drugs clinically. Tissue drug concentrations are not predicted by the model. However, plasma drug concentrations are predictable after any given dose once the parameters become known. Initial pharmacokinetic parameter estimation may be obtained from the literature using comparable age and weight for a specific individual.

*If physiologic models are better than compartment models, why not just use physiologic models?*

- A physiologic model is a detailed representation of drug disposition in the body. The model requires blood flow, extraction ratio, and specific tissue and organ size. This information is not often available for the individual. Thus, the less sophisticated compartment models are used more often.

*Since clearance is the term most often used in clinical pharmacy, why is it necessary to know the other pharmacokinetic parameters?*

- Clearance is used to calculate the steady-state drug concentration and to calculate the maintenance dose. However, clearance alone is not useful in determining the maximum and minimum drug concentrations in a multiple-dosing regimen.

---

[1]At steady state, the drug concentration in the central compartment (plasma) is in equilibrium to the drug concentration in the tissue compartment. At equilibrium, the drug concentrations in each compartment may not be equal due to drug protein binding and other factors.

*What is the significance of the apparent volume of distribution?*

- Apparent volumes of distribution are not real tissue volumes, but rather reflect the volume in which the drug is contained. For example,

$V_c$ = initial or plasma volume

$V_p$ = tissue or peripheral volume

$(V_D)_{ss}$ = steady-state volume of distribution (most often listed in the literature).

The steady-state drug concentration multiplied by $(V_D)_{ss}$ yields the amount of drug in the body. $(V_D)\beta$ is a volume usually determined from area under the curve (AUC), and differs from $(V_D)_{ss}$ somewhat in magnitude. $(V_D)\beta$ multiplied by $b$ gives clearance of the drug.

*What is the error assumed in a one-compartment model compared to a two-compartment or multicompartment model?*

- If the two-compartment model is ignored and the data are treated as a one-compartment model, the estimated values for the pharmacokinetic parameters are distorted. For example, during the distributive phase, the drug declines rapidly according to distribution $\alpha$ half-life, while in the elimination (terminal) part of the curve, the drug declines according to a $\beta$ elimination half-life.

*What kind of improvement in terms of patient care or drug therapy is made using the compartment model?*

- Compartment models have been used to develop dosage regimens and pharmacodynamic models. Compartment models have improved the dosing of drugs such as digoxin, gentamicin (Schentag et al 1977), lidocaine, and many others. The principal use of compartment models in dosing is to simulate a plasma drug concentration profile based on pharmacokinetic (PK) parameters. This information allows comparison of PK parameters in patients with only two or three points to a patient with full profiles using generated PK parameters.

## Learning Questions

1. Equation for the curve:

$$C = 52e^{-1.39t} + 18e^{-0.135t}$$

$$k_{10} = 0.41\ h^{-1}\quad k_{12} = 0.657\ h^{-1}\quad k_{21} = 0.458\ h^{-1}$$

2. Equation for the curve:

$$C = 28e^{-0.63t} + 10.5e^{-0.46t} + 14e^{-0.077t}$$

*Note:* When feathering curves by hand, a minimum of three points should be used to determine the line. Moreover, the rate constants and $y$ intercepts may vary according to the individual's skill. Therefore, values for $C$ should be checked by substitution of various times for $t$, using the derived equation. The theoretical curve should fit the observed data.

3. $C = 11.14\ \mu g/mL$.

4. The initial decline in the plasma drug concentration is due mainly to uptake of drug into tissues. During the initial distribution of drug, some drug elimination also takes place. After the drug has equilibrated with the tissues, the drug declines at a slower rate because of drug elimination.

5. A third compartment may indicate that the drug has a slow elimination component. If the drug is eliminated by a very slow elimination component, then drug accumulation may occur with multiple drug doses or long IV drug infusions. Depending on the blood sampling, a third compartment may be missed. However, some data may fit both a two-compartment and a three-compartment model. In this case, if the fit for each compartment model is very close statistically, the simpler compartment model should be used.

6. Because of the heterogeneity of the tissues, drug equilibrates into the tissues at different rates and different drug concentrations are usually observed in the different tissues. The drug concentration in the "tissue" compartment represents an "average" drug concentration and does not represent the drug concentration in any specific tissue.

7. $C = Ae^{-\alpha t} + Be^{-\beta t}$

   After substitution,

   $$C = 4.62e^{-8.94t} + 0.64e^{-0.19t}$$

   a. $V_c = \dfrac{X_0}{A+B} = \dfrac{75,000}{4.62+0.64} = 14,259 \text{ mL}$

   b. $V_p = \dfrac{V_e k_{12}}{k_{21}} = \dfrac{(14,259)(6.52)}{(1.25)} = 74,375 \text{ mL}$

   c. $k_{12} = \dfrac{AB(\beta - \alpha)^2}{(A+B)(A\beta + B\alpha)}$

   $$k_{12} = \dfrac{(4.62)(0.64)(0.19 - 8.94)^2}{(4.62+0.64)[(4.62)(0.19)+(0.64)(8.94)]}$$

   $$k_{12} = 6.52 \text{ h}^{-1}$$

   $$k_{21} = \dfrac{A\beta + B\alpha}{A+B} = \dfrac{(4.62)(0.19)(4.64)(8.94)}{4.62+0.64}$$

   $$k_{21} = 1.25 \text{ h}^{-1}$$

   d. $k = \dfrac{\alpha\beta(A+B)}{A\beta + B\alpha}$

   $$= \dfrac{(8.94)(0.19)(4.62+0.64)}{(4.62)(0.19)+(0.64)(8.94)}$$

   $$= 1.35 \text{ h}^{-1}$$

8. The tissue/peripheral compartments may not be sampled directly to obtain the drug concentration. Theoretical peripheral drug concentration, $C_p$, represents the average concentration in all the tissues outside the central compartment. The amount of drug in the tissue/peripheral $X_p$ represents the total amount of drug outside the central or plasma compartment. Occasionally $C_p$ may be equal to a particular tissue drug concentration in an organ. However, this $C_p$ may be equivalent by chance only.

9. The data were analyzed using computer software called RSTRIP, and found to fit a two-compartment model:

   $A(1) = 2.0049$   $A(2) = 6.0057$ (two preexponential values)

   $k(1) = 0.15053$   $k(2) = 7.0217$ (two exponential values)

   The equation that describes the data is:

   $$C = 2.0049e^{-0.15053t} + 6.0057e^{-7.0217t}$$

   The coefficient of correlation = 0.999 (very good fit).

   The model selection criterion = 11.27 (good model).

   The sum of squared deviations = $9.3 \times 10^{-5}$ (there is little deviation between the observed data and the theoretical value).

   $\alpha = 7.0217 \text{ h}^{-1}$, $\beta = 0.15053 \text{ h}^{-1}$.

10. a. Late-time samples were taken in some patients, yielding data that resulted in a monoexponential elimination profile. It is also possible that a patient's illness contributes to impaired drug distribution.

    b. The range of distribution half-lives is 30 to 45 minutes.

    c. None. Tissue concentrations are not generally well predicted from the two-compartment model. Only the amount of drug in the tissue compartment may be predicted.

    d. No. At steady state, the rate in and the rate out of the tissues are the same, but the drug concentrations are not necessarily the same. The plasma and each tissue may have different drug binding.

    e. None. Only the pooled tissue is simulated by the tissue compartment.

# REFERENCES

Avery JK: Routine procedure—bad outcome. *Tenn Med* **91**(7):280–281, 1998.

Eger E: In Papper EM, Kitz JR (eds). *Uptake and Distribution of Anesthetic Agents.* New York, McGraw-Hill, 1963, p. 76.

Eichler HG, Müller M: Drug distribution: The forgotten relative in clinical pharmacokinetics. *Clin Pharmacokinet* **34**(2):95–99, 1998.

Greenspon AJ, Mohiuddin S, Saksena S, et al: Comparison of intravenous tocainide with intravenous lidocaine for treating ventricular arrhythmias. *Cardiovasc Rev Rep* **10**:55–59, 1989.

Harron DWG: Digoxin pharmacokinetic modelling—10 years later. *Int J Pharm* **53**:181–188, 1989.

Hill HF, Coda BA, Tanaka A, Schaffer R: Multiple-dose evaluation of intravenous hydromorphone pharmacokinetics in normal human subjects. *Anesth Analg* **72**:330–336, 1991.

Jambhekar SS, Breen JP: Two compartment model. *Basic Pharmacokinetics*, 2nd ed. London, Chicago, Pharmaceutical Press, 2009, p. 269.

Jelliffe RW. The role of digitalis pharmacokinetics in converting atrial fibrillation and flutter to regular sinus rhythm. *Clin Pharmacokinet.* 2014 May;**53**(5):397–407. doi: 10.1007/s40262-014-0141-6. PMID: 24671885; PMCID: PMC4286389.

Mitenko PA, Ogilvie RI: Pharmacokinetics of intravenous theophylline. *Clin Pharmacol Ther* **14**:509, 1973.

Müller M: Monitoring tissue drug levels by clinical microdialysis. *Altern Lab Anim* **37**(suppl 1):57–59, 2009.

Pantuck AJ, Goldsmith JW, Kuriyan JB, Weiss RE: Seizures after ureteral stone manipulation with lidocaine. *J Urol* **157**(6):2248, 1997.

Parab PV, Ritschel WA, Coyle DE, Gree RV, Denson DD: Pharmacokinetics of hydromorphone after intravenous, peroral and rectal administration to human subjects. *Biopharm Drug Dispos* **9**:187–199, 1988.

Park GP, Kershner RP, Angellotti J, et al: Oral bioavailability and intravenous pharmacokinetics of amrinone in humans. *J Pharm Sci* **72**:817, 1983.

Reuning R, Sams R, Notari R: Role of pharmacokinetics in drug dosage adjustment. 1. Pharmacologic effects, kinetics, and apparent volume of distribution of digoxin. *J Clin Pharmacol* **13**:127–141, 1973.

Rochdi M, Sabouraud A, Baud FJ, Bismuth C, Scherrmann JM: Toxicokinetics of colchicine in humans: Analysis of tissue, plasma and urine data in ten cases. *Hum Exp Toxicol* **11**(6):510–516, 1992.

Schentag JJ, Jusko WJ, Plaut ME, Cumbo TJ, Vance JW, Abutyn E: Tissue persistence of gentamicin in man. *JAMA* **238**:327–329, 1977.

Swanson DJ, Reitberg DP, Smith IL, Wels PB, Schentag JJ: Steady-state moxalactam pharmacokinetics in patients: Noncompartmental versus two-compartmental analysis. *J Pharmacokinet-Biopharm* **11**(4):337–353, 1983.

Vallner JJ, Stewart JT, Kotzan JA, Kirsten EB, Honiger IL: Pharmacokinetics and bioavailability of hydromorphone following intravenous and oral administration to human subjects. *J Clin Pharmacol* **21**:152–156, 1981.

# BIBLIOGRAPHY

Dvorchick BH, Vessell ES: Significance of error associated with use of the one-compartment formula to calculate clearance of 38 drugs. *Clin Pharmacol Ther* **23**:617–623, 1978.

Jusko WJ, Gibaldi M: Effects of change in elimination on various parameters of the two-compartment open model. *J Pharm Sci* **61**:1270–1273, 1972.

Loughman PM, Sitar DS, Oglivie RI, Neims AH: The two-compartment open-system kinetic model: A review of its clinical implications and applications. *J Pediatr* **88**:869–873, 1976.

Mayersohn M, Gibaldi M: Mathematical methods in pharmacokinetics, II: Solution of the two-compartment open model. *Am J Pharm Ed* **35**:19–28, 1971.

Riegelman S, Loo JCK, Rowland M: Concept of a volume of distribution and possible errors in evaluation of this parameter. *J Pharm Sci* **57**:128–133, 1968.

Riegelman S, Loo JCK, Rowland M: Shortcomings in pharmacokinetics analysis by conceiving the body to exhibit properties of a single compartment. *J Pharm Sci* **57**:117–123, 1968.

# 14 Intravenous Infusion

HaiAn Zheng

## CHAPTER OBJECTIVES

- Describe the concept of steady state and how it relates to continuous dosing.

- Determine optimum dosing for an infused drug by calculating pharmacokinetic parameters from clinical data.

- Calculate loading doses to be used with an intravenous infusion.

- Describe the purpose of a loading dose.

- Compare the pharmacokinetic outcomes and clinical implications for a drug that follows a one-compartment model to a drug that follows a two-compartment model with or without a loading dose.

## INTRODUCTION

Drugs may be administered to patients by oral, topical, parenteral, or other various routes of administration. Examples of parenteral routes of administration include intravenous, subcutaneous, intramuscular, and other routes that require the drug to be given by sterile injection. Intravenous (IV) drug solutions may be either injected as a bolus dose (all at once) or infused slowly through a vein into the plasma at a constant rate (zero-order). The main advantage of giving a drug by IV infusion is that it allows precise control of plasma drug concentrations to fit the individual needs of the patient. For drugs with a narrow therapeutic window (eg, heparin), IV infusion maintains an effective constant plasma drug concentration by eliminating wide fluctuations between the peak (maximum) and trough (minimum) plasma drug concentration. Moreover, the IV infusion of drugs, such as antibiotics, may be given with IV fluids that include electrolytes and nutrients. Furthermore, the duration of drug therapy may be maintained or terminated as needed using IV infusion.

The plasma drug concentration–time curve of a drug given by constant IV infusion is shown in Fig. 14-1. Because no drug was present in the body at time zero, drug level rises from zero drug concentration and gradually becomes constant when a plateau or *steady-state* drug concentration is reached. At steady state, the rate of drug leaving the body (elimination rate) is equal to the rate of drug entering the body (infusion rate). Therefore, at steady state, the rate of change in the plasma drug concentration $dC_p/dt = 0$, and

$$\text{Rate of drug input} = \text{rate of drug output}$$
$$\text{(infusion rate)} \qquad \text{(elimination rate)}$$

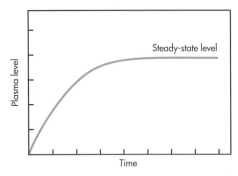

FIGURE 14-1 • Plasma level–time curve for constant IV infusion.

Based on this simple mass balance relationship, the following pharmacokinetic equation for infusion may be derived:

$$C_{ss} = \frac{R}{CL} \tag{14.1}$$

where $R$ is the infusion rate and $CL$ is the drug clearance. This equation is accurate and always valid regardless of the number of compartments characterizing the pharmacokinetic profile of the drug.

Should we want to define this equation using rate constants and volumes, its exact expression will then depend on the number of compartments that characterize the PK behavior of the drug under study. We will present examples for a drug whether it follows a one- or a two-compartment model.

## ONE-COMPARTMENT MODEL DRUGS

The pharmacokinetics of a drug given by constant IV infusion follows a zero-order input process in which the drug is directly infused into the systemic blood circulation. For most drugs, elimination of drug from the plasma is a first-order process. Drugs that are relatively polar, that are distributed in extracellular fluid volume (0.3 L/kg) and readily excreted by the kidney often display a monoexponential decline in terms of their pharmacokinetic profile. These drugs are well described by a one-compartment model. For them, the drug clearance is equal to the product of the total volume of distribution ($V_D$ or $V_{ss}$) with the elimination rate constant:

$$CL = k \cdot V_D \tag{14.2}$$

Therefore, in this one-compartment model, the infused drug follows zero-order input and

first-order output. The change in the amount of drug in the body at any time ($dD_B/dt$) during the infusion is the rate of input minus the rate of output.

$$\frac{dD_B}{dt} = R - kD_B \tag{14.3}$$

where $D_B$ is the amount of drug in the body, $R$ is the infusion rate (zero order), and $k$ is the elimination rate constant (first order).

Integration of Equation 14.3 and substitution of $D_B = C_p V_D$ gives:

$$C_p = \frac{R}{V_D k}(1 - e^{-kt}) \tag{14.4}$$

Equation 14.4 gives the plasma drug concentration $C_p$ at any time during the IV infusion where $t$ is the time for infusion, related to the volume of distribution ($V_D$). The graph for Equation 14.4 appears in Figs. 14-1 and 14-2. As the drug is infused, the value for certain time ($t$) increases in Equation 14.4. At infinite time $t = \infty$, $e^{-kt}$ approaches zero, and Equation 14.4 reduces to Equation 14.6, as the steady-state drug concentration ($C_{ss}$).

$$C_p = \frac{R}{V_D k}(1 - e^{-\infty}) \tag{14.5}$$

$$C_{ss} = \frac{R}{V_D k} \tag{14.6}$$

### Steady-State Drug Concentration ($C_{ss}$) and Time Needed to Reach $C_{ss}$

Once the steady state is reached, the rate of drug leaving the body (elimination rate) is equal to the rate

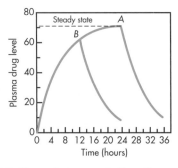

FIGURE 14-2 • Plasma drug concentrations–time profiles after IV infusion. IV infusion is stopped at steady state (A) or prior to steady state (B). In both cases, plasma drug concentrations decline exponentially (first order) according to a similar slope.

of drug entering the body (infusion rate). In other words, there is no *net* change in the amount of drug in the body, $D_B$, as a function of time during steady state. Drug elimination occurs according to first-order elimination kinetics. Whenever the infusion stops, either before or after steady state is reached, the drug concentration always declines according to first-order kinetics. The slope of the elimination curve is equal to $-k/2.3$ (Fig. 14-2). Even if the infusion is stopped before steady state is reached, the slope of the elimination curve remains the same (Fig. 14-2 (B)).

Mathematically, the time to reach true steady-state drug concentrations ($C_{ss}$) would take an infinite time. The time required to reach the steady-state drug concentration in the plasma is dependent on the elimination rate constant of the drug for a constant volume of distribution, as shown in Equation 14.6. Because drug elimination is exponential (first order), the plasma drug concentration becomes asymptotic to the theoretical steady-state plasma drug concentration. For zero-order elimination processes, if rate of input is greater than rate of elimination, plasma drug concentrations will keep increasing and no steady state will be reached. This is a potentially dangerous situation that will occur when saturation of metabolic process occurs. More on this can be found in Chapter 18 describing nonlinear pharmacokinetics.

In clinical practice, a plasma drug concentration prior to, but asymptotically approaching, the theoretical steady state is considered the steady-state plasma drug concentration ($C_{ss}$). In a constant IV infusion, the drug is infused at a constant or zero-order rate, $R$. During the IV infusion, the plasma drug concentration increases, and the rate of drug elimination increases because rate of elimination is concentration dependent (ie, rate of drug elimination = $kC_p$). $C_p$ keeps increasing until steady state is reached, at which time the rate of drug input (IV infusion rate) equals rate of drug output (elimination rate). The resulting plasma drug concentration at steady state ($C_{ss}$) is related to the rate of infusion and inversely related to the body clearance of the drug.

In clinical practice, the drug activity will be observed when the drug concentration is close to the desired plasma drug concentration, which is usually the *target* or *desired* steady-state drug concentration. For therapeutic purposes, the time for the

## TABLE 14-1 • Number of $t_{1/2}$ to Reach a Fraction of $C_{ss}$

| Percent of $C_{ss}$ Reached* | Number of Half-Lives |
|---|---|
| 90 | 3.32 |
| 95 | 4.32 |
| 99 | 6.65 |

*$C_{ss}$ is the steady-state drug concentration in plasma.

plasma drug concentration to reach more than 95% of the steady-state drug concentration in the plasma is often estimated. The time to reach 90%, 95%, and 99% of the steady-state drug concentration, $C_{ss}$, may be calculated. As detailed in Table 14-1, after IV infusion of the drug for five half-lives, the plasma drug concentration will be between 95% (4.32 $t_{1/2}$) and 99% (6.65 $t_{1/2}$) of the steady-state drug concentration. Thus, the time for a drug whose $t_{1/2}$ is 6 hours to reach 95% of the steady-state plasma drug concentration will be approximately 5 $t_{1/2}$, or 5 × 6 hours = 30 hours. The calculation of the values in Table 14-1 is given in the example that follows.

An increase in the infusion rate will not shorten the time to reach the steady-state drug concentration. If the drug is given at a more rapid infusion rate, a higher steady-state drug level will be obtained, but the time to reach steady state is the same (Fig. 14-3). This equation may also be obtained with the following approach. At steady state, the rate of infusion equals the rate of elimination. Therefore, the rate of change in the plasma drug concentration is equal to zero.

$$\frac{dC_p}{dt} = 0$$

$$\frac{dC_p}{dt} = \frac{R}{V_D} - kC_p = 0$$

$$(\text{Rate}_{in}) - (\text{Rate}_{out}) = 0 \qquad (14.7)$$

$$\frac{R}{V_D} = kC_p$$

$$C_{ss} = \frac{R}{V_D k}$$

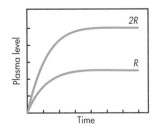

FIGURE 14-3 • Plasma level–time curve for IV infusions given at rates of R and 2R, respectively.

Equation 14.7 shows that the steady-state concentration $(C_{ss})$ is dependent on the volume of distribution, the elimination rate constant, and the infusion rate. Altering any one of these factors can affect steady-state concentration.

## EXAMPLE ▷ ▷ ▷

1. An antibiotic has a volume of distribution of 10 L and a k of 0.2 h$^{-1}$. A steady-state plasma concentration of 10 $\mu$g/mL is desired. The infusion rate needed to maintain this concentration can be determined as follows.
Equation 14.7 can be rewritten as

$$R = C_{ss}V_D k$$
$$= (10 \ \mu g/mL) \ (10) \ (1000 \ mL) \ (0.2 \ h^{-1})$$
$$= 20 \ mg/h$$

Assume the patient has a decreased renal function and the elimination rate constant has decreased to 0.1 h$^{-1}$. To maintain the steady-state concentration of 10 $\mu$g/mL, we must determine a new rate of infusion as follows.

$$R = (10 \ \mu g/mL) \ (10) \ (1000 \ mL) \ (0.1 \ h^{-1})$$
$$= 10 \ mg/h$$

When the elimination rate constant decreases, then the infusion rate must decrease proportionately to maintain the same $C_{ss}$. However, because the elimination rate constant is smaller (ie, the elimination $t_{1/2}$ is longer), the time to reach $C_{ss}$ will be longer.

2. An infinitely long period of time is needed to reach steady-state drug levels. However, in practice it is quite acceptable to reach 99% $C_{ss}$ (ie, 99% steady-state level). Using Equation 14.7, we know that the steady-state level is

$$C_{ss} = \frac{R}{V_D k}$$

and 99% steady-state level would be equal to

$$99\% \frac{R}{V_D k}$$

Substituting into Equation 14.4 for $C_p$, we can find out the time needed to reach steady state by solving for $t$.

$$99\% \frac{R}{V_D k} = \frac{R}{V_D k}(1 - e^{-kt})$$

$$99\% = 1 - e^{-kt}$$

$$e^{-kt} = 1\%$$

Take the natural logarithm on both sides:
$$-kt = \ln 0.01$$

$$t_{99\%ss} = \frac{\ln 0.01}{-k} = \frac{-4.61}{-k} = \frac{4.61}{k}$$

Substituting $(0.693/t_{1/2})$ for $k$,

$$t_{99\%ss} = \frac{4.61}{(0.693/t_{1/2})} = \frac{4.61}{0.693}t_{1/2}$$

$$t_{99\%ss} = 6.65 \cdot t_{1/2}$$

Notice that in the equation directly above, the time needed to reach steady state is not dependent on the rate of infusion, but only on the elimination half-life. Using similar calculations, the time needed to reach any percentage of the steady-state drug concentration may be obtained (Table 14.1).
IV infusion may be used to determine total body clearance if the infusion rate and steady-state level are known, as with Equation 14.1 repeated here:

$$C_{ss} = \frac{R}{CL} \tag{14.1}$$

$$CL_T = \frac{R}{C_{ss}} \tag{14.8}$$

**3.** A patient was given an antibiotic ($t_{1/2} = 6$ hours) by constant IV infusion at a rate of 2 mg/h. At the end of 2 days, the serum drug concentration was 10 mg/L. Calculate the total body clearance $CL$ for this antibiotic.

### Solution
The total body clearance may be estimated from rearrangement of Equation 14.1 (Equation 14.8). The serum sample was taken after 2 days or 48 hours of infusion, which time represents $8 \times t_{1/2}$, therefore, this serum drug concentration approximates the $C_{ss}$.

$$Cl_T = \frac{R}{C_{ss}} = \frac{2 \text{ mg/h}}{10 \text{ mg/L}} = 0.2 \text{ L/h}$$

---

### FREQUENTLY ASKED QUESTIONS

▶ How does one determine whether a patient has reached steady state during an IV infusion?

▶ What is the clinical relevance of steady state?

▶ How can the steady-state drug concentration be achieved more quickly?

---

## INFUSION METHOD FOR CALCULATING PATIENT ELIMINATION HALF-LIFE

The $C_p$-versus-time relationship that occurs during an IV infusion (Equation 14.4) may be used to calculate $k$, or indirectly the elimination half-life of the drug in a patient. Some information about the elimination half-life of the drug in the population must be known, and one or two plasma samples must be taken at a known time after infusion. Knowing the half-life in the general population helps determine if the sample is taken at steady state in the patient. To simplify calculation, Equation 14.4 is arranged to solve for $k$:

$$C_p = \frac{R}{V_D k}(1 - e^{-kt}) \qquad (14.4)$$

since

$$C_{ss} = \frac{R}{V_D k}$$

Substituting into Equation 14.4:

$$C_p = C_{ss}(1 - e^{-kt})$$

Rearranging and taking the log on both sides:

$$\log\left(\frac{C_{ss} - C_p}{C_{ss}}\right) = -\frac{kt}{2.3} \text{ and}$$

$$k = \frac{-2.3}{t}\log\left(\frac{C_{ss} - C_p}{C_{ss}}\right) \qquad (14.9)$$

where $C_p$ is the plasma drug concentration taken at time $t$, and $C_{ss}$ is the approximate steady-state plasma drug concentration in the patient.

---

## EXAMPLE 1 ▷ ▷ ▷

An antibiotic has an elimination half-life of 3 to 6 hours in the general population. A patient was given an IV infusion of an antibiotic at an infusion rate of 15 mg/h. Blood samples were taken at 8 and 24 hours, and plasma drug concentrations were 5.5 and 6.5 mg/L, respectively. Estimate the elimination half-life of the drug in this patient.

### Solution
Because the second plasma sample was taken at 24 hours, or $24/6 = 4$ half-lives after infusion, the plasma drug concentration in this sample is approaching 95% of the true plasma steady-state drug concentration assuming the extreme case of $t_{1/2} = 6$ hours.

By substitution into Equation 14.9:

$$\log\left(\frac{6.5 - 5.5}{6.5}\right) = -\frac{k(8)}{2.3}$$

$$k = 0.234 \text{ h}^{-1}$$

$$t_{1/2} = \frac{0.693}{0.234} = 2.96 \text{ hours}$$

The elimination half-life calculated in this manner is not as accurate as the calculation of $t_{1/2}$ using multiple plasma drug concentration time points after a single IV bolus dose or after stopping the IV infusion, or what one would get by *fitting* the concentrations to a one-compartment model. However, this method may be sufficient in clinical practice when no time is available for exact data fitting. If the second blood sample is taken closer to the time for steady state, the result is more accurate. At the 30th hour, for example, the plasma concentration would be 99% of the true steady-state value (corresponding to 30/6 or 5 elimination half-lives), and less error would result in applying Equation 14.9.

When Equation 14.9 was used in the example above to calculate the drug $t_{1/2}$ of the patient, the second plasma drug concentration was assumed to be the theoretical $C_{ss}$. As demonstrated below, when $k$ and the corresponding values are substituted,

$$\log\left(\frac{C_{ss} - 5.5}{C_{ss}}\right) = -\frac{(0.234)(8)}{2.3}$$

$$\frac{C_{ss} - 5.5}{C_{ss}} = 0.157$$

$$C_{ss} = 6.5 \text{ mg/L}$$

(Note that $C_{ss}$ is in fact the same as the concentration at 24 hours in the example above.) In clinical practice when time is not available to the pharmacist to do actual data fitting, before starting an IV infusion, an appropriate infusion rate ($R$) is generally calculated from Equation 14.9 using literature values for $C_{ss}$, $k$, and $V_D$ or $CL$. Two plasma samples are taken and the sampling times recorded. The second sample should be taken near the theoretical time for steady state, when possible. Equation 14.9 would then be used to calculate a $k$ and then $t_{1/2}$. If the elimination half-life calculated confirms that the second sample was taken at steady state, the plasma concentration is simply assumed as the steady-state concentration and a new infusion rate may be calculated.

## EXAMPLE 2 ▷ ▷ ▷

If the desired therapeutic plasma concentration is 8 mg/L for the above patient (Example 1), what is the suitable infusion rate for the patient?

### Solution

From Example 1, the trial infusion rate was 15 mg/h. Assuming the second blood sample is the steady-state level, 6.5 mg/mL, the clearance of the patient is

$$C_{ss} = \frac{R}{CL}$$

$$CL = \frac{R}{C_{ss}} = \frac{15}{6.5} = 2.31 \text{ L/h}$$

The new infusion rate should be

$$R = C_{ss} \cdot CL = 8 \cdot 2.31 = 18.48 \text{ mg/h}$$

In this example, the $t_{1/2}$ of this patient is a little shorter, about 3 hours compared to 3 to 6 hours reported for the general population. Therefore, the infusion rate should be a little greater in order to maintain the desired steady-state level of 15 mg/L.

Equation 14.8 is always accurate, regardless of the number of compartments, but is dependent on the error associated with its terms. For example, if the $C_{ss}$ used in the formula has a 5% deviation from the true $C_{ss}$, then the calculated $CL$ will be off by 5%.

## LOADING DOSE PLUS IV INFUSION— ONE-COMPARTMENT MODEL

The loading dose $D_L$, or initial bolus dose of a drug, is used to obtain desired concentrations as rapidly as possible. The concentration of drug in the body for a one-compartment model after an IV bolus dose is described by

$$C_1 = C_0 e^{-kt} = \frac{D_L}{V_D} e^{-kt} \qquad (14.10)$$

and concentration by infusion at the rate $R$ is

$$C_2 = \frac{R}{V_D k}(1 - e^{-kt}) \qquad (14.11)$$

Assume that an IV bolus dose $D_L$ of the drug is given and that an IV infusion is started at the same time. The total concentration $C_p$ at $t$ hours after the start of infusion would be equal to $C_1 + C_2$ due to the sum contributions of bolus and infusion, or

$$C_p = C_1 + C_2$$

$$C_p = \frac{D_L}{V_D}e^{-kt} + \frac{R}{V_D k}(1-e^{-kt})$$

$$\quad (14.12)$$

$$= \frac{D_L}{V_D}e^{-kt} + \frac{R}{V_D k} - \frac{R}{V_D k}e^{-kt}$$

$$= \frac{R}{V_D k} + \left(\frac{D_L}{V_D}e^{-kt} - \frac{R}{V_D k}e^{-kt}\right)$$

Let the loading dose ($D_L$) equal the amount of drug in the body at steady state

$$D_L = C_{ss}V_D$$

From Equation 14.6, $C_{ss}V_D = R/k$. Therefore,

$$D_L = R/k \quad (14.13)$$

Substituting $D_L = R/k$ in Equation 14.12 makes the expression in parentheses cancel out. Equation 14.12 reduces to Equation 14.14, which is the same expression for $C_{ss}$ or steady-state plasma concentrations (Equation 14.15 is identical to Equation 14.8):

$$C_p = \frac{R}{V_D k} \quad (14.14)$$

$$C_{ss} = \frac{R}{V_D k} \quad (14.15)$$

Therefore, if an IV loading dose of $R/k$ is given, followed by an IV infusion, steady-state plasma drug concentrations are obtained immediately and maintained (Fig. 14-4). In this situation, steady state is also achieved in a one-compartment model, since the rate in = rate out ($R = dD_B/dt$).

The loading dose needed to get immediate steady-state drug levels can also be found by the following approach.

Loading dose equation:

$$C_1 = \frac{D_L}{V_D}e^{-kt}$$

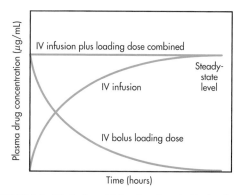

FIGURE 14-4 • IV Infusion with loading dose $D_L$. The loading dose is given by IV bolus injection at the start of the infusion. Plasma drug concentrations decline exponentially after $D_L$, whereas they increase exponentially during the infusion. The resulting plasma drug concentration–time curve is a straight line due to the summation of the two curves.

Infusion equation:

$$C_2 = \frac{R}{V_D k}(1-e^{-kt})$$

Adding up the two equations yields Equation 14.16, an equation describing simultaneous infusion after a loading dose.

$$C_p = \frac{D_L}{V_D}e^{-kt} + \frac{R}{V_D k}(1-e^{-kt}) \quad (14.16)$$

By differentiating this equation at steady state, we obtain:

$$\frac{dC_p}{dt} = 0 = \frac{-D_L k}{V_D}e^{-kt} + \frac{Rk}{V_D k}e^{-kt}$$

$$\quad (14.17)$$

$$0 = e^{-kt}\left(\frac{-D_L k}{V_D} + \frac{R}{V_D}\right)$$

$$\frac{D_L k}{V_D} = \frac{R}{V_D}$$

$$\quad (14.18)$$

$$D_L = \frac{R}{k} = \text{loading dose}$$

To maintain instant steady-state level ([dCp/dt] = 0), the loading dose should be equal to $R/k$.

For a one-compartment drug, if the $D_L$ and infusion rate are calculated such that $C_o$ and $C_{ss}$ are the same and both $D_L$ and infusion are started concurrently, then steady state and $C_{ss}$ will be achieved

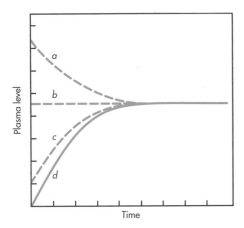

immediately after the loading dose is administered (Fig. 14-4). Similarly, in Fig. 14-5, curve *b* shows the blood level after a single loading dose of $R/k$ plus infusion from which the concentration desired at steady state is obtained. If the $D_L$ is not equal to $R/k$, then steady state will not occur immediately. If the loading dose given is larger than $R/k$, the plasma drug concentration takes longer to decline to the concentration desired at steady state (curve *a*). If the loading dose is lower than $R/k$, the plasma drug concentrations will increase slowly to desired drug levels (curve *c*), but more quickly than without any loading dose.

Another method for the calculation of loading dose $D_L$ is based on knowledge of the desired steady-state drug concentration $C_{ss}$ and the apparent volume of distribution $V_D$ for the drug, as shown in Equation 14.18.

$$D_L = C_{ss}V_D \qquad (14.19)$$

For many drugs, the desired $C_{ss}$ is reported in the literature as the effective therapeutic drug concentration. The $V_D$ and the elimination half-life are also available for these drugs.

## PRACTICE PROBLEMS

1. A physician wants to administer an anesthetic agent at a rate of 2 mg/h by IV infusion. The elimination rate constant is 0.1 h⁻¹ and the volume of distribution (one compartment) is 10 L.

How much is the drug plasma concentration at the steady state? What loading dose should be recommended to reach steady state immediately?

### Solution

$$C_{ss} = \frac{R}{V_D k} = \frac{2000}{(10 \times 10^3)(0.1)} = 2 \; \mu g/mL$$

To reach $C_{ss}$ instantly,

$$D_L = \frac{R}{k} = \frac{2 \; mg/h}{0.1/h} \qquad D_L = 20 \; mg$$

2. What is the concentration of a drug at 6 hours after infusion administration at 2 mg/h, with an initial loading dose of 10 mg (the drug has a $t_{1/2}$ of 3 hours and a volume of distribution of 10 L)?

### Solution

$$k = \frac{0.693}{3 \; h}$$

$$C_p = \frac{D_L}{V_D}e^{-kt} + \frac{R}{V_D k}(1 - e^{-kt})$$

$$C_p = \frac{10,000}{10,000}(e^{-(0.693/3)(6)})$$

$$+ \frac{2000}{(10,000)(0.693/3)}(1 - e^{-(0.693/3)(6)})$$

$$C_p = 0.90 \; \mu g/mL$$

3. Calculate the drug concentration in the blood after infusion has been stopped.

### Solution

This concentration can be calculated in two parts (see Fig. 14-2 (A)). First, calculate the concentration of drug during infusion, and second, calculate the concentration after the stop of the infusion, C. Then use the IV bolus dose equation ($C = C_0 e^{-kt}$) for calculations for any further point in time. For convenience, the two equations can be combined as follows:

$$C_p = \frac{R}{V_D k}(1 - e^{-kb})e^{-k(t-b)} \qquad (14.20)$$

where $b$ = length of time of infusion period, $t$ = total time (infusion and postinfusion), and $t - b$ = length of time after infusion has stopped. Here, we assume no bolus loading dose was given.

4. A patient was infused for 6 hours with a drug ($k = 0.01$ h$^{-1}$; $V_D = 10$ L) at a rate of 2 mg/h. What is the concentration of the drug in the body 2 hours after cessation of the infusion?

**Solution**

Using Equation 14.20,

$$C_p = \frac{2000}{(0.01)(10,000)}(1 - e^{-0.01(6)})e^{-0.01(8-6)}$$

$$C_p = 1.14 \ \mu g/mL$$

Alternatively, when infusion stops, $C_p'$ is calculated:

$$C_p' = \frac{R}{V_D k}(1 - e^{-kt})$$

$$C_p' = \frac{2000}{0.01 \times 10,000}(1 - e^{-0.01(6)})$$

$$C = C_p' e^{-0.01(2)}$$

$$C = 1.14 \ \mu g/mL$$

The two approaches should give the same answer.

5. An adult male asthmatic patient (78 kg, 48 years old) with a history of heavy smoking was given an IV infusion of aminophylline at a rate of 0.75 mg/kg/h. A loading dose of 6 mg/kg was given by IV bolus injection just prior to the start of the infusion. Two hours after the start of the IV infusion, the plasma theophylline concentration was measured and found to contain 5.8 $\mu$g/mL of theophylline. The apparent $V_D$ for theophylline is 0.45 L/kg. (Aminophylline is the ethylenediamine salt of theophylline and contains 80% of theophylline base.)

Because the patient was responding poorly to the aminophylline therapy, the physician wanted to increase the plasma theophylline concentration in the patient to 10 $\mu$g/mL. What dosage recommendation would you give the physician? Would you recommend another loading dose?

**Solution**

If no loading dose is given and the IV infusion rate is increased, the time to reach steady-state plasma drug concentrations will be about 4 to 5 $t_{1/2}$ to reach 95% of $C_{ss}$. Therefore, a second loading dose should be recommended to rapidly increase the plasma theophylline concentration to 10 $\mu$g/mL. The infusion rate must also be increased to maintain this desired $C_{ss}$.

The calculation of loading dose $D_L$ must consider the present plasma theophylline concentration.

$$D_L = \frac{V_D(C_{p,desired} - C_{p,present})}{(S)(F)} \tag{14.21}$$

where $S$ is the salt form of the drug and $F$ is the fraction of drug bioavailable. For aminophylline, $S$ is equal to 0.80 and for an IV bolus injection $F$ is equal to 1.

$$D_L = \frac{(0.45 \ L/kg)(78 \ kg)(10 - 5.8 \ mg/L)}{(0.8)(1)}$$

$$D_L = 184 \ mg \ aminophylline$$

The maintenance IV infusion rate may be calculated after estimation of the patient's clearance, $CL$. A loading dose and an IV infusion of 0.75 mg/h aminophylline (equivalent to $0.75 \cdot 0.8 = 0.6$ mg theophylline) per kg was given to the patient. For simplicity, if we assume the plasma theophylline concentration of 5.8 mg/L is close to the steady-state $C_{ss}$, total clearance may be estimated by

$$CL_T = \frac{R}{C_{ss,present}} = \frac{(0.6 \ mg/h/kg)(78 \ kg)}{5.8 \ mg/L}$$

$$CL_T = 8.07 \ L/h \ or \ 1.72 \ mL/min/kg$$

The usual $CL$ for adult, nonsmoking patients with uncomplicated asthma is approximately 0.65 mL/min/kg. Heavy smoking is known to increase $CL$ for theophylline.

The new IV infusion rate, $R'$ in terms of theophylline, is calculated by

$$R' = C_{ss}, \text{desired } CL$$

$$R' = 10 \ mg/L \cdot 8.07 \ L/h = 80.7 \ mg/h \ or$$
1.03 mg/h/kg of theophylline, which is equivalent to 1.29 mg/h/kg of aminophylline.

6. An adult male patient (43 years, 80 kg) is to be given an antibiotic by IV infusion. According to the literature, the antibiotic has an elimination

$t_{1/2}$ of 2 hours, $V_D$ of 1.25 L/kg, and is effective at a plasma drug concentration of 14 mg/L. The drug is supplied in 5-mL ampuls containing 150 mg/mL.

**a.** Recommend a starting infusion rate in milligrams per hour and liters per hour.

## Solution

Assume the effective plasma drug concentration is the target drug concentration or $C_{ss}$.

$$R = C_{ss} \cdot k \cdot V_D$$

$$= (14 \text{ mg/L}) (0.693/2 \text{ h}) (1.5 \text{ L/kg}) (80 \text{ kg})$$

$$= 485.1 \text{ mg/h}$$

Because the drug is supplied at a concentration of 150 mg/mL,

$$(485.1 \text{ mg})(\text{mL}/150 \text{ mg}) = 3.23 \text{ mL}$$

$$\text{Thus, } R = 3.23 \text{ mL/h}.$$

**b.** Blood samples were taken from the patient at 12, 16, and 24 hours after the start of the infusion. Plasma drug concentrations were as shown below:

| t (hour) | $C_p$ (mg/L) |
|----------|--------------|
| 12 | 16.1 |
| 16 | 16.3 |
| 24 | 16.5 |

From these additional data, calculate the total body clearance $CL_T$ for the drug in this patient.

## Solution

Because the plasma drug concentrations at 12, 16, and 24 hours were similar, steady state has essentially been reached. Assuming a $C_{ss}$ of 16.3 mg/mL, $CL_T$ is calculated.

$$CL_T = \frac{R}{C_{ss}} = \frac{485.1 \text{ mg/h}}{16.3 \text{ mg/L}} = 29.8 \text{ L/h}$$

**c.** From the above data, estimate the elimination half-life for the antibiotics in this patient.

## Solution

Generally, the apparent volume of distribution $(V_D)$ is less variable than $t_{1/2}$. Assuming that the literature value for $V_D$ is 1.25 L/kg, then $t_{1/2}$ may be estimated from the $CL$.

$$k = \frac{CL_T}{V_D} = \frac{29.9 \text{ L/h}}{(1.25 \text{ L/kg})(80 \text{ kg})} = 0.299 \text{ h}^{-1}$$

$$t_{1/2} = \frac{0.693}{0.299 \text{ h}^{-1}} = 2.32 \text{ h}$$

Thus, the $t_{1/2}$ for the antibiotic in this patient is 2.32 hours, which is in good agreement with the literature value of 2 hours.

**d.** After reviewing the pharmacokinetics of the antibiotic in this patient, should the infusion rate for the antibiotic be changed?

## Solution

To properly decide whether the infusion rate should be changed, the clinical pharmacist must consider the pharmacodynamics and toxicity of the drug. Assuming the drug has a wide therapeutic window and shows no sign of adverse drug toxicity, the infusion rate of 485.1 mg/h, calculated according to pharmacokinetic literature values for the drug, appears to be correct.

$$C_p = \frac{R}{Cl} (1 - e^{-(Cl/V_D)t})$$

## ESTIMATION OF DRUG CLEARANCE AND $V_D$ FROM INFUSION DATA

The plasma concentration of a drug during constant infusion was described in terms of volume of distribution $V_D$ and elimination constant $k$ in Equation 14.4. Alternatively, the equation may be described in terms of clearance by substituting for $k$ into Equation 14.4 with $k = CL/V_D$:

$$C_p = \frac{R}{CL} (1 - e^{-(CL/V_D)t}) \tag{14.22}$$

Physiologically we may be more interested in clearances and volumes, than in elimination rate constants. If that is the case, then the "independent" parameters that we would want to determine would be $CL$ and $V_D$, and $k$ would become an independent parameter. The time for steady state and the resulting steady-state concentration will be dependent on both clearance and volume of distribution. When PK is linear and clearances and volumes do not change over time, the time for steady state is then inversely related to clearance. Thus, drugs with small clearance will take a long time to reach steady state.

When evaluating clearance or elimination half-life with decreasing plasma concentrations, it is more robust to collect plasma samples that are separated in time by many half-lives. In contrast, calculating the elimination rate constant when concentrations are taken at time equivalent to less than 1 half-life will not be very discriminating due to the small change in the drug concentration, change which may be similar to the uncertainty related to each concentration that we measure. Blood samples taken at 3 to 4 half-lives will result in a large difference in concentration, which will then be much larger than the uncertainty related to the determination of these concentrations. So the $k$ or $CL$ will then be obtained with much better precision.

## INTRAVENOUS INFUSION OF TWO-COMPARTMENT MODEL DRUGS

Many drugs given by IV infusion follow two-compartment kinetics. For example, the respective distributions of theophylline and lidocaine in humans are described by the two-compartment open model. With two-compartment model drugs, IV infusion requires a distribution and equilibration of the drug before a stable blood level is reached. During a constant IV infusion, drug in the tissue compartment is in distribution equilibrium with the plasma; thus, constant $C_{ss}$ levels also result in constant drug concentrations in the tissue, that is, no *net* change in the amount of drug in the tissue occurs during steady state. Although some clinicians assume that tissue and plasma concentrations are equal when fully equilibrated, kinetic models only predict that the rate of drug transfer into and out of the compartments are equal at steady state. In other words, drug concentrations in the tissue can also remain constant, but may differ from plasma concentrations.

The time needed to reach a steady-state blood level depends entirely on the distribution half-life of the drug. The equation describing plasma drug concentration as a function of time is as follows:

$$C_p = \frac{R}{V_p k}\left[1 - \left(\frac{k-b}{a-b}\right)e^{-at} - \left(\frac{a-k}{a-b}\right)e^{-bt}\right] \quad (14.23)$$

where $a$ and $b$ are hybrid rate constants and $R$ is the rate of infusion. At steady state (ie, $t = \infty$), Equation 14.23 reduces to

$$C_{ss} = \frac{R}{V_p k} \quad (14.24)$$

By rearranging this equation, the infusion rate for a desired steady-state plasma drug concentration may be calculated.

$$R = C_{ss} V_p k \quad (14.25)$$

### Loading Dose for Two-Compartment Model Drugs

Drugs with long half-lives require a loading dose to more rapidly attain steady-state plasma drug levels. It is clinically desirable to achieve rapid therapeutic drug levels by using a loading dose. However, for a drug that follows the two-compartment pharmacokinetic model, the drug distributes slowly into extravascular tissues (compartment 2). Thus, drug equilibrium is not immediate. The plasma drug concentration of a drug that follows a two-compartment model after various loading doses is shown in Fig. 14-6. If a loading dose is given too rapidly, the drug may initially

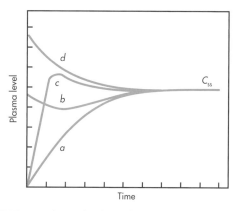

FIGURE 14-6 • Plasma drug level after various loading doses and rates of infusion for a drug that follows a two-compartment model: a, no loading dose; b, loading dose = R/k (rapid infusion); c, loading dose = R/b (slow infusion); d, loading dose = R/b (rapid infusion).

give excessively high concentrations in the plasma (central compartment), which then decreases as drug equilibrium is reached (Fig. 14-6). It is not possible to maintain an instantaneous, stable steady-state blood level for a two-compartment model drug with a zero-order rate of infusion. Therefore, a loading dose produces an initial blood level either slightly higher or lower than the steady-state blood level. To overcome this problem, several IV bolus injections given as short intermittent IV infusions may be used as a method for administering a loading dose to the patient (see Chapter 17).

## Total Volume of Distribution for Two-Compartment Model Drugs

After administration of any drug that follows two-compartment kinetics, plasma drug levels will decline due to elimination from the central compartment, and some redistribution will occur as drug in tissue diffuses back into the plasma fluid. The total volume of distribution $V_{ss}$, is the "hypothetical space" in which the drug is assumed to be distributed and is the sum of the volumes of the two compartments $V_c$ (central volume of distribution) and $V_p$ (peripheral volume of distribution), as shown by Equation 12.26. The product of the plasma drug concentration with $V_{ss}$ will give the total amount of drug in the body at that time, such that $C_{ss} \cdot V_{ss} =$ amount of drug in the body at steady state. At steady-state conditions, the rate of drug entry into the tissue compartment from the central compartment is equal to the rate of drug exit from the tissue compartment into the central compartment.

$$V_{ss} = V_c + V_p \qquad (14.26)$$

Because $V_p = V_c \cdot \dfrac{k_{12}}{k_{21}}$,

$V_{ss} = V_c + V_c \cdot \dfrac{k_{12}}{k_{21}}$; therefore,

$$V_{ss} = V_c \cdot \left(1 + \frac{k_{12}}{k_{21}}\right) \qquad (14.27)$$

In practice, Equation 14.27 is used to calculate $V_{ss}$. The $\underline{V}_D$ is a function of the transfer constants, $k_{12}$ and $k_{21}$, which represent the rate constants of drug going into and out of the tissue compartment,

respectively. The magnitude of $V_{ss}$ is dependent on the hemodynamic factors responsible for drug distribution and on the physical properties of the drug, properties which, in turn, determine the relative amount of intra- and extravascular drug.

Another volume term sometimes used and reported by PK software is the $V_\beta$, $V_z$, or $V_{area}$ (see Chapter 13). Although these terms are slightly different, they all represent the same volume but the terminology explains how they are calculated. $V_\beta$ or $V_z$ is the volume of distribution calculated using the clearance divided by the terminal rate constant (either denoted as $\beta$ or $\lambda_z$). $V_{area}$ is simply the same volume but calculated as Dose/$AUC_{inf}$.

$$V_\beta = CL/\beta$$

$$V_z = CL/\lambda_z$$

$$V_{area} = \text{Dose}/(AUC_{inf} \cdot \lambda_z)$$

The $V_\beta$, $V_z$, $V_{area}$ will be equal to the total volume of distribution only if the drug is well described by a one-compartment model. For drugs that are distributed in two compartments, the $V_\beta$, $V_z$, $V_{area}$ will be a hybrid volume, one that will not be equal to the $V_c$ nor the $V_{ss}$, but will be between the two. Some refer to this volume as the "volume during the terminal phase," as it is calculated as the ratio of $CL$ by the terminal rate constant.

It can be argued that the $V_\beta$, $V_z$, $V_{area}$ are not really useful. The total volume of distribution, $V_{ss}$, reflects the true distributional volume occupied by the plasma and the tissue pool. This volume, $V_{ss}$, multiplied by the steady-state plasma drug concentration, $C_{ss}$, yields the amount of drug in the body. The central volume of distribution, $V_c$, represents the volume into which the drug initially distributes when infused. That volume, $V_c$, is often used to determine the loading dose necessary to upload the body to a desired plasma drug concentration.

## PRACTICAL FOCUS

### Questions

1. Do you agree with the following statements for a drug that is described by a two-compartment pharmacokinetic model and given with a continuous IV infusion? At steady state, the drug is well equilibrated between the plasma and the tissue compartment,

$C_p = C_t$, and the rates of drug diffusion into and from the plasma compartment are equal

2. Azithromycin in plasma may be described by a central volume of distribution $(V_c)$ and a peripheral volume of distribution $(V_p)$ model. The steady-state volume of distribution $(V_{ss})$ is much larger than the initial volume of the $V_c$. Why?

3. "Rapid distribution of azithromycin into cells causes higher concentration in the tissues than in the plasma. . . ." Does this statement conflict with the steady-state concept? Why is the loading dose often calculated using the $V_{ss}$ instead of $V_c$?

4. Why is a loading dose used?

## Solutions

1. For a drug that follows a multiple-compartment model, the rates of drug diffusion into the tissues from the plasma and from the tissues into the plasma are equal at steady state. However, the tissue drug concentration is generally not equal to the plasma drug concentration.

2. When plasma drug concentration data are used alone to describe the disposition of the drug, no information on tissue drug concentration is known, and no model will predict actual tissue drug concentrations. To account for the mass balance (drug mass/volume = body drug concentration) of drug present in the body (tissue and plasma pool) at any time after dosing, the body drug concentration is assumed to be the plasma drug concentration. In reality, azithromycin tissue concentration is much higher. Therefore, the calculated volume of the tissue compartment is much bigger (31.1 L/kg) than its actual volume.

3. The product of the steady-state apparent $(V_D)_{ss}$ and the steady-state plasma drug concentration $C_{ss}$ estimates the amount of drug present in the body. The amount of drug present in the body may be important information for toxicity considerations, and may also be used as a therapeutic endpoint. In most cases, the therapeutic drug at the site of action accounts for only a small fraction of total drug in the tissue compartment. The pharmacodynamic profile may be described as a separate compartment (see effect compartment in Chapter 22). Based on pharmacokinetic and

biopharmaceutic studies, the factors that account for high tissue concentrations include diffusion constant, lipid solubility, and tissue binding to cell components. A ratio measuring the relative drug concentration in tissue and plasma is the partition coefficient, which is helpful in predicting the distribution of a drug into tissues. Ultimately, studies of tissue drug distribution using radiolabeled drug are much more useful.

The real tissue drug level will differ from the plasma drug concentration depending on the partitioning of drug in tissues and plasma. $(V_D)_\beta$ is a volume of distribution often calculated because it is easier to calculate than $(V_D)_{ss}$. This volume of distribution, $(V_D)_\beta$, allows the area under the curve to be calculated, an area which has been related to toxicities associated with many cancer chemotherapy agents. Many values for apparent volumes of distribution reported in the clinical literature are obtained using the area equation. Some early pharmacokinetic literature only includes the steady-state volume of distribution, which approximates the $(V_D)_\beta$ but is substantially smaller in many cases. In general, both volume terms reflect extravascular drug distribution. $(V_D)_\beta$ appears to be much more affected by the dynamics of drug disposition in the beta phase, whereas $(V_D)_{ss}$ reflects more accurately the inherent distribution of the drug.

4. When drugs are given in a multiple-dose regimen, a loading dose may be given to achieve steady-state drug concentrations more rapidly.

### FREQUENTLY ASKED QUESTIONS

▶ What is the main reason for giving a drug by slow IV infusion?

▶ Why do we use a loading dose to rapidly achieve therapeutic concentration for a drug with a long elimination half-life instead of increasing the rate of drug infusion or increasing the size of the infusion dose?

▶ Explain why the application of a loading dose as a single IV bolus injection may cause an adverse event or drug toxicity in the patient if the drug follows a two-compartment model with a slow elimination phase.

▶ What are some of the complications involved with IV infusion?

## CHAPTER SUMMARY

An IV bolus injection puts the drug into the systemic circulation almost instantaneously. For some drugs, IV bolus injections can result in immediate high plasma drug concentrations and drug toxicity. An IV drug infusion slowly inputs the drug into the circulation and can provide stable drug concentrations in the plasma for a longer time period. Constant IV drug infusions are considered to have zero-order drug absorption because of direct input. Once the drug is infused, the drug is eliminated by first-order elimination. Steady state is achieved when the rate of drug infusion (ie, rate of drug absorption) equals the rate of drug elimination. Four to five elimination half-lives are needed to achieve 95% of

steady state. A loading dose given as an IV bolus injection may be used at the start of an infusion to quickly achieve the desired steady-state plasma drug concentration. For drugs that follow a two-compartment model, multiple small loading doses or intermittent IV infusions may be needed to prevent plasma drug concentrations from becoming too high. Pharmacokinetic parameters may be calculated from samples taken during the IV infusion and after the infusion is stopped, regardless of whether steady state has been achieved. These calculated pharmacokinetic parameters are then used to optimize dosing for that patient when population estimates do not provide outcomes suitable for the patient.

## LEARNING QUESTIONS

1. A female patient (35 years old, 65 kg) with normal renal function is to be given a drug by IV infusion. According to the literature, the elimination half-life of this drug is 7 hours, it is well described by a one-compartment model, and the apparent $V_D$ is 23.1% of body weight. The pharmacokinetics of this drug assumes a first-order process. The desired steady-state plasma level for this antibiotic is 10 $\mu g/mL$.

   a. Assuming no loading dose, how long after the start of the IV infusion would it take to reach 95% of the $C_{ss}$?

   b. What is the proper loading dose for this antibiotic?

   c. What is the proper infusion rate for this drug?

   d. What is the total body clearance?

   e. If the patient suddenly develops partial renal failure, how long would it take for a new steady-state plasma level to be established (assume that 95% of the $C_{ss}$ is a reasonable approximation)?

   f. If the total body clearance declined 50% due to partial renal failure, what new infusion rate would you recommend to maintain the desired steady-state plasma level of 10 $\mu g/mL$.

2. An anticonvulsant drug was given as (a) a single IV dose and then (b) a constant IV infusion. The serum drug concentrations are as presented in Table 14-2.

   a. What is the steady-state plasma drug level?

   b. What is the time for 95% steady-state plasma drug level?

   c. What is the drug clearance?

**TABLE 14-2 • Serum Drug Concentrations for a Hypothetical Anticonvulsant Drug**

| Time (hour) | Single IV dose (1 mg/kg) | Constant IV Infusion (0.2 mg/kg per hour) |
|---|---|---|
| 0 | 10.0 | 0 |
| 2 | 6.7 | 3.3 |
| 4 | 4.5 | 5.5 |
| 6 | 3.0 | 7.0 |
| 8 | 2.0 | 8.0 |
| 10 | 1.35 | 8.6 |
| 12 | | 9.1 |
| 18 | | 9.7 |
| 24 | | 9.9 |

**d.** What is the plasma concentration of the drug 4 hours after stopping infusion (infusion was stopped after 24 hours)?

**e.** What is the infusion rate for a patient weighing 75 kg to maintain a steady-state drug level of 10 $\mu$g/mL?

**f.** What is the plasma drug concentration 4 hours after an IV dose of 1 mg/kg followed by a constant infusion of 0.2 mg/kg/h?

**3.** An antibiotic is to be given by IV infusion. How many milliliters per hour should a sterile drug solution (25 mg/mL) be given to a 75-kg adult male patient to achieve an infusion rate of 1 mg/kg/h?

**4.** An antibiotic drug is to be given to an adult male patient (75 kg, 58 years old) by IV infusion. The drug is supplied in sterile vials containing 30 mL of the antibiotic solution at a concentration of 125 mg/mL. What rate in milliliters per hour would you infuse this patient to obtain a steady-state concentration of 20 $\mu$g/mL? What loading dose would you suggest? Assume the drug follows the pharmacokinetics of a one-compartment open model. The apparent volume of distribution of this drug is 0.5 L/kg and the elimination half-life is 3 hours.

**5.** According to the manufacturer, a steady-state serum concentration of 17 mg/mL was measured when the antibiotic, cephradine (Velosef), was given by IV infusion to nine adult male volunteers (average weight, 71.7 kg) at a rate of 5.3 mg/kg/h for 4 hours.

**a.** Calculate the total body clearance for this drug.

**b.** When the IV infusion was discontinued, the cephradine serum concentration decreased exponentially, declining to 1.5 mg/mL at 6.5 hours after the start of the infusion. Calculate the elimination half-life.

**c.** From the information above, calculate the apparent volume of distribution.

**d.** Cephradine is completely excreted unchanged in the urine, and studies have shown that probenecid given concurrently causes elevation of the serum cephradine concentration. What is the probable mechanism for this interaction of probenecid with cephradine?

**6.** Calculate the excretion rate at steady state for a drug given by IV infusion at a rate of 30 mg/h. The $C_{ss}$ is 20 $\mu$g/mL. If the rate of infusion were increased to 40 mg/h, what would be the new steady-state drug concentration, $C_{ss}$? Would the excretion rate for the drug at the new steady state be the same? Assume first-order elimination kinetics and a one-compartment model.

**7.** An antibiotic is to be given to an adult male patient (58 years, 75 kg) by IV infusion. The elimination half-life is 8 hours and the apparent volume of distribution is 1.5 L/kg. The drug is supplied in 60-mL ampules at a drug concentration of 15 mg/mL. The desired steady-state drug concentration is 20 $\mu$g/mL.

**a.** What infusion rate in mg/h would you recommend for this patient?

**b.** What loading dose would you recommend for this patient? By what route of administration would you give the loading dose? When?

**c.** Why should a loading dose be recommended?

**d.** According to the manufacturer, the recommended starting infusion rate is 15 mL/h. Do you agree with this recommended infusion rate for your patient? Give a reason for your answer.

**e.** If you were to monitor the patient's serum drug concentration, when would you request a blood sample? Give a reason for your answer.

**f.** The observed serum drug concentration is higher than anticipated. Give two possible reasons based on sound pharmacokinetic principles that would account for this observation.

**8.** Which of the following statements **(a–e)** is/are true regarding the time to reach steady state for the three drugs below?

|  | Drug A | Drug B | Drug C |
|---|---|---|---|
| Rate of infusion (mg/h) | 10 | 20 | 15 |
| $k$ (h$^{-1}$) | 0.5 | 0.1 | 0.05 |
| $CL$ (L/h) | 5 | 20 | 5 |

**a.** Drug A takes the longest time to reach steady state.

**b.** Drug B takes the longest time to reach steady state.

  c. Drug C takes the longest time to reach steady state.

  d. Drug A takes 6.9 hours to reach steady state.

  e. None of the above is true.

9. If the steady-state drug concentration of a cephalosporin after constant infusion of 250 mg/h is 45 $\mu$g/mL, what is the drug clearance of this cephalosporin?

10. Some clinical pharmacists assumed that, at steady state when equilibration is reached between the plasma and the tissue, the tissue drug concentration would be the same as the plasma. Do you agree?

## ANSWERS

### Frequently Asked Questions

*How does one determine whether a patient has reached steady-state during an IV infusion?*

- In clinical practice, the drug activity will be observed when the drug concentration is close to the desired plasma drug concentration. For therapeutic purposes, the time for the plasma drug concentration to reach more than 95% of the steady-state drug concentration in the plasma is often estimated. After IV infusion of a drug for 5 half-lives, the plasma drug concentration will be between 95% (4.32 $t_{1/2}$) and 99% (6.65 $t_{1/2}$) of the steady-state drug concentration (Table 14-1). When necessary, blood-drug concentration can be measured and confirmed for clinical PK monitoring.

*What is the clinical relevance of steady-state?*

- In clinical practice, the drug steady-state concentration should be close to the desired plasma drug concentration within the therapeutic window of efficacy and safety. Once the steady state is reached, the rate of drug leaving the body (elimination rate) is equal to the rate of drug entering the body (infusion rate).

*How can the steady-state drug concentration be achieved more quickly?*

- An initial loading dose by bolus injection can be used to obtain desired concentration more quickly. But only increasing the infusion rate will not shorten the time to reach the steady-state drug concentration. If the drug is given at a more rapid infusion rate, a higher steady-state drug level will be obtained, but the time to reach steady state is the same.

*What is the main reason for giving a drug by slow IV infusion?*

- Slow IV infusion may be used to avoid side effects due to rapid drug administration. For example, intravenous immune globulin (human) may cause a rapid fall in blood pressure and possible anaphylactic shock in some patients when infused rapidly. Some antisense drugs also cause a rapid fall in blood pressure when injected via rapid IV into the body. The rate of infusion is particularly important in administering antiarrhythmic agents in patients. The rapid IV bolus injection of many drugs (eg, lidocaine) that follow the pharmacokinetics of multiple-compartment models may cause an adverse response due to the initial high drug concentration in the central (plasma) compartment before slow equilibration with the tissues.

*Why do we use a loading dose to rapidly achieve therapeutic concentration for a drug with a long elimination half-life instead of increasing the rate of drug infusion or increasing the size of the infusion dose?*

- The loading drug dose is used to rapidly attain the target drug concentration, which is approximately the steady-state drug concentration. However, the loading dose will not maintain the steady-state level unless an appropriate IV drug infusion rate or maintenance dose is also used. If a larger IV drug infusion rate or maintenance dose is given, the resulting steady-state drug concentration will be much higher and will remain sustained at the higher level. A higher infusion rate may be administered if the initial steady-state drug level is inadequate for the patient.

*What are some of the complications involved with IV infusion?*

▪ The common complications associated with intravenous infusion include phlebitis and infections at the infusion site caused by poor intravenous techniques or indwelling catheters.

## Learning Questions

**1. a.** To reach 95% of $C_{SS}$:

$$4.32t_{1/2} = (4.32)(7) = 30.2 \text{ h}$$

**b.** $D_L = C_{SS} V_D$

$$= (10)(0.231)(65,000) = 150 \text{ mg}$$

**c.** $R = C_{SS} V_D k = (10)(15,000)(0.099)$

$$= 14.85 \text{ mg/h}$$

**d.** $Cl_T = V_D k = (15,000)(0.099) = 1485 \text{ mL/h}$

**e.** To establish a new $C_{SS}$ will still take $4.32t_{1/2}$. However, the $t_{1/2}$ will be longer in renal failure.

**f.** If $Cl_T$ is decreased by 50%, then the infusion rate $R$ should be decreased proportionately:

$$R = 10(0.50)(1485) = 7.425 \text{ mg/h}$$

**2. a.** The steady-state level can be found by plotting the IV infusion data. The plasma drug–time curves plateau at 10 $\mu$g/mL. Alternatively, $V_D$ and $k$ can be found from the single IV dose data:

$$V_D = 100 \text{ mL/kg} \quad k = 0.2 \text{ h}^{-1}$$

**b.** Using equations developed in Example 2 in the first set of examples in Chapter 5:

$$0.95 \frac{R}{V_D k} = \frac{R}{V_D k}(1 - e^{-kt})$$

$$0.95 = 1 - e^{-0.2t}$$

$$0.05 = e^{-0.2t}$$

$$t_{95\% \text{ SS}} = \frac{\text{Ln } 0.05}{-0.2} = 15 \text{ h}$$

**c.** $Cl_T = V_D k \quad V_D = \dfrac{D_0}{C_P^0}$

$$Cl_T = 100 \times 0.2 \quad V_D = \frac{1000}{10} = \frac{100 \text{ mL}}{\text{kg}}$$

$$Cl_T = 20 \text{ mL/kg h}$$

**d.** The drug level 4 hours after stopping the IV infusion can be found by considering the drug concentration at the termination of infusion as $C_P^0$. At the termination of the infusion, the drug level will decline by a first-order process.

$$C_P = C_P^0 e^{-kt}$$

$$C_P = 9.9\, e^{-(0.2)(4)}$$

$$C_P = 4.5 \ \mu\text{g/mL}$$

**e.** The infusion rate to produce a $C_{SS}$ of 10 $\mu$g/mL is 0.2 mg/kg/h. Therefore, the infusion rate needed for this patient is

$$0.2 \text{ mg/kg h} \times 75 \text{ kg} = 15 \text{ mg/h}$$

**f.** From the data shown, at 4 hours after the start of the IV infusion, the drug concentration is 5.5 $\mu$g/mL; the drug concentration after an IV bolus of 1 mg/kg is 4.5 $\mu$g/mL. Therefore, if a 1-mg dose is given and the drug is then infused at 0.2 mg/kg/h, the plasma drug concentration will be 4.5 + 5.5 = 10 $\mu$g/mL.

**3.** Infusion rate $R$ for a 75-kg patient:

$$R = (1 \text{ mg/kg h})(75 \text{ kg}) = 75 \text{ mg/h}$$

Sterile drug solution contains 25 mg/mL. Therefore, 3 mL contains (3 mL) × (25 mg/mL), or 75 mg. The patient should receive 3 mL (75 mg)/h by IV infusion.

**4.** $C_{SS} = \dfrac{R}{V_D k} \quad R = C_{SS} V_D k$

$$R = (20 \text{ mg/L})(0.5 \text{ L/kg})(75 \text{ kg})\left(\frac{0.693}{3 \text{ h}}\right)$$

$$= 173.25 \text{ mg/h}$$

Drug is supplied as 125 mg/mL. Therefore,

$$125 \text{ mg/mL} = \frac{173.25 \text{ mg}}{X} \quad X = 1.386 \text{ mL}$$

$$R = 1.386 \text{ mL/h}$$

$$D_\text{L} = C_\text{SS} \, V_\text{D} = (20 \text{ mg/L})(0.5 \text{ L/kg})(75 \text{ kg})$$

$$= 750 \text{ mg}$$

**5.** $C_\text{SS} = \dfrac{R}{kV_\text{D}} = \dfrac{R}{Cl_\text{T}}$

**a.** $Cl_\text{T} = \dfrac{R}{C_\text{SS}} = \dfrac{5.3 \text{ mg/kg h} \times 71.71 \text{ kg}}{17 \text{ mg/L}}$

$$= 22.4 \text{ L/h}$$

**b.** At the end of IV infusion, $C_\text{p} = 17 \ \mu\text{g/mL}$. Assuming first-order elimination kinetics:

$$C_\text{p} = C_\text{p}^0 \, e^{-kt}$$

$$1.5 = 17 e^{-kt(2.5)}$$

$$0.0882 = e^{-2.5k}$$

$$\text{Ln } 0.0882 = -2.5 \, k$$

$$-2.43 = -2.5 \, k$$

$$k = 0.971 \text{ h}^{-1}$$

$$t_{1/2} = \frac{0.693}{0.971} = 0.714 \text{ h}$$

**c.** $Cl_\text{T} = kV_\text{D} \quad V_\text{D} = \dfrac{Cl_\text{T}}{k}$

$$V_\text{D} = \frac{22.4}{0.971} = 23.1 \text{ L}$$

**d.** Probenecid blocks active tubular secretion of cephradine.

**6.** At steady state, the rate of elimination should equal the rate of absorption. Therefore, the rate of elimination would be 30 mg/h. The $C_\text{SS}$ is directly proportional to the rate of infusion $R$, as shown by

$$C_\text{SS} = \frac{R}{kV_\text{D}} \quad kV_\text{D} = \frac{R}{C_\text{SS}}$$

$$\frac{R_\text{old}}{C_\text{SS,old}} = \frac{R_\text{new}}{C_\text{SS,new}}$$

$$\frac{30 \text{ mg/h}}{20 \ \mu\text{g/mL}} = \frac{40 \text{ mg/h}}{C_\text{SS,new}}$$

$$C_\text{SS,new} = 26.7 \ \mu\text{g/mL}$$

The new elimination rate will be 40 mg/h.

**7. a.** $R = C_\text{SS}kV_\text{D}$

$$R = (20 \text{ mg/L})(0.693/8 \text{ h})(1.5 \text{ L/kg})(75 \text{ kg})$$

$$= 194.9 \text{ mg/h}$$

$$R = 195 \text{ mg/h}/15 \text{ mg/mL} = 13 \text{ mL/h}$$

**b.** $D_\text{L} = C_\text{SS}V_\text{D} = (20) \ (1.5) \ (75) = 2250$ mg given by IV bolus injection

**c.** The loading dose is given to obtain steady-state drug concentrations as rapidly as possible.

**d.** 15 mL of the antibiotic solution contains 225 mg of drug. Thus, an IV infusion rate of 15 mL/h is equivalent to 225 mg/h. The $C_\text{SS}$ achieved by the manufacturer's recommendation is

$$C_\text{SS} = \frac{R}{kV_\text{D}} = \frac{225}{(0.0866)(112.5)} = 23.1 \text{ mg/L}$$

The theoretical $C_\text{SS}$ of 23.1 mg/L is close to the desired $C_\text{SS}$ of 20 mg/L. Assuming a reasonable therapeutic window, the manufacturer's suggested starting infusion rate is satisfactory.

**e.** Request a blood sample after reaching the steady-state, about 16 hours when loading dose is eliminated.

**f.** Possible reasons for higher-than-anticipated serum concentration: 1) real distribution volume is smaller; 2) drug elimination is slower.

**8.** C

**9.** $CL = R/C_{ss} = 250/45 = 5.56$ L/h

**10.** We only can assume this if there is no drug distribution barrier between plasma and tissue so that drug can freely access to the target tissue from plasma. Their concentration usually are not equal, depending on the distribution ratio between plasma and tissue.

## BIBLIOGRAPHY

Gibaldi M: Estimation of the pharmacokinetic parameters of the two-compartment open model from postinfusion plasma concentration data. *J Pharm Sci* **58**:1133–1135, 1969.

Hurley SF, McNeil JJ: A comparison of the accuracy of a least-squares regression, a Bayesian, Chiou's and the steady-state clearance method of individualizing theophylline dosage. *Clin Pharmacokinet* **14**:311–320, 1988.

Koup J, Greenblatt D, Jusko W, et al: Pharmacokinetics of digoxin in normal subjects after intravenous bolus and infusion dose. *J Pharmacokinet Biopharm* **3**:181–191, 1975.

Loo J, Riegelman S: Assessment of pharmacokinetic constants from postinfusion blood curves obtained after IV infusion. *J Pharm Sci* **59**:53–54, 1970.

Loughnam PM, Sitar DS, Ogilvie RI, Neims AH: The two-compartment open system kinetic model: A review of its clinical implications and applications. *J Pediatr* **88**:869–873, 1976.

Mitenko P, Ogilvie R: Rapidly achieved plasma concentration plateaus, with observations on theophylline kinetics. *Clin Pharmacol Ther* **13**:329–335, 1972.

Riegelman JS, Loo JC: Assessment of pharmacokinetic constants from postinfusion blood curves obtained after IV infusion. *J Pharm Sci* **59**:53, 1970.

Sawchuk RJ, Zaske DE: Pharmacokinetics of dosing regimens which utilize multiple intravenous infusions: Gentamicin in burn patients. *J Pharmacokinet Biopharm* **4**:183–195, 1976.

Wagner J: A safe method for rapidly achieving plasma concentration plateaus. *Clin Pharmacol Ther* **16**:691–700, 1974.

# 15

# Pharmacokinetic Calculations for Drug Elimination and Clearance

Murray P. Ducharme, Fang Wu, and Liang Zhao

## CHAPTER OBJECTIVES

■ Discuss the clinical role of clearance as a PK parameter.

■ Calculate clearance using different methods including the noncompartmental, compartmental, and "physiological" approaches.

■ Define clearance and its relationship to a corresponding half-life and a volume of distribution.

■ Differentiate between total, hepatic, and renal clearances.

■ Describe the processes for renal drug excretion and explain which renal excretion process predominates in the kidney for a specific drug given its renal clearance.

■ Describe the renal clearance model based on renal blood flow, glomerular filtration, and drug reabsorption.

■ Be able to calculate if a change in hepatic or renal clearance will have a significant effect or not.

■ Describe hepatic drug clearance in terms of blood flow and extraction using the "physiologic" well-stirred model.

■ Predict the impact of a drug–drug interaction on protein binding or intrinsic clearance on the liver and total drug clearances, unbound exposure, and oral bioavailability for low and highly extracted drugs using the "physiologic" well-stirred model.

## DRUG ELIMINATION

Chapter 6 discussed the physiologic aspects of drug elimination. This chapter will discuss the pharmacokinetic calculations of drug elimination including total body clearance, renal clearance, and hepatic clearance.

Drug elimination is a combination of different processes, interconnected with each other, that aim at removing the drug from the body. The major drug elimination processes include renal clearance through the kidney and hepatic clearance, which includes both biotransformation and biliary drug excretion. In general, hydrophilic, water-soluble drugs are eliminated more rapidly through the kidney than hydrophobic, lipid-soluble drugs. Many lipid-soluble drugs are metabolized in the liver by various oxidative reactions such as hydroxylation and then conjugated to form a glucuronide or sulfate metabolite. These metabolic processes transform the drug into more polar, water-soluble metabolites that are readily excreted into the urine or bile. Parent drugs may be also eliminated unchanged directly in the kidney or via biliary excretion through the liver. A clinician should consider all drug elimination processes and the importance of each process in the removal of the drug and its metabolites from the body.

In this chapter, we will focus on the diverse ways of calculating clearances, integrating liver and kidney functions, as well as understanding the elimination of parent compounds and metabolites.

## CLINICAL IMPORTANCE OF DRUG CLEARANCE

Drug elimination in the body involves many complex rate processes. Although organ systems have specific functions, the tissues within the organs are not structurally homogeneous, and elimination processes may vary in each organ.

The term *clearance* describes the process of drug elimination from the body or from a single organ without identifying the individual processes involved. *Clearance* may be defined as the volume of fluid removed of the drug from the body per unit of time. The units for clearance are volume/time, sometimes in milliliters per minute (mL/min) but most often reported in liters per hour (L/h). The volume concept is simple and convenient, because all drugs are dissolved and distributed in the fluids of the body.

Clearance directly relates to the systemic exposure of a drug (eg, $AUC_{inf}$) making it the most useful pharmacokinetic (PK) parameter clinically, as it will be used to calculate doses to administer in order to reach a therapeutic goal in terms of exposure. While the terminal half-life gives information only on the terminal phase of drug disposition, clearance takes into account all processes of drug elimination regardless of their mechanism.

The clearance of a drug ($CL$) is directly related to the dose administered and to the overall systemic exposure achieved with that dose as per the equation

$$CL = (F \times DOSE)/AUC_{0-inf}. \qquad (15.1)$$

Clinically, the overall systemic exposure ($AUC_{0-inf}$) resulting from an administered dose best correlates with the efficacy and toxicity of drugs. Drug clearance ($CL$) is therefore an important PK parameter to know in a given patient. If the therapeutic goal in terms of $AUC_{0-inf}$ is known for a drug, then the dose to administer to this patient is completely dictated by the clearance value ($CL$),

hence after IV administration

$$DOSE = CL \times AUC_{0-inf}$$

or more generally

$$DOSE = CL/F \times AUC_{0-inf} \qquad (15.2)$$

in which $CL/F$ can be called the "apparent clearance" when the absolute bioavailability ($F$) is unknown or not specified or assumed.

### FREQUENTLY ASKED QUESTIONS

▶ What is the difference between clearance and the rate of drug elimination?

▶ Why is clearance a clinically useful pharmacokinetic parameter?

## PRACTICE PROBLEM

An antibiotic against *Escherichia coli* is associated with a minimum inhibitory concentration ($MIC_{50}$) of 10 mcg/L and a minimum bactericidal concentration ($MBC_{50}$) of 20 mcg/L. Knowing that the $CL$ of the antibiotic in your patient is 1 L/h, and that the drug is bound to plasma proteins at 50%, calculate the daily IV bolus dose of the antibiotic that is needed to administer *minimally* per day to *inhibit* the growth of *E. coli* or to *kill* the *E. coli* in a patient who suffers from such a bacterial systemic infection.

### Solution

As discussed in Chapter 5, only free drug (not protein bound) is active and can inhibit or kill bacteria. The $MIC_{50}$ and $MBC_{50}$ are estimated *in vitro* using Mueller-Hinton broth that does not contain proteins such as albumin, and therefore represents "unbound" concentrations.

- Since the antibiotic is 50% bound to plasma proteins, then the unbound portion of the antibiotic is 50% or 0.5. Therefore, the target total concentrations for inhibiting or killing *E. coli* is 20 (ie, 10/0.5) and 40 (20/0.5) mcg/L, respectively.

- Once a target concentration is known (ie, here the MIC and MBC in terms of free drug concentrations), then the target AUC per day is simply this target concentration multiplied by 24 hours. The target $AUC_{0-24}$ for inhibiting or killing *E. coli* is therefore 480 mcg.h/L (ie, 20 × 24) and 960 mcg.h/L (ie, 40 × 24), respectively.

- The minimum IV daily dose to administer to a patient having a $CL$ of 1 l/h for inhibiting or killing *E. coli* is therefore 480 mcg and 960 mcg, respectively.

## PRINCIPLES OF CLEARANCE CALCULATIONS

*Drug clearance* is a pharmacokinetic term for describing irreversible drug elimination from the body without necessarily identifying the mechanism of the process. Drug clearance is also known as *body clearance* or *total body clearance* (abbreviated as $CL$ or $CL_T$) and considers the entire body as a single drug-eliminating system from which many unidentified elimination processes may occur.

There are several definitions of clearance, which are similarly based on volume of drug removed from the body per unit of time. The simplest concept of clearance regards the body as a space that contains a definite volume of apparent body fluid (apparent volume of distribution, $V$ or $V_D$) in which the drug is dissolved. Drug clearance is defined as the fixed volume of fluid (containing the drug) removed from the drug per unit of time. The units for clearance are volume/time (eg, mL/min, L/h). For example, if the $CL$ of penicillin is 15 mL/min in a patient and penicillin has a $V_D$ of 12 L, then from the clearance definition, 15 mL of the 12 L will be removed from the drug per minute.

Alternatively, $CL$ may be defined as the rate of drug elimination divided by the plasma drug concentration. This definition expresses drug elimination in terms of the volume of plasma eliminated of drug per unit time. This definition is a practical way to calculate clearance based on plasma drug concentration data.

$$CL = \text{elimination rate/plasma concentration} (C_p) \quad (15.3)$$

$$CL = (dD_E/dt)/C_p = (ug/min)/(ug/mL) = mL/min \quad (15.4)$$

where $D_E$ is the amount of drug eliminated and $dD_E/dt$ is the rate of elimination.

Rearrangement of Equation 15.4 gives Equation 15.5.

$$\text{Elimination rate} = dD_E/dt = C_p CL \quad (15.5)$$

The two definitions for clearance are similar because dividing the elimination rate by the $C_p$ yields the volume cleared of drug per minute, as shown in Equation 15.4.

As discussed in previous chapters, $CL = kV_D$ and the first-order elimination rate, $dD_E/dt$, is equal to $kD_B$ or $kC_p V_D$. Based on Equation 15.3, substituting elimination rate for $kC_p V_D$,

$$CL = KC_p V_D/C_p = KV_D \quad (15.6)$$

Equation 15.6 shows that clearance is the product of a volume of distribution, $V_D$, and a rate constant, $k$, both of which are constants when the PK is linear. As the plasma drug concentration decreases during elimination, the rate of drug elimination, $dD_E/dt$, decreases accordingly, but clearance remains constant. Clearance is constant as long as the rate of drug elimination is a first-order process (linear).

## EXAMPLE ▷ ▷ ▷

Penicillin has a $CL$ of 15 mL/min. Calculate the elimination rate for penicillin when the plasma drug concentration, $C_p$, is 2 $\mu g$/mL.

### Solution
Elimination rate $= C_p \times CL$ (from Equation 15.5)

$$\frac{dD_E}{dt} = 2\,\mu g/mL \times 15\ mL/min = 30\,\mu g/min$$

Assume that the plasma penicillin concentration is 10 $\mu g$/mL. From Equation 15.4, the rate of drug elimination is

$$\frac{dD_E}{dt} = 10\,\mu g/mL \times 15\ mL/min = 150\,\mu g/min$$

Thus, 150 $\mu g$/min of penicillin is eliminated from the body when the plasma penicillin concentration is 10 $\mu g$/mL.

Clearance may be used to estimate the rate of drug elimination at any given concentration. Using the same example, if the elimination rate of penicillin was measured as 150 $\mu g$/min when the plasma penicillin concentration was 10 $\mu g$/mL, then the clearance of penicillin is calculated from Equation 15.4:

$$CL = 150\ ug/min/10\ ug/mL = 15\ mL/min$$

### Additivity of Clearances
The elimination rate constant ($k$ or $kel$) represents the total sum of all of the different rate constants for drug elimination, including for example the renal ($k_R$) and liver ($k_H$) elimination rate constants. $CL$ is the total sum of all of the different clearance processes in the body that are occurring in parallel in terms of cardiac blood flow (therefore excepting lung clearance), including clearance through the kidney (renal clearance abbreviated as $CL_R$), and through the liver (hepatic clearance abbreviated as $CL_H$).

Elimination rate constant:

$$k \text{ or } kel \text{ where } \quad k = k_R + k_H + k_{other} \quad (15.7)$$

Clearance:

$$CL \text{ where } CL = CL_R + CL_H + CL_{other} \quad (15.8)$$

where

$$\text{Renal clearance: } CL_R = k_R \times V_D \quad (15.9)$$

$$\text{Hepatic clearance: } CL_H = k_H \times V_D \quad (15.10)$$

Total clearance:

$$CL = k \times V_D = (k_R + k_H + k_{other}) \times V_D \quad (15.11)$$

From Equation 15.11, for a one-compartment model (ie, where $V_D = V_c = V_{ss}$ and where $k = \lambda_z$), the total body clearance $CL$ of a drug is the product of two constants, $\lambda_z$ and $V_{ss}$, which reflect all the distribution and elimination processes of the drug in the body.

For a multi-compartment model (eg, where the total volume of distribution ($V_{ss}$) includes a central volume of distribution ($V_c$), and one ($V_p$) or more peripheral volumes of distributions), the total body clearance of a drug will be the product of the elimination rate constant from the central compartment ($K_{10}$) and $V_c$. The equations become:

$$\text{Renal clearance: } CL_R = k_R \times V_C \quad (15.12)$$

$$\text{Hepatic clearance: } CL_H = k_H \times V_C \quad (15.13)$$

Total clearance:

$$CL = k_{10} \times V_C = (k_R + k_H + k_{other}) \times V_C \quad (15.14)$$

Clearance values are often adjusted on a per-kilogram of actual body weight (ABW) or on a per-meter square of surface area basis, such as L/h per kilogram or per m², or normalized for a "typical" adult of 72 kg or 1.72 m². This approach is similar to the method for expressing $V$, because both pharmacokinetic parameters vary with body weight or body size. It has been found, however, that when expressing clearance between individuals of varying ABW such as predicting $CL$ between children and adults, $CL$ varies best allometrically (see Chapter 19) with actual body weight, meaning that $CL$ is best expressed with an allometric exponent (most often 0.75 is recommended; Holford et al, 2013) relating it to actual body weight as per the following expression:

$CL$ (predicted in a patient)

$$= CL_{(\text{population value for a 72 kg patient})} \times (ABW/72)^{0.75} \quad (15.15)$$

## EXAMPLE ▷ ▷ ▷

Determine the total body clearance for a drug in a 70-kg male patient. The drug follows the kinetics of a one-compartment model and has an elimination half-life of 3 hours with an apparent volume of distribution of 0.1 L/kg.

### Solution

First determine the elimination rate constant ($k$) and then substitute properly into Equation 15.11.

$$K = 0.693/3 = 0.231 \text{ h}^{-1}$$

$$CL = 0.231 \text{ h}^{-1} \times 0.1 \text{ L/kg} = 0.0231 \text{ L/h/kg}$$

For a 70-kg patient, $CL = 0.0231 \times 70 = 1.617$ L/h

## CLEARANCE MODELS

The various approaches for estimating drug clearance are described in Fig. 15-1 and will be explored in the following sections, starting with the compartmental approach, continuing with noncompartmental, and

**Compartmental model**

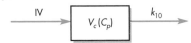

Static volume and first-order processes are assumed in simpler models. Here $Cl = k_{10} \times V_c$.

**Physiologic model**

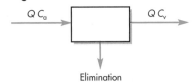

Elimination

Clearance is the product of the flow through an organ ($Q$) and the extraction ratio of that organ ($E$). For example, the hepatic clearance is $Cl_H = Q_H \times E_H$.

**Noncompartmental approach**

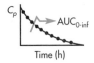

Volume of distribution does not need to be defined. $Cl = DOSE/AUC_{inf}$.

FIGURE 15-1 • Main approaches for calculating clearances.

finally with the physiological approach based on the well-stirred model.

## THE COMPARTMENTAL APPROACH

In compartmental PK, we use mathematical models made of diverse compartments to describe and characterize concentration time profiles that we observe for any given drug. The models that we use are therefore drug specific. Some drugs will have their PK characterized by a simple one-compartment model, while other drugs will need more complex models including two, three, or more compartments just for the parent drug. Software programs are used to fit concentration and time data to these diverse proposed models, and the PK model that best characterizes the data while also being the most parsimonious is retained. To this end, if both one- and two-compartment PK models fit equally well the data, the one-compartment model will be retained as it is the simplest. Software used in compartmental PK fitting will be described in more detail in Chapter 20.

Regardless of the number of compartments, clearance is always a direct measure of elimination from the central compartment. The central compartment consists of the plasma and highly perfused tissues in which drug equilibrates rapidly. The tissues for drug elimination, namely kidney and liver, are considered integral parts of the central compartment as they are very well perfused by cardiac blood flow.

Clearance is always the product of a rate constant and of a volume of distribution. Below are the different clearance formulas depending on the pharmacokinetic model that would describe appropriately the concentration-versus-time profiles of a drug product that would be administered intravenously and extravascularly from simple to more complicated scenarios.

### Clearance for Drugs that are Well Described Pharmacokinetically with a One-Compartment Model

After IV bolus administration, a drug that exhibits a concentration time profile that decreases in a straight line on a semi-log plot can be described by a mono-exponential decline. This decline in plasma drug concentrations with respect to time is illustrated in Fig. 15-2 (Panel C). A one-compartment model is the simplest model that can be used to describe the pharmacokinetics of this drug. Drugs that follow a one-compartment model are usually polar, distribute rapidly within the body, and are readily eliminated in the urine. Clinically, aminoglycosides antibiotics such as gentamicin, tobramycin, and amikacin are relatively well characterized and predicted by a one-compartment model.

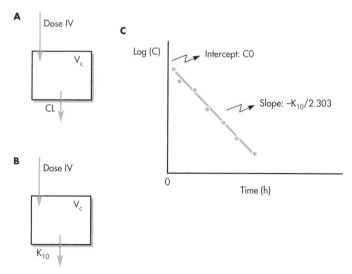

FIGURE 15-2 • One-compartment PK model parameterized in terms of clearance (Panel A), rate constant (Panel B), with its associated mono-exponential decline in concentration-versus-time relationship that would be expected on a semi-log plot (Panel C).

The one-compartment model can be parameterized in terms of clearance, by fitting $CL$ and $V_c$ (Panel A), or in terms of rate constant by fitting $K_{10}$ and $V_c$ (Panel B). This distinction in the parameters that are fitted by the model should not normally result in any difference overall in the obtained respective values of the three parameters ($K_{10}$, $V_c$, and $CL$). The third parameter will always be dependent on the other two. Parameterizing models either in terms of clearances or rate constants is usually dependent on the preferences of the pharmacokinetic scientist.

The equation for clearance in any compartment model is

$$CL = k_{10} \times V_c \qquad (15.16)$$

where $K_{10}$ is the elimination rate constant from the central compartment and $V_c$ is the central volume of distribution.

The total volume of distribution ($V_{ss}$) being equal to $V_c$ in a one-compartment model, and $k_{10}$ being also the "terminal" elimination rate constant, Equation 15.16 can also be written as:

$$CL = \lambda_z \times V_{ss} \qquad (15.17)$$

where $\lambda_z$ is the terminal elimination rate constant describing the fate of the concentration time profile and equivalent to $k_{10}$. The terminal elimination half-life, $t_{1/2}$, is obtained by dividing $\lambda_z$ by 0.693.

$$t_{1/2} = 0.693/\lambda_z \qquad (15.18)$$

After oral drug administration, clearance will be reported as $CL/F$ because the oral bioavailability is unknown when dose is divided by $AUC_{inf}$. If the absorption process is faster than the elimination process, the terminal rate constant, $\lambda_z$, will describe the elimination of the drug. If the drug exhibits a "flip-flop" profile because the absorption of the drug is much slower than the elimination process (eg, often the case with modified-release formulations), then the terminal rate constant, $\lambda_z$, will be reflective of the absorption rate constant and not the elimination rate constant. It is sometimes not possible to know if a drug exhibits a slower absorption than elimination. In these cases, it is always best to refer to $\lambda_z$ as the "terminal" rate constant instead of assuming it is the "elimination" rate constant.

## Clearance for Drugs that are Well Described Pharmacokinetically with a Two-Compartment Model

A drug follows the characteristics of a two-compartment model when after IV bolus administration, the observed concentration-time profile decreases in a curve that can be characterized by two different exponentials or two different straight lines when viewed on a semi-log plot. A two-compartment model is illustrated in Fig. 15-3 (Panel C). The two-compartment model describes the pharmacokinetics of drugs that are rapidly equilibrated in a central compartment but slowly distribute into a "peripheral" compartment, often called the "tissue" compartment. The second compartment is not as well perfused by blood or plasma. Clinically, the pharmacokinetic behavior of the antibiotic vancomycin is relatively well characterized and predicted by a two-compartment model.

The two-compartment model can be parameterized in terms of volumes and clearances, by fitting $CL$, $CL_d$ (distributional clearance), $V_c$, and $V_p$ (peripheral volume of distribution) (Panel A), or in terms of rate constant by fitting $K_{10}$, $k_{12}$, $k_{21}$, and $V_c$ (Panel B). This distinction in the parameters that are fitted by the model should not normally result in any differences overall in the obtained respective values of all parameters as the "non-fitted" parameter will simply be calculated using the other ones. Parameterizing models either in terms of clearances or rate constants is usually dependent on the preferences of the pharmacokinetic scientist.

As shown previously in Equation 15.16, the drug clearance is always the product of the elimination rate constant from the central compartment ($k_{10}$) and the central volume of distribution ($V_c$):

$$CL = k_{10} \times V_c \qquad (15.16)$$

The distributional clearance ($CL_d$) describes the clearance occurring between the central ($V_c$) and the peripheral compartment ($V_p$), and where the central compartment includes the plasma and the organs that are very well perfused, while the peripheral compartment includes organs that are less well perfused by cardiac blood flow.

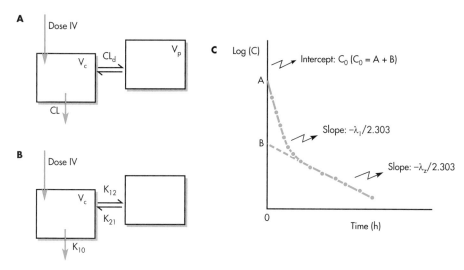

**FIGURE 15-3** • Two-compartment PK model parameterized in terms of clearances and volumes (Panel A), rate constants (Panel B), with its associated bi-exponential decline in concentration versus time relationship that would be expected on a semi-log plot (Panel C).

The relationships between the rate constants and clearances and volumes are:

$$CL_d = K_{12} \times V_c \qquad (15.19)$$

$$CL_d = K_{21} \times V_p \qquad (15.20)$$

which can be rearranged to provide an equation for $V_p$ using rate constants and the $V_c$:

$$V_p = V_c \times K_{12}/K_{21} \qquad (15.21)$$

The concentration time curve profile will follow a bi-exponential decline on a semi-log graph (Fig 15-3 Panel C) and the "distributional" rate constant $(\lambda_1)$ will be describing the rapid decline after IV administration that describes the distribution process, and the second and last exponential $(\lambda_z)$ will describe the terminal elimination phase. The relationship between the distributional and elimination half-lives and the obtained or fitted parameters by the model $(k_{10}, k_{12}, k_{21})$ are:

$$\lambda_1 = [(k_{10} + k_{12} + k_{21}) + \mathrm{SQRT}\,((k_{10} + k_{12} + k_{21})^2 - 4 \times (k_{10}{}^*k_{21}))]/2 \qquad (15.22)$$

$$\lambda_z = [(k_{10} + k_{12} + k_{21}) - \mathrm{SQRT}\,((k_{10} + k_{12} + k_{21})^2 - 4 \times (k_{10}{}^*k_{21}))]/2 \qquad (15.23)$$

The distribution $(t_{1/2}(\lambda_1))$ and terminal $(t_{1/2}(\lambda_z))$ half-lives are therefore:

$$t_{1/2}(\lambda_1) = 0.693/\lambda_1 \qquad (15.24)$$

$$t_{1/2}(\lambda_z) = 0.693/\lambda_z \qquad (15.25)$$

The total volume of distribution $V_{ss}$ will be the sum of the two volumes of distribution $V_c$ and $V_p$:

$$V_{ss} = V_c + V_p \qquad (15.26)$$

## RELATIONSHIP BETWEEN RATE CONSTANTS, VOLUMES OF DISTRIBUTION AND CLEARANCES

It is often stated that clearances and volumes are "independent" parameters, while rate constants are "dependent" parameters. Stated differently, a change in a patient in its drug clearance may not result in a change in its volume of distribution or vice versa, while a change in clearance or in the volume of distribution will result in a change in the appropriate rate constant (eg, $k_{10}$, $\lambda_z$). This statement is incorrect, as it is not always true. There are clinical instances where a change can lead to both volume of distribution and clearance changes, without a resulting

**TABLE 15-1** • Dependency between Clearance, Volume of Distribution, and Elimination Rate Constant

| Clinical Situation | | Parameter(s) Affected ("Dependent") | Parameter That May Not Be Affected ("Independent") | Adjustment to the Dosing Regimen |
|---|---|---|---|---|
| Abrupt weight change | Increased weight | $V_c$ and $CL$ increase | $K_{10}$ | Dose may have to be increased without adjusting the therapeutic interval |
| | Decreased weight | $V_c$ and $CL$ decrease | $K_{10}$ | |
| Abrupt change in renal function | Nephrotoxicity | $CL_R$ and $K_R$, resulting in decrease $CL$ and $K_{10}$ | $V_c$ | Therapeutic interval may have to be prolonged without adjusting the dose |
| | Recovery of renal function | $CL_R$ and $K_R$, resulting in increase $CL$ and $K_{10}$ | $V_c$ | |
| Abrupt change in liver function | Decrease enzymatic activity | $CL_H$ and $K_H$, resulting in decrease $CL$ and $K_{10}$ | $V_c$ | |
| | Decrease production of albumin | $V_c$ may increase (because drug protein binding may be affected) $CL_R$ and $K_R$ may increase due to increased filtration | --- | Dose and therapeutic interval may have to be adjusted |

change in the rate constant (eg, $k_{10}$, $\lambda_z$). A common example is a significant abrupt change in actual body weight (ABW) as both clearances and volumes of distribution correlate with ABW. A patient becoming suddenly edematous will not see his liver or renal function necessarily affected. In that example, both the patient's clearance and volume of distribution will be increased, while half-life or half-lives will remain relatively unchanged. In that situation, the dosing interval will not need to be changed, as the half-life will stay constant, but the dose to be given will need to be increased due to the greater volume of distribution and therefore clearance. It is therefore better to simply state that $K$, $V$, and $CL$ are parameters that are all linked with one another, and that a change in one parameter may induce a change in another one (that one would become "dependent") but not necessarily. To illustrate this point, some

examples of clinical situations inducing a change in one or more parameters are presented in Table 15-1.

### Renal Clearance

Renal clearance can be obtained with compartmental methods by simultaneously fitting and characterizing observed systemic drug concentrations and the amount of drug excreted into the urine over a period of ideally over three to four terminal half-lives or longer. As with any data modeling exercise, it is critical to use the simplest model that can explain all the data appropriately and to use a model that is identifiable.

Let us take the example of a drug administered orally and where the plasma drug concentration time data and excreted urinary drug amounts are simultaneously fitted to a two-compartment model

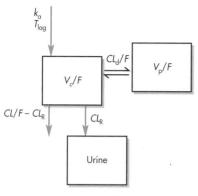

FIGURE 15-4 • Two-compartment PK model parameterized in terms of clearances and volumes, where plasma concentrations (central compartment) are fitted simultaneously with excreted urinary amounts in the urine.

after oral drug administration. A typical model that could be used is presented in Fig. 15-4.

Where the "fitted" pharmacokinetic parameters by the model would be:

- $T_{lag}$ is the time elapsed after dosing before the beginning of the absorption process
- ka is the first-order absorption rate constant
- Vc/F is the apparent central volume of distribution
- $(CL/F - CL_R)$ is the apparent total clearance that does not include the renal clearance
- $CL_R$ is the renal clearance
- $CL_d/F$ is the apparent distributional clearance between the central and peripheral volumes of distribution
- $V_p/F$ is the apparent peripheral volume of distribution

And where the subsequently "derived" or "calculated" pharmacokinetic parameters will be:

- The apparent total clearance, $CL/F$, which is the addition of $CL_R$ to the $(CL/F-CL_R)$
- The apparent total volume of distribution, $V_{ss}/F$, which is the addition of $V_c/F$ to the $V_p/F$
- The distribution $(\lambda_1)$ and terminal elimination $(\lambda_z)$ rate constants and half-lives which were already presented in equations 15.22 to 15.25.

Creatinine clearance (CrCL) may be calculated by diverse methods such as the Cockcroft and

Gault method (Cockcroft and Gault, 1976). In clinical practice, the estimation of the creatinine clearance allows clinicians to adjust dosage of drugs based on the patients' estimated renal function. Renal clearance, $CL_R$, is the summation of filtration, secretion, and reabsorption. $CL_R$ can be simplified to:

$$CL_R = \text{slope} \times CrCL + \text{intercept} \quad (15.27)$$

where the intercept reflects the reabsorption and secretion processes, assuming that the CrCL only reflects glomerular filtration rate (GFR).

Since

$$CL = CL_R + CL_{NR} \quad (15.28)$$

then

$$CL = (\text{slope} \times CrCL + \text{Intercept}) + CL_{NR} \quad (15.29)$$

An assumption that is often made when adjusting doses based on differing renal function is that decreasing renal function does not change the non-renal clearance (eg, hepatic and/or other clearances). This is a reasonable assumption to make until quite severe renal impairment is observed at which point changes in protein binding capacity and affinity as well as changes in enzymatic and transporter affinity may be seen. Because $CL_{NR}$ and the intercept are both constants, then the overall clearance formula can be simplified to:

$$CL = (\text{Slope} \times CrCL) + \text{Intercept} \quad (15.30)$$

This last intercept in Equation 15.30 is often simplified to being $CL_{NR}$, but in reality, if CrCL is assumed to only reflect the GFR function, then this intercept is really representative of the clearance from kidney secretion and reabsorption as well as that from non-renal routes.

## THE NONCOMPARTMENTAL APPROACH

Clearance estimated directly from the area under the curve of the plasma drug concentration–time curve using the noncompartmental method is often called a *model-independent* approach, as it does not need any assumption to be set in terms of number of compartments describing the kinetics or concentration time profile of the drug under study. It is not exactly true that this method is a model-independent one, though, as this method still assumes that the terminal phase decreases in a log-linear fashion which is model dependent, and many of its parameters can be calculated only when one assumes PK linearity. Referring to this method as "noncompartmental" is therefore more appropriate.

The *noncompartmental* approach is based on statistical moment theory and will be presented in more detail in Chapter 19. The main advantages of this approach are that clearance:

1. Can be easily calculated without making any assumptions related to rate constants (eg, distribution versus elimination rate constants) and volumes of distribution

2. Is presented in a clinically useful context as it is related to systemic exposure and the dose administered

3. Has a robust estimation in the context of rich sampling data as very little modeling is involved if any (eg, no modeling with steady-state data, and only very limited modeling by way of linear regression of the terminal phase after single dose administration)

Clearance can be determined directly from the time concentration curve by

$$CL = \text{Integral (0 to infinity) } D \times F/C(t) \, dt \quad (15.31)$$

where $D$ is the dose administered, $F$ is the bioavailability factor associated with the administration route used of the drug product, and $C(t)$ is an unknown function that describes the changing plasma drug concentrations.

Using the noncompartmental approach, the general equation uses the area under the curve of the drug concentration curve $[AUC]_0^\infty$ for the calculation of clearance.

$$CL = F \times D/AUC_{0\text{-inf}} \quad \text{(as presented earlier in Equation 15.2)}$$

where $AUC_{0\text{-inf}} = [AUC]_0^\infty = \int_0^\infty C_p \, dt$ and is the total systemic exposure obtained after a single dose $(D)$ until infinity.

Because $[AUC]_0^\infty$ is calculated from the drug concentration–time curve from zero to infinity using the trapezoidal rule, no model is assumed until the terminal phase after the last detectable concentration is obtained $(C_t)$. To extrapolate the data to infinity to obtain the residual $[AUC]_t^\infty$ or $(C_{Pt}/k)$, first-order elimination or linearity is usually assumed.

Equation 15.2 is used to calculate clearance after administration of a single dose, and where concentrations would be obtained in a rich sampling fashion until a last detectable concentration time point, $C_t$. The AUC from time zero to t $(AUC_{0\text{-}t})$ is often described as the "observed" AUC and calculated using the linear or mixed log-linear trapezoidal rule, while the AUC that needs to be extrapolated from time $t$ to infinity $(AUC_{t\text{-inf}})$ is often described as the "extrapolated" AUC. It is good PK practice for the clearance to be calculated robustly to never extrapolate the $AUC_{0\text{-}t}$ by more than 20%. It is also good PK practice for the $AUC_{0\text{-}t}$ to be calculated using a rich sampling strategy, meaning a minimum of 12 concentration time points across the concentration time curve from zero to $C_t$ after a single dose administration.

At steady state, when the concentration time profiles between administered doses become constant, the amount of drug administered over the dosing interval is exactly equal to the amount eliminated over that dosing interval $(\tau)$. The formula for clearance therefore becomes:

$$CL \text{ or } CL_{(ss)} = F \times D/AUC_{\tau(ss)} \quad (15.32)$$

If the drug exhibits linear pharmacokinetics in terms of time, then the clearance calculated after single dose administration $(CL)$ using formula 15.2 and the clearance calculated from steady state data $(CL_{(ss)})$ using formula 15.32 will be the same.

From equation 15.32, it can be derived that following a constant IV infusion, the steady-state concentration $(C_{ss})$ will then be equal to "rate in," the administration dosing rate $(R_0)$, divided by "rate out" or the clearance:

$$C_{ss} = F \times R_0/CL \text{ or } CL = F \times R_0/C_{ss} \quad (15.33)$$

where $R_0$ is the constant dosing rate (eg, in mg/h), $C_{ss}$ is the steady state concentration (eg, in mg/L), and $CL$ is the total body clearance (eg, in L/h).

## Renal Clearance

*Renal clearance*, $CL_R$, is defined as the volume in which the drug is dissolved that is removed from the drug per unit of time through the kidney. Renal clearance may be defined as a constant fraction of the central volume of distribution in which the drug is contained that is excreted by the kidney per unit of time. More simply, renal clearance is defined as the urinary drug excretion rate ($dD_u/dt$) divided by the plasma drug concentration ($C_p$).

$$CL_R = \text{excretion rate/plasma concentration}$$
$$= (dD_u/dt)/C_p \qquad (15.34)$$

As seen earlier in this chapter, most clearances besides that of the lungs are additive, and therefore the total body clearance can be defined as the sum of the renal clearance ($CL_R$) and of the non-renal clearance ($CL_{NR}$), whatever it may consist of (eg, hepatic or other):

$$CL = CL_R + CL_{NR} \qquad (15.35)$$

Therefore

$$CL_R = f_e \times CL \qquad (15.36)$$

where $f_e$ is the proportion of the bioavailable dose that is eliminated unchanged in the urine. Using the noncompartmental formula for $CL$ studied earlier (Equation 15.2) we obtain

$$CL_R = (f_e \times F \times \text{Dose})/AUC_{0\text{-inf}}$$

And consequently

$$CL_R = Ae_{0\text{-inf}}/AUC_{0\text{-inf}} \qquad (15.37)$$

$$f_e = Ae_{0\text{-inf}}/(F \times \text{Dose}) \qquad (15.38)$$

where $Ae_{0\text{-inf}}$ is the amount of drug eliminated unchanged in the urine from time 0 to infinity after a single dose. In practice, it is not possible to measure the amount of drug excreted unchanged in the urine until infinite time. In order to get a reasonable estimate of the renal clearance with this noncompartmental approach formula using the amount of drug excreted unchanged in the urine and the systemic drug exposure, one has to collect the urine and observe the AUC for the longest time

period possible. Ideally, sampling is collected over three to four terminal half-lives or more, so that the error made using this formula is less than 10%. For example, if a drug product has a terminal half-life of 12 hours, then one would need to collect the urine for a minimum of 48 hours and calculate the ratio of $Ae_{0\text{-}48}$ divided by $AUC_{0\text{-}48}$. For that particular drug product, $CL_R$ would be estimated as:

$$CL_R = Ae_{0\text{-inf}}/AUC_{0\text{-inf}} \sim Ae_{0\text{-}48}/AUC_{0\text{-}48}$$

It is easier to calculate renal clearance at steady state since the entire excreted drug eliminated unchanged in the urine from one dose will occur over one dosing interval. Equation 15.37 therefore becomes:

$$CL_{R(ss)} = Ae_{\tau(ss)}/AUC_{\tau(ss)} \qquad (15.39)$$

where $\tau$ is the dosing interval at which the drug is administered until steady state (ss) conditions are seen, and $Ae_{\tau(ss)}$ is the amount of drug excreted unchanged in the urine during a dosing interval at steady state and $AUC_{\tau(ss)}$ is the area under the systemic concentration time curve over the same dosing interval at steady state.

One important note is that by virtue of its method of calculation the relative bioavailability ($F$) of the drug is not present in the renal clearance calculation, while it always is for the total body clearance. Thus, if systemic drug concentrations and urinary drug excretion are collected after a drug product is administered extravascularly, then only an apparent clearance will be calculated (eg, $CL/F$):

Total clearance will be reported as an "apparent" clearance:

$CL/F = \text{Dose}/AUC_{0\text{-inf}}$ (after single dose administration)

$CL/F = \text{Dose}/AUC_{\tau(ss)}$ (at steady state during a dosing interval)

whereas the renal clearance will not be "apparent":

$CL_R = Ae_{0\text{-}x}/AUC_{0\text{-}x}$ (after single dose administration and where $x$ is the maximum length of time during which both urinary excreted amounts and the AUC can be observed; as mentioned earlier, it should be a minimum of three to four terminal half-lives).

$CL_R = Ae_{\tau(ss)}/AUC_{\tau(ss)}$ (at steady state over a dosing interval)

The non-renal clearance can be readily calculated when the drug product is administered intravenously, as $CL_{NR} = CL - CL_R$. This calculation is not possible with the noncompartmental approach after extravascular administration if the exact relative bioavailability is not known. The exact renal clearance can be calculated ($CL_R$), but only the apparent clearance can ($CL/F$). The non-renal clearance can only be estimated if the relative bioavailability, $F$, is assumed. For example, if the relative bioavailability is estimated to be hypothetically between 75 and 100%, then the non-renal clearance could be presented in the following manner:

$$CL/F = 10 \text{ L/h and } CL_R = 5 \text{ L/h}$$

Therefore:

If $F \sim 100\%$ then $CL_{NR} = 5$ L/h (eg, $CL_{NR} = (CL/F \times 1) - CL_R$)

But if $F \sim 75\%$ then $CL_{NR} = 2.5$ L/h (eg, $CL_{NR} = (CL/\times 0.75) - CL_R$)

An alternative approach to obtaining Equation 15.37 is to consider the mass balance of drug cleared by the kidney and ultimately excreted in the urine. For any drug cleared through the kidney, the rate of the drug passing through kidney (via filtration, reabsorption, and/or active secretion) must equal the rate of drug excreted in the urine.

Rate of drug passing through kidney = rate of drug excreted

$$CL_R \times C_p = Q_u \times C_u \qquad (15.40)$$

where $CL_R$ is renal clearance, $C_p$ is plasma drug concentration, $Q_u$ is the rate of urine flow, and $C_u$ is the urine drug concentration. Rearrangement of Equation 15.40 gives

$$CL_R = (Q_u \times C_u)/C_p = (\text{excretion rate})/C_p \qquad (15.41)$$

Because the excretion rate $= Q_u C_u = dD_u/dt$, Equation 15.41 is the equivalent of Equation 15.37.

Renal clearance is measured without regard to the physiologic mechanisms involved in the process. From a physiologic viewpoint, however, renal clearance may be considered the ratio of the sum of the glomerular filtration and active secretion rates less the reabsorption rate divided by the plasma drug concentration:

$$CL_R = (\text{filtration rate} + \text{secretion rate} + \text{reabsorption rate})/C_p \qquad (15.42)$$

The renal clearance of a drug is often related to the renal GFR, when reabsorption is negligible and the drug is not actively secreted. The renal clearance value for the drug is compared to that of a standard reference, such as inulin, which is cleared completely through the kidney by glomerular filtration only. The *clearance ratio*, which is the ratio of drug clearance to inulin clearance, may give an indication for the mechanism of renal excretion of the drug (Table 15-2). However, further renal drug excretion studies are necessary to confirm unambiguously the mechanism of excretion.

### Filtration Only

If glomerular filtration is the sole process for drug excretion and no drug is reabsorbed, then the amount of drug filtered at any time ($t$) will always be the product of the unbound concentration of the drug ($C_{p(u)}$) by the GFR, as drug bound to plasma proteins cannot be filtered. In the case of an unbound drug that is only filtered, not reabsorbed or secreted, the $CL_R$ of the drug will be equal to GFR. Otherwise, $CL_R$ represents all the processes by which the drug is cleared through the kidney, including any combination of filtration, reabsorption, and active secretion.

**TABLE 15-2 • Comparison of Clearance of a Sample Drug to Clearance of a Reference Drug, Inulin**

| Clearance Ratio | Probable Mechanism of Renal Excretion |
|---|---|
| $\dfrac{Cl_{drug}}{Cl_{inulin}} < 1$ | Drug is partially reabsorbed |
| $\dfrac{Cl_{drug}}{Cl_{inulin}} = 1$ | Drug is filtered only |
| $\dfrac{Cl_{drug}}{Cl_{inulin}} > 1$ | Drug is actively secreted |

## TABLE 15-3 • Urinary Drug Excretion Rate[*]

| Time (min) | $C_p$ (µg/mL) | Excretion Rate (µg/min) (Drug filtered by GFR per min) |
|---|---|---|
| 0 | $(C_{p(u)})_0$ | $(C_{p(u)})_0 \times 125$ |
| 1 | $(C_{p(u)})_1$ | $(C_{p(u)})_1 \times 125$ |
| 2 | $(Cp_{(u)})_2$ | $(C_{p(u)})_2 \times 125$ |
| T | $(Cp_{(u)})_t$ | $(C_{p(u)})_t = 125$ |

[*]Assumes that the drug is excreted by filtration only and that the GFR is 125 mL/min.
Note that the quantity of drug excreted per minute is always the unbound plasma concentration ($C_{p(u)}$) multiplied by the glomerular filtration rate, which here is a constant (eg, 125 mL/min).

### Filtration and Active Secretion

For a drug that is primarily filtered and secreted, with negligible reabsorption, the overall excretion rate may exceed GFR (Table 15-3). At low drug plasma concentrations, active secretion is not saturated, and the drug is excreted by filtration and active secretion. At high concentrations, the percentage of drug excreted by active secretion decreases due to saturation. Clearance decreases because excretion rate decreases (Fig. 15-5). Clearance decreases

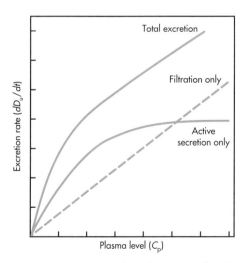

FIGURE 15-5 • Excretion rate–plasma level curves for a drug that demonstrates active tubular secretion and a drug that is secreted by glomerular filtration only.

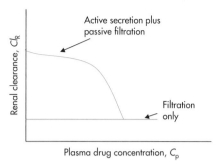

FIGURE 15-6 • Graph representing the decline of renal clearance. As the drug plasma level increases to a concentration that saturates the active tubular secretion, glomerular filtration becomes the major component for renal clearance.

because the total excretion rate of the drug increases to the point where it is approximately equal to the filtration rate (Fig. 15-6).

## EXAMPLES ▷ ▷ ▷

1. Two drugs, A and B, are entirely eliminated through the kidney by glomerular filtration (125 mL/min), with no reabsorption. The pharmacokinetics of Drugs A and B are well described by a one-compartment model. Drug A has half the distribution volume of drug B, and the $V_{ss}$ of drug B is 20 L. Both drugs are not bound to plasma proteins. What are the clearances of each drug?

### Solution

Since glomerular filtration of the two drugs is the same, and both drugs are not eliminated by other means, clearance for both drugs depends on renal plasma flow and extraction by the kidney only. Average clearance is equal to the GFR, 125 mL/min.

Basing the calculation on the elimination concept and applying Equation 15.14, $k_R$ and $\lambda z$ are easily determined, resulting indifferences in the elimination $t_{1/2}$ between the two drugs—in spite of similar drug clearance.

$$k_{R(drugA)} = k_{10(drug A)} = \lambda_{Z(drugA)} = CL/V_{ss}$$
$$= 125/(10 \times 1000) = 0.0125 \text{ min}^{-1}$$

$$k_{R(drugB)} = k_{10(drug B)} = \lambda_{Z(drugB)} = CL/V_{ss}$$
$$= 125/(20 \times 1000) = 0.00625 \text{ min}^{-1}$$

In spite of identical drug clearances, the $\lambda z$ for drug A is twice that of drug B. Drug A has an elimination half-life of 55.44 minutes, while that of drug B is 110.88 minutes—much longer because of the bigger volume of distribution.

2. In a subject with a normal GFR (eg, a CrCL of 125 mL/min), the renal clearance of a drug is 10 L/h, while its non-renal clearance is 5 L/h. Assuming no significant binding to plasma proteins, secretion, and reabsorption, how should we adjust the dosing regimen of the drug if the renal function and the GFR suddenly decreases in half (eg, CrCL = 62.5 mL/min)?

#### Solution

For a patient with "normal GFR"

$CL = CL_R + CL_{NR}$, so $CL = 15$ L/h

$CL_R = \text{slope} \times \text{CrCL}$,
therefore slope $= 10/(125 \times 60/1000) = 1.33$

For a patient with a GFR that decreases in half:

$CL_R = \text{slope} \times \text{CrCL} = 1.33 \times (62.5 \times 60/1000)$
$= 5$ L/h

$CL = CL_R + CL_{NR} = 5 + 5 = 10$ L/h

The clearance therefore decreased by 33%. In order to reach the same target exposure of the drug ($AUC_{inf}$), the dose per day will need to be decreased by 33% as Dose $= CL/AUC_{inf}$.

---

#### FREQUENTLY ASKED QUESTION

▶ What is the relationship between drug clearance and creatinine clearance?

---

#### Graphical Methods to Determine Renal Clearance

The clearance is given by the slope of the curve obtained by plotting the rate of drug excretion in urine ($dD_u/dt$) against $C_p$ (Equation 15.40). For a

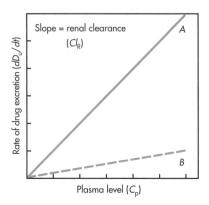

FIGURE 15-7 • Rate of drug excretion versus concentration of drug in the plasma. Drug A has a higher clearance than drug B, as shown by the slopes of line A and line B.

drug that is excreted rapidly, $dD_u/dt$ is large, the slope is steeper, and clearance is greater (Fig. 15-7, line A). For a drug that is excreted slowly through the kidney, the slope is smaller (Fig. 15-7, line B).

From Equation 15.40,

$$CL_R = (dD_u/dt)/C_p$$

Multiplying both sides by $C_p$ gives

$$CL_R \times C_p = dD_u/dt \qquad (15.43)$$

By rearranging Equation 15.43 and integrating, one obtains

$$[D_u]_{0-t} = CL_R \times AUC_{0-t} \qquad (15.44)$$

A graph is then plotted of cumulative drug excreted in the urine versus the area under the concentration–time curve (Fig. 15.8). Renal clearance is obtained from the slope of the curve. The AUC can be estimated by the trapezoidal rule or by other measurement methods. The disadvantage of this method is that if a data point is missing, the cumulative amount of drug excreted in the urine is difficult to obtain. However, if the data are complete, then the determination of clearance is accurate.

By plotting cumulative drug excreted in the urine from $t_1$ to $t_2$, versus, one obtains an equation similar to that presented previously:

$$[D_u]_{t_1-t_2} = CL_R \times AUC_{t_1-t_2} \qquad (15.45)$$

The slope is equal to the renal clearance (Fig. 15-9).

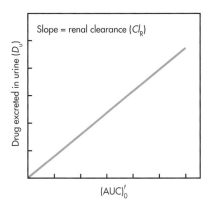

FIGURE 15-8 • Cumulative drug excretion versus AUC. The slope is equal to $CL_R$.

### The "Midpoint" Clearance Method

From Equation 15.41,

$$CL_R = (dD_u/dt)/C_p$$

which can be simplified to

$$CL_R = (X_{u(0-24)}/C_{p12})/24 \qquad (15.46)$$

where

$X_{u(0-24)}$ is the 24-hour excreted urinary amount of the drug obtained by multiplying the collected 24-hour urine volume ($V_{u(0-24)}$) by the measured urinary concentration ($C_{u(0-24)}$), and $C_{p12}$ is the mid-point plasma concentration of the drug measured at the mid-point of the collected interval, here at 12 hours.

This equation is obviously not very robust, as it is based on only one measured plasma concentration,

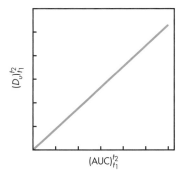

FIGURE 15-9 • Drug excreted versus $[AUC]_{t_1}^{t_2}$. The slope is equal to $CL_R$.

but it is often very useful in the clinic when very few plasma concentrations of drugs can be collected and measured. The overall duration of urinary collection is typically 24 hours, but different collection intervals can obviously be used.

The midpoint method is also commonly used in the clinic to calculate the creatinine clearance in patients, collecting how much creatinine is excreted in 24 hours and using the morning serum creatinine value that is assumed to be constant throughout the day in a given patient and therefore similar to the midpoint value.

## EXAMPLE ▷ ▷ ▷

The urine is collected for 24 hours in a patient in order to assess what his 24-hour creatinine clearance is. The following are obtained:

- 24-hour urine volume collected: 2 L
- Average creatinine concentration in the urine: 5500 $u$Mol/L
- Morning serum creatinine: 100 $u$Mol/L

What is the calculated creatinine clearance in that patient?

**Solution**

As per Equation 15.46, the clearance over 24 hours of creatinine will be the product of the urinary creatinine concentration by the volume excreted, and divided by the midpoint serum creatinine concentration.

CrCL (L/24 hours) = 2 × 5500/100 = 110 L per 24 hours

which can therefore be transformed to the usual mL/min units by dividing by 24 hours and 60 minutes and multiplying by 1000 mL:

CrCL (mL/min) = 110/24/60 × 1000 = 76.39 mL/min

### Metabolite(s) Clearance(s)

We have seen that

$$CL = CL_R + CL_{NR} \qquad (15.35)$$

which in the case of a drug eliminated unchanged in the urine and through biotransformation to a metabolite (m) in the liver

$$CL = CL_R + CL_{f(m)}$$

where $CL_{f(m)}$ is the formation clearance of a metabolite m from the parent drug. This equation can then be simplified to

$$CL_{f(m)} = f(m) \times CL = f(m) \times F \times DOSE/AUC_{inf}$$

And finally, assuming that the metabolite is only excreted unchanged in the urine, to:

$$CL_{f(m)} = Ae(m)_{0\text{-inf}}/AUC_{inf} \qquad (15.47)$$

where $Ae(m)_{0\text{-inf}}$ is the amount of metabolite excreted in the urine until infinity, while $AUC_{inf}$ is the total systemic exposure of the parent compound.

## PRACTICE PROBLEM

Consider a drug that is eliminated by first-order renal excretion and hepatic metabolism. The drug follows a one-compartment model and is given in a single IV or oral dose (Fig. 15-10). Working with the model presented in Fig. 15-10, assume that a single dose (100 mg) of this drug is given orally. The drug has a 90% oral bioavailability. The total amount of unchanged drug recovered in the urine is 60 mg, and the total amount of metabolite recovered in the urine is 30 mg (expressed as milligram equivalents to the parent drug). According to the literature, the elimination half-life for this drug is 3.3 hours and its apparent volume of distribution is 1000 L. From the

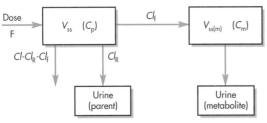

Dose, F → $V_{ss}$ ($C_p$) → $Cl_f$ → $V_{ss(m)}$ ($C_m$)
$Cl$-$Cl_R$-$Cl_f$     $Cl_R$
Urine (parent)     Urine (metabolite)

FIGURE 15-10 • Model of a drug eliminated by first-order renal excretion and hepatic transformation into a metabolite also excreted in the urine. ($CL_R$, renal clearance of parent drug; $CL_f$, formation clearance of parent drug to metabolite; $C_m$, plasma concentration of the metabolite; $C_p$, plasma concentration of the parent drug, $V_{ss}$, total volume of distribution of parent drug; $V_{ss(m)}$, apparent volume of distribution of metabolite; ($CL$-$CL_R$-$CL_f$), clearance of parent drug minus the renal and formation clearances; F, absolute bioavailability of parent drug.)

information given, find **(a)** the apparent clearance and the clearance, **(b)** the renal and non-renal clearance, **(c)** the formation clearance of the drug to the metabolite, and **(d)** if the drug undergoes another systemic metabolic or elimination route.

### Solution

**a.** Apparent clearance and clearance:

$$CL/F = k \times V/F$$

$$CL/F = 0.693/3.3 \times 1000 = 210 \text{ L/h}$$

$$CL = CL/F \times F = 210 \times 0.9 = 189 \text{ L/h}$$

**b.** Renal and non-renal clearance:

$$CL_R = Ae_{0\text{-inf}}/AUC_{0\text{-inf}}$$

and $AUC_{0\text{-inf}} = DOSE/CL/F = 100/210 = 0.4762 \text{ mg} \cdot \text{h}/\text{L}$

Therefore, $CL_R = 60/0.4762 = 126 \text{ L/h}$

$$CL_{NR} = 189 - 126 = 63 \text{ L/h}$$

**c.** Formation clearance of the parent drug to the metabolite

$$CL_f = Ae_{0\text{-inf}}/AUC_{0\text{-inf}} = 30/0.4762 = 63 \text{ L/h}$$

**d.** Does the drug undergo other elimination or metabolic routes?

$$CL/F = CL_R + CL_{NR} = CL_R + (CL_f + CL_{other})$$

Then, $CL_{other} = CL - CL_R - CL_f = 189 - 126 - 63$
$= 0 \text{ L/h}$

The drug does not undergo additional elimination or metabolic routes.

## PRACTICE PROBLEM

An antibiotic is given by IV bolus injection at a dose of 500 mg. The drug follows a one-compartment model. The total volume of distribution was 21 L and the elimination half-life was 6 hours. Urine was collected for 48 hours, and 400 mg of unchanged drug was recovered. What is the fraction of the dose excreted unchanged in the urine? Calculate $k$, $k_R$, $CL$, $CL_R$, and $CL_{NR}$.

## Solution

Since the elimination half-life, $t_{1/2}$, for this drug is 6 hours, a urine collection for 48 hours represents $8 \times t_{1/2}$, which allows for greater than 99% of the drug to be eliminated from the body. The fraction of drug excreted unchanged in the urine, $f_e$, is obtained by using Equation 15.38 and recalling that $F = 1$ for drugs given by IV bolus injection.

$$f_e = \frac{400}{500} = 0.8$$

Therefore, 80% of the bioavailable dose is excreted in the urine unchanged. Calculations for $k$, $k_R$, $CL_T$, $CL_R$, and $CL_{NR}$ are given here:

$$k = 0.693/6 = 0.1155 \text{ h}^{-1}$$

$$k_R = f_e \times k = 0.8 \times 0.1155 = 0.0924 \text{ h}^{-1}$$

$$CL = k \times V_{ss} = 0.1155 \times 21 = 2.43 \text{ L/h}$$

$$CL_R = k_R \times V_{ss} = 0.0924 \times 21 = 1.94 \text{ L/h}$$

$$CL_{NR} = CL - CL_R = 2.43 - 1.94 = 0.49 \text{ L/h}$$

## INTEGRATION OF COMPARTMENTAL AND NONCOMPARTMENTAL APPROACHES

A common area of confusion is the relationship between half-lives, volumes of distribution, clearances, and noncompartmental versus compartmental approaches.

As seen previously, clearances are always related to a rate constant ($k$) and to a volume of distribution ($V_d$) but these parameters will vary according to the mathematical model that describes appropriately the PK of the drug. Table 15-4 aims at reconciling this.

## THE PHYSIOLOGIC APPROACH USING THE "WELL-STIRRED MODEL" FOR LIVER (AND OTHER ORGANS) CLEARANCE

Clearance may be calculated for any organ involved in the irreversible removal of drug from the body using the "well-stirred" model. Many organs in the

## TABLE 15-4 • Relationships between Clearance, Volumes of Distribution, and Half-Lives

| Appearance of $C_p$ versus Time | Compartmental Method | Noncompartmental Method |
|---|---|---|
| Monoexponential decline | *Model after IV administration:* <br><br> $CL = k_{10} \times V_c$ <br> $V_{ss} = V_c$ as there is only one compartment <br> $\lambda_z = k_{10}$ as there is only one compartment <br> $CL = CL_R + CL_{NR}$ <br> $CL_R = K_R \times V_c$ <br> $t_{1/2} = 0.693/\lambda z$ | *Single-dose IV administration:* <br><br> $AUC_{0-t}$ typically calculated with linear or mixed linear/log linear trapezoidal rule <br> $C_t$ is the last detectable concentration time point <br> $\lambda_z$ is the negative slope using linear regression of the terminal log-linear phase of the concentration versus time profile. <br><br> $CL = DOSE/AUC_{0-inf}$ |
| Bi-exponential decline | *Model after IV administration:* <br><br> $CL = k_{10} \times V_c$ <br> $V_p = k_{12} \times V_c/k_{21}$ <br> $V_{ss} = V_c + V_p$ <br> $\lambda_1 = [((CL + CL_d)/V_c + CL_d/V_p) + \text{SQRT}(((CL + CL_d)/V_c + CL_d/V_p)^2 - 4 \times CL/V_c * CL_d/V_p))]/2$ <br> $\lambda_z = [((CL + CL_d)/V_c + CL_d/V_p) - \text{SQRT}(((CL + CL_d)/V_c + CL_d/V_p)^2 - 4 \times CL/V_c * CL_d/V_p))]/2$ <br> $t_{1/2}$ (distribution) $= 0.693/\lambda_1$ <br> $t_{1/2}$ (elimination) $= 0.693/\lambda_z$ | $AUC_{0-inf} = AUC_{0-t} + C_t/\lambda_z$ <br> $MRT = AUMC_{0-inf}/AUC_{0-inf} - (\text{Duration of infusion}/2)$ <br> $V_{ss} = CL \times MRT$ <br> $t_{1/2}$ (terminal) $= 0.693/\lambda_z$ |

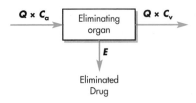

FIGURE 15-11 • The "well-stirred model" approach to clearance. ($Q$, blood flow; $C_a$, incoming drug concentration [usually arterial drug concentration]; $C_v$, outgoing drug concentration [venous drug concentration].)

body have the capacity for drug elimination, including drug excretion and biotransformation. The kidneys and liver are the most common organs involved in excretion and metabolism, respectively. Physiologic pharmacokinetic models are based on drug clearance through individual organs or tissue groups and often use the "well stirred" model to account for them (Fig. 15-11).

The "well-stirred" model assumes that there is a blood flow ($Q$) going through the organ, and the extraction ratio through that organ is denoted by the term $E$, which will be proportion of the arterial concentration ($C_a$) that has been removed as it goes through the organ, resulting in the drug venous concentration ($C_v$). The clearance of the organ will be the product of the blood flow by the extraction ratio. The equations are therefore:

$$CL = Q \times E \qquad (15.48)$$

$$E = (C_a - C_v)/C_a \qquad (15.49)$$

$E$ is an extraction ratio with no units. The value of $E$ may range from 0 (no drug removed by the organ) to 1 (100% of the drug is removed by the organ). An $E$ of 0.25 indicates that 25% of the incoming drug concentration is removed by the organ as the drug passes through it.

Substituting for E into Equation 15.48 yields

$$CL\ (organ) = Q\ (organ) \times (C_a - C_v)/C_a \qquad (15.50)$$

Equation 15.48 adapted for the liver as an organ yields the hepatic clearance ($CL_H$)

$$CL_H = Q_H \times E_H \qquad (15.51)$$

Therefore if $CL = CL_H + CL_{NH}$ (where $CL_{NH}$ is the non-hepatic clearance and would include as denoted above the renal clearance $CL_R$),

then $$CL = (Q_H \times E_H) + CL_{NH} \qquad (15.52)$$

For some drugs that are completely absorbed through the gut wall, that are not subject to gut wall metabolism, and are only eliminated by the liver, then $CL \sim CL_H$, and so $CL \sim Q_H \times E_H$.

The physiologic approach to organ clearance shows that the clearance from an organ depends on its blood flow and on its ability at eliminating the drug, whereas the total clearance is that of the volume in which the drug is distributed that is removed from the drug per unit of time.

It is important to note that the "well-stirred" model as presented above does not really appear physiologic or even plausible for the liver. For example, the well-stirred model assumes that enzymes in the liver are distributed uniformly, that the distribution of the drug within the liver is instantaneous, and that the liver is in fact "perfusion limited." This model was originally proposed and refined by the work of Gillette, Rowland, Benet, and Wilkinson (Gillette, 1971; Rowland et al, 1973; Wilkinson and Shand, 1975). Because the model did not appear "physiologically plausible," several other models were proposed, particularly through the work of Pang and Rowland (Pang and Rowland, 1977a; Pang and Rowland 1977b). A lot of subsequent models, although appearing more plausible physiologically, were shown to be worse at predicting drug–drug interactions (DDIs) occurring in the liver. Thus, the well-stirred model is still the model that is most often used (Pang et al, 2019), as it predicts DDIs relatively well. Pharmacists and clinicians should know that these equations are not "exact," however, and contrary to most PK equations presented in this book, such as $CL/F = Dose/AUC_{inf}$. In the future, a more appropriate model may be proposed.

Central to the well-stirred model is the equation:

$$E = f_u \times CL_{int(u)}/(f_u \times CL_{int(u)} + Q) \qquad (15.53)$$

where $f_u$ is the proportion of the drug concentration that is free from protein binding and can therefore be eliminated, and $CL_{int(u)}$ is the unbound intrinsic clearance of that organ.

For the liver, the following equations can therefore be proposed:

$$E_H = f_u \times CL_{int(u)}/(f_u \times CL_{int(u)} + Q_H) \quad (15.54)$$

$$CL_H = Q_H \times E_H \quad (15.51)$$

$$CL_H = Q_H \times f_u \times CL_{int(u)}/(f_u \times CL_{int(u)} + Q_H) \quad (15.55)$$

It should be noted that this equation, as it regards to the liver, uses the proposed hepatic blood flow ($Q_H$), which is whole-blood related, so the clearances calculated using this equation would be whole-blood clearances. These would be the correct formulas to use when we are looking at whole-blood concentrations, for example when estimating cyclosporine's PK, as the drug distributes in red blood cells. Clearances in PK are usually "plasma clearances" due to "plasma concentrations" being most often collected. Therefore, Equation 15.53 has to be modified to account for this if there is a difference in blood ($C_B$) and plasma ($C_p$) concentrations, as proposed by Yang et al. (2006):

$$CL_H = Q_H \times f_u \times CL_{int(u)}/(f_u \times CL_{int(u)}) \times C_p/C_B + Q_H) \quad (15.56)$$

Note that Equation 15.56 assumes that the free drug proportion in whole blood is the same as in plasma, which is not always the case (eg, cyclosporine is an example of such a drug, but its PK should anyway be assessed in whole blood because of the distribution of the drug in red blood cells).

## Relationship between Extraction and Bioavailability

The route of administration will affect how a drug will be metabolized prior to reaching the systemic circulation. Drugs given orally are often absorbed in the duodenal segment of the small intestine, transported via the mesenteric vessels to the hepatic portal vein, and then to the liver before entering the systemic circulation. Drugs that are highly metabolized by the liver or by the intestinal mucosal cells demonstrate poor systemic availability, or bioavailability, when given orally. This rapid metabolism of orally administered drugs before they reach the general circulation is termed *first-pass effect*

or *presystemic elimination*. In contrast, drugs given parenterally, transdermally, or by inhalation will avoid the "first-pass" effect.

The oral bioavailability of a drug is the ratio of the total systemic exposure seen after oral versus intravenous administration as per the following equation:

$$F = \frac{[AUC]_{0,oral}^{\infty} / D_{0,oral}}{[AUC]_{0,IV}^{\infty} / D_{0,IV}} \quad (15.57)$$

For drugs that undergo first-pass effects, $[AUC]_{0,oral}^{\infty}$ will be smaller than $[AUC]_{0,IV}^{\infty}$ and $F < 1$. Drugs such as propranolol, morphine, and nitroglycerin have $F$ values less than 1 because these drugs undergo significant first-pass effects.

The drug's oral bioavailability will be 100% minus everything that has been extracted via first pass ($E$):

$$F = 1 - E \quad (15.58)$$

The first pass extraction for an oral drug is defined by the following additions:

$$E = E_A + E_G + E_H \quad (15.59)$$

where $E_A$, $E_G$, and $E_H$ represent the extractions due to absorption, gut wall metabolism, and hepatic metabolism through "first pass." The first-pass effect is therefore not only hepatic ($E_H$) but also gut related.

Taking into account gut and hepatic first pass, the oral bioavailability can be defined as:

$$F = F_A \times F_G \times F_H \quad (15.60)$$

where $F_A$ is the proportion of the administered dose that is absorbed through the gut wall, $F_G$ is the absorbed dose that is not subject to gut wall metabolism, and $F_H$ is the absorbed dose not subject to gut wall metabolism that is not metabolized in the liver.

A common mistake is to interchange the term "absorption" and "bioavailability." They are not interchangeable, as absorption ($F_A$) is only one component of oral bioavailability ($F$). These terms are illustrated in Fig. 15-12, where the importance of the ABC efflux transporter P-gp, for example, will influence the overall absorption ($F_A$), the CYP3A enzymes in the gut wall will influence $F_G$, and all other enzymes and transporters in the liver will influence $F_H$.

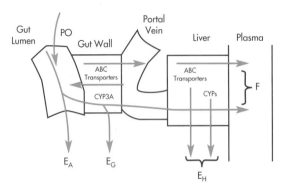

FIGURE 15-12 • Schematic description of the first-pass effect in terms of gut absorption, transport, metabolism, and hepatic metabolism and transport after oral administration (PO) of a drug.

Based on the well-stirred model (Benet et al, 2018), drugs that have high first-pass effect are historically called "high extraction" drugs (typically when $E > 0.7$), while drugs that have low first-pass effect have been called "low extraction" drugs (typically when $E < 0.3$).

To simplify the presentation of concepts, let us consider the liver as the main extraction organ responsible for the first-pass effect.

### Liver Extraction Ratio

The liver extraction ratio ($E_H$) provides a direct measurement of drug removal from the liver after oral administration of a drug. Based on the well-stirred model, the liver extraction ratio can be presented as being

$$E_H = (C_a - C_v)/C_a \qquad (15.49)$$

where $C_a$ is the drug concentration in the blood entering the liver and $C_v$ is the drug concentration leaving the liver.

$C_a$ is usually greater than $C_v$, and therefore $E_H$ will be less than 1. For example, for propranolol, $E_H$ is about 0.7—that is, about 70% of the drug is actually removed by liver first pass before it is available for general distribution to the body. By contrast, if the drug is injected intravenously, most of the drug would be distributed before reaching the liver, and less of the drug would be metabolized the first time the drug reaches the liver.

The $E_H$ may vary from 0 to 1.0. If both $E_H$ and the liver blood flow are known, then the hepatic clearance can be estimated using the well-stirred model as we have seen previously:

$$E_H = f_u \times CL_{int(u)}/(f_u \times CL_{int(u)} + Q_H) \qquad (15.54)$$

$$CL_H = Q_H \times E_H \qquad (15.51)$$

$$CL_H = Q_H \times f_u \times CL_{int(u)}/(f_u \times CL_{int(u)} + Q_H) \qquad (15.55)$$

Assuming a liver blood flow of 1.5 L/min (typical value in man), then for the previously presented example of propranolol having a $E_H$ of 70%, (or 0.7), we can estimate that its $CL_H$ would be 1.05 L/min (ie, $CL_H = Q_H \times E_H = 1.5 \times 0.7 = 1.05$ L/min).

We have seen that the oral bioavailability ($F$) depends on what is extracted by first pass, as per the equation $F = 1 - E$.

Let us assume that propranolol is well absorbed ($E_A \sim 0$) and not subject to gut wall metabolism ($E_G \sim 0$); then we can assume that $E \sim E_H$. The oral bioavailability of propranolol may therefore be estimated by $F = 1 - E_H$, and so it can be estimated to be 30% (ie, $F = 1 - 0.7$).

### Estimation of Reduced Bioavailability Due to Liver Metabolism and Variable Blood Flow

Blood flow to the liver plays an important role in the amount of drug metabolized after oral administration. Changes in blood flow to the liver may substantially alter the percentage of drug metabolized and therefore alter the percentage of bioavailable drug.

*Presystemic elimination* or *first-pass effect* is a very important consideration for drugs that have a high liver extraction ratio (Table 15-5). Drugs with low liver extraction ratios, such as theophylline, have very little presystemic elimination, as demonstrated by virtually complete oral bioavailability. In contrast, drugs with high liver extraction ratios have poor bioavailability when given orally. Therefore, the oral dose must be higher than the IV dose to achieve the same systemic exposure and therefore therapeutic response. In some cases, the oral administration of a drug with very high presystemic elimination, such as nitroglycerin or insulin, may be impractical due to very poor oral bioavailability. Thus, alternate routes of drug administration such as sublingual,

## TABLE 15-5 • Hepatic Extraction Ratios of Representative Drugs

| Extraction Ratios | | |
|---|---|---|
| Low (<0.3) | Intermediate (0.3–0.7) | High (>0.7) |
| **Hepatic Extraction** | | |
| Amobarbital | Aspirin | Arabinosyl-cytosine |
| Antipyrine | Quinidine | Encainide |
| Chloramphenicol | Desipramine | Isoproterenol |
| Chlordiazepoxide | Nortriptyline | Meperidine |
| Diazepam | | Morphine |
| Digitoxin | | Nitroglycerin |
| Erythromycin | | Pentazocine |
| Isoniazid | | Propoxyphene |
| Phenobarbital | | Propranolol |
| Phenylbutazone | | Salicylamide |
| Phenytoin | | Tocainide |
| Procainamide | | Verapamil |
| Salicylic acid | | |
| Theophylline | | |
| Tolbutamide | | |
| Warfarin | | |

*Data from Melmon K, Morelli HF: Clinical Pharmacology. New York, NY: Macmillan; 1978; Evans WE, Schentag JJ, Jusko WJ, et al: Principles of Therapeutic Drug Monitoring. Vancouver, WA: Applied Therapeutics; 1992.*

transdermal, parenteral, or nasal route of administration may be preferred in order to avoid the first-pass liver metabolisms.

Drugs with high presystemic elimination tend to demonstrate more intra- and intersubject variability in their oral bioavailability. The route of drug administration will impact the first-pass effect. As seen previously, drugs administered orally will be subject to gut and hepatic first pass. In contrast, drugs administered topically on the skin, given via inhalation, nasally, sublingually, vaginally, or rectally (in that particular case only if administered in the lower part of the rectum) will not go through the liver before being systemically absorbed and will therefore not be subject to the first-pass liver extraction, $E_H$. For example, nitroglycerin administered topically with a transdermal system will not be subject

to $E_H$ (the administration route bypasses the liver first-pass effect), but will be metabolized in the skin before reaching the systemic circulation (Auclair et al, 1998 a and b). The bioavailability of nitroglycerin given orally or transdermally will therefore be:

$$\text{Orally: } F = 1 - (E_A + E_G + E_H) \qquad (15.61)$$

$$\text{Transdermally: } F = 1 - E_S \qquad (15.62)$$

where $E_s$ is the extraction due to skin absorption and skin metabolism.

The quantity and type of metabolites formed may vary according to the route of drug administration and may be clinically important if one or more of the metabolites has pharmacologic or toxic activity.

## EXAMPLES ▷ ▷ ▷

1. A new propranolol 5-mg tablet was developed and tested in healthy volunteers. The relative bioavailability of propranolol from the tablet was 70%, compared to an oral solution of propranolol, and 21.6%, compared to an intravenous dose of propranolol. Calculate the relative and absolute bioavailability of the propranolol tablet. Comment on the feasibility of further improving the absolute bioavailability of the propranolol tablet.

### Solution

The relative bioavailability of propranolol from the tablet compared to the solution is 70% or 0.7. The absolute bioavailability, $F$, of propranolol from the tablet compared to the IV dose is 21.6%, or $F = 0.216$. From the table of E values (Table 15-6), the $E_H$ for propranolol ranges between 0.6 to 0.8. If the product is perfectly formulated, ie, the tablet dissolves completely and all the drug is released from the tablet, and propranolol is 100% absorbed ($F_A = 1$ or $E_A = 0$) and not subject to any gut wall metabolism ($F_G = 1$ or $E_G = 0$) the oral bioavailability of the drug will be what is remaining after liver first pass extraction

$$F = 1 - E_H$$
$$F = 1 - 0.7 \text{ (mean } E_H = 0.7)$$
$$F = 0.3$$

Thus, under normal conditions, total systemic bioavailability of propranolol from an oral tablet would be about 30% ($F = 0.3$). The measurement of relative bioavailability for propranolol is always conducted against a reference standard given by the same route of administration and can have a value greater than 100%.

The following shows a method for calculating the absolute bioavailability from the relative bioavailability provided that E is known. Using the above example,

Absolute bioavailability of the solution = $1 - E_H$
= $1 - 0.7 = 0.3 = 30\%$

Absolute bioavailability of the tablet = $x\%$

Relative bioavailability of the tablet to the solution = 70%

$$x = \frac{30 \times 70}{100} = 21\%$$

Therefore, this product has a theoretical absolute bioavailability of 21%. The small difference of calculated and actual (the difference between 21.6 and 21%) absolute bioavailability is due largely to liver extraction fluctuation. All calculations assumed linear pharmacokinetics, which is true for propranolol

2. Fluvastatin sodium (Lescol®, Novartis) is a drug used to lower cholesterol. The absolute bioavailability after an oral dose is reported to be 19% to 29%. The drug is rapidly and completely absorbed (manufacturer's product information). What are the reasons for the low oral bioavailability in spite of reportedly good absorption? What is the extraction ratio of fluvastatin? (The absolute bioavailability, $F$, is 46%, according to values reported in the literature.)

**Solution**

$$E = 1 - 0.46 = 0.54$$

Thus, 54% of the drug is lost due to first-pass effect because of potential absorption issues ($E_A$), gut wall metabolism ($E_G$), and liver first-pass metabolism ($E_H$). It is reported that the drug is 100% absorbed ($F_A$), so the extraction due to absorption $E_A$ is 0. The 46% extraction may therefore be due to first-pass gut ($E_G$) and liver ($E_H$) extraction.

**TABLE 15-6 •** Pharmacokinetic Classification of Drugs Eliminated Primarily by Hepatic Metabolism

| Drug Class | Liver Extraction Ratio (Approx.) | Percent Bound to Plasma Proteins |
|---|---|---|
| **High Extraction Drugs** | | |
| Lidocaine | 0.83 | 45–80[*] |
| Propranolol | 0.6–0.8 | 93 |
| Pethidine (meperidine) | 0.60–0.95 | 60 |
| Pentazocine | 0.8 | — |
| Propoxyphene | 0.95 | — |
| Nortriptyline | 0.5 | 95 |
| Morphine | 0.5–0.75 | 35 |
| **Low Extraction and Highly Bound Drugs** | | |
| Phenytoin | 0.03 | 90 |
| Diazepam | 0.03 | 98 |
| Tolbutamide | 0.02 | 98 |
| Warfarin | 0.003 | 99 |
| Chlorpromazine | 0.22 | 91–99 |
| Clindamycin | 0.23 | 94 |
| Quinidine | 0.27 | 82 |
| Digitoxin | 0.005 | 97 |
| **Low Extraction and Not Highly Bound Drugs** | | |
| Theophylline | 0.09 | 59 |
| Hexobarbital | 0.16 | — |
| Amobarbital | 0.03 | 61 |
| Antipyrine | 0.07 | 10 |
| Chlorampheni-col | 0.28 | 60–80 |
| Thiopental | 0.28 | 72 |
| Acetaminophen | 0.43 | 5[*] |

[*]Concentration dependent in part.
Reproduced with permission from Blaschke TF. Protein binding and kinetics of drugs in liver diseases, Clin Pharmacokinet 1977 Jan-Feb;2(1):32–44.

### Relationship between Blood Flow, Intrinsic Clearance, and Hepatic Clearance

Based on the well-stirred model and assuming that there is no difference between plasma and whole-blood concentrations for a drug, Equation 15.55

indicates whether the hepatic clearance of a drug will be affected by (1) liver blood flow ($Q_H$), (2) the unbound intrinsic clearance of the liver for that drug ($CL_{int(u)}$), and (3) the fraction of drug that is not bound to plasma proteins ($f_u$).

$$CL_H = Q_H \times fu \times CL_{int(u)}/(f_u \times CL_{int(u)} + Q_H) \quad (15.55)$$

### High-Extracted Drugs

For some drugs (such as isoproterenol, lidocaine, and nitroglycerin), and based on the well-stirred model, the extraction ratio is high (>0.7), and the drug is removed by the liver almost as rapidly as the organ is perfused by blood in which the drug is contained. For drugs with very high extraction ratios, the rate of drug metabolism is sensitive to changes in hepatic blood flow:

$E_H \sim 1$, therefore $CL_H = Q_H \times E_H$ is approximated to be $CL_H \sim Q_H$.

Thus, an increase in blood flow to the liver will increase the rate of drug removal by the organ. Propranolol, a β-adrenergic blocking agent, decreases hepatic blood flow by decreasing cardiac output. In such a case, the drug decreases its own clearance through the liver when given orally. Many drugs that demonstrate first-pass effects are drugs that have high extraction ratios with respect to the liver.

*Intrinsic clearance* ($CL_{int(U)}$) is used to describe the total ability of the liver to metabolize a drug in the absence of flow limitations, reflecting the inherent activities of the mixed-function oxidases and all other enzymes. Intrinsic clearance is a distinct characteristic of a particular drug, and as such, based on the well-stirred model, it aims at reflecting the inherent ability of the liver to metabolize the drug.

### Low-Extracted Drugs

Drugs with low liver extraction ratios (eg, theophylline, phenylbutazone, and procainamide) display a hepatic clearance that is less affected by hepatic blood flow:

- These drugs have much lower unbound intrinsic clearance, so $f_u \times CL_{int(U)} <<<< Q_H$
- Equation 15.53 shows that $CL_H = Q_H \times fu \times CL_{int(u)}/(f_u \times CL_{int(u)} + Q_H)$

- Because $f_u \times CL_{int(u)} <<<< Q_H$, the denominator ($f_u \times CL_{int(u)} + Q_H$) can be simplified to QH
- Therefore, $CL_H \sim f_u \times CL_{int(u)}$

The hepatic clearance of low-extracted drugs is more affected by the intrinsic activity of the mixed-function oxidases than by the liver blood flow. Cigarette or marijuana smoking, for example, induces enzymatic activity in the liver (CYP1A, CYP2A, and UGT enzymes among possibly others), thereby increasing the intrinsic and hepatic clearances of low-extracted drugs metabolized by these enzymatic pathways such as theophylline (a CYP1A2 substrate).

The overall relationship between the hepatic clearance of drugs and its liver extraction ratio is illustrated in Fig. 15.13.

Changes or alterations in mixed-function oxidase activity or biliary secretion can affect the intrinsic clearance and thus the rate of drug removal by the liver. Drugs that show low extraction ratios and are eliminated primarily by metabolism demonstrate marked variation in overall elimination half-lives within a given population. For example, the elimination half-life of theophylline varies from 3 to 9 hours. This variation in $t_{1/2}$ is thought to be due to genetic differences in intrinsic hepatic enzyme activity. Moreover, the elimination half-lives of these same drugs are also affected by enzyme induction,

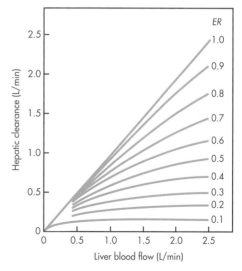

FIGURE 15-13 • The relationship between liver blood flow and total hepatic clearance for drugs with varying extraction rates (ER).

enzyme inhibition, age of the individual, nutritional, and pathologic factors.

## Impact of Protein-Binding or $CL_{int}(u)$ Changes on Hepatic Clearance

It is generally assumed that protein-bound drugs are not easily metabolized (*restrictive clearance*), while free (unbound) drugs can be subject to metabolism within the liver. Protein-bound drugs do not easily diffuse through cell membranes, while free drugs can reach the site of the mixed-function oxidase enzymes easily. Therefore, an increase in the unbound drug concentration in the blood will make more drug available for hepatic extraction.

According to the well-stirred model, hepatic clearance will be mostly dependent on liver blood flow for highly extracted drugs ($CL_H \sim Q_H$), whereas hepatic clearance will be mostly dependent on protein binding and unbound intrinsic clearance for low extracted drugs ($CL_H \sim f_u \times Cl_{int(u)}$). Highly extracted drugs have an "unrestricted clearance" and are "binding insensitive." In this case, the protein-bound drug is removed by the liver during hepatic clearance. Low-extracted compounds are drugs with a "restricted clearance" and are "binding sensitive." In this case, the drug is tightly bound to proteins and only the free or unbound drug is removed by the liver during hepatic clearance.

Most drugs are *restrictively* cleared—for example, diazepam, quinidine, tolbutamide, and warfarin. The clearance of these drugs is proportional to the fraction of unbound drug ($f_u$). However, some drugs, such as propranolol, morphine, and verapamil, are *nonrestrictively* extracted by the liver regardless of drug bound to protein or free. Kinetically, a drug is nonrestrictively cleared if its hepatic extraction ratio ($E_H$) is greater than the fraction of free drug ($f_u$), and the rate of drug clearance is unchanged when the drug is displaced from binding. Mechanistically, protein binding of a drug is a reversible process. For a nonrestrictively bound drug, the free drug fraction gets "stripped" from the protein relatively easily compared to a restrictively bound drug during the process of drug metabolism. The elimination half-life of a nonrestrictively cleared drug is not significantly affected by a change in the degree of protein binding. This is an analogous situation to a protein-bound drug that is actively secreted by the kidney.

For a low-extracted drug with restrictive clearance, $CL_H \sim f_u \times Cl_{int(u)}$, whereas for a highly extracted drug with unrestrictive clearance, $CL_H \sim Q_H$. A change in fu and $CL_{int(u)}$ will cause a proportional change in $CL_H$ for low extracted drugs but will have very little impact on highly extracted drugs.

## Impact of Protein Binding or $Cl_{int(u)}$ Changes on Total Clearance, Bioavailability, and Systemic Exposure

Drug protein binding displacements were historically thought to be the mechanism explaining changes in drug effect seen with many drug–drug interactions. Using the well-stirred model, we will see that this cannot be the case.

The clearance ($CL$, after IV administration where $F = 1$) or apparent clearance ($CL/F$) of a drug can be calculated after a single dose administration by the noncompartmental method (see Chapter 19) as the ratio of the administered dose divided by the total systemic exposure reflected by the area under the curve extrapolated to infinity ($AUC_{inf}$):

$$CL/F = DOSE/AUC_{inf} \quad \text{(from Equation 15.2)}$$

It can also be calculated after multiple dose and steady state conditions have been achieved as the ratio of the dose divided by the systemic exposure seen over the dosing interval at steady state ($AUC\tau_{(ss)}$):

$$CL/F = DOSE/AUC\,\tau_{(ss)} \quad (15.32)$$

For simplicity purposes, consider the situation of a drug that is only eliminated by the liver ($CL \sim CL_H$), is 100% absorbed ($F_A \sim 1$ or $E_A \sim 0$), and is not subject to any gut wall metabolism ($F_G \sim 1$ or $E_G \sim 0$). An example for a low extracted drug ($E \sim 0.1$) would be theophylline.

## Low Extracted Drugs

For a low extracted drug such as theophylline, $CL \sim CL_H \sim f_u \times Cl_{int(u)}$. What would happen if the free fraction of the drug would double by increasing from 40% to 80% due to presumed displacement from its protein binding sites by phenobarbital using the well stirred model?

1. Before being "displaced" from protein binding ($f_u$=40%):

- Considering a 100-mg dose of Theophylline and that $E_H$ ~0.1,
- Assuming a liver blood flow of 1.5 L/min,
- $CL \sim CL_H = Q_H \times E_H$, therefore $CL \sim CL_H$ = 0.15 L/min or 9 L/h
- $E_H = f_u \times CL_{int(U)}/(Q_H + f_u \times CL_{int(u)})$
- Which can be rearranged to:
  $CL_{int(u)} = -E_H \times Q_H/(E_H \times f_u - f_u)$
- Therefore $CL_{int(u)}$ = 0.41667 L/min
- $F = 1 - E_H$, therefore $F$ = 90%
- $AUC_{inf}$ after 100 mg IV dosing will be DOSE/$CL$ = 100/9 = 11.11 mg/L/h
- $AUC_{inf}$ after 100 mg PO dosing will be $F \times$ DOSE/$CL$ = 100 × 0.9/9 = 10 mg/L/h
- The "active" exposure will be the free drug exposure, so $AUC_{inf(u)}$ will be 11.11 * 0.4 = 4.44 mg/L/h and 10 × 0.4 = 4 mg/L/h after IV and PO administration, respectively.

2. After being "displaced" from protein binding ($f_u$ doubles at 80%):

- $E_H = f_u \times CL_{int(u)}/(Q_H + f_u \times CL_{int(u)})$ = 0.8 × 0.41667/(1.5+0.8 × 0.41667) = 0.182
- $CL \sim CL_H = Q_H \times E_H$, therefore $CL \sim CL_H$ = 0.273 L/min or 16.4 L/h
- $F = 1 - E_H$, therefore $F$ = 81.8%
- $AUC_{inf}$ after 100 mg IV dosing will be DOSE/$CL$ = 100/16.4 = 6.1 mg/L/h
- $AUC_{inf}$ after 100 mg PO dosing will be $F \times$ DOSE/$CL$ = 100 × 0.818/16.4 = 4.99 mg/L/h
- The "active" exposure will be the free exposure, so $AUC_{inf(u)}$ will be 6.1 × 0.8 = 4.88 mg/L/h and 4.99 × 0.8 = 3.9 mg/L/h after IV and PO administrations, respectively.

Because $f_u$ and $CL_{int(u)}$ are a product in the well-stirred model equations, doubling $f_u$ (via protein binding displacement) or doubling $CL_{int(u)}$ (enzymatic induction) will result in the same effect on oral bioavailability, clearance, and systemic drug exposure, but not on unbound systemic exposure, which

**TABLE 15-7 •** Effect of Doubling Free Drug Concentrations or Enzymatic Activity on Different PK Parameters for an Orally and Intravenously Administered Low-Extraction Drug ($E_H = 0.1$) Based on the Well-Stirred Model

| PK Parameter for a Low-Extraction Drug such as Theophylline ($E_H = 0.1$) | Doubling $f_u$ (Protein Displacement) | Doubling $Cl_{int(u)}$ (Enzyme Induction, eg, Smoking) |
|---|---|---|
| $f_u$ | Doubles | ---- |
| $CL_{int(u)}$ | ---- | Doubles |
| $CL_H \sim CL$ | ~Doubles | |
| $E_H \sim E$ | Decreases by 10% | |
| $F$ | ~Doubles | |
| $AUC_{inf}$ IV | ~Decreases in half | |
| $AUC_{inf(u)}$ IV | Similar | ~Decreases in half |
| $AUC_{inf}$ PO | ~Decreases in half | |
| $AUC_{inf(u)}$ PO | Similar | ~Decreases in half |

is normally responsible for pharmacologic activity. This is presented in Table 15-7.

From Table 15-7, for a low extraction drug, a displacement from protein binding sites will not lead to any significant change in unbound systemic exposure and therefore therapeutic effect. Should total drug concentrations be measured, though, a clinician may want to erroneously double the dose to reach the same exposure, which would be a mistake as only free drug concentrations are active and would double.

We can therefore appreciate that displacing a low extracted drug from its protein binding sites cannot be a mechanism explaining a difference in effect seen with a DDI, as unbound exposure will stay the same. Enzyme induction, on the other hand, will result in a decrease in half in the unbound concentrations (doubling will be seen with enzyme inhibition) and can therefore explain a difference in effect seen in a DDI.

### High Extracted Drugs

Consider what would now happen for a high extraction drug ($E_H = 0.9$) if the free fraction of the drug would also double by increasing from 5% to 10% due to presumed displacement from protein binding sites using the well stirred model:

3. Before being "displaced" from protein binding ($f_u = 5\%$):

- Considering a 100-mg dose and that $E_H \sim 0.90$,

- Assuming a liver blood flow of 1.5 L/min and an $f_u$ of 5%,

- $CL \sim CL_H = Q_H \times E_H$, therefore $CL \sim CL_H$ = 1.35 L/min or 81 L/h

- $E_H = f_u \times CL_{int(U)}/(Q_H + f_u \times CL_{int(u)})$

- Which can be rearranged to: $CL_{int(u)} = -E_H \times Q_H/(E_H \times f_u - f_u)$

- Therefore $CL_{int(u)}$ = 270 L/min

- $F = 1 - E_H$, therefore $F = 10\%$

- $AUC_{inf}$ after 100 mg IV dosing will be DOSE/$CL$ = 100/81 = 1.23 mg/L/h

- $AUC_{inf}$ after 100 mg PO dosing will be $F \times$ DOSE/$CL$ = 100 × 0.1/81 = 0.123 mg/L/h

- The "active" exposure will be the free exposure, so $AUC_{inf(u)}$ will be 1.23 × 0.04 = 0.0617 mg/L/h and 0.123 × 0.05 = 0.00617 mg/L/h after IV and PO administration, respectively.

4. After being "displaced" from protein binding ($f_{u\ doubles}$ at 10%):

- $E_H = f_u \times CL_{int(U)}/(Q_H + f_u \times CL_{int(u)})$ = 0.1 × 270/(1.5 + 0.1 × 270) = 0.947

- $CL \sim CL_H = Q_H \times E_H$, therefore $CL \sim CL_H$ = 1.421 L/min or 85.26 L/h

- $F = 1 - E_H$, therefore $F = 5.3\%$

- $AUC_{inf}$ after 100 mg IV dosing will be DOSE/$CL$ = 100/85.26 = 1.173 mg/L/h

- $AUC_{inf}$ after 100 mg PO dosing will be $F \times$ DOSE/$CL$ = 100 × 0.053/85.26 = 0.0622 mg/L/h

- The "active" exposure will be the free exposure, so $AUC_{inf(u)}$ will be 1.173 * 0.1 = 0.117 mg/L/h and 0.0622 × 0.1 = 0.0062 mg/L/h after IV and PO administrations, respectively.

Because $f_u$ and $CL_{int(u)}$ are a product in the well-stirred model equations, doubling $f_u$ (via protein binding displacement) or doubling $CL_{int(u)}$ (enzymatic induction) will result in the same effect on oral bioavailability, clearance and systemic drug exposure, but not on unbound systemic exposure which is normally responsible for pharmacologic activity. This is presented in Table 15-8.

As shown in Table 15-8, displacing a high extracted drug from protein binding sites will not lead to any significant change in the unbound systemic exposure and therapeutic effect, except after IV administration where it will double (see Table 15-8). DDI due to protein binding displacements are therefore only possible for high extracted drugs and only when they are administered IV.

### FREQUENTLY ASKED QUESTION

▶ Drug–drug interactions (DDIs) involving protein binding displacements and resulting in an increase in the free fraction of drugs are not considered to be clinically relevant, except for which type of drugs given by which administration route?

**TABLE 15-8 •** Effect of Doubling Free Drug Concentrations or Enzymatic Activity on Different PK Parameters for an Orally and Intravenously Administered High Extraction Drug (EH = 0.9) Based on the Well-Stirred Model

| PK parameters for a High-Extraction Drug (EH=0.9) | Doubling $f_u$ (Protein Displacement) | Doubling $Cl_{int(u)}$ (Enzyme Induction, eg, Smoking) |
|---|---|---|
| $f_u$ | Doubles | ---- |
| $CL_{int(u)}$ | ---- | Doubles |
| $CL_H \sim CL$ | | Similar (increases by 5%) |
| $E_H \sim E$ | | Similar (increases by 5%) |
| $F$ | | ~ Decreases in half |
| $AUC_{inf}$ IV | | ~Similar |
| $AUC_{inf(u)}$ IV | Doubles | ~Similar |
| $AUC_{inf}$ PO | | ~Decreases in half |
| $AUC_{inf(u)}$ PO | Similar | ~Decreases in half |

## CLEARANCE PREDICTIONS BASED ON THE FRACTIONS ELIMINATED THROUGH THE KIDNEY AND LIVER

We have seen in this chapter how to calculate renal and hepatic clearances, and that clearances, except for lung, are additive. A drug that is administered IV and that is eliminated by both kidney and liver can therefore have its clearance characterized by the following previously defined equations:

$$CL = CL_R + CL_H$$

$$CL_R = f_e \times CL$$

$$CL_H = f_m \times CL$$

where $f_e$ is the proportion of the bioavailable dose that is eliminated unchanged by the kidney, and $f_m$ is the proportion of the bioavailable dose that is eliminated by the liver through metabolism.

The renal clearance of a drug correlates with the calculated creatinine clearance according to the following:

$$CLR = slope \times CrCL + intercept$$

while the hepatic clearance of a drug can be estimated by the following equation assuming the well-stirred model:

$$CL_H = Q_H \times f_u \times CL_{int(u)}/(f_u \times CL_{int(u)}) \times (C_p/C_B + Q_H)$$

$$(15.56)$$

Using the above equations, we can therefore predict the impact of a change in the renal and/or hepatic clearance would have on the overall clearance, and therefore exposure of a drug.

## PRACTICE PROBLEM

From the product label, a drug is described to be eliminated unchanged in the urine at 50%, its oral bioavailability estimated to be 82%, and its total apparent clearance after oral dosing reported to be 1 L/h/kg. The typical dosing regimen of the drug is 100 mg given once a day.

1. What is the expected overall exposure ($AUC_{inf}$) of this drug in a typical 72-kg adult with a normal renal function (eg, CrCL = 125 mL/min)?
2. What is the fraction of the drug metabolized?
3. What would be the impact on the overall exposure if the renal function would decrease suddenly by 50%?

### Solution

1. The overall exposure of this drug in a typical 72-kg adult with normal renal function (eg, CrCL=125 mL/min) would be:

   $$CL/F = DOSE/AUC_{inf}$$

   Therefore, $AUC_{inf} = DOSE/CL/F = 100/(1 \times 72)$
   = 1.389 mg.h/L

2. The fraction of the drug metabolized is $f_m = 0.5$ (ie, $1 - f_e$)

3. In a typical 72-kg adult with a normal renal function, the renal clearance will be

   $$CL_R = f_e \times CL/F \times F = 0.5 \times (1 \times 72) \times 0.82$$
   = 29.52 L/h

   The value of hepatic clearance will be the same (CLH = 29.52), as $f_m$ in this case equals to $f_e$.

   With a 50% drop in renal function, the new clearance value would be:

   $$CL = CLR + CLH = (29.52 \times 0.5) + 29.52 = 44.28$$

   The oral bioavailability should not be affected by this drop in renal function, and so the total exposure would then become:

   $$AUC_{inf} = DOSE/(CL/F) = 100/(44.28/0.82)$$
   = 1.85 mg.h/L

   The total exposure is therefore increased by 33% (1.85/1.389) if the renal function decreases by 50%.

## CHAPTER SUMMARY

Clearance refers to the irreversible removal of drug from the systemic circulation of the body by all routes of elimination. Clearance may be defined as the volume of fluid containing drug that is removed from the body or organ per unit of time. The clearance of a drug is a clinically useful parameter as it is directly related to the systemic drug exposure of a drug, which dictates efficacy and safety of the administered dose. Clearance is a constant when the PK behavior of a drug is linear in terms of time and dose. Clearance can be calculated by many different methods, including noncompartmental, compartmental, and physiological using the well-stirred model.

In PK, clearance is typically calculated using compartmental or noncompartmental methods. Both methods will lead to the same results if there are enough data supporting the calculations. Assuming a specific compartment model, clearance will be the product of an elimination rate constant with a volume of distribution. In the simplest case, a one-compartment model for drugs whose concentration time profile decreases according to a monoexponential decline, the clearance will be the product of the terminal rate constant with the total volume of distribution. Clearance is inversely related to the elimination half-life of a drug. Organ clearances are additive, except for lung. The total body clearance is often described in terms of renal and nonrenal clearance. The renal clearance is dependent on renal blood flow, glomerular filtration, drug secretion, and reabsorption.

The physiological approach to drug clearance uses the assumptions of the "well-stirred model." The well-stirred model describes the relationship between hepatic clearance and changes in protein binding, liver blood flow, and enzymatic activity. While the well-stirred model does not appear to be physiologically plausible, its predictions are usually acceptable versus experimental data. More complex models developed over the last 40 years have not yet been proven to be better, let alone as good to predict DDIs as the well-stirred model. The physiological approach using the well-stirred model is currently used in PBPK models.

## LEARNING QUESTIONS

1. Explain why plasma protein binding will prolong the renal clearance of a drug that is excreted only by glomerular filtration but may not affect the renal clearance of a drug excreted by both glomerular filtration and active tubular secretion.

2. Theophylline is effective in the treatment of bronchitis at a blood level of 10 to 20 $\mu g/mL$. At therapeutic range, theophylline follows linear pharmacokinetics. The average $t_{1/2}$ is 3.4 hours, and the range is 1.8 to 6.8 hours. The average volume of distribution is 30 L.

   a. What are the average upper and lower clearance limits for theophylline assuming a one-compartment model?

   b. The renal clearance of theophylline is 0.36 L/h. What are the $k_{NR}$ and $k_{R}$?

3. A single 250-mg oral dose of an antibiotic is given to a young man (age 32 years, creatinine clearance CrCL = 122 mL/min, ABW=78 kg). From the literature, the drug is 50% bound to plasma proteins, and is known to have an apparent $V_{ss}$ equal to 21% of body weight and an elimination half-life of 2 hours. The dose is normally 90% bioavailable. Urinary excretion of the unchanged drug is equal to 70% of the bioavailable dose.

   a. What is the total body clearance for this drug assuming a one-compartment model?

   b. What is the renal clearance for this drug?

   c. What is the probable mechanism for renal clearance of this drug?

4. A drug with an elimination half-life of 1 hour was given to a male patient (80 kg) by intravenous infusion at a rate of 300 mg/h. At 7 hours after infusion, the plasma drug concentration was 11 $\mu g/mL$.

   a. What is the total body clearance for this drug?

   b. What is the apparent $V_{ss}$ for this drug assuming a one-compartment model?

   c. If the drug is not metabolized and is eliminated only by renal excretion, what is the renal clearance of this drug?

   d. What would then be the probable mechanism for renal clearance of this drug?

5. In order to rapidly estimate the renal clearance of a drug in a patient, a 2-hour postdose urine sample was collected and found to contain

200 mg of drug. A midpoint plasma sample was taken (1 hour postdose) and the drug concentration in plasma was found to be 2.5 mg/L. Estimate the renal clearance for this drug in this patient.

6. According to the manufacturer, an antibiotic given by IV infusion at a rate of 5.3 mg/kg/h to 9 adult male volunteers (average weight, 71.7 kg) resulted in a mean steady-state serum concentration of 17 $\mu$g/mL. Calculate the average clearance for this drug in the adult male volunteers.

7. This antibiotic is completely excreted unchanged in the urine, and studies have shown that probenecid given concurrently causes elevation of its serum concentrations. What is the probable mechanism for the interaction of probenecid?

8. When deciding on a dosing regimen of a drug to administer to a patient, what information can be obtained from knowing only the elimination half life? The clearance?

9. Ciprofloxacin hydrochloride (Cipro) is a fluoroquinolone antibacterial drug used to treat urinary tract infections. Ciprofloxacin contains several pKas (basic amine and carboxylic group) and may be considered a weak acid and eliminated primarily by renal excretion, although about 15% of a drug dose is metabolized. The serum elimination half-life in subjects with normal renal function is approximately 4 hours. The renal clearance of ciprofloxacin is approximately 300 mL/min. By what processes of renal excretion would you conclude that ciprofloxacin is excreted? Why?

10. A drug fitting a one-compartment model was found to be eliminated from the plasma by the following pathways with the corresponding elimination rate constants.

Metabolism: $k_H = 0.200 \text{ h}^{-1}$

Kidney excretion: $k_R = 0.250 \text{ h}^{-1}$

Biliary excretion: $k_B = 0.150 \text{ h}^{-1}$

a. What is the elimination half-life of this drug?

b. What would be the half-life of this drug if biliary secretion was completely blocked?

c. What would be the half-life of this drug if drug excretion through the kidney was completely impaired?

d. If drug-metabolizing enzymes were induced so that the rate of metabolism of this drug doubled, what would be the new elimination half-life?

11. A new broad-spectrum antibiotic was administered by rapid intravenous injection to a 50-kg woman at a dose of 3 mg/kg. The apparent volume of distribution of this drug was equivalent to 5% of body weight. The elimination half-life for this drug is 2 hours.

a. If 90% of the unchanged drug was recovered in the urine, what is the renal excretion rate constant?

b. Which is more important for the elimination of this drug, renal excretion or biotransformation? Why?

12. The bioavailability of propranolol is 26%. Propranolol is 87% bound to plasma proteins and has an elimination half-life of 3.9 hours. The apparent volume of distribution of propranolol is 4.3 L/kg. Less than 0.5% of the unchanged drug is excreted in the urine.

a. Assuming that the first-pass extraction of propranolol is only due to hepatic extraction, and using the approximate "well-stirred model", calculate the hepatic clearance for propranolol in an adult male patient (43 years old, 80 kg).

b. What would be the effect of hepatic disease such as cirrhosis on the (1) bioavailability of propranolol and (2) hepatic clearance of propranolol?

c. Explain how a change in (1) hepatic blood flow, (2) intrinsic clearance, or (3) plasma protein binding would affect hepatic clearance of propranolol.

d. What is meant by first-pass effects? From the data above, why is propranolol a drug with first-pass effects?

13. The following pharmacokinetic information for a specific oral formulation of erythromycin was reported:

Oral Bioavailability: 35%

Percent excreted unchanged in the urine: 12%

Plasma protein binding: 84%

Total volume of distribution after IV administration: 0.78 L/kg

Elimination half-life after IV administration: 1.6 hours

An adult male patient (41 years old, 81 kg) was prescribed 250 mg of this erythromycin formulation orally every 6 hours for 10 days. From the given data, calculate the following:

a. What is the Clearance?

b. What is the renal clearance?

c. What is the Hepatic clearance?

14. Which of the following statements describe(s) correctly the properties of a drug that follows linear pharmacokinetics?

a. The elimination half-life will change proportionally when the dose changes.

b. The area under the plasma curve (AUC) will increase proportionately with an increase in dose.

c. The clearance, half-life (half-lives), and volume of distribution(s) will remain constant, regardless of dose and time.

d. a) and b) are correct.

e. b) and c) are correct.

15. The unbound hepatic intrinsic clearance of two drugs ($f_u \times CL_{int(u)}$) are as follows:

Drug A: 13 L/min

Drug B: 0.026 L/min

Which drug is likely to show the greatest increase in hepatic clearance when hepatic blood flow is increased from 1 L/min to 1.5 mL/min? Which drug will likely be blood-flow limited?

## ANSWERS

### Learning Questions

1. Only the free fraction of a drug is filtered. Heavily bound drugs are thereby less filtered, and they have longer elimination half-lives. If a drug is mostly actively secreted, though, protein binding may not affect much its elimination half-life. Penicillin and cephalosporin antibiotics are great examples of drugs that are mostly filtered by the kidney and were developed and selected with greater protein binding characteristics in order to slow down their elimination half-life.

2. **a.** Using a one-compartment PK model, we can estimate the CL for these two limits of elimination half-lives:

   $CL = k_{10} \times V_c$, where in a one-compartment model, $V_c = V_{ss}$ and $k_{10} = \lambda_z$, and $t_{1/2} = 0.693/\lambda_z$.

   For $t_{1/2}$ of 1.8 h, $CL = 0.693/1.8 \times 30 = 11.55$ L/h.

   For $t_{1/2}$ of 6.8 h, $CL = 0.693/6.8 \times 30 = 3.06$ L/h.

   **b.** In a one-compartment PK model, $CL = K_{10} \times V_c$, where $V_c = V_{ss}$ and $K_{10} = \lambda_z$.

   Clearance is always the sum of renal and non-renal clearances, so $CL = CL_R + CL_{NR}$, and thereby $\lambda_z = k_R + k_{NR}$.

   For $t_{1/2}$ of 1.8 h: $CL = 11.55$. $CL_R = 0.36$ L/h, so $CL_{NR} = 11.55 - 0.36 = 11.19$ L/h. $k_{NR}$ therefore equals $CL_{NR}/V_c = 11.19/30 = 0.373$ h$^{-1}$ and $k_R$ equals $CL_R/V_c = 0.36/30 = 0.012$ h$^{-1}$.

   For $t_{1/2}$ of 6.8 h: $CL = 3.06$. $CL_R = 0.36$ L/h, so $CL_{NR} = 3.06 - 0.36 = 2.7$ L/h. $k_{NR}$ therefore equals $CL_{NR}/V_c = 2.7/30 = 0.09$ h$^{-1}$ and $k_R$ equals $CL_R/V_c = 0.36/30 = 0.012$ h$^{-1}$.

3. **a.** In a one-compartment model, $V_c = V_{ss}$ and $\lambda_z = k_{10}$. Because $CL/F = k_{10} \times V_c/F$, $CL/F$ then equals to $(0.693/2) \times (0.21 \times 78) = 5.68$ L/h

   **b.** $fe = 70\%$. Because $CL_R = fe \times (CL/F \times F)$, then $CL_R = (5.68 \times 0.9) \times 0.70 = 3.58$ L/h

   **c.** This patient has a normal renal function, with a GFR of approximately 122 mL/min. This translates into $122 \times 60/1000 = 7.32$ L/h.

   Only the free fraction of the drug is filtered by the kidney. Therefore, the filtration clearance would be equal to $7.32 \times 0.5 = 3.66$ L/h, which is almost equal to the renal clearance of the drug (3.58 L/h). Therefore, the drug is probably filtered by the kidney with little or insignificant secretion and reabsorption.

4. **a.** With a constant infusion, the steady-state concentration (Css) equals "rate in divided by rate out". So $C_{ss} = R_0/CL$. Therefore, $CL = R_0/C_{ss} = 300/11 = 27.27$ L/h

**b.** $CL = k_{10} \times V_c$. In a one-compartment model, $\lambda_z = k_{10}$ and $V_c = V_{ss}$.

Therefore $V_{ss} = CL/\lambda_z = 27.27/(0.693/1) = 39.35$ L

**c.** If $CL_{NR} = 0$, then $CL_R = CL$, therefore $CL_R = 27.27$ L/h

**d.** A patient with a normal renal function ($CL_{creat} \sim 120$ mL/min) will have a maximum clearance due to glomerular filtration of 7.2 L/h. The $CL_R$ being much larger than this at 27.27 L/h suggests that the drug is not only filtered but significantly secreted as well. It does not say anything about reabsorption, but if it undergoes any, then it is automatically much more secreted than it is reabsorbed.

**5.** The mid-point clearance formula is $CL_R = (U \times V)/P$, where $(U \times V)$ is the amount of drug excreted in the urine over two hours (200 mg/2 hours), and $P$ is the drug concentration in plasma at the mid-point time (2.5 mg/L).

$CL_R = (200/2)/2.5 = 40$ L/h

**6.** With a constant infusion, the steady-state concentration (Css) equals "rate in divided by rate out". So $C_{ss} = R_0/CL$. Therefore, $CL = R_0/C_{ss} = (5.3 \times 71.7)/17 = 22.35$ L/h

**7.** Probenecid has been reported to block the activities of the organic anion transporters OAT1 and OAT3 in the kidney. It is therefore probable that this drug is actively secreted by these transporters in the kidney.

**8.** From a simplistic point of view, the elimination half-life usually dictates how long the dosing interval will have to be, while the clearance will dictate the total daily dose that will need to be administered based on a target exposure (AUC).

**9.** The renal clearance of ciprofloxacin is much greater than the normal adult glomerular filtration rate (GFR $\sim 120$ mL/min or 7.2 L/h). It is therefore automatically heavily secreted, and may also be re-absorbed.

From a theoretical viewpoint, ciprofloxacin being a weak acid, its renal excretion could be increased with an alkaline pH, as the drug would become highly ionized, not lipid soluble, preventing its re-absorption process.

**10. a.** $k = k_H + k_R + k_B = 0.2 + 0.25 + 0.15 = 0.6$ h$^{-1}$

$t_{1/2} = 0.693/0.6 = 1.16$ h

**b.** $k = k_H + k_R + k_B = 0.2 + 0.25 + 0 = 0.45$ h$^{-1}$

$t_{1/2} = 0.693/0.45 = 1.54$ h

**c.** $k = k_H + k_R + k_B = 0.2 + 0 + 0.15 = 0.35$ h$^{-1}$

$t_{1/2} = 0.693/0.35 = 1.98$ h

**d.** $k = k_H + k_R + k_B = (0.2 \times 2) + 0.25 + 0.15 = 0.8$ h$^{-1}$

$t_{1/2} = 0.693/0.8 = 0.87$ h

**11. a.** $t_{1/2} = 2$ h, therefore $k = 0.693/2 = 0.3465$

$k_R = f_e \times k = 0.9 \times 0.3465 = 0.312$ h$^{-1}$

**b.** Biotransformation only accounts for 10% of the elimination of this drug $(1 - f_e)$, it is therefore a minor elimination pathway.

**12. a.** $F \sim F_H$, therefore $F_H = 0.26$ and $E_H = 1 - F_H = 0.74$

Because less than 0.5% of the drug is eliminated unchanged in the urine, we can also approximate that $CL \sim CL_H$

Based on the "well-stirred model", the hepatic clearance can be estimated to be:

$CL_H = Q_H \times E_H = 1.5 \times 0.74 = 1.11$ L/min

**b.** Assuming that the liver blood flow stays normal at 1.5 L/min, and that cirrhosis would <u>decrease in half</u>, the enzymatic activity of the liver ($Cl_{int(u)}$), the following can be estimated:

- Before cirrhosis:
  - $F = 0.26$ and $E \sim E_H = 0.74$
  - $CL \sim CL_H = 1.11$ L/min
  - $E_H = f_u \times CL_{int(u)}/(f_u \times CL_{int(u)} + Q_H)$
  - Therefore, $CL_{int(u)} = (E_H \times Q_H)/(f_u - f_u \times E_H) = (0.74 \times 1.5)/(0.13 - 0.13 \times 0.74)$ $CL_{int(u)} = 32.84$ L/min

- With cirrhosis (where enzymatic activity is decreased by half):
  - $CL_{int(u)}$ becomes 32.84/2 = 16.42 L/min
  - $E_H = f_u \times CL_{int(u)}/(F_u \times CL_{int(u)} + Q_H)$ $= 0.13 \times 16.42/(0.13 \times 16.42 + 1.5)$ $= 0.59$
  - $F \sim 1 - E_H = 1 - 0.59 = 0.41$
  - $CL \sim CL_H = Q_H \times E_H = 1.5 \times 0.59$ $= 0.885$ L/min

**c.**

- $CL_H = Q_H \times E_H$
  - A change in $Q_H$ will automatically affect $CL_H$

- $E_H$ is dependent on $CL_{int(u)}$ as per the following equation:
  - $E_H = f_u \times CL_{int(u)} / (f_u \times CL_{int(u)} + Q_H)$
  - For "High extraction drugs," the equation can almost be simplified to $E_H \sim 1$, and therefore a change in intrinsic clearance will have small effect on $CL_H$.
  - For all other drugs, a change in intrinsic clearance will affect $CL_H$, and more so for "low extraction drugs", where $E_H \sim f_u \times CL_{int(u)}$.
- A change in protein binding ($f_u$) will be similar to a change in $CL_{int(u)}$
  - $E_H = f_u \times CL_{int(u)} / (f_u \times CL_{int(u)} + Q_H)$
  - For "High extraction drugs," the equation can almost be simplified to $E_H \sim 1$, and therefore a change in protein binding will have small effect on $CL_H$.
  - For all other drugs, a change in protein binding will affect $CL_H$, and more so for "low extraction drugs", where $E_H \sim f_u \times CL_{int(u)}$.

d. A drug is considered to be subject to a first-pass effect when it is removed or metabolized within the body before it reaches the systemic circulation after an extra-vascular administration. For orally administered drugs, the extraction ratio ($E = E_A + E_G + E_H$) represents the fraction of the administered dose that does not reach the systemic circulation ($F = 1 - E$) and that is subject to this first-pass effect.

Propranolol has an oral bioavailability of 26%. The extraction ratio is therefore 74%, indicating that it is subject to the first-pass effect. In the preceding calculations, we assumed that most or all of this extraction was within the liver ($EH \sim E$), and not due significantly to either gut ($E_G$) or absorption ($E_A$) extraction.

13. $F = 0.35; f_e = 12\%; f_u = 0.16; V_{ss} = 81 \times 0.78 = 63.18$ L; $t_{1/2} = 1.6$ h; therefore, $\lambda_z = 0.693/1.6 = 0.433$ h$^{-1}$

a. The clearance cannot be calculated exactly with noncompartmental methods ($CL/F = Dose/AUC_{inf}$) as no exposure metrics are provided. Clearance can therefore be approximated using a one-compartment PK model, where $CL = k_{10} \times V_c$ and where we will approximate that $V_c \sim V_{ss}$, and $k_{10} \sim \lambda_z$:

$CL \sim \lambda_z \times V_{ss} = 0.433 \times 63.18 = 27.36$ L/h after IV administration

$CL/F \sim (\lambda_z \times V_{ss})/F = 27.36/0.35 = 78.16$ L/h after oral administration

b. $CL = CL_R + CL_{NR}$, where $CL_R = f_e \times CL$
$CL_R = f_e \times CL = 27.36 \times 0.12 = 3.28$ L/h

c. If we assume that $CL_{NR} \sim CL_H$ then
$CL_H = CL - CL_R = 27.36 - 3.28 = 24.08$ L/h

14. e) is correct. When a drug is said to exhibit linear pharmacokinetics, it usually means that its pharmacokinetic behavior is constant or linear as it regards to both time and dose. All PK parameters such as bioavailability ($F$), clearance ($CL$), volumes of distributions ($V_c$, $V_{ss}$), and half-lives ($t1/2abs$, $t1/2dist$, $t1/2el$) will be constant. Exposure PK metrics, such as $C_{max}$, AUC, and $C_{min}$ will increase or decrease proportionally with the doses administered.

15. According to the "well-stirred model", the hepatic clearance of a drug can be estimated with the following formula:

$CL_H = Q_H \times E_H$
Where, $E_H = f_u \times CL_{int(u)} / (f_u \times CL_{int(u)} + Q_H)$
When ($f_u \times CL_{int(u)}$) is much smaller than $Q_H$, the drug is considered to be a "Low extraction drug" and $CL_H \sim (f_u \times CL_{int(u)})$. For these drugs, $CL_H$ will therefore not increase or decrease as much with changes in $Q_H$. This is the case with Drug B.

Drug A on the other hand has a large ($f_u \times CL_{int(u)}$) compared to $Q_H$. The drug is therefore considered to be a "High extraction drug" and $CL_H \sim Q_H$. For these drugs, $CL_H$ will increase or decrease almost proportionally with changes in $Q_H$. We also commonly refer to these drugs as being "Blood-flow limited".

# REFERENCES

Auclair B, Sirois G, Ngoc AH, Ducharme MP: Novel pharmacokinetic modelling of transdermal nitroglycerin. *Pharm Res* **15**(4):612–617, 1998a.

Auclair B, Sirois G, Ngoc AH, Ducharme MP: Population pharmacokinetics of nitroglycerin and of its two metabolites after a single 24-hour application of a nitroglycerin transdermal matrix delivery system. *Ther Drug Monit* **20**(6):607–611, 1998b.

Benet LZ, Liu S, Wolfe AR: The universally unrecognized assumption in predicting drug clearance and organ extraction ratio. *Clin Pharmacol Ther* **103**(3):521–525, 2018.

Blaschke TF: Protein binding and kinetics of drugs in liver diseases. *Clin Pharmacokinet* **2**:32–44, 1977.

Brouwer KL, Dukes GE, Powell JR: Influence of liver function on drug disposition. Applied pharmacokinetics. In Evans WE, Schentag JJ, Jusko WJ, et al (eds). *Principles of Therapeutic Drug Monitoring*. Vancouver, WA, Applied Therapeutics, 1992, Chap 6.

Cockcroft DW, Gault MH: Prediction of creatinine clearance from serum creatinine. *Nephron* **16**(1):31–41, 1976.

Holford N, Heo YA, Anderson B: A pharmacokinetic standard for babies and adults. *J Pharm Sci* **102**(9):2941–2952, 2013.

Gillette JR: Factors affecting drug metabolism. *Ann N Y Acad Sci* **179**:43–66, 1971.

Pang KS, Rowland M: Hepatic clearance of drugs. I. Theoretical considerations of a "well-stirred" model and a "parallel tube" model. Influence of hepatic blood flow, plasma and blood cell binding, and the hepatocellular enzymatic activity on hepatic drug clearance. *J Pharmacokinet Biopharm* **5**(6):625–653, 1977a.

Pang KS, Rowland M: Hepatic clearance of drugs. II. Experimental evidence for acceptance of the "well-stirred" model over the "parallel tube" model using lidocaine in the perfused rat liver in situ preparation. *J Pharmacokinet Biopharm* **5**(6):655–680, 1977b.

Pang KS, Han YR, Noh K, Lee PI, Rowland M: Hepatic clearance concepts and misconceptions: Why the well-stirred model is still used even though it is not physiologic reality. *Biochem Pharmacol* **169**:1–17, 2019.

Rowland M, Benet LZ, Graham GG. Clearance concepts in pharmacokinetics. *J Pharmacokinet Biopharm* **1**:123–136, 1973.

Rowland M: Drug administration and regimens. In Melmon K, Morelli HF (eds). *Clinical Pharmacology*. New York, Macmillan, 1978, pp 25–70.

Wilkinson GR, Shand DG: A physiologic approach to hepatic drug clearance. *Clin Pharmacol Ther* **18**:377–390, 1975.

Yang J, Jamei M, Yeo KR, Rostami-Hodiegan, Tucker GT. Misuse of the well-stirred model of hepatic drug clearance. *Drug Metab Disp* **35**(3):501–502, 2006.

# BIBLIOGRAPHY

Benet LZ. Clearance (née Rowland) concepts: A downdate and an update. *J Pharmacokinet Pharmacodyn* **37**:529–539, 2010.

Cafruny EJ: Renal tubular handling of drugs. *Am J Med* **62**:490–496, 1977.

Hewitt WR, Hook JB: The renal excretion of drugs. In Bridges VW, Chasseaud LF (eds). *Progress in Drug Metabolism*, Vol 7. New York, Wiley, 1983, Chap 1.

Renkin EM, Robinson RR: Glomerular filtration. *N Engl J Med* **290**:785–792, 1974.

Smith H: *The Kidney: Structure and Function in Health and Disease*. New York, Oxford University Press, 1951.

Thomson P, Melmon K, Richardson J, et al: Lidocaine pharmacokinetics in advanced heart failure, liver disease and renal failure in humans. *Ann Intern Med* **78**:499–508, 1973.

Tucker GT: Measurement of the renal clearance of drugs. *Br J Clin Pharm* **12**:761–770, 1981.

Weiner IM, Mudge GH: Renal tubular mechanisms for excretion and organic acids and bases. *Am J Med* **36**:743–762, 1964.

Wilkinson GR: Clearance approaches in pharmacology. *Pharmacol Rev* **39**:1–47, 1987.

# 16

# Pharmacokinetics of Drug Absorption

Corinne Seng Yue and Dina Al-Numani

## CHAPTER OBJECTIVES

- Define oral drug absorption and its relevance.

- Describe different absorption rate processes (eg, first- and zero-order).

- Calculate the pharmacokinetic parameters of an orally administered drug that is described by a one-compartment model.

- Calculate the absorption rate constant for an orally administered drug that is described by a two-compartment pharmacokinetic model.

- Contrast current methods for characterizing absorption against historical methods.

- Describe flip-flop kinetics for oral extended-release drug products.

- Discuss the clinical implication of absorption half-life.

- Discuss how $k_a$ and $k_{el}$ influence $C_{max}$, $t_{max}$, and AUC.

- Discuss how changes in these parameters affect drug safety in a clinical situation.

## INTRODUCTION

Extravascular delivery routes are an important and popular means of drug administration and include all routes that are not intravenous (eg, oral, topical, intranasal, inhalation, intramuscular, and rectal). The route of drug administration that is chosen must be one that provides optimal therapeutic activity and safety for the patient (Chapter 7). With intravenous administration, the entire drug dose is injected directly into the systemic circulation. Drugs given by extravascular administration must first be absorbed from the site of administration. For example, after oral drug administration, the drug may be absorbed through the small intestine, whereas after inhalation, some of the drug will be absorbed after passing through the lung. The physiological aspects of drug absorption are discussed in Chapter 4. Pharmacokinetic characterization of drug absorption is important for the determination of drug exposure and the development of drug dosage regimens.

The oral route is the most common method of extravascular drug administration. The oral route is a safe, easy, and convenient method of drug administration. After drug products are given by the oral route, the drug must first be released from the drug product and dissolve in the fluids of the gastrointestinal (GI) tract for systemic drug absorption through the intestinal epithelium. In the case of oral drug solutions, this dissolution step is unnecessary as the drug is already in solution. Drug absorption is influenced by various physiological factors related to the GI tract (Chapter 4). The bioavailability of the drug is influenced by all the processes that allow the drug to reach the systemic circulation, including drug release from the drug product, dissolution into the fluids of the GI tract, transporters in the GI tract, passage of the drug through the gut wall, metabolism, and passage through

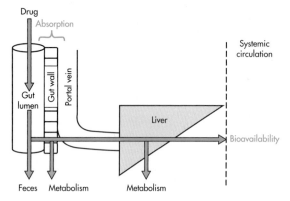

**FIGURE 16-1 •** Systemic drug absorption and bioavailability.

the liver via the hepatic portal vein and then into the systemic circulation (Fig. 16-1).

This chapter will focus on the pharmacokinetics of drug absorption following oral administration, explain the different methods that can be used to characterize and quantify drug absorption and bioavailability, and focus on the determination of absorption rate constants.

Oral drug administration is commonly thought to involve only the swallowing of drugs, but also includes buccal (gums and cheek), sublingual (under the tongue), orally disintegrating tablets, and chewable drug administration. Some drugs given by buccal and sublingual administration (eg, nitroglycerin, fentanyl) are absorbed in the buccal cavity of the mouth and bypass the GI tract. A portion of these doses may also be swallowed. Drugs given by orally disintegrating tablets or chewable tablets are swallowed and the drug is absorbed in the GI tract. Drug administration via intranasal and lung inhalation will be absorbed both in the lung and in the GI tract due to swallowing some of the drug. Although the focus of this chapter is on drug absorption following oral administration, the pharmacokinetic concepts presented here can be applied to other routes when drug absorption occurs prior to systemic drug delivery.

---

**FREQUENTLY ASKED QUESTION**

▶ Is systemic drug absorption the same as drug bioavailability?

---

## RELATIONSHIP BETWEEN ABSORPTION AND ELIMINATION PROCESSES FOLLOWING ORAL DRUG ADMINISTRATION

The rate of change in the amount of drug in the body at any given time is dependent on the relative rates of drug absorption and elimination. This is illustrated in Fig. 16-2 for an orally administered drug, where $D_{GI}$ is the amount of drug in the GI tract, $D_E$ is the amount of drug eliminated, $D_B$ is the amount of drug in body, and $V_c/F$ is the apparent volume of distribution.

This scheme shows the rate of amount of drug in the body at any time (t) (*exposure*) is equal to the rate of drug absorption minus the rate of drug elimination:

$$\frac{dD_B}{dt} = \frac{dD_{GI}}{dt} - \frac{dD_E}{dt} \qquad (16.1)$$

A plot of plasma concentration over time illustrates how absorption and elimination rates affect drug concentrations following a single oral dose of a drug product (Fig. 16-3).

After oral drug administration, drug is absorbed into the body and some of the drug is eliminated. At the beginning of the plasma concentration–time profile, drug in the body accumulates with time. This is the phase where the rate of drug absorption is greater than the rate of drug elimination. Note that during this phase, drug elimination occurs but drug absorption predominates.

$$\frac{dD_{GI}}{dt} > \frac{dD_E}{dt} \qquad (16.2)$$

At the *peak drug concentration* ($C_{max}$) in the plasma (Fig. 16-3), the rate of drug absorption is equal to the rate of drug elimination, and there is no net change in the amount of drug in the body.

$$\frac{dD_{GI}}{dt} = \frac{dD_E}{dt} \qquad (16.3)$$

Immediately after the time of peak drug absorption ($t_{max}$), some drug may still be at the absorption site (ie, in the GI tract or other site of administration).

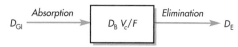

**FIGURE 16-2 •** Model of drug absorption from gastrointestinal tract and elimination from the body.

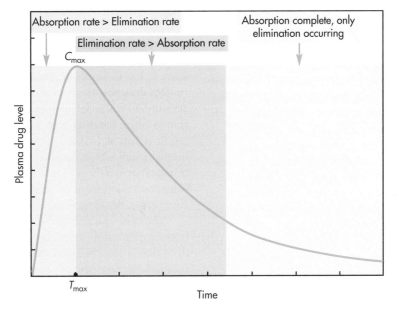

**FIGURE 16-3** • Example of a concentration–time profile following extravascular drug administration.

However, the rate of drug elimination at this time is faster than the rate of absorption, as represented by the *post-$C_{max}$ phase* which occurs just after peak drug absorption as shown in Fig. 16-3.

$$\frac{dD_{GI}}{dt} < \frac{dD_E}{dt} \tag{16.4}$$

When the drug at the absorption site becomes depleted, the rate of drug absorption approaches zero, or $dD_{GI}/dt = 0$. The tail end of the plasma concentration–time curve represents the *elimination phase*, where only the elimination of drug from the body occurs, and which is usually a first-order process. During the *elimination phase*, the rate of change in the amount of drug in the body is described as a first-order process, where $k_{el}$ is the first-order elimination rate constant:

$$\frac{dD_B}{dt} = -k_{el}D_B \tag{16.5}$$

## DRUG ABSORPTION PROCESSES— GENERAL CONCEPTS

As shown in Figs. 16-2 and 16-3, and in Equations 16.1–16.5, the amount of drug in the body at any given time depends on the relative rates of drug absorption and elimination. Both processes contribute to the drug concentrations in the body. Pharmacokinetic parameters associated with drug absorption, such as absorption rates, peak drug concentrations, and time to reach peak drug concentrations, are used to calculate drug exposure or predict drug effect. The determination of absorption and elimination rate constants are useful for developing multiple-dose regimens.

The calculation of the rate of systemic drug absorption from an orally administered drug product requires an estimate of the absorption rate constant, $k_a$. This absorption rate constant encompasses many individual rate processes, including dissolution of the drug, GI motility, blood flow, transport of the drug across the capillary membranes into the systemic circulation, and other factors.

The rate of drug absorption may be described by a single zero-order or first-order process. For most immediate-release (IR) dosage forms, drug absorption is a first-order process. If the drug, eg, ampicillin or amoxicillin, is absorbed by active diffusion (a saturable, carrier-mediated process), then the absorption rate may become constant or a *zero-order* process.

The overall rate of drug absorption for most IR drug products is a first-order rate process represented by an absorption rate constant, $k_a$. If the same drug is formulated as an extended-release (ER) drug product, the rate of drug release from the formulation is slowed. Ideally, the rate of drug release from an ER drug product is constant which can be described as a zero-order rate process. If the drug release from the ER drug product is the rate limiting step in absorption, then the rate of drug absorption may be described by a zero-order rate constant, $k_0$.

While many absorption processes can be described by a first-order or zero-order rate, some drugs have absorption processes that are described by more complicated systems. Absorption can sometimes be described by parallel processes (ie, more than one absorption rate happening at the same time). These drug absorption processes can include simultaneous first-order processes or a mixture of first-order and zero-order processes. Examples of drug products that are described by more complex absorption processes include transdermal nitroglycerin (Auclair et al, 1998a, 1998b), ciprofloxacin ophthalmic drops (DiMarco et al, 2004), extended-release methylphenidate (Teuscher et al, 2015; Jackson, 2019), and long-acting injectable paliperidone (Magnusson et al, 2017).

---

**FREQUENTLY ASKED QUESTION**

▶ What are the differences in the overall absorption process between an oral solution, an immediate release tablet formulation, or an extended-release formulation of the same drug?

---

## ZERO-ORDER DRUG ABSORPTION

Zero-order drug absorption occurs when the rate of drug absorption is constant. The zero-order rate constant, $k_0$ has the units of mass/time, eg, the amount (mg) of drug absorbed per unit of time. Examples of zero-order drug absorption include an IV drug infusion in which the drug is given at a constant rate, eg, mg/hr (Chapter 14), drug absorption from a transdermal patch which becomes zero order when the transport across the skin is the rate limiting step, and drug absorption from some ER drug products that have zero-order drug release.

The zero-order drug absorption process is illustrated in Fig. 16-4. In the left panel, the amount of drug that is absorbed and reaches the systemic circulation increases steadily regardless of the amount of drug that remains to be absorbed. The right panel illustrates the constancy in the amount that is absorbed as a function of time. Both panels are theoretical examples in which only absorption is depicted and where no elimination process occurs.

The change in the amount of drug in the GI tract ($D_{GI}$) with time can be represented as follows:

$$\frac{dD_{GI}}{dt} = -k_0 \qquad (16.6)$$

Zero-order drug absorption following oral drug administration can be related to nonlinear or saturable processes, such as a capacity-limited absorption (Chapter 18). If a drug relies on specific transporters to cross the GI lumen, zero-order absorption may

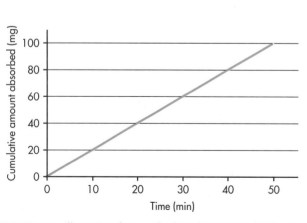

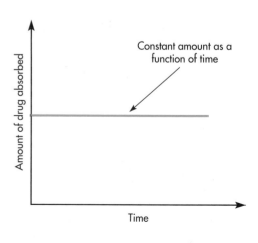

FIGURE 16-4 • Illustration of zero-order drug absorption in the absence of elimination.

be observed when these transporters become saturated. At drug concentrations that exceed the number of transporters available for drug absorption, the amount of drug that is absorbed will become constant, limited by the capacity of the transporters. As such, drugs may show first-order absorption at low doses but change to zero-order absorption at higher doses when the transporters are saturated.

Some drugs that are known to exhibit zero-order absorption include ethanol (Cooke, 1970), griseofulvin (Bates and Carrigan, 1975), and erythromycin (Colburn et al, 1977). Zero-order drug absorption can also be observed with controlled-release delivery systems, such as transdermal patches, as illustrated in the following example.

## CLINICAL APPLICATION— TRANSDERMAL DRUG DELIVERY

The stratum corneum (horny layer) of the epidermis of the skin acts as a barrier and rate-limiting step for systemic absorption of many drugs. After application of a transdermal system (patch), the drug dissolves into the outer layer of the skin and is absorbed by a pseudo first-order process due to high concentration in the skin. The drug is eliminated by a first-order process. Once the patch is removed, the residual drug concentrations in the skin continue to decline by a first-order process.

Ortho Evra® is a combination transdermal contraceptive patch with a contact surface area of 20 cm². Each patch contains 6.00 mg norelgestromin (NGMN) and 0.75 mg ethinyl estradiol (EE) and is designed to deliver 0.15 mg of NGMN and 0.02 mg EE to the systemic circulation daily. As shown in Fig. 16-5, serum EE is absorbed from the patch at a zero-order rate.

## FIRST-ORDER DRUG ABSORPTION

Systemic drug absorption after oral administration of a drug product (eg, solution, tablet, capsule) is often characterized by a first-order process. First-order absorption processes are those in which a constant proportion of drug is being absorbed per unit of time. This phenomenon is illustrated in Fig. 16-6 (elimination process is not occurring in this theoretical example).

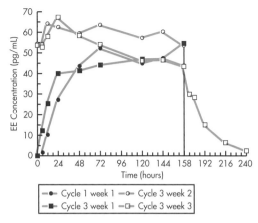

FIGURE 16-5 • Mean serum EE concentrations (pg/mL) in healthy female volunteers following application of Ortho Evra® on the buttock for three consecutive cycles (vertical line at 158 hours indicates time of patch removal). (Adapted with permission from approved label for Ortho Evra®, September, 2009.)

The left panel in Fig. 16-6 depicts the cumulative amount of drug absorbed as a function of time, showing that the cumulative amount increases with time, but tapers off when there is no drug left to be absorbed. A plot of the amount of drug absorbed (on the log scale) versus time is shown in the right panel, where a straight descending line describes this relationship, depicting that the rate at which the drug is being absorbed is constant. The cumulative amount of drug that is absorbed therefore depends on the absorption rate (which does not change) as well as the amount that remains to be absorbed, which decreases with time as drug absorption occurs. Therefore a tapering off of the cumulative amount absorbed is seen in the left panel.

For first-order absorption processes, the rate of change in the amount of drug in the GI tract ($D_{GI}$) with time depends on both the amount of drug in the GI tract at any given time and $k_a$, the first-order absorption rate constant (hr$^{-1}$).

$$\frac{dD_{GI}}{dt} = -k_a D_{GI} \qquad (16.7)$$

In many cases, the absorption of drug after a single oral dose does not start immediately, due to such physiologic factors as dissolution and release of the drug from the drug product, stomach-emptying time, and intestinal motility. The time delay prior to

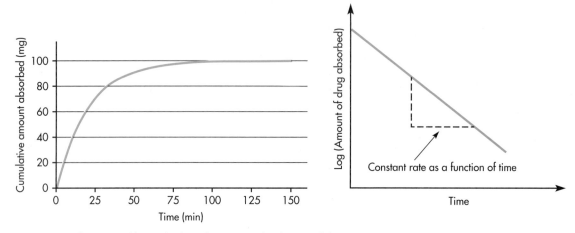

FIGURE 16-6 • Illustration of first-order drug absorption in the absence of elimination.

the commencement of drug absorption is known as the *lag time* ($T_{lag}$). This phenomenon is illustrated in Fig. 16-7.

## EQUATIONS DESCRIBING CONCENTRATION–TIME PROFILES FOLLOWING DRUG ABSORPTION

Previous sections have described the difference between zero-order and first-order absorption processes. As many absorption processes are associated with first-order processes, subsequent parts of this chapter will describe how first-order absorption rate constants can be estimated. Historical methods include the method of residuals and the Loo–Riegelman method. Other approaches include the Wagner–Nelson method as well as compartmental analyses. To better understand how absorption parameters can be calculated using these various approaches, some equations describing

the concentration–time profiles of drugs following oral administration are first reviewed. Equations for both one- and two-compartment models are presented.

### Zero-Order Oral Absorption, One-Compartment Model

In a one-compartment model, regardless of how the absorption rate is described, the amount of drug found in the body (in the blood or systemic circulation) at any given time is dependent on the absorption and elimination rates (Fig. 16-8), where $V_c/F$ is the apparent central volume of distribution.

Equation 16.8 describes the rate of change in the amount of drug in the body at any given time ($dD_B/dt$). This rate is a function of the absorption and elimination rates, and is also described as follows:

$$\frac{dD_B}{dt} = \text{rate in} - \text{rate out} \qquad (16.8)$$

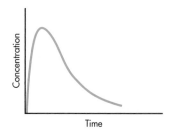

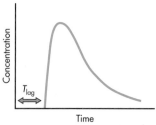

FIGURE 16-7 • Illustration of lag time in concentration–time profile.

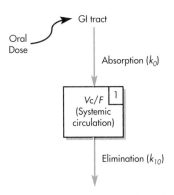

FIGURE 16-8 • One-compartment, zero-order oral absorption and first-order elimination model.

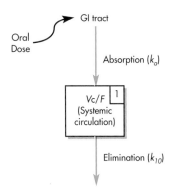

FIGURE 16-9 • One-compartment, first-order oral absorption and first-order elimination model.

For a zero-order absorption process, "rate in" is a function of the absorption rate constant ($k_0$). For most drugs, rate of drug elimination is described by a first-order rate constant ($k_{el}$ or $k_{10}$ for a one-compartment model). For a first-order elimination process, "rate out" is the product of the drug elimination rate constant ($k_{10}$) and amount of drug in the body ($D_B$). Equation 16.9 can be rewritten as follows:

$$\frac{dD_B}{dt} = k_0 - k_{10}D_B \qquad (16.9)$$

This equation can be integrated to present the drug amount, $D_B$, as a function of time.

$$D_B(t) = \frac{k_0}{k_{10}}(1 - e^{-k_{10} \cdot t}) \qquad (16.10)$$

Drug concentration, $C$, as a function of time, can be obtained by taking the above equation and dividing amount (mass) of drug by the apparent central volume of distribution ($V_c/F$).

$$C(t) = \frac{k_0}{V_c/F \cdot k_{10}}(1 - e^{-k_{10} \cdot t}) \qquad (16.11)$$

This equation describes the plasma drug concentration, $C$, at various times, $t$, for a drug whose pharmacokinetics is described by a one-compartment model with zero-order absorption and first-order elimination.

### First-Order Oral Absorption, One-Compartment Model

Figure 16-9 illustrates a one-compartment model with first-order absorption and elimination processes, where $V_c/F$ is the apparent central volume

of distribution. The plasma concentration–time curve that results from a model where absorption is described by a first-order process is depicted in Fig. 16-2 of the Introduction section.

As seen for the zero-order absorption process, the rate of change in the amount of drug in the body at any given time is a function of a "rate in" and a "rate out" (Equation 16.8). For a first-order absorption process, "rate in" is a function of the absorption rate constant ($k_a$) and the amount of drug in the GI tract ($D_{GI}$).

$$\frac{dD_B}{dt} = k_a D_{GI} - k_{10}D_B \qquad (16.12)$$

The amount of drug that leaves the GI tract (ie, the decrease in the amount of drug in the GI tract as it is absorbed into the bloodstream) can be described as follows:

$$\frac{dD_{GI}}{dt} = -k_a D_{GI} \qquad (16.13)$$

Integration of the differential equation gives:

$$D_{GI}(t) = D_{GI}^0 e^{-k_a t} \qquad (16.14)$$

where $D_{GI}^0$ is the initial amount of drug in the GI tract at time zero. The equation can also be rewritten in terms of dose and bioavailability.

$$D_{GI}(t) = D_0 \cdot F \cdot e^{-k_a t} \qquad (16.15)$$

The amount of drug that is initially found in the GI tract ($D_{GI}^0$) is essentially the amount of bioavailable drug, which can be represented as $D_0 {}^*F$, where $D_0$ is the oral dose of drug and $F$ is the bioavailability fraction. The value of $F$ may vary from 1 for a fully absorbed drug to 0 for a drug that is completely unabsorbed.

Equations 16.12 to 16.15 can be used to derive an equation describing the drug concentration ($C$) in the plasma at any time $t$.

$$C(t) = \frac{k_a D_0 F}{V_c (k_a - k_{10})}(e^{-k_{10}t} - e^{-k_a t}) \quad (16.16)$$

The maximal or peak concentration ($C_{max}$, Equation 16.18), and time at which this concentration occurs ($t_{max}$, Equation 16.17) can be estimated from Equation 16.16.

$$t_{max} = \frac{2.303 \cdot \log\left(\frac{k_a}{k_{10}}\right)}{k_a - k_{10}} \text{ or } t_{max} = \frac{\ln\left(\frac{k_a}{k_{10}}\right)}{k_a - k_{10}} \quad (16.17)$$

$$C_{max} = \frac{D_0}{V_c / F} e^{-k_{10} \cdot t_{max}} \quad (16.18)$$

The clinical relevance of $C_{max}$ and $t_{max}$ is discussed later in the chapter.

## CLINICAL APPLICATION

Manini et al (2005) reported an adverse drug reaction in a previously healthy young man who ingested a recommended dose of an over-the-counter cold remedy containing pseudoephedrine hydrochloride. Forty-five minutes later, he had an acute myocardial infarction. Elevations of cardiac-specific creatinine kinase and cardiac troponin I confirmed the diagnosis. Cardiac magnetic resonance imaging (MRI) confirmed a regional myocardial infarction. Cardiac catheterization 8 hours later revealed normal coronary arteries, suggesting a mechanism of vasospasm.

1. Could rapid drug absorption (large $k_a$) contribute to high-peak drug concentration of pseudoephedrine in this subject?

2. What is the effect of a small change in $k_{el}$ on the time and magnitude of $C_{max}$ (maximum plasma concentration)?

3. Can an adverse drug reaction occur before absorption is complete or before $C_{max}$ is reached?

## Discussion

As seen in Equations 16.17 and 16.18, peak concentrations are influenced by both $k_a$ and $k_{el}$. Therefore, an increase in the absorption rate (ie, increase in $k_a$) or a decrease in drug elimination (ie, decrease in $k_{el}$) can contribute to an increase in $C_{max}$.

Generally, transient high plasma drug concentrations are not considered unsafe as long as the plasma concentration remains within the recommended therapeutic range. This case highlights a potential danger of some sympathomimetic drugs such as pseudoephedrine hydrochloride that are formulated in an IR drug product. This adverse reaction would not have occurred if the patient had taken an ER pseudoephedrine hydrochloride product, since the drug absorption rate is intentionally slowed.

Nicotinic acid is an over-the-counter drug product that is available in an ER dosage form (Niaspan). If nicotinic acid is absorbed too rapidly, the patient will have adverse reactions such as vasodilatation, flushing, and possible fainting (Figge et al, 1988).

Adverse events can occur at any moment following drug administration, and their timing does not necessarily always coincide with the occurrence of $C_{max}$. The occurrence of the adverse event depends upon the relationship between the adverse event and drug concentrations. Some adverse events are more closely related to the drug dose or the extent of exposure (AUC), while other adverse events may not be related to drug exposure. For example, emesis may occur immediately after dosing due to drug interaction in the GI tract.

## PRACTICE PROBLEM

Two formulations of the same drug have been developed by a manufacturer. Formulation A is associated with a first-order absorption rate constant of 1/hr while Formulation B is associated with a first-order absorption rate constant of 0.45/hr. The drug follows a one-compartment model and has a first-order elimination rate constant ($k_{el}$) of 0.3 $h^{-1}$ and an apparent volume of distribution ($V_c/F$) of 0.4 L. If the goal of drug therapy is to reach maximal concentrations as quickly as possible, which formulation is preferred for patients?

1. The first step is to calculate $t_{max}$ for each formulation using Equation 16.17.

**2.** The maximal concentration is reached after approximately 1.7 hours for Formulation A, and at around 2.7 hours for Formulation B.

**3.** With Formulation A, maximal concentrations are reached 1 hour sooner than Formulation B and would therefore be the preferred formulation to administer to patients.

### Equations for Two-Compartment Models

A two-compartment model (Chapter 13) can be appropriate if after drug absorption, the drug is distributed to a central compartment (systemic circulation and rapidly drug equilibrating tissues) and a peripheral tissue compartment (slowly drug equilibrating tissues). Figure 16-10 depicts a two-compartment model with first-order absorption and first-order elimination, where $V_c/F$ is the apparent central volume of distribution and $V_p/F$ is the apparent volume of the peripheral (tissue) compartment; $k_{12}$ and $k_{21}$ are first-order rate constants representing drug transfer into the peripheral (tissue) compartment from the central compartment or from the peripheral (tissue) compartment into the central compartment. The elimination rate constant, $k_{10}$, represents drug elimination from the central compartment.

Using the two-compartment model depicted in Fig. 16-10, the plasma drug concentration, $C$, in the central compartment (systemic circulation or blood) at a given time $t$ following a single dose administration at time $t = 0$ is described by Equation 16.19.

$$C(t) = D_0 F \left[ Ae^{-\alpha \cdot t} + Be^{-\beta \cdot t} - (A + B)e^{-k_a \cdot t} \right] \quad (16.19)$$

The variables $\alpha$, $\beta$, $A$ and $B$ are hybrid first-order rate constants (Chapter 13) that can be determined with the relationships defined in Equations 16.20 to 16.23.

$$\alpha = \frac{k_{21} \cdot k_{10}}{\beta} \quad (16.20)$$

$$\beta = \frac{1}{2} \left[ k_{12} + k_{21} + k_{10} - \sqrt{(k_{12} + k_{21} + k_{10})^2 - 4 \cdot k_{21} \cdot k_{10}} \right] \quad (16.21)$$

$$A = \frac{k_a}{V_c/F} \cdot \frac{k_{21} - \alpha}{(k_a - \alpha) \cdot (\beta - \alpha)} \quad (16.22)$$

$$B = \frac{k_a}{V_c/F} \cdot \frac{k_{21} - \beta}{(k_a - \beta) \cdot (\alpha - \beta)} \quad (16.23)$$

In order to obtain accurate estimates of these hybrid rate constants, the drug must be given by an IV bolus injection and then the plasma drug concentration–versus time curve must be characterized.

In cases where the initial drug distribution phase is rapid, drug distribution occurs during drug absorption and the plasma drug concentration–versus time curve resembles a one-compartment model. After an IV bolus dose, the distribution phase can be observed, but after an oral dose, the resulting plasma drug concentration–versus time curve resembles a one-compartment model. For these situations, a drug that follows a two-compartment model after IV bolus resembles a one-compartment model after an oral dose. The error in using a one-compartment analysis for this two-compartment drug is very small.

> ### FREQUENTLY ASKED QUESTION
>
> ▶ If the pharmacokinetics of a drug are well characterized with a first-order absorption rate constant and a one-compartment model, would a larger absorption rate constant result in a greater amount of drug absorbed?

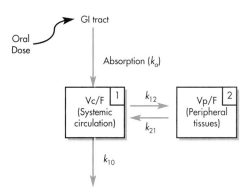

FIGURE 16-10 • Two-compartment, first-order oral absorption and first-order elimination model.

# METHODS FOR CALCULATING PHARMACOKINETIC PARAMETERS DESCRIBING DRUG ABSORPTION

Before the availability of computers, approaches including the method of residuals (also known as "curve stripping") and the Loo–Riegelman method were used to calculate absorption parameters. Although these methods are rarely used today, more details on the method of residuals and the Loo–Riegelman can be found in Appendices A and B, respectively, for the reader who is interested in these historical techniques. The only method for describing drug absorption that will be described here in more detail is the Wagner–Nelson method, as it has been found useful in developing in *in vitro*/*in vivo* correlations (IVIVC) (Chapter 7; FDA, 1997).

## Wagner–Nelson Method (One-Compartment Model)

The Wagner–Nelson method can be used to calculate $k_a$ for a drug exhibiting one-compartment kinetics with first-order absorption and elimination (Wagner and Nelson, 1963; Zhou 2003). This approach relies on characterizing absorption in terms of fraction of unabsorbed drug as a function of time.

This Wagner–Nelson method determines $k_a$ by calculating the fraction of unabsorbed drug with time, based only on plasma or serum drug concentration data. The amount of unabsorbed drug at any time is the amount of drug that remains in the gastrointestinal tract ($D_{GI}$), which is described as $D_{GI}(t) = D_0 e^{-k_a t}$ (Equation 16.14). When both sides of the equation are divided by dose ($D_0$), the fraction of unabsorbed drug can be calculated at any time using Equation 16.24:

$$\frac{D_{GI}(t)}{D_0} = e^{-k_a t} \qquad (16.24)$$

Log-transformation of both sides of Equation 16.24 gives Equation 16.25.

$$\mathrm{Log}\frac{D_{GI}(t)}{D_0} = \frac{-k_a t}{2.3} \qquad (16.25)$$

A plot of the amount drug unabsorbed versus time graphed on a semi-log scale (Fig. 16-11) yields a straight line with the slope $\frac{-k_a}{2.3}$.

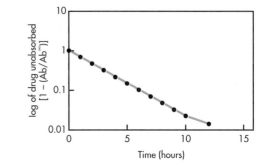

FIGURE 16-11 • Semi-log graph depicting the fraction of drug unabsorbed versus time using the Wagner–Nelson method.

The determination of the fraction of unabsorbed drug with respect to time provides an estimate for $k_a$ from the slope of the line. This method distinguishes between a first-order and a zero-order absorption process. If a linear graph is used, then the slope is the zero-order absorption process ($k_0$).

The fraction of unabsorbed drug ($\frac{D_{GI}}{D_0}$) is calculated indirectly by estimating the fraction of drug that is absorbed. The fraction of drug absorbed at any time is $\frac{Ab}{Ab^\infty}$, where $Ab$ is the amount of drug absorbed at any time $t$, and $Ab^\infty$ is the amount absorbed at $t = \infty$. The fraction of unabsorbed drug is therefore $1 - \frac{Ab}{Ab^\infty}$.

The amount of drug absorbed ($Ab$) is the sum of the amount of drug in the body ($D_b$) and the amount of drug excreted in the urine ($D_u$), as described in Equation 16.26.

$$Ab = D_b + D_u \qquad (16.26)$$

The amount of drug in the body ($D_b$) at any time is equal to $C_p V_c/F$, where $C_p$ is the plasma drug concentration and $V_c/F$ is the apparent volume of distribution. The amount of drug excreted in the urine at any time $t$ can be calculated as:

$$D_u(t) = k_{10} V_c/F [AUC]_0^t \qquad (16.27)$$

The amount of drug absorbed ($Ab$) at time $t$ can be represented by the following equation:

$$Ab(t) = C_p V_c/F + k_{10} V_c/F [AUC]_0^t \qquad (16.28)$$

At $t$ = infinity ($\infty$), $C_p$ = 0 (ie, plasma drug concentration is negligible), and the total amount of drug absorbed is defined by the second term in Equation 16.28 to yield Equation 16.29.

$$Ab^\infty = 0 + k_{10}V_c/F\,[AUC]_0^\infty \qquad (16.29)$$

Therefore, the fraction of drug absorbed at any given time can be obtained by dividing Equation 16.28 by Equation 16.29, to yield Equation 16.30 and its simplified version (Equation 16.31).

$$\frac{Ab}{Ab^\infty} = \frac{C_pV_c/F + k_{10}V_c/F[AUC]_0^t}{k_{10}V_c/F[AUC]_0^\infty} \qquad (16.30)$$

$$\frac{Ab}{Ab^\infty} = \frac{C_p + k_{10}[AUC]_0^t}{k_{10}[AUC]_0^\infty} \qquad (16.31)$$

The fraction unabsorbed at any time $t$ is given by Equation 16.32.

$$1 - \frac{Ab}{Ab^\infty} = 1 - \frac{C_p + k_{10}[AUC]_0^t}{k_{10}[AUC]_0^\infty} \qquad (16.32)$$

## PRACTICE PROBLEM

Calculate $k_a$ using the plasma drug concentration data time points in Table 16-1.

The steps are as follows, and the results are also shown in Table 16-1.

1. Calculate $k_{10}$ by plotting log concentrations of drug versus time. $K_{10}$ can be calculated from the slope of the terminal part (slope = $-k_{10}/2.3$).

## TABLE 16-1 • Data for Wagner–Nelson Method

| Time $t_n$ (h) | Concentration $C_p$ ($\mu$g/mL) | $[AUC]_{t_{n-1}}^{t_n}$ | $[AUC]_0^t$ | $k[AUC]_0^t$ | $C_p + k[AUC]_0^t$ | $\dfrac{Ab}{Ab^\infty}$ | $\left(1 - \dfrac{Ab}{Ab^\infty}\right)$ |
|---|---|---|---|---|---|---|---|
| 0 | 0 | 0 | 0 | | | | 1.000 |
| 1 | 3.13 | 1.57 | 1.57 | 0.157 | 3.287 | 0.328 | 0.672 |
| 2 | 4.93 | 4.03 | 5.60 | 0.560 | 5.490 | 0.548 | 0.452 |
| 3 | 5.86 | 5.40 | 10.99 | 1.099 | 6.959 | 0.695 | 0.305 |
| 4 | 6.25 | 6.06 | 17.05 | 1.705 | 7.955 | 0.794 | 0.205 |
| 5 | 6.28 | 6.26 | 23.31 | 2.331 | 8.610 | 0.856 | 0.140 |
| 6 | 6.11 | 6.20 | 29.51 | 2.951 | 9.061 | 0.905 | 0.095 |
| 7 | 5.81 | 5.96 | 35.47 | 3.547 | 9.357 | 0.934 | 0.066 |
| 8 | 5.45 | 5.63 | 41.10 | 4.110 | 9.560 | 0.955 | 0.045 |
| 9 | 5.06 | 5.26 | 46.35 | 4.635 | 9.695 | 0.968 | 0.032 |
| 10 | 4.66 | 4.86 | 51.21 | 5.121 | | | |
| 12 | 3.90 | 8.56 | 59.77 | 5.977 | | | |
| 14 | 3.24 | 7.14 | 66.91 | 6.691 | | | |
| 16 | 2.67 | 5.92 | 72.83 | 7.283 | | | |
| 18 | 2.19 | 4.86 | 77.69 | 7.769 | | | |
| 24 | 1.20 | 10.17 | 87.85 | 8.785 | | | |
| 28 | 0.81 | 4.02 | 91.87 | 9.187 | | | |
| 32 | 0.54 | 2.70 | 94.57 | 9.457 | | | |
| 36 | 0.36 | 1.80 | 96.37 | 9.637 | | | |
| 48 | 0.10 | 2.76 | 99.13 | 9.913 | | | |

A single drug dose is given orally. The plasma drug concentrations are measured at various times after the dose. $k = 0.1\ h^{-1}$ is obtained from the elimination portion of the curve.

2. Calculate $Ab$ $(C_p + k_{10}[\text{AUC}]_0^t)$ for each time point (see Chapter 2 for calculations of AUC from $t = n$ to $t = n + 1$).

   a. Calculate partial AUCs (column 3)

   b. Obtain $[\text{AUC}]_0^t$ at each time point (column 4)

   c. Multiply $[\text{AUC}]_0^t$ at each time point by $k$ (column 5)

   d. Add $Cp$ to $k_{10}[\text{AUC}]_0^t$ at each time point (column 6)

3. Calculate $Ab^\infty$ $(k_{10}[\text{AUC}]_0^\infty)$. $[\text{AUC}]_0^\infty$ can be calculated using the following formula: $[\text{AUC}]_0^\infty = [\text{AUC}]_0^t + \dfrac{C_t}{k_{10}}$, where $t$ is the time at the last measurable time point (Chapter 2) (ie, $[\text{AUC}]_0^\infty = 99.13 + 0.1/0.1 = 100.1 \ \mu g \cdot h/mL$).

4. Calculate $Ab/Ab^\infty$ at each time point (column 7).

5. Calculate $1 - Ab/Ab^\infty$ at each time point (column 8).

6. Plot the log of $(1 - Ab/Ab^\infty)$ versus time and find the slope to calculate $k_a$ (slope $= \dfrac{-k_a}{2.3}$). Use only the linear part of the plot to calculate the slope.

### FREQUENTLY ASKED QUESTIONS

▶ Can the Wagner–Nelson method be used to calculate $k_a$ for an orally administered drug that follows the pharmacokinetics of a two-compartment model?

▶ What is the absorption half-life of a drug and how is it determined?

▶ In switching a drug from IV to oral dosing, what is the most important consideration?

## Determination of Drug Absorption by Data Fitting

Various models and approaches have been used to predict drug absorption. Early approaches were developed by Wagner (1967) and Loo and Reigleman (1968). The availability of computer software (Chapter 20) has made deconvolution and convolution approaches popular to estimate drug absorption parameters. Compartmental model methods can also be used to estimate absorption parameters. These approaches are facilitated by the widespread availability of various software (Chapter 20). For example, if many plasma samples are collected in one individual following the intake of a single oral dose (as illustrated in Fig. 16-12), it would be possible to estimate pharmacokinetic parameters describing various processes, including drug absorption, distribution, and elimination.

The plasma drug concentration–time profile in Fig. 16-12 indicates that the pharmacokinetics of this drug can be characterized as a one-compartment model with first-order drug elimination (observed by the exponential decline in the semi-log scale). Therefore, it would be reasonable to first fit the data using a one-compartment model with parameters such as $k_a$, $V_c/F$, and $CL/F$. As described in Chapter 19, different methods could be used to obtain estimates for these parameters based on starting values provided by the user. Therefore, it would be possible to characterize the absorption process in this particular individual using such an approach.

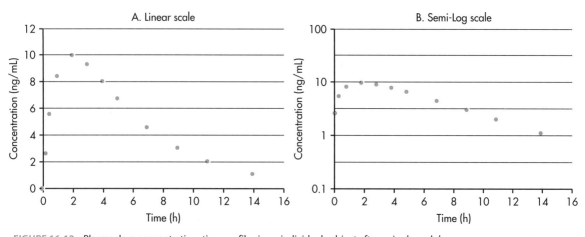

FIGURE 16-12 • Plasma drug concentration–time profiles in an individual subject after a single oral dose.

## RELATIONSHIP BETWEEN ABSORPTION RATE AND BIOAVAILABILITY PARAMETERS (AUC, $C_{max}$, $T_{max}$)

The rate of drug absorption and overall extent of drug exposure (measured by $C_{max}$ and AUC, respectively), are important parameters used to assess bioavailability and bioequivalence.

Equations 16.17 and 16.18 show how the absorption rate constant $(k_a)$ and the elimination rate constant $(k_{el})$ are related to the parameters $C_{max}$ and $t_{max}$. Table 16-2 illustrates changes in AUC, $C_{max}$, and $t_{max}$ as values for $k_a$ and $k_{el}$ are substituted into these equations.

If the values for $k_a$ and $k_{el}$ are reversed, then the same $t_{max}$ is obtained, but the $C_{max}$ and AUC are different. If the elimination rate constant is kept at 0.1 $h^{-1}$ and the $k_a$ changes from 0.2 to 0.6 $h^{-1}$ (absorption rate increases), then the $t_{max}$ becomes shorter (from 6.93 to 3.58 hours), the $C_{max}$ increases (from 5.00 to 6.99 $\mu$g/mL), but the AUC remains constant (100 $\mu$g h/mL). In contrast, when the absorption rate constant is kept at 0.3 $h^{-1}$ and $k_{el}$ changes from 0.1 to 0.5 $h^{-1}$ (elimination rate increases), then the $t_{max}$ decreases (from 5.49 to 2.55 hours), the $C_{max}$ decreases (from 5.77 to 2.79 $\mu$g/mL), and the AUC decreases (from

100 to 20 $\mu$g h/mL). Graphical representations of the effects of $k_a$ and $k_{el}$ on the time for peak absorption and the peak drug concentrations are shown in Fig. 16-13.

---

### FREQUENTLY ASKED QUESTION

▶ How does a larger absorption rate constant affect $C_{max}$, $t_{max}$, and AUC if the dose and elimination rate constant, $k_{el}$ remain constant?

---

### Flip-Flop Pharmacokinetics

The typical concentration–time profile for an orally administered drug illustrated in Fig. 16-3 is generally associated with IR drug products. For IR drug products, the absorption rate is generally faster than the elimination rate. The slower rate process is elimination. Once drug absorption is complete, the only remaining process is elimination, illustrated in the left panel of Fig. 16-14. The decrease in concentrations observed in the terminal phase of this concentration–time profile reflects the elimination of the drug, and this part of the profile is usually referred to as the *terminal elimination phase*.

Extended- or controlled-release drug products are designed to release drug slowly so that the

---

**TABLE 16-2 • Effects of the Absorption Rate Constant and Elimination Rate on $t_{max}$, $C_{max}$, and AUC**

| Absorption Rate Constant, $k_a$ ($h^{-1}$) | Elimination Rate Constant, $k_{el}$ ($h^{-1}$) | $t_{max}$ (h) | $C_{max}$ ($\mu$g/mL) | AUC ($\mu$g.h/mL) |
|---|---|---|---|---|
| 0.1 | 0.2 | 6.93 | 2.50 | 50 |
| 0.2 | 0.1 | 6.93 | 5.00 | 100 |
| 0.3 | 0.1 | 5.49 | 5.77 | 100 |
| 0.4 | 0.1 | 4.62 | 6.29 | 100 |
| 0.5 | 0.1 | 4.02 | 6.69 | 100 |
| 0.6 | 0.1 | 3.58 | 6.99 | 100 |
| 0.3 | 0.1 | 5.49 | 5.77 | 100 |
| 0.3 | 0.2 | 4.05 | 4.44 | 50 |
| 0.3 | 0.3 | 3.33 | 3.68 | 33.3 |
| 0.3 | 0.4 | 2.88 | 3.16 | 25 |
| 0.3 | 0.5 | 2.55 | 2.79 | 20 |

$t_{max}$ = peak plasma concentration, $C_{max}$ = peak drug concentration, AUC = area under the curve. Values are based on a single oral dose (100 mg) that is 100% bioavailable (F = 1) and has an apparent V of 10 L. The drug follows a one-compartment open model. $t_{max}$ is calculated by Equation 16.17 and $C_{max}$ is calculated by Equation 16.18. The AUC is calculated by the trapezoidal rule from 0 to 24 hours.

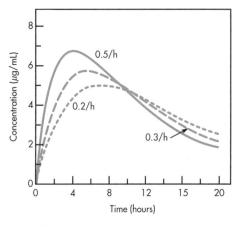 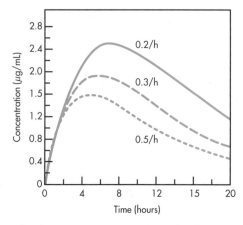

**FIGURE 16-13** • Effect of changes in the absorption rate constant, $k_a$ or the elimination rate constant, $k_{el}$, on the plasma drug concentration–time curve. *Left*: change in the absorption rate constant, $k_a$. Dose of drug is 100 mg, $V/F$ is 10 L, and $k_{el}$ is 0.1 h$^{-1}$. *Right*: change in the elimination rate constant. Dose of drug is 100 mg, $V/F$ is 10 L, and $k_a$ is 0.1 h$^{-1}$.

dissolution rate is the rate-limiting step and the rate of absorption is faster. The rate of absorption is slower than the rate of elimination. The right panel of Fig. 16-14 shows the shape of the concentration–time curve for an ER product that looks identical to its IR counterpart. However, an important difference is that the terminal portion of the ER concentration–time curve represents absorption rather than elimination. This is known as the *flip-flop* phenomenon.

In the case of flip-flop kinetics, the terminal phase parameter ($\lambda_z$) that is determined using standard noncompartmental methods actually represents absorption and not elimination. To determine the true elimination rate constant, data following intravenous administration of the drug must be obtained and the terminal elimination phase represents the true elimination rate constant.

Figure 16-15 illustrates the same profiles as in Fig. 16-14, but the concentration–time profiles of the drugs following IV administration have been superimposed to highlight differences.

As shown in Fig. 16-15 (left panel), for the IR drug where no flip-flop pharmacokinetics are present, the terminal phases of the concentration–time profiles are similar following both oral and IV administration. We can therefore state with confidence that the terminal phase following oral administration is truly representative of the elimination phase, as its slope is identical to the one seen after IV administration, which only reflects elimination. In contrast, the terminal slope of the ER drug following oral administration is very different from the slope that is observed following IV administration (Fig. 16-15, right panel). The decline in concentrations following

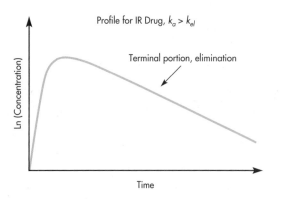 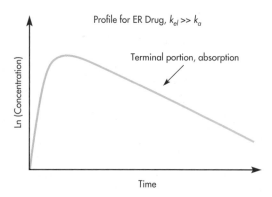

**FIGURE 16-14** • Semi-log concentration–time profiles of an IR and ER drug following oral administration.

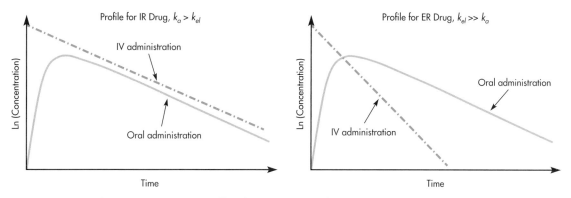

FIGURE 16-15 • Semi-log concentration–time profiles of an IR and ER drug following oral and intravenous administration.

IV administration is more rapid than the decline that is seen in the terminal phase of oral administration profile (ie, the slope is steeper following IV administration). This suggests that the slower decline observed in the terminal phase following oral administration is not related to elimination but rather to another process such as dissolution.

Most of the drugs observed to have flip-flop characteristics are drugs with fast elimination (ie, $k_{el} > k_a$). Drug absorption of most drug solutions or fast-dissolving products is essentially complete or at least half complete within an hour (ie, absorption half-life of 10 minutes, corresponding to a $k_a$ of 4.16 h$^{-1}$). Because most of the drugs used orally have longer elimination half-lives compared to absorption half-lives, the assumption that the smaller slope or smaller rate constant may be used as the elimination constant is generally correct.

For drugs that have a large elimination rate constant ($k_{el} > 0.69$ h$^{-1}$), the chance for flip-flop of $k_a$ and $k_{el}$ is much greater. The drug isoproterenol, for example, has an oral elimination half-life of only a few minutes, and flip-flop of $k_a$ and $k_{el}$ was noted early in time (Portmann, 1970). Similarly, the pharmacokinetics of salicyluric acid was flip-flopped when oral data were plotted. The $k_{el}$ for salicyluric acid was much larger than its $k_a$ (Levy et al, 1969). Many experimental drugs show flip-flop of $k_{el}$ and $k_a$, whereas few marketed oral drugs do. Drugs with a large $k_{el}$ are usually considered to be unsuitable for an oral drug product due to their large elimination rate constant, corresponding to a very short elimination half-life. In addition, as previously noted, an ER drug product may slow the absorption of a drug, such that the $k_a$ is smaller than the $k_{el}$ and thereby producing a flip-flop situation.

## CHAPTER SUMMARY

The pharmacokinetics of drug absorption can be characterized by a zero-order rate process, a first-order rate process, or a more complex process. As the drug is absorbed, the drug is also eliminated. For most drug products, the rate of drug absorption is faster than the rate of drug elimination. After drug absorption is complete, drug is generally eliminated by a first-order process. Absorption rate constants can be determined without computers using classical methods such as the method of residuals, Wagner–Nelson (one-compartment model), and Loo–Riegelman (two-compartment method).

Computers can also be used to characterize absorption, for example involving concentration–time data in a given patient that are fitted to compartmental equations. The choice of approach depends on the amount and quality of the available data, as well as the objective of the analysis. Changes in the absorption rate constant and the elimination rate constant can affect the $C_{max}$, $t_{max}$, and $AUC$. Proper characterization of the absorption processes can be used to develop multiple dosage regimens and IVIVC which allow the prediction of in vivo performance based on in vitro data.

## LEARNING QUESTIONS

1. Plasma samples from a patient were collected after an oral dose of 10 mg of a new benzodiazepine solution as follows:

| Time (hours) | Concentration (ng/mL) |
|---|---|
| 0.25 | 2.85 |
| 0.50 | 5.43 |
| 0.75 | 7.75 |
| 1.00 | 9.84 |
| 2.00 | 16.20 |
| 4.00 | 22.15 |
| 6.00 | 23.01 |
| 10.00 | 19.09 |
| 14.00 | 13.90 |
| 20.00 | 7.97 |

From the given data:

a. Determine the elimination rate constant of the drug and the elimination half-life.

b. Identify the maximal concentration and the time at which $C_{max}$ occurs.

2. For which types of pharmacokinetic models and routes of administration can the percentage of drug-unabsorbed method be used for the determination of absorption rate constant, $k_a$?

3. What are the main pharmacokinetic parameters that influence (a) time for peak drug concentration and (b) peak drug concentration?

4. Name a method of drug administration that will provide a zero-order input.

5. A single oral dose (100 mg) of an antibiotic was given to an adult male patient (43 years, 72 kg). From the literature, the pharmacokinetics of this drug fits a one-compartment open model and absolute bioavailability is 100%. The equation that best fits the pharmacokinetics of the drug is

$$C_p = 45(e^{-0.17t} - e^{-1.5t})$$

From the equation above, calculate (a) $t_{max}$, (b) $C_{max}$, and (c) $t_{1/2}$ for the drug in this patient. Assume $C_p$ is in $\mu g/mL$ and the first-order rate constants are in $h^{-1}$.

6. Two drugs, A and B, have the following pharmacokinetic parameters after a single oral dose of 500 mg:

| Drug | $k_a$ (h⁻¹) | $k_{el}$ (h⁻¹) | $V_c/F$(mL) |
|---|---|---|---|
| A | 1.0 | 0.2 | 10,000 |
| B | 0.2 | 1.0 | 20,000 |

Both drugs follow a one-compartment pharmacokinetic model and are 100% bioavailable.

a. Calculate the $t_{max}$ for each drug.

b. Calculate the $C_{max}$ for each drug.

7. The bioavailability of phenylpropanolamine hydrochloride was studied in 24 adult male subjects. The following data represent the mean blood phenylpropanolamine hydrochloride concentrations (ng/mL) after the oral administration of a single 25-mg dose of phenylpropanolamine hydrochloride solution:

| Time (hours) | Concentration (ng/mL) | Time (hours) | Concentration (ng/mL) |
|---|---|---|---|
| 0 | 0 | 3 | 62.98 |
| 0.25 | 51.33 | 4 | 52.32 |
| 0.5 | 74.05 | 6 | 36.08 |
| 0.75 | 82.91 | 8 | 24.88 |
| 1.0 | 85.11 | 12 | 11.83 |
| 1.5 | 81.76 | 18 | 3.88 |
| 2 | 75.51 | 24 | 1.27 |

a. From the above data, obtain the rate constant for absorption, $k_a$, and the rate constant for elimination, $k_{el}$, by the method of residuals.

b. Is it reasonable to assume that $k_a > k$ for a drug in a solution? How would you determine unequivocally which rate constant represents the elimination constant $k_{el}$?

c. From the data, which method, Wagner–Nelson or Loo–Riegelman, would be more appropriate to determine the order of the rate constant for absorption?

d. From your values, calculate the theoretical $t_{max}$. How does your value relate to the observed $t_{max}$ obtained from the subjects?

e. Would you consider the pharmacokinetics of phenylpropanolamine HCl to follow a one-compartment model? Why?

## ANSWERS

### Frequently Asked Questions

*Is systemic drug absorption the same as drug bioavailability?*

• Systemic drug absorption and drug bioavailability are not the same thing. The bioavailability of a drug reflects the amount of drug that reaches systemic circulation and is therefore available to exert its effect on target organs or tissues. While the absorption of the drug contributes to bioavailability, it is not the only factor that dictates bioavailability. Drugs that are well absorbed may not necessarily be associated with high bioavailability if pre-systemic metabolism transforms the products into metabolites before systemic circulation is attained.

*What is the difference in the overall absorption process between an oral solution, an immediate release tablet formulation, and an extended-release formulation of the same drug?*

• A drug that is in an immediate-release tablet formulation or extended-release formulation must first be dissolved into solution before it can be absorbed. This dissolution step is not required for a solution, therefore the absorption of a solution formulation is expected to start before the absorption of an immediate-release tablet formulation or extended-release formulation. The start of absorption, which would be signaled by the first detectable plasma or serum concentration, is therefore likely to be delayed for an immediate-release or extended-release formulation in comparison with a solution formulation. The absorption process of the immediate-release formulation is likely to be described by a first-order rate, while the absorption process of the extended-release formulation is more likely to be characterized by a zero-order rate.

*If the pharmacokinetics of a drug are well characterized with a first-order absorption rate constant and a one-compartment model, would a larger absorption rate constant result in a greater amount of drug absorbed?*

• The fraction of drug absorbed, $F$, and the absorption rate constant, $k_a$, are independent parameters. While both parameters are influenced by factors such as drug formulation, there is no direct link between the parameters. For example, a drug with a high $F$ can be associated with a slow or fast absorption rate constant. Similarly, a higher $k_a$ does not necessarily mean that more drug will be absorbed.

*Can the Wagner–Nelson method be used to calculate $k_a$ for an orally administered drug that follows the pharmacokinetics of a two-compartment model?*

• For a drug whose pharmacokinetics is described by a two-compartment model, the Loo–Riegelman method should generally be used rather than the Wagner–Nelson method. However, for drugs that are described by two-compartment models with a fast alpha (distribution) phase, the pharmacokinetic profile may resemble a one-compartment model. In such models, the distribution phase is masked by the absorption phase, and the Wagner–Nelson method for one-compartment drugs could still be used.

*What is the absorption half-life of a drug and how is it determined?*

• For drugs absorbed by a first-order process, the absorption half-life is $0.693/k_a$. The absorption half-life can give an indication of the time that is necessary for the absorption process to be completed. Absorption is generally considered to be complete after five to seven absorption half-lives.

*In switching a drug from IV to oral dosing, what is the most important consideration?*

• The fraction of drug absorbed may be less than 1 (ie, 100% bioavailable) after oral administration. In some cases, there may be a different salt form of the drug used for IV infusion compared to the salt form of the drug used orally. Therefore, a correction may be needed for the difference in molecular weight of the two salt forms as well as the fraction of drug absorbed. Furthermore, absorption processes that are not relevant to IV dosing must be taken into consideration following oral dosing. For instance, peak concentrations following oral dosing are attained later compared to an IV bolus.

Does a larger absorption rate constant affect $C_{max}$, $t_{max}$, and AUC if the dose and elimination rate constant, $k_{el}$, remains constant?

• The only parameters that are influenced by the absorption constant are $C_{max}$ and $t_{max}$. AUC is only influenced by dose, $F$, and $k_{el}$ or apparent clearance.

## Learning Questions

1. **a.** A semi-log figure of the data suggests that the last three data points (after 6 hours post-dose) would be suitable to use for the calculation of the elimination rate constant. The slope of the ln-transformed concentration data as a function of time is $-0.0878$ h$^{-1}$. This corresponds to an elimination rate constant of 0.0878 h$^{-1}$ ($t_{1/2} = 7.90$ h).

   **b.** By direct observation of the data, the $C_{max}$ is 23.01 ng/mL and it occurs at 6 hours post-dose.

2. The percent of drug-unabsorbed method is applicable to any model with first-order elimination, regardless of the process of drug input. If the drug is given by IV injection, the elimination rate constant, $k_{el}$, may be determined accurately. If the drug is administered orally, $k_{el}$ and $k_a$ may "flip-flop," resulting in an error unless IV data are available to determine $k_{el}$. For a drug that follows a two-compartment model, an IV bolus injection may be used to determine the rate constants for distribution and elimination.

3. The equations for a drug that follows the kinetics of a one-compartment model with first-order absorption and elimination are:

$$t_{max} = \frac{2.303 \cdot \log\left(\dfrac{k_a}{k_{el}}\right)}{k_a - k_{el}} \qquad C_{max} = \frac{FD_0 F}{V_c} e^{-k_{el} \cdot t_{max}}$$

As shown by these equations:

**a.** $t_{max}$ is influenced by $k_a$ and $k_{el}$ and not by $F$, $D_0$, or $V_c/F$.

**b.** $C_{max}$ is influenced by $F$, $D_0$, $V_c/F$, as well as the parameters that influenced $t_{max}$ ($k_a$ and $k_{el}$).

4. A drug product that might provide a zero-order input is an oral controlled-release tablet or a transdermal drug delivery system (patch). An IV drug infusion will also provide a zero-order drug input.

5. The general equation for a one-compartment open model with oral absorption is

$$C(t) = \frac{FD_0 Fk_a}{V_c(k_a - k_{10})} \left(e^{-k_{10}t} - e^{-k_a t}\right)$$

$$C(t) = 45\left(e^{-0.17t} - e^{-1.5t}\right)$$

$$\frac{FD_0 Fk_a}{V_c(k_a - k_{10})} = 45$$

$$k_{10} = 0.17 \text{ h}^{-1}$$

$$k_a = 1.5 \text{ h}^{-1}$$

**a.** $t_{max} = \dfrac{\ln(k_a/k_{10})}{k_a - k_{10}} = \dfrac{\ln(1.5/0.17)}{1.5 - 0.17} = 1.64$ h

**b.** $C_{max} = 45\left(e^{-(0.17)(1.64)} - e^{-(1.5)(1.64)}\right)$
$= 30.2 \ \mu g/mL$

**c.** $t_{1/2} = \dfrac{0.693}{k_{10}} = \dfrac{0.693}{0.17} = 4.08$ h

6. **a.** Drug A $t_{max} = \dfrac{\ln(1.0/0.2)}{1.0 - 1.2} = 2.01$ h

   Drug B $t_{max} = \dfrac{\ln(0.2/1.0)}{0.2 - 1.0} = 2.01$ h

   **b.** $C_{max} = \dfrac{FD_0 k_a}{V_c/F(k_a - k_{10})}\left(e^{-k_{10}t_{max}} - e^{-k_a t_{max}}\right)$

   Drug A $C_{max} = \dfrac{(1)\cdot(500)\cdot(1)}{10000\cdot(1.0 - 0.2)}\cdot\left(e^{-0.2 \cdot 2.01} - e^{-1 \cdot 2.01}\right)$

   $C_{max} = 0.0334$ mg/mL $= 33.4$ ug/mL

   Drug B $C_{max} = \dfrac{(1)\cdot(500)\cdot(0.2)}{20000\cdot(0.2 - 1)}\cdot\left(e^{-1 \cdot 2.01} - e^{-0.2 \cdot 2.01}\right)$

   $C_{max} = 0.00334$ mg/mL $= 3.34$ ug/mL

**7. a.** Values obtained using Microsoft Excel gave the following estimates:

$$k_a = 2.84 \text{ h}^{-1} \quad k_{10} = 0.186 \text{ h}^{-1} \quad t_{1/2} = 3.73 \text{ h}$$

**b.** A drug in an aqueous solution is in the most absorbable form compared to other oral dosage forms. The assumption that $k_a > k_{10}$ is generally true for drug solutions and immediate-release oral dosage forms such as compressed tablets and capsules. Drug absorption from extended-release dosage forms may have $k_a < k_{10}$. To demonstrate unequivocally which slope represents the true $k_{10}$, the drug must be given by IV bolus or IV infusion, and the slope of the elimination portion of the curve can be obtained from this data.

**c.** The Loo–Riegelman method requires IV data. Therefore, only the Wagner–Nelson method may be used on these data.

**d.** Observed $t_{max}$ and $C_{max}$ values are taken directly from the experimental data. In this example, $C_{max}$ is 85.11 ng/mL, which occurred at a $t_{max}$ of 1 hour. The theoretical $t_{max}$ and $C_{max}$ are obtained as follows (using equations for the one-compartment model):

$$t_{max} = \frac{2.3 \log(k_a/k_{10})}{k_a - k_{10}}$$

$$= \frac{2.3 \log(2.84/0.186)}{2.84 - 0.186} = 1.03 \text{ h}$$

$$C_{max} = \frac{FD_0 k_a}{V_c(k_a - k_{10})} (e^{-k_{10}t_{max}} - e^{-k_a t_{max}})$$

where $FD_0 k_a/V_c (k_a - k_{10})$ is the $y$ intercept equal to 110 ng/mL and $t_{max} = 1.03$ h.

$$C_{max} = (110)(e^{-(1.186)(1.0)} - e^{-(2.84)(1.03)})$$

$$C_{max} = 85 \text{ ng/mL}$$

**e.** When the data is plotted on a semi-log scale, concentrations appear to decline in a monoexponential manner following the attainment of $C_{max}$. Therefore, the pharmacokinetics of phenylpropanolamine HCl can likely be described by a one-compartment model. This could be confirmed by fitting the data using a program such as NONMEM˚ or ADAPT˚.

## REFERENCES

Auclair B, Sirois G, Ngoc AH, Ducharme MP: Novel pharmacokinetic modelling of transdermal nitroglycerin. *Pharm Res* 15(4):614–619, 1998a.

Auclair B, Sirois G, Ngoc AH, Ducharme MP: Population pharmacokinetics of nitroglycerin and of its two metabolites after a single 24-hour application of a nitroglycerin transdermal matrix delivery system. *Ther Drug Monit* 20(6):607–611, 1998b.

Bates TR, Carrigan PJ: Apparent absorption kinetics of micronized griseofulvin after its oral administration on single- and multiple-dose regimens to rats as a corn oil-in-water emulsion and aqueous suspension. *J Pharm Sci* 64(9):1475–1481, 1975.

Cooke AR: The simultaneous emptying and absorption of ethanol from the human stomach. *Am J Dig Dis* 15:449–454, 1970.

Colburn WA, Di Santo AR, Gibaldi M: Pharmacokinetics of erythromycin on repetitive dosing. *J Clin Pharmacol* 17(10 Pt 1):592–600, 1977.

DiMarco MP, Chen J, Wainer IW, Ducharme MP: A population pharmacokinetic-metabolism model for individualizing ciprofloxacin therapy in ophthalmology. *Ther Drug Monit* 26(4):401–407, 2004.

FDA, Center for Drug Evaluation and Research. Guidance for Industry: Extended Release Oral Dosage Forms: Development, Evaluation, and Application of In Vitro/In Vivo Correlations. September 1997.

Figge HL, Figge V, Souney PF, Sacks FM, Shargel L, Kaul AF: Comparison of excretion of nicotinuric acid after ingestion of two controlled release nicotinic acid preparations in man. *J Clin Pharmacol* 28:1136–1140, 1988.

Jackson AJ: A Semi-physiologically based model for methylphenidate pharmacokinetics in adult humans. *J Bioequiv Bioavail* 11(2):390, 2019.

Loo JCK, Riegelman S: New method for calculating the intrinsic absorption rate of drugs. *J Pharm Sci* 57:918–928, 1968.

Levy G, Amsel LP, Elliot HC: Kinetics of salicyluric acid elimination in man. *J Pharm Sci* 58:827–829, 1969.

Magnusson MO, Samtani MN, Plan EL, Jonsson EN, Rossenu S, Vermeulen A, et al. Population pharmacokinetics of a novel once-every 3 months intramuscular formulation of paliperidone palmitate in patients with schizophrenia. *Clin Pharmacokinet* 56(4):421–433, 2017.

Manini AF, Kabrhel C, Thomsen TW: Acute myocardial infarction after over-the-counter use of pseudoephedrine. *Ann Emerg Med* 45(2):213–216, 2005.

Portmann G: Pharmacokinetics. In Swarbrick J (ed). *Current Concepts in the Pharmaceutical Sciences*, vol 1. Philadelphia, Lea & Febiger, 1970, Chap 1.

Teuscher NS, Adjei A, Findling RL, Greenhill LL, Kupper RJ, Wigal S: Population Pharmacokinetics of methylphenidate hydrochloride extended-release multiple-layer beads in pediatric subjects with attention deficit hyperactivity disorder. *Drug Des Devel Ther* **9**:2767–2775, 2015.

Wagner JG: Use of computers in pharmacokinetics. *Clin Pharmacol Ther* **8**:201–218, 1967.

Wagner JG, Nelson E: Percent absorbed time plots derived from blood level and/or urinary excretion data. *J Pharm Sci* **52**:610–611, 1963.

Zhou H: Pharmacokinetic strategies in deciphering atypical drug absorption profiles. *J Clin Pharmacol* **43**:211–227, 2003.

## BIBLIOGRAPHY

Boxenbaum HG, Kaplan SA: Potential source of error in absorption rate calculations. *J Pharmacokinet Biopharm* **3**:257–264, 1975.

Boyes R, Adams H, Duce B: Oral absorption and disposition kinetics of lidocaine hydrochloride in dogs. *J Pharmacol Exp Ther* **174**:1–8, 1970.

Dvorchik BH, Vessel ES: Significance of error associated with use of the one-compartment formula to calculate clearance of 38 drugs. *Clin Pharmacol Ther* **23**:617–623, 1978.

Veng-Pedersen P, Gobburu JVS, Meyer MC, Straughn AB: Carbamazepine level-A in vivo–in vitro correlation (IVIVC): A scaled convolution based predictive approach. *Biopharm Drug Dispos* **21**:1–6, 2000.

Wagner JG, Nelson E: Kinetic analysis of blood levels and urinary excretion in the absorptive phase after single doses of drug. *J Pharm Sci* **53**:1392, 1964.

## APPENDIX A

### Method of Residuals

The method of residuals is rarely used nowadays given the availability of computers. It allows the scientist to determine the absorption rate constant $k_a$ using semi-log graphs and a technique also known as "curve stripping." This method relies on the determination of the elimination rate constant ($k_{10}$), which is conducted in the same manner as described in Chapter 12. An example of this approach for a drug whose pharmacokinetics is described by a one-compartment model (with no lag time associated with a first-order absorption rate) is described herein.

Equation 16.16 describes systemic drug concentration as a function of time for a one-compartment model which includes one exponential term for the first-order absorption ($e^{-k_a t}$) and one for the first-order elimination ($e^{-k_{10} t}$). When absorption is almost complete, $t$ becomes bigger and the term $e^{-k_a t}$ approaches zero. Equation 16.16 can be reduced to Equation A.1:

$$C_p(t) = \frac{F k_a D_0}{V_c (k_a - k_{10})} e^{-k_{10} t} \qquad (A.1)$$

The log transformation of both sides of Equation A.1 yields Equation A.2:

$$\text{Log}(C_p(t)) = \text{Log}\left(\frac{F k_a D_0}{V_c (k_a - k_{10})}\right) - \frac{k_{10} t}{2.303} \qquad (A.2)$$

where $-\dfrac{k_{10}}{2.303}$ is a slope and the first term is an intercept. This relationship is illustrated in Fig. A-1, which represents a plot of the plasma drug concentration versus time with the $y$-axis (plasma concentration) on the logarithm scale.

As seen in Fig. A-1, the post-absorptive phase (after 5 hours post-dose) is a straight line. The slope of this line is equal to $-\dfrac{k_{10}}{2.303}$ while the intercept is a constant that depends on dose, relative bioavailability, and both $k_a$ and $k_{10}$.

It should be noted that performing a natural-log transformation of Equation A.1 would yield an equation that is similar to Equation A.2, but the slope of the terminal phase of the concentration–time profile

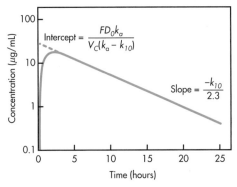

**FIGURE A-1** •Plasma drug concentration versus time, single oral dose.

## TABLE A-1 • Determination of Residual Concentrations

| Time (hours) | Observed Concentration (ug/mL) | Extrapolated Concentration (ug/mL) | Residual Concentration (ug/mL) |
|---|---|---|---|
| 0.5 | 9.1 | 97.7 | 88.6 |
| 1 | 16.4 | 92.9 | 76.5 |
| 2 | 27.0 | 83.9 | 56.9 |
| 4 | 36.9 | 68.5 | 31.6 |
| 8 | 35.9 | 45.7 | 9.8 |
| 12 | 27.4 | 30.5 | 3.1 |
| 18 | 16.1 | 16.6 | 0.5 |
| 24 | 9.0 | | |
| 36 | 2.7 | | |
| 48 | 0.8 | | |
| 72 | 0.07 | | |

would correspond directly to $-k_{10}$ rather than $-\dfrac{k_{10}}{2.303}$. This is shown in Equation A.3.

$$Ln(C(t)) = Ln\left(\frac{Fk_a D_0}{V_c(k_a - k_{10})}\right) - k_{10}t \qquad \text{(A.3)}$$

Therefore, assuming that the terminal portion of the concentration–time curve represents mainly elimination, as absorption is complete at this stage, the slope of the ln-transformed concentrations versus time can be used to determine the elimination rate constant ($k_{10}$). Extrapolating the line to time zero yields the y-intercept, which is $\log\left(\dfrac{Fk_a D_0}{V_c(k_a - k_{10})}\right)$.

The linear relationship described in Equations A.2 and A.3 is critical to applying the "method of residuals" (introduced in Chapter 5 for a two-compartment IV bolus model) which can then be used to quantify $k_a$.

A step-by-step explanation of how to apply the method of residuals to estimate $k_a$ for a one-compartment model, assuming $k_a \gg k_{10}$, is described in more detail below. Data from Table A-1 are used as an example and the approach is also illustrated in Fig. A-2. Each of the steps described below can be done manually or with the help of a computer program such as Microsoft Excel.

1. Create a plot of the observed concentrations as a function of time (solid blue line in Fig. A-2), on a semi-log scale (ie, where y-axis is on a log or natural log scale).

2. Using plot created in Step 1, identify data points that are in the post-absorptive phase, as those occurring shortly after $t_{max}$ may still reflect drug absorption.

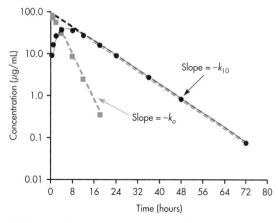

FIGURE A-2 • Illustration of method of residuals to determine $k_a$.

3. Create a regression line with the log-transformed or ln-transformed concentrations identified in Step 2 (in this example, concentrations at 24, 36, 48, and 72 hours) as a function of time. A minimum of three data points should be used. The slope of the regression reflecting drug elimination is equal to $-k_{10}$ (or $-k_{10}/2.3$ if concentration data was log-transformed instead of naturally-log transformed).

4. Using the regression equation (ie, slope), estimate the $y$-intercept (manually or using built-in computer functions).

5. Use the regression equation to calculate extrapolated concentrations for the time points that were not included in the determination of the equation. Extrapolated concentrations are presented in Table A-1, and the regression line (including extrapolated time points) is represented by the dashed black line in Fig. A-2.

6. Calculate the "residual concentration" for each time point by subtracting the observed value (solid blue line) from the extrapolated value (dashed black line). Plot the residual concentrations as a function of time with concentrations on a semi-log scale.

7. The equation for the residual values (dashed blue line) can be described by subtracting Equation 16.11 (representing the equation that describes drug concentration in plasma at any time $t$) from Equation A.1 (representing the equation that describes drug concentration in plasma when absorption is almost complete), which gives:

$$C_p(t) = \frac{Fk_a D_0}{V_c(k_a - k_{10})} e^{-k_a t} \quad (A.4)$$

The log transformation of both sides of Equation A.4 yields Equation A.5:

$$Log(C(t)) = Log\left(\frac{Fk_a D_0}{V_c(k_a - k_{10})}\right) - \frac{k_a t}{2.303} \quad (A.5)$$

8. As can be seen from Equation A.5, the linear regression that relates the log-transformed residual concentrations to time has the same $y$-intercept as the regression line associated with elimination. The slope of Equation A.5 (dashed blue line in Figure A-2) is equal to $-k_a/2.3$ (or $-k_a$ if concentration data was naturally-log transformed).

Thus, using the method of residuals, it is possible to calculate the parameter $k_a$ by determining the slope of a regression line that includes residual concentrations.

## Method of Residuals in the Presence of a Lag Time

The method of residuals can also be applied to drugs that are associated with a delay (lag time) prior to the start of absorption. A lag time can occur when there is a delay in gastric emptying or with enteric-coated rug products. The lag time must be taken into consideration in the calculations, by subtracting the lag time from each time point as described in Equation A.6.

$$C(t) = \frac{Fk_a D_0}{V_c(k_a - k_{10})} [e^{-k_{10}(t - t_{lag})} - e^{-k_a(t - t_{lag})}] \quad (A.6)$$

Once this adjustment has been made, the other steps described in the preceding section can be applied to determine $k_a$.

## APPENDIX B

### Loo–Riegelman Method (Two-Compartment Model)

When the concentration–time curve suggests multi-exponential decay of a drug, the Loo–Riegelman method can be used instead. This method also relies on the determination of the portion of unabsorbed drug, and requires data following IV administration (in addition to oral data).

First it is necessary to determine the amount of drug that is absorbed. Equation 16.28 for the amount of drug absorbed ($Ab$) is modified as follows, such that the amount of drug in the body ($D_b$) is partitioned into an amount that is found in systemic circulation or central compartment ($D_c$) and an amount that is in tissue ($D_t$):

$$Ab = D_c + D_t + D_u \quad (B.1)$$

In Equation B.1, $D_c$ is the amount of drug in the central (plasma) compartment, $D_t$ is the amount of drug in the tissue compartment, and $D_u$ is the amount of drug excreted in urine. Based on Equation 16.30, the amount of absorbed drug can be rewritten as follows (where $C_p$ represents drug concentration in the central compartment):

$$Ab = C_p V_c / F + D_t + k_{10} V_c / F [AUC]_0^t \quad (B.2)$$

Using Equation 16.31 and Equation B.2, the fraction of absorbed drug can be expressed by Equation B.3.

$$\frac{Ab}{Ab^\infty} = \frac{C_p V_c / F + D_t + k_{10} V_c / F [AUC]_0^t}{k_{10} V_c / F [AUC]_0^\infty} \quad (B.3)$$

If the right-hand side of Equation B.3 is simplified by dividing all terms by a volume of distribution, the equation can be re-written as follows:

$$\frac{Ab}{Ab^\infty} = \frac{C_p + \left(\dfrac{D_t}{V_p}\right) + k_{10}[AUC]_0^t}{k_{10}[AUC]_0^\infty} \quad (B.4)$$

The second term in the numerator on the right side of the equation represents tissue concentration $(\frac{D_t}{V_p})$, which can be estimated using the Loo–Riegelman method as follows:

$$(C_t)_{t_n} = \frac{k_{12} \Delta C_p \Delta t}{2} + \frac{k_{12}}{k_{21}} (C_p)_{t_{n-1}} (1 - e^{-k_{21}\Delta t}) + (C_t)_{t_{n-1}} e^{-k_{21}\Delta t}$$

$$(B.5)$$

Where $C_t$ is $\frac{D_t}{V_p}$, or apparent tissue concentration, $t$ = time of sampling for sample $n$, $t_{n-1}$ = time of sampling for the sampling point preceding sample $n$, and $(C_t)t_{n-1}$ = concentration of drug at central compartment for sample $n - 1$. The rate constants $k_{12}$ and $k_{21}$ can be calculated from the IV data, using the method of residuals that is described in Chapter 13.

Finally, a plot of the fraction of drug unabsorbed $(1 - \frac{Ab}{Ab^\infty})$ versus time (with the y-axis on a natural log-transformed scale) gives $-k_a$ in the linear portion as the slope from which the value for $k_a$ is obtained.

# 17 Multiple-Dosage Regimens

Rodney C. Siwale and Shabnam N. Sani

## CHAPTER OBJECTIVES

- Define the index for measuring drug accumulation.

- Define drug accumulation and drug accumulation $t_{1/2}$.

- Explain the principle of superposition and its assumptions in multiple-dose regimens.

- Calculate the steady-state $C_{max}$ and $C_{min}$ after multiple IV bolus dosing of drugs.

- Calculate $k$ and $V_D$ of aminoglycosides in multiple-dose regimens.

- Adjust the steady-state $C_{max}$ and $C_{min}$ in the event the last dose is given too early, too late, or totally missed following multiple IV dosing.

Earlier chapters of this book discussed single-dose drug and constant-rate drug administration. By far though, most drugs are given in several doses, for example, multiple doses to treat chronic disease such as arthritis, hypertension, etc. After single-dose drug administration, the plasma drug level rises above and then falls below the *minimum effective concentration* (MEC), resulting in a decline in therapeutic effect. To treat chronic disease, multiple-dosage or IV infusion regimens are used to maintain the plasma drug levels within the narrow limits of the therapeutic window (eg, plasma drug concentrations above the MEC but below the *minimum toxic concentration* or MTC) to achieve optimal clinical effectiveness. These drugs may include antibacterials, cardiotonics, anticonvulsants, hypoglycemics, antihypertensives, hormones, and others. Ideally, a dosage regimen is established for each drug to provide the appropriate plasma level without excessive fluctuation and drug accumulation outside the desired therapeutic window.

For certain drugs, such as antibiotics, a desirable MEC can be determined. For drugs that have a narrow therapeutic range (eg, digoxin and phenytoin), there is a need to define the therapeutic minimum and maximum nontoxic plasma concentrations (MEC and MTC, respectively). In calculating a multiple-dose regimen, the desired or *target* plasma drug concentration must be related to a therapeutic response, and the multiple-dose regimen must be designed to produce plasma concentrations within the therapeutic window.

There are two main parameters that can be adjusted in developing a dosage regimen: (1) the size of the drug dose and (2) $\tau$, the frequency of drug administration (ie, the time interval between doses).

## DRUG ACCUMULATION

To calculate a multiple-dose regimen for a patient or patients, pharmacokinetic parameters are first obtained from the plasma level–time curve generated by single-dose drug studies. With these pharmacokinetic parameters and knowledge of the size of the dose and dosage interval ($\tau$), the complete plasma level–time curve or the plasma level may be predicted at any time and any number of doses after the beginning of the dosage regimen. For simplicity, this chapter assumes a one-compartment model and linear pharmacokinetics. For a multicompartmental drug, pharmacokinetic parameters are calculated simply using a pharmacokinetic model and software to predict the drug concentrations.

For calculation of multiple-dose regimens, it is necessary to determine whether successive doses of drug will have any effect on the previous dose. The principle of *superposition* assumes linear pharmacokinetics in which early doses of drug behave independently and do not affect the pharmacokinetics of subsequent doses. Therefore, the systemic profiles after the second, third, or $n$th dose will overlay or superimpose the systemic level attained after the $(n-1)$th dose. In addition, the $\mathrm{AUC} = (\int_0^\infty C_p\, dt)$ for the first dose is equal to the steady-state area between doses, that is, $(\int_{t_1}^{t_2} C_p\, dt)$ as shown in Fig. 17-1.

The principle of *superposition* empowers the pharmacokineticist to project the plasma drug concentration–time curve of a drug after multiple consecutive doses based on the plasma drug concentration–time curve obtained after a single dose.

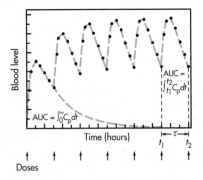

The basic assumptions are (1) a one-compartment model, (2) that the drug is eliminated by first-order kinetics, and (3) that the pharmacokinetics of the drug after a single dose (first dose) are not altered after taking multiple doses, hence that the PK is linear as it regards to dose and time.

The plasma drug concentrations after multiple doses may be predicted from the plasma drug concentrations obtained after a single dose. In Table 17-1, the plasma drug concentrations from 0 to 24 hours are measured after a single dose. A constant dose of drug is given every 4 hours and plasma drug concentrations after each dose are generated using the data after the first dose. Thus, the *predicted* plasma drug concentration in the patient is the total drug concentration obtained by adding the residual drug concentration obtained from each previous dose. The superposition principle may be used to predict drug concentrations after multiple doses of many drugs. Because the superposition principle is an overlay method, it may be used to predict drug concentrations after multiple doses given at either *equal* or *unequal* dosage intervals. For example, the plasma drug concentrations may be predicted after a drug dose is given every 8 hours, or 3 times a day before meals at 8 AM, 12 noon, and 6 PM.

There are situations, however, in which the superposition principle does not apply. In these cases, the pharmacokinetics of the drug change after multiple dosing due to various factors, including changing pathophysiology in the patient, saturation of a drug carrier system, enzyme induction, and enzyme inhibition. Drugs that follow nonlinear pharmacokinetics (see Chapter 18) will not have predictable plasma drug concentrations after multiple doses using the superposition principle.

If the drug is administered at a fixed dose and a fixed dosage interval, as is the common case with many multiple-dose regimens, the amount of drug in the body will increase and then plateau to a mean plasma level higher than the peak $C_p$ obtained from the initial dose (Figs. 17-1 and 17-2). When the second dose is given after a time interval shorter than the time required to "completely" eliminate the previous dose, *drug accumulation* will occur in the body. In other words, the plasma concentrations following the second dose will be higher than corresponding

**TABLE 17-1 •** Predicted Plasma Drug Concentrations for Multiple-Dose Regimen Using the Superposition Principle*

| Dose Number | Time (h) | Plasma Drug Concentration (µg/mL) | | | | | | Total |
|---|---|---|---|---|---|---|---|---|
| | | Dose 1 | Dose 2 | Dose 3 | Dose 4 | Dose 5 | Dose 6 | |
| 1 | 0 | 0 | | | | | | 0 |
| | 1 | 21.0 | | | | | | 21.0 |
| | 2 | 22.3 | | | | | | 22.3 |
| | 3 | 19.8 | | | | | | 19.8 |
| 2 | 4 | 16.9 | 0 | | | | | 16.9 |
| | 5 | 14.3 | 21.0 | | | | | 35.3 |
| | 6 | 12.0 | 22.3 | | | | | 34.3 |
| | 7 | 10.1 | 19.8 | | | | | 29.9 |
| 3 | 8 | 8.50 | 16.9 | 0 | | | | 25.4 |
| | 9 | 7.15 | 14.3 | 21.0 | | | | 42.5 |
| | 10 | 6.01 | 12.0 | 22.3 | | | | 40.3 |
| | 11 | 5.06 | 10.1 | 19.8 | | | | 35.0 |
| 4 | 12 | 4.25 | 8.50 | 16.9 | 0 | | | 29.7 |
| | 13 | 3.58 | 7.15 | 14.3 | 21.0 | | | 46.0 |
| | 14 | 3.01 | 6.01 | 12.0 | 22.3 | | | 43.3 |
| | 15 | 2.53 | 5.06 | 10.1 | 19.8 | | | 37.5 |
| 5 | 16 | 2.13 | 4.25 | 8.50 | 16.9 | 0 | | 31.8 |
| | 17 | 1.79 | 3.58 | 7.15 | 14.3 | 21.0 | | 47.8 |
| | 18 | 1.51 | 3.01 | 6.01 | 12.0 | 22.3 | | 44.8 |
| | 19 | 1.27 | 2.53 | 5.06 | 10.1 | 19.8 | | 38.8 |
| 6 | 20 | 1.07 | 2.13 | 4.25 | 8.50 | 16.9 | 0 | 32.9 |
| | 21 | 0.90 | 1.79 | 3.58 | 7.15 | 14.3 | 21.0 | 48.7 |
| | 22 | 0.75 | 1.51 | 3.01 | 6.01 | 12.0 | 22.3 | 45.6 |
| | 23 | 0.63 | 1.27 | 2.53 | 5.06 | 10.1 | 19.8 | 39.4 |
| | 24 | 0.53 | 1.07 | 2.13 | 4.25 | 8.50 | 16.9 | 33.4 |

*A single oral dose of 350 mg was given and the plasma drug concentrations were measured for 0–24 h. The same plasma drug concentrations are assumed to occur after doses 2–6. The total plasma drug concentration is the sum of the plasma drug concentrations due to each dose. For this example, $V_D = 10 L$, $t_{1/2} = 4 h$, and $k_a = 1.5 h^{-1}$. The drug is 100% bioavailable and follows the pharmacokinetics of a one-compartment open model.

plasma concentrations immediately following the first dose. However, if the second dose is given after a time interval longer than the time required to eliminate the previous dose, drug will not accumulate (see Table 17-1).

As repetitive equal doses are given at a constant frequency, the plasma level–time curve plateaus after a certain time period based on the terminal half-life of the drug. It is important to emphasize that for novel drug dosage forms nowadays, such as

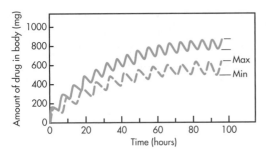

**FIGURE 17-2** • Amount of drug in the body as a function of time. Equal doses of drug were given every 6 hours (upper curve) and every 8 hours (lower curve). $k_a$ and $k$ remain constant.

sustained-release formulations, the absorption half-life is longer and so the terminal half-life (longest of all half-lives) is the one dictating accumulation. (drugs with shorter terminal half-life reach steady state faster compared to those with longer half-life) and a steady state is obtained. At steady state, the plasma drug levels fluctuate between $C_{max}^{\infty}$ and $C_{min}^{\infty}$ Once steady state is obtained, $C_{max}^{\infty}$ and $C_{min}^{\infty}$ are constant and remain unchanged from dose to dose. In addition, the AUC between ($\int_{t_1}^{t_2} C_p\, dt$) is constant during a dosing interval at steady state (see Fig. 17-1). The $C_{max}^{\infty}$ is important in determining drug safety. The $C_{max}^{\infty}$ should always remain below the MTC. The $C_{max}^{\infty}$ is also a good indication of drug accumulation. If a drug produces the same $C_{max}^{\infty}$ at steady state, compared with the $(C_{n-1})_{max}$ after the first dose, then there is no drug accumulation. If $C_{max}^{\infty}$ is much larger than $(C_{n-1})_{max}$ then there is significant accumulation during the multiple-dose regimen. Accumulation is affected by the relationship between the terminal half-life of the drug and the dosing interval. The index for measuring drug accumulation $R$ is

$$R = \frac{(C^{\infty})_{max}}{(C_{n=1})_{max}} \qquad (17.1)$$

Substituting for $C_{max}$ after the first dose and at steady state yields

$$R = \frac{D_0/V_D\,[1/(1-e^{-k\tau})]}{D_0/V_D} \qquad (17.2)$$

$$R = \frac{1}{1-e^{-k\tau}}$$

Equation 17.2 shows that drug accumulation measured with the $R$ index depends on the terminal

rate constant, and the dosing interval and is independent of the dose. For a drug given in repetitive oral doses, the time required to reach steady state is dependent ONLY on the terminal half-life of the drug and is independent of the size of the dose, the length of the dosing interval, and the number of doses. For example, if the dose or dosage interval of the drug is altered, as shown in Fig. 17-2, the time required for the drug to reach steady state is the same, but the final steady-state plasma level changes proportionately.

Furthermore, if the drug is given at the same dosing rate but as an infusion (eg, 25 mg/h), the average plasma drug concentrations ($C_{av}^{\infty}$) will be the same but the fluctuations between $C_{max}^{\infty}$ and $C_{min}^{\infty}$ will vary (Fig. 17-3). An average steady-state plasma drug concentration is obtained by dividing the area under the curve (AUC) for a dosing period (ie, $\int_{t_1}^{t_2} C_p\, dt$) by the dosing interval $\tau$, at steady state.

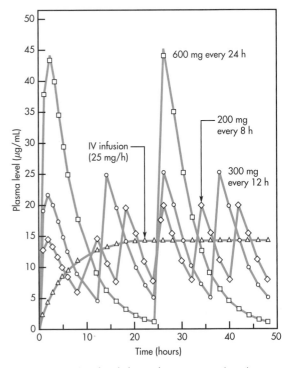

**FIGURE 17-3** • Simulated plasma drug concentration–time curves after IV infusion and oral multiple doses for a drug with an elimination half-life of 4 hours and apparent $V_D$ of 10 L. IV infusion given at a rate of 25 mg/h, oral multiple doses are 200 mg every 8 hours, 300 mg every 12 hours, and 600 mg every 24 hours.

An equation for the estimation of the time to reach one-half of the steady-state plasma levels or the accumulation half-life has been described by van Rossum and Tomey (1968).

$$\text{Accumulation } t_{1/2} = t_{1/2}\left(1 + 3.3\log\frac{k_a}{k_a - k}\right) \quad (17.3)$$

For IV administration, $k_a$ is very rapid (approaches $\infty$); $k$ is very small in comparison to $k_a$ and can be omitted in the denominator of Equation 17.3. Thus, Equation 17.3 reduces to

$$\text{Accumulation } t_{1/2} = t_{1/2}\left(1 + 3.3\log\frac{k_a}{k_a}\right) \quad (17.4)$$

Since $k_a/k_a = 1$ and $\log 1 = 0$, the accumulation $t_{1/2}$ of a drug administered intravenously is the elimination $t_{1/2}$ of the drug. From this relationship, the time to reach 50% steady-state drug concentrations is dependent only on the terminal $t_{1/2}$ and not on the dose or dosage interval.

As shown in Equation 17.4, the accumulation $t_{1/2}$ is directly proportional to the elimination $t_{1/2}$. Table 17-2 gives the accumulation $t_{1/2}$ of drugs with various terminal half-lives given by multiple oral doses (see Table 17-2).

From a clinical viewpoint, the time needed to reach 90% of the steady-state plasma concentration is 3.3 times the terminal half-life, whereas the time required to reach 99% of the steady-state plasma concentration is 6.6 times the terminal half-life (Table 17-3). It should be noted from Table 17-3 that at a constant dose size, the shorter the dosage interval, the larger the dosing rate (mg/h), and the higher the steady-state drug level.

The number of doses for a given drug to reach steady state is dependent on the terminal half-life of the drug and the dosage interval $\tau$ (see Table 17-3). If the drug is given at a dosage interval equal to the half-life of the drug, then 6.6 doses are required to reach 99% of the theoretical steady-state plasma drug concentration. The number of doses needed to reach steady state is $6.6t_{1/2}/\tau$, as calculated in the far right column of Table 17-3. As discussed in Chapter 14, Table 14-1, it takes 4.32 half-lives to reach 95% of steady state.

## CLINICAL EXAMPLE

Paroxetine (Prozac) is an antidepressant drug with a long terminal half-life of 21 hours. Paroxetine is well absorbed after oral administration and has a $t_{max}$ of about 5 hours, longer than most drugs.

**TABLE 17-2 •** Effect of Elimination Half-Life and Absorption Rate Constant on Accumulation Half-Life after Oral Administration*

| Elimination Half-Life (h) | Elimination Rate Constant (1/h) | Absorption Rate Constant (1/h) | Accumulation Half-Life (h) |
|---|---|---|---|
| 4 | 0.173 | 1.50 | 4.70 |
| 8 | 0.0866 | 1.50 | 8.67 |
| 12 | 0.0578 | 1.50 | 12.8 |
| 24 | 0.0289 | 1.50 | 24.7 |
| 4 | 0.173 | 1.00 | 5.09 |
| 8 | 0.0866 | 1.00 | 8.99 |
| 12 | 0.0578 | 1.00 | 13.0 |
| 24 | 0.0289 | 1.00 | 25.0 |

*Accumulation half-life is calculated by Equation 17.3, and is the half-time for accumulation of the drug to 90% of the steady-state plasma drug concentration.

**TABLE 17-3** • Interrelation of Elimination Half-Life, Dosage Interval, Maximum Plasma Concentration, and Time to Reach Steady-State Plasma Concentration*

| Elimination Half-Life (h) | Dosage Interval, $\tau$(h) | $C_{max}^{\infty}$ ($\mu$g/mL) | Time for $C_{av}^{\infty b\dagger}$ (h) | No. Doses to Reach 99% Steady State |
|---|---|---|---|---|
| 0.5 | 0.5 | 200 | 3.3 | 6.6 |
| 0.5 | 1.0 | 133 | 3.3 | 3.3 |
| 1.0 | 0.5 | 341 | 6.6 | 13.2 |
| 1.0 | 1.0 | 200 | 6.6 | 6.6 |
| 1.0 | 2.0 | 133 | 6.6 | 3.3 |
| 1.0 | 4.0 | 107 | 6.6 | 1.65 |
| 1.0 | 10.0 | 100$^{\ddagger}$ | 6.6 | 0.66 |
| 2.0 | 1.0 | 341 | 13.2 | 13.2 |
| 2.0 | 2.0 | 200 | 13.2 | 6.1 |

*A single dose of 1000 mg of three hypothetical drugs with various elimination half-lives but equal volumes of distribution ($V_D$ = 10 L) were given by multiple IV doses at various dosing intervals. All time values are in hours; $C_{max}^{\infty}$ = maximum steady-state concentration; ($C_{av}^{\infty b}$) = average steady-state plasma concentration; the maximum plasma drug concentration after the first dose of the drug is ($C_{n=1}$)$_{max}$ = 100 $\mu$g/mL.
$^{\dagger}$Time to reach 99% of steady-state plasma concentration.
$^{\ddagger}$Since the dosage interval, $\tau$, is very large compared to the elimination half-life, no accumulation of drug occurs.

Slow elimination may cause the plasma curve to peak slowly. The $t_{max}$ is affected by $k$ and $k_a$, as discussed in Chapter 16. The $C_{max}$ for paroxetine after multiple dosing of 30 mg of paroxetine for 30 days in one study ranged from 8.6 to 105 ng/mL among 15 subjects. Clinically it is important to achieve a stable steady-state level in multiple dosing that does not "underdose" or overdose the patient. The pharmacist should advise the patient to follow the prescribed dosing interval and dose as accurately as possible. Taking a dose too early or too late contributes to variation. Individual variation in metabolism rate can also cause variable blood levels, as discussed later in Chapter 21.

## REPETITIVE INTRAVENOUS INJECTIONS

The maximum amount of drug in the body following a single rapid IV injection is equal to the dose of the drug. For a one-compartment open model, the drug will be eliminated according to first-order kinetics.

$$D_B = D_0 e^{-k\tau} \qquad (17.5)$$

where $D_B$ is the amount of drug remaining in the body. If $\tau$ is equal to the dosage interval (ie, the time between the first dose and the next dose), then the amount of drug remaining in the body after several hours can be determined with

$$D_B = D_0 e^{-k\tau} \qquad (17.6)$$

The fraction ($f$) of the dose remaining in the body is related to the elimination constant ($k$) and the dosage interval ($\tau$) as follows:

$$f = \frac{D_B}{D_0} = e^{-k\tau} \qquad (17.7)$$

With any given dose, $f$ depends on $k$ and $\tau$. If $\tau$ is large, $f$ will be smaller because $D_B$ is smaller.

## EXAMPLE ▷ ▷ ▷

1. A patient receives 1000 mg every 6 hours by repetitive IV injection of an antibiotic with a terminal half-life of 3 hours. Assume the drug is distributed according to a one-compartment model and the volume of distribution is 20 L.
   a. Find the maximum and minimum amounts of drug in the body.
   b. Determine the maximum and minimum plasma concentrations of the drug.

## Solution

**a.** The fraction of drug remaining in the body is estimated by Equation 17.7. The concentration of the drug declines to one-half after 3 hours ($t_{1/2} = 3$ h), after which the amount of drug will again decline by one-half at the end of the next 3 hours. Therefore, at the end of 6 hours, only one-quarter, or 0.25, of the original dose remains in the body. Thus $f$ is equal to 0.25. To use Equation 17.7, we must first find the value of $k$ from the $t_{1/2}$.

$$k = \frac{0.693}{t_{1/2}} = \frac{0.693}{3} = 0.231\ \text{h}^{-1}$$

The time interval $\tau$ is equal to 6 hours. From Equation 17.7,

$$f = e^{-(0.231)(6)}$$

$$f = 0.25$$

In this example, 1000 mg of drug is given intravenously, so the amount of drug in the body is immediately increased by 1000 mg. At the end of the dosage interval (ie, before the next dose), the amount of drug remaining in the body is 25% of the amount of drug present just after the previous dose, because $f = 0.25$. Thus, if the value of $f$ is known, a table can be constructed relating the fraction of the dose in the body before and after rapid IV injection (Table 17-4).

From Table 17-4 the maximum amount of drug in the body is 1333 mg and the minimum amount of drug in the body is 333 mg. The difference between the maximum and minimum values, $D_0$, will always equal the injected dose.

$$D_{\text{max}} - D_{\text{min}} = D_0 \qquad (17.8)$$

In this example,

$$1333 - 333 = 1000\ \text{mg}$$

$D_{\text{max}}^{\infty}$ can also be calculated directly by the relationship

$$D_{\text{max}}^{\infty} = \frac{D_0}{1 - f} \qquad (17.9)$$

**TABLE 17-4 •** Fraction of the Dose in the Body before and after Intravenous Injections of a 1000-mg Dose*

| Number of Doses | Amount of Drug in Body | |
|---|---|---|
| | Before Dose | After Dose |
| 1 | 0 | 1000 |
| 2 | 250 | 1250 |
| 3 | 312 | 1312 |
| 4 | 328 | 1328 |
| 5 | 332 | 1332 |
| 6 | 333 | 1333 |
| 7 | 333 | 1333 |
| ∞ | 333 | 1333 |

*$f = 0.25$.

Substituting known data, we obtain

$$D_{\text{max}}^{\infty} = \frac{1000}{1 - 0.25} = 1333\ \text{mg}$$

Then, from Equation 17.8,

$$D_{\text{min}}^{\infty} = 1333 - 1000 = 333\ \text{mg}$$

The average amount of drug in the body at steady state, $D_{\text{av}}^{\infty}$ can be found by Equation 17.10 or Equation 17.11. $F$ is the fraction of dose absorbed. For an IV injection, $F$ is equal to 1.0.

$$D_{\text{av}}^{\infty} = \frac{FD_0}{k\tau} \qquad (17.10)$$

$$D_{\text{av}}^{\infty} = \frac{FD_0 1.44 t_{1/2}}{\tau} \qquad (17.11)$$

Equations 17.10 and 17.11 can be used for repetitive dosing at constant time intervals and for any route of administration as long as elimination occurs from the central compartment. Substitution of values from the example into Equation 17.11 gives

$$D_{\text{av}}^{\infty} = \frac{(1)(1000)(1.44)(3)}{6} = 720\ \text{mg}$$

Since the drug in the body declines exponentially (ie, first-order drug elimination), the value $D_{av}^{\infty}$ is not the arithmetic mean of $D_{max}^{\infty}$ and $D_{min}^{\infty}$. The limitation of using $D_{av}^{\infty}$ is that the fluctuations of $D_{max}^{\infty}$ and $D_{min}^{\infty}$ are not known.

**b.** To determine the concentration of drug in the body after multiple doses, divide the amount of drug in the body by the volume in which it is dissolved. For a one-compartment model, the maximum, minimum, and steady-state concentrations of drug in the plasma are found by the following equations:

$$C_{max}^{\infty} = \frac{D_{max}^{\infty}}{V_D} \qquad (17.12)$$

$$C_{min}^{\infty} = \frac{D_{min}^{\infty}}{V_D} \qquad (17.13)$$

$$C_{av}^{\infty} = \frac{D_{av}^{\infty}}{V_D} \qquad (17.14)$$

A more direct approach to finding $C_{max}^{\infty}$ and $C_{min}^{\infty}$, is $C_{av}^{\infty}$:

$$C_{max}^{\infty} = \frac{C_p^0}{1 - e^{-k\tau}} \qquad (17.15)$$

where $C_p^0$ is equal to $D_0/V_D$.

$$C_{min}^{\infty} = \frac{C_p^0 e^{-k\tau}}{1 - e^{-k\tau}} \qquad (17.16)$$

$$C_{av}^{\infty} = \frac{FD_0}{V_D k\tau} \qquad (17.17)$$

For this example, the values for $C_{max}^{\infty}$ and $C_{min}^{\infty}$, is $C_{av}^{\infty}$ are 66.7, 16.7, and 36.1 $\mu$g/mL, respectively.

As mentioned, $C_{av}^{\infty}$ is not the arithmetic mean of $C_{max}^{\infty}$ and $C_{min}^{\infty}$ because plasma drug concentration declines exponentially. The $C_{av}^{\infty}$ is equal to $[AUC]_{t_1}^{t_2}$ or $(\int_{t_1}^{t_2} C_p \, dt)$ for a dosage interval at steady state divided by the dosage interval $\tau$.

$$C_{av}^{\infty} = \frac{[AUC]_{t_1}^{t_2}}{\tau} \qquad (17.18)$$

$C_{av}^{\infty}$ gives an estimate of the mean plasma drug concentration at steady state. The $C_{av}^{\infty}$ is often the target drug concentration for optimal therapeutic effect and gives an indication as to how long this plasma drug concentration is maintained during the dosing interval (between doses). The $C_{av}^{\infty}$ is dependent on both AUC and $\tau$. The $C_{av}^{\infty}$ reflects drug exposure after multiple doses. Drug exposure is often related to drug safety and efficacy as discussed later in Chapter 22. For example, drug exposure is closely monitored when a cytotoxic or immunosuppressive, anticancer drug is administered during therapy. AUC may be estimated by sampling several plasma drug concentrations over time. Theoretically, AUC is superior to sampling just the $C_{max}$ or $C_{min}$. For example, when cyclosporine dosing is clinically evaluated using AUC, the AUC is approximately estimated by two or three points. Dosing error is less than using AUC compared to the trough method alone (Primmett et al, 1998). In general, $C_{min}^{\infty}$, or trough level, is more frequently used than $C_{max}^{\infty}$. $C_{min}$ is the drug concentration just before the next dose is given and is less variable than peak drug concentration, $C_{max}^{\infty}$. The sample time for $C_{max}^{\infty}$ is approximated and the true $C_{max}^{\infty}$ may not be accurately estimated. In some cases, the plasma trough level, $C_{min}^{\infty}$, is considered by some investigators as a more reliable sample to describe total amount of drug in the body or exposure at that particular time as the drug may have equilibrated with the surrounding tissues, assuming that the drug is eliminated from the central compartment, which is usually true.

The AUC is related to the amount of drug absorbed divided by total body clearance ($CL$), as shown in the following equation:

$$[AUC]_{t_1}^{t_2} = \frac{FD_0}{CL} = \frac{FD_0}{kV_D} \qquad (17.19)$$

Substitution of $FD_0/kV_D$ for AUC in Equation 17.18 gives Equation 17.17, assuming a one-compartment model. Equation 17.17 or 17.18 can be used to obtain $C_{av}^{\infty}$ after a multiple-dose regimen regardless of the route of administration.

It is sometimes desirable to know the plasma drug concentration at any time after the administration of $n$ doses of drug. The general expression for calculating this plasma drug concentration assuming a one-compartment model is

$$C_p = \frac{D_0}{V_D} \left( \frac{1 - e^{-nk\tau}}{1 - e^{-k\tau}} \right) e^{-kt} \qquad (17.20)$$

where $n$ is the number of doses given and $t$ is the time after the $n$th dose.

At steady state, $e^{-nk\tau}$ approaches zero and Equation 17.20 reduces to

$$C_p^\infty = \frac{D_0}{V_D}\left(\frac{1}{1-e^{-k\tau}}\right)e^{-kt} \qquad (17.21)$$

where $C_p^\infty$ is the steady-state drug concentration at time $t$ after the dose.

2. The patient in the previous example received 1000 mg of an antibiotic every 6 hours by repetitive IV injection. The drug has an apparent volume of distribution of 20 L and terminal half-life of 3 hours. Calculate (a) the plasma drug concentration, $C_p$ at 3 hours after the second dose, (b) the steady-state plasma drug concentration, $C_p^\infty$ at 3 hours after the last dose, (c) $C_{max}^\infty$ (d) $C_{min}^\infty$, and (e) $C_{SS}$ assuming a one-compartment model.

### Solution

a. The $C_p$ at 3 hours after the second dose—use Equation 17.20 and let $n = 2$, $t = 3$ hours, and make other appropriate substitutions.

$$C_p = \frac{1000}{20}\left(\frac{1-e^{-(2)(0.231)(6)}}{1-e^{-(0.231)(6)}}\right)e^{-0.231(3)}$$

$$C_p = 31.3 \text{ mg/L}$$

b. The $C_p^\infty$ at 3 hours after the last dose—because steady state is reached, use Equation 17.21 and perform the following calculation:

$$C_p^\infty = \frac{1000}{20}\left(\frac{1}{1-e^{-0.231(6)}}\right)e^{-0.231(3)}$$

$$C_p^\infty = 33.3 \text{ mg/L}$$

c. The $C_{max}^\infty$ is calculated from Equation 17.15.

$$C_{max}^\infty = \frac{1000/20}{1-e^{-(0.231)(6)}} = 66.7 \text{ mg/L}$$

d. The $C_{min}^\infty$ may be estimated as the drug concentration after the dosage interval $\tau$, or just before the next dose.

$$C_{min}^\infty = C_{max}^\infty e^{-kt} = 66.7e^{-(0.231)(6)} = 16.7 \text{ mg/L}$$

e. The $C_{av}^\infty$ is estimated by Equation 17.17— because the drug is given by IV bolus injections, $F = 1$.

$$C_{av}^\infty = \frac{1000}{(0.231)(20)(6)} = 36.1 \text{ mg/L}$$

$C_{av}^\infty$ is represented as $C_{SS}$ in some references.

### Problem of a Missed Dose

Equation 17.22 describes the plasma drug concentration $t$ hours after the $n$th dose is administered; the doses are administered $\tau$ hours apart according to a multiple-dose regimen assuming a one-compartment model:

$$C_p = \frac{D_0}{V_D}\left(\frac{1-e^{-nk\tau}}{1-e^{-k\tau}}\right)e^{-kt} \qquad (17.22)$$

Concentration contributed by the missing dose is

$$C_p' = \frac{D_0}{V_D}e^{-kt_{miss}} \qquad (17.23)$$

in which $t_{miss}$ = time elapsed since the scheduled dose was missed. Subtracting Equation 17.23 from Equation 17.20 corrects for the missing dose as shown in Equation 17.24.

$$C_p = \frac{D_0}{V_D}\left[\left(\frac{1-e^{-nk\tau}}{1-e^{-k\tau}}\right)e^{-kt} - e^{-kt_{miss}}\right] \qquad (17.24)$$

*Note:* If steady state is reached (ie, either $n$ = large or after many doses), the equation simplifies to Equation 17.25. Equation 17.25 is useful when steady state is reached.

$$C_p = \frac{D_0}{V_D}\left(\frac{e^{-kt}}{1-e^{-kt}}\right) - e^{-kt_{miss}} \qquad (17.25)$$

Generally, if the missing dose is recent ($<<5t_{1/2}$), it will affect the present drug level more. If the missing dose is several half-lives later ($>5t_{1/2}$), the missing dose may be omitted because it will be very small. Equation 17.24 accounts for one missing dose, but several missing doses can be subtracted in a similar way if necessary.

## EXAMPLE ▷ ▷ ▷

A cephalosporin ($k = 0.2$ h$^{-1}$, $V_D = 10$ L) was administered by IV multiple dosing; 100 mg was injected every 6 hours for six doses. What was the plasma drug concentration 4 hours after the sixth dose (ie, 40 hours later) if (a) the fifth dose was omitted, (b) the sixth dose was omitted, and (c) the fourth dose was omitted, assuming a one-compartment model?

### Solution

**Substitute** $k = 0.2$ h$^{-1}$, $V_D = 10$ L, $D = 100$ mg, $n = 6$, $t = 4$ hours, and $\tau = 6$ hours into Equation 17.20 and evaluate:

$$C_p = 6.425 \text{ mg/L}$$

If no dose was omitted, then 4 hours after the sixth injection, $C_p$ would be 6.425 mg/L.

**a.** Missing the fifth dose, its contribution must be subtracted off, $t_{miss} = 6 + 4 = 10$ hours (the time elapsed since missing the dose) using the steady-state equation:

$$C_p' = \frac{D_0}{V_D} e^{-kt_{miss}} = \frac{100}{10} e^{-(0.2 \times 10)}$$

Drug concentration correcting for the missing dose = $6.425 - 1.353 = 5.072$ mg/L.

**b.** If the sixth dose is missing, $t_{miss} = 4$ hours:

$$C_p' = \frac{D_0}{V_D} e^{-kt_{miss}} = \frac{100}{10} e^{-(0.2 \times 4)} = 4.493 \text{ mg/L}$$

Drug concentration correcting for the missing dose = $6.425 - 4.493 = 1.932$ mg/L.

**c.** If the fourth dose is missing, $t_{miss} = 12 + 4 = 16$ hours:

$$C_p' = \frac{D_0}{V_D} e^{-kt_{miss}} = \frac{100}{10} e^{-(0.2 \times 16)} = 0.408 \text{ mg/L}$$

The drug concentration corrected for the missing dose = $6.425 - 0.408 = 6.017$ mg/L.

*Note:* The effect of a missing dose becomes less pronounced at a later time. A strict dose regimen compliance is advised for all drugs. With some drugs, missing a dose can have a serious effect on therapy. For example, compliance is important for the anti-HIV1 drugs such as the protease inhibitors.

### Early or Late Dose Administration during Multiple Dosing

When one of the drug doses is taken earlier or later than scheduled, the resulting plasma drug concentration can still be calculated based on the principle of superposition, and assuming a one-compartment model. The dose can be treated as missing, with the late or early dose added back to take into account the actual time of dosing, using Equation 17.26.

$$C_p = \frac{D_0}{V_D} \left( \frac{1 - e^{-k\tau}}{1 - e^{-k\tau}} e^{-k\tau} - e^{-k\tau_{miss}} + e^{-k\tau_{actual}} \right) \quad (17.26)$$

in which $t_{miss}$ = time elapsed since the dose (late or early) is scheduled, and $t_{actual}$ = time elapsed since the dose (late or early) is actually taken. Using a similar approach, a second missed dose can be subtracted from Equation 17.20. Similarly, a second late/early dose may be corrected by subtracting the scheduled dose followed by adding the actual dose. Similarly, if a different dose is given, the regular dose may be subtracted and the new dose added back.

## EXAMPLE ▷ ▷ ▷

Assume the same drug as above (ie, $k = 0.2$ h$^{-1}$, $V_D = 10$ L) was given by multiple IV bolus injections and that at a dose of 100 mg every 6 hours for 6 doses. What is the plasma drug concentration 4 hours after the sixth dose, if the fifth dose were given an hour late?

Substitute into Equation 17.26 for all unknowns: $k = 0.2$ h$^{-1}$, $V_D = 10$ L, $D = 100$ mg, $n = 6$, $\tau = 4$ h, $\tau = 6$ h, $t_{miss} = 6 + 4 = 10$ hours, $t_{actual} = 9$ hours (taken 1 hour late, ie, 5 hours before the sixth dose).

$$C_p = \frac{D_0}{V_D} \left( \frac{1 - e^{-nk\tau}}{1 - e^{-k\tau}} e^{-k\tau} - e^{-k\tau_{miss}} + e^{-k\tau_{actual}} \right)$$

$$C_p = 6.425 - 1.353 + 1.653 = 6.725 \text{ mg/L}$$

*Note:* 1.353 mg/L was subtracted and 1.653 mg/mL was added because the fifth dose was not given as planned, but was given 1 hour later.

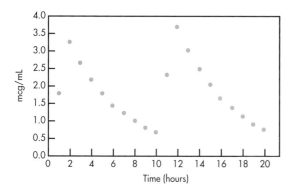

FIGURE 17-4 • Plasma drug concentration after two doses by IV infusion. Data from Table 17-5.

## INTERMITTENT INTRAVENOUS INFUSION

Intermittent IV infusion is a method of successive short IV drug infusions in which the drug is given by IV infusion for a short period of time followed by a drug elimination period, then followed by another short IV infusion mostly to minimize adverse effects (Fig. 17-4). In drug regimens involving short IV infusion, the drug may not reach steady state. The rationale for intermittent IV infusion is to prevent transient high drug concentrations and accompanying side effects. Many drugs are better tolerated when infused slowly over time compared to IV bolus dosing.

### Administering One or More Doses by Constant Infusion: Superposition of Several IV Infusion Doses

For a continuous IV infusion (see Chapter 14):

$$C_p = \frac{R}{CL}(1 - e^{-k\tau}) = \frac{R}{kV_D}(1 - e^{-k\tau}) \quad (17.27)$$

Equation 17.27 may be modified to determine drug concentration after one or more short IV infusions for a specified time period (Equation 17.28).

$$C_p = \frac{D}{t_{inf}V_D k}(1 - e^{-k\tau}) \quad (17.28)$$

where $R$ = rate of infusion = $D/t_{inf}$, $D$ = size of infusion dose, and $t_{inf}$ = infusion period.

After the infusion is stopped, the drug concentration post-IV infusion is obtained using the first-order equation for drug elimination:

$$C_p = C_{stop}e^{-kt} \quad (17.29)$$

where $C_{stop}$ = concentration when infusion stops, and $t$ = time elapsed since infusion stopped.

## EXAMPLE ▷ ▷ ▷

An antibiotic was infused with a 40-mg IV dose over 2 hours. Ten hours later, a second dose of 40 mg was infused, again over 2 hours. **(a)** What is the plasma drug concentration 2 hours after the start of the first infusion? **(b)** What is the plasma drug concentration 5 hours after the second dose infusion was started? Assume $k = 0.2$ h$^{-1}$ and $V_D = 10$ L for the antibiotic.

### Solution

The predicted plasma drug concentrations after the first and second IV infusions are shown in Table 17-5. Using the principle of superposition, the total plasma drug concentration is the sum of the residual drug concentrations due to the first IV infusion (column 3) and the drug concentrations due to the second IV infusion (column 4). A graphical representation of these data is shown in Fig. 17-4.

a. The plasma drug concentration at 2 hours after the first IV infusion starts is calculated from Equation 17.28.

$$C_p = \frac{40/2}{10 \times 0.2}(1 - e^{-0.2 \times 2}) = 3.30 \text{ mg/L}$$

b. From Table 17-5, the plasma drug concentration at 15 hours (ie, 5 hours after the start of the second IV infusion) is 2.06 $\mu$g/mL. At 5 hours after the second IV infusion starts, the plasma drug concentration is the sum of the residual plasma drug concentrations from the first 2-hour infusion according to first-order elimination and the residual plasma

**TABLE 17-5 • Drug Concentration after Two Intravenous Infusions***

|  | Time(h) | Plasma Drug Concentration after Infusion 1 | Plasma Drug Concentration after Infusion 2 | Total Plasma Drug Concentration |
|---|---|---|---|---|
| Infusion 1 begins | 0 | 0 |  | 0 |
|  | 1 | 1.81 |  | 1.81 |
| Infusion 1 stopped | 2 | 3.30 |  | 3.30 |
|  | 3 | 2.70 |  | 2.70 |
|  | 4 | 2.21 |  | 2.21 |
|  | 5 | 1.81 |  | 1.81 |
|  | 6 | 1.48 |  | 1.48 |
|  | 7 | 1.21 |  | 1.21 |
|  | 8 | 0.99 |  | 0.99 |
|  | 9 | 0.81 |  | 0.81 |
| Infusion 2 begins | 10 | 0.67 | 0 | 0.67 |
|  | 11 | 0.55 | 1.81 | 2.36 |
| Infusion 2 stopped | 12 | 0.45 | 3.30 | 3.74 |
|  | 13 | 0.37 | 2.70 | 3.07 |
|  | 14 | 0.30 | 2.21 | 2.51 |
|  | 15 | 0.25 | 1.81 | 2.06 |

*Drug is given by a 2-hour infusion separated by a 10-hour drug elimination interval. All drug concentrations are in μg/mL. The declining drug concentration after the first infusion dose and the drug concentration after the second infusion dose give the total plasma drug concentration.

drug concentrations from the second 2-hour IV infusion as shown in the following scheme:

| ← | 10 hours → | ← | 10 hours → |
|---|---|---|---|
| First infusion for 2 hours | Stopped (no infusion for 8 hours) | Second infusion for 2 hours | Stopped (no infusion for 8 hours) |

The plasma drug concentration is calculated using the first-order elimination equation, where $C_{stop}$ is the plasma drug concentration at the stop of the 2-hour IV infusion.

The plasma drug concentration after the completion of the first IV infusion when $t = 15$ hours is

$$C_p = C_{stop} e^{-kt} = 3.30 e^{-0.2 \times 15} = 0.25 \ \mu g/L$$

The plasma drug concentration 5 hours after the second IV infusion is

$$C_p = C_{stop} e^{-kt} = 3.30 e^{-0.2 \times 3} = 1.81 \ \mu g/mL$$

The total plasma drug concentration 5 hours after the start of the second IV infusion is

$$0.25 \ mg/L + 1.81 \ mg/L = 2.06 \ mg/L.$$

## CLINICAL EXAMPLE

Gentamicin sulfate was given to an adult male patient (57 years old, 70 kg) by intermittent IV infusions. One-hour IV infusions of 90 mg of gentamicin were given at 8-hour intervals. Gentamicin clearance is similar to creatinine clearance and was estimated as 7.2 L/h with an elimination half-life of 3 hours. Assuming a one-compartment model,

**a.** What is the plasma drug concentration after the first IV infusion?

**b.** What is the peak plasma drug concentration, $C_{max}$, and the trough plasma drug concentration, $C_{min}$, at steady state?

**Solution**

**a.** The plasma drug concentration directly after the first infusion is calculated from Equation 17.27, where $R$ = 90 mg/h, $CL$ = 7.2 L/h, and $k$ = 0.231 h$^{-1}$. The time for infusion, $t_{int}$, is 1 hour.

$$C_p = \frac{90}{7.2}(1 - e^{-(0.231)(1)}) = 2.58 \text{ mg/L}$$

**b.** The $C_{max}^\infty$ at steady state may be obtained from Equation 17.30.

$$C_{max}^\infty = \frac{R(1 - e^{kt_{inf}})}{CL} \frac{1}{(1 - e^{-kt})} \qquad (17.30)$$

where $C_{max}$ is the peak drug concentration following the $n$th infusion, at steady state, $t_{inf}$ is the time period of infusion, and $\tau$ is the dosage interval. The term $1/(1 - e^{-k\tau})$ is the accumulation factor for repeated drug administration.

Substitution in Equation 17.30 gives

$$C_{max}^\infty = \frac{90(1 - e^{-(0.231)(1)})}{7.2} \times \frac{1}{(1 - e^{-(0.231)(8)})}$$

$$= 3.06 \text{ mg/L}$$

The plasma drug concentration $C_p^\infty$ at any time $t$ after the last infusion ends when steady state is obtained by Equation 17.31 and assumes that plasma drug concentrations decline according to first-order elimination kinetics.

$$C_p^\infty = \frac{R(1 - e^{-kt_{inf}})}{CL} \times \frac{1}{(1 - e^{-kt})} \times e^{-k(t)} \qquad (17.31)$$

where $t_{inf}$ is the time for infusion and $t$ is the time period after the end of the infusion.

The trough plasma drug concentration, $C_{min}^\infty$ at steady state is the drug concentration just before the start of the next IV infusion or after a dosage interval equal to 8 hours after the last infusion stopped. Equation 17.31 can be used to determine the plasma drug concentration at any time after the last infusion is stopped (after steady state has been reached).

$$C_{min}^\infty = \frac{90(1 - e^{-(0.231)(1)})}{7.2} \times \frac{e^{-(0.231)(8)}}{(1 - e^{-(0.231)(8)})}$$

$$= 0.48 \text{ mg/L}$$

## ESTIMATION OF $k$ AND $V_D$ OF AMINOGLYCOSIDES IN CLINICAL SITUATIONS

As illustrated above, antibiotics are often infused intravenously by multiple doses, so it is desirable to adjust the recommended starting dose based on the patient's individual $k$ and $V_D$ values. According to Sawchuk and Zaske (1976), individual parameters for aminoglycoside pharmacokinetics may be determined in a patient by using a limited number of plasma drug samples taken at appropriate time intervals. The equation was simplified by replacing an elaborate model with the one-compartment model to describe drug elimination and appropriately avoiding the distributive phase. The plasma sample should be collected 15 to 30 minutes post-infusion (with infusion lasting about 60 minutes) and, in patients with poor renal function, 1 to 2 hours post-infusion, to allow adequate tissue distribution. The second and third blood samples should be collected about two to three half-lives later, in order to get a good estimation of the slope. The data may be determined graphically or by regression analysis using a scientific calculator or computer program.

$$V_D = \frac{R(1 - e^{-kt_{inf}})}{[C_{max}^\infty - C_{min}^\infty e^{-kt_{inf}}]} \qquad (17.32)$$

The dose of aminoglycoside is generally fixed by the desirable peak, $C_{max}^\infty$ and trough plasma concentration, $C_{min}^\infty$. For example, $C_{max}^\infty$ for gentamicin may be set at 6 to 10 $\mu$g/mL with the steady-state trough level, $C_{min}^\infty$ generally about 0.5 to 2 $\mu$g/mL, depending on the severity of the infection and renal considerations. The upper range is used only for life-threatening infections. The infusion rate for any desired peak drug concentration may be calculated using Equation 17.33, assuming a one-compartment model.

$$R = \frac{V_{D}kC_{max}^{\infty}(1-e^{-k\tau})}{(1-e^{-kt_{inf}})} \quad (17.33)$$

The dosing interval $\tau$ between infusions may be adjusted to obtain a desired concentration.

---

**FREQUENTLY ASKED QUESTION**

▶ Is the drug accumulation index (R) applicable to any drug given by multiple doses or only to drugs that are eliminated slowly from the body?

▶ What are the advantages/disadvantages of giving a drug by a constant IV infusion, intermittent IV infusion, or multiple IV bolus injections? What drugs would most likely be given by each route of administration? Why?

▶ Why is the accumulation index, R, not affected by the dose or clearance of a drug? Would it be possible for a drug with a short half-life to have R much greater than 1?

---

## MULTIPLE-ORAL-DOSE REGIMEN

Figures 17-1 and 17-2 present typical cumulation curves for the concentration of drug in the body after multiple oral doses given at a constant dosage interval. The plasma concentration at any time during an oral or extravascular multiple-dose regimen, assuming a one-compartment model and constant doses and dose interval, can be determined as follows:

$$C_{p} = \frac{Fk_{a}D_{0}}{V_{D}(k-k_{a})}\left[\left(\frac{1-e^{-nk_{a}\tau}}{1-e^{-k_{a}\tau}}\right)e^{-k_{a}t} - \left(\frac{1-e^{-nk\tau}}{1-e^{-k\tau}}\right)e^{-kt}\right] \quad (17.34)$$

where $n$ = number of doses, $\tau$ = dosage interval, $F$ = fraction of dose absorbed, and $t$ = time after administration of $n$ doses.

The mean plasma level at steady state, $C_{av}^{\infty}$, is determined by a similar method to that employed for repeat IV injections. Equation 17.17 can be used for finding $C_{av}^{\infty}$ for any route of administration.

$$C_{av}^{\infty} = \frac{FD_{0}}{V_{D}k\tau} \quad (17.17)$$

Because proper evaluation of $F$ and $V_{D}$ requires IV data, the AUC of a dosing interval at steady state may be substituted in Equation 17.17 to obtain

$$C_{av}^{\infty} = \frac{\int_{0}^{\infty}C_{p}\,dt}{\tau} = \frac{[AUC]_{0}^{\infty}}{\tau} \quad (17.35)$$

One can see from Equation 17.17 that the magnitude of $C_{av}^{\infty}$ is directly proportional to the size of the dose and the extent of drug absorbed. Furthermore, if the dosage interval ($\tau$) is shortened, then the value for $C_{av}^{\infty}$ will increase. The $C_{av}^{\infty}$ will be predictably higher for drugs distributed in a small $V_{D}$ (eg, plasma water) or that have long terminal half-lives than for drugs distributed in a large $V_{D}$ (eg, total body water) or that have very short elimination half-lives. Because body clearance ($CL_{r}$) is equal to $kV_{D}$, substitution into Equation 17.17 yields

$$C_{av}^{\infty} = \frac{FD_{0}}{CL_{T}\tau} \quad (17.36)$$

Thus, if $CL_{T}$ decreases, $C_{av}^{\infty}$ will increase.

The $C_{av}^{\infty}$ does not give information concerning the fluctuations in plasma concentration $C_{max}^{\infty}$ and $C_{min}^{\infty}$. In multiple-dose regimens, $C_{p}$ at any time can be obtained using Equation 17.34, where $n = n$th dose. At steady state, the drug concentration can be determined by letting $n$ equal infinity. Therefore, $e^{-nk\tau}$ becomes approximately equal to zero and Equation 17.22 becomes

$$C_{p} = \frac{k_{a}FD_{0}}{V_{D}(k_{a}-k)}\left[\left(\frac{1}{1-e^{-k\tau}}\right)e^{-kt} - \left(\frac{1}{1-e^{k_{a}\tau}}\right)e^{-k_{a}t}\right] \quad (17.37)$$

The maximum and minimum drug concentrations ($C_{max}^{\infty}$ and $C_{min}^{\infty}$) can be obtained with the following equations:

$$C_{max}^{\infty} = \frac{FD_{0}}{V_{D}}\left(\frac{1}{1-e^{-k\tau}}\right)e^{-kt_{p}} \quad (17.38)$$

$$C_{min}^{\infty} = \frac{k_{a}FD_{0}}{V_{D}(k_{a}-k)}\left(\frac{1}{1-e^{-k\tau}}\right)e^{-k\tau} \quad (17.39)$$

The time at which maximum (peak) plasma concentration (or $t_{max}$) occurs following a single oral dose is

$$t_{max} = \frac{2.3}{k_a - k} \log \frac{k_a}{k} \qquad (17.40)$$

whereas the peak plasma concentration, $t_p$, following multiple doses is given by Equation 17.41.

$$t_p = \frac{1}{k_a - k} \ln \left[ \frac{k_a (1 - e^{-k\tau})}{k (1 - e^{-k_a \tau})} \right] \qquad (17.41)$$

Large fluctuations between $C_{max}^{\infty}$ and $C_{min}^{\infty}$ can be hazardous, particularly with drugs that have a narrow therapeutic index. The larger the number of divided doses, the smaller the fluctuations in the plasma drug concentrations. For example, a 500-mg dose of drug given every 6 hours will produce the same $C_{av}^{\infty}$ value as a 250-mg dose of the same drug given every 3 hours, while the $C_{max}^{\infty}$ and $C_{min}^{\infty}$ fluctuations for the latter dose will be decreased by one-half (see Fig. 17-3). With drugs that have a narrow therapeutic index, the dosage interval should not be longer than the terminal half-life.

## EXAMPLE ▷ ▷ ▷

An adult male patient (46 years old, 81 kg) was given 250 mg of tetracycline hydrochloride orally every 8 hours for 2 weeks. From the literature, tetracycline hydrochloride is about 75% bioavailable and has an apparent volume of distribution of 1.5 L/kg. The elimination half-life is about 10 hours. The absorption rate constant is 0.9 h$^{-1}$. From this information, calculate (a) $C_{max}$ after the first dose, (b) $C_{min}$ after the first dose, (c) plasma drug concentration $C_p$ at 4 hours after the seventh dose, (d) maximum plasma drug concentration at steady state, $C_{max}^{\infty}$ (e) minimum plasma drug concentration at steady state, $C_{min}^{\infty}$ and (f) average plasma drug concentration at steady state, $C_{av}^{\infty}$

### Solution

**a.** $C_{max}$ after the first dose occurs at $t_{max}$—therefore, using Equation 17.40,

$$t_{max} = \frac{2.3}{0.9 - 0.07} \log \left( \frac{0.9}{0.07} \right)$$

$$t_{max} = 3.07$$

Then substitute $t_{max}$ into the following equation for a single oral dose (one-compartment model) to obtain $C_{max}$.

$$C_{max} = \frac{F D_0 k_a}{V_D (k_a - k)} (e^{-k t_{max}} - e^{-k_a t_{max}})$$

$$C_{max} = \frac{(0.75)(250)(0.9)}{(121.5)(0.9 - 0.07)} (e^{-0.07(3.07)} - e^{-0.9(3.07)})$$

$$C_{max} = 1.28 \text{ mg/L}$$

**b.** $C_{min}$ after the first dose occurs just before the administration of the next dose of drug—therefore, set $t = 8$ hours and solve for $C_{min}$.

$$C_{min} = \frac{(0.75)(250)(0.9)}{(121.5)(0.9 - 0.07)} (e^{-0.07(8)} - e^{-0.9(8)})$$

$$C_{min} = 0.95 \text{ mg/L}$$

**c.** $C_p$ at 4 hours after the seventh dose may be calculated using Equation 17.34, letting $n = 7$, $t = 4$, $\tau = 8$, and making the appropriate substitutions.

$$C_p = \frac{(0.75)(250)(0.9)}{(121.5)(0.07 - 0.9)}$$

$$\times \left[ \left( \frac{1 - e^{-(7)(0.9)(8)}}{1 - e^{-0.9(8)}} \right) e^{-0.9(4)} - \left( \frac{1 - e^{-(7)(0.07)(8)}}{1 - e^{-(0.07)(8)}} \right) e^{-0.07(4)} \right]$$

$$C_p = 2.86 \text{ mg/L}$$

**d.** $C_{max}^{\infty}$ at steady state: $t_p$ at steady state is obtained from Equation 17.41.

$$t_p = \frac{1}{k_a - k} \ln \left[ \frac{k_a (1 - e^{-k\tau})}{k (1 - e^{-k_a \tau})} \right]$$

$$t_p = \frac{1}{0.9 - 0.07} \ln \left[ \frac{0.9 (1 - e^{-(0.07)(8)})}{0.07 (1 - e^{-(0.9)(8)})} \right]$$

$$t_p = 2.05 \text{ hours}$$

Then $C_{max}^{\infty}$ is obtained using Equation 17.38.

$$C_{max}^{\infty} = \frac{0.75(250)}{121.5}\left(\frac{1}{1-e^{-0.07(8)}}\right)e^{-0.07(2.05)}$$

$$C_{min}^{\infty} = 3.12 \text{ mg/L}$$

e. $C_{min}^{\infty}$ at steady state is calculated from Equation 17.39.

$$C_{min}^{\infty} = \frac{(0.9)(0.75)(250)}{(121.5)(0.9-0.07)}\left(\frac{1}{1-e^{-0.07(8)}}\right)e^{-(0.7)(8)}$$

$$C_{max}^{\infty} = 2.23 \text{ mg/L}$$

f. $C_{av}^{\infty}$ at steady state is calculated from Equation 17.17.

$$C_{av}^{\infty} = \frac{(0.75)(250)}{(121.5)(0.07)(8)}$$

$$C_{av}^{\infty} = 2.76 \text{ mg/L}$$

## LOADING DOSE

Since extravascular doses require time for absorption into the plasma to occur, therapeutic effects are delayed until sufficient plasma concentrations are achieved. To reduce the onset time of the drug—that is, the time it takes to achieve the minimum effective concentration (assumed to be equivalent to the $C_{av}^{\infty}$)—a loading (priming) or initial dose of drug is given. The main objective of the loading dose is to achieve desired plasma concentrations, $C_{av}^{\infty}$, as quickly as possible. If the drug follows one-compartment pharmacokinetics, then in theory, steady state is also achieved immediately following the loading dose. Thereafter, a maintenance dose is given to maintain $C_{av}^{\infty}$ at steady state so that the therapeutic effect is also maintained. In practice, a loading dose may be given as a bolus dose or a short-term loading IV infusion.

As discussed earlier, the time required for the drug to accumulate to a steady-state plasma level is dependent mainly on its terminal half-life. The time needed to reach 90% of $C_{av}^{\infty}$ is approximately 3.3 half-lives, and the time required to reach 99% of $C_{av}^{\infty}$ is equal to approximately 6.6 half-lives. For a drug with a half-life of 4 hours, it will take approximately 13 and 26 hours to reach 90% and 99% of $C_{av}^{\infty}$, respectively.

For drugs absorbed rapidly in relation to elimination ($k_a \gg k$) and that are distributed rapidly, the loading dose $D_L$ can be calculated as follows:

$$\frac{D_L}{D_0} = \frac{1}{(1-e^{-k_a\tau})(1-e^{-k\tau})} \quad (17.42)$$

For extremely rapid absorption, as when the product of $k_a\tau$ is large or in the case of IV infusion, $e^{-k_a\tau}$ becomes approximately zero and Equation 17.42 reduces to

$$\frac{D_L}{D_0} = \frac{1}{1-e^{-k\tau}} \quad (17.43)$$

The loading dose should approximate the amount of drug contained in the body at steady state. The dose ratio is equal to the loading dose divided by the maintenance dose.

$$\text{Dose ratio} = \frac{D_L}{D_0} \quad (17.44)$$

As a general rule of thumb, if the selected dosage interval is equal to the drug's terminal half-life, then the dose ratio calculated from Equation 17.44 should be equal to 2.0. In other words, the loading dose will be equal to double the initial drug dose. Figure 17-5 shows the plasma level–time curve for dosage regimens with equal maintenance doses but different loading doses. A rapid approximation of loading dose, $D_L$, may be estimated from

$$D_L = \frac{V_D C_{av}^{\infty}}{(S)(F)} \quad (17.45)$$

where $C_{av}^{\infty}$ is the desired plasma drug concentration, $S$ is the salt factor of the drug, and $F$ is the fraction of drug bioavailability.

Equation 17.45 assumes very rapid drug absorption from an immediate-release dosage form. The $D_L$ calculated by this method has been used in clinical situations for which only an approximation of the $D_L$ is needed.

These calculations for loading doses are not applicable to drugs that demonstrate multicompartment kinetics. Such drugs distribute slowly into extravascular tissues, and drug equilibration and steady state may not occur until after the apparent plateau is reached in the vascular (central) compartment.

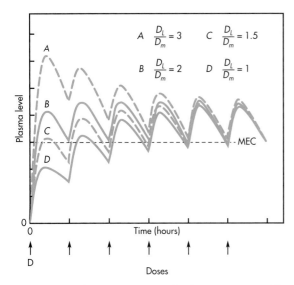

FIGURE 17-5 • Concentration curves for dosage regimens with equal maintenance doses (D) and dosage intervals (τ) and different dose ratios. (Reproduced with permission from Ariens EJ: Physico-Chemical Aspects of Drug Action. New York, NY: Pergamon; 1968.)

## DOSAGE REGIMEN SCHEDULES

Predictions of steady-state plasma drug concentrations usually assume the drug is given at a constant dosage interval throughout a 24-hour day. Very often, however, the drug is given only during the waking hours (Fig. 17-6). Niebergall et al (1974)

discussed the problem of scheduling dosage regimens and particularly warned against improper timing of the drug dosage. For drugs with a narrow therapeutic index such as theophylline (Fig. 17-6), large fluctuation between the maximum and minimum plasma levels are undesirable and may lead to subtherapeutic plasma drug concentrations and/or too high, possibly toxic, drug concentrations. These wide fluctuations occur if larger doses are given at wider dosage intervals (see Fig. 17-3). For example, Fig. 17-7 shows procainamide given with a 1.0-g loading dose on the first day followed by maintenance doses of 0.5 g four times a day. On the second, third, and subsequent days, the procainamide plasma levels did not reach the therapeutic range until after the second dose of drug.

Ideally, drug doses should be given at evenly spaced intervals. However, to improve patient compliance, dosage regimens may be designed to fit with the lifestyle of the patient. For example, the patient is directed to take a drug such as amoxicillin four times a day (QID), before meals and at bedtime, for a systemic infection. This dosage regimen will produce unequal dosage intervals during the day, because the patient takes the drug before breakfast, at 0800 hours (8 AM); before lunch, at 1200 hours (12 noon); before dinner, at 1800 hours (6 PM); and before bedtime, at 2300 hours (11 PM). For these drugs, evenly spaced dosage intervals are not that critical to the

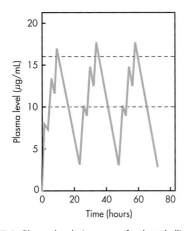

FIGURE 17-6 • Plasma level–time curve for theophylline given in doses of 160 mg 3 times a day. Dashed lines indicate the therapeutic range. (Reproduced with permission from Niebergall PJ, Sugita ET, Schnaare RL. Potential dangers of common drug dosing regimens, *Am J Hosp Pharm*. 1974 Jan;31(1):53–58.)

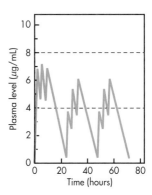

FIGURE 17-7 • Plasma level–time curve for procainamide given in an initial dose of 1.0 g followed by doses of 0.5 g 4 times a day. Dashed lines indicate the therapeutic range. (Reproduced with permission from Niebergall PJ, Sugita ET, Schnaare RL. Potential dangers of common drug dosing regimens, *Am J Hosp Pharm*. 1974 Jan;31(1):53–58.)

effectiveness of the antibiotic as long as the plasma drug concentrations are maintained above the *minimum inhibitory concentration* (MIC) for the microorganism. In some cases, a drug may be given at a larger dose allowing for a longer duration above MIC if fluctuation is less critical. In Augmentin BID-875 (amoxicillin/clavulanate tablets), the amoxicillin/clavulanate tablet is administered twice daily.

Patient compliance with multiple-dose regimens may be a problem for the patient in following the prescribed dosage regimen. Occasionally, a patient may miss taking the drug dose at the prescribed dosage interval. For drugs with long terminal half-lives (eg, levothyroxine sodium or oral contraceptives), the consequences of one missed dose are minimal, since only a small fraction of drug is lost between daily dosing intervals. The patient should either take the next drug dose as soon as the patient remembers or continue the dosing schedule starting at the next prescribed dosing period. If it is almost time for the next dose, then the skipped dose should not be taken and the regular dosing schedule should be maintained. Generally, the patient should not double the dose of the medication. For specific drug information on missed doses, USP DI II, *Advice for the Patient*, published annually by the United States Pharmacopeia, is a good source of information.

The problems of widely fluctuating plasma drug concentrations may be prevented by using a controlled-release formulation of the drug, or a drug in the same therapeutic class that has a long terminal half-life. The use of extended-release dosage forms allows for less frequent dosing and prevents undermedication between the last evening dose and the first morning dose. Extended-release drug products may improve patient compliance by decreasing the number of doses within a 24-hour period that the patient needs to take. Patients generally show better compliance with a twice-a-day (BID) dosage regimen compared to a three-times-a-day (TID) dosage schedule.

## CLINICAL EXAMPLE

Bupropion hydrochloride (Wellbutrin) is a noradrenergic/dopaminergic antidepressant. Jefferson et al (2005) have reviewed the pharmacokinetic properties of bupropion and its various formulations and clinical applications, the goal of which is optimization

of major depressive disorder treatment. Bupropion hydrochloride is available in three oral formulations. The immediate-release (IR) tablet is given three times a day, the sustained-release tablet (Wellbutrin SR) is given twice a day, and the extended-release tablet (Wellbutrin XL) is given once a day.

The total daily dose was 300 mg bupropion HCl. The AUC for each dose treatment was similar, showing that the formulations were bioequivalent based on extent of absorption. The fluctuations between peak and trough levels were greatest for the IR product given three times a day and least for the once-a-day XL product. According to the manufacturer, all three dosage regimens provide equivalent clinical efficacy. The advantage of the extended-release product is that the patient needs only to take the drug once a day. Often, IR drug products are less expensive compared to an extended-release drug product. In this case, the fluctuating plasma drug levels for buproprion IR tablet given three times a day are not a safety issue, and the tablet is equally efficacious as the 150-mg SR tablet given twice a day or the 300-mg XL tablet given once a day. The patient may also consider the cost of the medication.

## PRACTICE PROBLEMS

1. Patient C.S. is a 35-year-old man weighing 76.6 kg. The patient is to be given multiple IV bolus injections of an antibiotic every 6 hours. The effective concentration of this drug is 15 $\mu$g/mL. After the patient is given a single IV dose, the elimination half-life for the drug is determined to be 3.0 hours and the apparent $V_D$ is 196 mL/kg. Determine a multiple IV dose regimen for this drug (assume drug is given every 6 hours).

**Solution**

$$C_{av}^\infty = \frac{FD_0}{V_D k \tau}$$

For IV dose, $F = 1$,

$$D_0 = (15\ \mu g/mL)\left(\frac{0.693}{3\ h}\right)(196\ mL/kg)(6\ h)$$

$$D_0 = 4.07\ mg/kg\ every\ 6\ hours$$

Since patient C.S. weighs 76.6 kg, the dose should be as shown:

$$D_0 = (4.07 \text{ mg/kg})(76.6 \text{ kg})$$

$$D_0 = 312 \text{ mg every 6 hours}$$

After the condition of this patient has stabilized, the patient is to be given the drug orally for convenience of drug administration. The objective is to design an oral dosage regimen that will produce the same steady-state blood level as the multiple IV doses. The drug dose will depend on the bioavailability of the drug from the drug product, the desired therapeutic drug level, and the dosage interval chosen. Assume that the antibiotic is 90% bioavailable and that the physician would like to continue oral medication every 6 hours.

The average or steady-state plasma drug level is given by

$$C_{av}^{\infty} = \frac{FD_0}{V_D k \tau}$$

$$D_0 = \frac{(15 \ \mu g/mL)(193 \text{ mL/kg})(0.693)(6 \text{ h})}{(0.9)(3 \text{ h})}$$

$$D_0 = 454 \text{ mg/kg}$$

Because patient C.S. weighs 76.6 kg, he should be given the following dose:

$$D_0 = (4.54 \text{ mg/kg})(76.6 \text{ kg})$$

$$D_0 = 348 \text{ mg every 6 hours}$$

For drugs with equal absorption but slower absorption rates ($F$ is the same but $k_a$ is smaller), the initial dosing period may show a lower blood level; however, the steady-state blood level will be unchanged.

2. In practice, drug products are usually commercially available in certain specified strengths. Using the information provided in the preceding problem, assume that the antibiotic is available in 125-, 250-, and 500-mg tablets. Therefore, the pharmacist or prescriber must now decide which tablets are to be given to the patient. In this case, it may be possible to give the patient 375 mg (eg, one 125-mg tablet and one 250-mg tablet)

every 6 hours. However, the $C_{av}^{\infty}$ should be calculated to determine if the plasma level is approaching a toxic value. Alternatively, a new dosage interval might be appropriate for the patient. It is very important to design the dosage interval and the dose to be as simple as possible, so that the patient will not be confused and will be able to comply with the medication program properly.

**a.** What is the new $C_{av}^{\infty}$ if the patient is given 375 mg every 6 hours?

**Solution**

$$C_{av}^{\infty} = \frac{(0.9)(375,000)(3)}{(196)(76.6)(6)(0.693)}$$

$$C_{av}^{\infty} = 16.2 \ \mu g/mL$$

Because the therapeutic objective was to achieve a minimum effective concentration (MEC) of 15 $\mu g/mL$, a value of 16.2 $\mu g/mL$ is reasonable.

**b.** The patient has difficulty in distinguishing tablets of different strengths. Can the patient take a 500-mg dose (eg, two 250-mg tablets)?

**Solution**

The dosage interval ($\tau$) for the 500-mg tablet would have to be calculated as follows:

$$\tau = \frac{(0.9)(500,000)(3)}{(196)(76.6)(15)(0.693)}$$

$$\tau = 8.63 \text{ h}$$

**c.** A dosage interval of 8.63 hours is difficult to remember. Is a dosage regimen of 500 mg every 8 hours reasonable?

**Solution**

$$C_{av}^{\infty} = \frac{(0.9)(500,000)(3)}{(196)(76.6)(8)(0.693)}$$

$$C_{av}^{\infty} = 16.2 \ \mu g/mL$$

Notice that a larger dose is necessary if the drug is given at longer intervals.

**TABLE 17-6** • Effect of Dosing Schedule on Predicted Steady-State Plasma Drug Concentrations*

| Dosing Schedule | | | Steady-State Drug Concentration (µg/mL) | | |
|---|---|---|---|---|---|
| Dose (mg) | 1 (h) | Dosing Rate, $D_0/\tau$ (mg/h) | $C_{max}^{\infty}$ | $C_{av}^{\infty}$ | $C_{min}^{\infty}$ |
| — | — | 25† | 14.5 | 14.5 | 14.5 |
| 100 | 4 | 25 | 16.2 | 14.5 | 11.6 |
| 200 | 8 | 25 | 20.2 | 14.5 | 7.81 |
| 300 | 12 | 25 | 25.3 | 14.5 | 5.03 |
| 600 | 24 | 25 | 44.1 | 14.5 | 1.12 |
| 400 | 8 | 50 | 40.4 | 28.9 | 15.6 |
| 600 | 8 | 75 | 60.6 | 43.4 | 23.4 |

*Drug has an elimination half-life of 4 hours and an apparent $V_D$ of 10 L.
†Drug given by IV infusion. The first-order absorption rate constant $k_a$ is 1.2 h⁻¹ and the drug follows a one-compartment open model.

In designing a dosage regimen, one should consider a regimen that is practical and convenient for the patient. For example, for good compliance, the dosage interval should be spaced conveniently for the patient. In addition, one should consider the commercially available dosage strengths of the prescribed drug product.

The use of Equation 17.17 to estimate a dosage regimen initially has wide utility. The $C_{av}^{\infty}$ is equal to the dosing rate divided by the total body clearance of the drug in the patient:

$$C_{av}^{\infty} = \frac{FD_0}{\tau} \frac{1}{CL_T} \qquad (17.47)$$

where $FD_0/\tau$ is equal to the dosing rate R, and $1/CL_T$ is equal to $1/kV_D$.

In designing dosage regimens, the dosing rate $D_0/\tau$ is adjusted for the patient's drug clearance to obtain the desired $C_{av}^{\infty}$. For an IV infusion, the zero-order rate of infusion (R) is used to obtain the desired steady-state plasma drug concentration $C_{SS}$. If R is substituted for $FD_0/\tau$ in Equation 17.47, then the following equation for estimating $C_{SS}$ after an IV infusion is obtained:

$$C_{ss} = \frac{R}{CL_T} \qquad (17.48)$$

From Equations 17.47 and 17.48, all dosage schedules having the same dosing rate $D_0/\tau$, or R, will have the same $C_{av}^{\infty}$ or $C_{SS}$, whether the drug is given by multiple doses or by IV infusion. For example, dosage schedules of 100 mg every 4 hours, 200 mg every 8 hours, 300 mg every 12 hours, and 600 mg every 24 hours will yield the same $C_{av}^{\infty}$ in the patient. An IV infusion rate of 25 mg/h in the same patient will give a $C_{SS}$ equal to the $C_{av}^{\infty}$ obtained with the multiple-dose schedule (see Fig. 17-3; Table 17-6).

**FREQUENTLY ASKED QUESTION**

▶ Why is the steady-state peak plasma drug concentration measured sometime after an IV dose is given in a clinical situation?

▶ Why is the $C_{min}$ value at steady state less variable than the $C_{max}$ value at steady state?

▶ Is it possible to take a single blood sample to measure the $C_{av}$ value at steady state?

## CHAPTER SUMMARY

The purpose of giving a loading dose is to achieve desired (therapeutic) plasma concentrations as quickly as possible. For a drug with long terminal half-life, it may take a long time (several half-lives) to achieve steady-state levels. The loading dose must be calculated appropriately based on pharmacokinetic parameters to avoid overdosing. When several doses are administered for a drug with linear kinetics, drug accumulation may occur according to the principle of superposition. Superposition allows the derivation of equations that predict the plasma drug peak and trough concentrations of a drug at steady state and the theoretical drug concentrations at any time after the dose is given. The principle of superposition is used to examine the effect of an early, late, or missing dose on steady-state drug concentration.

$C_{max}^{\infty}$, $C_{min}^{\infty}$, and $C_{av}^{\infty}$ are useful parameters for monitoring the safety and efficacy of a drug during multiple dosing. A clinical example of multiple dosing using short, intermittent intravenous infusions has been applied to the aminoglycosides and is based on pharmacokinetics and clinical factors for safer dosing. The index for measuring drug accumulation during multiple dosing, $R$, is related to the dosing interval and the half-life of the drug, but not the dose. This parameter compares the steady-state concentration with drug concentration after the initial dose. The plasma concentration at any time during an oral or extravascular multiple-dose regimen, for a one-compartment model and constant doses and dose interval, is dependent on $n$ = number of doses, $\tau$ = dosage interval, $F$ = fraction of dose absorbed, and $t$ = time after administration of $n$ doses.

$$C_p = \frac{F k_a D_0}{V_D(k - k_a)}\left(\frac{1 - e^{nk_a\tau}}{1 - e^{-k_a\tau}}\right)e^{-k_a t} - \left(\frac{1 - e^{-nk\tau}}{1 - e^{-k\tau}}\right)e^{-kt}$$

The trough steady-state concentration after multiple oral dosing is

$$C_{min}^{\infty} = \frac{k_a F D_0}{V_D(k_a - k)}\left(\frac{1}{1 - e^{-k\tau}}\right)e^{-kt}$$

The relationship between average steady-state concentration, the AUC, and dosing interval is

$$C_{av}^{\infty} = \frac{\int_0^{\infty} C_p\, dt}{\tau} = \frac{[AUC]_0^{\infty}}{\tau}$$

This parameter is a good measure of drug exposure.

## LEARNING QUESTIONS

1. Gentamicin has an average terminal half-life of approximately 2 hours and an apparent volume of distribution of 20% of body weight. It is necessary to give gentamicin, 1 mg/kg every 8 hours by multiple IV injections, to a 50-kg woman with normal renal function. Calculate (a) $C_{max}$, (b) $C_{min}$, and (c) $C_{av}^{\infty}$.

2. A physician wants to give theophylline to a young male asthmatic patient (age 29 years, 80 kg). According to the literature, the terminal half-life for theophylline is 5 hours and the apparent $V_D$ is equal to 50% of the body weight. The plasma level of theophylline required to provide adequate airway ventilation is approximately 10 $\mu$g/mL.

   a. The physician wants the patient to take medication every 6 hours around the clock. What dose of theophylline would you recommend (assume theophylline is 100% bioavailable)?

   b. If you were to find that theophylline is available to you only in 225-mg capsules, what dosage regimen would you recommend?

3. What pharmacokinetic parameter is most important in determining the time at which the steady-state plasma drug level ($C_{av}^{\infty}$) is reached?

4. Name two ways in which the fluctuations of plasma concentrations (between $C_{max}^{\infty}$ and $C_{min}^{\infty}$) can be minimized for a person on a multiple-dose drug regimen without altering the $C_{av}^{\infty}$.

5. What is the purpose of giving a loading dose?

6. What is the loading dose for an antibiotic ($k = 0.23$ h$^{-1}$) with a maintenance dose of 200 mg every 3 hours?

7. What is the main advantage of giving a potent drug by IV infusion as opposed to multiple IV injections?

8. A drug has an terminal half-life of 2 hours and a volume of distribution of 40 L. The drug is given at a dose of 200 mg every 4 hours by multiple IV bolus injections. Predict the plasma drug concentration at 1 hour after the third dose.

9. The terminal half-life of an antibiotic is 3 hours and the apparent volume of distribution is 20% of the body weight. The therapeutic window for this drug is from 2 to 10 $\mu$g/mL. Adverse toxicity is often observed at drug concentrations above 15 $\mu$g/mL. The drug will be given by multiple IV bolus injections.

   a. Calculate the dose for an adult male patient (68 years old, 82 kg) with normal renal function to be given every 8 hours.

   b. Calculate the anticipated $C_{max}^{\infty}$ and $C_{min}^{\infty}$ values.

   c. Calculate the $C_{av}^{\infty}$ value.

   d. Comment on the adequacy of your dosage regimen.

10. Tetracycline hydrochloride (Achromycin V, Lederle) is prescribed for a young adult male patient (28 years old, 78 kg) suffering from gonorrhea. According to the literature, tetracycline HCl is 77% orally absorbed, is 65% bound to plasma proteins, has an apparent volume of distribution of 0.5 L/kg, has an terminal half-life of 10.6 hours, and is 58% excreted unchanged in the urine. The minimum inhibitory drug concentration (MIC) for gonorrhea is 25–30 $\mu$g/mL.

   a. Calculate an *exact* maintenance dose for this patient to be given every 6 hours around the clock.

   b. Achromycin V is available in 250- and 500-mg capsules. How many capsules (state dose) should the patient take every 6 hours?

   c. What loading dose using the above capsules would you recommend for this patient?

11. The body clearance of sumatriptan (Imitrex) is 250 mL/min. The drug is about 14% bioavailable. What would be the average plasma drug concentration after 5 doses of 100 mg PO every 8 hours in a patient? (Assume steady state was reached.)

12. Cefotaxime has a volume of distribution of 0.17 L/kg and an terminal half-life of 1.5 hours. What is the peak plasma drug concentration in a patient weighing 75 kg after receiving 1 g IV of the drug 3 times daily for 3 days?

## ANSWERS

### Frequently Asked Questions

*Is the drug accumulation index (R) applicable to any drug given by multiple doses or only to drugs that are eliminated slowly from the body?*

- Accumulation index, R, is a ratio that indicates steady-state drug concentration to the drug concentration after the first dose. The accumulation index does not measure the absolute size of overdosing; it measures the amount of drug cumulation that can occur due to frequent drug administration. Factors that affect R are the elimination rate constant, k, and the dosing interval, $\tau$. If the first dose is not chosen appropriately, the steady-state level may still be incorrect. Therefore, the first dose and the dosing interval must be determined correctly to avoid any significant drug accumulation. The accumulation index is a good indication of accumulation due to frequent drug dosing, applicable to any drug, regardless of whether the drug is bound to tissues.

*What are the advantages/disadvantages for giving a drug by constant IV infusion, intermittent IV infusion, or multiple IV bolus injections? What drugs would most likely be given by each route of administration? Why?*

- Some of the advantages of administering a drug by constant IV infusion include the following: (1) A drug may be infused continuously for many hours without disturbing the patient. (2) Constant infusion provides a stable blood drug level for drugs that have a narrow therapeutic index. (3) Some drugs are better tolerated when infused slowly. (4) Some drugs may be infused simultaneously with electrolytes or other infusion media in an acute-care setting. Disadvantages of administering a drug by constant IV infusion include the following: (1) Some drugs are more suitable to be administered as an IV bolus injection. For example, some reports show that an aminoglycoside given once daily resulted in fewer side effects compared with dividing the dose into two or three doses daily. Due to drug accumulation in the kidney and adverse toxicity, aminoglycosides are generally not given by prolonged IV infusions. In contrast, a prolonged period of low drug level for penicillins and tetracyclines may not be so efficacious and may result in a longer cure time for an infection. The pharmacodynamics of the individual drug must be studied to determine the best course of action. (2) Drugs such as nitroglycerin are less likely to produce tolerance when administered intermittently versus continuously.

*Why is the steady-state peak plasma drug concentration often measured sometime after an IV dose is given in a clinical situation?*

■ After an IV bolus drug injection, the drug is well distributed within a few minutes. In practice, however, an IV bolus dose may be administered slowly over several minutes or the drug may have a slow distribution phase. Therefore, clinicians often prefer to take a blood sample 15 minutes or 30 minutes after IV bolus injection and refer to that drug concentration as the peak concentration. In some cases, a blood sample is taken an hour later to avoid the fluctuating concentration in the distributive phase. The error due to changing sampling time can be large for a drug with a short elimination half-life.

*Is a loading dose always necessary when placing a patient on a multiple-dose regimen? What are the determining factors?*

■ A loading or priming dose is used to rapidly raise the plasma drug concentration to therapeutic drug levels to obtain a more rapid pharmacodynamic response. In addition, the loading dose

along with the maintenance dose allows the drug to reach steady-state concentration quickly, particularly for drugs with long terminal half-lives.

An alternative way of explaining the loading dose is based on clearance. After multiple IV dosing, the maintenance dose required is based on $CL$, $C_{ss}$, and $\tau$.

$$C_{SS} = \frac{\text{Dose}}{\tau CL}$$

$$\text{Dose} = C_{SS} \tau CL$$

If $C_{ss}$ and $\tau$ are fixed, a drug with a smaller clearance requires a smaller maintenance dose. In practice, the dosing interval is adjustable and may be longer for drugs with a small $CL$ if the drug does not need to be dosed frequently. The steady-state drug level is generally determined by the desired therapeutic drug.

*Does a loading dose significantly affect the steady-state concentration of a drug given by a constant multiple-dose regimen?*

■ The loading dose will affect only the initial drug concentrations in the body. Steady-state drug levels are obtained after several terminal half-lives (eg, $4.32t_{1/2}$ for 95% steady-state level). Only 5% of the drug contributed by the loading dose will remain at 95% steady state. At 99% steady-state level, only 1% of the loading dose will remain.

## Learning Questions

1. $V_D = 0.20(50 \text{ kg}) = 10,000 \text{ mL}$

a. $D_{max} = \dfrac{D_0}{1-f} = \dfrac{50 \text{ mg}}{1-e^{-(0.693/2)(8)}} = 53.3 \text{ mg}$

$C_{max} = \dfrac{D_{max}}{V_D} = \dfrac{53.3 \text{ mg}}{10,000 \text{ mL}} = 5.33 \ \mu\text{g/mL}$

b. $D_{min} = 53.3 - 50 = 3.3 \text{ mg}$

$C_{min} = \dfrac{3.3 \text{ mg}}{10,000 \text{ mL}} = 0.33 \ \mu\text{g/mL}$

c. $C_{av}^{\infty} = \dfrac{FD_0 1.44t_{1/2}}{V_D \tau}$

$= \dfrac{(50)(1.44)(2)}{(10,000)(8)} = 1.8 \ \mu\text{g/mL}$

**2. a.** $D_0 = \dfrac{C_{av}^{\infty} V_D \tau}{1.44 t_{1/2}}$

$= \dfrac{(10)(40,000)(6)}{(1.44)(5)}$

$= 333$ mg every 6 h

**b.** $\tau = \dfrac{FD_0 1.44 t_{1/2}}{V_D C_{av}^{\infty}}$

$= \dfrac{(225,000)(1.44)(5)}{(40,000)(10)} = 4.05$ h

**6.** Dose the patient with 200 mg every 3 hours.

$D_L = \dfrac{D_0}{1 - e^{-k\tau}} = \dfrac{200}{1 - e^{-(0.23)(3)}} = 400$ mg

Notice that $D_L$ is twice the maintenance dose, because the drug is given at a dosage interval equal approximately to the $t_{1/2}$ of 3 hours.

**8.** The plasma drug concentration, $C_p$, may be calculated at any time after $n$ doses by Equation 17.21 and proper substitution.

$C_p = \dfrac{D_0}{V_D} \left( \dfrac{1 - e^{-nk\tau}}{1 - e^{-k\tau}} \right) e^{-kt}$

$C_p = \dfrac{200}{40} \left( \dfrac{1 - e^{-(3)(0.347)(4)}}{1 - e^{-(0.347)(4)}} \right) e^{-(0.347)(1)}$

$= 4.63$ mg/L

Alternatively, one may conclude that for a drug whose terminal $t_{1/2}$ is 2 hours, the predicted plasma drug concentration is approximately at steady state after 3 doses or 12 hours. Therefore, the above calculation may be simplified to the following:

$C_p = \dfrac{D_0}{V_D} \left( \dfrac{1}{1 - e^{-k\tau}} \right) e^{-k\tau}$

$C_p = \left( \dfrac{200}{40} \right) \left( \dfrac{1}{1 - e^{-(0.347)(4)}} \right) e^{-(0.347)(1)}$

$= 4.71$ mg/L

**9.** $C_{max}^{\infty} = \dfrac{D_0 / V_D}{1 - e^{-k\tau}}$

where

$V_D = 20\%$ of 82 kg $= (0.2)(82) = 16.4$ L

$k = (0.693/3) = 0.231$ h$^{-1}$

$D_0 = V_D C_{max}^{\infty} (1 - e^{-k\tau}) = (16.4)(10)(1 - e^{-(0.231)(8)})$

**a.** $D_0 = 138.16$ mg to be given every 8 hours

**b.** $C_{min}^{\infty} = C_{max}^{\infty} (e^{-k\tau}) = (10)(e^{-(0.231)(8)})$

$= 1.58$ mg/L

**c.** $C_{av}^{\infty} = \dfrac{D_0}{kV_D \tau} = \dfrac{138.16}{(0.231)(16.4)(8)}$

$= 4.56$ mg/L

**d.** In the above dosage regimen, the $C_{min}^{\infty}$ of 1.59 mg/L is below the desired $C_{min}^{\infty}$ of 2 mg/L. Alternatively, the dosage interval, $\tau$, could be changed to 6 hours.

$D_0 = V_D C_{max}^{\infty} (1 - e^{-k\tau}) = (16.4)(10)(1 - e^{-(0.231)(6)})$

$D_0 = 123$ mg to be given every 6 h

$C_{min}^{\infty} = C_{max}^{\infty} (e^{-k\tau}) = (10)(e^{-(0.231)(6)}) = 2.5$ mg/L

$C_{av}^{\infty} = \dfrac{D_0}{kV_D \tau} = \dfrac{123}{(0.231)(16.4)(6)} = 5.41$ mg/L

**10. a.**    $C_{av}^{\infty} = \dfrac{FD_0}{kV_D \tau}$

Let $C_{av}^{\infty} = 27.5$ mg/L

$D_0 = \dfrac{C_{av}^{\infty} kV_D \tau}{F} = \dfrac{(27.5)(0.693/10.6)(0.5)(78)(6)}{0.77}$

$= 546.3$ mg

$D_0 = 546.3$ mg every 6 h

**b.** If a 500-mg capsule is given every 6 hours,

$C_{av}^{\infty} = \dfrac{FD_0}{kV_D \tau} = \dfrac{(0.77)(500)}{(0.693/10.6)(0.5)(78)(6)}$

$= 25.2$ mg/L

**c.** $D_L = \dfrac{D_M}{1 - e^{-k\tau}} = \dfrac{500}{1 - e^{(0.654)(6)}} = 1543$ mg

$D_L = 3 \times 500$ mg capsules $= 1500$ mg

# REFERENCES

Jefferson JW, Pradko JF, Muir KT: Bupropion for major depressive disorder: Pharmacokinetic and formulation considerations. *Clin Ther* **27**(11):1685–1695, 2005.

Kruger-Thiemer E: Pharmacokinetics and dose-concentration relationships. In Ariens EJ (ed). *Physico-Chemical Aspects of Drug Action.* New York, Pergamon, 1968, p 97.

Niebergall PJ, Sugita ET, Schnaare RC: Potential dangers of common drug dosing regimens. *Am J Hosp Pharm* **31**:53–59, 1974.

Primmett D, Levine M, Kovarik, J, Mueller E, Keown P: Cyclosporine monitoring in patients with renal transplants: Two- or three-point methods that estimate area under the curve are superior to trough levels in predicting drug exposure. *Ther Drug Monit* **20**(3):276–283, June 1998.

Sawchuk RJ, Zaske DE: Pharmacokinetics of dosing regimens which utilize multiple intravenous infusions: Gentamycin in burn patients. *J Pharmacokin Biopharm* **4**(2):183–195, 1976.

van Rossum JM, Tomey AHM: Rate of accumulation and plateau concentration of drugs after chronic medication. *J Pharm Pharmacol* **30**:390–392, 1968.

Volume II Advice for the Patient: Drug information in Lay Language (USP DI Vol II: Advice for the Patient). Thomson MICROMEDEX Physicians Desk Reference (PDR) Author

# BIBLIOGRAPHY

Gibaldi M, Perrier D: *Pharmacokinetics,* 2nd ed. New York, Marcel Dekker, 1962, pp 451–457.

Levy G: Kinetics of pharmacologic effect. *Clin Pharmacol Ther* **7**:362, 1966.

van Rossum JM: Pharmacokinetics of accumulation. *J Pharm Sci* **75**:2162–2164, 1968.

Wagner JG: Kinetics of pharmacological response, I: Proposed relationship between response and drug concentration in the intact animal and man. *J Theor Biol* **20**:173, 1968.

Wagner JG: Relations between drug concentrations and response. *J Mond Pharm* **14**:279–310, 1971.

# 18

# Nonlinear Pharmacokinetics

Leon Shargel and Murray P. Ducharme

## CHAPTER OBJECTIVES

- Compare the difference between linear pharmacokinetics and nonlinear pharmacokinetics.

- Explain why nonlinear pharmacokinetics occurs with enzyme mediated or drug carrier systems. Discuss potential risks in dosing drugs that follow nonlinear kinetics.

- Demonstrate how to detect nonlinear kinetics using AUC-versus-doses plots.

- Use the appropriate equation and graphical methods to calculate the $V_{max}$ and $K_M$ parameters after multiple dosing in a patient.

- Describe the use of the Michaelis–Menten equation to simulate the elimination of a drug by a saturable enzymatic process.

- Estimate the dose for a nonlinear drug such as phenytoin in multiple-dose regimens.

- Describe chronopharmacokinetics (time-dependent pharmacokinetics) and its influence on drug disposition.

Previous chapters discussed linear pharmacokinetic models using first-order kinetics to describe the course of drug disposition and action. These linear pharmacokinetic models assumed that the pharmacokinetic parameters for a drug does not change when different doses or multiple doses of a drug are given to the patient. For some drugs, increased doses or chronic multiple doses can cause deviations from the linear pharmacokinetic profile observed with single low doses of the same drug. This *nonlinear* pharmacokinetic behavior is also termed *dose-dependent pharmacokinetics/nonlinearity* when it is related to dose, and *time-dependent pharmacokinetics/nonlinearity* when it is related to time.

Many of the processes of drug absorption, distribution, biotransformation, and excretion involve enzymes or carrier-mediated systems. For some drugs given at therapeutic levels, one of these specialized processes may become saturated. As shown in Table 18-1, various causes of nonlinear pharmacokinetic behavior are theoretically possible. In addition to drug saturation of plasma protein–binding or carrier-mediated systems, drugs may demonstrate nonlinear pharmacokinetics due to a pathologic alteration in drug absorption, distribution, and elimination. For example, aminoglycosides may cause renal nephrotoxicity, thereby altering their own renal drug excretion. In addition, gallstone obstruction of the bile duct will alter biliary drug excretion. In these cases, the main pharmacokinetic outcome will be a change in the apparent elimination rate constant which will cause a change in the systemic exposure (AUC).

Many drugs demonstrate *saturation* or *capacity-limited metabolism/absorption*. These drugs will result in dose-dependent nonlinearity. Examples of saturable metabolic processes include glycine conjugation of salicylate, sulfate conjugation of salicylamide, acetylation of *p*-aminobenzoic acid, and the elimination of phenytoin

## TABLE 18-1 • Examples of Drugs Showing Nonlinear Kinetics

| Cause* | Drug |
|---|---|
| **GI Absorption** | |
| Saturable transport in gut wall | Riboflavin, gebapentin, L-dopa, baclofen, ceftibuten |
| Intestinal metabolism | Salicylamide, propranolol |
| Drugs with low solubility in GI given in relatively high dose | Chlorothiazide, griseofulvin, danazol |
| Saturable gastric or GI decomposition | Penicillin G, omeprazole, saquinavir |
| **Distribution** | |
| Saturable plasma protein binding | Phenylbutazone, lidocaine, salicylic acid, ceftriaxone, diazoxide, phenytoin, warfarin, disopyramide |
| Cellular uptake | Methicillin (rabbit) |
| Tissue binding | Imipramine (rat) |
| CSF transport | Benzylpenicillins |
| Saturable transport into or out of tissues | Methotrexate |
| **Renal Elimination** | |
| Active secretion | Mezlocillin, para-aminohippuric acid |
| Tubular reabsorption | Riboflavin, ascorbic acid, cephapirin |
| Change in urine pH | Salicylic acid, dextroamphetamine |
| **Metabolism** | |
| Saturable metabolism | Phenytoin, salicylic acid, theophylline, valproic acid[†] |
| Cofactor or enzyme limitation | Acetaminophen, alcohol |
| Enzyme induction | Carbamazepine |
| Altered hepatic blood flow | Propranolol, verapamil |
| Metabolite inhibition | Diazepam |
| **Biliary Excretion** | |
| Biliary secretion | Iodipamide, sulfobromophthalein sodium |
| Enterohepatic recycling | Cimetidine, isotretinoin |

*Hypothermia, metabolic acidosis, altered cardiovascular function, and coma are additional causes of dose and time dependencies in drug overdose.
[†]In guinea pig and probably in some younger subjects.
Data from Evans WE, Schentag JJ, Jusko WJ: Applied Pharmacokinetics, 3rd ed, Vancouver, WA: Applied Therapeutics; 1992.

(Tozer et al, 1981). Levodopa is an example of a drug that displays saturable absorption. Drugs that demonstrate saturation kinetics may show the following characteristics:

1. Elimination or absorption of drug does not follow simple first-order kinetics—that is, the elimination or absorption kinetics are nonlinear and may be a combination of zero-order and first-order processes.

2. The elimination or absorption half-lives change as doses are increased. The half-life increases with increased dose due to saturation of an enzyme/transporter system important for drug elimination or absorption.

3. The area under the curve (AUC) does not increase in a proportional manner to the administered dose of the drug.

4. The saturation or capacity-limited processes may be affected by other drugs that require the same enzyme or carrier-mediated system (eg, competition effects).

5. The composition and/or ratio of the metabolites of a drug may be affected by a change in the dose.

Some drugs will display nonlinearity that is dependent on time, instead of on the dose. Carbamazepine is an example of such a drug. By inducing its own metabolism and transport over time (induction of CYP3A enzymes and P-gp transporters) (Owen et al, 2006; Lutz et al, 2018) Carbamazepine dosing regimens have to be changed over time, by giving the drug more frequently in order to have the same effective systemic exposure. Dosing regimens are typically started by administering the drug twice a day, and after a few weeks, the drug is given three times a day and finally four times a day in order to keep the systemic exposure within the therapeutic range.

The prediction of plasma drug concentration, whether for the first dose or for an adjusted dosing regimen, is difficult for drugs with dose-dependent nonlinearity. Drug concentrations in the blood can increase rapidly once an elimination process is saturated. In general, metabolism (biotransformation) in the liver and active tubular secretion by the kidney are the processes most often saturated.

Figure 18-1 shows plasma level–time curves for two drugs given by IV bolus injection that are described by a one-compartment pharmacokinetic model. Curves A and B is for a drug that demonstrates *saturable* kinetics at a higher dose. When a large dose is given, the plasma level–time shows an initial slow elimination phase followed by a much more rapid elimination phase at lower blood concentrations (Curve A). The initial slow decline of drug concentrations in Curve A is due to saturation of an elimination process; as the drug concentration declines, the elimination process is no longer saturated and a first-order elimination resembling the same elimination half-life as Curve B. Curve C is for a drug that follow nonlinear kinetics at all dose levels.

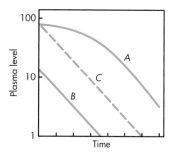

FIGURE 18-1 • Plasma level–time curves for a drug that exhibits a saturable elimination process. Curves A and B represent high and low doses of drug, respectively, given in a single IV bolus. The terminal slopes of curves A and B are the same. Curve C represents the normal first-order elimination of a different drug.

After a small dose of the drug is given, apparent first-order kinetics are observed, because no saturation kinetics occur (curve B). If the pharmacokinetic data were estimated only from the blood levels described by curve B, then a 2-fold increase in the dose would give the blood profile presented in curve C, which considerably underestimates the drug concentration as well as the duration of action.

To determine whether a drug is following dose-dependent kinetics, the drug is given at various dosage levels, and a plasma level–time curve is obtained for each dose. The curves should exhibit parallel slopes if the drug follows dose-independent kinetics. Alternatively, a plot of the areas under the plasma level–time curves at various doses should be linear (Fig. 18-2).

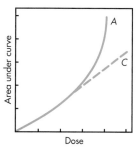

FIGURE 18-2 • Area under the plasma level–time curve versus dose for a drug that exhibits a saturable elimination process. Curve A represents dose-dependent or saturable elimination kinetics. Curve C represents dose-independent kinetics.

## SATURABLE ENZYME ELIMINATION PROCESSES

The elimination of drug by a saturable enzymatic process can be described by *Michaelis–Menten kinetics*.

$$\text{Elimination rate} = \frac{dC_p}{dt} = \frac{V_{max}C_p}{K_M + C_p} \quad (18.1)$$

where $C_p$ is the concentration of drug in the plasma, $V_{max}$ is the maximum elimination rate, and $K_M$ is the Michaelis constant that reflects the *capacity* of the enzyme system. $K_M$ is not an elimination constant but is actually a hybrid rate constant in enzyme kinetics, representing both the forward and backward reaction rates. $K_M$ is equal to the drug concentration or amount of drug in the body at $0.5V_{max}$. The values for $K_M$ and $V_{max}$ are dependent on the nature of the drug and the enzymatic process involved.

The elimination rate of a hypothetical drug with a $K_M$ of 0.1 $\mu$g/mL and a $V_{max}$ of 0.5 $\mu$g/mL per hour is calculated in Table 18-2 by using Equation 18.1.

### TABLE 18-2 • Effect of Drug Concentration on the Elimination Rate and Rate Constant*

| Drug Concentration ($\mu$g/mL) | Elimination Rate ($\mu$g/mL/h) | Elimination Rate/ Concentration† ($h^{-1}$) |
|---|---|---|
| 0.4 | 0.400 | 1.000 |
| 0.8 | 0.444 | 0.556 |
| 1.2 | 0.462 | 0.385 |
| 1.6 | 0.472 | 0.294 |
| 2.0 | 0.476 | 0.238 |
| 2.4 | 0.480 | 0.200 |
| 2.8 | 0.483 | 0.172 |
| 3.2 | 0.485 | 0.152 |
| 10.0 | 0.495 | 0.0495 |
| 10.4 | 0.495 | 0.0476 |
| 10.8 | 0.495 | 0.0459 |
| 11.2 | 0.496 | 0.0442 |
| 11.6 | 0.496 | 0.0427 |

*$K_M = 0.1$ $\mu$g/mL, $V_{max} = 0.5$ $\mu$g/mL/h.
†The ratio of the elimination rate to the concentration is equal to the rate constant.

Because the ratio of the elimination rate to drug concentration changes as the drug concentration changes (ie, $dC_p/dt$ is not constant, Equation 18.1), the rate of drug elimination also changes and is not a first-order or linear process. A first-order elimination process would yield the same elimination rate constant at all plasma drug concentrations. At drug concentrations of 0.4–10 $\mu$g/mL, the enzyme system is not saturated, and the rate of elimination is a mixed or nonlinear process (Table 18-2). At higher drug concentrations, 10.0 $\mu$g/mL and above, the elimination rate approaches the maximum velocity ($V_{max}$) of approximately 0.5 (0.496) $\mu$g/mL per hour. At $V_{max}$, the elimination rate is a constant and is considered a zero-order process.

Equation 18.1 describes a nonlinear enzyme process that encompasses a broad range of drug concentrations. When the drug concentration $C_p$ is large in relation to $K_M$ ($C_p \gg K_M$), saturation of the enzymes occurs and the value for $K_M$ is negligible. The rate of elimination proceeds at a fixed or constant rate equal to $V_{max}$. The elimination of drug becomes a zero-order process and Equation 18.1 becomes:

$$-\frac{dC_p}{dt} = \frac{V_{max}C_p}{C_p} = V_{max} \quad (18.2)$$

### PRACTICE PROBLEM

Using the hypothetical drug considered in Table 18-2 ($V_{max} = 0.5$ $\mu$g/mL per hour, $K_M = 0.1$ $\mu$g/mL), how long would it take for the plasma drug concentration to decrease from 20 to 12 $\mu$g/mL?

### Solution

Because 12 $\mu$g/mL is above the saturable level, as indicated in Table 18-2, elimination occurs at a zero-order rate of approximately 0.5 $\mu$g/mL per hour.

Time needed for the drug to decrease to

$$12 \ \mu g/mL = \frac{20 - 12 \ \mu g}{0.5 \ \mu g/h} = 16 \ h$$

A saturable process can also exhibit linear elimination when drug concentrations are much less than enzyme concentrations. When the drug concentration $C_p$ is small in relation to the $K_M$, the rate of drug elimination becomes a first-order process. The data generated from Equation 18.2 ($C_p \leq 0.05\ \mu g/mL$, Table 18-3) using $K_M = 0.8\ \mu g/mL$ and $V_{max} = 0.9\ \mu g/mL$ per hour shows that enzymatic drug elimination can change from a nonlinear to a linear process over a restricted concentration range. This is evident because the rate constant (or elimination rate/drug concentration) values are constant. At drug concentrations below 0.05 $\mu g/mL$, the ratio of elimination rate to drug concentration has a constant value of 1.1 $h^{-1}$. Mathematically, when $C_p$ is much smaller than $K_M$, $C_p$ in the denominator is negligible and the elimination rate becomes first order.

$$-\frac{dC_p}{dt} = \frac{V_{max}\,C_p}{C_p + K_M} = \frac{V_{max}}{K_M}\,C_p$$

$$-\frac{dC_p}{dt} = k'C_p$$ 

(18.3)

The first-order rate constant for a saturable process, $k'$, can be calculated from Equation 18.3:

$$k' = \frac{V_{max}}{K_M} = \frac{0.9}{0.8} = 1.1\ h^{-1}$$

This calculation confirms the data in Table 18-3, because enzymatic drug elimination at drug concentrations below 0.05 $\mu g/mL$ resembles a first-order rate process with a rate constant of 1.1 $h^{-1}$. Therefore, the $t_{1/2}$ due to enzymatic elimination can be calculated:

$$t_{1/2} = \frac{0.693}{1.1} = 0.63\ h$$

## PRACTICE PROBLEM

How long would it take for the plasma concentration of the drug in Table 18-3 to decline from 0.05 to 0.005 $\mu g/mL$?

### Solution

Drug elimination approximates a first-order process for the specified concentrations,

$$C_p = C_p^0 e^{-kt}$$

$$\log C_p = C_p^0 - \frac{kt}{2.3}$$

$$t = \frac{\log C - \log C_p^0}{k}$$

$C_p^0 = 0.05\ \mu g/mL$, $k = 1.1\ h^{-1}$, and $C_p = 0.005\ \mu g/mL$.

$$t = \frac{2.3\,(\log 0.05 - \log 0.005)}{1.1}$$

$$= \frac{2.3\,(-1.30 + 2.3)}{1.1}$$

$$= \frac{2.3}{1.1} = 2.09\ h$$

When given in therapeutic doses, most drugs produce plasma drug concentrations well below $K_M$ for carrier-mediated enzyme systems affecting the pharmacokinetics of the drug. Therefore, most drugs at normal therapeutic concentrations follow first-order rate processes. Only a few drugs, such as salicylate and phenytoin, tend to saturate hepatic enzyme activity at higher therapeutic doses. With these drugs, elimination kinetics is first order with very small doses, is mixed order at higher doses, and may approach zero order with very high therapeutic doses.

| **TABLE 18-3** • Effect of Drug Concentration on the Elimination Rate and Rate Constant* | | |
|---|---|---|
| **Drug Concentration ($C_p$) ($\mu g/mL$)** | **Elimination Rate ($\mu g/mL/h$)** | **Elimination Rate Concentration ($h^{-1}$)†** |
| 0.01 | 0.011 | 1.1 |
| 0.02 | 0.022 | 1.1 |
| 0.03 | 0.033 | 1.1 |
| 0.04 | 0.043 | 1.1 |
| 0.05 | 0.053 | 1.1 |
| 0.06 | 0.063 | 1.0 |
| 0.07 | 0.072 | 1.0 |
| 0.08 | 0.082 | 1.0 |
| 0.09 | 0.091 | 1.0 |

*$K_M = 0.8\ \mu g/mL$, $V_{max} = 0.9\ \mu g/mL/h$.
†The ratio of the elimination rate to the concentration is equal to the rate constant.

## DRUG ELIMINATION BY CAPACITY-LIMITED PHARMACOKINETICS: ONE-COMPARTMENT MODEL, IV BOLUS INJECTION

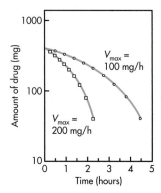

FIGURE 18-3 • Amount of drug in the body versus time for a capacity-limited drug following an IV dose. Data generated using $V_{max}$ of 100 (O) and 200 mg/h (□). $K_M$ is kept constant.

The rate of elimination of a drug that follows capacity-limited pharmacokinetics is governed by the $V_{max}$ and $K_M$ of the drug. Equation 18.1 describes the elimination of a drug that distributes in the body as a single compartment and is eliminated by Michaelis–Menten or capacity-limited pharmacokinetics. If a single IV bolus injection of drug ($D_0$) is given at $t = 0$, the drug concentration ($C_p$) in the plasma at any time $t$ may be calculated by an integrated form of Equation 18.1 described by

$$\frac{C_0 - C_p}{t} = V_{max} - \frac{K_M}{t} \ln \frac{C_0}{C_p} \qquad (18.4)$$

Alternatively, the amount of drug in the body after an IV bolus injection may be calculated by the following relationship. Equation 18.5 may be used to simulate the decline of drug in the body after various size doses are given, provided the $K_M$ and $V_{max}$ of drug are known.

$$\frac{D_0 - D_t}{t} = V_{max} - \frac{K_M}{t} \ln \frac{D_0}{D_t} \qquad (18.5)$$

where $D_0$ is the amount of drug in the body at $t = 0$. In order to calculate the time for the dose of the drug to decline to a certain amount of drug in the body, Equation 18.5 must be rearranged and solved for time $t$:

$$t = \frac{1}{V_{max}} \left( D_0 - D_t + K_M \ln \frac{D_0}{D_t} \right) \qquad (18.6)$$

The relationship of $K_M$ and $V_{max}$ to the time for an IV bolus injection of drug to decline to a given

amount of drug in the body is illustrated in Figs. 18-3 and 18-4. Using Equation 18.6, the time for a single 400-mg dose given by IV bolus injection to decline to 20 mg was calculated for a drug with a $K_M$ of 38 mg/L and a $V_{max}$ that varied from 200 to 100 mg/h (Table 18-4). With a $V_{max}$ of 200 mg/h, the time for the 400-mg dose to decline to 20 mg in the body is 2.46 hours, whereas when the $V_{max}$ is decreased to 100 mg/h, the time for the 400-mg dose to decrease to 20 mg is increased to 4.93 hours (see Fig. 18-3). Thus, there is an inverse relationship between the time for the dose to decline to a certain amount of drug in the body and the $V_{max}$ as shown in Equation 18.6.

Using a similar example, the effect of $K_M$ on the time for a single 400-mg dose given by IV bolus injection to decline to 20 mg in the body

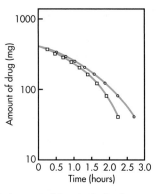

FIGURE 18-4 • Amount of drug in the body versus time for a capacity-limited drug following an IV dose. Data generated using $K_M$ of 38 mg/L (□) and 76 mg/L (O). $V_{max}$ is kept constant.

## TABLE 18-4 • Capacity-Limited Pharmacokinetics: Effect of $V_{max}$ on the Elimination of Drug*

| Amount of Drug in Body (mg) | Time for Drug Elimination (h) | |
|---|---|---|
| | $V_{max} = 200$ mg/h | $V_{max} = 100$ mg/h |
| 400 | 0 | 0 |
| 380 | 0.109 | 0.219 |
| 360 | 0.220 | 0.440 |
| 340 | 0.330 | 0.661 |
| 320 | 0.442 | 0.884 |
| 300 | 0.554 | 1.10 |
| 280 | 0.667 | 1.33 |
| 260 | 0.781 | 1.56 |
| 240 | 0.897 | 1.79 |
| 220 | 1.01 | 2.02 |
| 200 | 1.13 | 2.26 |
| 180 | 1.25 | 2.50 |
| 160 | 1.37 | 2.74 |
| 140 | 1.49 | 2.99 |
| 120 | 1.62 | 3.25 |
| 100 | 1.76 | 3.52 |
| 80 | 1.90 | 3.81 |
| 60 | 2.06 | 4.12 |
| 40 | 2.23 | 4.47 |
| 20 | 2.46 | 4.93 |

*A single 400-mg dose is given by IV bolus injection. The drug is distributed into a single compartment and is eliminated by capacity-limited pharmacokinetics. $K_M$ is 38 mg/L. The time for drug to decline from 400 to 20 mg is calculated from Equation 18.6 assuming the drug has $V_{max} = 200$ mg/h or $V_{max} = 100$ mg/h.

## TABLE 18-5 • Capacity-Limited Pharmacokinetics: Effects of $K_M$ on the Elimination of Drug*

| Amount of Drug in Body (mg) | Time for Drug Elimination (h) | |
|---|---|---|
| | $K_M = 38$ mg/L | $K_M = 76$ mg/L |
| 400 | 0 | 0 |
| 380 | 0.109 | 0.119 |
| 360 | 0.220 | 0.240 |
| 340 | 0.330 | 0.361 |
| 320 | 0.442 | 0.484 |
| 300 | 0.554 | 0.609 |
| 280 | 0.667 | 0.735 |
| 260 | 0.781 | 0.863 |
| 240 | 0.897 | 0.994 |
| 220 | 1.01 | 1.12 |
| 200 | 1.13 | 1.26 |
| 180 | 1.25 | 1.40 |
| 160 | 1.37 | 1.54 |
| 140 | 1.49 | 1.69 |
| 120 | 1.62 | 1.85 |
| 100 | 1.76 | 2.02 |
| 80 | 1.90 | 2.21 |
| 60 | 2.06 | 2.42 |
| 40 | 2.23 | 2.67 |
| 20 | 2.46 | 3.03 |

*A single 400-mg dose is given by IV bolus injection. The drug is distributed into a single compartment and is eliminated by capacity-limited pharmacokinetics. $V_{max}$ is 200 mg/h. The time for drug to decline from 400 to 20 mg is calculated from Equation 18.6 assuming the drug has $K_M = 38$ mg/L or $K_M = 76$ mg/L.

is described in Table 18-5 and Fig. 18-4. Assuming $V_{max}$ is constant at 200 mg/h, the time for the drug to decline from 400 to 20 mg is 2.46 hours when $K_M$ is 38 mg/L, whereas when $K_M$ is 76 mg/L, the time for the drug dose to decline to 20 mg is 3.03 hours. Thus, an increase in $K_M$ (with no change in $V_{max}$) will increase the time for the drug to be eliminated from the body.

The one-compartment open model with capacity-limited elimination pharmacokinetics adequately describes the plasma drug concentration–time profiles for some drugs. The mathematics needed to describe nonlinear pharmacokinetic behavior of drugs that follow two-compartment or more complex models need to be solved by a computer. A one-compartment model is often utilized for quick calculations when computer software is not readily available.

## PRACTICE PROBLEMS

1. A drug eliminated from the body by capacity-limited pharmacokinetics has a $K_M$ of 100 mg/L and a $V_{max}$ of 50 mg/h. If 400 mg of the drug is given to a patient by IV bolus injection, calculate the time for the drug to be 50% eliminated. If 320 mg of the drug is to be given by IV bolus injection, calculate the time for 50% of the dose to be eliminated. Explain why there is a difference in the time for 50% elimination of a 400-mg dose compared to a 320-mg dose.

### Solution

Use Equation 18.6 to calculate the time for the dose to decline to a given amount of drug in the body. For this problem, $D_t$ is equal to 50% of the dose $D_0$.

If the dose is 400 mg,

$$t = \frac{1}{50}\left(400 - 200 + 100\ln\frac{400}{200}\right) = 5.39 \text{ h}$$

If the dose is 320 mg,

$$t = \frac{1}{50}\left(320 - 160 + 100\ln\frac{320}{160}\right) = 4.59 \text{ h}$$

For capacity-limited elimination, the elimination half-life is dose dependent, because the drug elimination process is partially saturated. Therefore, small changes in the dose will produce large differences in the time for 50% drug elimination. The parameters $K_M$ and $V_{max}$ determine when the dose is saturated.

2. Using the same drug as in Problem 1, calculate the time for 50% elimination of the dose when the doses are 10 and 5 mg. Explain why the times for 50% drug elimination are similar even though the dose is reduced by one-half.

### Solution

As in Practice Problem 1, use Equation 18.6 to calculate the time for the amount of drug in the body at zero time ($D_0$) to decline 50%.

If the dose is 10 mg,

$$t = \frac{1}{50}\left(10 - 5 + \ln\frac{10}{5}\right) = 1.49 \text{ h}$$

If the dose is 5 mg,

$$t = \frac{1}{50}\left(5 - 2.5 + 100\ln\frac{5}{2.5}\right) = 1.44 \text{ h}$$

Whether the patient is given a 10-mg or a 5-mg dose by IV bolus injection, the times for the amount of drug to decline 50% are approximately the same. For 10- and 5-mg doses, the amount of drug in the body is much less than the $K_M$ of 100 mg. Therefore, the amount of drug in the body is well below saturation of the elimination process and the drug declines at a first-order rate.

## Determination of $K_M$ and $V_{max}$

Equation 18.1 relates the rate of drug biotransformation to the concentration of the drug in the body. The same equation may be applied to determine the rate of enzymatic reaction of a drug *in vitro* (Equation 18.7). When an experiment is performed with solutions of various concentration of drug $C$, a series of reaction rates ($v$) may be measured for each concentration. Special plots may then be used to determine $K_M$ and $V_{max}$.

Equation 18.7 may be rearranged into Equation 18.8.

$$v = \frac{V_{max}C}{K_M + C} \tag{18.7}$$

$$\frac{1}{v} = \frac{K_M}{V_{max}}\frac{1}{C} + \frac{1}{V_{max}} \tag{18.8}$$

Equation 18.8 is a linear equation when $1/v$ is plotted against $1/C$. The $y$ intercept for the line is $1/V_{max}$, and the slope is $K_M/V_{max}$. An example of a drug reacting enzymatically with rate ($v$) at various concentrations $C$ is shown in Table 18-6 and Fig. 18-5. A plot of $1/v$ versus $1/C$ is shown in Fig. 18-6. A plot of $1/v$ versus $1/C$ is linear with an intercept of 0.33 mmol. Therefore,

$$\frac{1}{V_{max}} = 0.33 \text{ min} \cdot \text{mL}/\mu\text{mol}$$

$$V_{max} = 3 \ \mu\text{mol}/\text{mL} \cdot \text{min}$$

| TABLE 18-6 • Information Necessary for Graphic Determination of $V_{max}$ and $K_M$ | | | | |
|---|---|---|---|---|
| Observation Number | C (µM/mL) | V (µM/mL/min) | 1/V (mL/min/µM) | 1/C (mL/µM) |
| 1 | 1 | 0.500 | 2.000 | 1.000 |
| 2 | 6 | 1.636 | 0.611 | 0.166 |
| 3 | 11 | 2.062 | 0.484 | 0.090 |
| 4 | 16 | 2.285 | 0.437 | 0.062 |
| 5 | 21 | 2.423 | 0.412 | 0.047 |
| 6 | 26 | 2.516 | 0.397 | 0.038 |
| 7 | 31 | 2.583 | 0.337 | 0.032 |
| 8 | 36 | 2.63 | 0.379 | 0.027 |
| 9 | 41 | 2.673 | 0.373 | 0.024 |
| 10 | 46 | 2.705 | 0.369 | 0.021 |

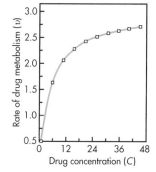

FIGURE 18-5 • Plot of rate of drug metabolism at various drug concentrations. ($K_M = 0.5$ µmol/mL, $V_{max} = 3$ µmol/mL/min.)

the slope = 1.65 = $K_M/V_{max}$ = $K_M/3$ or $K_M = 3 \times 1.65$ µ mol/mL = 5 µ mol/mL. Alternatively, $K_M$ may be found from the x intercept, where $-1/K_M$ is equal to the x intercept. (This may be seen by extending the graph to intercept the x axis in the negative region.)

With this plot (Fig. 18-6), the points are clustered. Other methods are available that may spread the points more evenly. These methods are derived from rearranging Equation 18.8 into Equations 18.9 and 18.10.

$$\frac{C}{v} = \frac{1}{V_{max}}C + \frac{K_M}{V_{max}} \qquad (18.9)$$

$$v = -K_M\frac{v}{C} + V_{max} \qquad (18.10)$$

A plot of $C/v$ versus $C$ would yield a straight line with $1/V_{max}$ as slope and $K_M/V_{max}$ as intercept (Equation 18.9). A plot of $v$ versus $v/C$ would yield a slope of $-K_M$ and an intercept of $V_{max}$ (Equation 18.10).

The necessary calculations for making the above plots are shown in Table 18-7. The plots are shown in Figs. 18-7 and 18-8. It should be noted that the data are spread out better by the two latter plots. Calculations from the slope show that the same $K_M$ and $V_{max}$ are obtained as in Fig. 18-6. When the data are more scattered, one method may be more accurate than the other. A simple approach is to graph the data and examine the linearity of the graphs. The same basic type of plot is used in the clinical literature to

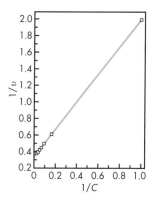

FIGURE 18-6 • Plot of 1/v versus 1/C for determining $K_M$ and $V_{max}$.

**TABLE 18-7** • Calculations Necessary for Graphic Determination of $K_M$ and $V_{max}$

| C (µM/mL) | V (µM/mL/min) | C/V (min) | V/C (1/min) |
|---|---|---|---|
| 1 | 0.500 | 2.000 | 0.500 |
| 6 | 1.636 | 3.666 | 0.272 |
| 11 | 2.062 | 5.333 | 0.187 |
| 16 | 2.285 | 7.000 | 0.142 |
| 21 | 2.423 | 8.666 | 0.115 |
| 26 | 2.516 | 10.333 | 0.096 |
| 31 | 2.583 | 12.000 | 0.083 |
| 36 | 2.634 | 13.666 | 0.073 |
| 41 | 2.673 | 15.333 | 0.065 |
| 46 | 2.705 | 17.000 | 0.058 |

determine $K_M$ and $V_{max}$ for individual patients for drugs that undergo capacity-limited kinetics.

### Determination of $K_M$ and $V_{max}$ in Patients

Equation 18.7 shows that the rate of drug metabolism ($v$) is dependent on the concentration of the drug ($C$). This same basic concept may be applied to the rate of drug metabolism of a capacity-limited drug in the body. The body may be regarded as a single compartment in which the drug is dissolved. The rate of drug metabolism will vary depending on the concentration of drug $C_p$ as well as on the metabolic rate constants $K_M$ and $V_{max}$ of the drug in each individual.

An example for the determination of $K_M$ and $V_{max}$ is given for the drug phenytoin. Phenytoin undergoes capacity-limited kinetics at therapeutic drug concentrations in the body. To determine $K_M$

and $V_{max}$, two different dose regimens are given at different times, until steady state is reached. The steady-state plasma drug concentrations are then measured by assay. At steady state, the rate of drug metabolism ($v$) is assumed to be the same as the rate of drug input $R$ (dose/day). Therefore, Equation 18.11 may be written for the rate of drug metabolism in the body (Equation 18.7). Steady state will not be reached if the drug input rate, $R$, is greater than the $V_{max}$ and drug accumulation will continue to occur without reaching a steady-state plateau.

$$R = \frac{V_{max} C_{ss}}{K_M + C_{ss}} \qquad (18.11)$$

where $R$ = dose/day or dosing rate, $C_{ss}$ = steady-state plasma drug concentration, $V_{max}$ = maximum metabolic rate constant in the body, and $K_M$ = Michaelis–Menten constant of the drug in the body.

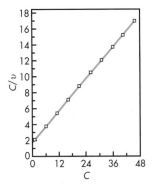

FIGURE 18-7 • Plot of $C/v$ versus $C$ for determining $K_M$ and $V_{max}$.

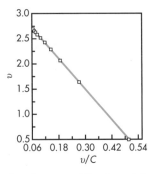

FIGURE 18-8 • Plot of $v$ versus $v/C$ for determining $K_M$ and $V_{max}$.

## EXAMPLE ▷ ▷ ▷

Phenytoin was administered to a patient at dosing rates of 150 and 300 mg/d, respectively. The steady-state plasma drug concentrations were 8.6 and 25.1 mg/L, respectively. Find the $K_M$ and $V_{max}$ of this patient. What dose is needed to achieve a steady-state plasma drug concentration of 11.3 mg/L?

### SOLUTION

There are three methods for solving this problem, all based on the same basic equation (Equation 18.11).

### Method A

Inverting Equation 18.11 on both sides yields

$$\frac{1}{R} = \frac{K_M}{V_{max}} \frac{1}{C_{ss}} + \frac{1}{V_{max}} \qquad (18.12)$$

Multiply both sides by $C_{ss} V_{max}$,

$$\frac{V_{max} C_{ss}}{R} = K_M + C_{ss}$$

Rearranging

$$C_{ss} = \frac{V_{max} C_{ss}}{R} - K_M \qquad (18.13)$$

A plot of $C_{ss}$ versus $C_{ss}/R$ is shown in Fig. 18-9. $V_{max}$ is equal to the slope, 630 mg/d, and $K_M$ is found from the $y$ intercept, 27.6 mg/L (note the negative intercept).

### Method B

From Equation 18.11,

$$RK_M + RC_{ss} = V_{max} C_{ss}$$

Dividing both sides by $C_{ss}$ yields

$$R = V_{max} - \frac{K_M R}{C_{ss}} \qquad (18.14)$$

A plot of $R$ versus $R/C_{ss}$ is shown in Fig. 18-10. The $K_M$ and $V_{max}$ found are similar to those calculated by the previous method (Fig. 18-9).

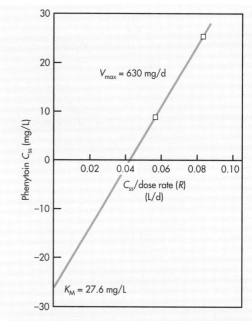

FIGURE 18-9 • Plot of $C_{ss}$ versus $C_{ss}/R$ (method A). (Reproduced with permission from Witmer DR, Ritschel WA. Phenytoin-isoniazid interaction: a kinetic approach to management. Drug Intell Clin Pharm. 1984 Jun;18(6):483–486.)

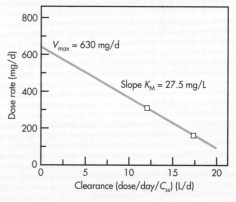

FIGURE 18-10 • Plot of $R$ versus $R/C_{ss}$ or clearance (method B). (Reproduced with permission from Witmer DR, Ritschel WA. Phenytoin-isoniazid interaction: a kinetic approach to management. Drug Intell Clin Pharm. 1984 Jun;18(6):483–486.)

### Method C

A plot of $R$ versus $C_{ss}$ is shown in Fig. 18-11. To determine $K_M$ and $V_{max}$:

1. Mark points for $R$ of 300 mg/d and $C_{ss}$ of 25.1 mg/L as shown. Connect with a straight line.
2. Mark points for $R$ of 150 mg/d and $C_{ss}$ of 8.6 mg/L as shown. Connect with a straight line.

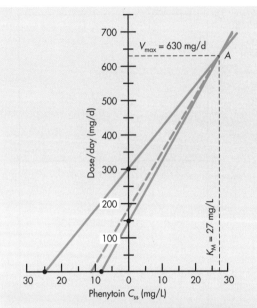

**FIGURE 18-11** • Plot of R versus $C_{ss}$ (method C). (Reproduced with permission from Witmer DR, Ritschel WA. Phenytoin-isoniazid interaction: a kinetic approach to management. *Drug Intell Clin Pharm.* 1984 Jun;18(6):483–486.)

3. The point where lines from the first two steps cross is called point A.
4. From point A, read $V_{max}$ on the y axis and $K_M$ on the x axis. (Again, $V_{max}$ of 630 mg/d and $K_M$ of 27 mg/L are found.)

This $V_{max}$ and $K_M$ can be used in Equation 18.11 to find an R to produce the desired $C_{ss}$ of 11.3 mg/L. Alternatively, join point A on the graph to meet 11.3 mg/L on the x axis; R can be read where this line meets the y axis (190 mg/d).

To calculate the dose needed to keep steady-state phenytoin concentration of 11.3 mg/L in this patient, use Equation 18.7.

$$R = \frac{(630 \text{ mg/d})(11.3 \text{ mg/L})}{27 \text{ mg/L} + 11.3 \text{ mg/L}}$$

$$= \frac{7119}{38.3} = 186 \text{ mg/d}$$

This answer compares very closely with the value obtained by the graphic method. All three methods have been used clinically. Vozeh et al (1981) introduced a method that allows for an estimation of phenytoin dose based on steady-state concentration resulting from one dose. This method is based on a statistically compiled nomogram that makes it possible to project a most likely dose for the patient.

### Determination of $K_M$ and $V_{max}$ by Direct Method

When steady-state concentrations of phenytoin are known at only two dose levels, there is no advantage in using the graphical method. $K_M$ and $V_{max}$ may be calculated by solving two simultaneous equations formed by substituting $C_{ss}$ and R (Equation 18.11) with $C_1$, $R_1$, $C_2$, and $R_2$. The equations contain two unknowns, $K_M$ and $V_{max}$, and may be solved easily.

$$R_1 = \frac{V_{max} C_1}{K_M + C_1}$$

$$R_2 = \frac{V_{max} C_2}{K_M + C_2}$$

Combining the two equations yields Equation 18.15.

$$K_M = \frac{R_2 - R_1}{(R_1/C_1) - (R_2/C_2)} \qquad (18.15)$$

where $C_1$ is steady-state plasma drug concentration after dose 1, $C_2$ is steady-state plasma drug concentration after dose 2, $R_1$ is the first dosing rate, and $R_2$ is the second dosing rate. To calculate $K_M$ and $V_{max}$, use Equation 18.15 with the values $C_1 = 8.6$ mg/L, $C_2 = 25.1$ mg/L, $R_1 = 150$ mg/d, and $R_2 = 300$ mg/d. The results are

$$K_M = \frac{300 - 150}{(150/8.6) - (300/25.1)} = 27.3 \text{ mg/L}$$

Substitute $K_M$ into either of the two simultaneous equations to solve for $V_{max}$.

$$150 = \frac{V_{max}(8.6)}{27.3 + 8.6}$$

$$V_{max} = 626 \text{ mg/d}$$

### Interpretation of $K_M$ and $V_{max}$

An understanding of Michaelis–Menten kinetics provides insight into the nonlinear kinetics and helps avoid dosing a drug at a concentration near enzyme saturation. In the above phenytoin dosing example, since $K_M$ occurs at $0.5 V_{max}$, $K_M = 27.3$ mg/L, implying that at a plasma drug concentration of 27.3 mg/L, enzymes responsible for phenytoin metabolism are eliminating the drug at 50% $V_{max}$, that

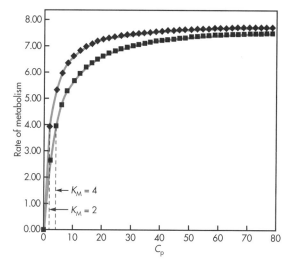

FIGURE 18-12 • Diagram showing the rate of metabolism when $V_{max}$ is constant (8 μg/mL/h) and $K_M$ is changed ($K_M = 2$ μg/mL for top curve and $K_M = 4$ μg/mL for bottom curve). Note the rate of metabolism is faster for the lower $K_M$, but saturation starts at lower concentration.

is, 0.5 × 626 mg/d or 313 mg/d. When the subject is receiving 300 mg of phenytoin per day, the plasma drug concentration of phenytoin is 8.6 mg/L, which is considerably below the $K_M$ of 27.3 mg/L. In practice, the $K_M$ in patients can range from 1 to 15 mg/L, and $V_{max}$ can range from 100 to 1000 mg/d. Patients with a low $K_M$ tend to have greater changes in plasma concentrations during dosing adjustments. Patients with a smaller $K_M$ (same $V_{max}$) will show a greater change in the rate of elimination when plasma drug concentration changes compared to subjects with a higher $K_M$. A subject with the same $V_{max}$ but different $K_M$ is shown in Fig. 18-12. (For another example, see the slopes of the two curves generated in Fig. 18-4.)

### Dependence of Elimination Half-Life on Dose

For drugs that follow linear kinetics, the elimination half-life is constant and does not change with therapeutic dose, time, or drug concentration. For a drug that follows dose-dependent nonlinear kinetics, the elimination half-life and drug clearance both change with dose and drug concentration. Generally, the elimination half-life becomes longer, clearance becomes smaller, and the AUC becomes disproportionately larger with increasing dose. The relationship between elimination half-life and drug

concentration is shown in Equation 18.16. The elimination half-life is dependent on the Michaelis–Menten parameters and concentration.

$$t_{1/2} = \frac{0.693}{V_{max}}(K_M + C_p) \qquad (18.16)$$

Some pharmacokineticists prefer not to calculate the elimination half-life of a nonlinear drug because the elimination half-life is not constant. Clinically, if the half-life is increasing as plasma concentration increases and there is no apparent change in metabolic or renal function, then there is a good possibility that the drug may be metabolized by nonlinear kinetics.

### Dependence of Clearance on Dose

The total body clearance of a drug given by IV bolus injection that follows a one-compartment model with Michaelis–Menten elimination kinetics changes with respect to time and plasma drug concentration. Within a certain drug concentration range, an average or mean clearance ($CL_{av}$) may be determined. Because the drug follows Michaelis–Menten kinetics, $CL_{av}$ is dose dependent. $CL_{av}$ may be estimated from the AUC and the dose given (Wagner et al, 1985).

According to the Michaelis–Menten equation,

$$\frac{dC_p}{dt} = \frac{V_{max}C_p}{K_M + C_p} \qquad (18.17)$$

Inverting Equation 18.17 and rearranging yields

$$C_p dt = \frac{K_M}{V'_{max}}dC_p - \frac{C_p}{V'_{max}}dC_p \qquad (18.18)$$

The area under the curve, $[AUC]_0^\infty$ is obtained by integration of Equation 18.18 $[AUC]_0^\infty = \int_0^\infty C_p\,dt$)

$$\int_0^\infty C_p dt = \int_{C_p^0}^\infty \frac{K_M}{V'_{max}}dC_p + \int_{C_p^0}^\infty \frac{C_p}{V'_{max}}dC_p \qquad (18.19)$$

where $V'_{max}$ is the maximum velocity for metabolism. Units for $V'_{max}$ are mass/compartment volume per unit time. $V'_{max} = V_{max}/V_D$; Wagner et al (1985) used $V_{max}$ in Equation 18.20 as mass/time to be consistent with biochemistry literature, which considers the initial mass of the substrate reacting with the enzyme.

Integration of Equation 18.18 from time 0 to infinity gives Equation 18.20.

$$[AUC]_0^\infty = \frac{C_p^0}{V_{max}/V_D}\left(\frac{C_p^0}{2} + K_M\right) \quad (18.20)$$

where $V_D$ is the apparent volume of distribution.

Because the dose $D_0 = C_p^0 V_D$ Equation 18.20 may be expressed as

$$[AUC]_0^\infty = \frac{D_0}{V_{max}}\left(\frac{C_p^0}{2} + K_M\right) \quad (18.21)$$

To obtain mean body clearance, $CL_{av}$ is then calculated from the dose and the AUC.

$$CL_{av} = \frac{D_0}{[AUC]_0^\infty} = \frac{V_{max}}{(C_p^0/2) + K_M} \quad (18.22)$$

$$CL_{av} = \frac{V_{max}}{(D_0/2V_D) + K_M} \quad (18.23)$$

Alternatively, dividing Equation 18.17 by $C_p$ gives Equation 18.24, which shows that the clearance of a drug that follows nonlinear pharmacokinetics is dependent on the plasma drug concentration $C_p$, $K_M$, and $V_{max}$.

$$CL = \frac{V_D(dC_p/dt)}{C_p} = \frac{V_{max}}{K_M + C_p} \quad (18.24)$$

Equation 18.22 or 18.23 calculates the average clearance $CL_{av}$ for the drug after a single IV bolus dose over the entire time course of the drug in the body. For any time period, clearance may be calculated (see Chapter 15) as

$$CL_T = \frac{dD_E/dt}{C_p} \quad (18.25)$$

In Chapter 15, the physiologic model based on blood flow and intrinsic clearance is used to describe drug metabolism. The extraction ratios of many drugs are listed in the literature. Actually, extraction ratios are dependent on dose, enzymatic system, and blood flow. For practical purposes, they are often assumed to be constant at normal doses.

Except for phenytoin, there is a lack of $K_M$ and $V_{max}$ data defining the nature of nonlinear drug elimination in patients. However, abundant information is available supporting variable metabolism due to genetic polymorphism (Chapter 21). The clearance (apparent) of many of these drugs in patients who are slow metabolizers changes with dose, although these drugs may exhibit linear kinetics in subjects with the "normal" phenotype. Metoprolol and many β-adrenergic antagonists are extensively metabolized. The plasma levels of metoprolol in slow metabolizers (Lennard et al, 1986) were much greater than other patients, and the AUC, after equal doses, is several times greater among slow metabolizers of metoprolol (Fig. 18-13). A similar picture is observed

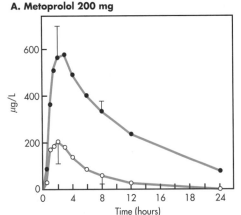

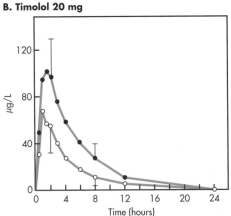

FIGURE 18-13 • Mean plasma drug concentration-versus-time profiles following administration of single oral doses of (A) metoprolol tartrate 200 mg to 6 extensive metabolizers (EMs) and 6 poor metabolizers (PMs) and (B) timolol maleate 20 mg to six EMs (O) and four PMs (•). (Data from Lennard MS, et al: Oxidation phenotype—A major determinant of metoprolol metabolism and response. *NEJM* **307**:1558–1560, 1982; Lennard MS, et al: The relationship between debrisoquine oxidation phenotype and the pharmacokinetics and pharmacodynamics of propranolol. *Br J Clin Pharmac* **17**(6):679–685, 1984; Lewis RV: Timolol and atenolol: Relationships between oxidation phenotype, pharmacokinetics and pharmacodynamics. *Br J Clin Pharmac* **19**(3):329–333, 1985.)

with another $\beta$-adrenergic antagonist, timolol. These drugs have smaller clearance than normal.

## Nonlinearity in Protein Binding

Valproic acid is a drug that has nonlinear protein binding. At high concentrations, drug binding to albumin becomes saturated, and drug concentrations thereby do not increase in a linear fashion with dose (Gómez Bellver MJ, et al 1993). The pharmacokinetics of valproic acid are, however, linear when free drug concentrations are followed so it is not associated with saturation of enzymatic metabolism.

---

**FREQUENTLY ASKED QUESTION**

▶ What is the Michaelis–Menten equation? How are $V_{max}$ and $K_M$ obtained? What are the units for $V_{max}$ and $K_M$? What is the relevance of $V_{max}$ and $K_M$?

▶ What are the main differences in pharmacokinetic parameters between a drug that follows linear pharmacokinetics and a drug that follows nonlinear pharmacokinetics?

---

## CLINICAL FOCUS

Paroxetine hydrochloride (Paxil) is an orally administered psychotropic drug. Paroxetine is extensively metabolized, and the metabolites are considered to be inactive. Nonlinearity in pharmacokinetics is observed with increasing doses. The major pathway for paroxetine metabolism is via CYP2D6 enzymes. The elimination half-life is about 21 hours, but saturation of this enzyme at clinical doses appears to account for the nonlinearity of paroxetine kinetics with increasing dose and increasing duration of treatment. The role of this enzyme in paroxetine metabolism also suggests potential drug–drug interactions. Clinical drug interaction studies have been performed with substrates of CYP2D6 and show that paroxetine can inhibit the metabolism of many drugs metabolized by CYP2D6 including itself, desipramine, risperidone, and atomoxetine.

Paroxetine hydrochloride is known to also inhibit the metabolism of selective serotonin reuptake inhibitors (SSRIs) and monoamine oxidase inhibitors (MAOIs), producing the "serotonin syndrome" (hyperthermia, muscle rigidity, and rapid changes in vital signs). Many cases of accidental overdosing with paroxetine hydrochloride have been reported since 1998 (Vermeulen, 1998). In the case of overdose, high liver drug concentrations and an extensive tissue distribution (large $V_D$) made the drug difficult to remove. Vermeulen (1998) reported that saturation of CYP2D6 could result in a disproportionally higher plasma level than could be expected from an increase in dosage. The CYP2D6 enzymes are polymorphically expressed, in that among Caucasians, for example, 5 to 10% have a lower activity of CYP2D6 and are called "slow metabolizers." More on this topic is presented in Chapter 21.

---

**FREQUENTLY ASKED QUESTION**

▶ Would you expect paroxetine (Paxil) plasma drug concentrations, $C_p$, to be higher or lower after multiple doses?

---

## DRUGS DISTRIBUTED AS ONE-COMPARTMENT MODEL AND ELIMINATED BY NONLINEAR PHARMACOKINETICS

The equations presented thus far are for drugs given by IV bolus, distributed as a one-compartment model, and eliminated only by nonlinear pharmacokinetics. The following equations describe other routes of drug administration and including mixed drug elimination, by which the drug may be eliminated by both nonlinear (Michaelis–Menten) and linear (first-order) processes.

### Mixed Drug Elimination

Drugs may be metabolized to several different metabolites by parallel pathways. At low drug doses corresponding to low drug concentrations at the site of the biotransformation enzymes, the rates of formation of metabolites are first order. However, with higher doses of drug, more drug is absorbed and higher drug concentrations are presented to the biotransformation enzymes. At higher drug concentrations, the enzyme involved in metabolite formation may become saturated, and the rate of metabolite formation becomes nonlinear and approaches zero order. For example, sodium salicylate is metabolized to both a glucuronide and a glycine conjugate (hippurate). The rate of formation of the glycine conjugate is limited by the amount of glycine available. Thus, the rate of formation of the glucuronide continues as a first-order process, whereas the rate of conjugation with glycine is capacity limited.

The equation that describes a drug that is eliminated by both first-order and Michaelis–Menten kinetics after IV bolus injection is given by

$$\frac{dC_p}{dt} = -kC_p - \frac{V_{max}}{(K_M + C_p)V}C_p \quad (18.26)$$

Or, in terms of drug amount ($X_p$) in the central compartment, the equation can be described as:

$$\frac{dX_p}{dt} = -kX_p - \frac{V_{max}}{(K_M + C_p)V}X_p$$

where $k$ is the first-order rate constant representing the sum of all first-order elimination processes, while the second term of Equation 18.26 represents the saturable or capacity limited process, and where V is the volume of distribution of that compartment.

## CLINICAL FOCUS

The pharmacokinetic profile of niacin is complicated due to extensive first-pass metabolism that is dosing-rate specific. In humans, one metabolic pathway is through a conjugation step with glycine to form nicotinuric acid (NUA). NUA is excreted in the urine, although there may be a small amount of reversible metabolism back to niacin. The other metabolic pathway results in the formation of nicotinamide adenine dinucleotide (NAD). It is unclear whether nicotinamide is formed as a precursor to, or following the synthesis of NAD. Nicotinamide is further metabolized to at least N-methylnicotinamide (MNA) and nicotinamide-N-oxide (NNO). MNA is further metabolized to two other compounds, N-methyl-2-pyridone-5-carboxamide (2PY) and N-methyl-4-pyridone-5-carboxamide (4PY). The formation of 2PY appears to predominate over 4PY in humans. At doses used to treat hyperlipidemia, these metabolic pathways are saturable, which explains the nonlinear relationship between niacin dose and plasma drug concentrations following multiple doses of Niaspan (niacin) extended-release tablets (Niaspan, FDA-approved label, 2009).

### Zero-Order Input and Nonlinear Elimination

The usual example of zero-order input is constant IV infusion. If the drug is given by constant IV infusion and is eliminated only by nonlinear pharmacokinetics from the central compartment, then the following equation describes the rate of change of the plasma drug concentration:

$$\frac{dC_p}{dt} = \frac{k_0}{V_D} - \frac{V'_{max}C_p}{K_M + C_p} \quad (18.27)$$

Or, in terms of drug amount ($X_p$) in the central compartment, the equation can be described as:

$$\frac{dX_p}{dt} = k_0 - \frac{V_{max}}{K_M V + X_p}X_p$$

where $k_0$ is the dosing rate of the constant IV infusion in the central compartment, and V is the volume of distribution of the central compartment.

### First-Order Absorption and Nonlinear Elimination

The relationship that describes the rate of change in the amount of drug in the central compartment for a drug that is given extravascularly (eg, orally), absorbed by first-order absorption from a depot compartment (eg, gut), and eliminated only by nonlinear pharmacokinetics, is given by the following equations. $X_{GI}$ is amount of drug remaining to be absorbed in the GI tract.

$$\frac{dX_{GI}}{dt} = +dose - k_a X_{GI}$$

$$\frac{dX_p}{dt} = +KaXgi - \frac{V_{max}}{(K_M V + X_p)}X_p$$

$$C_p = X_p/V \quad (18.28)$$

where $k_a$ is the first-order absorption rate constant.

If the drug is eliminated by parallel pathways consisting of both linear and nonlinear pharmacokinetics, Equation 18.28 may be extended to Equation 18.29.

$$\frac{dC_p}{dt} = K_a C_{GI} e^{-k_a t} - \frac{V'_{max} C_p}{K_M + C_p} - kC_p \qquad (18.29)$$

where $k$ is the first-order elimination rate constant.

## CHRONOPHARMACOKINETICS AND TIME-DEPENDENT PHARMACOKINETICS

*Chronopharmacokinetics* broadly refers to changes in pharmacokinetics that are related to time. Many drugs will display small changes in their pharmacokinetic behavior during the day, mainly due to the "inactive" (sleep) versus the "active" part of the day. During the day we exercise and eat. These activities will affect how quickly drugs become bioavailable from extravascular dosing, and how they are renally and hepatically eliminated due in part to differences in cardiac output and organ blood flow. The maximum ($C_{max}$) and overall (AUCτ) exposures observed with a drug may be different when it is administered in the morning versus just before bedtime. This explains why drugs should be given consistently at the same time of the day in patients as much as possible. Chronopharmacokinetics is therefore an important consideration during drug therapy.

*Time-dependent pharmacokinetics* or *time-dependent nonlinearity* generally refers to a change in the drug absorption, distribution, or elimination over a period of time (Table 18-8). Unlike dose-dependent pharmacokinetics or dose-dependent nonlinearity, which involves a pharmacokinetic change when the dose is changed, time-dependent nonlinearity may be the result of alteration in the physiology or biochemistry in an organ or a region in the body that influences drug disposition (Levy, 1983).

Time-dependent pharmacokinetics is often due to *autoinduction* or sometimes *autoinhibition* of enzymatic and transporter activities. For example,

Pitlick and Levy (1977) showed that repeated doses of carbamazepine induced the enzymes responsible for its elimination (ie, auto-induction), thereby increasing the clearance of the drug. This increased clearance is due to induction of CYP3A and P-gp activity (Owen et al, 2006; Lutz et al, 2018). Autoinduction also occurs with anticancer agents, such as cyclophosphamide and ifosfamide (Williams et al, 1999; Pasternyk DiMarco et al, 2000). The phenomenon of autoinduction is caused by the protective effects of CYP enzymes, whose role is to detoxify compounds and transform them into more water-soluble analytes that are more readily eliminated by the kidney or the bile. Many anticancer agents are "toxic" not only to cancer but normal cells. Repeated administration of these anticancer drugs induces the expression of enzymes and transporters, leading to a faster elimination. The steady-state concentration of a drug that causes autoinduction will be lower than would be expected from the first single dose administration, due to the increased clearance over time.

Autoinhibition is more rare but may occur during the course of metabolism of certain drugs such as troleandomycin. Troleandomycin is metabolized by CYP3A enzymes, but the metabolite formed inhibits the activity of these same enzymes by complexing with them (Sekiguchi, 2009). In this case, the metabolites formed increase in concentration and further inhibit metabolism of the parent drug. In biochemistry, this phenomenon is known as *product inhibition.*

Many different CYP enzymes are involved in drug metabolism, and drug–drug interactions may explain observed nonlinearity in the pharmacokinetics of a drug. Two drugs that are substrates for the same CYP enzymes and transported by the same transporter may interact with each other, simply by competition, even though they are not considered strong inhibitors or inducers of that pathway. Drug metabolism and pharmacogenetics are discussed more extensively in Chapter 21.

## TABLE 18-8 • Drugs Showing Circadian or Time-Dependent Disposition

| | | | |
|---|---|---|---|
| Cefodizime | Fluorouracil | Ketoprofen | Theophylline |
| Cisplatin | Heparin | Mequitazine | |

*Data from Hrushesky WJM, Langer R, Theeuwes F: Temporal Control of Drug Delivery, vol 618. New York, NY: Annals of the Academy of Science; 1991.*

## Circadian Rhythms and Influence on Drug Response

*Circadian rhythms* are rhythmic or cyclical changes in plasma drug concentrations that may occur daily due to normal changes in body functions. Some rhythmic changes that influence body functions and drug response are controlled by genes and subject to modification by environmental factors. The mammalian circadian clock is a self-sustaining oscillator, usually within a period of ~24 hours, that cyclically controls many physiological and behavioral systems. The biological clock attempts to synchronize and respond to changes in length of the daylight cycle and optimize body functions.

Circadian rhythms are regulated through periodic activation of transcription by a set of clock genes. For example, melatonin onset is associated with onset of the quiescent period of cortisol secretion that regulates many functions. Some well-known circadian physiologic parameters are core body temperature, heart rate, and other cardiovascular parameters. These fundamental physiologic factors can affect disease states as well as toxicity and therapeutic response to drug therapy. The toxic dose of a drug may vary as much as several-fold, depending on the time of drug administration—during either sleep or wake cycle.

An example of circadian changes on drug response involves observations with chronic obstructive pulmonary disease (COPD) patients. Symptoms of hypoxemia may be aggravated in some COPD patients due to changes in respiration during the sleep cycle. Circadian variations have been reported involving the incidence of acute myocardial infarction, sudden cardiac death, and stroke. Platelet aggregation favoring coagulation is increased after arising in the early morning hours, coincident with the peak incidence of these cardiovascular events, although much remains to be elucidated.

Time-dependent pharmacokinetics and physiologic functions are important considerations in the treatment of certain hypertensive subjects, in whom early-morning rise in blood pressure may increase the risk of stroke or hypertensive crisis. Verapamil is a commonly used antihypertensive. The diurnal pattern of forearm vascular resistance (FVR) between hypertensive and normotensive volunteers was studied at 9 PM on 24-hour ambulatory blood

pressure monitoring, and the early-morning blood pressure rise was studied in 23 untreated hypertensives and 10 matched, normotensive controls. The diurnal pattern of FVR differed between hypertensives and normotensives, with normotensives exhibiting an FVR decline between 2 PM and 9 PM, while FVR rose at 9 PM in hypertensives. Verapamil appeared to minimize the diurnal variation in FVR in hypertensives, although there were no significant differences at any single time point. Verapamil effectively reduced ambulatory blood pressure throughout the 24-hour period, but it did not blunt the early-morning rate of blood pressure rise despite peak S-verapamil concentrations in the early morning (Nguyen et al, 2000).

## CLINICAL FOCUS

Hypertensive patients are sometimes characterized as "dippers" if their nocturnal blood pressure drops below their daytime pressure. Non-dipping patients appear to be at an increased risk of cardiovascular morbidity. Blood pressure and cardiovascular events have a diurnal rhythm, with a peak of both in the morning hours, and a decrease during the night. The circadian variation of blood pressure provides assistance in predicting cardiovascular outcome (de la Sierra et al, 2011; Muxfeldt, et al, 2009).

The pharmacokinetics of many cardiovascular acting drugs have a circadian phase dependency (Lemmer, 2006). Examples include beta-blockers, calcium channel blockers, oral nitrates, and ACE inhibitors. There is clinical evidence that antihypertensive drugs should be dosed in the early morning in patients who are hypertensive "dippers," whereas for patients who are non-dippers, it may be necessary to add an evening dose or even to use a single evening dose not only to reduce high blood pressure (BP) but also to normalize a disturbed non-dipping 24-hour BP profile. However, for practical purposes, some investigators found diurnal BP monitoring in many individuals too variable to distinguish between dippers and non-dippers (Lemmer, 2006).

The issue of time-dependent pharmacokinetics/pharmacodynamics (PK/PD) may be an important issue in some antihypertensive care. Pharmacists should recognize drugs that exhibit this type of time-dependent PK/PD.

## Clinical and Adverse Toxicity Due to Nonlinear Pharmacokinetics

The presence of nonlinear or dose-dependent pharmacokinetics, whether due to saturation of a process involving absorption, first-pass metabolism, binding, or renal excretion, can have significant clinical consequences. However, nonlinear pharmacokinetics may not be noticed in drug studies that use a narrow dosing range in patients. In the case of nonlinear dose-dependent elimination, underpredicting the systemic exposure of higher dosing regimen may result in disproportionate increases in adverse reactions affecting the harm–benefit ratio.

Nonlinear dose response relationships can be detected (Hashimoto et al, 1994, 1995; Jonsson et al, 2000; Pasternyk DiMarco 2000) or even ruled out (Auclair et al, 1999) by population pharmacokinetic analyses. For example, nonlinear fluvoxamine pharmacokinetics was reported (Jonsson et al, 2000) to be present even at subtherapeutic doses. By using simulated data and applying nonlinear mixed-effect models using NONMEM, the authors also demonstrated that use of nonlinear mixed-effect models in population pharmacokinetics had an important application in the detection and characterization of nonlinear processes (pharmacokinetic and pharmacodynamic). In contrast, nonlinear pharmacokinetics was reported for piperacillin/tazobactam, but a population pharmacokinetic analysis using all of the clinical studies conducted for approval indicated that the pharmacokinetics were instead linear (Auclair et al, 1999). Population pharmacokinetics is discussed further in Chapter 20.

## BIOAVAILABILITY OF DRUGS THAT FOLLOW NONLINEAR PHARMACOKINETICS

The bioavailability of drugs that follow nonlinear pharmacokinetics is difficult to estimate accurately. As shown in Table 18-1, each process of drug absorption, distribution, and elimination is potentially saturable. Drugs that follow linear pharmacokinetics, and that are not affected by variable absorption lag times, follow the principle of superposition (Chapter 17). The assumption in applying the rule of superposition

is that each dose of drug superimposes on the previous dose. Consequently, the systemic exposure associated with subsequent doses is predictable. In the presence of a saturable pathway for drug absorption, distribution, or elimination, the drug's pharmacokinetic behavior will change within a single dose or with subsequent (multiple) doses. Levodopa, a drug commonly used to treat Parkinson disease, is absorbed in the intestine through amino acid transporters (Merck & Co, Inc., 2020) and is therefore thought to have a potential saturable absorption process in man.

The extent of bioavailability or exposure is generally estimated using $[\text{AUC}]_0^\infty$. If drug absorption is saturation limited in the gastrointestinal tract, then a smaller fraction of drug is absorbed systemically when the gastrointestinal drug concentration is high. A drug with a saturable elimination pathway may also have a concentration-dependent AUC affected by the magnitude of $K_M$ and $V_{max}$ of the enzymes involved in drug elimination (Equation 18.21). At low $C_p$, the rate of elimination is first order, even at the beginning of drug absorption from the gastrointestinal tract. As more drug is absorbed, either from a single dose or after multiple doses, systemic drug concentrations increase to levels that saturate the enzymes involved in drug elimination. The body drug clearance changes and the AUC increases disproportionately to the increase in dose (see Fig. 18-2).

## NONLINEAR PHARMACOKINETICS DUE TO DRUG–PROTEIN BINDING

Greater protein binding typically prolongs the elimination half-life of otherwise relatively similar drugs at the same time as it decreases their apparent central volume of distribution. Drugs that are protein bound must first dissociate into the free or nonbound form in order to be eliminated by glomerular filtration or to be metabolized by enzymes. This explains the prolongation of their elimination half-life when the rate limiting step becomes the dissociation from their protein binding state, and not their elimination. This is seen with penicillins and beta-lactam compounds that are typically eliminated by the kidney, and where the higher their albumin binding is, the longer their

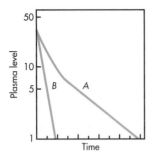

FIGURE 18-14 • Plasma curve comparing the elimination of two drugs given in equal IV doses. Curve *A* represents a drug 90% bound to plasma protein. Curve *B* represents a drug not bound to plasma protein.

elimination half-life becomes. Their apparent central volume of distribution will also appear smaller as their protein binding becomes greater, as the drug will be forced to distribute only within the plasma where albumin is ($V \sim 0.05$ L/kg), instead of within the extracellular fluid volume ($V_c \sim 0.3$ L/kg) for a hydrophilic drug not bound appreciably to proteins. These two phenomena are illustrated in Fig. 18-14, where two hypothetical drugs with very different protein binding, but otherwise relatively similar

and eliminated solely by glomerular filtration, are administered intravenously in equal doses. The drug with greater protein binding (A) will be associated with a much higher maximum plasma concentration, because it is distributed in a smaller apparent volume, and will have a longer elimination half-life than the drug that does not bind to plasma proteins, because less free drug is available for glomerular filtration in the course of renal excretion. The pharmacokinetics of relevant antibiotic examples are also presented in Table 18-9.

The concentration of free drug, $C_f$, can be calculated at any time as follows:

$$C_f = C_p (1 - \text{fraction bound}) \qquad (18.30)$$

For any protein-bound drug, the free drug concentration ($C_f$) will always be less than the total drug concentration ($C_p$).

When binding to plasma proteins is nonlinear, the percent of drug bound decreases when saturation of binding sites occurs. This means that the percent bound will increase once saturation disappears and as the plasma drug concentration decreases (Chapter 5). Albumin contains many different

**TABLE 18-9 •** Pharmacokinetic Behavior after IV Administration of Several Penicillins, Carbapenem, Monobactam, and Cephalosporins in Terms of Their Protein Binding, Volumes of Distribution, and Elimination Half-Lives

| Drug Name | Protein (Albumin) Binding (%) | Volume of Distribution, V (L/Kg) | Terminal Half-Life (h) |
|---|---|---|---|
| Ampicillin | 20 | 0.28 | 1 |
| Aztreonam | 56 | 0.2 | 2 |
| Cefazolin | 80 | 0.12 | 2 |
| Cefotaxime | 36 | 0.23 | 1.7 |
| Ceftriaxone | 90 | 0.16 | 80 |
| Cephalexine | 10 | 0.26 | 1 |
| Imipenem | 20 | 0.23 | 1 |
| Penicillin | 65 | 0.3 | 0.5 |
| Piperacillin | 32 | 0.18 | 1.2 |
| Ticarcillin | 45 | 0.21 | 1.2 |

*Reproduced with permission from Calop J, Limat S, Fernandez C: Pharmacie Clinique et Therapeutique, 3rd ed. Paris: Elsevier Masson; 2008.*

binding sites and is considered a "high-capacity, low affinity" binding protein. This signifies that saturation of binding sites is extremely rare, and only when drugs are administered in very high amounts (ie, in "grams"). As mentioned, two examples of drugs that can saturate albumin binding sites because they are administered in very high amounts ("grams") on a daily basis are Valproic acid (Depakene®) and acetylsalicylic acid (aspirin). Since saturable protein binding of drug can cause nonlinear drug elimination rates, pharmacokinetic fitting of "total" concentration data (includes concentrations of drug that are bound and not bound ("free") to plasma proteins) to a simple one-compartment model without accounting for binding will result in erroneous estimates of all pharmacokinetic parameters, including the clearance, volume of distribution, and elimination half-life.

Valproic acid (Depakene) shows nonlinear pharmacokinetics that are understood to be due to saturation of albumin protein binding sites at high concentrations. The free fraction of valproic acid is 10% at a plasma drug concentration of 40 $\mu$g/mL, but almost double at 18.5% at a plasma drug level of 130 $\mu$g/mL. The pharmacokinetics of valproic acid will therefore appear to be nonlinear using "total" plasma concentrations over this range but will appear to be linear when using "free" plasma concentrations.

### One-Compartment Model Drug with Saturable Protein Binding

The process of elimination of a drug distributed in a single compartment with saturable protein binding is hypothetically illustrated in Fig. 18-15. The one compartment contains both free drug and bound drug, which are dynamically interconverted with rate constants $k_1$ and $k_2$. Elimination of drug occurs only with the free drug, at a first-order rate. The bound drug is not eliminated. Assuming a saturable and instantly reversible drug-binding process, where $P$ = protein concentration in plasma, $C_f$ = plasma concentration of free drug, $k_d = k_2/k_1 =$

dissociation constant of the protein drug complex, $C_p$ = total plasma drug concentration, and $C_b$ = plasma concentration of bound drug,

$$\frac{C_b}{P} = \frac{(1/k_d)C_f}{1+(1/k_d)C_f} \tag{18.31}$$

This equation can be rearranged as follows:

$$C_b = \frac{PC_f}{k_d + C_f} = C_p - C_f \tag{18.32}$$

Solving for $C_f$,

$$C_f = \frac{1}{2}\left[-(P+k_d-C_p)+\sqrt{(P+k_d-C_p)^2+4k_dC_p}\right] \tag{18.33}$$

Because the rate of drug elimination is $dC_p/dt$,

$$\frac{dC_p}{dt} = -kC_f \tag{18.34}$$

$$\frac{dC_p}{dt} = \frac{-k}{2}\left[-(P+k_d-C_p)+\sqrt{(P+k_d-C_p)^2+4k_dC_p}\right]$$

This differential equation describes the relationship of changing plasma drug concentrations during elimination. The equation is not easily integrated but can be solved using a numerical method. Figure 18-16 shows the plasma drug concentration curves for a one-compartment protein-bound drug having a volume of distribution of 50 mL/kg and an elimination

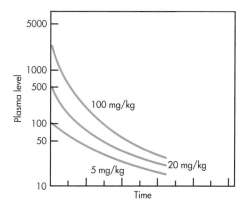

FIGURE 18-16 • Plasma drug concentrations for various doses of a one-compartment model drug with protein binding. (Adapted with permission from Coffey JJ, Bullock FJ, Schoenemann PT. Numerical solution of nonlinear pharmacokinetic equations: effects of plasma protein binding on drug distribution and elimination, *J Pharm Sci.* 1971 Nov;60(11):1623–1628.)

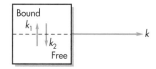

FIGURE 18-15 • One-compartment model with drug–protein binding.

half-life of 30 minutes. The protein concentration is 4.4% and the molecular weight of the protein is 67,000 Da. At various doses, the pharmacokinetics of elimination of the drug, as shown by the plasma curves, ranges from linear to nonlinear, depending on the total plasma drug concentration.

Nonlinear drug elimination pharmacokinetics occurs at higher doses. Because more free drug is available at higher doses, initial drug elimination occurs more rapidly. For drugs demonstrating nonlinear pharmacokinetics, the free drug concentration may increase slowly at first, but when the dose of drug is raised beyond the protein-bound saturation point, free plasma drug concentrations may rise abruptly. Therefore, the concentration of free drug should always be measured or calculated to make sure the patient receives a proper dose when nonlinear protein binding occurs for a drug administered at its conventional indicated dosing regimens.

### Determination of Linearity in Data Analysis

During new drug development, the pharmacokinetics of the drug are studied. A common approach is to give several graded doses to human volunteers and obtain plasma drug concentration curves for each dose. From these data, a graph of AUC versus dose is generated as shown in Fig. 18-2. The drug follows linear kinetics if AUC versus dose for various doses is proportional (ie, linear relationship). In practice, the experimental data may not be very clear, especially after oral drug administration and there is considerable variability in the data. For example, the AUC versus three-graded doses of a new drug is shown in Fig. 18-17. A linear regression line was drawn through the three data points. The conclusion is that the drug follows dose-independent (linear) kinetics based upon a linear regression line through the data and a correlation coefficient, $R^2 = 0.97$.

### Analysis of the Data in Figure 18-17

As stated above, Fig. 18-17 shows that the drug follows dose-independent (linear) kinetics based upon a linear regression line through the data and a correlation coefficient, $R^2 = 0.97$.

- *Do you agree with this conclusion after inspecting the graph?*

The conclusion for linear pharmacokinetics in Fig. 18-17 seems reasonable based on the estimated regression line drawn through the data points.

However, another pharmacokineticist noticed that the regression line in Fig. 18-17 does not pass through the origin point (0,0). This pharmacokineticist considered the following questions:

- Are the patients in the study receiving the drug doses well separated by a washout period during the trial such that no residual drug remained in the body and carried to the present dose when plasma samples are collected?
- Is the method for assaying the samples validated? Could a high sample blank or interfering material be artificially adding to elevate 0 time drug concentrations?
- How does the trend line look if the point (0,0) is included?

When the third AUC point is above the trend line, it is risky to draw a conclusion. One should verify that the high AUC is not due to a lower elimination or clearance due to saturation.

In Fig. 18-18, a regression line was obtained by forcing the same data through point (0,0). The linear

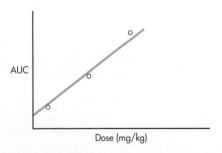

**FIGURE 18-17 ·** Plot of AUC versus dose to determine linearity. The regression line is based on the three doses of the drug.

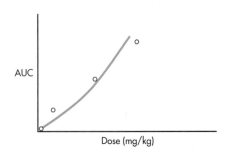

**FIGURE 18-18 ·** Plot of AUC versus dose to determine linearity.

regression analysis and estimated $R^2$ appears to show that the drug followed nonlinear pharmacokinetics. The line appears to have a curvature upward and the possibility of some saturation at higher doses. This pharmacokineticist recommends additional study by adding a higher dose to more clearly check for dose dependency.

- *What is your conclusion?*

Considerations

- The experimental data are composed of three different drug doses.
- The regression line shows that the drug follows linear pharmacokinetics from the low dose to the high dose.
- The use of a (0.0) value may provide additional information concerning the linearity of the pharmacokinetics. However, extrapolation of curves beyond the actual experimental data can be misleading.
- The conclusion in using the (0.0) time point shows that the pharmacokinetics is nonlinear below the lowest drug dose. This may occur after oral dosing because at very low drug doses some of the drug is decomposed in the gastrointestinal tract or metabolized prior to systemic absorption. With higher doses, the small amount of drug loss is not observed systemically.

Some common issues during data analysis for linearity are listed in Table 18-10.

*Note:* In some cases the oral absorption mechanism is unique and drug clearance by the oral route may involve absorption site-specific enzymes or transporters located on the brush border of the small intestine. Extrapolating pharmacokinetic information from IV dose data should be done cautiously only after a careful consideration of these factors. It is helpful to know whether nonlinearity is caused by distribution, elimination, or absorption factors.

---

**FREQUENTLY ASKED QUESTION**

▶ What is the cause of nonlinear pharmacokinetics that is not dose related?

▶ For drugs that have several metabolic pathways, must all the metabolic pathways be saturated for the drug to exhibit nonlinear pharmacokinetics?

---

**TABLE 18-10 • Some Common Issues during Data Analysis for Linearity**

| Oral Data | Issues during Data Analysis | Comments |
|---|---|---|
| | Last data point may be below the LOD or limit of detection. What should the AUC tailpiece be? | Last sample point scheduled too late in the study protocol. |
| | Last data point still very high, much above the LOD. What should be the AUC tailpiece? | Last sample point scheduled too early. A substantial number of data points may be incorrectly estimated by the tailpiece method. |
| | Incomplete sample spacing around peak. | Total AUC estimated may be quite variable or unreliable. |
| | Oral AUC data are influenced by $F$, $D$, and $Cl$. | When examining $D_0/Cl$ vs $D_0$, $F$ must be held constant. Any factor causing change in $F$ during the trial will introduce uncertainty to AUC. |
| | $F$ may be affected by efflux, transporters (see Chapter 13), and GI CYP enzymes. An increase in $F$ and decrease in $Cl$ or vice versa overdoses may mask each other. | Nonlinearity of AUC vs $D_0$ may not be evident and one may incorrectly conclude a drug follows linear kinetics when it does not. |
| IV data | AUC data by IV are influenced by $D_0$ and $Cl$ only. | When examining $D_0/Cl$ vs $D_0$, $F$ is always constant. Therefore, it is easier to see changes in AUC when $Cl$ changes by IV route. |

LOD, limit of detection.

# DOSE-DEPENDENT PHARMACOKINETICS

## Role of Transporters

In classical pharmacokinetics, we study whether the pharmacokinetics of a drug is linear or not by examining the area under plasma drug concentration curve obtained from various doses administered, whether intravenously or extravenously. The method is simple and definitive. The method is useful revealing the kinetics in the body as a whole. However, more detailed information is obtained by the careful characterization of the complete pharmacokinetic behavior of the drug, not just its overall exposure. *Regional pharmacokinetics* is aimed at carefully studying the pharmacokinetic behavior of a drug in a specific region, for example, a better characterization of the absorption process through different techniques which can help highlight the roles of certain transporters. Over the last few decades, transporters have been characterized in individual cells or in various types of cells. These transporters may critically enhance or reduce local cell drug concentrations, allowing influx of drugs into the cell or removing drug from the cell by efflux transporters, a defensive mechanism of the body. Many of the cells express transporters genetically, which may also be triggered on or turned off in disease state. Whether the overall pharmacokinetic process is linear or nonlinear may be explained by certain "local" processes. The knowledge of the local effects of transporters and how they can be influence can help optimize the safe and effective use of drug. The impact of transporters is discussed by various authors in a review book edited by You and Morris (2014). Table 18-11 summarizes some of the transporters that play an important role in drug disposition and how they may impact drug linearity.

## TABLE 18-11 • Drug Transports and Comments on Roles in Altering Linearity of Absorption or Elimination

| Transporters | Comments |
| --- | --- |
| Xenobiotic transporter expression | Transporters may be age and gender related. These differences may change the linearity of a drug through saturation. |
| Polymorphisms of drug transporters | Polymorphisms may have a clinical relevance affecting toxicity and efficacy in a similar way through change in pharmacokinetics. |
| Interplay of drug transporters and enzymes in liver | The role of transporters on hepatic drug is profound and may greatly change the overall linearity of a drug systemically.<br>The concept of drug clearance, $Cl$, and intrinsic clearance has to be reexamined as a result of the translocation of transporters, at cellular membranes as suggested in a recent review. |
| Drug–drug interaction change due to transporters | Clinical relevance, pharmacokinetics, pharmacodynamics, and toxicity may decrease or increase if a drug is a transporter substrate or inhibitor. Less clear is the change from linear to nonlinear kinetics due to drug–drug interaction. |
| Drug transporters in the intestine | ABC transporters are very common and this can alter the absorption nature of a drug product, for example, the bioavailability and linearity of drug absorption. Bile acid transporters affect drug movement and elimination by biliary excretion. The nature of the process must be studied. |
| Drug transport in the kidney | Various organic anion and cation drug transporters have been described. These transporters may alter the linearity of systemic drug elimination if present in large quantity. |
| Multidrug resistance protein: P-glycoprotein | These proteins may affect drug concentration in a cell or group of cells. Hence, they are important elements in determining PK linearity. |
| Mammalian oligopeptide transporters | These transporters play a role in drug absorption and distribution. |
| Breast cancer resistance protein | These transporters play a role in drug linearity and dosing in cancer therapy. |

## CHAPTER SUMMARY

Nonlinear pharmacokinetics refers to kinetic processes that result in disproportional changes in plasma drug concentrations when the dose is changed ("dose-dependent nonlinearity"), or over time ("time-dependent nonlinearity"). Dose-dependent pharmacokinetics is typically seen when the clearance or the elimination rate constant is decreased at higher doses because of saturation of the metabolism or elimination processes. A classic example is the anticonvulsant phenytoin which saturates its own metabolism through CYP2C9 enzymes at standard clinical doses (eg, 300 mg per day or more). More than proportional increases in systemic exposure will be seen with increasing dosages. Dose-dependent pharmacokinetics can also be seen with saturation of the absorption process (eg, Levodopa) or protein binding sites (eg, valproic acid). In both of these cases, the increase in systemic exposure will be less than the increasing dosages, as bioavailability will be decreased for the former, while the percentage of free drug will increase for the latter resulting in a greater elimination process. Time-dependent pharmacokinetics is observed with continuous administrations of carbamazepine. Over time, carbamazepine induces its own metabolism via CYP3A enzymes and must be given more frequently (ie, from bid to tid and then qid regimens for the immediate-release formulations). Dose-dependent pharmacokinetics is also often seen with anticancer agents that are toxic to normal cells as well as cancer cells. Examples are ifosfamide and cyclosphophamide, which are eliminated more rapidly after 5 days of daily administrations, presumably because of CYP induction, a normal defense from the organism to try to get rid of a perceived toxic agent.

The Michaelis–Menten kinetic equation may be applied in vitro or in vivo to describe nonlinear drug disposition. Phenytoin, for example, is commonly followed pharmacokinetically by pharmacists using a Michalis–Menten elimination process.

An approach to determine nonlinear pharmacokinetics is to plot AUC versus doses and observe whether the AUC increases in a proportional fashion with the administered dosages. Drug overdosing in clinical practice may be due to undetected saturation of a metabolic enzyme due to genotype difference in a subject (eg, CYP2D6). Another cause of overdosing in clinical practice is due to undetected saturation of a metabolic enzyme due to coadministration of a second drug/agent that alters the original linear elimination process (eg, drug–drug interaction). Drug transporters play an important role in the body. Membrane-located transporters may cause uneven drug distribution at cellular level, and hiding concentration-dependent kinetics may occur at the local level within body organs. These processes include absorption, distribution, and elimination, and are important in drug therapy. Some transporters are triggered by disease or expressed differently in individuals and should be recognized by pharmacists during dosing regimen recommendation.

## LEARNING QUESTIONS

1. Define *nonlinear pharmacokinetics*. How do drugs that follow nonlinear pharmacokinetics differ from drugs that follow linear pharmacokinetics?

   a. What is the rate of change in the plasma drug concentration with respect to time, $dC_p/dt$, when $C_p << K_M$?

   b. What is the rate of change in the plasma drug concentration with respect to time, $dC_p/dt$, when $C_p >> K_M$?

2. What processes of drug absorption, distribution, and elimination may be considered "capacity limited," "saturated," or "dose dependent"?

3. Drugs such as phenytoin and salicylates have been reported to follow dose-dependent elimination kinetics. What changes in pharmacokinetic parameters, including $t_{1/2}$, $V_D$, AUC, and $C_p$, could be predicted if the amounts of these drugs administered were increased from low pharmacologic doses to high therapeutic doses?

4. A given drug is metabolized by capacity-limited pharmacokinetics. Assume $K_M$ is 50 $\mu$g/mL, $V_{max}$ is 20 $\mu$g/mL per hour, and the apparent $V_D$ is 20 L/kg.

   a. What is the reaction order for the metabolism of this drug when given in a single intravenous dose of 10 mg/kg?

   b. How much time is necessary for the drug to be 50% metabolized?

5. How would induction or inhibition of the hepatic enzymes involved in drug biotransformation theoretically affect the pharmacokinetics of a drug that demonstrates nonlinear pharmacokinetics due to saturation of its hepatic elimination pathway?

6. Assume that both the active parent drug and its inactive metabolites are excreted by active tubular secretion. What might be the consequences of increasing the dosage of the drug on its elimination half-life?

7. The drug isoniazid was reported to interfere with the metabolism of phenytoin. Patients taking both drugs together show higher phenytoin levels in the body. Using the basic principles in this chapter, do you expect $K_M$ to increase or decrease in patients taking both drugs? (*Hint:* see Fig. 18-4.)

8. Explain why $K_M$ sometimes has units of mM/mL and sometimes mg/L.

9. The $V_{max}$ for metabolizing a drug is 10 mmol/h. The rate of metabolism ($v$) is 5 $\mu$mol/h when drug concentration is 4 $\mu$mol. Which of the following statements is/are true?

   a. $K_M$ is 5 $\mu$mol for this drug.

   b. $K_M$ cannot be determined from the information given.

   c. $K_M$ is 4 $\mu$mol for this drug.

10. Which of the following statements is/are true regarding the pharmacokinetics of diazepam (98% protein bound) and propranolol (87% protein bound)?

    a. Diazepam has a long elimination half-life because it is difficult to be metabolized due to extensive plasma–protein binding.

    b. Propranolol is an example of a drug with high protein binding but unrestricted (unaffected) metabolic clearance.

    c. Diazepam is an example of a drug with low hepatic extraction.

    d. All of the above.

    e. a and c.

    f. b and c.

11. Which of the following statements describe(s) correctly the properties of a drug that follows nonlinear or capacity-limited pharmacokinetics?

    a. The elimination half-life will remain constant when the dose changes.

    b. The area under the plasma curve (AUC) will increase proportionally as dose increases.

    c. The rate of drug elimination = $C_p \times K_M$.

    d. All of the above.

    e. a and b.

    f. None of the above.

12. The hepatic intrinsic clearances of two drugs are

    drug A: 1300 mL/min

    drug B: 26 mL/min

    Which drug is likely to show the greatest increase in hepatic clearance when hepatic blood flow is increased from 1 L/min to 1.5 L/min?

    a. Drug A

    b. Drug B

    c. No change for both drugs

## ANSWERS

### Frequently Asked Questions

*Why is it important to monitor drug levels carefully for dose dependency?*

■ A patient with concomitant hepatic disease may have decreased biotransformation enzyme activity. Infants and young subjects may have immature hepatic enzyme systems. Alcoholic subjects may have liver cirrhosis and lack certain coenzymes. Other patients may experience enzyme saturation at normal doses due to genetic polymorphism. Pharmacokinetics provides a simple way to identify nonlinear kinetics in these patients and to estimate an appropriate dose. Finally, concomitant use of other drugs may cause nonlinear pharmacokinetics at lower drug doses due to enzyme inhibition.

*What are the main differences in pharmacokinetic parameters between a drug that follows linear pharmacokinetics and a drug that follows nonlinear pharmacokinetics?*

■ A drug that follows linear pharmacokinetics will display constant elimination half-life, clearance, and volumes of distributions. The steady-state drug concentrations and AUCs will be proportional to the size of the doses administered. Nonlinear pharmacokinetics, on the other hand, will result in different pharmacokinetic behavior over time ("time-dependent nonlinearity") or over ranges of administered doses ("dose-dependent nonlinearity"). Time-dependent pharmacokinetics is often the result of autoinduction by increasing the metabolism and elimination of a drug over time, while dose-dependent pharmacokinetics is often the result of saturation of drug metabolism and/or transport when doses are administered above a certain threshold. This type of nonlinear pharmacokinetics is often described using the Michaelis–Menten equations, where $V_{max}$ and $K_M$ become important parameters to determine.

*What is the cause of nonlinear pharmacokinetics that is not dose related?*

■ *Chronopharmacokinetics* is the study of nonlinear pharmacokinetics that is time related. The time-dependent or temporal process of drug elimination can be the result of rhythmic changes in the body. For example, nortriptyline and theophylline levels are higher when administered between 7 and 9 AM compared to between 7 and 9 PM after the same dose. Other factors that cause nonlinear pharmacokinetics over time may result from enzyme induction (eg, carbamazepine inducing CYP3A enzymes) or enzyme inhibition (eg, troleandomycin inhibiting CYP3A enzymes) after multiple doses of the drug. Furthermore,

the drug or a metabolite may accumulate following multiple dosing and affect the metabolism or renal elimination of the drug.

*What are the main differences between a model based on Michaelis–Menten kinetic ($V_{max}$ and $K_M$) and the physiologic model that describes hepatic metabolism based on clearance?*

■ Physiologic models are often based on organ drug clearances that are described nonlinearly in terms of blood flow and intrinsic clearances (Chapter 15). The Michaelis–Menten equation describes the clearance in terms of maximum velocity ($V_{max}$) and of a constant that relates concentrations with half of the maximum velocity ($K_M$). Besides its use in pharmacokinetics (eg, for phenytoin), the Michaelis–Menten equations are routinely applied to describe *in vitro* enzymatic reactions. These two model equations, although both relatively similar and resulting in nonlinear clearances, are therefore completely different, as one is based on organ blood flow and intrinsic clearance ("physiologic" model), while the other is based on enzymatic parameters (Michaelis–Menten). In clinical practice, the physiologic model has limited use in dosing patients because blood flow and intrinsic clearance organ data are not available or measurable.

### Learning Questions

2. Capacity-limited processes for drugs include:

    ■ Absorption
      Active transport
      Intestinal and gut wall metabolism
    ■ Distribution
      Protein binding
    ■ Elimination
      Biotransformation in the liver or other organs
      Active biliary secretion
      Active tubular secretion in the kidney
      Active tubular reabsorption in the kidney

4.  $C_P^0 = \dfrac{\text{dose}}{V_D} = \dfrac{10{,}000\ \mu g}{20{,}000\ \text{mL}} = 0.5\ \mu g/\text{mL}$

From Equation 18.1,

$$\text{Elimination rate} = -\dfrac{dC_P}{dt} = \dfrac{V_{max}C_P}{K_M + C_P}$$

Because $K_M = 50$ $\mu$g/mL, $C_p << K_M$ and the reaction rate is first order. Thus, the above equation reduces to Equation 18.3.

$$-\frac{dC_p}{dt} = \frac{V_{max}C_p}{K_M} = k'C_p$$

$$k' = \frac{V_{max}}{K_M} = \frac{20\ \mu g/h}{50\ \mu g} = 0.4\ h^{-1}$$

For first-order reactions,

$$t_{1/2} = \frac{0.693}{k'} = \frac{0.693}{0.4} = 1.73\ h$$

The drug will be 50% metabolized in 1.73 hours.

7. When isoniazid is coadministered, plasma phenytoin concentrations are increased due to a reduction in its metabolic rate $v$. Equation 18.1 shows that $v$ and $K_M$ are inversely related ($K_M$ in denominator). An increase in $K_M$ will be accompanied by an increase in plasma drug concentration. Figure 18-4 shows that an increase in $K_M$ is accompanied by an increase in the amount of drug in the body at any time $t$. Equation 18.4 relates drug concentration to $K_M$, and it can be seen that the two are proportionally related, although they are not linearly proportional to each other due to the complexity of the equation. An actual study in the literature shows that $k$ is increased several-fold in the presence of INH in the body.

8. The $K_M$ has the units of concentration. In laboratory studies, $K_M$ is expressed in moles per liter, or micromoles per milliliter, because reactions are expressed in moles and not milligrams. In dosing, drugs are given in milligrams and plasma drug concentrations are expressed as milligrams per liter or micrograms per milliliter. The units of $K_M$ for pharmacokinetic models are estimated from *in vivo* data. They are therefore commonly expressed as milligrams per liter, which is preferred over micrograms per milliliter because dose is usually expressed in milligrams. The two terms may be shown to be equivalent and convertible. Occasionally, when simulating amount of drug metabolized in the body as a function of time, the amount of drug in the body has been assumed to follow Michaelis–Menten kinetics, and $K_M$ assumes the unit of $D_0$ (eg, mg). In this case, $K_M$ takes on a very different meaning.

## REFERENCES

Coffey J, Bullock FJ, Schoenemann PT: Numerical solution of nonlinear pharmacokinetic equations: Effect of plasma protein binding on drug distribution and elimination. *J Pharm Sci* **60**:1623, 1971.

de la Sierra A, Segura J, Banegas JR, et al: Clinical features of 8295 patients with resistant hypertension classified on the basis of ambulatory blood pressure monitoring. *Hypertension* **57**(5):898–902, 2011.

Ducharme MP: Principes d'utilisation des antibiotiques. In: Calop J, Limat S, Fernandez C, eds. *Pharmacie Clinique et Therapeutique*, 3rd ed. Masson, Paris, 2008, pp 935–958.

Gómez Bellver MJ, Garcéa Sánchez AC, Alonso Gonzalez D, Santos Buelga A, Dominguez–Gil: Plasma: Protein Binding Kinetics of Valproic Acid Over a Broad Dosage Range: Therapeutic Implications, Journal of Clinical Pharmacy and Therapeutics, 1365-2710, 1993 (https://onlinelibrary.wiley.com/doi/abs/10.1111/j.1365-2710.1993.tb00612.x)

Hashimoto Y, Odani A, Tanigawara Y, Yasuhara M, Okuno T, Hori R: Population analysis of the dose-dependent pharmacokinetics of zonisamide in epileptic patients. *Biol Pharm Bull* **17**:323–326, 1994.

Hashimoto Y, Koue T, Otsuki Y, Yasuhara M, Hori R, Inui K: Simulation for population analysis of Michaelis–Menten kinetics. *J Pharmacokinet Biopharmacol* **23**:205–216, 1995.

Jonsson EN, Wade JR, Karlsson MO: Nonlinearity detection: Advantages of nonlinear mixed-effects modeling. *AAPS Pharmsci* **2**(3), article 32, 2000.

Lemmer B: The importance of circadian rhythms on drug response in hypertension and coronary heart disease—From mice and man. *Pharmacol Ther* **111**(3):629–651, 2006.

Lennard MS, Tucker GT, Woods HF: The polymorphic oxidation of beta-adrenoceptor antagonists—Clinical pharmacokinetic considerations. *Clin Pharmacol* **11**:1–17, 1986.

Lutz JD, Kirby BJ, Wang L, et al. Cytochrome P450 3A induction predicts P-glycoprotein induction; Part 2: Prediction of decreased substrate exposure after rifabutin or carbamazepine. *Clin Pharmacol Ther* **104**(6):1191–1198, 2018.

Levy RH: Time-dependent pharmacokinetics. *Pharmacol Ther* **17**:383–392, 1983.

Merck & Co., Inc. Sinemet® US approved FDA label. Revised 03/2020. Last accessed: 20 July 2020 at: https://www.accessdata.fda.gov/scripts/cder/daf/index.cfm?event=overview.process&ApplNo=017555.

Muxfeldt ES, Cardoso CRL, Salles F: Prognostic value of nocturnal blood pressure reduction in resistant hypertension. *Arch Intern Med* **169**(9):874–880, 2009.

Nguyen BN, Parker RB, Noujedehi M, Sullivan JM, Johnson JA: Effects of COER-verapamil on circadian pattern of forearm vascular resistance and blood pressure. *J Clin Pharmacol* **40** (suppl):1480–1487, 2000.

Owen A, Goldring C, Morgan P, Park BK, Pirmohamed M: Induction of P-glycoprotein in lymphocytes by carbamazepine and rifampicin: The role of nuclear hormone response elements. *Br J Clin Pharmacol* **62**(2):237–242, 2006.

Pasternyk DiMarco M, Wainer IW, Granvil CP, Batist G, Ducharme MP: New insights into the pharmacokinetics and metabolism of (R,S)-ifosfamide in cancer patients using a population pharmacokinetic-metabolism model. *Pharm Res* **17**(6):645–652, 2000.

Pitlick WH, Levy RH: Time-dependent kinetics, I. Exponential autoinduction of carbamazepine in monkeys. *J Pharm Sci* **66**:647, 1977.

Reinberg AE: Concepts of circadian chronopharmacology. In Hrushesky WJM, Langer R, Theeuwes F (eds). *Temporal Control of Drug Delivery.* New York, Annals of the Academy of Science, 1991, vol 618, p 102.

Sekiguchi N, Higashida A, Kato M, et al: Prediction of drug–drug interactions based on time-dependent inhibition from high throughput screening of cytochrome P450 3A4 inhibition. *Drug Metab Pharmacokinet* **24**(6):500–510, 2009.

Vermeulen T: Distribution of paroxetine in three postmortem cases. *J Analytical Toxicology* **22**:541–544, 1998.

Vozeh S, Muir KT, Sheiner LB: Predicting phenytoin dosage. *J Pharm Biopharm* **9**:131–146, 1981.

Wagner JG, Szpunar GJ, Ferry JJ: Michaelis–Menten elimination kinetics: Areas under curves, steady-state concentrations, and clearances for compartment models with different types of input. *Biopharm Drug Disp* **6**:177–200, 1985.

Williams ML, Wainer IW, Granvil CP, Gerhcke B, Bernstein ML, Ducharme MP: Population pharmacokinetics of (R)- and (S)-cyclophosphamide and their dechloroethylated metabolites in cancer patients. *Chirality* **11**:301–308, 1999.

Witmer DR, Ritschel WA: Phenytoin isoniazid interaction: A kinetic approach to management. *Drug Intell Clin Pharm* **18**:483–486, 1984.

You G, Morris ME: *Drug Transporters: Molecular Characterization and Role in Drug Disposition.* John Wiley and Sons, 2014.

## BIBLIOGRAPHY

AbbVie Inc. Depakene (Valproic acid) US FDA approved label. Last accessed 13 July 2020 at: https://www.accessdata.fda.gov/drugsatfda_docs/label/2020/018081s071,018082s054lbl.pdf.

Amsel LP, Levy G: Drug biotransformation interactions in man, II. A pharmacokinetic study of the simultaneous conjugation of benzoic and salicylic acids with glycine. *J Pharm Sci* **58**:321–326, 1969.

Auclair B, Ducharme MP: Piperacillin and tazobactam exhibit linear pharmacokinetics after multiple standard clinical doses. *Antimicrob Agents Chemother* **43**(6):1465–1468, 1999.

Dutta S, Matsumoto Y, Ebling WF: Is it possible to estimate the parameters of the sigmoid $E_{max}$ model with truncated data typical of clinical studies? *J Pharm Sci* **85**:232–239, 1996.

Evans WE, Schentag JJ, Jusko WJ: *Applied Pharmacokinetics,* 3rd ed, Vancouver, WA, Applied Therapeutics, 1992.

Gibaldi M: Pharmacokinetic aspects of drug metabolism. *Ann N Y State Acad Sci* **179**:19, 1971.

Kruger-Theimer E: Nonlinear dose concentration relationships. *Il Farmaco* **23**:718–756, 1968.

Levy G: Pharmacokinetics of salicylate in man. *Drug Metab Rev* **9**:3–19, 1979.

Levy G, Tsuchiya T: Salicylate accumulation kinetics in man. *N Engl J Med* **287**:430–432, 1972.

Ludden TM: Nonlinear pharmacokinetics. Clinical applications. *Clin Pharmacokinet* **20**:429–446, 1991.

Ludden TM, Hawkins DW, Allen JP, Hoffman SF: Optimum phenytoin dosage regimen. *Lancet* **1**:307–308, 1979.

Mehvar R: Principles of nonlinear pharmacokinetics: *Am J Pharm Edu* **65**:178–184, 2001.

Mullen PW: Optimal phenytoin therapy: A new technique for individualizing dosage. *Clin Pharm Ther* **23**:228–232, 1978.

Mullen PW, Foster RW: Comparative evaluation of six techniques for determining the Michaelis–Menten parameters relating phenytoin dose and steady state serum concentrations. *J Pharm Pharmacol* **31**:100–104, 1979.

Perrier D, Ashley JJ, Levy G: Effect of product inhibition in kinetics of drug elimination. *J Pharmacokinet Biopharmacol* **1**:231, 1973.

Prins JM, Weverling GJ, van Ketel RJ, Speelman P: Circadian variations in serum levels and the renal toxicity of aminoglycosides in patients. *Clin Pharmacol Ther* **62**:106–111, 1997.

Sarveshwer Rao VV, Rambhau D, Ramesh Rao B, Srinivasu P: Circadian variation in urinary excretion of ciprofloxacin after a single dose oral administration at 1000 and 2200 hours in human subjects. *India Antimicrob Agents Chemother (USA)* **41**:1802–1804, 1997.

Von Roemeling R: The therapeutic index of cytotoxic chemotherapy depends upon circadian drug timing. In Hrushesky WJM, Langer R, Theeuwes F (eds). *Temporal Control of Drug Delivery.* New York, Annals of the Academy of Science, 1991, vol 618, pp 292–311.

Van Rossum JM, van Lingen G, Burgers JPT: Dose-dependent pharmacokinetics. *Pharmacol Ther* **21**:77–99, 1983.

Wagner J: Properties of the Michaelis–Menten equation and its integrated form which are useful in pharmacokinetics. *J Pharm Biopharm* **1**:103, 1973.

# Empirical Models, Mechanistic Models, Statistical Moments, and Noncompartmental PK/PD Analyses

Corinne Seng Yue, Philippe Colucci, and Murray P. Ducharme

## CHAPTER OBJECTIVES

- Describe the differences between empirical and mechanistic models.

- Understand the differences between different types of compartmental analyses.

- Describe the physiologic pharmacokinetic (PBPK) model with equations and underlying assumptions.

- List the advantages and disadvantages related to the use of PBPK, population PK, and the noncompartmental PK approaches for data analyses and predictions.

- Describe *interspecies scaling* and its application in pharmacokinetics and toxicokinetics.

- Describe statistical moment theory and explain how it provides a unique way to study time-related changes in *macroscopic events.*

- Define *mean residence time* (MRT) and how it can be calculated.

- Define *mean transit time* (MTT) and how it can be used to calculate the *mean dissolution time* (MDT), or *in vivo* mean dissolution time, for a solid drug product given orally.

- Estimate other PK parameters such as mean absorption time and total volume of distribution using MRT

The introductory chapter to this section (Chapter 11) presented the three main methods that can be used to calculate, predict, and simulate PK and PK/PD. The subsequent chapters provided the main equations used to describe and characterize PK profiles for drugs and biologics that display linear and nonlinear characteristics. All these equations can be used to describe individual and population PK and PK/PD data by incorporating them in a complete PK and PK/PD model. This chapter will first show how to conduct model-independent analyses (noncompartmental PK analyses), which can be used to scientifically describe and quantify the PK of drugs when a large number of observations are made after a drug dose. The latter method is crucial for drug and biologic development because of its simplicity and is also recognized for its robustness. While noncompartmental approaches are frequently used by undergraduate students, clinicians, and researchers, more elaborate model-based methods are often employed in drug development to characterize PK and/or PK/PD. For students or researchers interested in data fitting, the remainder of the chapter will focus on how to specify the PK and/or PK/PD models that can be derived from equations described in previous chapters. Simple models, such as those used to conduct allometric scaling from animals to humans, will be examined as well as more complicated ones, from population compartmental models to physiologically-based models.

## NONCOMPARTMENTAL ANALYSIS

Noncompartmental analyses provide an alternative method for describing drug pharmacokinetics without having to assign a particular compartmental model to the drug. Although this method is often considered to be *model independent*, there are still a few assumptions and key considerations that must not be overlooked.

This approach is therefore better referred to as "noncompartmental" as it does assume a "model," in that, among other things reviewed below, the PK needs to be linear and the terminal phase must be log-linear.

The first assumption is that the drug in question displays linear pharmacokinetics (DiStefano and Landaw, 1984; Gibaldi and Perrier, 2007). In other words, exposure increases in proportion with increasing dose and PK parameters are stable through time. A second important assumption is that the drug is eliminated from the body strictly from the pool in which it is being measured—the plasma, for example (Benet and Ronfeld, 1969; DiStefano and Landaw, 1984). Finally, this approach assumes that all sources of the drug are direct and unique to the measured pool (DiStefano and Landaw, 1984). If these assumptions hold true, noncompartmental analyses can be conducted if sufficient concentration–time data are available (eg, if there are rich data). In most circumstances, "rich data" following parenteral drug administration are considered to be a minimum of 12 different concentration–time points (eg, include the predose concentration) associated with a single-dose administration. Any less data may provide inaccurate estimations of pharmacokinetic parameters using the noncompartmental approach.

## Statistical Moment Theory

Noncompartmental analyses are based on statistical moment theory, which provides a unique way to study time-related changes in *macroscopic events*. A macroscopic event is considered the overall event brought about by the constitutive elements involved. For example, in chemical processing, a dose of tracer molecules may be injected into a reactor tank to track the transit time (residence time) of materials that stay in the tank. The constitutive elements in this example are the tracer molecules, and the macroscopic events are the residence times shared by groups of tracer molecules. Each tracer molecule is well mixed and distributes noninteractively and randomly in the tank. In the case of all the molecules ($\int_0^{D_0} d\mathrm{De} = D_0$) that exit from the tank, the rate of exit of tracer molecules ($-d\mathrm{De}/dt$) divided by $D_0$ yields the probability of a molecule having a given residence time $t$. A mathematical formula describing the probability of

a tracer molecule exited at any time is a probability density function. *Mean residence time* (MRT) is the expected value or mean of the distribution.

MRT provides a fundamentally different approach than classical pharmacokinetic models, which involve the concept of dose, half-life, clearance, volume, and concentration. The classical approach does not account for the observation that molecules in a cluster move individually through space and are more appropriately tracked as statistical distribution based on residence–time considerations. Consistent with the concept of mass and the dynamic movement of molecules within a region or "space," MRT is an alternative concept to describe how drug molecules move in and out of a system. The concept is well established in chemical kinetics, where the relationships between MRT and rate constants for different systems are known.

A probability density function $f(t)$ multiplied by $t^m$ and integrated over time yields the moment curve (Equation 19.1). The moment curve shows the characteristics of the distribution.

$$\mu_m \text{ or } m\text{th moment} = \int_0^\infty t^m f(t)\,dt \qquad (19.1)$$

where $f(t)$ is the probability density function, $t$ is time, and $m$ is the $m$th moment.

For example, when $m = 0$, substituting for $m = 0$ yields Equation 19.2, called the *zero moment*, $\mu_0$:

$$\mu_0 = \int_0^\infty f(t)\,dt \qquad (19.2)$$

If the distribution is a true probability function, the area under the zero-moment curve is 1. When $f(t)$ represents drug concentration that is a function of time, the zero moment is referred to as area under the curve (AUC). The AUC can be obtained through integration of $f(t)$ or using the trapezoidal method, as described in Chapter 2. The trapezoidal methods most commonly used include the linear or the mixed linear/ln-linear methods. The linear trapezoidal method entails calculating the areas between two concentrations ($C_1$ and $C_2$) at two time points ($t_1$ and $t_2$) with Equation 19.3.

$$AUC_{t_1-t_2} = 0.5 \times (C_1 + C_2) \times (t_2 - t_1) \quad (19.3)$$

The linear trapezoidal rule is the most commonly used approach within noncompartmental analyses to estimate the AUC, and is by default the method that is used in Phase I and BE type PK studies. The second most common approach for estimating AUCs is the mixed linear/ln-linear trapezoidal rule. With this approach, the linear trapezoidal rule is used for increasing concentrations (up to the $C_{max}$), and the ln-linear trapezoidal rule is used for concentrations that are in the descending phase (after $C_{max}$). This approach may be superior to the linear trapezoidal rule for estimating AUCs for drugs with a long terminal half-life where less observations are obtained to characterize the whole profiles, or when the time intervals between observations are long (eg, many days or weeks). Equation 19.4 describes calculation of an area following the ln-linear trapezoidal rule:

$$AUC_{t_1-t_2} = (C_1-C_2) \times (t_2-t_1)/(\ln(C_1) - \ln(C_2)) \quad (19.4)$$

The first moment can be obtained by substituting into Equation 19.1 with $m = 1$, giving the first moment $\mu_1$ as shown in Equation 19.5:

$$\mu_1 = \int_0^\infty t^1 f(t)dt \quad (19.5)$$

The area under the curve $f(t)$ times $t$ is called the AUMC, or the *area under the first moment curve*. The *first moment*, $\mu_1$, defines the *mean* of the distribution.

Similarly, when $m = 2$, Equation 19.1 becomes the *second moment*, $\mu_2$:

$$\mu_2 = \int_0^\infty t^2 f(t)dt \quad (19.6)$$

where $\mu_2$ defines the variance of the distribution. Higher moments, such as $\mu_3$ or $\mu_4$, represent skewness and kurtosis of the distribution. Equation 19.1 is therefore useful in characterizing families of moment curves of a distribution.

The principal use of the moment curve is the calculation of the MRT of a drug in the body. It does not have much meaning on its own. The elements of the distribution curve describe the distribution of drug molecules after administration and the residence time of the drug molecules in the body.

## Mean Residence Time

According to statistical moment theory, MRT is the expected value or mean of the distribution of a probability density function. However, MRT can also be viewed from the perspective of the disposition of drug molecules. After an intravenous (IV) bolus drug dose ($D_0$), the drug molecules distribute throughout the body. These molecules stay (reside) in the body for various time periods. Some drug molecules leave the body almost immediately after entering, whereas other drug molecules leave the body at a much later time period. The term MRT describes the average time that drug molecules stay in the body or in a kinetic space.

The equation to calculate the MRT following IV bolus or constant infusion administrations is described in Equation 19.7:

$$MRT = \frac{AUCM_{inf}}{AUC_{inf}} - \frac{Duration}{2} \quad (19.7)$$

where $AUMC_{inf}$ is the area under the (first) moment-versus-time curve from $t = 0$ to infinity, $AUC_{inf}$ (or zero moment curve) is the area under the concentration-versus-time curve from $t = 0$ to infinity, and Duration is the duration of the drug infusion.

The $AUMC_{0-t}$ can be extrapolated to infinity using the following equation and assuming a log-linear terminal phase:

$$AUMC_{inf} = AUMC_{0-t} + \frac{C_{last} \cdot t}{\lambda_z} + \frac{C_{last}}{\lambda_z^2} \quad (19.8)$$

In this equation, $C_{last}$ represents the last detectable concentration. One major limitation of the $AUMC_{inf}$ calculation is that it can only be calculated after a single-dose administration, and not at steady-state conditions like the $AUC_{inf}$. This is because the superposition principle of the AUC (eg, that the $AUC_{inf}$ after a single dose is exactly equal to the $AUC_{tau(ss)}$ for a drug product exhibiting linear pharmacokinetics, see Chapter 15 for additional details) does not apply to the AUMC calculation. So the AUMC cannot be calculated easily at steady state over a dosing interval like the AUC. In practical terms, it means that the AUMC, and therefore the MRT, can only be calculated readily with the noncompartmental approach after a drug is administered as a single dose.

---

### FREQUENTLY ASKED QUESTIONS

▶ Why is statistical moment used in pharmacokinetics?

▶ Why is MRT used in pharmacokinetics? How is MRT related to the total volume of distribution ($V_{ss}$)?

# EXAMPLE ▷ ▷ ▷

An antibiotic was given to two subjects by an IV bolus dose of 1000 mg. Assume that the drug's pharmacokinetics is well described by a one-compartment model. The drug has a volume of distribution of 10 L and follows a one-compartment model with an elimination constant ($\lambda_z$) of (1) 0.1 $h^{-1}$ and (2) 0.2 $h^{-1}$ in the two subjects. Assume that the concentration at time zero was 100 mg/L in each subject. Determine the CL and the MRT for each subject based on the concentrations listed in Table 19-1 using the noncompartmental approach.

## SOLUTION

### Noncompartmental Approach

1. From Table 19-1, multiply each time point with the corresponding plasma $C_p$ to obtain points for the moment curve. Use the linear trapezoidal rule and sum the area to obtain the area under the concentration–time curve ($AUC_{0-t}$) and the area under the moment curve ($AUMC_{0-t}$) for each subject, as demonstrated in Table 19-2.

## TABLE 19-1 • Simulated Plasma Data after an IV Bolus Dose, Illustrating Calculation of MRT

| Time (h) | $C_p$ (mg/L) Subject 1 | $C_p$ (mg/L) Subject 2 |
|---|---|---|
| 0 | 100 | 100 |
| 1 | 90.484 | 81.873 |
| 2 | 81.873 | 67.032 |
| 3 | 74.082 | 54.881 |
| 4 | 67.032 | 44.933 |
| 6 | 54.881 | 30.119 |
| 8 | 44.933 | 20.19 |
| 12 | 30.119 | 9.072 |
| 16 | 20.19 | 4.076 |
| 24 | 9.072 | 0.823 |
| 30 | 4.979 | 0.248 |

The $AUC_{0-t}$ (area from time zero to 30 hours) for subject 1 is 961.6 mg·h/L while it is 509.2 mg·h/L for subject 2. We can then calculate the $AUC_{inf}$:

$$AUC_{inf} = AUC_{0-t} + C_{last}/\lambda_z$$

so $AUC_{inf} = 961.605 + 4.979/0.1 = 1011.395$ mg·h/L (subject 1)

$AUC_{inf} = 509.243 + 0.248/0.2 = 510.483$ mg · h/L (subject 2)

The CL is therefore: $CL = Dose/AUC_{inf}$

So $CL = 1000/1011.395 = 0.99$ L/h (subject 1)

$CL = 1000/510.483 = 1.96$ L/h (subject 2)

The $AUMC_{0-t}$ may be calculated by using Equation 19.8:

$$AUMC_{inf} = 7971.79 + 149.37/0.1 + 4.979/0.1^2$$
$$= 9963.4 \text{ (subject 1)}$$

$$AUMC_{inf} = 2483.502 + 7.44/0.2 + 0.248/0.2^2$$
$$= 2526.9 \text{ (subject 2)}$$

And, finally the MRT:

$$MRT = AUMC_{inf}/AUC_{inf} - Duration/2$$

So $MRT = 9963.4/1011.395 = 9.85$ h (subject 1)

$MRT = 2526.9/510.483 = 4.95$ h (subject 2)

## Mean Transit Time, Mean Absorption Time, and Mean Dissolution Time

After IV administration, the rate of systemic drug absorption is zero, because the drug is placed directly into the bloodstream. The MRT calculated for a drug after IV administration basically reflects the elimination processes in the body, and therefore the time that molecules stay in the systemic circulation. When drugs are administered extravascularly, such as after oral administration, the ratio of AUMC to AUC reflects not only the residence time of such molecules once they are in the systemic circulation (MRT) but the duration of the time during which they are absorbed (MAT). The AUMC/AUC ratio therefore

## TABLE 19-2 • Example of Calculation of MRT

| | | Subject 1 | | | | Subject 2 | | |
|---|---|---|---|---|---|---|---|---|
| Time (h) | $C_p$ (mg/L) | AUC (mg/L*h) | $C_p \times t$ (mg/L*h) | AUMC (mg/L*h²) | $C_p$ (mg/L) | AUC (mg/L*h) | $C_p \times t$ (mg/L*h) | AUMC (mg/L*h²) |
| 0 | 100 | | 0 | | 100 | | 0 | |
| 1 | 90.484 | 95.242 | 90.484 | 45.242 | 81.873 | 90.9365 | 81.873 | 40.9365 |
| 2 | 81.873 | 86.1785 | 163.746 | 127.115 | 67.032 | 74.4525 | 134.064 | 107.9685 |
| 3 | 74.082 | 77.9775 | 222.246 | 192.996 | 54.881 | 60.9565 | 164.643 | 149.3535 |
| 4 | 67.032 | 70.557 | 268.128 | 245.187 | 44.933 | 49.907 | 179.732 | 172.1875 |
| 6 | 54.881 | 121.913 | 329.286 | 597.414 | 30.119 | 75.052 | 180.714 | 360.446 |
| 8 | 44.933 | 99.814 | 359.464 | 688.75 | 20.19 | 50.309 | 161.52 | 342.234 |
| 12 | 30.119 | 150.104 | 361.428 | 1441.784 | 9.072 | 58.524 | 108.864 | 540.768 |
| 16 | 20.19 | 100.618 | 323.04 | 1368.936 | 4.076 | 26.296 | 65.216 | 348.16 |
| 24 | 9.072 | 117.048 | 217.728 | 2163.072 | 0.823 | 19.596 | 19.752 | 339.872 |
| 30 | 4.979 | 42.153 | 149.37 | 1101.294 | 0.248 | 3.213 | 7.44 | 81.576 |
| | Sum | 961.605 | | 7971.79 | | 509.2425 | | 2483.502 |

changes depending on how the drug is administered. Hence many refer to this ratio as $MRT_{PO}$ when the drug is orally administered, $MRT_{inh}$ when the drug is administered via inhalation, $MRT_{IM}$ when the drug is administered intramuscularly, and so on. This method of reporting the MRT suggests that the duration of time that drug molecules stay in the systemic circulation changes with the method of administration, which is incorrect if the drug displays linear pharmacokinetic properties. In addition, it creates confusion when other parameters need to be calculated, such as the $V_{ss}$, as shown later. Although it is not incorrect to label the ratio of AUMC/AUC by calling it a MRT with specification of the administration route, it is recommended to avoid confusion by referring to this ratio as the mean transit time (MTT):

$$MTT = AUMC_{inf}/AUC_{inf} \text{ after extravascular}$$
administration    (19.9)

and as we have seen earlier,

$$MRT = AUMC_{inf}/AUC_{inf} - \text{Duration}/2 \text{ after IV}$$
administration

such that

$$MTT = MAT + MRT \qquad (19.10)$$

where MAT is the mean absorption time or the average time it takes for drug molecules to be absorbed into the systemic circulation.

With this nomenclature, the MRT is always obtained after IV administration, and the MTT always represents the total transit time, which is the sum of the MAT and the MRT. MAT will be dictated by the route of administration, and in turn, this value will influence the MTT, but the MRT will remain constant regardless of the route of administration.

Therefore, after oral administration $MTT_{PO} = MAT_{PO} + MRT$, after IM administration $MTT_{IM} = MAT_{IM} + MRT$, and so on.

In some cases, IV data are not available and an MTT for a solution may be calculated. The mean dissolution time (MDT), or *in vivo* mean dissolution time, for an immediate-release (IR) solid drug product (tablet, capsule) given orally is described by Equation 19.11:

$$MDT_{PO(IR)} = MTT_{PO(IR)} - MTT_{PO(solution)} \qquad (19.11)$$

MDT reflects the time for the drug to dissolve *in vivo*, and it has been evaluated for a number of drug products. MDT is most readily estimated for immediate-release type products, because the absorption process (or MAT) may be influenced by certain types of modified-release drug products.

## EXAMPLE ▷ ▷ ▷

Data for ibuprofen (Gillespie et al, 1982) are shown in Tables 19-3 and 19-4. Serum concentrations for ibuprofen after administration of a capsule and a solution are tabulated as a function of time in Tables 19-3 and 19-4, respectively.

As listed in Table 19-5, the MTT for the solution was 2.65 hours and for the capsule was 4.04 hours. Therefore, MDT for the product is 4.04 − 2.65 = 1.39 hours.

### Other Pharmacokinetic Parameters Calculated by Noncompartmental Analysis

For a more detailed explanation on how to derive drug clearance (*CL*) using the noncompartmental approach, the reader is referred to Chapter 15. In essence, using the AUC value (zero-moment curve) obtained with the trapezoidal method, total apparent clearance (*CL/F*) can be determined as follows:

$$CL/F = \frac{\text{Dose}}{\text{AUC}_{\text{inf}}}$$

In addition, absolute bioavailability (*F*) can also be determined using concentration data obtained following IV and oral administration of a drug (Gibaldi and Perrier, 2007).

$$F = \frac{\text{Dose}_{\text{IV}} \cdot \text{AUC}_{\text{oral}}}{\text{Dose}_{\text{oral}} \cdot \text{AUC}_{\text{IV}}} \tag{19.12}$$

**TABLE 19-3 • Serum Concentrations for Ibuprofen Capsule**

| Time (h) | $C_p$ | $C_p t$ | $tC_p \Delta t$ |
|---|---|---|---|
| 0 | 0 | 0 | |
| 0.167 | 0.06 | 0.01002 | 0.000836 |
| 0.333 | 3.59 | 1.195 | 0.1000 |
| 0.50 | 7.79 | 3.895 | 0.425 |
| 1 | 13.3 | 13.300 | 4.298 |
| 1.5 | 14.5 | 21.750 | 8.762 |
| 2 | 16.9 | 33.80 | 13.887 |
| 3 | 16.6 | 49.80 | 41.80 |
| 4 | 11.9 | 47.60 | 48.70 |
| 6 | 6.31 | 37.86 | 85.46 |
| 8 | 3.54 | 28.32 | 66.18 |
| 10 | 1.36 | 13.60 | 41.92 |
| 12 | 0.63 | 7.56 | 21.16 |
| | | | Total AUMC = 332.695 |

$k = 0.347 \text{ h}^{-1}$, $\text{AUC}_{\text{inf}} = 89.1$

AUMC of tail piece (extrapolation to ∞) $= \dfrac{C_p \cdot t}{k} + \dfrac{C_p}{k^2} = \dfrac{0.63 \cdot 12}{0.347} + \dfrac{0.63}{0.347^2} = 27.02$

$\text{AUMC}_{\text{inf}} = 332.695 + 27.02 = 359.715$

$\text{MTT}_{\text{capsule}} = \dfrac{359.715}{89.1} = 4.04 \text{ h}$

*Data from Gillespie WR, DiSanto AR, Monovich RE, Albert KS. Relative bioavailability of commercially available ibuprofen oral dosage forms in humans, J Pharm Sci. 1982 Sep;71(9):1034–1038.*

## TABLE 19-4 • Serum Concentrations for Ibuprofen Solution

| Time (h) | $C_p$ | $C_p t$ | $tC_p \Delta t$ |
|---|---|---|---|
| 0 | 0 | 0 | |
| 0.167 | 17.8 | 2.973 | 0.248 |
| 0.333 | 29.0 | 9.657 | 1.048 |
| 0.5 | 29.7 | 14.85 | 2.046 |
| 1 | 25.7 | 25.7 | 10.14 |
| 1.5 | 19.7 | 29.55 | 13.81 |
| 2 | 17.0 | 34.0 | 15.88 |
| 3 | 11.0 | 33.0 | 33.50 |
| 4 | 7.1 | 28.4 | 30.70 |
| 6 | 3.82 | 22.92 | 51.33 |
| 8 | 1.44 | 11.52 | 34.45 |
| 10 | 0.57 | 5.70 | 17.22 |
| 12 | 0.38 | 4.56 | 10.26 |
| | | | Total AUMC = 220.64 |

$k = 0.455$ h$^{-1}$, AUC$_{inf}$ = 87.7

AUMC of tail piece (extrapolation to $\infty$) $= \dfrac{C_p \cdot t}{k} + \dfrac{C_p}{k^2} = \dfrac{0.38 \cdot 12}{0.455} + \dfrac{0.38}{0.455^2} = 11.86$

AUMC$_{inf}$ = 220.64 + 11.86 = 232.478

MTT$_{solution} = \dfrac{232.478}{87.7} = 2.65$ h

*Data from Gillespie WR, DiSanto AR, Monovich RE, Albert KS. Relative bioavailability of commercially available ibuprofen oral dosage forms in humans, J Pharm Sci. 1982 Sep;71(9):1034–1038.*

MRT is useful in calculating other pharmacokinetic parameters, particularly the total volume of distribution ($V_{ss}$).

$$V_{ss} = CL \times MRT \qquad (19.13)$$

We have previously seen that the AUMC cannot be readily calculated with the noncompartmental method, unless it is after a single-dose administration. In addition, the MRT can only be calculated after IV administration, as otherwise the MTT is calculated (when an extravascular administration is used) and this parameter includes the MAT in addition to the MRT. This means that the total volume of distribution ($V_{ss}$) can therefore only be readily calculated after a

## TABLE 19-5 • Parameters for Capsule and Solution Ibuprofen

| Parameter | Units | Capsule | Solution |
|---|---|---|---|
| AUC$_{inf}$ | µg/mL·h | 89.1 | 87.7 |
| AUMC$_{inf}$ | µg/mL·h$^2$ | 359.7 | 232.5 |
| $k_a$ | h$^{-1}$ | 0.46 | 4.90 |
| $K$ | h$^{-1}$ | 0.347 | 0.455 |
| MTT | Hours | 4.04 | 2.65 |

*Data from Gillespie WR, DiSanto AR, Monovich RE, Albert KS. Relative bioavailability of commercially available ibuprofen oral dosage forms in humans, J Pharm Sci. 1982 Sep;71(9):1034–1038.*

single-dose IV administration. This is a major limitation of the noncompartmental approach, compared to the compartmental approach when the total volume of distribution can always be calculated, but obviously only if a valid compartmental model is used.

## CLINICAL EXAMPLE ▷ ▷ ▷

Aripiprazole is an atypical antipsychotic drug used in the treatment of schizophrenia, among other indications. Efficacy for schizophrenia in adults has been demonstrated for doses of 10 mg, 15 mg, 20 mg, and 30 mg, as described in the product label (Otsuka Pharmaceutical Co. Ltd, 2019). The clearance of aripiprazole in healthy adult volunteers was found to be approximately 63 mL/h.kg (Belmonte et al, 2018).

1. If the clearance in adult schizophrenic patients is assumed to be similar to what is estimated in healthy adult volunteers, what is the minimal efficacious exposure ($AUC_{inf}$) that can be determined for aripiprazole?

   Answer: If $CL/F = Dose/AUC_{inf}$, then $AUC_{inf}$ can be calculated by dividing dose by apparent clearance. For a typical subject weighing 70 kg, clearance would be 63 mL/h × 70 kg, or 4.41 L/h. The efficacious $AUC_{inf}$ that would be associated with a dose of 15 mg would therefore be 15 mg divided by 4.41 L/h, or 3.40 mg.h/L.

2. What dose would be appropriate for patients who are poor metabolizers of CYP2D6 and whose mean clearance is 36.7 mL/h.kg, if the intended exposure is the one that is associated with a dose of 15 mg?

   Answer: The previous calculation demonstrated that a dose of 15 mg is associated with an $AUC_{inf}$ of 3.40 mg.h/L. To determine an appropriate dose for a patient with a specific clearance, one could simply multiply the apparent clearance by the desired $AUC_{inf}$. In this case, a mean clearance of 36.7 mL/h.kg is equivalent to a value of approximately 2.57 L/h for a patient weighing 70 kg. An appropriate dose would therefore be approximately 8.7 mg (2.57 L/h × 3.40 mg.h/L), or roughly half the typical dose of 15 mg.

## MODEL DEVELOPMENT CONSIDERATIONS

The noncompartmental method is a simple and robust approach that can be used to describe the absorption, distribution, and elimination of a drug and its metabolites in quantitative terms (see Chapter 1). However, some researchers or clinicians may be interested in developing a PK model to describe the observed time course for drug concentrations in the body. The model can use observed data to estimate various pharmacokinetic parameters and predict drug dosing outcomes, pharmacodynamics, and toxicity.

When developing a model, certain underlying assumptions are made by the pharmacokineticist as to the type of pharmacokinetic model, the order of the rate processes, tissue blood flow, the method for the estimation of the plasma or tissue volume, and other factors. Even with a more general approach such as the noncompartmental method, first-order drug elimination is assumed in the calculation of $AUC_{inf}$. In selecting a model for data analysis, the pharmacokineticist may choose more than one method of modeling, depending on many factors, including analysis objectives, experimental conditions, study design, and completeness of data. The goodness-of-fit of the model and the desired pharmacokinetic parameters are other considerations. Each estimated PK parameter has an inherent variability because of the variability of the biological system and of the observed data.

Despite challenges in the construction of these PK models, such models have been extremely useful in describing the time course of drug action, improving drug therapy by enhancing drug efficacy, and minimizing adverse reactions through more accurate dosing regimens. PK models are used routinely in the development process of new molecules or drug delivery systems.

Models can be broadly categorized as empirical or mechanistic. *Empirical models* are focused on describing the data with the specification of very few assumptions about the data being analyzed. An example of an empirical model is one that is used for allometric scaling, a type of prediction of PK parameters across diverse species. On the other hand, *mechanistic models* specify assumptions and attempt to incorporate known factors about the systems surrounding the data into the model, while describing the available data (Bonate, 2011). Both physiological modeling and compartmental modeling fall into the latter category, and each will be described in more detail later in this chapter. PK parameters can also be calculated without the specification of compartments in an almost model-independent manner, using noncompartmental analysis derived from statistical moment theory. This chapter will touch upon the aforementioned types of PK models but will also provide the essentials of the noncompartmental PK approach.

## EMPIRICAL MODELS

### Allometric Scaling

Various approaches have been used to compare and predict the pharmacokinetics of a drug among different species. *Interspecies scaling* is a method used in toxicokinetics and for the extrapolation of therapeutic drug doses in humans from nonclinical animal drug studies. *Toxicokinetics* is the application of pharmacokinetics to toxicology for interpolation and extrapolation based on anatomic, physiologic, and biochemical similarities (Mordenti and Chappell, 1989; Bonate and Howard, 2000; Mahmood, 2000, 2007; Hu and Hayton, 2001; Evans et al, 2006).

The basic assumption in interspecies scaling is that physiologic variables, such as clearance, heart rate, organ weight, and biochemical processes, are related to the weight or body surface area of the animal species (including humans). It is commonly assumed that all mammals use the same energy source (oxygen) and energy transport systems across animal species (Hu and Hayton, 2001). Interspecies scaling uses a physiologic variable, $y$, that is graphed against the body weight of the species on log–log axes to transform the data into a linear relationship (Fig. 19-1).

The general allometric equation obtained by this method is

$$y = bW^a \qquad (19.14)$$

where $y$ is the pharmacokinetic or physiologic property of interest, $b$ is an allometric coefficient, $W$ is the weight or surface area of the animal species, and $a$ is the allometric exponent. *Allometry* is the study of size.

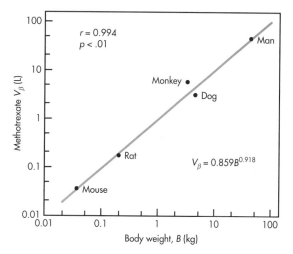

**FIGURE 19-1** • Interspecies correlation between methotrexate volume of distribution $V_\beta$ and body weight. Linear regression analysis was performed on logarithmically transformed data. (Reproduced with permission from Boxenbaum H. Interspecies scaling, allometry, physiological time, and the ground plan of pharmacokinetics. *J Pharmacokinet Biopharm.* 1982 Apr;10(2):201–227.)

Both $a$ and $b$ vary with the drug. Examples of various pharmacokinetic or physiologic properties that demonstrate allometric relationships are listed in Table 19-6.

In the example shown in Fig. 19-1, the apparent methotrexate volume of distribution is related to body weight $B$ of five animal species by the equation $V_\beta = 0.859B^{0.918}$.

The allometric method gives an empirical relationship that allows for approximate interspecies scaling based on the size of the species. Not considered in the method are certain specific interspecies differences related to gender, nutrition, pathophysiology, route of drug administration, protein binding, transporters, and polymorphisms. Some of these more specific cases, such as the pathophysiologic condition of the animal or human, may preclude pharmacokinetic or allometric predictions. Allometric scaling is only useful to predict parameters that are related to size, so in essence, this means clearances and volumes. This approach is not as useful to estimate rate constants such as the elimination rate constant $k_{el}$, as $k_{el}$ is the result of a clearance divided by a volume. Where clearances and volumes are related to size in the exact same manner (eg, *CL* in

**TABLE 19-6 •** Examples of Allometric Relationship for Interspecies Parameters

| Physiologic or Pharmacokinetic Property | Allometric Exponent[a] | Allometric Coefficient[b] |
|---|---|---|
| Basal $O_2$ consumption (mL/h) | 0.734 | 3.8 |
| Endogenous N output (g/h) | 0.72 | 0.000042 |
| $O_2$ consumption by liver slices (mL/h) | 0.77 | 3.3 |
| Clearance | | |
|    Creatinine (mL/h) | 0.69 | 8.72 |
|    Inulin (mL/h) | 0.77 | 5.36 |
|    PAH (mL/h) | 0.80 | 22.6 |
|    Antipyrine (mL/h) | 0.89 | 8.16 |
|    Methotrexate (mL/h) | 0.69 | 10.9 |
|    Phenytoin (mL/h) | 0.92 | 47.1 |
|    Aztreonam (mL/h) | 0.66 | 4.45 |
|    Ara-C and Ara-U (mL/h) | 0.79 | 3.93 |
| Volume of distribution (V) | | |
|    Methotrexate (L/kg) | 0.92 | 0.859 |
|    Cyclophosphamide (L/kg) | 0.99 | 0.883 |
|    Antipyrine (L/kg) | 0.96 | 0.756 |
|    Aztreonam (L/kg) | 0.91 | 0.234 |
| Kidney weight (g) | 0.85 | 0.0212 |
| Liver weight (g) | 0.87 | 0.082 |
| Heart weight (g) | 0.98 | 0.0066 |
| Stomach and intestines weight (g) | 0.94 | 0.112 |
| Blood weight (g) | 0.99 | 0.055 |
| Tidal volume (mL) | 1.01 | 0.0062 |
| Elimination half-life | | |
|    Methotrexate (min) | 0.23 | 54.6 |
|    Cyclophosphamide (min) | 0.24 | 36.6 |
|    Digoxin (min) | 0.23 | 98.3 |
|    Hexobarbital (min) | 0.35 | 80.0 |
|    Antipyrine (min) | 0.07 | 74.5 |
| Turnover times | | |
|    Serum albumin (1/day) | 0.30 | 5.68 |
|    Total body water (1/day) | 0.16 | 6.01 |
|    RBC (1/day) | 0.10 | 68.4 |
|    Cardiac circulation (min) | 0.21 | 0.44 |

*Data from Ritschel WA, Banerjee PS. Physiological pharmacokinetic models: principles, applications, limitations and outlook, Methods Find Exp Clin Pharmacol. 1986 Oct;8(10):603–614.*

L/h/kg and $V$ in L/h/kg), the rate constant will not differ at all with size.

Interspecies scaling has been refined by considering the aging rate and life span of species. In terms of physiologic time, each species has a characteristic life span, its maximum life-span potential (MLP), which is controlled genetically (Boxenbaum, 1982). Because many energy-consuming biochemical processes, including drug metabolism, vary inversely with the aging rate or life span of the animal, this allometric approach has been used for drugs that are eliminated mainly by hepatic intrinsic clearance.

Through the study of various species in handling several drugs that are metabolized predominantly by the liver, some empirical relationships regarding drug clearance of several drugs have been related mathematically in a single equation. For example, the hepatic intrinsic clearance of biperiden in rat, rabbit, and dog was extrapolated to humans (Nakashima et al, 1987). Equation 19.15 describes the relationship between biperiden intrinsic clearance with body weight and MLP:

$$CL_{int} \times MLP = 1.36 \times 10^7 \times B^{0.892} \quad (19.15)$$

where MLP is the maximum life-span potential of the species, $B$ is the body weight of the species, and $CL_{int}$ is the hepatic intrinsic clearance of the free drug.

Although further model improvements are needed before accurate prediction of pharmacokinetic parameters can be made from animal data, some interesting results were obtained by Sawada et al (1985) on nine acid and six basic drugs. When interspecies differences in protein–drug binding are properly considered, the volume of distribution of many drugs may be predicted with 50% deviation from experimental values (Table 19-7).

The application of MLP to pharmacokinetics has been described by Boxenbaum (1982). Initially, hepatic intrinsic clearance was considered to be related to volume or body weight. Indeed, a

**TABLE 19-7 • Relationship between Predicted and Observed Values of Various Pharmacokinetic Parameters in Humans for 15 Drugs**

| Drug | V (L/kg) | | | CL (mL/min per kg) | | | $t_{1/2}$ (min) | | |
|------|----------|-----------|----------|----------|-----------|----------|----------|-----------|----------|
| | Observed | Predicted | Percent* | Observed | Predicted | Percent* | Observed | Predicted | Percent* |
| Phenytoin | 0.640 | 0.573 | 10.5 | 0.574 | 0.483 | 15.9 | 792 | 822 | 3.79 |
| Quinidine | 3.20 | 3.69 | 22.2 | 2.91 | 3.25 | 11.7 | 470 | 785 | 67.0 |
| Hexobarbital | 1.27 | 0.735 | 42.1 | 3.57 | 4.25 | 19.0 | 261 | 120 | 54.0 |
| Pentobarbital | 0.999 | 1.57 | 57.2 | 0.524 | 0.964 | 84.0 | 1340 | 1126 | 16.0 |
| Phenylbutazone | 0.122[†] | 0.0839[‡] | 31.2 | 0.0205 | 0.0162 | 21.0 | 4110 | 3590 | 12.7 |
| Warfarin | 0.108 | 0.109 | 0.926 | 0.0367 | 0.0165 | 55.0 | 2040 | 4560 | 124 |
| Tolbutamide | 0.112 | 0.116 | 3.57 | 0.180 | 0.0589 | 67.3 | 434 | 1360 | 214 |
| Chlorpromazine | 11.2[†] | 9.05[‡] | 19.2 | 4.29 | 4.63 | 7.93 | 1810 | 1350 | 25.2 |
| Propranolol | 3.62 | 3.77 | 4.14 | 11.2 | 15.56 | 38.9 | 167 | 135 | 19.2 |
| Pentazocine | 5.56 | 7.19 | 29.3 | 18.3 | 11.6 | 36.6 | 203 | 408 | 101 |
| Valproate | 0.151 | 0.482 | 219 | 0.110 | 0.159 | 44.5 | 954 | 2110 | 121 |
| Diazepam | 0.950 | 1.44 | 51.6 | 0.350 | 2.13 | 509 | 1970 | 469 | 76.2 |
| Antipyrine | 0.869 | 0.878 | 1.04 | 0.662 | 0.664 | 3.02 | 654 | 917 | 40.2 |
| Phenobarbital | 0.649 | 0.817 | 25.9 | 0.0530 | 0.0825 | 55.7 | 6600 | 5870 | 11.0 |
| Amobarbital | 1.04 | 1.21 | 16.3 | 0.556 | 1.01 | 81.7 | 1360 | 827 | 39.2 |

*Absolute percent of error.
[†]The value of $V_{ss}$.
[‡]Predicted from the value of $V_{ss}$ in the rat.
Data from Sawada Y, Hanano M, Sugiyama Y, et al: Prediction of the disposition of nine weakly acidic and six weakly basic drugs in humans from pharmacokinetic parameters in rats, J Pharmacokinet Biopharm. 1985 Oct;13(5):477–492.

plot of the log drug clearance versus body weight for various animal species resulted in an approximately linear correlation (ie, a straight line). However, after correcting intrinsic clearance by MLP, an improved log–linear relationship was achieved between free drug $CL_{int}$ and body weight for many drugs. A possible explanation for this relationship is that the biochemical processes, including $CL_{int}$, in each animal species are related to the animal's normal life expectancy (estimated by MLP) through the evolutionary process. Animals with a shorter MLP have higher basal metabolic rates and tend to have higher intrinsic hepatic clearance and thus metabolize drugs faster. Boxenbaum (1982, 1983) postulated a constant "life stuff" in each species, such that the faster the life stuff is consumed, the more quickly the life stuff is used up. In the fourth-dimension scale (after correcting for MLP), all species share the same intrinsic clearance for the free drug.

$$\frac{(MLP) \cdot (CL_{int})}{B} = constant \qquad (19.16)$$

$$CL_{int} = aB^x \qquad (19.17)$$

Extensive work with caffeine in five species (mouse, rat, rabbit, monkey, and humans) by Bonati et al (1985) verified this approach. Caffeine is a drug that is metabolized predominantly by the liver. For caffeine,

$$Q_H = 0.0554 \times B^{0.894}$$

$$Liver\ weight = 0.0370 \times B^{0.849}$$

where $B$ is body weight and $Q_H$ is the liver blood flow.

Hepatic clearance for the unbound drug did not show a direct correlation among the five species. After intrinsic clearance was corrected for MLP (calculation based on brain weight), an excellent relationship was obtained among the five species (Fig. 19-2).

The subject of interspecies scaling was investigated using $CL$ values for 91 substances for several species by Hu and Hayton (2001). These investigators used $Y = a\ (BW)b$ in their analysis, similar to Equation 19.1 above but with different symbols: $Y$ = biological variable dependent on the body weight of the species, $a$ = allometric coefficient, $b$ = allometric exponent, and $BW$ = body weight of the species.

One issue discussed by Hu and Hayton is the uncertainty in the allometric exponent ($b$) of xenobiotic clearance ($CL$). Published literature has focused on whether the basal metabolic rate scale is a 2/3 or 3/4 power of the body mass. When the uncertainty in the determination of a $b$ value is relatively large, a fixed-exponent approach might be feasible according to Hu and Hayton. In this regard, 0.75 might be used for substances that are eliminated mainly by metabolism or by metabolism and excretion combined, whereas 0.67 might apply for drugs that are eliminated mainly by renal excretion. The researchers pointed out that genetic (intersubject) difference may be a limitation for using a single universal constant.

More recently, Anderson and Holford (2009) proposed various models for predicting clearance in humans as a function of size or organ maturation. They suggested that allometric scaling using a fixed exponent and body weight is superior to scaling using body surface area and proposed an exponent of 0.75 regardless of route of elimination, in contrast with the findings of Hu and Hayton. The use of the exponent of 0.75 is based on the linear relationship that is seen between log of basal metabolic rate and log-transformed weight, across a variety of species that were studied (including humans). In this linear

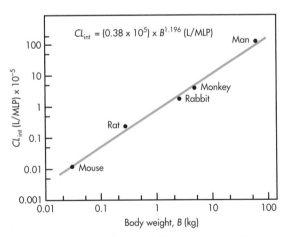

**FIGURE 19-2** • Caffeine (free drug) $CL_{int}$ per maximum life-span potential (MLP) in mammalian species as a function of body weight. MLP values were calculated for monkeys, rabbits, rats, and mice employing the following numeric values: MLP = $10.389 \times (brain\ weight)^{0.636} \times (body\ weight)^{0.225}$. (Data from Boxenbaum H. Interspecies scaling, allometry, physiological time, and the ground plan of pharmacokinetics. *J Pharmacokinet Biopharm.* 1982 Apr;10(2):201–227.)

relationship, a slope of 0.75 was observed. In addition, Anderson and Holford pooled data from eight publications and conducted an analysis of glomerular filtration data to determine the predictors and exponent that best described the data. The best predictor of body size was normal fat mass (a variable that distinguishes the contribution of fat-free mass and normal fat mass towards drug clearance) and the most appropriate exponent was 0.75.

Allometry is also frequently used for establishing doses to use in first-in-human studies based on preclinical data. With this approach, the drug clearance values calculated for different species, along with corresponding animal weights, can be used to predict the drug clearance in humans weighing 70 kg. It should be noted that this approach assumes that size is the most important determinant for predicting drug clearance, therefore it considers that all other factors are similar between humans and animals. The human clearance values obtained from allometry can be used to predict potentially efficacious doses in humans and define safe starting doses for first-in-human studies. The FDA has published a guidance on how to estimate the maximum safe starting dose in initial clinical trials in healthy volunteers (US FDA, 2005), and the EMA also provides some guidelines on dose selection in first-in-human trials (EMA, 2018a). In particular, the FDA guidance describes how PK parameters can be scaled between species by estimating an allometric exponent based on weight. While human equivalent doses can be estimated in this manner, safe starting doses are generally considered to be equivalent to 1/10 of the human equivalent dose. To further facilitate the calculation of the human equivalent dose, the FDA also provides a table of predetermined conversion factors that can be used with the "no observed adverse event level" in the most sensitive species to calculate a human equivalent dose. The values in this table were predetermined from allometric principles relating body surface area to parameters using an exponent of 2/3. Although the methods described in the FDA guidance are a quick and convenient way to calculate starting doses in humans, PBPK models have vastly improved and now offer an alternative method of predicting human PK from preclinical data. Additional description of the PBPK approach can be found later in this chapter.

Allometric scaling has also been useful for predicting drug clearance in children based on values that are estimated in adults. For instance, drug clearance in children could be estimated using the following general equation:

$$CL_{child} = CL_{adult} \times \left( \frac{Weight_{child}}{Weight_{adult}} \right)^{0.75} \quad (19.18)$$

The reader is referred to Chapter 24 for more considerations related to PK in pediatric populations.

## MECHANISTIC MODELS

### Historical Perspective

As previously described, mechanistic models include both compartmental and PBPK approaches. Although an in-depth review of the development of these approaches is beyond the scope of this chapter, a few key moments in the history of mechanistic modeling are described below.

In the 1950s, Gerhard Levy studied drug dissolution properties and developed some of the earliest fitting methods. He developed the Levy–Beaker method to test drug dissolution and formulation properties, which led to better understanding of key PK principles such as terminal half-life, clearance, and bioavailability (Levy, 1961; Levy and Hollister, 1965).

Additional fitting methods evolved over the next two decades, thanks in part to the work conducted by Wagner, Loo, Rigelman, Gibaldi, and Chiou, among others. This led to the creation of one- and two-compartment models that described the time course of drug concentrations in various matrices (Wagner and Nelson, 1963, 1964). Until the 1970s, model-based approaches relied on curve-fitting and stripping methods (see Chapter 16 for more details), but this changed when personal computers become readily available and more affordable. Wagner was one of the first researchers to promote the use of computers for PK analysis, because they could analyze data rapidly (Wagner, 1967). Despite the use of early computing technologies, PK models were mostly individually based such that each individual's data was fitted separately from other individuals' data. An important milestone in the history of compartmental analysis was achieved when the population approach was born in the 1970s, mostly thanks to the efforts of Lewis Sheiner and Stuart Beal, who developed the software called NONMEM® (Beal et al, 2009). This software is still used today and remains one of the gold standards for compartmental PK analyses in academia and in the industry.

## Compartmental Models

The essence of compartmental analysis is to create a mathematical and statistical model defined by integrated, matrix, and/or differential equations that describe the PK and/or PD behavior of a drug.

A model can be used to fit data using individual (eg, weighted least squares, maximum likelihood, maximum *a posteriori* probability) or population techniques (eg, first-order conditional estimation (FOCE), expectation maximization (EM)) so that mean parameter estimates along with their variability are obtained in an individual or population (most often nowadays) along with a residual variability or error component. An illustration of a compartmental model developed to describe the PK of sodium ferric gluconate complex is presented in Fig. 19-3 (Seng Yue et al, 2013).

Although a compartmental model can never explain the "true" mechanisms underlying PK and/or PD behavior, important correlations between covariates and parameters may point the way to further

studies or provide deeper mechanistic understanding (Sheiner, 1984). Among other advantages of the population compartmental method are its use in special populations (such as pediatric or hepatic impairment patients) and its potential partitioning of variability into interindividual, intraindividual, interoccasion, and other potential residual sources (Ette and Williams, 2004).

Various types of compartmental analyses exist, ranging from individual analysis to population PK modeling including the naïve pooled data approach, the standard two-stage approach, and nonlinear mixed-effect modeling. The latter includes, among others, the iterative two-stage, the FOCE and with interaction (FOCEI), the Laplace method, and EM approaches such as the maximum likelihood expectation maximization method (Sheiner, 1984; Steimer et al, 1984; Rodman et al, 2006; Wang et al, 2007). In these last approaches, all data are modeled simultaneously while retaining individual information in order to obtain estimates of population mean and variance as well as quantify sources of variability (Ludden, 1988; Ette and Williams, 2004). These types of compartmental analyses will be described in this chapter, and the software and general approaches that can be used to conduct these analyses are discussed in Chapter 20.

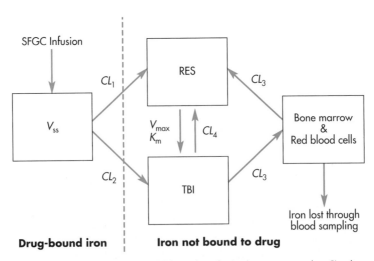

FIGURE 19-3 • Final compartmental pharmacokinetic model for sodium ferric gluconate complex. $CL_1$: clearance of sodium ferric gluconate complex iron (SFGC-I) to the reticuloendothelial system (RES) compartment; $CL_2$: clearance of SFGC-I directly to transferrin, $V_{ss}$ the apparent steady-state volume of distribution of SFGC-I; $CL_3$: clearance of iron entering and exiting the marrow and red blood cell compartment; $CL_4$: clearance of TBI to the RES; $K_m$: iron concentration associated with half of the maximal rate of exchange between the RES and TBI compartments; $V_{max}$: maximal rate of exchange between the RES and TBI compartments.

Important to data fitting are nonlinear regressions. In contrast with linear regression, where data are being fitted with a straight line defined by a slope and intercept, nonlinear regression depends on equations whose partial derivatives (with respect to each of the parameters) involve other model parameters (Gabrielsson and Weiner, 2006). The equations used to describe the model depicted in Fig. 19-3 are presented in Table 19-8.

Another important difference between the two types of regressions is that linear regressions have analytical solutions such that the functions can be manipulated to obtain a specific equation for the solution, while only numerical solutions exist for nonlinear regressions. For nonlinear equations, only approximate solutions to the equations can be obtained through iterative processes that are described in further detail below.

## Algorithms for Numerical Problem Solving

Many combinations of parameter estimates must be evaluated in order to find the parameters that best describe the data, and many algorithms have been developed to systematically do so. Each algorithm uses its own set of criteria to determine which set of parameter estimates is the most appropriate. This section will first describe some approaches used by

algorithms to reach a numerical solution, after which the algorithms themselves will be compared.

The aim of model development is to minimize the differences between the predicted and observed values, and generally the least-squares and maximum likelihood approaches are used to quantify these differences (Bonate, 2011). Various least-squares metrics (often termed "residual sum of squares") exist, and they are outlined in Table 19-9 (Gabrielsson and Weiner, 2006; Bonate, 2011).

The ordinary least-squares method is inherently biased because it tends to favor model estimates that provide better predictions for larger observations compared to smaller ones. The weighted least squares and ML/ELS (Extended Least Squares) approaches are an improvement over the ordinary least-squares method since they account for the magnitude of observations (and their relative variability) by incorporating a weighting factor into their formulas. The ML/ELS approaches differ from the weighted least-squares approach because they deal with the probability of observing the actual data given the model and its parameter estimates. In these methods, the function that is being minimized is the log likelihood, or the probability of observing the actual concentration values given a set of model parameter estimates. The function for log likelihood is presented in Equation 19.19. It should be noted that the only difference between

## TABLE 19-8 • Differential Equations Describing Compartmental Pharmacokinetic Model for Sodium Ferric Gluconate Complex

| Compartment | Equation |
|---|---|
| Serum | $\dfrac{dX(1)}{dt} = R(1) - \dfrac{Cl_1 + Cl_2}{V_{ss}} \cdot X(1)$ |
| Reticuloendothelial system | $\dfrac{dX(2)}{dt} = \dfrac{Cl_1}{V_{ss}} \cdot X(1) + \dfrac{Cl_3}{V\_RBC} \cdot X(4) + \dfrac{Cl_4}{V\_TBI} \cdot X(3) - \dfrac{V_{max}}{Km \cdot V\_RBC + X(2)} \cdot X(2)$ |
| Transferrin bound iron | $\dfrac{dX(3)}{dt} = \dfrac{Cl_2}{V_{ss}} \cdot X(1) + \dfrac{V_{max}}{Km \cdot V\_RBC + X(2)} \cdot X(2) - \dfrac{Cl_4}{V\_TBI} \cdot X(3) - \dfrac{Cl_3}{V\_TBI} \cdot X(3)$ |
| Red blood cells (marrow) | $\dfrac{dX(4)}{dt} = \dfrac{Cl_3}{V\_TBI} \cdot X(3) - \dfrac{Cl_3}{V\_RBC} \cdot X(4) - K0 \cdot R(2)$ |

$CL_1$: clearance of SFGC-I to the reticuloendothelial system (RES) compartment; $CL_2$: clearance of SFGC-I directly to transferrin; $V_{ss}$: the apparent steady-state volume of distribution of SFGC-I; $V_{TBI}$: volume of distribution associated with TBI; $CL_3$: clearance of iron entering and exiting the marrow and red blood cell compartment; $V_{RBC}$: marrow and red blood cell compartment; $CL_4$: clearance of TBI to the RES; Km: iron concentration associated with half of the maximal rate of exchange between the RES and TBI compartments; $V_{max}$: maximal rate of exchange between the RES and TBI compartments.

## TABLE 19-9 • Comparison of Least-Squares Methods

| Method | Objective Function Formula | Characteristics |
|---|---|---|
| Ordinary least squares | $O_{OLS} = \sum_{i=1}^{n}(C_i - \hat{C}_i)^2$ | No weighting |
| Weighted least squares | $O_{WLS} = \sum_{i=1}^{n}W_i(C_i - \hat{C}_i)^2$ | Model and parameters must be defined and stated empirically |
| Extended least squares or maximum likelihood | $O_{ELS} = \sum_{i=1}^{n}[W_i(C_i - \hat{C}_i)^2 + \ln(\text{var}(\hat{C}_i))]$ | Models can be defined, but parameters of the models are fitted within the procedure, eg, $W_i = 1/\text{var}(\hat{C}_i)$ |

$\hat{C}_i$ = predicted ith concentration value, $C_i$ = observed ith concentration value, $W_i$ = weighting factor, n = number of observations, var = variance

ELS and ML is in the assumptions that are specified about the distribution of the variance parameters. In the ML approach, the distribution is assumed to be normal, while no such assumption is made when the term "ELS" is used (Beal and Sheiner, 1989).

$$LL(C|\theta) = -\frac{n}{2}\ln(2\pi) - \frac{n}{2}\ln\left[\frac{\sum(C_i - \hat{C}_i)^2}{n}\right] - \frac{n}{2} \quad (19.19)$$

Because it is easier to minimize a positive number rather than a negative one, the log likelihood is often multiplied by –2 to obtain a positive number called the "–2 log likelihood."

Some algorithms apply linearization techniques to approximate the model using linear equations and they aim to minimize values such as the "–2 log likelihood," for example. For individual population analyses, Cauchy's method employs a first-order Taylor series expansion, Newton- or Newton–Raphson-based methods utilize a second-order Taylor series expansion, while the Gauss–Newton method iteratively uses multiple linear regressions via first-order Taylor series expansion. The Levenberg–Marquardt method is another algorithm that includes a modification of the Gauss–Newton method. Finally, in contrast with the algorithms previously described, the Nelder–Mead simplex approach does not involve linearization procedures. This technique is thought to be the most robust and involves the examination of the response surface (to find the lowest point) using a series of moving and contracting or expanding polyhedra (three-dimensional objects composed of flat polygonal faces joined by vertices). The

latter approach has always been implemented in the ADAPT® software series by D'Argenio and Schmitzky, a software that has been constantly improved for the last 40 years and is currently available as ADAPT5®.

Some of the algorithms used in the context of population compartmental analyses include the first-order (FO) method, FOCE approach, the stochastic approximation of expectation maximization, and the maximum likelihood expectation maximization method, to name a few. In both the FO and FOCE algorithms as implemented within NONMEM, the minimum objective function (which is related to the sum of squares) is sought out by linearization of the model through a series of first-order Taylor series expansions of the error model. The difference between the FO and FOCE algorithms is that in the former, interindividual variability for PK parameters is estimated using estimates of the population mean and variance in a *post hoc* step, while in the latter, interindividual variability is estimated simultaneously with the population mean and variance (Beal and Sheiner, 1998). In other words, within NONMEM the FO algorithm uses a linearization technique that first assumes $\eta = 0$, contrary to the FOCE algorithm which uses the posterior mode of $\eta$ (that relies on conditional estimates) (Bonate, 2011). A modification of the FOCE algorithm, known as the Laplacian FOCE method, exists also within NONMEM whereby a second-order Taylor series is performed instead of the first-order expansion (Beal and Sheiner, 1998).

The maximum likelihood expectation maximization algorithm is different from the previous methods because it does not rely on any linearization techniques (D'Argenio et al, 2009). This algorithm involves maximizing a likelihood function through an iterative series of two steps that are repeated until convergence. In the first step, termed the expectation step, or "E-step," the conditional mean and covariance for each individual's data are computed and the expected likelihood function associated with these parameters is obtained. In the second step, the maximization step, or "M-step," the population mean, covariance, and error variance parameters are updated to maximize the likelihood from the previous step (D'Argenio et al, 2009; Bonate, 2011).

### Individual and Population Analyses

As its name implies, individual analysis involves the development of a model using data from one source (such as one human or one animal). Because of the error that is always inherent in data, whether related to the collection procedures themselves or to analytical assays, a model can never perfectly predict the observed data. The relationship between observed and predicted concentration values must therefore account for this error, as defined in Equation 19.20. In this equation, $X_i$ represents a vector of known values (such as dose and sampling times), $C_i$ represents the vector of observed concentrations, $\varepsilon_i$ represents the measurement errors, $\phi_j$ represents the vector of model parameters (in other words the PK parameters), and $f_i$ is the function that relates $C_i$ to $\phi_j$ and $X_i$. The subscript $i$ represents the total number of observations or values.

$$C_i = f_i(\phi_j, X_i) + \varepsilon_i \qquad (19.20)$$

Population analysis can be viewed as an extension of individual analyses, since it attempts to develop a model that predicts concentration data associated with different individuals or animals. The general concept is similar to that embraced by individual analysis, except that the model must also take into consideration interindividual variability. The resulting model is therefore able to predict concentration values for each individual within the population, but it also provides an "overall" (mean or population) set of predictions. In other words, the model describes the behavior of the whole population as well as the behavior of each individual

within this population. Another distinction is that a population analysis will always use the same structural model (eg, a two-compartment model) to fit all individuals' data for a specific drug under study, while individual analyses could theoretically use different models to fit data from different subjects (eg, a one-compartment model for some subjects and a two-compartment model for others).

In a population analysis, observed concentrations must be ascribed to specific subjects, as defined in Equation 19.21, which is analogous to Equation 19.20. In this equation, $X_{ij}$ represents a vector of known values (represented by $i$) for the $j$th subject, $C_{ij}$ represents the vector of observed concentrations for the $j$th subject, $\varepsilon_{ij}$ represents the measurement errors for the $j$th subject, $\phi_j$ represents the vector of model parameters for the $j$th subject, and $f_{ij}$ is the function that relates $C_{ij}$ to $\phi_j$ and $X_{ij}$.

$$C_{ij} = f_{ij}(\phi_j, X_{ij}) + \varepsilon_{ij} \qquad (19.21)$$

Each individual has a distinct set of PK model parameters ($\phi_j$) that will provide the best predicted values for that individual's observed data. However, as previously mentioned, there is also a typical profile of "population predictions" that is associated with population PK model parameters ($\theta$) that can be regarded as mean values. The relationship between the mean PK parameters and individual PK parameters is described by Equation 19.22, where $g$ is a known function that relates $\phi_j$ to $\theta$ using the individual's characteristics such as height or weight, denoted by $z_j$. The last term, $\eta_j$, represents random (unexplained or uncontrollable) variability that also causes $\phi_j$ to deviate from $\theta$.

$$\phi_j = g(\theta, z_j) + \eta_j \qquad (19.22)$$

There are various types of population compartmental analyses, but the most basic type is the "naïve-average data" method, where the average concentration values at given time points are computed from the entire dataset, and then a model is developed using these average values. A similar method is the "naïve pooled data" approach, where data from different individuals are treated as though they were obtained from a single individual, and then analyzed using the individual approach.

The two-stage approach to population compartmental analyses offers some improvement over the previous ones. In essence, data from each subject are first fitted individually (in other words, using the individual approach but using the same structural model to fit each individual's data), and in the second step, population parameter estimates are obtained. Different types of two-stage approaches exist, such as the standard two-stage approach, the global two-stage approach, and finally a mixed-effect modeling approach known as the iterative two-stage approach, which has been abbreviated as IT2S (Forrest et al, 1991), ITS (ADAPT5) or IT2B (Pmetrics®). In the standard two-stage approach, the population parameter estimates (for mean and variance) are determined by calculating the mean and variance of the individual PK parameters, while the global two-stage approach actually estimates expectations for the mean and variance through an iterative process. The iterative two-stage method is a nonlinear mixed-effect modeling technique that uses a more refined iterative approach utilizing a mixture of ML and maximum *a posteriori* probability techniques. Within each population iteration, prior values are used to estimate individual PK parameters in the first step, while individual values are then used in the second step to recalculate a newer, more probable set of population parameters. Steps one and two are subsequently repeated until there is little to no difference between the new and old prior distributions (eg, until the algorithm "converges").

In contrast with the iterative two-stage approach, other types of nonlinear mixed-effect modeling techniques, such as that of the FO or FOCE methods implemented by NONMEM, proceed by first fitting the data in a reverse manner so they obtain population mean estimates followed in a second step with individual data estimates (therefore called "*post hocs*"). The fixed effects (variables that can be controlled, such as dose or pharmacokinetic parameters) and random effects (uncontrollable factors like interoccasion variability) are fitted simultaneously with respect to population mean and variability estimates as well as the residual variability.

All of the nonlinear mixed effect modeling techniques discussed thus far in this chapter estimate the approximate likelihood of the results given the data. A significant advancement in the field was the introduction of EM methods within PK/PD analyses using either nonparametric (Schumitzky, 1991) or parametric distributions (Schumitzky, 1995). These EM methods use exact maximum likelihood estimation and may therefore be more accurate than the previously described methods which use linear approximation. Many different EM methods are currently available in PKPD software (see Chapter 20). Some use Monte Carlo integration and others employ importance sampling. The latter is considered preferable and has been implemented in the maximum likelihood expectation maximization algorithm of ADAPT5 (Wang et al, 2007; D'Argenio et al, 2009). Colucci et al (2011) have suggested, using simulated datasets, that the maximum likelihood expectation maximization algorithm appears to perform at least as well as FOCE while presenting much fewer shrinkage issues.

## Parametric versus Nonparametric Modeling

The vast majority of population PK/PD tools available use parametric modeling, which means that they assume a distribution, typically a normal or a ln-normal distribution of PK and/or PD parameters. PK parameters such as those related to exposure (eg, $C_{max}$, $AUC_s$) or those calculated from such parameters (eg, $CL/F$) are known to be ln-normally distributed. On the other hand, PD parameters occasionally follow a normal distribution. NONMEM is a software program that was originally meant for population PK analysis and therefore assumes by default a ln-normal distribution (eg, population means are geometric means). ADAPT5 gives the user the possibility of choosing normal or ln-normal distribution with its algorithms such as maximum likelihood expectation maximization.

The main drawback of parametric approaches to population PK/PD assessments is the assumption of this distribution. Even if a parameter truly follows a ln-normal distribution, for example $CL/F$, the distribution in one dataset may not be unimodal, meaning that there may be more than one distinct group within that population. The addition of covariates and mixture models in population PK may solve this issue and provide a good characterization of the overall population, but doing so is quite complex. A simpler approach would naturally be not to assume a distribution *per se*, and fit the data using nonparametric approaches. This approach was first proposed by Mallet (1986) and was included in his proposed tool "NPML." Jelliffe and his colleagues have championed for many years the use of a nonparametric EM population tool, originally called NPEM (Kisor et al, 1992) and part of the USC pack (Jelliffe, 1991), which is now implemented within the Pmetrics software (Neely et al, 2012). Although there are certainly theoretical advantages that favor the use of nonparametric population PK modeling, in practice this approach has never been popular among scientists.

More details about software available to conduct population PK and PK/PD analyses, as well as general approaches, can be found in Chapter 20.

---

### FREQUENTLY ASKED QUESTIONS

▶ How can we tell if we are using the right model to describe our data?

▶ Are certain algorithms better than others?

▶ When should individual compartmental analysis be used rather than population analysis?

---

### Applications of Compartmental Modeling

Compartmental modeling is an extremely versatile tool that allows researchers to do much more than simply estimate pharmacokinetic and/or pharmacodynamic parameters and quantify their variability. In some cases, it may be of interest to better understand the sources of variability by attributing variability to specific patient characteristics. For example, compartmental models can evaluate whether demographic factors (weight, age, laboratory values, drug polymorphism), drug-related factors (formulation, manufacturer), or other potential variables (disease variables, use of concomitant medication) contribute to interindividual variability in certain parameters. Not only does compartmental modeling allow the identification of important covariates, but it can also quantify their relative importance.

Compartmental models are often used to relate a drug's PK to its response (PD), whether it be efficacy, toxicity, or both. PK-PD modeling can also be used to link preclinical (animal) data to data collected from human subjects by providing a common framework for understanding the data. A well-constructed compartmental model can also be used to answer a wide variety of questions through simulations. Throughout drug development, questions arise at various stages, and compartmental models can be used at all stages to answer these questions. For instance, in Phase 1, questions regarding optimal dosing for Phase 2 can be answered using PK/PD modeling. Among other uses, compartmental modeling can be used to support proof-of-concept claims, select optimal dosing regimens, optimize dosing schedule, and refine study designs (FDA guidance; Chien et al, 2005).

An example of how PK/PD modeling was helpful in making key decisions surrounding the development of a drug is described by Nieforth and colleagues. Interferons are used to treat various viral infections and malignancies. Despite their therapeutic benefits, their short half-life requires frequent administration (three times per week) and they can be highly antigenic. PEGylation of interferons is thought to increase the circulating half-life as well as decrease immunogenicity. In this example, a PK/PD model was constructed to relate the exposure to PEG-modified interferon alfa-2a to its effect on the induction of the production of MX protein (Nieforth et al, 1996). Because of their many effects, MX proteins were considered to be a useful PD probe. The goal of model development was to provide information to improve dosing strategies as well as guide the drug development of future modified molecules.

The PK/PD model was based on data from a randomized single ascending dose study that included 45 healthy adult male subjects receiving one of four subcutaneous doses of PEG-modified interferon alfa-2a or interferon alfa-2a. The PK of the interferon products, described by a one-compartment model with first-order absorption and elimination, was related to the PD through an indirect model. The drug stimulated the production of MX protein via an $E_{max}$ function.

The simulations obtained from the PK/PD modeling exercise indicated that, although the addition of a PEG moiety to interferon alfa-2a did indeed prolong the half-life of the drug, the PD properties associated with the PEG-modified interferon alfa-2a would still necessitate a twice-weekly dosing regimen in order to attain a comparable response to the unmodified product. This was a far cry from the anticipated once-weekly dosing for the PEG-modified product and these predictions were confirmed by two Phase II trials.

In conclusion, PK/PD modeling demonstrated that the PEG-modified interferon alfa-2a provided little therapeutic benefit over its unmodified counterpart, which proved to be consistent with Phase II findings. These findings contributed to the decision to discontinue the development of this product for this indication.

Modeling and simulations are not only being used and further developed by the pharmaceutical industry or academia but, from a regulatory perspective, have also been used to enhance decision making and contribute to product labeling (pertaining to dosage and administration, safety, or clinical pharmacology) (Bhattaram et al, 2007). In some submissions to the FDA, drug companies benefitted from modeling and simulations performed by reviewers who were able to extract information from the data that had not otherwise been presented (Bhattaram et al, 2005, 2007). Lee et al (2011) found that over an 8-year period (2000 to 2008), modeling and simulations contributed to the approval of 64% of products while it influenced the labeling of 67% of products.

## Physiologic Pharmacokinetic Models

PBPK models are fundamentally different from compartmental PK models, as they rely on our detailed knowledge and understanding of the physiologic processes that govern the passage of drugs in the body. The human body is composed of organ systems containing living cells bathed in an extracellular aqueous fluid (see Chapter 13). Both drugs and endogenous substances, such as hormones, nutrients, and oxygen, are transported to the organs by the same network of blood vessels (arteries). The drug concentration within a target organ therefore depends on plasma drug concentration, plasma versus tissue protein binding, the rate of blood flow to an organ, and the rate of drug uptake into the tissue. Physiologically, uptake (accumulation) of drug by organ tissues occurs from the extracellular fluid, which equilibrates rapidly with the capillary blood in the organ. Some drugs cross the plasma membrane into the interior fluid (intracellular water) of the cell (Fig. 19-4).

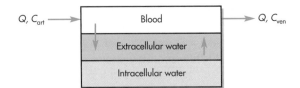

FIGURE 19-4 • In describing drug transfer, the physiologic pharmacokinetic model divides a body organ into three parts: capillary vessels, extracellular space, and intracellular space.

In addition to drug accumulation, some organs of the body are involved in drug elimination, either by excretion (eg, kidney) or by metabolism (eg, liver). The elimination of drug by an organ may be described by drug clearance in the organ (see Chapter 15). The liver is an example of an organ with drug metabolism and drug uptake (accumulation). PBPK modeling aims to consider as much as possible all processes of drug uptake, distribution, and elimination.

In PBPK models, drugs are carried by blood flow from the administration (input) site to various body organs, where the drug rapidly equilibrates with the interstitial water in the organ. PBPK models are mathematical models describing drug movement and disposition in the body based on organ blood flow and the organ spaces penetrated by the drug. In its simplest form, a PBPK model considers the drug to be blood flow limited. Drugs are carried to organs by arterial blood and leave organs by venous blood (Fig. 19-5).

In such a model, transmembrane movement of drug is rapid, and the capillary membrane does not offer any resistance to drug permeation. Uptake of drug into the tissues is rapid, and a constant ratio of drug concentrations between the organ and the venous blood is quickly established. This ratio is the tissue/blood partition coefficient:

$$P_{\text{tissue}} = \frac{C_{\text{tissue}}}{C_{\text{blood}}} \qquad (19.23)$$

where $P$ is the partition coefficient.

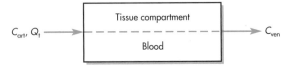

FIGURE 19-5 • Noneliminating tissue organ. The extracellular water is merged with the plasma water in the blood.

The magnitude of the partition coefficient can vary depending on the drug and on the type of tissue. Adipose tissue, for example, has a high partition for lipophilic drugs. The rate of drug carried to a tissue organ and tissue drug uptake depends on the rate of blood flow to the organ and the tissue/blood partition coefficient, respectively.

The rate of blood flow to the tissue is expressed as $Q_t$ (mL/min), and the rate of change in the drug concentration with respect to time within a given tissue organ is expressed as

$$\frac{d(V_{tissue}C_{tissue})}{dt} = Q_t(C_{in} - C_{out}) \quad (19.24)$$

$$\frac{d(V_{tissue}C_{tissue})}{dt} = Q_t(C_{art} - C_{ven}) \quad (19.25)$$

where $C_{art}$ is the arterial blood drug concentration and $C_{ven}$ is the venous blood drug concentration. $Q_t$ is blood flow and represents the volume of blood flowing through a typical tissue organ per unit of time.

If drug uptake occurs in the tissue, the incoming concentration, $C_{art}$, is higher than the outgoing venous concentration, $C_{ven}$. The rate of change in the tissue drug concentration is equal to the rate of blood flow multiplied by the difference between the blood drug concentrations entering and leaving the tissue organ. In the *blood flow–limited model,* drug concentration in the blood leaving the tissue and the drug concentration within the tissue are in equilibrium, and $C_{ven}$ may be estimated from the tissue/blood partition coefficient in Equation 19.23. Substituting in Equation 19.25 with $C_{ven} = C_{tissue}/P_{tissue}$ yields

$$\frac{d(V_{tissue}C_{tissue})}{dt} = Q_t\left(C_{art} - \frac{C_{tissue}}{P_{tissue}}\right) \quad (19.26)$$

Equation 19.26 describes drug distribution in a noneliminating organ or tissue group. For example, drug distribution to muscle, adipose tissue, and skin can be represented in a similar manner by Equations 19.27, 19.28, and 19.29, respectively, as shown below. For tissue organs in which drug is eliminated (Fig. 19-6), parameters representing drug elimination from the liver ($k_{LIV}$) and kidney ($k_{KID}$) are added to account for drug removal through metabolism or excretion. Equations 19.30 and 19.31 are derived similarly to those for the non-eliminating organs above.

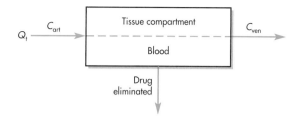

FIGURE 19-6 • A typical eliminating tissue organ.

Removal of drug from any organ is described by drug clearance (*CL*) from that organ. The rate of drug elimination is the product of the drug concentration in the organ and the organ clearance.

$$\text{Rate of drug elimination} = \frac{V_{tissue}\,dC_{tissue}}{dt}$$

$$= C_{tissue} \times Cl_{tissue}$$

The rate of drug elimination may be described for each organ or tissue (Fig. 19-7).

Muscle: $\dfrac{d(V_{MUS}C_{MUS})}{dt} = Q_{MUS}\left(C_{MUS} - \dfrac{C_{MUS}}{P_{MUS}}\right)$ (19.27)

Adipose tissue: $\dfrac{d(V_{FAT}C_{FAT})}{dt} = Q_{FAT}\left(C_{FAT} - \dfrac{C_{FAT}}{P_{FAT}}\right)$

$$(19.28)$$

Skin: $\dfrac{d(V_{SKIN}C_{SKIN})}{dt} = Q_{SKIN}\left(C_{SKIN} - \dfrac{C_{SKIN}}{P_{SKIN}}\right)$ (19.29)

Liver: $\dfrac{d(V_{LIV}C_{LIV})}{dt} = C_{LIV}(Q_{LIV} - Q_{GI} - Q_{SP})$

$$+ Q_{GI}\left(\frac{C_{GI}}{P_{GI}}\right) + Q_{SP}\left(\frac{C_{SP}}{P_{SP}}\right) - Q_{LIV}\left(\frac{C_{LIV}}{P_{LIV}}\right)$$

$$- C_{LIV}\left(\frac{Cl_{int}}{P_{LIV}}\right)$$

$$(19.30)$$

Kidney: $\dfrac{d(V_{KID}C_{KID})}{dt}$

$$= Q_{KID}\left(C_{KID} - \frac{C_{KID}}{P_{KID}}\right) - C_{KID}\left(\frac{Cl_{KID}}{P_{KID}}\right)$$

$$(19.31)$$

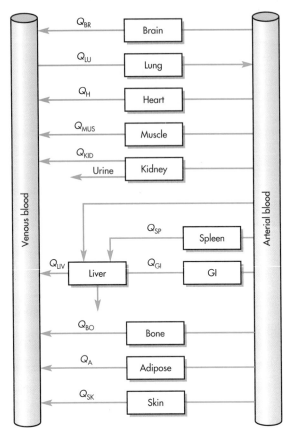

Lung: $\dfrac{d(V_{LU}C_{LU})}{dt} = Q_{LU}\left(\dfrac{C_{LU}}{P_{LU}}\right)$    (19.32)

where LIV = liver, SP = spleen, GI = gastrointestinal tract, KID = kidney, LU = lung, FAT = adipose, SKIN = skin, and MUS = muscle.

The mass balance for the rate of change in drug concentration in the blood pool is

$$\dfrac{d(V_b C_b)}{dt} = Q_{MUS}\left(\dfrac{C_{MUS}}{P_{MUS}}\right) + Q_{LIV}\left(\dfrac{C_{LIV}}{P_{LIV}}\right) + Q_{KID}\left(\dfrac{C_{KID}}{P_{KID}}\right)$$

(muscle)        (liver)        (kidney)

$$+ Q_{SKIN}\left(\dfrac{C_{SKIN}}{P_{SKIN}}\right) + Q_{FAT}\left(\dfrac{C_{FAT}}{P_{FAT}}\right) - Q_b C_b$$

(skin)        (adipose)    (blood)

(19.33)

Lung perfusion is unique because the pulmonary artery returns venous blood flow to the lung, where carbon dioxide is exchanged for oxygen and the blood becomes oxygenated. Equation 19.32 presents the equation for the lung. The blood from the lungs flows back to the heart (into the left atrium) through the pulmonary vein, and the quantity of blood that perfuses the pulmonary system ultimately passes through the remainder of the body. In describing drug clearance through the lung, perfusion from the heart (right ventricle) to the lung is considered venous blood (Fig. 19-7). With some drugs, the lung is a clearing organ besides serving as a merging pool for venous blood. In those cases, a lung clearance term could be included in the general model.

After IV drug administration, drug uptake in the lungs may be very significant if the drug has high affinity for lung tissue. If actual drug clearance is at a much higher rate than the drug clearance accounted for by renal and hepatic clearance, then lung clearance of the drug should be suspected, and a lung clearance term should be included in the equation in addition to lung tissue distribution.

The system of differential equations used to describe the blood flow–limited model is usually solved through computer programs in an analogous manner to what is used with compartmental modeling. Because of the large number of parameters involved in the mass balance, and because "true" solutions to a set of differential equations may not solely exist, more than one set of parameters often fit the experimental data. This is common with human data, in which many of the organ tissue data items are not available. The lack of sufficient tissue data sometimes leads to unconstrained models. As additional data become available, new or refined models are adopted. For example, methotrexate was initially described by a flow-limited model, but later work described the model as a *diffusion-limited model*.

Because invasive methods are available for animals, tissue/blood ratios or partition coefficients can be determined accurately by direct measurement. Using experimental pharmacokinetic data from animals, PBPK models may yield more reliable predictions.

## Physiologic Pharmacokinetic Model with Binding

The PBPK model described above assumed flow-limited drug distribution without drug binding to either plasma or tissues. In reality, many drugs are bound to a variable extent in either plasma or tissues. With most physiologic models, drug binding is assumed to be linear (not saturable or concentration dependent). Moreover, bound and free drug in both tissue and plasma are in equilibrium. Further, the free drug in the plasma and in the tissue equilibrates rapidly. Therefore, the free drug concentration in the tissue and the free drug concentration in the emerging blood are equal:

$$[C_b]_f = [C_t]_f \tag{19.34}$$

$$[C_b]_f = f_b[C_b] \tag{19.35}$$

$$[C_t]_f = f_t[C_t] \tag{19.36}$$

where $f_b$ is the blood-free drug fraction, $f_t$ is the tissue-free drug fraction, $C_t$ is the total drug concentration in tissue, and $C_b$ is the total drug concentration in blood.

Therefore, the partition ratio, $P_t$, of the tissue drug concentration to that of the plasma drug concentration is

$$\frac{f_b}{f_t} = \frac{[C_t]}{[C_b]} = P_t \tag{19.37}$$

By assuming linear drug binding and rapid drug equilibration, the free drug fraction in tissue and blood may be incorporated into the partition ratio and the differential equations. These equations are similar to those above except that free drug concentrations are substituted for $C_b$. Drug clearance in the liver is assumed to occur only with the free drug. The inherent capacity for drug metabolism (and elimination) is described by the term $CL_{int}$ (see Chapter 6). General mass balance of various tissues is described by Equation 19.38:

$$\frac{d(V_{tissue}C_{tissue})}{dt} = Q_t(C_{art} - C_{ven})$$

$$\frac{d(V_{tissue}C_{tissue})}{dt} = Q_t\left(C_{art} - \frac{C_t}{P_t}\right) \tag{19.38}$$

or

$$\frac{d(V_{tissue}C_{tissue})}{dt} = Q_t\left(C_{art} - \frac{C_t f_t}{f_b}\right)$$

For liver metabolism,

$$\frac{d(V_{LIV}C_{LIV})}{dt} = C_b(Q_{LIV} - Q_{GI} - Q_{SP}) - Q_{LIV}\left(\frac{C_{LIV}}{P_{LIV}}\right)$$

(hepatic drug elimination)

$$+ Q_{GI}\left(\frac{C_{GI}}{P_{GI}}\right) + Q_{SP}\left(\frac{C_{SP}}{P_{SP}}\right) \tag{19.39}$$

The mass balance for the drug in the blood pool is

$$\frac{d(V_b C_b)}{dt} = Q_{MUS}C_{MUS} + Q_{LIV}\left(\frac{C_{LIV}}{P_{LIV}}\right)$$

(muscle)        (liver)

$$+ Q_{KID}\left(\frac{C_{KID}}{P_{KID}}\right) + Q_{SKIN}\left(\frac{C_{SKIN}}{P_{SKIN}}\right) \tag{19.40}$$

(kidney)        (skin)

$$+ Q_{FAT}\left(\frac{C_{FAT}}{P_{FAT}}\right) - Q_b C_b$$

(adipose)    (blood)

The influence of binding on drug distribution is an important factor in interspecies differences in pharmacokinetics. In some instances, animal data may predict drug distribution in humans by taking into account the differences in drug binding. For the most part, extrapolations from animals to humans or between species are rough estimates only, and there are many instances in which species differences are not entirely attributable to drug binding and metabolism.

## Blood Flow–Limited versus Diffusion-Limited Model

Most PBPK models assume rapid drug distribution between tissue and venous blood. Rapid drug equilibrium assumes that drug diffusion is extremely fast and that the cell membrane offers no barrier to drug permeation. If no drug binding is involved, the tissue drug concentration is the same as that of

**TABLE 19-10** • Drugs Described by Physiologic Pharmacokinetic Model

| Drug | Category | Comment | Reference |
|------|----------|---------|-----------|
| Thiopental | Anesthetic | Blood, flow limited | Chen and Andrade (1976) |
| BSP | Diagnostic | Plasma, flow limited | Luecke and Thomason (1980) |
| Nicotine | Stimulant | Blood, flow limited | Gabrielsson and Bondesson (1987) |
| Lidocaine | Antiarrhythmic | Blood, flow limited | Benowitz et al (1974) |
| Methotrexate | Antineoplastic | Plasma, flow limited | Bischoff et al (1970) |
| Biperiden | Anticholinergic | Blood, flow limited | Nakashima and Benet (1988) |
| Cisplatin | Antineoplastic | Plasma, multiple metabolite, binding | King et al (1986) |

the venous blood leaving the tissue. This assumption greatly simplifies the mathematics involved. Table 19-10 lists some of the drugs that have been described by a flow-limited model. This model is also referred to as the *perfusion model*. A more complex type of PBPK model is called the *diffusion-limited model* or the *membrane-limited model*. In the diffusion-limited model, the cell membrane acts as a barrier for the drug, which gradually permeates by diffusion. Because blood flow is very rapid and drug permeation is slow, a drug concentration gradient is established between the tissue and the venous blood (Lutz and Dedrick, 1985). The rate-limiting step of drug diffusion into the tissue depends on the permeation across the cell membrane rather than blood flow. Because of the time lag in equilibration between blood and tissue, the pharmacokinetic equation for the diffusion-limited model is very complicated.

## Physiologic Pharmacokinetic Model Incorporating Hepatic Transporter-Mediated Clearance

It is now well recognized that drug transporters play important roles in the processes of absorption, distribution, and excretion and should be accounted for in PBPK models. Predicting human drug disposition, especially when involving hepatic transport, is difficult during drug development. However, drug transport may be a critical process in overall drug disposition in the body such that without a realistic description of transport processes in the body,

model accuracy may be deficient. As it was noted when the allometric approach was described, simple approaches often assume that body size is the most important factor that is predictive of pharmacokinetics. In contrast, PBK modeling can take more factors into consideration when making predictions.

Watanabe et al (2009) describe a model with hepatobiliary excretion mediated by transporters, organic anion-transporting polypeptide (OATP) 1B1, and multidrug resistance–associated protein (MRP) 2, for the HMG-CoA reductase inhibitor drug, pravastatin. While the classical blood flow–based PBPK models developed 40 years ago using systems of differential equations are still useful in describing the mass balance and transfer of drug within major organs, the models are inadequate in light of new discoveries in molecular biology and pharmacogenomics. Drug disposition and drug targeting are better understood based upon using influx/efflux and binding mechanisms in microstructures such as interior cellular structures, membrane transporters, surface receptors, genomes, and enzymes. The liver is a complex organ intimately connected to drug transport and bile movement. Compartment concepts are needed to track the mass of drug transfer in and out of those fine structures as shown by the example in Fig. 19-8. Human liver microsomes are used to help predict the metabolic clearance of drugs in the body.

The PBPK model with pravastatin (Watanabe et al, 2009) is used to evaluate the concentration–time profiles for drugs in the plasma and peripheral

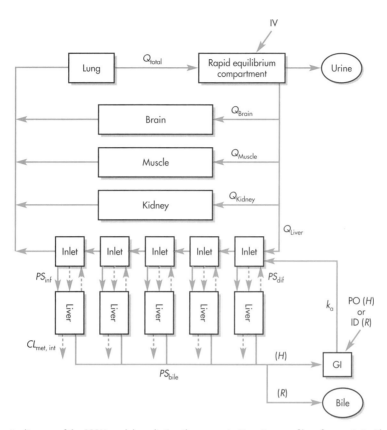

FIGURE 19-8 • Schematic diagram of the PBPK model predicting the concentration–time profiles of pravastatin. The liver compartment was divided into five compartments to mimic the dispersion model. Indicated are blood flow ($Q$), active hepatic uptake clearance ($PS_{inf}$), passive diffusion clearance ($PS_{dif}$), biliary clearance ($PS_{bile}$), and metabolic clearance ($Cl_{met, int}$), human ($H$), and rat ($R$). The enterohepatic circulation was incorporated in the case of humans. (Reproduced with permission from Watanabe T, Kusuhara H, Maeda K, et al: Physiologically based pharmacokinetic modeling to predict transporter-mediated clearance and distribution of pravastatin in humans, *J Pharmacol Exp Ther.* 2009 Feb;328(2):652–662.)

organs in humans using physiological parameters, subcellular fractions (cells lysed and contents fractionated based on density), and drug-related parameters (unbound fraction and metabolic and membrane transport clearances extrapolated from *in vitro* experiments). The principle of the prediction was as follows. First, subcellular fractions were obtained by comparing *in vitro* and *in vivo* parameters in rats. Then, the *in vitro* human parameters were extrapolated *in vivo* using the subcellular fractions obtained in rats. Pravastatin was selected as the model compound because many studies have investigated the mechanisms involved in the drug disposition in rodents, and clinical data after IV and oral administration are available.

When multiple drug metabolites are involved, the physiologic model of the cascade events can be quite complicated, and an abbreviated approach may be used. St-Pierre et al (1988) developed a simple one-compartment open model, based on the liver as the only organ of drug disappearance and metabolite formation. The model was used to illustrate the metabolism of a drug to its primary, secondary, and tertiary metabolites. The model encompassed the cascading effects of sequential metabolism (Fig. 19-9).

The concentration–time profiles of the drug and metabolites were examined for both oral and IV drug administration. Formation of the primary metabolite from drug in the gut lumen, with or without further absorption, and metabolite formation arising from first-pass metabolism of the drug and the primary metabolite during oral absorption were

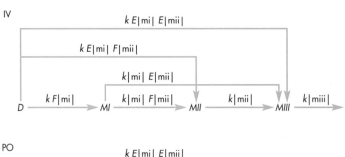

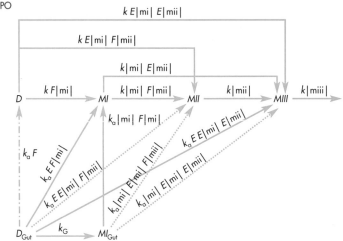

**FIGURE 19-9** • A schematic representation of the one-compartment open model for drug (*D*) and its primary (MI), secondary (MII), and tertiary (MIII) metabolites after intravenous (IV) and (po) drug dosing (scheme II) The effective rate constants contributing to the appearance of the metabolites in the systemic circulation are presented. The solid lines denote sources pertaining to drug or metabolite species in the circulation; the uneven dashed lines represent sources arising from absorption of drug or the primary metabolite from the gut lumen; and the stippled lines denote sources arising from first-pass metabolism of the drug or primary metabolite. D, MI, MII, and MIII are drug and primary, secondary, and tertiary metabolites, respectively; {mi}, {mii}, and {miii} define parameters associated with the primary, secondary, and tertiary metabolites, respectively; $D_{Gut}$ and $MI_{Gut}$ denote the amounts of drug and primary metabolite in gut, respectively. *k*, $k_a$, and $k_G$ are the total elimination rate constant, the absorption rate constant, and the elimination rate constant of drug from the gut lumen, respectively, under first-order conditions. *F* is the effective availability by the first-pass organs. *E* is the effective extraction ratio by the first-pass organs. (Reproduced with permission from St-Pierre MV, Xu X, Pang KS. Primary, secondary, and tertiary metabolite kinetics, *J Pharmacokinet Biopharm*. 1988 Oct;16(5):493–527.)

considered. Mass balance equations, incorporating modifications of the various absorption and conversion rate constants, were integrated to provide the explicit solutions.

## FREQUENTLY ASKED QUESTIONS

▶ Why are differential equations used to describe physiologic models?

▶ Why do we assume that drug concentrations in venous and arterial blood are the same in pharmacokinetics?

▶ Why should transporters be considered in physiological models?

## Application and Limitations of Physiologic Pharmacokinetic Models

The PBPK model is related to drug concentration and tissue distribution using physiologic and anatomic information. For example, the effect of a change in blood flow on the drug concentration in a given tissue may be estimated once the model is characterized. Similarly, the effect of a change in mass size of different tissue organs on the redistribution of drug may also be evaluated using the system of physiologic model differential equations generated. When several species are involved, the physiologic model may predict the pharmacokinetics of a drug in humans when only animal data are available.

Changes in drug–protein binding, tissue organ–drug partition ratios, and intrinsic hepatic clearance may be inserted into the PBPK model.

Most pharmacokinetic studies are modeled based on blood samples drawn from various venous sites after either IV or oral dosing. Physiologists have long recognized the unique difference between arterial and venous blood. For example, arterial tension (pressure) of oxygen drives the distribution of oxygen to vital organs. Chiou (1989) and Mather (2001) have discussed the pharmacokinetic issues when differences in drug concentrations in arterial and venous are considered (see Chapter 13). The implication of venous versus arterial sampling is hard to estimate and may be more drug dependent. Most pharmacokinetic models are based on sampling of venous data. In theory, mixing occurs quickly when venous blood returns to the heart and becomes reoxygenated again in the lung. Chiou (1989) has estimated that for drugs that are highly extracted, the discrepancies may be substantial between actual concentration and concentration estimated from well-stirred pharmacokinetic models. Therefore, PBPK models can account for these discrepancies to further improve predictions.

As previously described, PBPK modeling is being used more extensively to predict the PK of drugs in humans based solely on physicochemical properties or preclinical data. Recently, the US FDA and the EMA have published guidance documents on the format and content of PBPK analyses that are submitted for review (US FDA, 2016; EMA, 2018a). The availability of PBPK software such as Gastroplus® and Simcyp® has made these types of analyses even more accessible than before. One of the challenges with PBPK modeling has always been the determination of rate constants and other values needed to describe pharmacological and physiological processes, and these software programs include predetermined values based on literature and past experience.

Currently, PBPK models are often used to understand or predict drug–drug interactions (using validated models) and to select doses for first-in-human trials or appropriate initial doses for pediatric patients (EMA, 2018b). Other uses for the PBPK approach are also being explored, such as the capacity of such models to predict the effect of food or oral drug absorption (Li et al, 2018); however, additional work is required before clinical trials can be waived solely on the basis of PBPK modeling results.

## COMPARISON OF DIFFERENT APPROACHES

### Physiological versus Compartmental Approach

Both physiological and compartmental models aim to incorporate as much information as possible about the system (biological or other) that encompasses the data being modeled. Both approaches rely on differential equations or partial differential equations to ensure that laws of mass balance are respected.

While physiological models take into consideration biological processes at very specific molecular levels, compartmental models may lump various organs or tissues into groups. For example, a one-compartment model "groups" together all components of the human body such that they are represented by a single box. Thus, compartmental models can be viewed as more simplistic in comparison with their physiologic model counterparts.

The major advantage of compartmental models is that the time course of drug in the body may be monitored quantitatively with a limited amount of data. Generally, only plasma drug concentrations and limited urinary drug excretion data are available. Compartmental models have been applied successfully for the prediction of drug pharmacokinetics and the development of dosage regimens. Moreover, compartmental models are very useful in relating plasma drug levels to pharmacodynamic and toxic effects in the body.

The simplicity and flexibility of the compartmental model is the principal reason for its wide application. In many cases, the compartmental model may be used to extract some information about the underlying physiologic mechanism through model testing of the data. Thus, compartmental analysis may lead to a more accurate description of the underlying physiological processes and the kinetics involved. In this regard, compartmental models are sometimes misunderstood, overstretched, and even abused. For example, the tissue drug levels predicted by a compartmental model represent only a composite pool for drug equilibration between all tissue and the circulatory system (plasma compartment).

However, extrapolation to a specific tissue drug concentration is inaccurate and analogous to making predictions without experimental data. Although specific tissue drug concentration data are missing, many investigators may make general predictions about average tissue drug levels.

The compartmental model is particularly useful for comparing the pharmacokinetics of related therapeutic agents (Chapter 22). In the clinical pharmacokinetic literature, drug data comparisons are based on compartmental models. Though alternative pharmacokinetic models have been available for approximately 20 years, the simplicity of the compartment model allows easy tabulation of parameters such as $V_{ss}$, the distribution $t_{1/2}$, and the terminal $t_{1/2}$.

Because the PBPK model is more detailed, accounting for processes of drug distribution, drug binding, metabolism, and drug flow to the body organs, disease-related changes in specific physiologic processes are more readily related to changes in the pharmacokinetics of the drug. Furthermore, organ mass, volumes, and blood perfusion rates are often scalable, based on size, among different individuals, and even among different species. This allows a perturbation in one parameter and the prediction of the effect of changing physiology on drug distribution and elimination. The physiological pharmacokinetic model can also be modified to include a specific feature of a drug. For example, for an antitumor agent that penetrates into the cell, both the drug level in the interstitial water and the intracellular water may be considered in the model. Blood flow and tumor size may even be included in the model to study any change in the drug uptake at that site.

PBPK models can also take into consideration physicochemical properties of the drug as well as characteristics related to its formulation. Formulation experts often use PBPK models to determine the potential impact of formulation changes on various PK processes. They can also be used to calculate the amount of drug in the blood and in any tissues for any time period if the initial amount of drug in the blood is known. In contrast, the tissue compartment in the multicompartmental model is not related to any actual anatomic tissue groups, and therefore it is not possible to predict the drug concentrations in a specific tissue.

While both types of analyses can be challenging, there are also difficulties specific to each method.

In PBPK modeling, obtaining the necessary rates and constants to describe molecular processes is not always obvious or easy. Those who perform compartmental modeling must deal with the challenges of noisy data, or data whose behavior is not easily described by simple models, making the determination of the "best model" more difficult and time consuming.

The compartmental approach also raises concerns about "identifiability," which means that a process should not be fitted if it cannot be "identified" or supported by the data, while in the PBPK approach most of the parameters are not identifiable and are "fixed." For example, a compartmental model will not predict an oral bioavailability parameter if concentration data are only available following IV administration. Predicting an oral bioavailability parameter would then be "unidentifiable." This is in direct contrast to the PBPK modeling approach in which a bioavailability parameter may still be included the model, even though there are no data to support it. Although "unidentifiable" parameters may be estimated using a PBPK approach, this does not necessarily mean the parameter is robust or reliable, and so scientists should be careful in interpreting data that comes from such a PBPK model.

A common descriptor of the compartmental versus the PBPK approach is to describe the former as a "top-down" approach, while the latter is a "bottom-up" approach. A "top-down" approach means that the compartmental model is created from the data, and the model will therefore need to be identifiable from these data, and ideally will be shown to be perfectly capable of explaining these data. A "bottom-up" approach means that the PBPK model may be created before actual data are obtained in order to predict what concentration–time profiles may look like. It is with this simple comparison, "top-down" versus "bottom-up," that it is easier to reconcile both methods and see when it may be useful to use one rather than the other. When a lot of data are available, compartmental modeling should be prioritized. In contrast, when no data are available yet for a drug product, then PBPK may be extremely useful to potentially predict what may happen. For scenarios that are somewhere between these two extreme situations (no data or a lot of data), then both models may coexist and be useful. It is important to note

**TABLE 19-11 •** Advantages and Disadvantages of Noncompartmental versus Compartmental Population Analyses

|  | Advantages | Disadvantages |
|---|---|---|
| **Noncompartmental analysis** | – Easy and quick to perform<br>– No special software is needed<br>– Robust and easily reproducible | – Requires rich sampling<br>– Makes assumptions regarding linearity |
| **Compartmental population analysis** | – Can be performed with rich or sparse data<br>– Can be performed using data from heterogeneous sources or special populations<br>– Can deal with both linearity and nonlinearity | – Requires experienced analyst<br>– Time consuming and labor intensive<br>– Software is not user friendly |

as well that a mixture of the two approaches can be used. For example, compartmental modeling can use "physiological" parameters to predict or explain CYP enzyme activity when drug–drug interaction data are being modeled (Pasternyk Di Marco et al, 2000).

### Noncompartmental versus Compartmental Approach

Noncompartmental and compartmental analyses are both excellent methods that can be used to characterize the PK, PD, and/or PK/PD of a drug, when used in their appropriate context. The disadvantages of each method highlight the advantages of the others, but when utilized correctly, each approach has its own merits. Table 19-11 summarizes the key advantages and disadvantages of each approach (Tett et al, 1998; Ette and Williams, 2004; Seng Yue et al, 2019).

For additional information, the reader is also referred to the section in Chapter 15 that describes the relationships between clearance, volume of distribution, and rate constants between the noncompartmental and compartmental approaches.

### SELECTION OF PHARMACOKINETIC MODELS

Many factors should be considered when using mathematical models to study rate processes (eg, pharmacokinetics of a drug). Ultimately, the type of model used will depend on the questions that need to be answered as well as the nature of the available data.

Indeed, adequate experimental design and the availability of valid data are important considerations in model selection and testing. More details on model selection and testing can be found in Chapter 20. For example, the experimental design can determine whether a drug is being eliminated by saturable (dose-dependent) or simple linear kinetics. A plot of metabolic rate versus drug concentration can be used to determine dose dependence, as in Fig. 19-10.

Metabolic rate can be measured at various drug concentrations using an *in vitro* system (see Chapter 6). In Fig. 19-10, curve *B*, saturation occurs at higher drug concentration.

For illustration, consider the drug concentration–time profile for a drug given by IV bolus. The combined metabolic and distribution processes may result in profiles like those in Fig. 19-11.

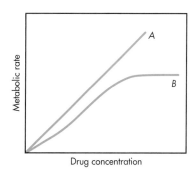

FIGURE 19-10 • Metabolic rate versus drug concentration. Drug *A* follows first-order pharmacokinetics, whereas drug *B* follows nonlinear pharmacokinetics and saturation occurs at higher drug concentrations.

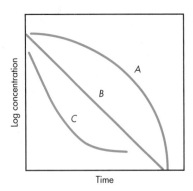

**FIGURE 19-11** • Plasma drug concentration profiles due to distribution and metabolic process. (See text for description of A, B, and C.)

Curve *A* represents a slow initial decline due to saturation and a faster terminal decline as drug concentration decreases. Curve *C* represents a dominating distributive phase masking the effect of nonlinear metabolism. Finally, a combination of *A* and *C* may approximate a rough overall linear decline (curve *B*). Notice that the drug concentration–time profile is shared by many different processes and that the goodness-of-fit is not an adequate criterion

for adopting a model. For example, concluding linear metabolism based only on curve *B* would be incorrect. Contrary to common belief, complex models tend to mask opposing variables that must be isolated and tested through better experimental designs. In this case, a constant infusion until steady-state experiment would yield information on saturation without the influence of initial drug distribution.

The use of pharmacokinetic models has been critically reviewed by Rescigno and Beck (1987) and by Riggs (1963). These authors emphasize the difference between model building and simulation. A model is a secondary system designed to test the primary system (real and unknown). The assumptions made by a model must be realistic and consistent with physical observations. On the other hand, a simulation may emulate the phenomenon without resembling the true physical process. A simulation without identifiable support of the physical system does little to aid understanding of the basic mechanism, and the computation has only hypothetical meaning.

## CHAPTER SUMMARY

PK data can be described using model-independent (noncompartmental) or model-dependent approaches. Noncompartmental analyses are based on statistical moment theory. The latter is a statistical approach that treats drug molecules as individual units that move through organ and body spaces according to kinetic principles. This permits model-independent development of many equations and parameters that are familiar to classical kineticists. This approach allows the determination of the time for mean residence of the molecules (eg, dose administered) in the body according to the route of administration. The variance of the residence time can also be determined using statistical moment theory based on probability density function. This approach allows another way of computing the volume of distribution of a drug through the derived equations. The noncompartmental approach assumes that a drug possesses linear PK, elimination, and that

sampling occurs from the same compartment. Various types of models can be used to describe PK data. These include empirical, data-driven models such as allometric scaling. The latter is used to predict pharmacokinetic parameter values for humans based on animal data. Another model category is the mechanistic one, in which models aim to include as much information as possible about the system that surrounds the data being studied. Physiologically based PK models are mechanistic models that use a system of differential equations to describe drug transfer and accumulation in various tissues or organs in the body. Published data in the physiology literature regarding size (mass) of organs and blood flow to each organ and body mass are used. Compartmental models are also mechanistic models that use a system of differential equations to describe drug disposition. In contrast with PBPK models, molecular processes are not specifically modeled; thus a compartment does not usually represent one specific actual organ or tissue. Because they do not include physiological data (organ size, blood flow, etc), compartmental models can be applied to sparse data obtained from individual subjects or groups of subjects. Model-dependent pharmacokinetic parameters can thus be determined with different approaches. The decision to use one approach versus another depends on the objective of the analysis and the available data.

## LEARNING QUESTIONS

1. After an IV bolus dose (500 mg) of an antibiotic, plasma–time concentration data were collected and the area under the curve was computed to be 25 mg/L·h. The area under the first moment-versus-time curve was found to be 100 mg/L·h$^2$.

   a. What is the mean residence time of this drug?

   b. What is the clearance of this drug?

   c. What is the total volume of distribution of this drug?

2. If the data in Question 1 are fit to a one-compartment model with an elimination $k$ that is found to be 0.25 h$^{-1}$, MRT may be calculated compartmentally simply as $1/k$. What different assumptions are used in here versus Question 1?

3. What are the principal considerations in interspecies scaling?

4. What are the key considerations in fitting plasma drug data to a pharmacokinetic model?

5. What assumptions must hold true in order to conduct noncompartmental analyses?

## ANSWERS

### Frequently Asked Questions

*How can we tell if we are using the right model to describe our data?*

- In reality, there is no "right" model, because different combinations of pharmacokinetic parameter estimates can often describe the same set of data using a given model. There can be a model that is superior to another according to predefined criteria, but it is not necessarily the "right" model. The most appropriate model also depends on the objectives of the modeling exercise, as well as the nature of the data that were collected.

*Are certain algorithms better than others?*

- Each algorithm has its strengths and weaknesses and depending on the nature of the data being fitted, some algorithms may present certain advantages over others. For example, some of the algorithms that employ linearization may converge more quickly than those that perform no linearization; therefore, results could possibly be obtained more quickly.

*When should individual compartmental analysis be used rather than population analysis?*

- Besides being used when data are only available from one subject, individual compartmental analysis can be used to perform naïve pooled data analysis with data from a larger population. For example, data from a group of subjects can be pooled together such that a mean concentration–time profile is created from this group. The mean profile can then be fitted using a compartmental PK model, and the results can be used as initial estimates to perform population PK analyses if desired.

*Why are differential equations used to describe physiologic models?*

- Differential equations are used to describe the rate of drug transfer between different tissues and the blood. Differential equations have the advantage of being very adaptable to computer simulation without a lot of mathematical manipulations.

*Why do we assume that drug concentrations in venous and arterial blood are the same in pharmacokinetics?*

- After an IV bolus drug injection, a drug is diluted rapidly in the venous pool. The venous blood is oxygenated in the lung and becomes arterial blood. The arterial blood containing the diluted drug then perfuses all the body organs through the systemic circulation. Some drug molecules diffuse into the tissue and others are eliminated. In cycling through the body for the first time, the blood leaving a tissue (venous) generally has a lower drug concentration than the perfusing blood (arterial). Drug concentration in the venous blood rapidly equilibrates with the tissue and will become arterial blood in the next perfusion cycle (seconds later) through the body. In practice, only venous blood is sampled and assayed but since equilibrium is rapidly attained between tissue, arterial blood, and venous blood, it is generally assumed that drug concentrations in venous blood are equivalent to those found in arterial blood.

*Why should transporters be considered in physiological models?*

- Drug transporters play important roles in the processes of absorption, distribution, and excretion, and if they are not considered in physiological models, the models may not be as accurate as they should be.

*Why is statistical moment used in pharmacokinetics?*

- Statistical moment is adaptable to mean residence time calculation and is widely used in pharmacokinetics because of its simplicity and robustness.

*Why is MRT used in pharmacokinetics?*

- Mean residence time (MRT) represents the average staying time of the drug in a body organ or compartment as the molecules diffuse in and out. MRT is an alternative concept used to describe how long a drug stays in the body. The main advantage of MRT is that it is based on probability and is consistent with how drug molecules behave in the physical world. Concentration in a heterogeneous region of the body may be hard to pinpoint.

*How is MRT related to the total volume of distribution ($V_{ss}$)?*

- The $V_{ss}$ can be determined from MRT according to the following equation: $V_{ss} = CL \times MRT$, using data obtained following single-dose IV drug administration.

**Learning Questions**

1. **a.** $MRT = AUMC/AUC = 100/25 = 4$ hours

   **b.** $CL = Dose/AUC = 500/25 = 20$ L/h

   **c.** $V_{ss} = CL \times MRT = 20 \times 4 = 80$ L

2. $MRT = 1/0.25 = 4$ hours. In this case, the one-compartment model must be assumed.

3. The principal considerations are size, drug-protein binding, and maximum life span potential of the species.

4. The objectives of the modeling must always be kept in mind, and the simplest model that best explains the data should always be retained.

5. Linear kinetics are assumed, and it is also assumed that drug loss (elimination) only occurs from the compartment from which samples are being collected.

## REFERENCES

Anderson BJ, Holford NHG: Mechanistic basis of using body size and maturation to predict clearance in humans. *Drug Metab Pharmacokinet* **24**(1):25–36, 2009.

Beal SL, Sheiner LB: Part I, Users basic guide. In *NONMEM Users Guide*. San Francisco, CA, University of California, 1989.

Beal SL, Sheiner LB: Part VII, Conditional Estimation Methods. In *NONMEM Users Guide*. San Francisco, CA, University of California, 1988.

Beal SL, Sheiner LB, Boeckmann A, Bauer R: In *NONMEM User's Guides (1989-2009)*. Icon Development Solutions, Ellicott City, MD, 2009.

Belmonte C, Ochoa D, Román M, et al: Influence of *CYP2D6*, *CYP3A4*, *CYP3A5* and *ABCB1* polymorphisms on pharmacokinetics and safety of aripiprazole in healthy volunteers. *Basic Clin Pharmacol Toxicol* **122**:596–605, 2018.

Benet LZ, Ronfeld RA: Volume terms in pharmacokinetics. *J Pharm Sci* **58**(5):639–641, 1969.

Benowitz N, Forsyth RP, Melmon KL, Rowland M: Lidocaine disposition kinetics in monkey and man, 1. Prediction by a perfusion model. *Clin Pharmacol Ther* **16**:87–98, 1974.

Bhattaram VA, Booth BP, Ramchandani RP, et al: Impact of pharmacometrics on drug approval and labeling decisions: A survey of 42 new drug applications. *AAPS J* **7**(3):E503–E512, 2005.

Bhattaram VA, Bonapace C, Chilukuri DM, et al: Impact of pharmacometric reviews on new drug approval and labeling decisions—A survey of 31 new drug applications submitted between 2005 and 2006. *Clin Pharmacol Ther* **81**(2):213–221, 2007.

Bischoff KB, Dedrick RL, Zaharko DS: Preliminary model for methotrexate pharmacokinetics. *J Pharm Sci* **59**:149–154, 1970.

Bonate PL: *Pharmacokinetic-Pharmacodynamic Modeling and Simulation*. 2nd ed. New York, NY: Springer; 2011.

Bonate PL, Howard D: Prospective allometric scaling: Does the emperor have clothes? *J Clin Pharmacol* **40**:665–670, 2000.

Bonati M, Latini R, Tognoni G, et al: Interspecies comparison of in vivo caffeine pharmacokinetics in man, monkey, rabbit, rat, and mouse. *Drug Metab Rev* **15**:1355–1383, 1985.

Boxenbaum H: Interspecies scaling, allometry, physiological time, and the ground plan of pharmacokinetics. *J Pharmacokinet Biopharm* **10**:201–227, 1982.

Boxenbaum H: Evolution biology, animal behavior, fourth-dimensional space, and the raison d'etre of drug metabolism and pharmacokinetics. *Drug Metab Rev* **14**:1057–1097, 1983.

Chen CN, Andrade JD: Pharmacokinetic model for simultaneous determination of drug levels in organs and tissues. *J Pharm Sci* **65**:717–724, 1976.

Chien JY, Friedrich S, Heathman MA, de Alwis DP, Sinha V: Pharmacokinetics/Pharmacodynamics and the stages of drug development: Role of modeling and simulation. *AAPS J* **7**(3):E544–E559, 2005.

Chiou WL: The phenomenon and rationale of marked dependence of drug concentration on blood sampling site: Implication in pharmacokinetics, pharmacodynamics, toxicology and therapeutics. Part I, *Clin Pharmacokinet* **17**(3):175–199, 1989; Part II, *Clin Pharmacokinet* **17**(3):275–290, 1989.

Colucci P, Grenier J, Seng Yue C, Turgeon J, Ducharme MP. Performance of different population pharmacokinetic algorithms. *Ther Drug Monit* **33**:583–591, 2011.

D'Argenio DZ, Schumitzky A, Wang X: *ADAPT 5 User's Guide: Pharmacokinetic/Pharmacodynamic Systems Analysis Software*. Los Angeles, CA: Biomedical Simulations Resource; 2009.

DiStefano JI, Landaw E. Multiexponential, multicompartmental, and noncompartmental modeling. I. Methodological limitations and physiological interpretations. *Am J Physiol* **264**:R651–R664, 1984.

European Medicines Agency (EMA): Guideline on strategies to identify and mitigate risks for first-in-human and early clinical trials with investigational medicinal products. London, UK, February 2018a.

European Medicines Agency (EMA): Guideline on the reporting of physiologically based pharmacokinetic (PBPK) modeling and simulation. London, UK: December 2018b.

Ette EI, Williams PJ: Population pharmacokinetics I: Background, concepts, and models. *Ann Pharmacother* **38**(10):1702–1706, 2004.

Evans CA, Jolivette LJ, Nagilla R, et al: Extrapolation of preclinical pharmacokinetics and molecular feature analysis of "discovery-like" molecules to predict human pharmacokinetics. *Drug Metab Disp* **34**(7):1255–1265, 2006.

Forrest A, Drusano GL, Plaisance I, Kroll G, Gonzalez MA: Evaluation of a new program for population PK/PD analysis: Applied to simulated phase I data. *Clin Pharmacol Ther* **49**:153, 1991.

Gabrielsson J, Bondesson U: Constant-rate infusion of nicotine and cotinine, I. A physiological pharmacokinetic analysis of the cotinine disposition, and effects on clearance and distribution in the rat. *J Pharmacokinet Biopharm* **15**:583–599, 1987.

Gabrielsson J, Weiner D: Parameter Estimation. *Pharmacokinetic & Pharmacodynamic Data Analysis: Concepts and Applications*. 4th ed. Stockholm, Swedish Pharmaceutical Press, 2006.

Gibaldi M, Perrier D: Noncompartmental analysis based on statistical moment theory. In Gibaldi M, Perrier M (eds). *Pharmacokinetics*, 2nd ed. New York, NY, Informa Healthcare, 2007, pp 409–417.

Gillespie WR, Disanto AR, Monovich RE, Albert DS: Relative bioavailability of commercially available ibuprofen oral dosage forms in humans. *J Pharm Sci* **71**:1034–1038, 1982.

Hu T-M, Hayton WL: Allometric scaling of xenobiotic clearance: Uncertainty versus universality. *AAPS PharmSci* **3**(4):30–34, article 29, 2001 (www.pharmsci.org).

Jelliffe RW. The USC*PACK PC programs for population pharmacokinetic modeling, modeling of large kinetic/dynamic systems, and adaptive control of drug dosage regimens. *Proc Annu Symp Comput Appl Med Care* 992–994, 1991.

King FG, Dedrick RL, Farris FF: Physiological pharmacokinetic modeling of *cis*-dichlorodiammineplatinum(II) (DDP) in several species. *J Pharmacokinet Biopharm* **14**:131–157, 1986.

Kisor DF, Waitling SM, Zarowitz BJ, Jelliffe RW. Population pharmacokinetics of gentamicin. Use of the nonparametric expectation maximization (NPEM) algorithm. *Clin Pharmacokinet* **23**(1):62–68, 1992.

Lee JY, Garnett CE, Gobburu JV, et al: Impact of pharmacometric analyses on new drug approval and labelling decisions: A review of 198 submissions between 2000 and 2008. *Clin Pharmacokinet* **50**(10):627–635, 2011.

Levy G: Comparison of dissolution and absorption rates of different commercial aspirin tablets. *J Pharm Sci* **50**:388–392, 1961.

Levy LG, Hollister LE: Dissolution rate limited absorption in man. Factors influencing drug absorption from prolonged-release dosage form. *J Pharm Sci* **54**:1121–1125, 1965.

Li M, Zhao P, Pan Y, Wagner C: Predictive performance of physiologically based pharmacokinetic models for the effect of food on oral drug absorption: Current status. *CPT Pharmacometrics Syst Pharmacol* **7**:82–89, 2018.

Ludden TM: Population pharmacokinetics. *J Clin Pharmacol* **28**(12):1059–1063, 1988.

Luecke RH, Thomason LE: Physiological flow model for drug elimination interactions in the rat. *Comput Prog Biomed* **11**:88–89, 1980.

Lutz RJ, Dedrick RL: Physiological pharmacokinetics: Relevance to human risk assessment. In Li AP (ed). *New Approaches in Toxicity Testing and Their Application in Human Risk Assessment.* New York, Raven, 1985, pp 129–149.

Mahmood I: Critique of prospective allometric scaling: Does the emperor have clothes? *J Clin Pharmacol* **40**:671–674, 2000.

Mahmood I: Application of allometric principles for the prediction of pharmacokinetics in human and veterinary drug development. *Adv Drug Deliv Rev* **59**(11):1177–1192, 2007.

Mallet A: A maximum likelihood estimation method for random coefficient regression models. *Biometrika* **73**:645–656, 1986.

Mather LE: Anatomical-physiological approaches in pharmacokinetics and pharmacodynamics. *Clin Pharmacokinet* **40**(10):707–722, 2001.

Mordenti J, Chappell W: The use of interspecies scaling in toxicology. In Yacobi A, Skelly JP, Batra VK (eds). *Toxicokinetic and New Drug Development.* New York, Pergamon, 1989, pp 42–96.

Nakashima E, Benet LZ: General treatment of mean residence time, clearance, and volume parameters in linear mammillary models with elimination from any compartment. *J Pharmacokinet Biopharm* **16**:475–492, 1988.

Nakashima E, Yokogawa K, Ichimura F, et al: A physiologically based pharmacokinetic model for biperiden in animals and its extrapolation to humans. *Chem Pharm Bull* **35**:718–725, 1987.

Neely MN, van Guilder MG, Yamada WM, Schumitzky A, Jelliffe RW: Accurate detection of outliers and subpopulations with Pmetrics, a nonparametric and parametric pharmacometric modeling and simulation package for R. *Ther Drug Monit* **34**:467–476, 2012

Nieforth KA, Nadeau R, Patel IH, et al: Use of an indirect pharmacodynamic stimulation model of MX protein induction to compare in vivo activity of interferon alfa-2a and a polyethylene glycol-modified derivative in healthy subjects. *Clin Pharmacol Ther* **59**:636–646, 1996.

Otsuka Pharmaceutical Co., Ltd., ABILIFY FDA product label, August 2019.

Pasternyk Di Marco M, Wainer IW, Granvil CL, Batist G, Ducharme MP: New insights into the pharmacokinetics and metabolism of (R,S)-Ifosfamide in cancer patients using a population pharmacokinetic-metabolism model. *Pharm Res* **17**(6):645–652, 2000.

Rescigno A, Beck JS: Perspective in pharmacokinetics and the use and abuses of models. *J Pharmacokinet Biopharm* **15**:327–344, 1987.

Riggs DS: *A Mathematical Approach to Physiological Problems.* Baltimore, Williams & Wilkins, 1963.

Ritschel WA, Banerjee PS: Physiological pharmacokinetic models: Principles, applications, limitations and outlook. *Meth Find Exp Clin Pharmacol* **8**:603–614, 1986.

Rodman JH, D'Argenio DZ, Peck CC: Analysis of pharmacokinetic data for individualizing drug dosage regimens. In Burton ME, Shaw LM, Schentag JJ, Evans WE (eds). *Applied Pharmacokinetics & Pharmacodynamics: Principles of Therapeutic Drug Monitoring.* 4th ed. Baltimore, MD: Lippincott Williams & Wilkins, 2006.

Sawada Y, Hanano M, Sugiyama Y, Iga T: Prediction of the disposition of nine weakly acidic and six weakly basic drugs in humans from pharmacokinetic parameters in rats. *J Pharmacokinet Biopharm* **13**:477–492, 1985.

Schumitzky A. Nonparametric EM algorithms for estimating prior distributions. *Appl Math Comput* **45**:143–157, 1991.

Schumitzky A. EM Algorithms and two safe methods in pharmacokinetic population analysis. In D'Argenio DZ (ed). *Advanced Methods of Pharmacokinetic and Pharmacodynamic Systems Analysis.* Vol. II. Plenum Press; New York: 1995, pp 145–160.

Seng Yue C, Gallicano K, Labbé L, Ducharme MP: Novel population pharmacokinetic method compared to the standard noncompartmental approach to assess bioequivalence of iron gluconate formulations. *J Pharm Pharm Sci* **16**(3):424–440, 2013.

Seng Yue C, Ozdin D, Selber-Hnatiw S, Ducharme M: Opportunities and challenges related to the implementation of model-based bioequivalence criteria. *Clin Pharm Ther* **105**(2):350–362, 2019.

Sheiner LB: The population approach to pharmacokinetic data analysis: Rationale and standard data analysis methods. *Drug Metab Rev* **15**(1–2):153–171, 1984.

Steimer JL, Mallet A, Golmard JL, Boisvieux JF: Alternative approaches to estimation of population pharmacokinetic parameters: comparison with the nonlinear mixed-effect model. *Drug Metab Rev* **15**(1–2):265–92, 1984.

St-Pierre MV, Xu Xin, Pang KS: Primary, secondary, and tertiary metabolite kinetics. *Pharmacokinet Biopharm* **16**(5):493–527, 1988.

Tett SE, Holford NHG, McLachlan AJ. Population pharmacokinetics and pharmacodynamics: An underutilized resource. *Drug Info J* **32**:693–710, 1998.

US FDA (U.S. Department of Health and Human Services, Food and Drug Administration, Center for Drug Evaluation and Research): Guidance for Industry – Estimating the Maximum Safe Starting Dose in Initial Clinical Trials for Therapeutics in Adult Healthy Volunteers. Rockville, MD. July 2005.

US FDA (U.S. Department of Health and Human Services, Food and Drug Administration, Center for Drug Evaluation and Research): Guidance for Industry – Physiologically Based Pharmacokinetic Analyses – Format and Content. Silver Springs, MD. December 2016.

US FDA (U.S. Department of Health and Human Services, Food and Drug Administration, Center for Drug Evaluation and Research): Guidance for Industry – Population Pharmacokinetics. Rockville, MD. July 2019.

Wagner JG, Nelson E: Per cent absorbed time plots derived from blood level and/or urinary excretion data. *J Pharm Sci* **52**:610–611, 1963.

Wagner JG, Nelson E: Kinetic analysis of blood levels and urinary excretion in the absorptive phase after single doses of drug. *J Pharm Sci* **53**:1392–1403, 1964.

Wagner JG: Use of computers in pharmacokinetics. *Clin Pharmacol Ther* **8**:201–218, 1967.

Wang X, Schumitzky A, D'Argenio DZ. Nonlinear random effects mixture models: Maximum likelihood estimation via the EM algorithm. *Comput Stat Data Anal* **51**(12):6614-6623, 2007.

Watanabe T, Kusuhara H, Maeda K, Shitara Y, Sugiyama Y: Physiologically based pharmacokinetic modeling to predict transporter-mediated clearance and distribution of pravastatin in humans. *J Pharmacol Exper Therap* **328**(2):652–662, 2009.

## BIBLIOGRAPHY

Banakar UV, Block LH: Beyond bioavailability testing. *Pharm Technol* 7:107–117, 1983.

Benet LZ, Galeazzi RL: Noncompartmental determination of the steady-state volume of distribution. *J Pharm Sci* **68**: 1071–1073, 1979.

Benet LZ: Mean residence time in the body versus mean residence time in the central compartment. *J Pharmacokinet Biopharm* **13**:555–558, 1985.

Bischoff KB, Dedrick RL, Zaharko DS, Longstreth JA: Methotrexate pharmacokinetics. *J Pharm Sci* **60**:1128–1133, 1971.

Boxenbaum H, D'Souza RW: Interspecies pharmacokinetics scaling, biological design and neoteny. In Testa B, D'Souza WD (eds). *Advances in Drug Research*, vol 19. New York, Academic, 1990, pp 139–196.

Chanter DO: The determination of mean residence time using statistical moments: Is it correct? *J Pharmacokinet Biopharm* **13**:93–100, 1985.

Colburn WA: Pharmacokinetic/pharmacodynamic model: What it is! *J Pharmacokinet Biopharm* **15**:545–555, 1987.

Himmelstein KJ, Lutz RJ: A review of the applications of physiologically based pharmacokinetic modeling. *J Pharmacokinet Biopharm* 7:127–145, 1979.

Kasuya Y, Hirayama H, Kubota N, Pang KS: Interpretation and estimation of mean residence time with statistical moment theory. *Biopharm Drug Disp* **8**:223–234, 1987.

Mayer PR, Brazzell R: Application of statistical moment theory to pharmacokinetics. *J Clin Pharmacol* **28**:481-483, 1988.

Sawada Y, Hanano M, Sugiyama Y, Iga T: Prediction of the disposition of nine weakly acidic and six weakly basic drugs in humans from pharmacokinetic parameters in rats. *J Pharmacokinet Biopharm* **13**:477–492, 1985.

Smallwood RH, Mihaly GW, Smallwood RA, Morgan DJ: Effect of a protein binding change on unbound and total plasma concentrations for drugs of intermediate hepatic extraction. *J Pharmacokinet Biopharm* **16**(5):529–542, 1988.

Veng-Pedersen P, Gillespie W: The mean residence time of drugs in the systemic circulation. *J Pharm Sci* **74**:791–792, 1985.

Wagner JG: Do you need a pharmacokinetic model, and, if so, which one? *J Pharmacokinet Biopharm* **3**:457–478, 1975.

Wagner JG: Dosage intervals based on mean residence times. *J Pharm Sci* **76**:35–38, 1987.

Wagner JG: Types of mean residence times. *Biopharm Drug Disp* **9**:41–57, 1988.

West GB: The origin of universal scaling laws in biology. *Physica A* **263**:104–113, 1999.

# 20

# Applications of Software Packages in Pharmacokinetics

Philippe Colucci, Corinne Seng Yue, and Murray P. Ducharme

## CHAPTER OBJECTIVES

- Describe the types of computer software programs that are available for use in pharmacokinetics.

- Provide one-compartment equations to optimize aminoglycoside antibiotic treatment.

- Discuss the limitations of computer software programs in simulating PK models.

- Explain the concept of "goodness-of-fit" and the relationship between observed, experimental data, and theoretical data derived by the computer.

- Differentiate the software and tools available to scientists to conduct individual or population PK analyses and physiologically based PK analyses.

- Provides a brief outline of how to design, complete, and report population PK/PD analyses.

## INTRODUCTION

The use of computers and software packages is now mainstream for clinicians, undergraduate students, and researchers. Chapter 19 introduced the concepts of how to conduct model-independent PK analyses and described how PK and PK/PD models are derived using known algorithms. This chapter is a continuation of that chapter and introduces different software packages that are available. This chapter discusses objectives or applications of software packages with a review of the different approaches that are utilized in software packages, and examples of how equations for noncompartmental and compartmental analyses can be used to optimize the therapy in patients.

With the increase in number of pharmacokinetic software packages, it is important to understand what analyses can be accomplished by each PK software package and its limitations. For example, will the software allow the user to calculate noncompartmental, individual, or population analyses? Various computer software packages are presented along with the required input and the resulting output. These examples will help the reader to recognize and interpret the results that are presented in the literature. Finally, this chapter provides a brief description of how to design, complete, and report population PK analyses.

## SOFTWARE APPLICATIONS

The available PK or PK/PD software can be used to accomplish various objectives. For clinicians, clinical PK software is used to improve or facilitate patient drug therapy. For example, software programs are available for the clinical monitoring of narrow-therapeutic-index drugs (ie, critical-dose drugs) such as the aminoglycosides, theophylline, phenytoin, cyclosporine, tacrolimus, lithium, or others. These programs may include calculations for creatinine clearance using the Cockcroft–Gault method (Chapter 23) or other equations, dosage estimation, PK parameter estimation, and simulation of predicted drug concentrations for the individual patient. Clinical PK software packages are available for guiding clinicians using the patient's PK. Personalized tools can also be used by the clinician to rapidly provide the required PK information (for example, on a smartphone) and help guide the treatment of their patients in real time. Sound clinical judgment must be considered when using clinical PK software programs to guide drug therapy in patients.

Software packages are available to describe the pharmacokinetics of individual drugs. Although these software packages can be used indirectly to improve patient care at the clinical level, they normally require computers and are more predominately used for research. These software packages allow the user to answer hypothetical questions through modeling and simulation. PK data from clinical trials can be simulated to determine the impact of different pathologic conditions. For example, simulations can predict drug concentration–time profiles in renally impaired patients versus normal subjects. Simulations can be done for a multitude of different clinical scenarios. In practice, experimental data would be difficult if not impossible to obtain from subjects under all possible conditions. Computer simulations lead to better understanding of drug therapy, which in turn provides better guidelines of how to care for patients. Often, dosing guidelines on drug labels are determined through these simulations and not necessarily a specific clinical study. An improved understanding of the software's requirements, applications, outputs, and limitations will improve the understanding of related pharmacokinetic information.

Software packages are available to predict/simulate *in vivo* drug concentration–time profiles based on the *in vitro* drug dissolution and other *in vitro* characteristics. Some of these software packages use physiologically based pharmacokinetics (PBPK). These software packages often use models based on data including physiologic, dissolution, preclinical data, etc to predict *in vivo* PK including *in vitro–in vivo* correlation (IVIVC). IVIVC can be used to predict potential drug concentration–time profiles in the population based on changes in the *in vitro* dissolution parameters.

Some computer program applications created for teaching PK are available for faculty and students. Some of these applications use spreadsheets which can incorporate many of the PK formulas described in this book (Charles and Duffull, 2001; Gabrielsson et al, 2014; Zolt and Holt, 2017).

## OVERVIEW OF THE DIFFERENT APPROACHES IN SOFTWARE PACKAGES

The different software applications described in the previous section use PK and PK/PD analysis approaches that include noncompartment, individual compartment, population compartment, Bayesian, and PBPK. Table 20-1 provides a list of the software applications, their analysis approaches, and some common software packages that are offered for these different applications. More details are provided in the following sections. The mention of a software package within this text does not mean that it has been endorsed by the authors.

The most frequent computer software packages applied by clinicians or pharmacists are clinical PK applications for developing dosage regimens and patient monitoring. For example, Bayesian analysis to predict an expected concentration–time profile using limited blood samples and the patient's characteristics is used for therapeutic drug monitoring (TDM). Doses and dosing frequency can be adjusted for the individual patient according to the predicted results. The Bayesian method requires prior information on the parameters being predicted or fitted. Fortunately, the PK for most drugs prescribed clinically are described in the literature, making a Bayesian or TDM analysis accessible. Examples of how these can be applied to improve patient care are provided later in this chapter.

Many different approaches can be used to describe the PK of a drug. A well-known approach is the noncompartmental method, which is introduced in Chapter 11 and described in Chapter 19. As the name implies, the noncompartmental approach does not require the specification of the number of compartments or exponentials that characterize the shape of the concentration-versus-time curve

## TABLE 20-1 • Software Packages and Their Applications

| Application | Approach | Description | Examples | Comment |
|---|---|---|---|---|
| Clinical pharmacokinetic | Bayesian | Clinical monitoring of narrow-therapeutic-index drugs (i.e., critical-dose drugs) | | May include calculations for CL, dosage estimation, PK parameter estimation, and PK simulations for individual patient. |
| Describe and Simulate PK | Noncompartmental analyses | Model independent analyses | • Excel spreadsheet<br>• Bear (to be used with R)<br>• Phoenix WinNonlin® | WinNonlin® is popular in the pharmaceutical industry for its ease of use |
| | Individual compartmental analyses | Built-in PK models | • Phoenix WinNonlin®<br>• PK-SIM® | Fitting drug concentration–time data |
| | | User can define the individual PK or PD model | • ADAPT 5®<br>• NONMEM®<br>• Phoenix WinNonlin® | Different algorithms are available |
| | • Population compartmental analyses<br>• Bayesian<br>• PBPK | User can define the population PK or PD model | • ADAPT 5®<br>• Berkeley Madonna®<br>• Monolix®<br>• NONMEM®<br>• Phoenix NLME®<br>• Pmetrics® (to be used with R)<br>• PK-SIM®<br>• NLINMIX (used with SAS) | Fitting data into a pharmacokinetic or pharmacodynamic model |
| In Vivo Simulations from In Vitro data | • PBPK<br>• IVIVC | Model uses various data including physiologic, dissolution, etc., to predict in vivo PK | • GastroPlus®<br>• SimCYP®<br>• Berkeley Madonna®<br>• Phoenix® NLME (IVIVC) | For industry or research |

(Yamaoka et al, 1978; Riegelman and Collier, 1980; Gibaldi et al, 2007). The method utilizes simple analyses that require very little computer power if any. In most cases, a spreadsheet such as Excel can be used to calculate the PK parameters associated with this analysis. Although a simple spreadsheet can be used, computer software programs that offer noncompartmental analysis simplify the management of the input data and the output tables and profiles from a large number of subjects or patients. These programs facilitate the determination of additional PK parameters such as initial drug concentration, $C_0$, after bolus administration, or the elimination rate constant ($k_{el}$). Moreover, these software packages provide the ability to use predefined PK parameter equations, which improves the precision in the parameter calculations. It is incumbent upon the scientist to ensure that these predefined parameters are appropriate for their study and data.

Another method to describe drug PK is the mechanistic *compartmental approach*, which is considered a classical PK approach. It is introduced in Chapter 11 and discussed in all subsequent chapters up to Chapter 19. The compartmental approach is used for any type of drug, whether the drug exhibits linear or nonlinear characteristics. The compartmental approach can be used with varying quantities of data including data collected after single-dose or under steady-state conditions. The compartment model can characterize all routes of drug administration. Compartmental analyses rely on models that have both a mathematical and a statistical basis. For this reason, specialized PK software packages must be used. The main methodological approaches to compartmental analyses include individual or population-based approaches.

For individual PK analysis, a model is written to explain the observed concentrations in an individual. The PK models use nonlinear equations that may have no definite numerical solutions (Chapter 19). PK models are often written mathematically with differential equations, and have to be solved according to the software algorithms. Multiple functions/algorithms have been used to best minimize the error between the observed and predicted drug concentrations. The algorithm often used to minimize the error between the observed and predicted drug concentrations is termed the *least squares* method. Most software programs give the user the opportunity to utilize ordinary least squares, weighted least squares, or maximum likelihood. The model does not attempt to determine the population PK parameters but only individual PK parameters. This type of analysis is relatively quick to perform, although longer than the noncompartmental analysis.

The *population compartmental approach* involves the simultaneous analysis of data from multiple individuals. This analysis is superior to the individual compartmental analysis in terms of robustness and is the preferred approach when performing compartmental analyses since computing power is not a limiting factor. Population compartmental analyses estimate the expected average PK parameters for the population, along with their inter-individual and residual variability. Many algorithms have been proposed to perform population compartmental analysis in Chapter 19. These algorithms include parametric and nonparametric approaches. Numerous methods and software packages perform population PK analyses. The most common software packages are described in the following sections of this chapter and include some examples. The excellent book by Bonate (2011) provides more in-depth explanations and techniques regarding population compartment analyses.

PBPK models are more complex than population pharmacokinetic models. PBPK models are based on known physiologic processes (Chapter 19). They require a large amount of information related to the anatomical, physiological, physical, and chemical descriptions of the phenomena. For example, *in vitro* data such as the physicochemical properties of the drug are included in the PBPK model to describe the drug absorption process. These PBPK software programs are complex and computation-heavy and require users to be extremely well versed in the technique. This approach is used in research and drug development in the pharmaceutical industry. This methodology is expected to increase in popularity as the predictions become more reliable and accepted by regulatory agencies.

IVIVC is an analysis that attempts to relate *in vitro* data, usually drug dissolution, to *in vivo* observations, usually the percent of drug absorbed (Chapter 7).

Both *in vitro* drug dissolution data and *in vivo* bioavailability data from different formulations of the same drug are needed to perform an IVIVC. If an IVIVC is achieved, the pharmaceutical manufacturer does not need to conduct additional bioequivalence studies when making a change to a formulation. IVIVC may be used in the development of an extended-release version of an immediate-release drug product. If the *in vivo* PK characteristics of the immediate-release formulation are well described, the characteristics of the extended-release drug may be predicted by correlating the changes in the dissolution pattern of the new formulation to the changes in the *in vivo* PK characteristics. Regulatory agencies require several different extended-release formulations (ie, slow-release, intermediate-release, and fast extended-release formulations) be tested in an *in vivo* bioequivalence study. A correlation model is then built to relate the *in vitro* dissolution curves from the different immediate-release and extended-release products to their respective *in vivo* PK characteristics. If the *in vivo* PK characteristics can be predicted by the model according to specific predefined criteria, then future modifications to an extended release formulation of the same drug can be predicted simply based on the new dissolution curve without having to conduct an *in vivo* study. The FDA and EMA have published guidelines on how these types of IVIVC should be conducted (FDA 1997, EMA 2014).

## SOFTWARE PACKAGES

### Clinical Pharmacokinetics

Many clinical PK software packages are available with built-in models for the most common narrow therapeutic drugs. TDM is the practice of sampling blood and measuring plasma drug concentrations from an individual to optimize drug therapy for that patient. For example, TDM will ensure that the plasma drug concentrations of a narrow therapeutic drug remain within a safe and efficacious range. Only limited, sparse blood samples (one or two) are taken at strategic times. With these strategic limited plasma drug concentration data collected from the patient, the clinician can use the software to predict the patient's plasma drug concentration profile for different dosing regimens and to provide the clinician with more information to select the most appropriate dosing regimen for their patient. This software can also take into consideration other factors that can influence drug exposure. For example, changes in the patient's pathophysiology such as a change in renal clearance can be input into the software and a new plasma drug concentration profile can be predicted. Thorough reviews of the available software packages are provided by Fuchs et al (2013) and Sager et al (2015).

Although software applications are available, clinicians and pharmacists can use their smartphones with a spreadsheet application such as Excel and develop PK formulas to optimize

patient therapy. For example, aminoglycosides (eg, gentamicin), a class of antibiotics used in the treatment of aerobic gram-negative bacilli infections, are dosed carefully to optimize the efficacy and limit potential nephrotoxicity and ototoxicity. Because aminoglycosides are drug concentration–dependent in their bactericidal effect, the drug concentrations must be maintained within a narrow therapeutic range. The pharmacokinetics of gentamicin can be predicted using an Excel spreadsheet. The PK of gentamicin is adequately estimated by a one-compartment model. The volume of distribution can be estimated using lean body weight, and the elimination is a function of glomerular filtration. Using the patient's lean body weight and glomerular filtration rate, gentamicin concentrations following the administration of a specific dose can be predicted. Table 20-2A provides an example of a spreadsheet that can be used to select an appropriate starting dose for their patient (ie, predict potential expected gentamicin plasma concentrations prior to collecting any TDM concentration). Using this spreadsheet, a physician or pharmacist can enter the eight input values at the top and the expected gentamicin concentrations will be calculated in the bottom table. Based on these predicted drug concentrations, a dosing regimen may be optimized to obtain the desired peak and trough gentamicin concentrations (based on minimum inhibitory concentration). Once the first dose is administered, concentrations at approximately $C_{max}$ and end of dosing interval are obtained to determine the elimination rate as well the volume of distribution. Table 20-2B is a spreadsheet that allows the clinicians to enter the TDM concentrations to obtain PK parameters ($V_c$ and $k_{el}$) specific to their patient. The subsequent doses can be adjusted according to these specific patient's parameters.

### Software to Describe and Predict Pharmacokinetics

Each software package is specialized for certain applications. Their specific advantages and disadvantages can favor the use of different software packages depending upon the specific situations. The type of software package to be used is based on

**TABLE 20-2A** • EXCEL® Spreadsheet of Expected Gentamicin or Tobramycin Concentrations Prior to TDM Concentrations

| Input category | Value | |
|---|---|---|
| Actual body weight (kg) | 70 | |
| Height (inches) | 70 | |
| Gender<br>(1 = male; 2 = female) | 1 | |
| Age (yrs) | 50 | |
| Scr ($\mu$mol/L) | 90 | |
| Dosing interval; t (h) | 12 | |
| Dose (mg) | 250 | |
| Infusion time; $T_{inf}$ (h) | 1 | |
| **Calculated Weight Category** | **Value** | **Formula** |
| IBW (kg) | 73 | IF("Gender"=1,50+2.3*(Height-60),45.5+2.3*(Height-60)) |
| Lean Body Weight (kg) | 71.8 | IBW+(ABW-IBW)*0.4 |
| **Calculated PK Parameters** | **Value** | **Formula** |
| $V_c$ (L) | 21.5 | 0.3*LBW |
| $K_{el}$ | 0.283 | IF("Gender"=1,0.01+0.003*(140-AGE)/(Scr*0.011),<br>0.01+0.003*(140-AGE)/(Scr*0.011)*0.85) |
| **Expected Plasma Concentrations** | | |
| Plasma 1st dose $C_{max}$ (mg/L) | 10.1 | $(Dose/(V_c*K_{el}*T_{inf}))*(1-\exp(-K_{el}*T_{inf}))$ |
| Plasma 1st dose $C_{min}$ (mg/L) | 0.45 | $C_{max}*\exp(-K_{el}*(t-T_{inf}))$ |
| Plasma SS $C_{max}$ (mg/L) | 10.6 | $C_{max}$ 1st dose / $(1-\exp(-K_{el}*(tau-T_{inf})))$ |
| Plasma SS $C_{min}$ (mg/L) | 0.47 | $C_{max}$ SS dose * $\exp(-K_{el}*(tau-T_{inf}))$ |

the objectives of the PK analyses, the available data, and past experiences of users. Some software packages are free and some are commercially available at a cost. Some free programs may require additional (paid) programs in order to work. For example, the software may require a Fortran compiler to compile PK and PD models. Because software packages may have different functionalities, different results (eg, PK parameter estimates) may be obtained. Various software packages are available that have different applications, ranging from simple PK calculations (noncompartmental calculations) to the more complicated PK calculations (PBPK). The listing of a software package within this chapter does not mean that the software has been endorsed by the authors. Furthermore, the descriptions may not reflect the latest versions of software, as features are often added or improved. The user is encouraged to contact the program vendors directly for the most recent information.

### Noncompartmental Pharmacokinetic Software Packages

Noncompartmental PK analysis is considered model independent; ie, no model is required. Spreadsheets (eg, Excel) can calculate various PK parameters. For example, Excel can determine the elimination rate constant, $k_{el}$ which is the slope of the ln-transformed drug concentrations-versus-time curve.

**TABLE 20-2B • EXCEL® Spreadsheet of Expected Gentamicin or Tobramycin Concentrations based on Patient's TDM Concentrations**

| Original Patient Information | Value | TDM Information | Value |
|---|---|---|---|
| Actual body weight (kg) | 70 | Time of concentration 1 (hours after dosing) | 1.5 |
| Height (inches) | 70 | Time of concentration 2 (hours after dosing) | 11.5 |
| Gender (1 = male; 2 = female) | 1 | Concentration 1 (mg/L) | 10.0 |
| Age (yrs) | 50 | Concentration 12 (mg/L) | 0.2 |
| Scr ($\mu$mol/L) | 90 | | |
| Dosing interval; t (h) | 12 | | |
| Dose (mg) | 250 | | |
| Infusion time; $T_{inf}$ (h) | 1 | | |

| Calculated Weight Category | Value | Formula | |
|---|---|---|---|
| IBW (kg) | 73 | IF("Gender"=1,50+2.3*(Height-60),45.5+2.3*(Height-60)) | |
| Lean body weight (kg) | 71.8 | IBW+(ABW-IBW)*0.4 | |

| Calculated PK Parameters from TDM Concentrations | Value | Formula | |
|---|---|---|---|
| $V_c$ (L) | 18.9 | Dose*(1-exp(-$K_{el}$*T1))/(C1*T1*$K_{el}$) | |
| $K_{el}$ | 0.391 | (ln(C1)-ln(C2))/(T2-T1) | |

| Expected Plasma Concentrations | | | |
|---|---|---|---|
| Plasma 1st dose $C_{max}$ (mg/L) | 10.9 | (Dose/($V_c$ * $K_{el}$ *$T_{inf}$))*(1-exp(-$K_{el}$ *$T_{inf}$)) | |
| Plasma 1st dose $C_{min}$ (mg/L) | 0.15 | $C_{max}$ *exp(-$K_{el}$ *(t-$T_{inf}$)) | |
| Plasma SS $C_{max}$ (mg/L) | 11.1 | $C_{max}$ 1st dose / (1-exp(-$K_{el}$ *(tau-$T_{inf}$))) | |
| Plasma SS $C_{min}$ (mg/L) | 0.15 | $C_{max}$ SS dose * exp(-$K_{el}$ *(tau-$T_{inf}$)) | |

**Commercial Software Packages** Commercial software packages are available with easy-to-use interface for data management, creation of graphs, noncompartmental analysis, and bioequivalence testing. A popular software package for this type of analysis is the Phoenix WinNonlin® software package. Phoenix WinNonlin is easy to use with just some basic instructions or training. PK parameters such as AUCs, $C_{max}$, CL, and $V_{ss}$ are predefined with the software. The software package also allows the user to define additional PK parameters such as partial AUCs. An advantage of noncompartment software packages is the rapid determination of the elimination rate constant for all subjects included in the dataset. The software can handle small or large numbers of subjects or drug concentration versus time profiles. Some modules within Phoenix allow for easy tabulation of results, creation of figures and validation of the software. WinNonlin's input and output data may be managed via Excel (Microsoft)-compatible spreadsheet files. Another important advantage is that the software tracks changes made to files and ensures the necessary traceability and transparency critical for all data analyses. The dataset includes the subject number, the nominal and/or exact blood collection times, and the drug concentrations. Additional information can be provided such as the period, formulation, and sequence associated with the data. An example of the data input file read by WinNonlin is in Table 20-3.

## TABLE 20-3 • Example of WinNonlin® Input File

| Subject | Period | Formulation | Sch_Time h | Act_Time h | Concentration pg/mL |
|---------|--------|-------------|------------|------------|---------------------|
| 1 | 1 | 2 | 0 | 0.00 | 0 |
| 1 | 1 | 2 | 0.5 | 0.50 | 305 |
| 1 | 1 | 2 | 1 | 1.00 | 362 |
| 1 | 1 | 2 | 2 | 2.00 | 588 |
| 1 | 1 | 2 | 3 | 3.00 | 675 |
| 1 | 1 | 2 | 4 | 4.00 | 969 |
| 1 | 1 | 2 | 6 | 6.00 | 1037 |
| 1 | 1 | 2 | 8 | 8.00 | 1043 |
| 1 | 1 | 2 | 12 | 12.02 | 928 |
| 1 | 1 | 2 | 24 | 24.00 | 1106 |
| 1 | 1 | 2 | 36 | 36.02 | 884 |
| 1 | 1 | 2 | 48 | 48.02 | 941 |
| 1 | 1 | 2 | 60 | 60.00 | 1019 |
| 1 | 1 | 2 | 72 | 72.03 | 969 |
| 1 | 1 | 2 | 96 | 96.15 | 1007 |
| 1 | 1 | 2 | 120 | 120.00 | 950 |
| 1 | 1 | 2 | 144 | 144.02 | 879 |
| 1 | 1 | 2 | 168 | 168.02 | 805 |
| 1 | 1 | 2 | 216 | 216.00 | 643 |
| 1 | 1 | 2 | 288 | 288.02 | 646 |
| 1 | 1 | 2 | 360 | 360.02 | 513 |
| 1 | 1 | 2 | 456 | 456.02 | 283 |
| 1 | 1 | 2 | 552 | 552.00 | 241 |
| 1 | 1 | 2 | 720 | 720.10 | 154 |
| 2 | 1 | 1 | 0 | 0.00 | 0 |
| 2 | 1 | 1 | 0.5 | 0.50 | 154 |
| 2 | 1 | 1 | 1 | 1.00 | 218 |
| 2 | 1 | 1 | 2 | 2.00 | 293 |
| 2 | 1 | 1 | 3 | 3.00 | 405 |
| 2 | 1 | 1 | 4 | 4.00 | 438 |
| 2 | 1 | 1 | 6 | 6.02 | 434 |
| 2 | 1 | 1 | 8 | 8.00 | 416 |
| 2 | 1 | 1 | 12 | 12.00 | 382 |
| 2 | 1 | 1 | 24 | 24.00 | 483 |

*(Continiued)*

**TABLE 20-3 • Example of WinNonlin® Input File (Continued)**

| Subject | Period | Formulation | Sch_Time h | Act_Time h | Concentration pg/mL |
|---------|--------|-------------|------------|------------|---------------------|
| 2 | 1 | 1 | 36 | 36.00 | 379 |
| 2 | 1 | 1 | 48 | 48.00 | 430 |
| 2 | 1 | 1 | 60 | 60.00 | 327 |
| 2 | 1 | 1 | 72 | 72.00 | 400 |
| 2 | 1 | 1 | 96 | 96.18 | 455 |
| 2 | 1 | 1 | 120 | 120.00 | 314 |
| 2 | 1 | 1 | 144 | 144.00 | 333 |
| 2 | 1 | 1 | 168 | 168.00 | 314 |
| 2 | 1 | 1 | 216 | 216.00 | 310 |
| 2 | 1 | 1 | 288 | 288.00 | 272 |
| 2 | 1 | 1 | 360 | 360.00 | 220 |
| 2 | 1 | 1 | 456 | 456.48 | 203 |
| 2 | 1 | 1 | 552 | 552.65 | 155 |
| 2 | 1 | 1 | 720 | 720.13 | 154 |

The software also allows the user to conduct some pre-defined statistical analyses. Table 20-4 and Fig. 20-1 provide examples of some PK results and figures that are outputted.

Other software packages offer similar possibilities. An example of a free tool that may be used is "Bear," which is a software package designed to work with R. Bear stands for bioequivalence/bioavailability (BE/BA) for R (Lee and Lee, 2020). Bear can calculate typical noncompartmental PK parameters for a bioequivalence study and calculate the 90% confidence intervals for the ratio of the test to reference products for pivotal BE parameters such as AUC and $C_{max}$. This software may not be as user-friendly as WinNonlin but its association with a free programming language (R) and its availability at no cost makes it appealing.

**Compartment Pharmacokinetic Software** Several PK software packages for individual and population compartmental analyses are available. Some have built-in PK or PK/PD models while others require the user to specify these models to obtain PK parameter estimates. The built-in PK models are easy to use but provide little flexibility. PK parameters for drugs that are described by complicated PK processes can only be estimated using the software packages that allow the user to define the models. Two of the most common software packages for compartmental analyses include NONMEM® (Nonlinear Mixed Effects Model) and ADAPT 5®. These packages are very flexible, as the user is required to provide the nonlinear mixed-effects models.

Since 1985, ADAPT-II® followed by ADAPT 5 has been developed and supported by the Biomedical Simulations Resource (BMSR) in the Department of Biomedical Engineering at the University of Southern California, under support from the National Institute for Biomedical Imaging and Bioengineering and the National Center for Research Resources of the National Institutes of Health (NIH). ADAPT 5 is a free computational modeling platform (although it does require the user to have a valid Intel® Visual Fortran compiler, which can be costly). ADAPT 5 is intended for basic and advanced clinical research

**TABLE 20-4 • Example of WinNonlin® Output Files**

**PK Parameter Output**

| Subject | Formulation | $C_{max}$ pg/mL | $AUC_{last}$ h*pg/mL | $AUC_{INF\_obs}$ h*pg/mL |
|---|---|---|---|---|
| 1 | 2 | 1106 | 431284 | 436154 |
| 2 | 1 | 483 | 326797 | 405731 |

**ANVA Output**

| FormRef | RefLSM | RefLSM_ SE | Ref- GeoLSM | Test | TestLSM | TestLSM_ SE | TestGeoLSM | Difference | Diff_ SE | Diff_ DF | Ratio _%Ref_ | CI_90_ Lower | CI_90_ Upper |
|---|---|---|---|---|---|---|---|---|---|---|---|---|---|
| 1 | 6.28 | 0.21 | 532.8 | 2 | 6.92 | 0.21 | 1014.8 | 0.64 | 0.30 | 4 | 190.45 | 100.13 | 362.25 |
| 1 | 12.63 | 0.19 | 305552.5 | 2 | 12.65 | 0.19 | 312425.3 | 0.02 | 0.28 | 4 | 102.25 | 56.83 | 183.98 |
| 1 | 12.78 | 0.19 | 355724.9 | 2 | 12.67 | 0.19 | 317698.5 | -0.11 | 0.27 | 4 | 89.31 | 50.01 | 159.49 |

*Tables output separately in WinNonlin.*

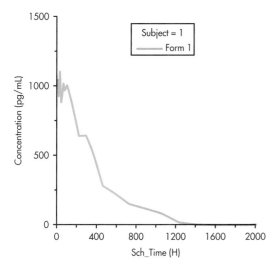

FIGURE 20-1 • Example of WinNonlin individual concentration–time profile.

and has been developed under the direction of David Z. D'Argenio in collaboration with Alan Schumitzky and Xiaoning Wang (D'Argenio et al, 2009). ADAPT 5 allows the user to choose from numerous algorithms both for individual [eg, weighted least squares (WLS), maximum likelihood (ML), generalized least squares (GLS), maximum *a posteriori* (MAP) Bayesian estimation] and population analyses [eg, maximum likelihood estimation via the EM algorithm with importance sampling (MLEM), iterative two-stage (ITS), standard two-stage (STS), and naive-pooled data (NPD) modeling]. Other important features of ADAPT 5 includes a module for simulations (SIM) and for determining optimal samples needed for a PK study. A free tool named AMGET, written to work with R (see description of the R software), is available to help automate certain analyses users will want to conduct with results from ADAPT 5. For example, AMGET allows users to simply and rapidly create informative diagnostic plots for ADAPT 5 models.

NONMEM, developed originally by S. L. Beal and L. B. Sheiner and the NONMEM Project Group at the University of California, is a program used to estimate PK/PD parameters. NONMEM is one of the first PK/PD modeling software programs and is considered by many scientists as the standard for population compartmental PK and PK/PD analyses.

The program first appeared in 1979, and numerous papers featuring NONMEM have been published. NONMEM versions 1 through 6 were developed by Sheiner and Beal and were the property of the Regents of the University of California. ICON Development Solutions acquired exclusive rights to NONMEM and has made significant updates for their first version, which was named NONMEM 7. The current version is 7.4. In addition to its basic applications to population PK and/or PD analysis, NONMEM is useful for evaluating relationships between pharmacokinetic parameters and demographic data (often referred to as covariates) such as age, weight, and disease state. Different algorithms are available in NONMEM to perform population compartmental analyses. The original algorithm implemented in NONMEM is the First Order (FO) method. After robustness issues were discovered with the FO method, Stuart and Beal added several additional algorithms in NONMEM version IV (1992): the First Order Conditional Estimation methods with (FOCEI) and without (FOCE) interaction, and the Laplace method. Starting with version 7, ITS, and Monte Carlo expectation-maximization and Markov Chain Monte Carlo Bayesian methods have been added. NONMEM can be used to simulate data as well as fit data. NONMEM requires a Fortran compiler, although it is compatible with a free Fortran compiler that is easily found online.

The software packages for compartmental analyses require entering multiple information to obtain estimates of PK parameters. The input files require the following data at a minimum: subject ID, dosing times, dose administered, sample collection times, drug concentrations, and when applicable other information such as covariate information. Table 20-5 provides an example of a NONMEM input file for an analysis of theophylline, which is included as part of the software package (only first 2 subjects out of 12 are presented). The software requires the model to be specified, the algorithm to be used, and if a population analysis is conducted, prior information of the PK parameters, including inter-subject variabilities and residual variability. Figure 20-2 provides NONMEM output for the same theophylline example (only partial output is presented as full output has numerous pages of information). Each software program has different

## TABLE 20-5 • NONMEM® Theophylline Input File

| #ID | DOSE | TIME | DV | WT |
|-----|------|------|------|------|
| 1 | 4.02 | 0 | . | 79.6 |
| 1 | . | 0 | 0.74 | . |
| 1 | . | 0.25 | 2.84 | . |
| 1 | . | 0.57 | 6.57 | . |
| 1 | . | 1.12 | 10.5 | . |
| 1 | . | 2.02 | 9.66 | . |
| 1 | . | 3.82 | 8.58 | . |
| 1 | . | 5.1 | 8.36 | . |
| 1 | . | 7.03 | 7.47 | . |
| 1 | . | 9.05 | 6.89 | . |
| 1 | . | 12.12 | 5.94 | . |
| 1 | . | 24.37 | 3.28 | . |
| 2 | 4.4 | 0 | . | 72.4 |
| 2 | . | 0 | 0 | . |
| 2 | . | 0.27 | 1.72 | . |
| 2 | . | 0.52 | 7.91 | . |
| 2 | . | 1 | 8.31 | . |
| 2 | . | 1.92 | 8.33 | . |
| 2 | . | 3.5 | 6.85 | . |
| 2 | . | 5.02 | 6.08 | . |
| 2 | . | 7.03 | 5.4 | . |
| 2 | . | 9 | 4.55 | . |
| 2 | . | 12 | 3.01 | . |
| 2 | . | 24.3 | 0.9 | . |

DV, dependent variable (in this example this refers to plasma concentration); WT, patient's weight.

requirements for inputting relevant data and the user is referred to each software's manual or user guide for details.

Other software packages include Monolix, Nlinmix (SAS), Phoenix NLME®, and Pmetrics. Phoenix NLME is an example of a software with built-in packages. This software package can be used for population PK and PK/PD analyses and multiple different nonlinear mixed-effects modeling algorithms.

Although these algorithms are based on the same mathematical principles as those found in more common PK software packages, different algorithms can deliver different results compared to other packages. This software is relatively user-friendly compared to some other programs available. Monolix allows users to apply nonlinear mixed-effect models for advanced population analysis, PK/PD, and preclinical and clinical trial modeling and simulation. The primary algorithm utilized by this software is the Stochastic Approximation of EM (SAEM) algorithm coupled with Monte Carlo and Markov Chains (MCMC) for maximum likelihood estimation (Delyon et al, 1999).

Pmetrics is a free software package developed by the Laboratory of Applied Pharmacokinetics at the University of Southern California (USC) that is used within R. Pmetrics is the latest evolution of the USC pack developed from Roger Jelliffe's laboratory at USC, the first available academic package designed for PK analyses and clinical therapeutic drug monitoring. In contrast to most other compartment PK software packages discussed in this chapter, this program provides a nonparametric approach to determine PK and PD parameters and is therefore of special interest. The available algorithms include the ITS Bayesian parametric population PK modeling (IT2B) in order to provide better initial estimates, nonparametric adaptive grid (NPAG) to estimate the population PK parameters from a nonparametric distribution, and a semiparametric Monte Carlo simulator for further simulations. The nonparametric population PK tool NPAG was formerly known as NPEM and NPEM2 and includes an EM algorithm initially developed by Alan Schumitzky. It has the advantage of calculating the true likelihood like other EM methods, but it provides the population results without artificially assuming a parametric distribution (most commonly linear or ln-linear).

R is a language and environment within which statistical computing and graphics are implemented. R is available as free software under the terms of the Free Software Foundation's GNU General Public License in source code form. R is not a PK software per se but provides a wide variety of statistical (linear and nonlinear modeling, classical statistical tests, time-series analysis, classification, clustering, etc) and graphical techniques for data handling and model analysis.

```
$PROB   THEOPHYLLINE   POPULATION DATA
$INPUT       ID DOSE=AMT TIME CP=DV WT
$DATA        THEOPP

$SUBROUTINES  ADVAN2

$PK
;THETA(1)=MEAN ABSORPTION RATE CONSTANT (1/HR)
;THETA(2)=MEAN ELIMINATION RATE CONSTANT (1/HR)
;THETA(3)=SLOPE OF CLEARANCE VS WEIGHT RELATIONSHIP (LITERS/HR/KG)
;SCALING PARAMETER=VOLUME/WT SINCE DOSE IS WEIGHT-ADJUSTED
    CALLFL=1
    KA=THETA(1)+ETA(1)
    K=THETA(2)+ETA(2)
    CL=THETA(3)*WT+ETA(3)
    SC=CL/K/WT

$THETA  (.1,3,5) (.008,.08,.5) (.004,.04,.9)
$OMEGA BLOCK(3)  6 .005 .0002 .3 .006 .4
$ERROR
    Y=F+EPS(1)

$SIGMA  .4

$EST    MAXEVAL=450  PRINT=5

 ONE COMPARTMENT MODEL WITH FIRST-ORDER ABSORPTION (ADVAN2)
0MAXIMUM NO. OF BASIC PK PARAMETERS:   3
0BASIC PK PARAMETERS (AFTER TRANSLATION):
   ELIMINATION RATE (K) IS BASIC PK PARAMETER NO.:  1
   ABSORPTION RATE (KA) IS BASIC PK PARAMETER NO.:  3


 #TERM:
0MINIMIZATION SUCCESSFUL
 NO. OF FUNCTION EVALUATIONS USED:      149
 NO. OF SIG. DIGITS IN FINAL EST.:  4.7




 ********************************************************************************************
 ********************                       FIRST ORDER
 ********************
 #OBJT:**************            MINIMUM VALUE OF OBJECTIVE FUNCTION
 ********************
 ********************************************************************************************
 *********************
 ********************           104.561        *******************************
 ********************************************************************************************
 ********************                       FIRST ORDER
 ********************                    FINAL PARAMETER ESTIMATE
 ********************************************************************************************

 THETA - VECTOR OF FIXED EFFECTS PARAMETERS   *********
         TH 1     TH 2     TH 3
         2.77E+00 7.81E-02 3.63E-02

 OMEGA - COV MATRIX FOR RANDOM EFFECTS - ETAS  ********

         ETA1     ETA2     ETA3
 ETA1
 +       5.55E+00
 ETA2
 +       5.24E-03 2.40E-04
 ETA3
 +      -1.28E-01 9.11E-03 5.15E-01

 SIGMA - COV MATRIX FOR RANDOM EFFECTS - EPSILONS  ****
         EPS1
 EPS1
 +       3.88E-01
```

FIGURE 20-2 • NONMEM Control file for theophylline

## *In Vivo* Simulations from *In Vitro* Data

*In vivo* simulations from *in vitro* data analyses are complicated and are typically used by pharmaceutical scientists. Software allowing PBPK analysis and *in vivo* simulations from *in vitro* data include Berkeley Madonna, GastroPlus®, PK-Sim®, and Simcyp®. Recent advancements have made these software packages more accessible and include user-friendly interfaces. These analyses require data from *in vitro* to *in vivo* information. If these data are not available, then the analyses may rely on too many assumptions, which decreases the ability of the model to make accurate predictions. The predictive capability of these software packages becomes more accurate as more data is collected and more information becomes available. For example, information on liver enzymes and transporters is being included in the software package so that predictions improve over time. These software packages are used to predict the expected PK parameter values in humans and other species. The improved capability of the software has encouraged regulatory agencies to accept waiving drug–drug interaction (DDI) studies using these software packages. The FDA has recently issued a guidance on the content and format of PBPK analyses (FDA, 2018). It should be noted, though, that the analyses are not straightforward, can be time-consuming, and must be properly validated in order for agencies to waive these DDI studies. Furthermore, some of these software packages can be quite costly.

Berkeley Madonna is a commercially available, general-purpose differential equation solver for constructing mathematical models. It was developed on the Berkeley campus under the sponsorship of the National Science Foundation (NSF) and the NIH. The software package offers much flexibility to the PBPK model developer, but more advanced modeling and programming skills and experience are required. Berkeley Madonna has a relatively user-friendly graphical interface that allows the user to modify the model by modifying a diagram rather than writing equations. Berkeley Madonna has been used extensively in the development of PBPK models (Khalil and Läer, 2011; Lin et al, 2017).

GastroPlus, Simcyp, and PK-Sim are PBPK-based simulation software packages that predict expected drug concentrations from multiple different administration routes based on the physicochemical properties, *in vitro* assessments, and preclinical data of these drugs. Features of the software include a variety of dosage forms: intravenous (bolus or infusion), immediate release, and controlled release. IVIVC can also be conducted for immediate- or controlled-release formulations. These software packages perform *in vitro–in vivo* extrapolation (IVIVE). These software packages also allow simulations in an array of populations such as pediatrics, oncology patients, and data from animal studies.

These software packages and WinNonlin may have predefined functions to conduct IVIVC analyses. However, with sufficient scientific knowledge in fitting *in vitro* dissolution curves and correlations with *in vivo* PK characteristics, other software packages such as ADAPT 5 and NONMEM can be used to conduct these IVIVC analyses.

## Design, Analysis, and Reporting of Population Compartmental PK/PD Analyses

Most new drug submissions to regulatory agencies include some population compartmental PK or PK/PD analyses. The pharmaceutical industry uses this analysis to better characterize their drug product, plan for upcoming studies, predict future study outcomes, avoid costly *in vivo* studies, and confirm safety and efficacy of the proposed dosage regimen. These analyses are also increasingly used in the development of generic drug products. For example, to market a generic version of an albuterol inhaled product in the United States, an *in vivo* dose-scale bioequivalence study is required to prove equivalence, using the forced expiratory volume, $FEV_1$ in 1 second as a clinical endpoint (FDA, 2018).

These analyses are being used more frequently. Standards in data collection, analyses, and reporting are essential to ensure the validity of the results. The results of these analyses must be reproducible by other scientists. FDA and EMA have produced guidances on population PK/PD analyses and reporting (EMA, 2007; FDA, 2019). Multiple steps are required to ensure a successful population compartmental analysis with a well-documented report. This report includes the identification of the analysis objectives, selection of an appropriate study design, thorough data collection, appropriate methodology, and accurate reporting. Each element is described in more detail below.

## Identification of Analysis Objectives

Before planning a population PK or PK/PD analysis, it is important to understand the purpose of the analysis and identify what one hopes to gain from the results. Analyses can be conducted to describe and quantify the PK in a particular group of healthy volunteers or patients. Some analyses are intended to develop models that can be used to simulate data in different groups. Population PK analyses are often used to understand the impact of covariates on a drug's PK/PD, especially in a patient population. The population PK approach is a flexible approach that can be customized based on the analysis objectives. The objectives must be clearly stated to properly plan the analyses.

## Data Collection

The ability of a PK/PD analysis to meet its objectives (whether descriptive or predictive in nature) is dependent on the quality of the data that is included in the analysis. The data is a critical element that must be considered before undertaking a population PK or PK/PD analysis. The design of the study (or studies) will depend upon the objectives and the available data. The study design depends upon the objectives of the study, which may not be the same objectives as those of the compartmental analyses. For example, the main objective of the study may be to demonstrate proof of concept for the drug in a Phase II protocol. In contrast, the compartmental analysis may aim to construct a model using previous data collected in Phase I studies as well as data collected in the Phase II study. From this analysis, the objective is to develop a potential dose-exposure-effect relationship for optimization of the dose for Phase III. The main objective of the study may not require any PK blood sample collection; however, for the compartmental analysis, some samples will be required.

While PK data collection may not be a primary assessment in study design, it is important to ensure that the data required for the PK analyses will be collected. These data include dosing information (doses and dosing times), concentration data with sampling times, demographics, and other information that could influence PK or PD, such as disease status.

For PK analyses, the collection of concentration data is very important. Blood samples must be collected at time points that are the most informative. In some cases, the study design or population does not permit intensive PK sample collection such as those collected in a typical Phase I study. The collection of trough PK samples (collected prior to subsequent doses) is fairly easy to accomplish, but additional PK samples are often required.

The timing of the PK sample collections and clinical observations can be influenced by various factors. The mechanism of action of the drug can provide suggestions on the blood sampling schedule along with timing of clinical observations. For example, to study whether there is a direct immediate relationship between the plasma drug concentrations and the intended effect, blood samples could be collected at the same time as measurements of drug response. Blood samples can also be taken if the patient or subject has an adverse response to the drug. If the pharmacodynamic (PD) effect is delayed or observed long after dosing, then there may not be a direct link between plasma drug concentration and PD effect and it may not be relevant to characterize plasma drug concentrations and PD effect at the same time. In such scenarios, the PK/PD relationship may be linked to other parameters such as AUC (extent of exposure) or time above a certain drug concentration.

A question often arises as to how many subjects need to provide blood samples. There is no absolute number, and the desired quantity of data can vary from study to study. The desired number of samples depends upon the expected variability in the parameters. In studies where intensive samples cannot be collected in patients, fewer samples are collected at optimized times in all randomized patients. More blood samples may be collected from a subset of patients. In this way, the PK can be predicted for all patients and plasma drug concentrations can then be linked to the individual measures of efficacy.

The main objectives of the study may not only be to develop a compartmental PK/PD model for the drug. For instance, the main study objectives could be to assess the safety and tolerability of a drug in a patient population, or to determine how drug response evolves over time. However, the study should still be designed to collect the necessary data to meet all objectives, including the development of the PK/PD model, given the constraints of each study or population. The objectives of the study and known information on the drug will help to develop a study design that provides insight into which data should be collected and how the data should be analyzed for both the study objectives and the PK/PD modeling.

## Pharmacokinetic Analysis Plan

A pharmacokinetic analysis plan should contain information including the objectives of the analyses, the data to be used, how the dataset will be constructed, what models will be tested, model discrimination criteria, covariate analysis (if required), model validation, and simulation scenarios if pertinent. The objectives of the analysis dictate the study design and data analyses. For example, if an analysis is to develop a population PK model for predictive purposes, the model will require a more vigorous validation process than a model that is purely descriptive in nature.

### Analysis Objectives and Data

Clear objectives in the analysis plan guide the methodology and the information to be reported. The required data should also be clearly identified. For example, will data from patients who do not complete the study be included? In most cases, partial data from patients may be useful in the population compartmental analysis, and are included. The study protocol should provide the rationale for which data can or cannot be included. The study protocol should be agreed upon prior to initiation of the study. For example, a scientist may want to analyze only data collected under fasted conditions. In this case, the study protocol should explicitly state that the data from patients having eaten within 2 hours of dosing will not be considered as fasting data and will be excluded. Another example is a study that is designed to evaluate different drug formulations. After study initiation, a decision is made not to further develop one drug formulation. To avoid introducing additional variability and complexity to the

modeling, the data from this one drug formulation may be excluded from the analysis.

A description of the construction of the dataset is common practice and is linked to the data to be used in the analysis and some standards should be applied. A description of how plasma concentrations, urine concentrations, or PD measures reported as missing or below the limit of quantitation will be handled in the dataset is important. An indication if actual or nominal times used in the analysis should be mentioned. The plan should describe how continuous and discrete covariates are entered in the dataset, and what is done if a patient does not have the information provided. In that case, it is common to either set the covariate to missing for that patient or set it to the median or mean value of the other patients with similar characteristics. If there are covariates that will be derived from other covariates, such as body mass index (BMI) from weight and body surface area (BSA), the equation to obtain that covariate can be described in advance. The plan should describe all intended treatment of data and the report should account for any deviations from this plan.

### Exploratory Data Analysis

Prior to starting any population compartmental analyses, an examination of the observed data should be conducted. This may be done using tables, figures, or some correlations. This will help reveal certain trends or features in the population data that can help dictate the modeling analysis.

### Structural Model Determination

The next step of the analysis that should be described in the plan is the structural model determination. The typical PK structural models are tested are one-, two-, and three-compartment models. If the drug is administered extravascularly (eg, oral drug administration), different absorption processes may be tested (Chapter 16). To select the most appropriate structural model, models that are simpler and more complicated than the final chosen model must be tested to confirm the choice. The structural model that is retained should be "sandwiched" between a simpler model that does not explain the data as well and a more complex model that does not provide additional benefits compared to the chosen model. For example, a two-compartment model may be found to be better than the one-compartment model. If these are the only models tested, it is impossible to know whether a more complex model such as a three-compartment model would provide even better results. Therefore, the three-compartment should be tested and if it is not significantly better than the two-compartment model, then the two-compartment model can be chosen with more confidence.

Beyond the testing of models with different numbers of compartments and different types of absorption processes, other elements must be considered as well. For instance, if data from different formulations or periods are collected in the same patients, it may be important to state how this will be handled. There may be the need for a relative bioavailability parameter or inter-occasion variability parameters. If inter-occasion variability is included in the model, the plan should specify how this will be coded and how occasions will be defined. If metabolite data were collected, a description of how parent and metabolite data will be fitted should be provided. The plan should specify if the metabolite data will be simultaneously modeled with the parent data or separately. In addition, the plan can detail if the parent drug is analyzed first and the PK parameters for the parent drug to be fixed when the metabolite data is analyzed. The plan can state that one approach may be preferred but that if adequate results cannot be obtained, a different approach will be used.

If a PK/PD analysis is the objective of the analysis, most analyses will typically start with the PK analysis first and then fix the PK parameters to the individual parameters for each patient while analyzing the PD data. This type of analysis is often called a *sequential analysis*. The PD effect could be described by direct or indirect effect models (the PK/PD relationship is discussed in Chapter 22). If placebo data is available, the analysis should contain some information on how placebo data or baseline results will be handled in the analysis.

## Assumptions and Error Model

All model assumptions must be predefined. For example, PK parameters may be assumed to follow a log-normal distribution and the model can be assumed so without doing any tests. In addition, PD parameters may be assumed to follow a normal distribution instead of a log-normal distribution.

The PK analysis plan should describe how the error model or residual variability (eg, epsilons in NONMEM) will be coded. Types of error models include proportional error models, additive error models, or a combination of both.

## Criteria for Model Selection

Model discrimination criteria must be described as various criteria exist. One criterion used to compare models is the *Akaike information criterion* (AIC) which is an estimator of the relative quality of a model for a given set of data. AIC is calculated as the likelihood objection function plus a penalty for the number of parameters. The AIC values are compared directly to the AIC of another model that was fitted using the same dataset. Another comparator that is often used is the *minimum objection function* (MOF). The MOF does not provide any information on the quality of fit but can be compared to the MOF of a different model that was fitted using the same dataset. Assuming a *chi-square distribution*, a new model may be considered an improvement over the reference model if the MOF decreases (upon the addition of parameters to the model) or does not increase (upon the removal of parameters from the model) by a certain significant value. For example, if one parameter is added to the model and the MOF decreases by more than 6.63 (*p*-value < 0.01 for 1 degree of freedom), then this will indicate a statistically significant improvement in the quality of the fit. The *p*-value criteria will need to be specified *a priori*.

Attributes are usually monitored to ensure a better quality of fit such as improved predicted drug concentrations versus observed drug concentrations over time.

Additional attributes include a lower value of the residual variability, the plausibility of the PK parameters for both the population model and the individual fitted estimates, and an improvement in a different quality-of-fit representations. Quality-of-fit representations include population predictions versus observed concentrations, weighted residuals versus predicted concentrations, and weighted residuals versus time. For example, a model with a greater number of compartments may have a better AIC or MOF. However, even though the model has a better MOF or AIC, it may be rejected if the parameter estimates do not make sense such as in the case where the estimated half-life that is not physiologically possible with the data being analyzed.

### Covariate Analyses

Once the structural PK model is selected, covariate analysis can be conducted. The covariates to be tested should be listed in the analysis plan. Covariates that should be considered for testing include those which are believed to have a potential influence on PK or PD variability. Only covariates with sufficient data should be tested. For example, if the study only includes Caucasians, it will not be possible to test the influence of race on PK or PD.

Results of the analysis may suggest other covariates to be tested which were not originally listed in the plan. The testing of additional covariates is not an issue. However, it is important to describe how all covariates will be chosen and retained in the model. For example, if the patients in the study all had weights below 70 kg, then weight is not an acceptable covariate to make inferential simulations for a population with much higher weights (eg, above 100 kg).

Covariates may be first explored visually by creating graphs of covariates versus individually fitted PK parameters associated with the final structural model. This will provide an indication of which covariates could be of importance. Correlations between the covariate and individual PK parameters may be performed to determine which covariates have the strongest relationship with the parameters. Some people use the one-at-a-time stepwise approach, and others include everything at once, and then remove them one by one. Covariate testing should be envisioned if a stepwise process is used. For example, the addition of covariates related to size (eg, actual body weight (ABW), height, BMI, BSA) can first be tested on the most identifiable PK parameters (eg, $V_c/F$; $CL/F$, or $k_{10}$). ABW may be added on $CL/F$ and $V_c/F$ using known principles of allometry (Chapter 19) without requiring additional model parameters (eg, fitting volumes in L/kg and clearances to ABW/median value with an allometric exponent of 0.75). As a next step, other covariates could be tested on the most identifiable parameters. Identifiable parameters are those that uniquely estimate the true values for those parameters. Once the covariates on parameters such as $CL/F$ and $V_c/F$ have been sufficiently tested, the addition of covariates on other parameters, such as those related to rate of absorption ($k_a$) and lag times, can be tested. Finally, covariates can be tested on parameters that are not as robustly identifiable such as distributional clearance, peripheral volume, and distributional rate constants (eg, $CL_d/F$, $V_p/F$, $k_{12}$, $k_{21}$).

Criteria used to accept or reject covariate models should also be clearly defined in the analysis plan. This could include a similar approach to the structural model discrimination process using MOF, based on a chi-square distribution and a critical $p$-value of 0.01. If more than one covariate is added to the final structural model, a deconstruction step should be conducted to ensure that all clinical covariates that have been added are still needed and that covariates were not made superfluous by the addition of others. Criteria for model deconstruction must also be defined, and they can be similar to the criteria used for covariate selection.

The addition of covariates is particularly important if the model is required to simulate the outcome for future studies. The inclusion of covariates in a model allows the user to make predictions that can vary according to different levels of covariates. A model that includes gender should be able to make predictions for both males and females. A model that includes weight should be able to make predictions for individuals with a specific weight or range of weights. In covariate analysis, particular attention is given to the predicted drug concentrations or PD response marker versus the observed values. Inclusion of covariates in a model allows quantitating the variability associated with certain parameters. Knowing the intersubject variability leads to a better understanding of why the PK parameter of one subject is different from that of another subject. Care must be taken regarding the number of covariates added to the model. If the structural model did not fit the data from the individual subjects adequately, it is possible that this will be compensated by the addition of many covariates, which is not the goal of this step. If this is the case, then the structural model discrimination should be reviewed.

## Model Refinement and Validation

The determination of the population PK or PK/PD model may or may not include covariates. Additional analyses may be conducted to determine whether the model could be further improved or simplified. Analyses may be conducted to detect the presence of covariances or correlations between PK or PD parameters. Additional models may be tested if warranted by the results, using MOF values and assuming a chi-square distribution and a critical *p*-value of 0.01.

Once a model is chosen, it should be validated. There are two types of validation—internal validation and external validation. *Internal validation* uses established criteria to test the model by using the data included in the analysis. No new data are required for this validation. *External validation* consists of predicting the expected outcome for each individual from an external validation dataset. External validation requires data that have not been included in the analyses. These data can be obtained from different sources. Data from a separate study

can be obtained, data from the literature can be used, or data from the ongoing analyses can be set aside from the dataset and used exclusively for the external validation. Models are usually validated internally since no additional data are required. Multiple approaches are often employed to validate a model internally. At a minimum, *goodness-of-fit* plots should be presented. Goodness-of-fit plots, including population or individual predicted concentrations versus observed concentration and residuals versus time or concentrations, may be created and inspected closely to ensure that there are no obvious trends or biases in the predictions. For example, the predicted versus observed data points are clustered around the line of identity. If low concentrations are always overestimated and high concentrations are always underestimated, then the model is probably not valid and is only predicting concentrations in the middle of what is observed. Figure 20-3 presents a goodness-of-fit figure illustrating predicted versus observed concentrations for a model that predicts the concentrations well (A) and a model that has unsatisfactory predictions of the concentrations (B).

Figures should also be created with predicted data or residuals that are presented as a function of time. These figures can detect time-dependent issues with the model, such as nonlinearity that is not accounted for. A second validation is verification that the individual fitted parameters are

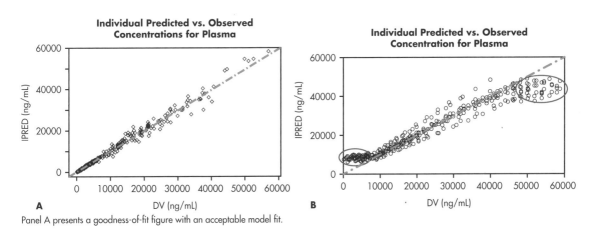

Panel A presents a goodness-of-fit figure with an acceptable model fit.

Panel B presents a model that should be rejected as the lower concentrations are overestimated and higher concentrations are underestimated (circles).

FIGURE 20-3 • Example of goodness-of-fit figures.

in line with the observed PK results (often called "posterior predictive checks"). This verification can be performed by comparing individual fitted predicted AUC and $C_{max}$ parameters to those obtained using individual observed data and standard noncompartmental methods. If the dataset contains data from multiple studies or dose strengths, verification can be done by study or dose level, to ensure that the model characterizes the observed data correctly at the individual data level and at the study or dose level. If the model is to be used to predict future populations, then a comparison of summary statistics based on population predicted PK parameters and fitted individual PK parameters should be shown. If these results are comparable, the individual PK parameters accurately reflect the observed values. Therefore, it can be considered that the mean predicted PK parameters and their variabilities are consistent with the observed data. These results along with goodness-of-fit data suggest that the final population PK model can simulate other studies. An additional tool often used is visual predictive checks (Bergstrand et al, 2011). For this validation step, the final PK model is used to simulate concentration–time profiles for each subject included in the population compartmental analysis. Using these predicted concentrations, median and 90% confidence intervals are constructed (using a percentile approach) and overlaid on the observed data. The percentage of observed values outside of the predicted 90% confidence intervals is calculated. Theoretically, approximately 10% of these values must fall outside the 90% confidence intervals. These graphs will also show if trends in the fitted data are unacceptable, such as a poor fit in a subset of patients or for a certain range of values.

Additional internal validation tools exist. For example, bootstraps can be done with the final model to obtain 90% confidence intervals around the population PK parameter estimates and their expected variability estimates. If the population PK parameter estimated with the final model falls outside this range or is skewed to one extremity, then the results obtained from the final model may be from a local minima (ie, a solution that is not the optimal solution). In that case, the final model should be re-run using different priors to see if this would fix the problem. This could also indicate that there are some

subjects that are influential in the estimation of the population PK parameters.

External validation differs from internal validation and predicts the expected outcome for each individual from the external validation dataset based on their covariates. If the model can correctly predict the concentrations or PD outcome for the different patients, then the model is considered to be accurate at predicting different populations.

The choice of using an internal or external validation procedure depends on several factors. Excluding data from the original dataset to conduct an external validation may make it more challenging for the model to accurately estimate the population PK/PD parameters, as less data are available for the analysis. Splitting the data into two datasets, one for analysis and one for validation, is not a good strategy if there is little data to begin with. Data from the literature that can be used for external validation may not always provide all of the necessary information to simulate according to the covariates that were important in the model, and therefore some assumptions may be required which may invalidate the outcome. Using a new study, probably obtained after the model was completed, to determine if the model is accurate at predicting new data is optimal. This is similar to Sheiner's "learn and confirm" paradigm (Sheiner, 1997). This consists of learning from your current data and predicting future outcomes. If the outcome is different, then as a scientist, you need to go back and determine what assumptions that were included in the model are inaccurate, and improve the model.

### Simulations

If simulations are required, then the analysis plan should specify which populations will be simulated, the size of the populations, the general study design, and the dose or dosing regimen(s). If parameters are to be calculated from the simulated concentrations, the parameters and the method of calculations should be described.

### Software

The software packages including their versions, the computer operating system, and chip should be included. Population compartmental analyses often require long and complex mathematical and statistical computational analyses which could differ slightly from one computer to the other.

## Compartment PK/PD Reporting

While the successful completion of a population PK or PK/PD analysis is the ultimate goal, if the results are not presented in a clear and comprehensive manner, the importance of the findings may not be fully appreciated. Some regulatory agencies have emitted guidances (EMA, 2007; FDA, 2019) on population compartmental analysis. They describe what type of information they expect to see in reports, and state that the following sections should be presented:

*(1) an executive summary, (2) a synopsis, (3) an introduction, (4) data, (5) the methods, (6) the results, (7) a discussion, (8) conclusions, and (9) an appendix (if applicable).*

These sections are relatively standard for any report; however, before 1999, no guidance on population PK analyses existed. The 1999 FDA guidance was recently updated in July 2019 to include more details on what should be presented in reports, as well as what types of files should be submitted to the agency. This demonstrates that population PK analyses are now becoming more mainstream, requiring agencies to outline a standard approach for the presentation of the results.

The report presents the analysis that was planned and describes all results, including any deviations from the original plan. The methodology and results sections will therefore include details as described in the previous sections. The report must provide sufficient details on how the final model was chosen. The different structural models that were tested and their results should be presented. Results for models that were accepted and rejected should be shown for full transparency. This kind of information should be presented for the different steps (eg, structural, covariates, covariance). Finally, the final structural model should be clearly described. An illustration of the final model in the report can also be helpful to the reader.

Table 20-6 presents an example of what could be described for the model discrimination steps, and Fig. 20-4 presents how the model could be

## TABLE 20-6 • Example of a Model Discrimination Table

| Model Number | Description | Reference Model | MOF | # Of Fitted Parameters | Minimum MOF Reduction to Accept Model (p<0.05) | Difference | Residual Variability | Comments |
|---|---|---|---|---|---|---|---|---|
| 1 | 1cpt, $k_a$, CL/F | NA | 6509 | 3 | NA | NA | 24 | |
| 2 | 2cpt, $k_a$, CL/F | 1 | 6118 | 5 | −5.99 | −391 | 17 | |
| 3 | 3cpt, $k_a$, CL/F | 2 | 6117 | 7 | −5.99 | −1 | 17 | |
| **4** | **2cpt, $k_a$, Abs Lag, CL/F** | **2** | **5998** | **6** | **−3.84** | **−119** | **10** | **Final structural model** |
| 5 | 2cpt, $k_0$, Abs Lag, CL/F | 4 | 6136 | 6 | 0.00 | 19 | 13 | |
| 6 | 2cpt, $k_a$, Abs Lag, Non-linear elimination | 4 | 5998 | 7 | −3.84 | 0 | 10 | |

*Cpt = compartment; $k_a$ = absorption rate constant; Abs Lag = lag time before start of absorption; CL/F = apparent clearance; MOF = minimum objective function; shaded row = significant model improvement; **shaded and bolded row** = final structural model.*

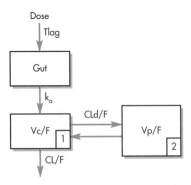

FIGURE 20-4 • Depiction of a final model. $k_a$ = Absorption rate constant; Gut = Oral depot compartment; CLd/F = Apparent distributional clearance; CL/F = Apparent clearance; Vc/F = Apparent central volume of distribution; Vp/F = Apparent peripheral volume of distribution; Tlag = Lag time before start of absorption.

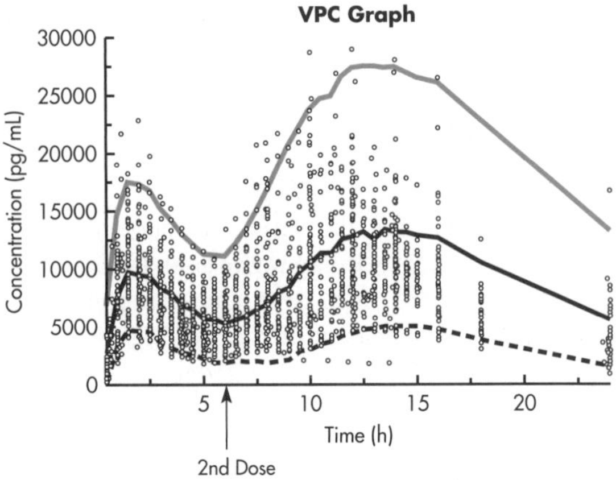

**VPC Graph**

FIGURE 20-5 • Visual predictive check figure. Dashed line = 5th percentile of the predicted concentrations from 1000 simulated subjects; Black line = 50th percentile of the predicted concentrations from 1000 simulated subjects; Blue line = 95th percentile of the predicted concentrations from 1000 simulated subjects; Black circle = Observed data.

depicted graphically. As we can see from the table, some models were accepted, as they improved the overall quality of the predictions while others were rejected, as they did not. A narrative to explain the different steps is also required so that the reader can understand the steps that led from one model to another.

As mentioned in the analysis plan section, model validation is crucial. Regulatory agencies stipulate that the validation of the model must be carefully described. Figures 20-3A and 20-5 provide examples of goodness-of-fit figures and visual predictive check (VPC) figures for an acceptable final model. In the example illustrated by Fig. 20-3A, the data are equally distributed or spread around the line of identity and there are no trends in the individual predicted figures that would suggest any issues with the structural model. The VPC figures show that the model has good predictive performance, as simulated results and observed results are consistent with one another.

Simulations of future studies need to be well described if such simulations were conducted. Why the fitted model is appropriate to use for simulations should be discussed. If the model must be modified to conduct simulations, the rationale behind these modifications must be explained. For example, if

the model was developed from a specific population (eg, adults) and then used to simulate expected concentrations in completely different populations (eg, newborns, toddlers, and young children), there needs to be a justification that explains why the model can be used to simulate those populations. If the clearance and volume of distribution estimates do not include weight as a covariate, then the simulations will likely be inaccurate for all children. Other aspects of the model will need to be considered. For example, if the drug is metabolized by CYP3A or is known to be eliminated renally, the model must consider that children do not have the same enzymatic or renal capacity as adults. Without these considerations, the simulations will be inaccurate and must be rejected. The results of the simulations will not be applicable to any decision-making process for future studies.

FDA and EMA provide guidance on the contents of population PK/PD reports. Investigators must provide information in the report to allow reviewers to reproduce the work. All pivotal models (including input and output files) should be provided. This does not mean that all models should be provided, but certainly the final structural and covariate model should be provided. Some files can be provided electronically, as described in the guidance documents. Electronic information includes the datasets used for the analyses of all pivotal models and the individual fitted results for at least the final model.

## CHAPTER SUMMARY

Various software packages are available to conduct population PK/PD compartmental analyses. A description of the more popular computer software packages has been presented. Each software package analyzes the data differently according to its own functions and algorithms. Some software packages calculate PK/PD parameters using a noncompartmental approach; others use empirical models to obtain individual or population PK/PD parameters. Software packages are also available to conduct physiologically-based pharmacokinetic analyses.

The strengths and weaknesses of each software package are presented for the selection of the most appropriate software package to conduct analysis. No software is necessarily better than another.

Different software packages can even be used at different stages of an analyses to provide different perspectives on the same data.

No matter which software package is used, proper planning and reporting of the analyses is required to ensure that the analysis will be accurate, reproducible, and acceptable. The objectives of the modeling are critical for the determination of what data is needed, when to collect the data, and how the data is to be analyzed. The final report should present the results in a clear and structured way so that scientists and regulatory agencies can review it for completeness and validity. Regulatory agencies are more stringent with their expectations surrounding these analyses, and the final report should reflect this.

## EXAMPLE 1 ▷ ▷ ▷

From a series of plasma drug concentration versus time data (Table 20-7, columns A and B), determine the elimination rate constant using the regression feature of MS Excel.

### TABLE 20-7 • Concentration–Time Data for Example 1

| A | B | C | D | E |
|---|---|---|---|---|
| Time (hours) | Conc | Ln (Conc) | | |
| 0 | 0 | | | |
| 2 | 7049.53 | 8.86 | | |
| 4 | 7194.95 | 8.88 | | |
| 6 | 6178.08 | 8.73 | | |
| 8 | 5116.2 | 8.54 | | |
| 10 | 4200.5 | 8.34 | | |
| 12 | 3441.45 | 8.14 | Slope | -0.1 |
| 14 | 2818.09 | 7.94 | | |
| 16 | 2307.36 | 7.74 | | |

### Solution

a. Type in the time and concentration data shown in columns A and B (see Fig. 20-6).

b. In column C, log-transform all concentration data found in column B. Data point #1 may be omitted because ln of zero cannot be determined.

c. From the main menu, select Insert:

Select function

SLOPE

Y data range (select last 4 value)

X data range (select last 4 value)

The slope, given in column E of Fig. 20-6, is –0.1. In this case, the ln concentration is plotted versus time, and the slope is simply the elimination rate constant.

*Note*: To check this result, students may be interested in simulating the data with dose = 10,000 $\mu$g/kg, $V_D$ = 1000 mL/kg, $k_a$ = 0.8 h$^{-1}$, and $k$ = 0.1 h$^{-1}$.

# EXAMPLE 2 ▷ ▷ ▷

Generate data for a two-compartment model using two differential equations. Initial conditions are dose = 1, $V_{ss} = 1$, $k_{12} = 0.2$, $k_{21} = 1$, and $k_{el} = 3$.

**Solution**

The data may be generated with ADAPT 5 (Fig. 20-6).

```
            ADAPT 5      SIM --   MODEL SIMULATION
Enter file name for storing session run (*.run) : Run1.run
          -----MODEL INPUT INFORMATION -----
Data file name (*.dat) : C: \pt1.csv
          ** This is a population data file: C:\pt1.csv
              Will analyze 1st subject

  The number of model inputs:     0
  The number of bolus inputs:     1
  Enter the compartment number for each bolus input (e.g.  1, 3, ...):  1)
  The number of input event times:    1

        Input Event Information
              Time Value for all Inputs
  Event        Units,       B(1)
     1.        0.000        1.000


            ----- MODEL OUTPUT INFORMATION------
  The number of model output equations:    2
  The number of observations:     15
              ----- SIMULATION SELECTION ------
  The following simulation options are availble:
        1.  Individual simulation
        2.  Individual simulation with output error
        3.  Population simulation
        4.  Population simulation with output error
  Enter option number: 1
            ----- ENTER PARAMETER INFORMATION ------
  Parameter file name: C:\Priors1.prm
  Enter values for indicated parameters:
   Parameter   Old Value    New Valvue  (<Enter> if no change)
      K         3.000
      K12        .2000
      K21       1.000
      Vc        1.000
      Vp        1.000
```

FIGURE 20-6 • A sample of the ADAPT 5 program used to solve the two differential equations describing a two-compartment model after IV bolus dose. (The first 15 data points are shown. Time is in hours.)

```
Enter Initial Conditions:
  Parameter    Old Value    New Valvue   (<Enter> if no change)
     IC( 1)    0.000
     IC( 2)    0.000


          ----- RESULTS -----
          --- A. Parameter Summary ---
  Individual simulation
  Parameter       Value
     K            3.000
     K12          0.2000
     K21          1.000
     Vc           1.000
     Vp           1.000
     IC( 1)       0.000
     IC( 2)       0.000
          ----- B. Simulation Summary -----
  Model: 2-cpt model;  example 2           Individual simulation
       Obs. Num.     Time           Y(1),  ...    ,Y( 2)
            1        0.000          0.000
            2        0.1700E-01     0.9471        0.000
            3        0.3300E-01     0.8999        0.3281E-02
            4        0.50000E-01    0.8524        0.6160E-02
            5        0.6700E-01     0.8074        0.9008E-02
            6        0.8300E-01     0.7673        0.1165E-01
            7        0.1000         0.7269        0.1397E-01
            8        0.1170         0.6887        0.1836E-01
            9        0.1330         0.6547        0.2020E-01
           10        0.1500         0.6203        0.2201E-01
           11        0.1670         0.5879        0.2367E-01
           12        1.000          0.5076E-01    0.3067E-01
           13        2.000          0.7278E-02    0.1346E-01
           14        3.000          0.2433E-02    0.5446E-02
           15        4.000          0.9586E-03    0.2188E-02
```

FIGURE 20-6 • (Continued)

## EXAMPLE 3  ▷ ▷ ▷

After a drug is administered orally, plasma drug concentration–time data may be fitted to a one- or two-compartment model, to estimate the absorption rate constant, elimination rate constant, and volume of distribution. Based on the results of these models, it is possible to determine which model best explains the results using the minimum objective function (MOF). Results from NONMEM (one-, two-compartment models) are shown in Fig. 20-7A and B. In this case, the plasma concentrations were better fitted using a two-compartment model than a one-compartment model. The MOF was significantly lower with the two-compartment model versus a one-compartment model.

```
$PROBLEM Run1; Book Chapter 1CPT Oral plasma
$INPUT ID, TIME, RATE, DOSE=AMT, DV, EVID, MDV
$DATA NM1.CSV
$SUBROUTINES ADVAN2 TRANS2
$PK

   ALAG1 = THETA(1)*EXP(ETA(1))
   KA = THETA(2)*EXP(ETA(2))
   CL = THETA(3)*EXP(ETA(3))
   V = THETA(4)*EXP(ETA(4))

   SC = V

    K10 = CL/V
    HALF=LOG(2)/K10

$THETA
      (0    0.3   ) ; ALAG
      (0    10    ) ; KA
      (0    1     ) ; CL
      (0    4     ) ; VC

$OMEGA 0.05    ; ALAG
       0.05    ; KA
       0.05    ; CL
       0.05    ; VC

$ERROR
      IPRED = F
      IF(F.GT.0)THEN
        W = F
      ELSE
        W = 1
      END IF
      IRES = DV - IPRED
      IWRES = IRES/W

      Y = F + F*EPS(1) + EPS(2)

$SIGMA 0.05 0.05

$ESTIMATION METHOD=1 NOABORT SIGDIGITS=3 MAXEVAL=9999 PRINT=0 POSTHOC

NM-TRAN MESSAGES

WARNINGS AND ERRORS (IF ANY) FOR PROBLEM 1
```

FIGURE 20-7 · **(A)** Sample output from NONMEM showing oral data fitted to a one-compartment model with first-order absorption and first-order elimination (ADVAN2, TRANS2).

```
(WARNING 2) NM-TRAN INFERS THAT THE DATA ARE POPULATION.
CREATING MUMODEL ROUTINE...


 PROBLEM NO.: 1
 Run1; Book Chapter 1CPT Oral plasma
0DATA CHECKOUT RUN: NO
 DATA SET LOCATED ON UNIT NO.: 2
 THIS UNIT TO BE REWOUND: NO
 NO. OF DATA RECS IN DATA SET: 378
 NO. OF DATA ITEMS IN DATA SET: 7
 ID DATA ITEM IS DATA ITEM NO.: 1
 DEP VARIABLE IS DATA ITEM NO.: 5
 MDV DATA ITEM IS DATA ITEM NO.: 7
0INDICES PASSED TO SUBROUTINE PRED:
   6 2 4 3 0 0 0 0 0 0
0LABELS FOR DATA ITEMS:
 ID TIME RATE DOSE DV EVID MDV
0FORMAT FOR DATA:
 (7E7.0)


 TOT. NO. OF OBS RECS: 340
 TOT. NO. OF INDIVIDUALS: 18
0LENGTH OF THETA: 4
0DEFAULT THETA BOUNDARY TEST OMITTED: NO
0OMEGA HAS SIMPLE DIAGONAL FORM WITH DIMENSION: 4
0DEFAULT OMEGA BOUNDARY TEST OMITTED: NO
0SIGMA HAS SIMPLE DIAGONAL FORM WITH DIMENSION: 2
0DEFAULT SIGMA BOUNDARY TEST OMITTED: NO
0INITIAL ESTIMATE OF THETA:
 LOWER BOUND INITIAL EST UPPER BOUND
  0.0000E+00 0.3000E+00 0.1000E+07
  0.0000E+00 0.1000E+02 0.1000E+07
  0.0000E+00 0.1000E+01 0.1000E+07
  0.0000E+00 0.4000E+01 0.1000E+07
0INITIAL ESTIMATE OF OMEGA:
  0.5000E-01
  0.0000E+00 0.5000E-01
  0.0000E+00 0.0000E+00 0.5000E-01
  0.0000E+00 0.0000E+00 0.0000E+00 0.5000E-01
0INITIAL ESTIMATE OF SIGMA:
  0.5000E-01
  0.0000E+00 0.5000E-01
0ESTIMATION STEP OMITTED: NO
  CONDITIONAL ESTIMATES USED: YES
  CENTERED ETA: NO
  EPS-ETA INTERACTION: NO
  LAPLACIAN OBJ. FUNC.: NO
  NO. OF FUNCT. EVALS. ALLOWED: 9999
```

FIGURE 20-7A • (*Continued*)

```
 NO. OF SIG. FIGURES REQUIRED: 3
 INTERMEDIATE PRINTOUT: NO
 ESTIMATE OUTPUT TO MSF: NO
 ABORT WITH PRED EXIT CODE 1: NO
 IND. OBJ. FUNC. VALUES SORTED: NO
 THE FOLLOWING LABELS ARE EQUIVALENT
 PRED=NPRED
 RES=NRES
 WRES=NWRES
 1DOUBLE PRECISION PREDPP VERSION 7.2.0


 ONE COMPARTMENT MODEL WITH FIRST-ORDER ABSORPTION (ADVAN2)
0MAXIMUM NO. OF BASIC PK PARAMETERS: 3
0BASIC PK PARAMETERS (AFTER TRANSLATION):
  ELIMINATION RATE (K) IS BASIC PK PARAMETER NO.: 1
  ABSORPTION RATE (KA) IS BASIC PK PARAMETER NO.: 3


  TRANSLATOR WILL CONVERT PARAMETERS
  CLEARANCE (CL) AND VOLUME (V) TO K (TRANS2)
0COMPARTMENT ATTRIBUTES
  COMPT. NO. FUNCTION  INITIAL   ON/OFF    DOSE D    EFAULT    DEFAULT
                       STATUS    ALLOWED   ALLOWED   FOR DOSE  FOR OBS.
     1        DEPOT    OFF       YES       YES       YES       NO
     2        CENTRAL  ON        NO        YES       NO        YES
     3        OUTPUT   OFF       YES       NO        NO        NO

1
  ADDITIONAL PK PARAMETERS - ASSIGNMENT OF ROWS IN GG
  COMPT. NO.      INDICES
             SCALE   BIOAVAIL.  ZERO-ORDER  ZERO-ORDER   ABSORB
                     FRACTION   RATE        DURATION     LAG
     1        *       *          *           *            4
     2        5       *          *           *            *
     3        *       -          -           -            -
             - PARAMETER IS NOT ALLOWED FOR THIS MODEL
             * PARAMETER IS NOT SUPPLIED BY PK SUBROUTINE;
               WILL DEFAULT TO ONE IF APPLICABLE
0DATA ITEM INDICES USED BY PRED ARE:
 EVENT ID DATA ITEM IS DATA ITEM NO.: 6
 TIME DATA ITEM IS DATA ITEM NO.: 2
 DOSE AMOUNT DATA ITEM IS DATA ITEM NO.: 4
 DOSE RATE DATA ITEM IS DATA ITEM NO.: 3

0PK SUBROUTINE CALLED WITH EVERY EVENT RECORD.
 PK SUBROUTINE NOT CALLED AT NONEVENT (ADDITIONAL OR LAGGED) DOSE TIMES.
0ERROR SUBROUTINE CALLED WITH EVERY EVENT RECORD.
1
 #TBLN: 1
 #METH: First Order Conditional Estimation
```

FIGURE 20-7A • (*Continued*)

```
 #TERM:
0MINIMIZATION SUCCESSFUL
 NO. OF FUNCTION EVALUATIONS USED: 359
 NO. OF SIG. DIGITS IN FINAL EST.: 3.4
0PARAMETER ESTIMATE IS NEAR ITS BOUNDARY
 THIS MUST BE ADDRESSED BEFORE THE COVARIANCE STEP CAN BE IMPLEMENTED

 ETABAR IS THE ARITHMETIC MEAN OF THE ETA-ESTIMATES,
 AND THE P-VALUE IS GIVEN FOR THE NULL HYPOTHESIS THAT THE TRUE MEAN IS 0.

 ETABAR: -2.4682E-06 1.3091E-06 -9.0175E-03 1.6093E-03
 SE: 9.5606E-06 5.0353E-06 3.3000E-02 1.8596E-02

 P VAL.: 7.9628E-01 7.9487E-01 7.8465E-01 9.3104E-01

 ETAshrink(%): 9.8133E+01 9.9017E+01 -2.1777E-01 7.8698E+00
 EPSshrink(%): 5.9519E+00 4.7599E+00

 #TERE:
 Elapsed estimation time in seconds: 1.68
1

 ********************************************************************************
 *****************
  *****************
 *****************
  *****************                    FIRST ORDER CONDITIONAL ESTIMATION
 *****************
 #OBJT:*************                   MINIMUM VALUE OF OBJECTIVE FUNCTION
 *****************
  ******************
 *****************
  ********************************************************************************
 *****************

#OBJV:****************************    1497.827    ************************
 **********************
1
 ********************************************************************************
 *****************
  *****************
 *****************
  *****************                    FIRST ORDER CONDITIONAL ESTIMATION
 *****************
  *****************                    FINAL PARAMETER ESTIMATE
 *****************
  *******************
 *****************
  ********************************************************************************
 *****************
```

FIGURE 20-7A • (Continued)

```
 THETA - VECTOR OF FIXED EFFECTS PARAMETERS *********

        TH 1          TH 2          TH 3          TH 4
        3.36E-01      5.56E+00      1.28E+00      4.30E+00
 OMEGA - COV MATRIX FOR RANDOM EFFECTS - ETAS ********

        ETA1          ETA2          ETA3          ETA4

 ETA1
 +      5.00E-06

 ETA2
 +      0.00E+00      5.00E-06

 ETA3
 +      0.00E+00      0.00E+00      2.07E-02

 ETA4
 +      0.00E+00      0.00E+00      0.00E+00      7.76E-03

 SIGMA - COV MATRIX FOR RANDOM EFFECTS - EPSILONS ****

        EPS1          EPS2

 EPS1
 + 1.13E-02

 EPS2
 +      0.00E+00      1.80E+00

1

 OMEGA - CORR MATRIX FOR RANDOM EFFECTS - ETAS *******

        ETA1          ETA2          ETA3          ETA4

 ETA1
 +      2.24E-03

 ETA2
 +      0.00E+00      2.24E-03

 ETA3
 +      0.00E+00      0.00E+00      1.44E-01

 ETA4
 +      0.00E+00      0.00E+00      0.00E+00      8.81E-02
 SIGMA - CORR MATRIX FOR RANDOM EFFECTS - EPSILONS ***

        EPS1          EPS2

 EPS1
 +      1.06E-01
 EPS2
 +      0.00E+00      1.34E+00
```

FIGURE 20-7A • *(Continued)*

```
$PROBLEM Run1; Book Chapter 2CPT Oral plasma
$INPUT ID, TIME, RATE, DOSE=AMT, DV, EVID, MDV
$DATA NM1.CSV
$SUBROUTINES ADVAN4 TRANS4
$PK

   ALAG1 = THETA(1)*EXP(ETA(1))
   KA    = THETA(2)*EXP(ETA(2))
   CL    = THETA(3)*EXP(ETA(3))
   V2    = THETA(4)*EXP(ETA(4))
   Q     = THETA(5)*EXP(ETA(5))
   V3    = THETA(6)*EXP(ETA(6))

   SC = V2

      K12 = Q/V2
      K21 = Q/V3
      K10 = CL/V2

      C1 = K12 + K21 + K10
      C2 = K21*K10

      Lambda = 0.5*(C1 - SQRT(C1*C1 - 4*C2))

      HALF=LOG(2)/Lambda

$THETA
      (0    0.3   ) ; ALAG
      (0    10    ) ; KA
      (0    1     ) ; CL
      (0    4     ) ; VC
      (0    0.2   ) ; CLD
      (0    5     ) ; VP

$OMEGA 0.05    ; ALAG
       0.05    ; KA
       0.05    ; CL
       0.05    ; VC
       0.05    ; CLD
       0.05    ; VP
$ERROR
      IPRED = F
      IF(F.GT.0)THEN
        W = F
      ELSE
        W = 1
      END IF
      IRES = DV - IPRED
      IWRES = IRES/W
```

FIGURE 20-7 • (B) Sample output from NONMEM showing oral data fitted to a two-compartment model with first-order absorption and first-order elimination (ADVAN4, TRANS4).

```
        Y = F + F*EPS(1) + EPS(2)

$SIGMA 0.05 0.05

$ESTIMATION METHOD=1 NOABORT SIGDIGITS=3 MAXEVAL=9999 PRINT=0 POSTHOC

NM-TRAN MESSAGES

 WARNINGS AND ERRORS (IF ANY) FOR PROBLEM 1
 (WARNING 2) NM-TRAN INFERS THAT THE DATA ARE POPULATION.
 CREATING MUMODEL ROUTINE...


 PROBLEM NO.:         1
Run1; Book Chapter 2CPT Oral plasma
0DATA CHECKOUT RUN:             NO
 DATA SET LOCATED ON UNIT NO.:   2
 THIS UNIT TO BE REWOUND:       NO
 NO. OF DATA RECS IN DATA SET:   378
 NO. OF DATA ITEMS IN DATA SET:  7
 ID DATA ITEM IS DATA ITEM NO.:  1
 DEP VARIABLE IS DATA ITEM NO.:  5
 MDV DATA ITEM IS DATA ITEM NO.: 7
0INDICES PASSED TO SUBROUTINE PRED:
   6   2   4   3   0   0   0   0   0   0   0
0LABELS FOR DATA ITEMS:
 ID TIME RATE DOSE DV EVID MDV
0FORMAT FOR DATA:
 (7E7.0)


 TOT. NO. OF OBS RECS:      340
 TOT. NO. OF INDIVIDUALS:  18
0LENGTH OF THETA:    6
0DEFAULT THETA BOUNDARY TEST OMITTED:    NO
0OMEGA HAS SIMPLE DIAGONAL FORM WITH DIMENSION:       6
0DEFAULT OMEGA BOUNDARY TEST OMITTED:    NO
0SIGMA HAS SIMPLE DIAGONAL FORM WITH DIMENSION:       2
0DEFAULT SIGMA BOUNDARY TEST OMITTED: NO
0INITIAL ESTIMATE OF THETA:
 LOWER BOUND    INITIAL EST    UPPER BOUND
  0.0000E+00    0.3000E+00    0.1000E+07
  0.0000E+00    0.1000E+02    0.1000E+07
  0.0000E+00    0.1000E+01    0.1000E+07
  0.0000E+00    0.4000E+01    0.1000E+07
  0.0000E+00    0.2000E+00    0.1000E+07
  0.0000E+00    0.5000E+01    0.1000E+07
0INITIAL ESTIMATE OF OMEGA:
 0.5000E-01
```

**FIGURE 20-7B** • (*Continued*)

```
 0.0000E+00    0.5000E-01
 0.0000E+00    0.0000E+00    0.5000E-01
 0.0000E+00    0.0000E+00    0.0000E+00    0.5000E-01
 0.0000E+00    0.0000E+00    0.0000E+00    0.0000E+00    0.5000E-01
 0.0000E+00    0.0000E+00    0.0000E+00    0.0000E+00    0.0000E+00    0.5000E-01
0INITIAL ESTIMATE OF SIGMA:
 0.5000E-01
 0.0000E+00    0.5000E-01
0ESTIMATION STEP OMITTED:            NO
 CONDITIONAL ESTIMATES USED:        YES
 CENTERED ETA:                      NO
 EPS-ETA INTERACTION:               NO
 LAPLACIAN OBJ. FUNC.:              NO
 NO. OF FUNCT. EVALS. ALLOWED:      9999
 NO. OF SIG. FIGURES REQUIRED:      3
 INTERMEDIATE PRINTOUT:             NO
 ESTIMATE OUTPUT TO MSF:            NO
 ABORT WITH PRED EXIT CODE 1:       NO
 IND. OBJ. FUNC. VALUES SORTED:     NO


 THE FOLLOWING LABELS ARE EQUIVALENT
 PRED=NPRED
 RES=NRES
 WRES=NWRES
1DOUBLE PRECISION PREDPP VERSION 7.2.0


 TWO COMPARTMENT MODEL WITH FIRST-ORDER ABSORPTION (ADVAN4)
0MAXIMUM NO. OF BASIC PK PARAMETERS:     5
0BASIC PK PARAMETERS (AFTER TRANSLATION):
 BASIC PK PARAMETER NO. 1: ELIMINATION RATE (K)
 BASIC PK PARAMETER NO. 2: CENTRAL-TO-PERIPH. RATE (K23)
 BASIC PK PARAMETER NO. 3: PERIPH.-TO-CENTRAL RATE (K32)
 BASIC PK PARAMETER NO. 5: ABSORPTION RATE (KA)
 TRANSLATOR WILL CONVERT PARAMETERS
 CL, V2, Q, V3 TO K, K23, K32 (TRANS4)
0COMPARTMENT ATTRIBUTES
 COMPT. NO.    FUNCTION    INITIAL    ON/OFF    DOSE      DEFAULT    DEFAULT
                           STATUS     ALLOWED   ALLOWED   FOR DOSE   FOR OBS.
    1          DEPOT       OFF        YES       YES       YES        NO
    2          CENTRAL     ON         NO        YES       NO         YES
    3          PERIPH.     ON         NO        YES       NO         NO
    4          OUTPUT      OFF        YES       NO        NO         NO
1
 ADDITIONAL PK PARAMETERS - ASSIGNMENT OF ROWS IN GG
 COMPT. NO.                               INDICES
               SCALE       BIOAVAIL.    ZERO-ORDER   ZERO-ORDER   ABSORB
                           FRACTION     RATE         DURATION     LAG
    1          *           *            *            *            6
    2          7           *            *            *            *
    3          *           *            *            *            *
    4          *           -            -            -            -
```

FIGURE 20-7B · (*Continued*)

```
                 - PARAMETER IS NOT ALLOWED FOR THIS MODEL
                 * PARAMETER IS NOT SUPPLIED BY PK SUBROUTINE;
                   WILL DEFAULT TO ONE IF APPLICABLE
0DATA ITEM INDICES USED BY PRED ARE:
 EVENT ID DATA ITEM IS DATA ITEM NO.:           6
 TIME DATA ITEM IS DATA ITEM NO.:               2
 DOSE AMOUNT DATA ITEM IS DATA ITEM NO.:        4
 DOSE RATE DATA ITEM IS DATA ITEM NO.:          3


0PK SUBROUTINE CALLED WITH EVERY EVENT RECORD.
 PK SUBROUTINE NOT CALLED AT NONEVENT (ADDITIONAL OR LAGGED) DOSE TIMES.
0ERROR SUBROUTINE CALLED WITH EVERY EVENT RECORD.
1



 #TBLN: 1
 #METH: First Order Conditional Estimation


 #TERM:
0MINIMIZATION SUCCESSFUL
 NO. OF FUNCTION EVALUATIONS USED:        462
 NO. OF SIG. DIGITS IN FINAL EST.:        3.2
0PARAMETER ESTIMATE IS NEAR ITS BOUNDARY
 THIS MUST BE ADDRESSED BEFORE THE COVARIANCE STEP CAN BE IMPLEMENTED

 ETABAR IS THE ARITHMETIC MEAN OF THE ETA-ESTIMATES,
 AND THE P-VALUE IS GIVEN FOR THE NULL HYPOTHESIS THAT THE TRUE MEAN IS 0.

 ETABAR: -1.8435E-06 1.5359E-06 -1.9829E-02 2.6382E-03 1.0060E-06 -6.2575E-07
 SE:      8.2275E-06 6.3126E-06  3.7159E-02 1.8238E-02 7.1168E-06  2.5343E-06

 P VAL.: 8.2271E-01 8.0777E-01 5.9361E-01 8.8498E-01 8.8758E-01 8.0497E-01

 ETAshrink(%): 9.8394E+01 9.8768E+01 -4.3824E-01 7.8343E+00 9.8611E+01 9.9505E+01
 EPSshrink(%): 1.6718E+01 4.8067E+00

 #TERE:
 Elapsed estimation time in seconds:     3.38
1
 *****************************************************************************
***************
 ***************
***************
 ***************                     FIRST ORDER CONDITIONAL ESTIMATION
***************
 #OBJT:*************                 MINIMUM VALUE OF OBJECTIVE FUNCTION
***************
 ***************
```

FIGURE 20-7B • (Continued)

```
* * * * * * * * * * * * * *
 * * * * * * * * * * * * * * * * * * * * * * * * * * * * * * * * * * * * * * * * * * * * * * * * * * * * * * * * * * * * * * *
* * * * * * * * * * * * * *
 #OBJV:* * * * * * * * * * * * * * * * * * * * * * * * * * * *   1260.882   * * * * * * * * * * * * * * * * * * * * * * *
* * * * * * * * * * * * * *
1
 * * * * * * * * * * * * * * * * * * * * * * * * * * * * * * * * * * * * * * * * * * * * * * * * * * * * * * * * * * * * * * *
* * * * * * * * * * * * * *
 * * * * * * * * * * * * * *
* * * * * * * * * * * * * *
 * * * * * * * * * * * * * *                        FIRST ORDER CONDITIONAL ESTIMATION
* * * * * * * * * * * * * *
 #OBJT:* * * * * * * * * * * * *            FINAL PARAMETER ESTIMATE
* * * * * * * * * * * * * *
 * * * * * * * * * * * * * *
* * * * * * * * * * * * * *
 * * * * * * * * * * * * * * * * * * * * * * * * * * * * * * * * * * * * * * * * * * * * * * * * * * * * * * * * * * * * * * *
* * * * * * * * * * * * * *

 THETA - VECTOR OF FIXED EFFECTS PARAMETERS * * * * * * * * *


         TH 1        TH 2        TH 3        TH 4        TH 5        TH 6

         3.00E-01    4.25E+00    1.17E+00    4.06E+00    1.60E-01    4.61E+00

 OMEGA - COV MATRIX FOR RANDOM EFFECTS - ETAS * * * * * * * *

         ETA1        ETA2        ETA3        ETA4        ETA5        ETA6

 ETA1
 +       5.00E-06


 ETA2
 +       0.00E+00    5.00E-06


 ETA3
 +       0.00E+00    0.00E+00    2.61E-02
 ETA4
 +       0.00E+00    0.00E+00    0.00E+00    7.46E-03


 ETA5
 +       0.00E+00    0.00E+00    0.00E+00    0.00E+00    5.00E-06


 ETA6
 +       0.00E+00    0.00E+00    0.00E+00    0.00E+00    0.00E+00    5.00E-06
```

FIGURE 20-7B • (Continued)

```
SIGMA - COV MATRIX FOR RANDOM EFFECTS - EPSILONS ****


              EPS1             EPS2


EPS1
+        1.06E-02


EPS2
+        0.00E+00      2.50E-01


 OMEGA - CORR MATRIX FOR RANDOM EFFECTS - ETAS *******

        ETA1          ETA2          ETA3          ETA4          ETA5          ETA6


ETA1
+        2.24E-03


ETA2
+        0.00E+00      2.24E-03


ETA3
+        0.00E+00      0.00E+00      1.62E-01


ETA4
+        0.00E+00      0.00E+00      0.00E+00      8.64E-02


ETA5
+        0.00E+00      0.00E+00      0.00E+00      0.00E+00      2.24E-03


ETA6
+        0.00E+00      0.00E+00      0.00E+00      0.00E+00      0.00E+00      2.24E-03


 SIGMA - CORR MATRIX FOR RANDOM EFFECTS - EPSILONS ***


              EPS1             EPS2


EPS1
+        1.03E-01


EPS2
+        0.00E+00 5.00E-01
```

FIGURE 20-7B • (*Continued*)

## LEARNING QUESTIONS

1. What types of objectives can be met using a population compartmental PK/PD analysis?

2. Data are collected in two different studies for the same drug. Study 1 is a Phase I study where a single dose is administered in healthy volunteers. Plasma samples are collected prior to dosing and at 0.25, 0.5, 0.75, 1, 1.5, 2, 2.5, 3, 4, 6, 8, 10, 12, 16, and 24 hours after drug administration. Study 2 is a Phase II study in patients. Patients receive a dose twice a day for 7 days. Plasma samples are collected on Day 1 prior to

dosing and at 1, 4, and 12 hours after dosing, Day 3 prior to dosing and at 2 hours after dosing, and on Day 7 prior to dosing and at 0.5, 2, 6, and 24 hours after dosing.

   **a.** What type of software could you use to calculate the AUC and $C_{max}$ in each study?

   **b.** What PK analyses would you use?

3. For a drug under development, the pharmacokineticist has *in vitro* data and animal PK data only. What type of clinical PK analysis can be done and what software could be used?

## ANSWERS

1. Population PK/PD analysis can describe the PK and PD of a drug. Using this approach, population PK and PD parameters are obtained, including the intersubject variability for each parameter. Furthermore, the individual fitted PK and PD parameters can be obtained. The population PK/PD approach is be used to better understand the factors that influence a drug's PK/PD, and the effects of various covariates can be quantified. In addition to describing the PK/PD in a specific population, this approach can simulate future studies in different populations or investigate the exposure and response associated with different dosing regimens.

2. **a.** For the Phase I study, a rich sampling scheme was used since many data are available. AUC and $C_{max}$ can be calculated using observed concentrations using Excel or other user-friendly software packages such as Phoenix WinNonlin. For the Phase II study, there are not many samples collected post-dose and so it is not possible to use observed concentration data to calculate AUC and $C_{max}$ (insufficient data). Therefore, one would first have to use a PK software package such as ADAPT 5 or NONMEM to fit a model and estimate the PK parameters (eg, $k_a$, CL). Using these estimating parameters and the final model, predicted concentrations can be used to calculate the AUC and $C_{max}$.

   **b.** For the Phase I study, many options are available. As there is a rich sampling scheme, a noncompartmental approach can suffice. However, if a model could be obtained from these Phase I data, then the model could be used to plan subsequent studies. In that case, an individual or population compartmental PK analysis would be recommended. For the Phase II study, noncompartmental analysis is not recommended as there is enough data to conduct a robust noncompartmental analysis. Fitting the data using individual or population PK analysis is the preferred method of analysis. However, if a model from the Phase I study was developed, then a Bayesian PK analysis can be also used to obtain the PK parameters for each individual.

3. Although initial noncompartment pharmacokinetics can be estimated from animal data, no clinical data have been collected in humans, and therefore standard noncompartment PK or compartmental analyses cannot be done in humans. This could only be done when sufficient data in humans are available. However, a physiologically based PK analysis could be attempted to predict the concentration profile that could be expected in humans. For this type of analysis, a software package such as GastroPlus, PK-Sim, or Simcyp could be used. Physicochemical properties of the drug can be input into the software as well as relevant *in vitro* characteristics. Preclinical data can be used to validate the model before predicting clinical results.

## REFERENCES

Beal SL, Sheiner LB: Estimating population kinetics. *Crit Rev Biomed Eng* **8**(3):195–222, 1982.

Bergstrand M, Hooker AC, Wallin JE, Karlsson MO: Prediction-corrected visual predictive checks for diagnosing nonlinear mixed-effects models. *AAPS J* **13**(2):143–151, 2011.

Bonate PL: *Pharmacokinetic-Pharmacodynamic Modeling and Simulation*, 2nd ed. New York, Springer, 2011.

Charles BG, Duffull SB: Pharmacokinetic software for the health sciences: Choosing the right package for teaching purposes. *Clin Pharmacokinet* **40**(6):395–403, 2001.

D'Argenio DZ, Schumitzky A, Wang X: *ADAPT 5 User's Guide: Pharmacokinetic/Pharmacodynamic Systems Analysis Software*. Los Angeles, Biomedical Simulations Resource, 2009.

Delyon B, Lavielle M, Moulines E: Convergence of a stochastic approximation version of the EM algorithm. *Ann Statis* **27**(1):94–128, 1999.

EMA. Guideline on the pharmacokinetic and clinical evaluation of modified release dosage forms. 20 November 2014. https://www.ema.europa.eu/en/documents/scientific-guideline/guideline-pharmacokinetic-clinical-evaluation-modified-release-dosage-forms_en.pdf (retrieved Sep 13, 2020).

EMA. Guideline on reporting the results of population pharmacokinetic analyses. 21 June 2007. https://www.ema.europa.eu/en/documents/scientific-guideline/guideline-reporting-results-population-pharmacokinetic-analyses_en.pdf (retrieved Nov 2, 2019).

FDA CDER. Albuterol sulfate metered powder; inhalation product specific guidance. (https://www.accessdata.fda.gov/drugsatfda_docs/psg/PSG_205636.pdf (recommended Sept 2018, revised Mar 2020).

FDA. Extended-release oral dosage forms: Development, evaluation, and application of in vitro/in vivo correlations. September 1997. https://www.fda.gov/media/70939/download (retrieved Sep 13, 2020).

FDA. Physiologically based pharmacokinetic analyses – Format and content guidance for industry. August 2018. file:///C:/Users/Murray%20Ducharme/Documents /LAC_PC/LAC_PC_Current/Regulatory%20agency%20documents/PBPK%20guidance_2018.pdf (retrieved Nov 3, 2019).

FDA. Population Pharmacokinetics Guidance for Industry. July 2019. https://www.fda.gov/regulatory-information/search-fda-guidance-documents/population-pharmacokinetics (retrieved Nov 1, 2019).

Fuchs A, Csajka C, Thoma Y, Buclin T, Widmer N: Benchmarking therapeutic drug monitoring software: A review of available computer tools. *Clin Pharmacokinet* **52**(1):9–22, Jan 2013.

Gabrielsson J, Andersson K, Tobin G, Ingvast-Larsson C, Jirstrand M: Maxsim2 - Real-time interactive simulations for computer-assisted teaching of pharmacokinetics and pharmacodynamics. *Comput Methods Programs Biomed* **113**(3):815–829, Mar 2014.

Gibaldi M, Perrier D: *Pharmacokinetics*. 2nd ed. New York, Informa Healthcare, 2007.

Khalil F, Läer S: Physiologically based pharmacokinetic modeling: methodology, applications, and limitations with a focus on its role in pediatric drug development. *J Biomed Biotechnol* 2011; 2011.

Lee HY, Lee YJ: Bear v2.8.9 (built for R v4.0.x). the data analysis tool for average bioequivalence (ABE) and bioavailability (BA). http://pkpd.kmu.edu.tw/bear/ (retrieved Oct 2020).

Lin Z, Jaberi-Douraki M, He C, et al: Performance assessment and translation of physiologically based pharmacokinetic models from acslX to Berkeley Madonna, MATLAB, and R language: Oxytetracycline and gold nanoparticles as case examples. *Toxicol Sci* **158**(1):23–35, Jul 1 2017.

Riegelman S, Collier P: The application of statistical moment theory to the evaluation of in vivo dissolution time and absorption time. *J Pharmacokinet Biopharm* **8**(5):509–534, Oct 1980.

Sager JE, Yu J, Ragueneau-Majlessi I, Isoherranen N: Physiologically based pharmacokinetic (PBPK) modeling and simulation approaches: A systematic review of published models, applications, and model verification. *Drug Metab Dispos* **43**(11):1823–1837, Nov 2015.

Sheiner LB: Learning versus confirming in clinical drug development. *Clin Pharmacol Ther* **61**(3):275–291, Mar 1997.

Yamaoka K, Nakagawa T, Uno T: Statistical moments in pharmacokinetics. *J Pharmacokinet Biopharm* **6**(6):547–558, Dec 1978.

Zuna I, Holt A. ADAM, a hands-on patient simulator for teaching principles of drug disposition and compartmental pharmacokinetics. *Br J Clin Pharmacol* **83**(11), Nov 2017.

## BIBLIOGRAPHY

Bourne DWA: Mathematical modeling of pharmaceutical data. In Swarbrick J, Boylan JC (eds). *Encyclopedia of Pharmaceutical Technology*, Vol 9. New York, Marcel Dekker, 1994.

Cutler DJ. Theory of the mean absorption time, an adjunct to conventional bioavailability studies. *J Pharm Pharmacol* **30**(8):476–478, 1978.

Ette EI, PJ Williams: *Pharmacometrics the Science of Quantitative Pharmacology*, 1st ed. New Jersey, John Wiley & Sons, 2007.

Gabrielsson J, Weiner D: Non-compartmental analysis. *Methods Mol Biol* **929**:377–389, 2012.

Gabrielsson J, Weiner D: *Pharmacokinetics and Pharmacodynamic Data Analysis: Concepts and Applications*, 2nd ed. Stockholm, Swedish Pharmaceutical Press, 1998.

Gex-Fabry M, Balant LP: Consideration on data analysis using computer methods and currently available software for personal computers. In Welling PG, Balant LP (eds). *Handbook of Experimental Pharmacology, Vol 110, Pharmacokinetics of Drugs*. Berlin, Springer-Verlag, 1994.

Karol M, Gillespie WR, Veng-Pederson P: *AAPS Short Course: Convolution, Deconvolution and Linear Systems*. Washington, DC, AAPS, 1991.

Maronda R (ed): Clinical applications of pharmacokinetics and control theory: Planning, monitoring, and adjusting dosage regiments of aminoglycosides, lidocaine, digoxitin, and digoxin. In Jelliffe RW (ed). *Selected Topics in Clinical Pharmacology*. New York, Springer-Verlag, 1986, Chap 3.

Rowland M, Tozer TN: *Clinical Pharmacokinetics Concepts and Applications*, 3rd ed. Philadelphia, Lippincott Williams & Wilkins, 1995.

Schumitzky A: Nonparametric EM algorithms for estimating prior distributions. *Appl Math Comput* **45**:143–157, 1991.

Tanswell P, Koup J: TopFit: a PC-based pharmacokinetic/pharmacodynamic data analysis program. *Int J Clin Pharmacol Ther Toxicol* **31**(10): 514–420, 1993.

# Pharmacodynamics and Clinical Pharmacokinetics

# 21

# Pharmacogenetics, Drug Metabolism, Transporters, and Individualization of Drug Therapy

Brianne Raccor and Michael L. Adams

## CHAPTER OBJECTIVES

- Define pharmacogenetics and pharmacogenomics.

- Define genetic polymorphism and explain the difference between genotype and phenotype.

- Explain with relevant examples how genetic variability influences drug response, pharmacokinetics, and dosing regimen design.

- Describe the relevance of CYP enzymes and their genetic variability to pharmacokinetics and dosing.

- List the major drug transporters and describe how their genetic variability can impact pharmacokinetics.

- Discuss the main issues in applying genomic data to patient care; for example, clinical interpretation of data from various laboratories and accuracy of record keeping of large amounts of genomic data.

Variable response to a drug in the general population is thought to follow a normal or Gaussian distribution about a mean or average dose, $ED_{50}$ (Fig. 21-1). Patients who fall within region A of the curve may be described as hyper-responders while those in region B may be characterized as poor or hypo-responders. While pharmacokinetic and pharmacodynamic differences are thought to be primarily responsible for this Gaussian variation in drug response, the extremes in drug response may be due to unique interindividual genetic variability. Modern genetic methods have identified alterations in drug-metabolizing enzymes, drug transporters, and drug receptors that, at least in part, explain many of these extremes in drug response. This has given birth to the field of *pharmacogenomics*, which the FDA defines as "the study of variations of DNA and RNA characteristics as related to drug response." Pharmacogenomics seeks to characterize inter-individual drug-response variability at the genetic level (Ventola, 2011). A related term, *pharmacogenetics*, is often used interchangeably but is defined by the FDA as "the study of variations in DNA sequence as related to drug response" (Ventola, 2011).

Advances in pharmacogenetics have been enabled by high-throughput technology that allows for the screening of tens of thousands to a million genetic variants rapidly and simultaneously. These technologies usually rely on target enrichment, hybridization, or amplification-based strategies. For example, the DNA chip is a microchip that uses hybridization technology to concurrently detect the presence of tens of thousands of sequence variants in a small sample. The probes (of known sequence) are spotted onto discreet locations on the chip, so that complementary DNA hybridization from the patient's sample to a probe residing in a defined location indicates the presence of a specific sequence (Mancinelli et al, 2000; Dodgan et al, 2013). In contrast to searching for only

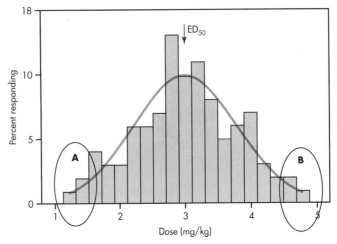

**FIGURE 21-1** • Simulated Gaussian distribution of population response to a hypothetical drug. $ED_{50}$ indicates the mean dose producing a therapeutic outcome, while regions **A** and **B** highlight patients who are hyper- or hypo-responders to the drug effect, respectively.

known common genetic variants, next generation sequencing technology can provide sequencing of entire genes or exomes (Schwarz et al, 2019). This technology enables the identification of novel and rare variants in an individual or population.

Application of pharmacogenetics to pharmacokinetics and pharmacodynamics helps in development of models that may predict an individual's risk to an adverse drug event and therapeutic response (Fernandez-Rozadilla et al, 2013; Meyer et al, 2013). The promise of such modeling efforts is that more individualized dosing regimens may be developed, resulting in more "personalized medicine" with fewer adverse events and better therapeutic outcomes (Phillips et al, 2001). This chapter will focus on variations in pharmacokinetic components due to pharmacogenetic factors. Variations in drug response due to genetic variations in the drug's receptor or downstream processes can also be identified using pharmacogenetic principles and screening; however, that is beyond the scope of this chapter.

## GENETIC POLYMORPHISMS

Historically, population variability in drug metabolism or therapeutic response was described in terms of the observed phenotype; for example, slow metabolizers or sensitive responders. With our understanding of genetics, we are often able to ascribe specific alterations in gene sequence, or genotype, to explain such observed effects. *Genetic polymorphisms* are variations in gene sequences that occur in at least 1% of the general population, resulting in multiple alleles or variants of a gene sequence. Polymorphisms are distinct from *mutations* that occur in less than 1% of the population. The most commonly occurring form of genetic variability is the *single nucleotide polymorphism* (SNP, often called "snip"), resulting from a change in a single nucleotide base pair within the gene sequence (Ahles and Engelhardt, 2014). Synonymous SNPs in the coding region of a gene generally result in no change in the amino acid sequence of the eventual protein product. Non-synonymous SNPs in the coding region will result in a change in the amino acid sequence of the protein. In some cases, this alteration may have little effect on the protein's structure and function; for example, if one acidic amino acid is replaced by another. However, nonsynonymous SNPs have the potential to drastically alter the function of protein (Ahles and Engelhardt, 2014). An example of such an effect occurs if nucleotide position 2935 of the *CYP2D6* gene has a C instead of an A (c.2935A>C). During translation, this results in the insertion of a proline instead of histidine at amino acid position 324 (H324P) generating the *CYP2D6\*7* allele, with no drug metabolizing activity (Ingelman-Sundberg et al, 2014). Genetic variants that result from the insertion or deletion of a nucleotide in the coding region are also classified as SNPs. Since the mRNAs from genes are translated to protein in 3-nucleotide codons, such insertions or deletions can have a significant effect on the eventual protein product. An example of such a polymorphism is the *CYP2D6\*3* allele where a single nucleotide deletion ($A_{2637}$) results in a frame shift in translation that produces an enzyme with no catalytic activity (Ingelman-Sundberg et al, 2014). Each variant of gene is designated using a star (\*) naming system, and each gene could potentially contain multiple variants. A grouping of select variants is called a haplotype and results in unique combinations of polymorphisms with potentially novel phenotypes.

SNPs outside the coding region of the gene can result in altered levels of protein activity as well. Polymorphisms in the promoter sequence of a gene can influence gene transcription rates resulting in greater or lesser amounts of mRNA, and consequently protein expression. Alternatively, SNPs in a splicing control region of the gene can result in the production of a unique protein often missing one or more exons and resulting in a unique (often truncated or inactive) protein. In some cases, multiple copies of a gene on a chromosome can result in increased levels of protein being expressed, and once again the *CYP2D6* gene serves as a relevant example. The *CYP2D6xN* variant (where N = 2–12 copies) results in very high expression of the functional enzyme in patients who are considered ultrarapid metabolizers of certain drugs (Ingelman-Sundberg et al, 2014; see below). Polymorphic induction of gene expression is distinct from that induced by drugs such as phenytoin, barbiturates, etc. However, it is not difficult to see that a mixed form of CYP gene expression due to genetics and drug induction could increase metabolic activity to an even greater extent. Deletion or inversion of entire genes on the chromosome would obviously have the opposite effect on enzyme activity and drug metabolism.

## Genetic Polymorphism in Drug Metabolism

As discussed in Chapter 6, drug metabolism is responsible for the chemical modification of drugs or other xenobiotics that usually results in increased polarity to enhance elimination from the body.

The enzymes that perform drug metabolism are classified as either phase I or phase II enzymes, and their relative contributions to drug metabolism are highlighted in Fig. 21-2. Phase I enzymes perform oxidation, reduction, and hydrolysis reactions while phase II enzymes perform conjugation reactions. Polymorphisms have been reported in both phases of drug-metabolizing enzymes and can affect the pharmacokinetic profile of a drug for a given patient. Understanding a patient's genetic determinants of drug metabolism and the consequences of these polymorphisms could be used to design optimum, personalized dosing regimens in the clinic that would avoid adverse reactions or treatment failures due to subtherapeutic doses. While this may appear perfectly logical, the redundancy of drug metabolism and potential contribution from numerous other factors (such as diet, other drugs, age, weight, etc) make it difficult to translate enzyme status data to a clinical decision. For example, warfarin therapy is complicated by a combination of metabolic (*CYP2C9* polymorphisms contribute 2%–10%), pharmacodynamic (*VKORC1* polymorphisms contribute 10%–25%), and environmental factors (20%–25%) (PharmGKB, 2019). Several algorithms that take into account genetic information have been developed for warfarin dosing, and some are available online (Warfarin Dosing, 2014; PharmGKB, 2019). While these appear to be useful tools to account for genetic differences, the reported effectiveness of achieving an optimal anticoagulant dose of warfarin using algorithms is variable, especially among blacks (Caraco et al, 2008; Wang et al, 2012; Kimmel et al, 2013; Pirmohamed et al, 2013). These confounding results demonstrate the need for more investigation into the factors (including pharmacokinetic and pharmacodynamic factors) that contribute to variable responses, as well as robust clinical investigations to validate these observations.

As of 2019, there are 268 FDA approved drugs that contain pharmacogenetic information in their drug label related to polymorphisms in drug-metabolizing enzymes that contribute to variable drug response (PharmGKB, 2019). Drugs that are thought to be affected by the polymorphisms, the clinical consequences associated with their overdosing, and specific label information are included in Table 21-1 (Evans and Relling, 1999; PharmGKB, 2019).

**TABLE 21-1** • Clinically Important Genetic Polymorphisms of Drug Metabolism and Transporters That Influence Drug Response

| | Drug | Drug Effect/Side Effect | FDA Label Information* (10-Pharmacogenetics Knowledge Base, 2019) |
|---|---|---|---|
| CYP2C9 | Warfarin | Hemorrhage | Actionable |
| | Celecoxib | Enhanced Toxicity | Actionable |
| | Sulfonylureas | Hypoglycemia | - |
| | Phenytoin | Phenytoin toxicity | - |
| | Dronabinol | CNS effects | Actionable |
| | Siponimod | Enhanced Toxicity | Testing Required |
| CYP2D6 | Antiarrhythmics | Proarrhythmic and other toxic effects in poor metabolizers | - |
| | Antidepressants | Inefficacy in ultrarapid metabolizers | Actionable/Information[†] |
| | Antipsychotics | Tardive dyskinesia | Actionable/Information[†] |
| | Eliglustat | Inefficacy in ultrarapid metabolizers | Testing required |
| | Opioids | Inefficacy of codeine as analgesic, narcotic side effects, dependence | Actionable |
| | Pimozide | Toxicity with high dose in poor metabolizers | Testing required |
| | Tamoxifen | Lower efficacy | Actionable |
| | Tetrabenazine | Toxicity with high dose in poor metabolizers or inefficacy in ultrarapid metabolizers | Testing recommended |
| | Warfarin | Higher risk of hemorrhage | - |
| | β-Adrenoceptor antagonists | Increased blockade | Actionable/Information[†] |
| CYP2C19 | Omeprazole/ Esomeprazole | Higher exposure | Actionable |
| | Citalopram | QT prolongation | Actionable |
| | Diazepam | Prolonged sedation | Actionable |
| | Clopidogrel | Inefficacy in poor metabolizers | Actionable |
| Dihydropyrimidine dehydrogenase | Fluorouracil | Myelotoxicity, neurotoxicity | Actionable |
| | Capecitabine | Myelotoxicity, neurotoxicity | Actionable |
| Plasma pseudo-cholinesterase | Succinylcholine | Prolonged apnea | - |
| N-acetyltransferase | Sulfamethoxazole | Hypersensitivity | Actionable |
| | Sulfasalazine | Drug Accumulation | Actionable |
| | Procainamide | Drug-induced lupus erythematosus | - |

*(Continiued)*

**TABLE 21-1 •** Clinically Important Genetic Polymorphisms of Drug Metabolism and Transporters That Influence Drug Response (*Continued*)

| | Drug | Drug Effect/Side Effect | FDA Label Information* (10-Pharmacogenetics Knowledge Base, 2019) |
|---|---|---|---|
| | Hydralazine | Drug-induced lupus erythematosus | Information |
| | Isoniazid | Drug-induced lupus erythematosus | Information |
| Thiopurine methyltransferase | Mercaptopurine | Myelotoxicity | Testing recommended |
| | Thioguanine | Myelotoxicity | Testing recommended |
| | Azathioprine | Myelotoxicity | Testing recommended |
| UDP-**G**lucuronosyl-transferase | Irinotecan | Diarrhea, Myelotoxicity | Actionable |
| Multidrug-resistance gene (*MDR1*) | Digoxin | Increased concentrations of digoxin in plasma | - |
| Organic anion transporter protein (*SLCO1B1*) | Simvastatin | Myopathy | - |
| | Rosuvastatin | Higher exposure | Actionable |

*Information/Informative: Drug label contains information on gene or protein responsible for drug metabolism that are not clinically significant
Actionable: Drug label contains information about changes in efficacy, dosage, or toxicity of a drug due to gene variants but does not suggest or require genetic or other testing.
Testing recommended: Drug label recommends testing or states testing should be performed for specific gene or protein variants prior to use, sometimes in a specific population.
Testing required: Drug label implies genetic or other testing should be performed prior to use, sometimes in a specific population.
†Depends upon the specific drug agent.
Data from Evans WE, Relling MV. Pharmacogenomics: translating functional genomics into rational therapeutics, Science. 1999 Oct 15;286(5439): 487–491.

Further examples of polymorphism affecting drugs among different race and special subject groups are shown in Table 21-2.

### CYP Enzymes

CYP enzymes (formerly referred to as Cytochrome P-450 isozymes) are the primary phase I oxidative enzymes that are found in many species with functionality in the metabolism of xenobiotics and endogenous biochemical processes. CYPs are divided into families identified with numbers (CYP1, CYP2, CYP3, etc) and subfamilies identified with letters (CYP2A, CYP2B, etc) based on amino acid similarities. The major drug-metabolizing CYP families are CYP1, CYP2, and CYP3 (see Fig. 21-2), and those will be the focus of this section.

### CYP2D6

CYP2D6 is the most highly polymorphic CYP enzyme, with more than 70 allelic variants reported (Ingelman-Sundberg et al, 2014). Many of these allelic variants are clinically important because although CYP2D6 only makes up about 5% of hepatic CYP activity, it is responsible for the metabolism of as much as 25% of commonly prescribed drugs (Fig. 21-2). These drugs include antidepressants, antiarrhythmics, beta-adrenergic antagonists, and opioids, which frequently have narrow therapeutic indices. While we now have more detailed information on the genotypes, the phenotypic differences in CYP2D6 were originally observed with debrisoquine, resulting in the more general descriptions of poor metabolizer (PM), extensive metabolizer (EM),

**TABLE 21-2** • Examples of Polymorphisms Affecting Drug Receptors and Enzymes Showing Frequency of Occurrence

| Enzyme/Receptor | Frequency of Polymorphism | Drug | Drug Effect/Side Effect |
|---|---|---|---|
| CYP2C9 | 14%–28% (heterozygotes) | Warfarin | Hemorrhage |
| | | Tolbutamide | Hypoglycemia |
| | 0.2%–1% (homozygotes) | Phenytoin | Phenytoin toxicity |
| | | Glipizide | Hypoglycemia |
| | | Losartan | Decreased antihypertensive effect |
| CYP2D6 | 5%–10% (poor metabolizers) | Antiarrhythmics | Proarrhythmic and other toxic effects |
| | | | Toxicity in poor metabolizers |
| | 1%–10% (ultrarapid metabolizers) | Antidepressants | Inefficacy in ultrarapid metabolizers |
| | | Antipsychotics | Tardive dyskinesia |
| | | Opioids | Inefficacy of codeine as analgesic, narcotic side effects, dependence |
| | | Warfarin | Higher risk of hemorrhage |
| | | β-Adrenoceptor antagonists | Increased—blockade |
| CYP2C19 | 3%–6% (Whites) | Omeprazole | Higher cure rates when given with clarithromycin |
| | 8%–23% (Asians) | Diazepam | Prolonged sedation |
| Dihydropyrimidine dehydrogenase | 0.1% | Fluorouracil | Myelotoxicity, Neurotoxicity |
| Plasma pseudo-cholinesterase | 1.5% | Succinylcholine | Prolonged apnea |
| N-acetyltransferase | 40%–70% (Whites) | Sulphonamides | Hypersensitivity |
| | 10%–20% (Asians) | Amonafide | Myelotoxicity (rapid acetylators) |
| | | Procainamide, hydralazine, isoniazid | Drug-induced lupus erythematosus |
| Thiopurine methyltransferase | 0.3% | Mercaptopurine, thioguanine, azothioprine | Myelotoxicity |
| UDP-glucuronosyltransferase | 10%–15% | Irinotecan | Diarrhea, myelosuppression |
| ACE | | Enalapril, lisinapril, captopril | Renoprotective effect, cardiac indexes, blood pressure |
| Potassium channels | | Quinidine | Drug-induced QT syndrome |

(Continiued)

## TABLE 21-2 • Examples of Polymorphisms Affecting Drug Receptors and Enzymes Showing Frequency of Occurrence (*Continued*)

| Enzyme/Receptor | Frequency of Polymorphism | Drug | Drug Effect/Side Effect |
|---|---|---|---|
| HERG | | Cisapride | Drug-induced torsade de pointes |
| KvLQT1 | | Terfenadine disopyramide | Drug-induced long-QT syndrome |
| VKORC | | Warfarin | Over-anticoagulation |
| Epidermal growth factor receptor (EGFR) | | Gefitinib | Certain polymorphs susceptible |
| HKCNE2 | | Meflaquine clarithromycin | Drug-induced arrhythmia |

*Data from Meyer (2000), Evans and Relling (1999), and Limdi and Veenstra (2010).*

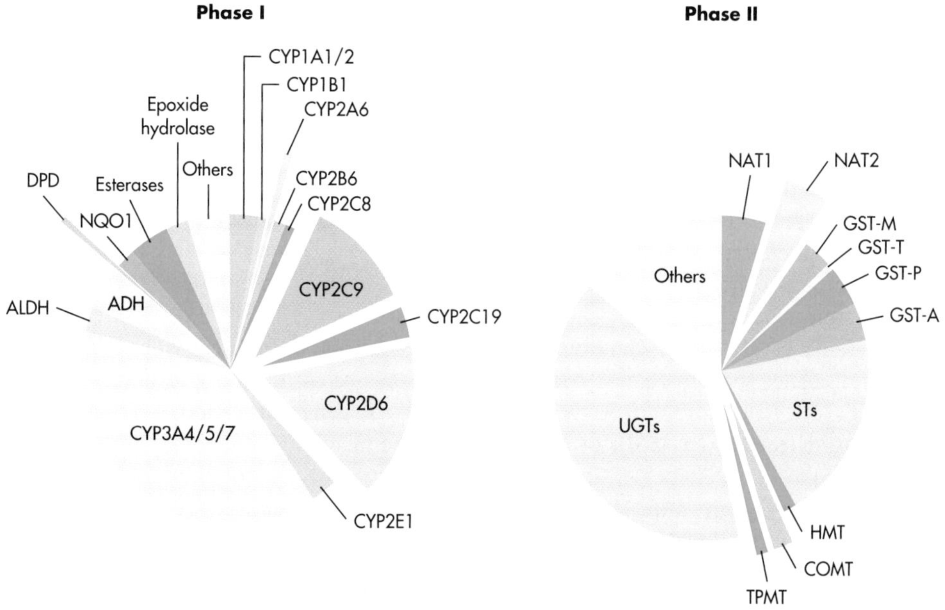

FIGURE 21-2 • Drug-metabolizing enzymes that exhibit clinically relevant genetic polymorphisms. Essentially all of the major human enzymes responsible for modification of functional groups (classified as phase I reactions [left]) or conjugation with endogenous substituents (classified as phase II reactions [right]) exhibit common polymorphisms at the genomic level; those enzyme polymorphisms that have already been associated with changes in drug effects are separated from the corresponding pie charts. The percentage of phase I and phase II metabolism of drugs that each enzyme contributes is estimated by the relative size of each section of the corresponding chart. ADH, alcohol dehydrogenase; ALDH, aldehyde dehydrogenase; CYP, cytochrome P-450; DPD, dihydropyrimidine dehydrogenase; NQO1, NADPH, quinone oxidoreductase or DT diaphorase; COMT, catechol O-methyltransferase; GST, glutathione S-transferase; HMT, histamine methyltransferase; NAT, N-acetyltransferase; STs, sulfotransferases; TPMT, thiopurine methyltransferase; UGTs, uridine 5′-triphosphate glucuronosyltransferases. (Adapted with permission from Evans WE, Relling MV. Pharmacogenomics: translating functional genomics into rational therapeutics. Science. 1999 Oct 15; 286(5439):487–491.)

and ultrarapid metabolizer (UM) (Mahgoub et al, 1977; Idle et al, 1978).

It is estimated that approximately 10% of the Caucasian population, 1% of the Asian population, and between 0% and 19% of the African population have a PM phenotype of CYP2D6 (McGraw and Waller, 2012), resulting in increased plasma concentration of the parent drug due to decreased metabolic clearance. In the case of debrisoquine, the increased plasma concentration results in an exaggerated hypotensive response. When a patient with a PM phenotype is administered a tricyclic antidepressant, the increased plasma concentration increases the potential for CNS depression. Tricyclic antidepressants such as imipramine form active metabolites (eg, desmethylimipramine), which contribute to both the therapeutic and the adverse effects of these compounds. If metabolism is required for a drug to have activity, the patient with a PM phenotype is more likely to have a treatment failure than an adverse event. This has been reported with the breast cancer agent tamoxifen (Rolla et al, 2012). Tamoxifen has an active metabolite (endoxifen) produced by CYP2D6 that is thought to be responsible for much of its antiestrogenic activities. The patient with the PM phenotype would not metabolize tamoxifen to the active metabolite and therefore does not benefit from clinically relevant endoxifen concentrations (Rolla et al, 2012). Genotypically, PM have two null alleles, which do not code for functional CYP2D6 due to a frame shift (CYP2D6*3 and *6), a splicing defect (CYP2D6*4), or a gene deletion (CYP2D6*5).

The UM have very high rates of CYP2D6 enzymatic activity resulting in low plasma concentrations of drugs with consequent lower efficacy. Active drugs like the tricyclic antidepressant amitriptyline may require doses several-fold higher than standard doses to achieve therapeutic activity when the patient is a UM. On the other hand, drugs that require metabolism to an active metabolite are extremely active, with potentially serious consequences. Codeine is converted to morphine by a CYP2D6 O-demethylation reaction to provide analgesic effects, and morphine-associated toxicity has been reported after codeine administration in patients who are UM (Gasche et al, 2004). The UM phenotype is the result of multiple copies (up to 12

copies) of either the wild-type CYP2D6*1 or the *2 gene on a single chromosome, resulting in greatly enhanced functional CYP2D6 activity (Ingelman-Sundberg et al, 2014). The UM phenotype is found in Caucasian populations (1%–10%) but is more common in others such as Saudi Arabians (20%) and Ethiopians (29%) (Samer et al, 2013).

CYP2D6 EM phenotype includes 60%–85% of the Caucasian population and has normal enzymatic activity (CYP2D6*1). In addition to PM, EM, and UM, an intermediate metabolizer (IM) phenotype has also been identified. The IM phenotype is a result of either one null allele or two deficient alleles and is prevalent in up to 50% of Asians, 30% of Africans, and around 10%–15% of Caucasians (Samer et al, 2013). The deficient alleles include CYP2D6*2, *10, and *17, each of which has enzymatic activity that is less than the wild-type enzyme (CYP2D6*1).

Understanding this complex interplay between all the different alleles of CYP2D6 and the many drugs that it metabolizes provides a great opportunity for accurate genotyping to provide for sound clinical decisions to prevent adverse events and prevent therapeutic failures.

### CYP1A2

CYP1A2 activity varies widely with genetic polymorphisms contributing to observed differences in levels of gene expression. CYP1A2 is responsible for the metabolism of about 5% of marketed drugs, including the fluoroquinolones, fluvoxamine, clozapine, olanzapine, and theophylline. Approximately 15% of the Japanese, 5% of the Chinese, and 5% of the Australian non-smoker populations are classified as CYP1A2 poor metabolizers. CYP1A activity is induced by smoking status, with smokers having an approximate 40% higher theophylline clearance than nonsmokers. A common cause of an altered phenotype is due to the allelic variant, CYP1A2*1F, which results in an increased expression caused by an SNP in the upstream promoter region. Enhanced enzyme levels are thought to cause faster substrate clearance, which has been associated with treatment failures for clozapine in smokers with the *1F allele (Eap et al, 2004). CYP1A2*1C is also an SNP in the upstream promoter region that results in decreased enzyme expression and has a prevalence up to 25% in Asian populations (McGraw and Waller, 2012).

## CYP2A6

Smoking rates have been on the decline in many parts of the world, but the World Health Organization estimates that there are still 1.1 billion smokers worldwide (https://www.who.int/news-room/fact-sheets/detail/tobacco). Nicotine is the main cause of the addictive nature of cigarettes. The enzyme responsible for the inactivation of nicotine is CYP2A6 (Nakajima et al, 1996b). CYP2A6 is a highly polymorphic enzyme whose activity varies between the sexes. It produces cotinine, which it further metabolizes to 3-hydroxycotinine. The ratio of 3-hydroxycotinine to cotinine is known as the nicotine metabolite ratio and is a phenotypic marker of CYP2A6 activity. The nicotine metabolite ratio has been used as a predictor of smoking related activities. For instance, reduced CYP2A6 function has been associated with lower cigarette consumption and a higher likelihood of smoking cessation (Schoedel et al, 2004; Lerman et al, 2006). The most common alleles associated with a reduced function phenotype of CYP2A6 are *2,*4, *9, and *12. The *2 and *4 are associated with a complete loss of function and the *9 and *12 with decreased (PharmGKB, 2019). An increase in CYP2A6 enzyme activity is due to either gene duplication or the *1B allele that leads to an increase in protein expression (Wang et al, 2006).

## CYP2C9

CYP2C9 has at least 60 different allelic variants, with the two most common variants being CYP2C9*2 and *3. Both of these variants result in reduced CYP2C9 activity and are carried by about 35% of the Caucasian population. CYP2C9 is a major contributor to the metabolism of the active enantiomer (S-) of the narrow therapeutic index blood thinner warfarin (PharmGKB, 2019). When a patient has one of these two polymorphisms, the dose of warfarin needed for clinically relevant anticoagulation is generally much less since drug clearance is reduced. If the dose of warfarin is not appropriately lowered, then there is an increased risk of bleeding. There are several other drugs affected by the polymorphisms of CYP2C9, including many nonsteroidal anti-inflammatory drugs, sulfonylureas, angiotensin II receptor antagonists, and phenytoin. For each of these, the CYP2C9*2 and *3 polymorphisms result in higher plasma concentrations but, because of their high therapeutic indices (except phenytoin), do not usually result in adverse effects. In the case of phenytoin, the polymorphisms result in drug accumulation and require dose reduction to prevent toxicity (ie, dizziness, nystagmus, ataxia).

## CYP2C19

CYP2C19 is a highly polymorphic drug-metabolizing enzyme with at least 35 variants reported (Ingelman-Sundberg et al, 2014). Polymorphisms in CYP2C19 result in variable drug response to clopidogrel and several antidepressants. The PM phenotype is often the result of two null alleles, CYP2C19*2 and *3. Both alleles produce truncated, nonfunctional CYP2C19 through the introduction of a stop codon. The stop codon in the CYP2C19*2 allele is the result of a splicing defect that introduces a frame shift, while in the CYP2C19*3 allele, an SNP introduces the early stop codon (de Morais et al, 1994). The allelic frequency of CYP2C19*2 has been shown to be 15% in Africans, 29%–35% in Asians, 12%–15% in Caucasians, and 61% in Oceanians. CYP2C19*3 is mainly found in Asians (5%–9%) with very low frequency in Caucasians (0.5%) (Samer et al, 2013).

The CYP2C19 PM phenotype results in a lack of efficacy for the antiplatelet prodrug clopidogrel. For activation, clopidogrel requires a two-step metabolism by several different CYPs with CYP2C19 being a significant contributor. Studies have demonstrated, and the FDA has added to the label, that deficiencies in CYP2C19 activity may result in the increased risk of adverse cardiovascular outcomes because the PM does not activate clopidogrel sufficiently (Scott et al, 2011). With omeprazole, the opposite occurs, since metabolism inactivates the drug. The PM phenotype results in higher plasma concentrations, larger AUC values, and greater efficacy in lowering gastric pH than extensive metabolizers with CYP2C19*1 alleles (Ogawaa and Echizen, 2010). The higher plasma concentration of omeprazole is particularly useful in the multiple-drug treatment of Helicobacter pylori. In the PM patients treated with omeprazole, the H. pylori eradication rate is higher when they have one or more of the null alleles (Shi and Klotz, 2008).

The *CYP2C19*17* allele results in a gain of function and therefore has more metabolic capacity than the wild-type enzyme, *CYP2C19*1*, because of an SNP in the upstream noncoding region that induces transcription (Sim et al, 2006). Patients who have this UM phenotype are either heterozygous or homozygous for *CYP2C19*17*. Carriers of this allele are associated with higher risk for bleeding due to the increased metabolism of clopidogrel to the active metabolite (Sibbing et al, 2010; Zabalza et al, 2012). These examples demonstrate that both loss and gain of function alleles can have significant effects on patient outcomes depending upon the blood levels and activity of the parent drug and the metabolite.

### CYP3A

CYP3A4 is the most abundant CYP in the liver and metabolizes over 50% of the clinically used drugs (Fig. 21-2). In addition, the liver expression of CYP3A4 is variable between individuals. To date, over 30 allelic variants of CYP3A4 have been identified (Ingelman-Sundberg et al, 2014). Despite the large number of variants, there are limited data demonstrating any clinical significance for CYP3A4 substrates. Some of the variability may be caused by allelic variants that influence the upstream noncoding region of the gene, specifically in *CYP3A4*1B* allele, which may influence gene expression, although the exact transcription factor binding site has not been identified (Sata et al, 2000). The *CYP3A4*2* allele has a non-synonymous SNP that is found in about 2.7% of the Caucasian population and has some decreased clearance for the calcium channel blocker nifedipine but not for testosterone 6β-hydroxylation (Sata et al, 2000). The effects of the polymorphisms in *CYP3A4* are still under investigation but currently there are no null phenotypes.

CYP3A5 is structurally similar to CYP3A4, metabolizes a significant number of CYP3A4 substrates, but has common genetic polymorphisms that are clinically relevant. To date, 25 allelic variants of CYP3A5 have been identified; the most common being *CYP3A5*3* (Lamba et al, 2012). *CYP3A5*3* is a SNP that results in an alternative RNA splice site producing a transcript that contains a premature stop codon. This results in a nonfunctional enzyme product. *CYP3A5*3* expression is common among many ethnic groups, and allelic frequencies range from 82% to 95% in white populations to 33% in African American populations (Lamba et al, 2012). Individuals that express *CYP3A5*3* are termed non-expressors, and individuals who express the wild-type, *CYP3A5*1*, are termed expressors. CYP3A5 expression directly impacts the metabolism of tacrolimus, which is a narrow therapeutic index drug used as an immunosuppressant to prevent organ rejection after transplantation. CYP3A5 expression can increase the clearance of tacrolimus and directly impact dosing requirements (Passey et al, 2011).

### Other Phase I Enzymes

While the CYPs are the most abundant and extensively studied phase I drug-metabolizing enzymes, others have polymorphisms that have an effect on the clearance (or activation) of drugs and therefore affect the clinical outcomes of patients secondary to, at least partially, changes in pharmacokinetics.

### Plasma Pseudocholinesterase or Serum Butyrylcholinesterase

Plasma pseudocholinesterase is responsible for the inactivation through ester hydrolysis of the neuromuscular blockers succinylcholine and mivacurium. While mivacurium is no longer marketed in the U.S. market, succinylcholine is used to provide skeletal muscle relaxation or paralysis for surgery or mechanical ventilation. There are at least 65 allelic variants of pseudocholinesterase that have been identified in approximately 1.5% of the population that result in various levels of pseudocholinesterase deficiencies (Soliday et al, 2010). These allelic variants include non-synonymous point mutations or frame shift mutations that result in a PM phenotype for succinylcholine. Patients with slowed metabolism of succinylcholine have elevated blood levels, prolonged duration of action, and prolonged apnea compared to patients with fully functional pseudocholinesterase.

### Dihydropyrimidine Dehydrogenase

Dihydropyrimidine dehydrogenase (DPD) is the first reduction and rate-limited step in breakdown of the pyrimidine nucleic acids and their analogs.

Polymorphisms in DPD coding gene (*DPYD*) may result in a loss of enzymatic activity leading to the accumulation of the chemotherapeutic agent 5-fluorouracil (5-FU), which leads to significant toxicity including leukopenia, thrombocytopenia, and stomatitis. It is estimated that approximately 3%–5% of population has low or deficient DPD activity (Lu et al, 1993; Etienne et al, 1994). There are four alleles, each with low frequency, that appear to account for the majority of the deficient DPD activity observed. *DPYD*2A* and *13* both result in loss of function, while the other two result in decreased enzymatic activity (Amstutz et al, 2018). Many other allelic variants have been identified to date but have only been found in very small numbers or have unknown clinical consequences. Two additional well-characterized allelic variants, *DPYD*5* and *DPY-D*9A*, result in normal enzymatic function (Amstutz et al, 2018).

## PHASE II ENZYMES

As discussed in the chapter on drug metabolism (Chapter 6), phase II drug-metabolizing enzymes are commonly referred to as transferases and perform conjugation reactions that add a biochemical compound to a xenobiotic to facilitate its elimination. Just like the phase I reactions, there are genetic variations in the several phase II enzymes that influence the pharmacokinetics of drugs.

### Thiopurine S-Methyltransferase

Thiopurine drugs including 6-mercaptopurine (MP) and azathioprine are used for their anticancer and immunosuppressive properties but can have significant adverse effects, including myelosuppression. MP and the MP pro-drug azathioprine (it forms MP in the body) require enzymatic activation to active metabolites before they exert their mechanism of action. The phase II metabolizing enzyme thiopurine S-methyltransferase (TPMT) is involved in the degradation of thiopurine drugs (Colombel et al, 2000; Ansari et al, 2002; PharmGKB, 2019). At least 28 allelic variants in the coding and splicing region of TPMT have been identified, with most of the null phenotypes being associated with *TPMT*2*, *TPMT*3A*, and *TPMT*3B* alleles

resulting in non-synonymous mutations that lead to the production of an unstable enzyme and reduced activity overall. Individuals who are homozygous for these null phenotypes are at a substantially higher risk of life-threatening myelosuppression using conventional starting dosages for MP and azathioprine for the treatment of inflammatory and malignant diseases (Relling et al, 2011). A dosage reduction or alternative treatment plan should be considered with these individuals. Individuals who are heterozygous for TPMT deficiency may tolerate conventional doses due to the lower levels of active metabolites in the body. The most common variant in Caucasians that results in loss of TPMT function is *TPMT*3A*, which is present in about 5% of the population and may result in the accumulation of MP and active metabolites leading to an increased risk for adverse effects (Ameyaw et al, 1999; Schaeffeler et al, 2008).

### Uridine Diphosphate-Glucuronosyltransferase

Uridine diphosphate (UDP)-glucuronosyltransferase (UGT) is a superfamily of phase II drug-metabolizing enzymes that produce glucuronidation metabolites through conjugation reactions (see Chapter 6). Like the CYPs, the UGTs are divided into families identified with numbers (UGT1, UGT2, etc) and subfamilies identified with letters (UGT1A, UGT2B, etc) based on amino acid similarities. Drug metabolism is catalyzed almost exclusively by UGT1 and UGT2 (Meech et al, 2012). Multiple alleles for UGT1 gene families have been reported causing changes in enzymatic activity or expression levels that may contribute to individual variations in drug response (UGT Nomenclature Committee, 2005). One of the most frequently studied genetic variations in Caucasians is the *UGT1A1*28* allele (32%) (Stingl et al, 2014) due to changes in the promoter region that decrease the expression of UGT1A1 (Beutler et al, 1998). The *UGT1A1*6* allele is found most frequently in the Asian population (18%) and contains a non-synonymous SNP in the coding region that results in decreased UGT1A1 activity (Stingl et al, 2014).

The potential effect of variable activity of UGT is dependent on the relationship between parent drug and metabolite. While most UGT metabolites are inactive, there are examples of activation including morphine metabolism to the active 6-glucuronide metabolite and various carboxylic acids metabolism to reactive, potentially toxic acylglucuronides (Stingl et al, 2014). The potential effects of these changes have been reported for over 22 different drugs with various changes to pharmacokinetic profiles including AUC and clearance (Stingl et al, 2014). A summary of the pharmacogenetics for all 22 drugs is beyond the scope of this chapter, but one example of a drug that includes FDA labeling related to UGT polymorphisms, irinotecan, will be briefly discussed.

Irinotecan is a prodrug topoisomerase-1 inhibitor that is approved to treat metastatic colon or rectal cancer. The active metabolite of irinotecan, SN-38, is produced by ester hydrolysis and is primarily cleared through biliary excretion after inactivation by UGT (Rothenberg, 1998). The accumulation of SN-38 is associated with dose- and treatment-limiting adverse effects including bone marrow toxicity and diarrhea. The FDA-approved label for irinotecan recommends a dosage reduction in patients who are homozygous for *UGT1A1*28* due to an increased risk of neutropenia (FDA, 2019). In Asian populations, the *UGT1A1*6* allele is associated with increased irinotecan toxicity and decreased clearance compared to the *UGT1A1*1* (wild-type) allele (Han et al, 2009). Other UGT enzymes involved in SN-38 glucuronidation and are known to be polymorphic, such as UGT1A7 and UGT1A9. Polymorphisms in these enzymes may contribute to irinotecan toxicity, and their inclusion may improve prediction in patient populations (Lankisch et al, 2008; Lévesque et al, 2013).

Multiple UGTs are involved in the inactivation of tobacco-related chemical compounds. Research is ongoing to detect differences due to genetic variability in the UGT-mediated inactivation of tobacco-derived carcinogenic nitrosamines (Wassenaar et al, 2015).

### N-Acetyltransferase

N-acetyltransferase (NAT) was identified as a polymorphic enzyme through phenotypic observations of fast or slow acetylators of the antituberculosis drug, isoniazid (Evans and White, 1964). There are two different human genes, *NAT1* and *NAT2*, that code for functional NAT activity. While both NAT1 and NAT2 are polymorphic, polymorphisms within NAT2 display a greater range of effects on enzyme activity. Although some publications only refer to the slow and fast or "rapid" acetylator phenotype for NAT2, an intermediate phenotype is recognized as occurring when an individual carries one copy of a slow allele and one copy of fast or "rapid" (PharmGKB, 2019). Several NAT2 alleles, *5, *6, *7, *10, and *14, are either null genes or encode of defective enzymes that contribute to the slow phenotype (PharmGKB, 2019). Patients who are slow metabolizers of isoniazid exhibit increased blood levels of the drug, which results in an increased incidence of neurotoxicity (PharmGKB, 2019). The metabolism of both procainamide and hydralazine is also dependent upon the activity of NAT2 such that slow metabolizers are associated with an increased risk of lupus erythematosus (Chen et al, 2007). With fast metabolizers, there can also be an increased toxicity of the topoisomerase II inhibitor, amonafide, which is associated with a higher incidence of myelosuppression (Innocenti et al, 2001).

## TRANSPORTERS

Several membrane transporter proteins are involved in drug absorption from the intestinal tract and distribution through the body. The two major superfamilies of transporters are the ATP-binding cassette (ABC) transporters and the solute carrier (SLC) transporters. Since the identification of P-glycoprotein, an ABC transporter, an increased appreciation of the influence of these transporters on pharmacokinetic parameters has developed and has only grown more as the study of the impact of pharmacogenetics on these transporters has evolved. It is likely that significant issues in oral drug bioavailability and variable pharmacokinetics result from genetic polymorphisms in transporters. The current understanding of transporter pharmacogenetics is advancing and here we outline several polymorphisms with difference levels of confidence in their clinical significance.

### ABC Transporters

#### P-Glycoprotein (MDR1, ABCB1)

The ATP binding cassette subfamily B member 1 (*ABCB1*) gene codes for the efflux protein

P-glycoprotein (P-gp), also known as multiple drug resistant protein 1 (MDR1), that is frequently associated with drug resistance to antineoplastic agents including vincristine and doxorubicin. In cancers that express P-gp, the drug is transported out of the cells, keeping the drug concentrations inside the target cell low. In addition to this resistance function, expression of P-gp also contributes to the efflux of some drugs from various tissues that affect the pharmacokinetics and clinical efficacy of these compounds. There are many P-gp substrates and inhibitors. At least 66 SNPs in the *ABCB1* gene have been reported, and the three most studied SNPs include two synonymous and one non-synonymous variants (Brambila-Tapia, 2013). The synonymous SNPs are reported to result in decreased expression of P-gp due to decreased mRNA expression, unstable mRNA, or alterations in protein folding (Sissung et al, 2012). The effects of these SNPs on drug serum levels have been examined in multiple studies with substrates including digoxin and docetaxel. The reported results on the pharmacokinetic profile of these two drugs have been inconsistent, with studies showing increased blood levels or no change compared to the wild-type gene (Sissung et al, 2012). These results highlight the dependency on the individual substrate, the complexity, and the effect of specific tissue transporter expression, which contributes to the pharmacokinetic profile of each drug. Additionally, there are also known inhibitors to P-gp that complicate the prediction of the pharmacokinetic profile in patients that are administered multiple drugs.

*Other ABC Transporters*

The multidrug resistance-associated proteins (MRPs) are members of the ATP-binding cassette (ABC) superfamily with six members currently, of which MRP1 (ABCC1), MRP2 (ABCC2), and MRP3 (ABCC3) are commonly known to effect drug disposition. Like MDR, these transporters can also be expressed in cancer cells, which confer resistance to the chemotherapeutic agent tamoxifen. It appears that polymorphisms in this family are rare and occur at different frequencies among different populations. Despite numerous studies, the functional importance of these polymorphisms remains unclear (Sissung et al, 2012).

ABCG2, also known as breast cancer resistance protein (BCRP), is polymorphic with one well-characterized SNP (c.421C>A) results in a glutamine substitution for a lysine at residue 1411 (Q141K) and is associated with a decreased function compared to the wild-type (Imai et al, 2002; Yee et al, 2018). This variant (c.421C>A) is clinically associated with increased diarrhea in patients treated with gefitinib, an anticancer epidermal growth factor inhibitor (Li et al, 2007). The International Transporter Consortium highlighted the c.421C>A polymorphism of *ABCG2* as clinically important based on the strength of the current literature (Giacomini et al, 2013; Yee et al, 2018). Future studies with specific substrates and polymorphisms may ultimately provide additional information on the variable responses or adverse effects of drugs.

### Solute Carrier Transporters

Another important class of drug transporters is the solute carriers (SLCs) such as the organic anion transporter polypeptide (OATP) and organic cation transporter (OCT). These transporters are located throughout the body and have various roles in the transport of many different drugs. OATP1B1 (coded by the *SLCO1B1* gene) is a hepatic influx transporter with at least 40 non-synonymous SNPs identified that result in either an altered expression or activity of OATP1B1 (Wassenaar et al, 2015). While the clinical consequences of all of these SNPs are unknown, one SNP (c.521T>C) causes an amino acid substitution, alanine for a valine, at residue 174 (V174A) and has been associated with an increased risk of simvastatin-induced myopathy (Yee et al, 2018; Ramesy et al, 2014). This non-synonymous SNP is associated with a lower plasma clearance of simvastatin and is found in the *SLCO1B1*5*, **15*, and **17* alleles (Ramesy et al, 2014). These alleles are present in most populations with a frequency between 5% and 20% and warrant the avoidance of high-dose simvastatin (>40 mg) or treatment with another statin to decrease the risk of simvastatin-induced myopathies (Sissung et al, 2012). The International Transporter Consortium highlighted the c.521T>C polymorphism of *SLCO1B1* as clinically important (Giacomini et al, 2013).

## GLOSSARY

**Allele:** An alternative form of a gene at a given locus.

**Biological marker (biomarker):** A characteristic that is objectively measured and evaluated as an indicator of normal biologic processes, pathogenic processes, or pharmacologic responses to a therapeutic intervention.

**Genetic polymorphism:** Minor allele frequency of ≥1% in the population.

**Genome:** The complete DNA sequence of an organism.

**Genotype:** The alleles at a specific locus an individual carries.

**Haplotype:** A group of alleles from two or more loci on a chromosome, inherited as a unit.

**Minor allele:** A less common allele at a polymorphic locus.

**Pharmacogenetic test:** An assay intended to determine interindividual variations in DNA sequence related to drug absorption and disposition (pharmacokinetics) or drug action (pharmacodynamics), including polymorphic variation in the genes that encode the functions of transporters, metabolizing enzymes, receptors, and other proteins.

**Pharmacogenetics:** The study of variations in DNA sequence as related to drug response. In this chapter, the term "pharmacogenetics" is interchangeable with "pharmacogenomics."

**Pharmacogenomic test:** An assay intended to study interindividual variations in whole-genome or candidate gene, single-nucleotide polymorphism (SNP) maps, haplotype markers, or alterations in gene expression or inactivation that may be correlated with pharmacological function and therapeutic response. In some cases, the *pattern or profile of change* is the relevant biomarker, rather than changes in individual markers.

**Pharmacogenomics:** The study of variations of DNA and RNA characteristics as related to drug response. Pharmacogenetics focuses on a single gene while pharmacogenomics studies multiple genes.

**Phenotype:** Observable expression of a particular gene or genes.

**Promoter:** A segment of DNA sequence that controls initiation of transcription of the gene and is usually located upstream of the gene.

**Single-nucleotide polymorphism:** A DNA sequence variation occurring when a single nucleotide—A, T, C, or G—in the gene (or other shared sequence) is altered.

## CHAPTER SUMMARY

The overarching theme for the effects of polymorphisms in drug-metabolizing enzymes and transporters is that they have the potential to modify the pharmacokinetic profile by influencing drug clearance or activation, secondary to metabolism. While the pharmacogenetics of these pharmacokinetic determinants can account for some of this variability, it is not able to explain all therapeutic or adverse event variations. So currently the FDA only recommends pharmacogenetic testing, due to pharmacokinetic factors, in a limited number of drug therapy regimens (see Table 21-1). One instance where genetic testing is required (based on pharmacokinetic parameters) is in the use of tetrabenazine for the treatment of Huntington's disease chorea, where daily dosing is guided by CYP2D6 phenotypes to prevent adverse events and achieve therapeutic efficacy. A second instance is genotyping for polymorphisms in *CYP2C19*, which is responsible for the bioactivation of clopidogrel, an antiplatelet agent. In either case, the clinician's decision to order a genetic test prior to drug therapy may be predicated on multiple factors such as whether there are alternative drug choices, whether the test results can be obtained in an appropriate time frame, and whether the insurance or patient is willing to pay for the test. In the two examples above, a genetic test may be ordered prior to tetrabenazine dose exceeding 50 mg per day, while prasugrel or ticagrelor may be selected instead of clopidogrel as they are not affected by *CYP2C19* variants. Genetic polymorphisms that affect pharmacodynamic interactions also contribute to the variability of drug response, and genetic testing is required in multiple instances where such variations alter the response to drug therapy; for example, imatinib for c-KIT-positive tumors. Additionally, there are many other factors including concomitant medications that may act as metabolism inducers or inhibitors, disease states, and age that cannot be accounted for by genetics alone. It is these observations that temper the excitement of personalized medicine in preventing all adverse effects and therapeutic failures.

## CASE STUDY

During a routine dental cleaning, JM complains to her dentist about a recent discomfort that she has been experiencing. Her dentist examines her teeth and recommends having her wisdom teeth removed. Two weeks later, she has her wisdom teeth removed without complications. To help alleviate the pain her dentist prescribed acetaminophen with codeine (Tylenol #3), taken as needed every 4 hours for pain. The next day, JM has no pain relief using the medication as prescribed by her dentist. After hours of focusing on the pain, JM recalls the consumer DNA test kit that her cousin gave her last year as a gift and remembered it saying something about codeine in the commentary on the results. The report states that she may experience adverse reactions with some antidepressants (ie, tricyclic antidepressants) and not feel pain relief with codeine. Explain the genetic explanation behind this statement in the report.

### Answer

The DNA test revealed that JM is a carrier of alleles that make her a poor CYP2D6 metabolizer. She does not feel relief from the combination of drugs that she is on because codeine requires CYP2D6 to convert codeine to morphine in the liver for effective management of pain. She may experience adverse effects with the use of certain antidepressants, such as some of the tricyclic antidepressants, because she is not able to metabolize these drugs for removal from the body.

## FREQUENTLY ASKED QUESTIONS

▶ What is the difference between pharmacogenetics and pharmacogenomics? How are pharmacogenetics and pharmacogenomics used to improve healthcare?

▶ What is the difference between a mutation, polymorphism, SNP, and haplotype? Why are these distinctions important for individualizing drug therapy?

▶ What types of genes are important to drug therapy? How would variability in these genes impact drug therapy?

▶ How common and clinically relevant are metabolic polymorphisms?

▶ How can genetic information be used to improve drug therapy for individuals and/or groups of patients?

## ANSWERS

### Frequently Asked Questions

*What is the difference between pharmacogenetics and pharmacogenomics? How are pharmacogenetics and pharmacogenomics used to improve healthcare?*

■ The study of pharmacogenomics involves characterizing the broad variation across the entire genome to explain drug response, but pharmacogenetics usually focuses on a single genetic marker as a predictor of drug response. In either case, understanding the role of genetic variation in drug response could be used to predict an individual's risk to an adverse drug event and/or therapeutic response.

*What is the difference between a mutation, polymorphism, SNP, and haplotype? Why are these distinctions important for individualizing drug therapy?*

■ *Genetic polymorphisms* are variations in gene sequences that occur in at least 1% of the general population, resulting in multiple alleles or variants of a gene sequence. Polymorphisms are distinct from *mutations* that occur in less than 1% of the population. A *single nucleotide polymorphism*

(SNP) is the result of a change in a single nucleotide base pair within the gene sequence. A grouping of select variants is called a haplotype and results in unique combinations of polymorphisms with potentially novel phenotypes. These terms are used to characterize the frequency of an allelic variant or the types of variation observed in a DNA sequence. Novel phenotypes may be observed due to the type of genetic variation, which is important for predicting an individual's drug response.

*What types of genes are important to drug therapy? How would variability in these genes impact drug therapy?*

- Genes that code for drug-metabolizing enzymes or transporters can affect the pharmacokinetics of a drug and lead to variations in drug response. Changes in pharmacodynamics due to genetic variations in the drug's receptor or downstream processes could also lead to an alteration in drug response.

*How common and clinically relevant are metabolic polymorphisms?*

- For a specific drug-metabolizing enzyme, the frequencies of the allelic variants within a population will vary. The redundancy of drug metabolism and potential contribution from numerous other factors (such as diet, other drugs, age, weight, etc) make it difficult to translate enzyme status data to a clinical decision. However, there are 268 FDA-approved drugs that contain pharmacogenetic information in their drug label, which could be used in clinical decision making.

*How can genetic information be used to improve drug therapy for individuals and/or groups of patients?*

- Understanding a patient's genetic determinants of drug metabolism and the consequences of these polymorphisms could be used to design optimum, personalized dosing regimens in the clinic that would avoid adverse reactions or treatment failures due to subtherapeutic doses.

## REFERENCES

Ahles A, Engelhardt S: Polymorphic variants of adrenoceptors: Pharmacology, physiology, and role in diseases. *Pharmacol Rev* **66**:598, 2014.

Ameyaw MM, Collie-Duguid ES, Powrie RH, Ofori-Adjei D, Mcleod HL: Thiopurine methyltransferase alleles in British and Ghanaian populations. *Hum Mol Genet* **8**:367, 1999.

Amstutz U, Henricks LM, Offer SM, et al: Clinical pharmacogenetics implementation consortium (CPIC) guideline for dihydropyrimidine dehydrogenase genotype and fluoropyrimidine dosing: 2017 update. *Clin Pharmacol Ther* **102**:210, 2018.

Ansari A, Hassan C, Duley J, et al: Thiopurine methyltransferase activity and the use of azathioprine in inflammatory bowel disease. *Aliment Pharmacol Ther* **16**:1743, 2002.

Beutler E, Gelbart T, Demina A: Racial variability in the UDP-glucuronosyltransferase 1 (UGT1A1) promoter: A balanced polymorphism for regulation of bilirubin metabolism? *Proc Natl Acad Sci U S A* **95**:8170, 1998.

Brambila-Tapia AJL: MDR1 (ABCB1) polymorphisms: Functional effects and clinical implications. *Revista de Investigacion Clinicia* **65**:445, 2013.

Caraco Y, Blotnick, S, Muszkat M: CYP2C9 genotype-guided warfarin prescribing enhances the efficacy and safety of anticoagulation: A prospective randomized controlled study. *Clin Pharmacol Ther* **83**:460, 2008.

Chen M, Xiz B, Chen B, et al: N-acetyltransferase 2 slow acetylator genotype associated with adverse effects of sulphasalazine

in the treatment of inflammatory bowel disease. *Can J Gastroenterol* **21**:155, 2007.

Colombel JF, Ferrari N, Debuysere H, et al: Genotypic analysis of thiopurine S-methyltransferase in patients with Crohn's disease and severe myelosuppression during azathioprine therapy. *Gastroenterology* **118**:1025, 2000.

de Morais SM, Wilkinson GR, Blaisdell J, Nakamura K, Meyer UA, Goldstein JA: The major genetic defect responsible for the polymorphism of S-mephenytoin metabolism in humans. *J Biol Chem* **269**:15419, 1994.

Dodgan TM, Hochfeld WE, Fickl H, et al: Introduction of the AmpliChip CYP450 test to a South African cohort: A platform comparative prospective cohort study. *BMC Med Genetics* **14**:20, 2013.

Eap CB, Bender S, Jaquenoud Siront E, et al: Nonresponse to clozapine and ultrarapid CYP1A2 activity: Clinical data and analysis of *CYP1A2* gene. *J Clin Psychopharmacol* **24**:214, 2004.

Etienne MC, Lagrange JL, Dassonville O, et al: Population study of dihydropyrimidine dehydrogenase in cancer-patients. *J Clin Oncol* **12**:2248, 1994.

Evans DAP, White TA: Human acetylation polymorphism. *J Lab Clin Med* **63**:394, 1964.

Evans WE, Relling MV: Pharmacogenomics: Translating functional genomics into rational therapeutics. *Science* **286**:487, 1999.

FDA (US Food and Drug Administration): Drugs at FDA: FDA-approved drugs. Silver Spring, MD, 2019. http://www.fda.gov/drugsatfda/.

Fernandez-Rozadilla C, Cazier JB, Moreno V, et al: Pharmacogenomics in colorectal cancer: A genome-wide association study to predict toxicity after 5-fluorouracil or FOLFOX administration. *Pharmacogen J* **13**:209, 2013.

Gasche Y, Daali R, Fathi M, et al: Codeine intoxication associated with ultrarapid CYP2D6 metabolism. *N Engl J Med* **351**:2827, 2004.

Giacomini KM, Balimane PV, Cho SK, et al: International Transporter Consortium Commentary on clinically important transporter polymorphisms. *Clin Pharmacol Ther* **94**:23, 2013.

Han JY, Lim HS, Park YH, Lee SY, Lee JS: Integrated pharmacogenetic prediction of irinotecan pharmacokinetics and toxicity in patients with advanced non-small cell lung cancer. *Lung Cancer* **63**:115, 2009.

Idle JR, Mahgoub A, Lancaster R, Smith RL: Hypotensive response to debrisoquine and hydroxylation phenotype. *Life Sci* **11**:979, 1978.

Ingelman-Sundberg M, Daly AK, Nebert DW (eds): The Human Cytochrome P450 Allele Nomenclature Database. Stockholm, Sweden, 2014. http://www.cypalleles.ki.se/.

Innocenti F, Iyer L, Ratain MJ: Pharmacogenetics of anticancer agents: Lessons from amonafide and irinotecan. *Drug Metab Dispos* **26**:596, 2001.

Imai Y, Nakane M, Kage K, Tsukahara S, Ishikawa E, Tsuruo T, et al: C421A polymorphism in the human breast cancer resistance protein gene is associated with low expression of q141k protein and low-level drug resistance. *Mol Cancer Ther* **1**:611–6, 2002.

Kimmel SE, French B, Kasner SE, et al: A pharmacogenetic versus a clinical algorithm for warfarin dosing. *N Engl J Med* **369**:2283, 2013.

Lamba, J, Hebert JM, Schuetz EG, et al: PharmGKB summary: Very important pharmacogene information for CYP3A5. *Pharmacogenet Genomics* **22**:555, 2012.

Lankisch TO, Schulz C, Zwingers T, et al: Gilbert's syndrome and irinotecan toxicity: Combination with UDP-glucuronosyltransferase 1A7 variants increases risk. *Cancer Epidemiol Biomarkers Prev* **17**:695, 2008.

Lerman C, Tyndale R, Patterson F, et al: Nicotine metabolite ratio predicts efficacy of transdermal nicotine for smoking cessation. *Clin Pharmacol Ther* **79**:600, 2006.

Lévesque E, Bélanger AS, Harvey M, et al: Refining the UGT1A haplotype associated with irinotecan-induced hematological toxicity in metastatic colorectal cancer patients treated with 5-fluorouracil/irinotecan-based regiments. *J Pharmacol Exp Ther* **345**:95, 2013.

Li J, Cusatis G, Brahmer J, et al: Association of variant ABCG2 and the pharmacokinetics of epidermal growth factor receptor tyrosine kinase inhibitors in cancer patients. *Cancer Biol Ther* **6**:432–8, 2007.

Limdi NA, Veenstra DL: Expectations, validity, and reality in pharmacogenetics. *J Clin Epidemiol* **63**:960, 2010.

Lu ZH, Zhang RW, Diasio RB: Dihydropyrimidine dehydrogenase-activity in human peripheral-blood mononuclear-cells and liver-population characteristics, newly identified deficient patients, and clinical implication in 5-fluorouracil chemotherapy. *Cancer Res* **53**:5433, 1993.

Mahgoub A, Idle JR, Dring LG, Lancaster R, Smith RL: Polymorphic hydroxylation of debrisoquine in man. *Lancet* **ii**:584, 1977.

Mancinelli L, Cronin M, Sadee W: Pharmacogenomics: The promise of personalized medicine. *AAPS PharmSci* **2**(1):29, 2000.

McGraw J, Waller D: Cytochrome P450 variations in different ethnic populations. *Expert Opin Drug Metab Toxicol* **8**:371, 2012.

Meech R, Miners JO, Lewis BC, Mackenzie PI: The glycosidation of xenobiotics and endogenous compounds: Versatility and redundancy in the UDP glycosyltransferase superfamily. *Pharmacol Ther* **134**:200, 2012.

Meyer UA, Zanger UM, Schwab M: Omics and drug response. *Ann Rev Pharm Tox* **53**:475, 2013.

Meyer US: Pharmacogenetics and adverse drug reactions. *Lancet* **356**:1667, 2000.

Nakajima M, Yamamoto T, Nunoya K, et al. Characterization of CYP2A6 involved in 3′-hydroxylation of cotinine in human liver microsomes. *J Pharmacol Exp Ther* **277**:1010, 1996b.

Ogawaa E, Echizen H: Drug-drug interaction profiles of proton pump inhibitors. *Clin Pharmacokinet* **49**:509, 2010.

Passey C, Birnbaum AK, Brundage RC, et al: Dosing equation for tacrolimus using genetic variants and clinical factors. *Br J Clin Pharmacol* **72**:948, 2011.

Pharm GKB: Pharmacogenetics Knowledge Base, Palo Alto, California, 2019. http://www.pharmgkb.org/.

Phillips KA, Veenstra DL, Ores E, et al: Potential role of pharmacogenetics in reducing adverse drug reactions-A systematic review. *JAMA* **286**:2270, 2001.

Pirmohamed MA, Burnside G, Eriksson N, et al: A randomized trial of genotype-guided dosing of warfarin. *N Engl J Med* **369**:2294, 2013.

Ramesy LB, Johnson SG, Caudle KE, et al: The Clinical Pharmacogenetics Implementation Consortium guideline for SLCO1B1 and simvastatin-induced myopathy: 2014 update. *Clin Pharmacol Ther* **96**:423, 2014.

Relling MV, Gardner EE, Sandborn WJ, et al: Clinical Pharmacogenetics Implementation Consortium guidelines for thiopurine methyltransferase genotype and thiopurine dosing. *Clin Pharmacol Ther* **89**:387, 2011.

Rolla R, Vidali M, Meola S, et al: Side effects associated with ultrarapid cytochrome P450 2D6 genotype among women with early-stage breast cancer treated with tamoxifen. *Clin Lab* **58**:1211, 2012.

Rothenberg ML: Efficacy and toxicity of irinotecan in patients with colorectal cancer. *Semin Oncol* **25**:39, 1998.

Samer CF, Ing Lorenzini K, Rollason V, Daali Y, Desmeules JA: Applications of CYP450 testing in the clinical setting. *Mol Diagn Ther* **17**:165, 2013.

Sata F, Sapone A, Elizondo G, et al: CYP3A4 allelic variants with amino acid substitutions in exons 7 and 12: Evidence for an allelic variant with altered catalytic activity. *Clin Pharmacol Ther* **67**:45, 2000.

Schaeffeler E, Zanger UM, Eichelbaum M, Asante-Poku S, Shin JG, Schwab M: Highly multiplexed genotyping of thiopurine S-methyltransferase variants using MALD-TOF mass spectrometry: Reliable genotyping in different ethnic groups. *Clin Chem* **54**:1637, 2008.

Schoedel KA, Hoffmann EB, Rao Y, et al: Ethnic variation in CYP2A6 and association of genetically slow nicotine metabolism and smoking in adult Caucasians. *Pharmacogenetics* **14**:615, 2004.

Schwarz UI, Gulilat M, Kim RB: The role of next-generation sequencing in pharmacogenetics and pharmacogenomics. *Cold Spring Harb Perspect Med* **9**: a033027, 2019.

Scott SA, Sangkuhl K, Gardner EE, et al: Clinical pharmacogenetics implementation consortium guidelines for cytochrome P450-2C19 (CYP2C19) genotype and clopidogrel therapy. *Clin Pharmacol Ther* **90**:328, 2011.

Shi S, Klotz U: Proton pump inhibitors: An update of their clinical use and pharmacokinetics. *Eur J Clin Pharmacol* **64**:935, 2008.

Sibbing D, Koch W, Gebhard D, et al: Cytochrome 2C19*17 allelic variant, platelet aggregation, bleeding events and stent thrombosis in clopidogrel-treated patients with coronary stent placement. *Circulation* **121**:512, 2010.

Sim SC, Risinger, C, Dahl ML, et al: A common novel CYP2C19 gene variant causes ultrarapid drug metabolism relevant for the drug response to proton pump inhibitors and antidepressants. *Clin Pharmacol Ther* **79**:103, 2006.

Sissung TM, Troutman SM, Campbell TJ, et al: Transporter pharmacogenetics: Transporter polymorphisms affect normal physiology, diseases, and pharmacotherapy. *Discov Med* **13**:19, 2012.

Soliday FK, Conley YP, Henker R: Pseudocholinesterase deficiency: A comprehensive review of genetic, acquired, and drug influences. *AANA J* **78**:313, 2010.

Stingl JC, Bartels H, Viviani R, Lehmann ML, Brockmoller J: Relevance of UDP-glucuronosyltransferase polymorphisms for drug dosing: A quantitative systematic review. *Pharmacol Ther* **141**:92, 2014.

UGT Nomenclature Committee: Alleles Nomenclature Home Page. June 2005. https://www.pharmacogenomics.pha.ulaval.ca/ugt-alleles-nomenclature/ (accessed May 17, 2019).

Ventola CL: Pharmacogenomics in clinical practice: Reality and expectations. *P T* **36**:412, 2011.

Wang M, Lang X, Cui S, et al: Clinical application of pharmacogenetic-based warfarin-dosing algorithm in patients of Han nationality after rheumatic valve replacement: A randomized and controlled trial. *Int J Med Sci* **9**:472, 2012.

Wang J, Pitarque M, Ingelman-Sundberg M: 3'-UTR polymorphism in the human CYP2A6 gene affects mRNA stability and enzyme expression. *Biochem Biophys Res Commun* **340**:491, 2006.

Warfarin Dosing. St. Louis, MO, 2014. http://www.warfarindosing.org/Source/Home.aspx.

Wassenaar CA, Conti DV, Das S, et al: UGT1A and UGT2B genetic variation alters nicotine and nitrosamine glucuronidation in European and African American smokers. *Cancer Epidemiol Biomarkers Prev* **24**:94, 2015.

Yee SW, Brackman, DJ, Ennis EA, et al: Influence of transporter polymorphisms on drug disposition and response: A perspective from the International Transporter Consortium. *Clin Pharmacol Ther* **104**:803, 2018.

Zabalza M, Subirana I, Sala J, et al: Meta-analyses of the association between cytochrome CYP2C19 loss- and gain-of-function polymorphisms and cardiovascular outcomes in patients with coronary artery disease treated with clopidogrel. *Heart* **98**:100, 2012.

# 22 Relationship between Pharmacokinetics and Pharmacodynamics

Mathangi Gopalakrishnan, Vipul Kumar Gupta, and Manish Issar

## CHAPTER OBJECTIVES

- Quantitatively describe the relationship between drug, receptor, and the pharmacologic response.

- Explain why the intensity of the pharmacologic response increases with drug concentrations and/or dose up to a maximum response.

- Explain the difference between an agonist, a partial agonist, and an antagonist.

- Describe the difference between a reversible and a non-reversible pharmacologic response.

- Define the term biomarker and explain how biomarkers can be used in the clinical development of drugs.

- Show how the $E_{max}$ and sigmoidal $E_{max}$ model describe the relationship of the pharmacodynamic response to drug concentration.

- Define the term pharmacokinetic–pharmacodynamic model and provide an equation that quantitatively simulates the time course of drug action.

- Explain the effect compartment in the pharmacodynamic model and name the underlying assumptions.

- Describe the effect of changing drug dose and/or drug elimination half-life on the duration of drug response.

- Describe how observed drug tolerance or unusual hysteresis-type drug response can be explained using PD models based on simple drug receptor theory.

- Define the term drug exposure and explain how drug exposure relates to drug therapy

## PHARMACOKINETICS AND PHARMACODYNAMICS

The role of pharmacokinetics (PK) to derive dosing regimens to achieve therapeutic drug concentrations for optimal safety and efficacy was described in the previous chapters. A rational approach for designing a drug's dosing regimen would be to link the exposure of the drug within the body to the desirable (efficacy) and undesirable (safety/toxicity) effects of the drug. At the site of action, the drug interacts with a receptor, and this drug–receptor interaction initiates a cascade of events resulting in a pharmacodynamic response or effect. Thus, *pharmacodynamics* (PD) refers to the relationship between drug concentration at the site of action (receptor) and the observed pharmacologic response. This chapter describes how the exposures of a drug over time (dose, concentrations, dosing regimens) can be related to the desirable and undesirable effects of the drug. Just as the PK of a drug has been described via mathematical models, the relationship between drug concentration and pharmacological effect can be described using mathematical models, which can be applied for simulations and predictions. The chapter is organized as follows: first, a definition of terms that are often used interchangeably in the pharmacodynamic-pharmacokinetic (PK–PD) literature is provided. Second, the reader is introduced to how the PK–PD information is integrated in drug development. Third, the chapter briefly describes the drug–receptor theory and the use of biomarkers, followed by the theoretical basis of PK–PD relationship. Lastly, the chapter describes the different types of possible PK–PD relationships with real examples. The examples and case studies provided in the chapter integrate the concepts from a drug development perspective.

### Definitions for Exposure, Response, and Effect

In the study of PK and PD, it is important to use correct terminology, as terms are often used interchangeably and incorrectly. This section provides definitions of the terms that will be used throughout this chapter.

The relationship between PK and PD is referred to as *exposure–response relationship*, drug concentration–response relationship, or drug concentration–effect relationship. Exposure–response information is used to determine the safety and efficacy of drugs in the process of drug development and FDA approval. It is important to understand the benefit-risk of drugs during the drug approval process and to provide essential information for pharmacists and clinicians so that they can ensure that dosing is optimized in patients.

#### Exposure

*Exposure* is defined as any dose or drug input into the body or as a measure of acute or integrated drug concentrations in plasma or other biological fluid (eg, $C_{max}$, $C_{min}$, $C_{ss}$, AUC). Commonly used exposure measures are dose of a drug and plasma concentrations ($C_p$). Any input to characterize the pharmacokinetic aspect of the drug is a measure of exposure.

#### Response

A *response (R)* refers to a direct measure of the pharmacologic observation. For example, measure of diastolic blood pressure (DBP) at some time point is considered as a response.

$R(t)$ = Response at time, $t$: = Diastolic blood pressure
   = 92 mm Hg

#### Effect

*Effect (E)* refers to a change in the biological response from one time to another. An effect is a derived or calculated value from an observed response. For example, a change from a

$E$ = Effect: = Change from baseline in DBP at 8 weeks

To further illustrate, let us consider the DBP measured at the beginning of a clinical trial in a subject as 92 mm Hg, denoted as $R(t = 0)$, and DBP measured at the end of 8 weeks of the trial, $R(t = 8)$, is 82 mm Hg. Here, $R(t = 0)$ and $R(t = 8)$ are the responses. The effect, $E$, which is of interest, is change from baseline in DBP at 8 weeks calculated as −10 mm Hg is denoted below:

$E = R(t = 8) - R(t = 0) = 82$ mm Hg − 92 mm Hg
   = −10 mm Hg

Effects include a broad range of endpoints or biomarkers ranging from clinically remote biomarkers (eg, receptor occupancy) to a presumed mechanistic effect (eg, % angiotensin-converting enzyme (ACE) inhibition) to a potential surrogate (eg, change from baseline in blood pressure or change in lipids, etc). The scientific community often uses response and effect interchangeably, but for the purpose of this chapter, we refer to *response* as something which is measured directly and *effect* as something derived from measuring the response.

### PK–PD Information Flow in Drug Development

The role of PK and PD in the drug development process is impactful, and several drug developers and scientists have discussed its importance in drug development and decision making (Derendorf et al, 2000; Sheiner and Steimer, 2000; Gobburu and Marroum, 2001; Kimko and Pinheiro, 2014). In general, the new drug development process is series of developmental and evaluative steps carried out from the stage of an investigational new drug application (IND) leading to the submission of new drug application (NDA). The regulatory bodies such as the Food and Drug Administration (FDA) and European Medicines Agency (EMA) review the NDA and provide approval/disapproval for the new drugs to be marketed. This process as it pertains to the US FDA is illustrated as an example in Fig. 22-1.

There are predominantly four phases in the drug development process, as shown in Fig. 22-1.

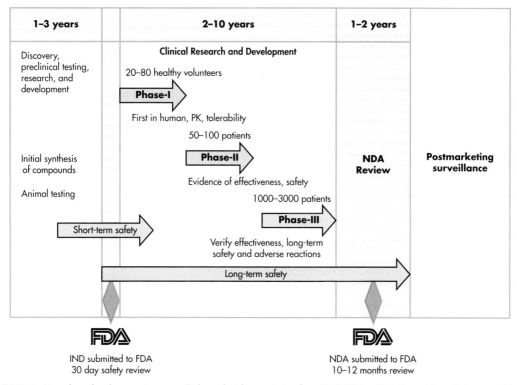

| 1–3 years | 2–10 years | 1–2 years | |
|---|---|---|---|
| Discovery, preclinical testing, research, and development | **Clinical Research and Development**  20–80 healthy volunteers  **Phase-I**  First in human, PK, tolerability  50–100 patients  **Phase-II**  Evidence of effectiveness, safety | **NDA Review** | **Postmarketing surveillance** |
| Initial synthesis of compounds  Animal testing | 1000–3000 patients  **Phase-III** | | |
| Short-term safety | Verify effectiveness, long-term safety and adverse reactions | | |
| | Long-term safety | | |

FDA

IND submitted to FDA
30 day safety review

FDA

NDA submitted to FDA
10–12 months review

FIGURE 22-1 • New drug development process. (Adapted with permission from Peck CC, Barr WH, Benet LZ, et al. Opportunities for integration of pharmacokinetics, pharmacodynamics, and toxicokinetics in rational drug development, J Clin Pharmacol. 1994 Feb; 34(2):111–119.)

The details of the four phases in drug development and how the PK–PD information at each of the phases can be useful are described briefly here and shown in Fig. 22-2. The initial phase is the preclinical testing phase. During this phase, the new molecular entities are tested for biological activity in experimental animals from mice to primate models. The toxicity and safety data available at this stage are used to proceed for safety evaluation in humans at the IND stage. The preclinical PK-safety information is helpful in deriving first in human (FIH) doses or maximum recommended starting dose (MRSD) by means of allometric scaling. Moreover, preclinical studies on pharmacodynamic activity from different exposures/doses may indicate the likely steepness of the dose–response curves in humans.

After discovery and preclinical testing, the new molecular entity (NME) enters the clinical testing phase. Typically, the clinical testing phase consists of early-phase (Phases I and II) and late-phase clinical trials (Phase III). During Phase I studies, the PK and

tolerability of the NME is studied in healthy volunteers by means of dose escalation. Information on initial parameters of toxicity, maximum tolerated dose, and PK characteristics of the drug and metabolite (if any) are obtained. The initial Phase I studies help establish the appropriate dosing program for Phase II studies by means of the observed dose/exposure–safety relationship.

Phase II studies are conducted in a small group of patients to assess whether the drug exhibits anticipated therapeutic benefit in the intended patient population. The principal goal of Phase II studies is to provide evidence for the efficacy or proof of effect of the investigational drug. Additional PK–PD information gained in Phase II studies are used to build dose-exposure-response relationships to obtain a rational dosing strategy for Phase III studies. The exposure-response relationships can be used to design strategies for dose optimization and individualized dosing in Phase III trials. In order to avoid failure in the Phase III trials mainly due to an incorrect dose/dosing

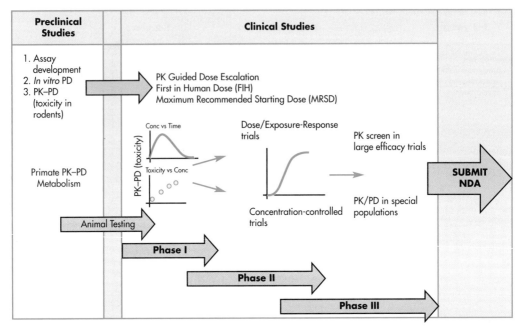

FIGURE 22-2 • PK, PD, and toxicity information during the drug development process. (Adapted with permission from Peck CC, Barr WH, Benet LZ, et al. Opportunities for integration of pharmacokinetics, pharmacodynamics, and toxicokinetics in rational drug development, J Clin Pharmacol. 1994 Feb;34(2):111–119.)

regimen selection, it is imperative to accrue/leverage valuable information that is gained in Phase II studies and apply this information to design Phase III trials to increase the likelihood of success.

Phase III studies used for drug approval are considered pivotal clinical trials. Typically, two adequate and well-controlled clinical trials are submitted for drug approval. Phase III studies are conducted in a larger patient population and are designed to document the clinical efficacy and safety of the investigational drug and further refine the dose-exposure-response relationship. The information gained in preclinical and clinical studies becomes part of the regulatory body approved drug label that ultimately reaches the prescriber and hence the patient.

The preceding section discussed the implications of PK–PD relationship in the drug development process. To understand how a drug elicits a response, it is necessary to understand the process at a cellular and a molecular level. The following section describes the interaction of a drug molecule with a receptor, resulting in a pharmacodynamic response.

## Drug–Receptor Interaction

Receptors are cellular proteins that interact with endogenous ligands (such as neurotransmitters and hormones) to elicit a physiological response, thereby regulating cellular functions (Blumenthal and Garrison, 2011). Understanding the role of receptor–endogenous ligand interaction in physiology and pathophysiology enables targeting of specific receptors for therapeutic benefit. There are different types of receptors that are located either outside or inside of cell membranes. Various types of receptors, their localization, and some representative examples are listed in Table 22-1.

The drug–receptor interactions involve weak chemical forces or bonds (eg, hydrogen bonding, ionic electrostatic bonds, Van der Waals forces). Typically, the drug–receptor interaction results in a cascade of downstream events eliciting a PD response. The interaction of drug with a receptor follows the *law of mass action* (Clark, 1927) which can be described as the *receptor occupancy theory* and is described in greater detail under $E_{max}$ drug–concentration effect model.

**TABLE 22-1 •** Selected Examples of Drug Receptors

| Type | Description | Examples |
|------|-------------|----------|
| Ion channels | Located on cell surface or transmembrane; governs ion flux | Acetylcholine (nicotinic) |
| G-protein coupled receptor | Located on cell surface or transmembrane; GTP involved in receptor action | Acetylcholine (muscarinic) α- and β-adrenergic receptor Proteins Eicosanoids |
| Transcription factors | Within cell in cytoplasm, activate or suppress DNA transcription | Steroid hormones Thyroid hormone |

Data from Moroney AC: The MERCK Manual of Diagnosis and Therapy. Whitehouse Station, NJ: Merck Sharp & Dohme; 2011; Katzung BG, Masters SB, Trevor AJ: Basic and Clinical Pharmacology. New York, NY: McGraw Hill; 2011.

Typically, a single drug molecule interacts with a receptor with a single binding site to produce a pharmacologic response, as illustrated below.

[Drug] + [Receptor]
⟺ [Drug – receptor complex] → response

where the parentheses [ ] denote molar concentrations.

This scheme illustrates the *occupation theory* for the interaction of a drug molecule with a receptor. More recent schemes consider a drug that binds to macromolecules as a *ligand*. Thus, the reversible interaction of a ligand (drug) with a receptor may be written as (Neubig et al, 2003).

$$L + R \underset{}{\overset{k_1}{\rightleftharpoons}} LR \underset{}{\overset{k_2}{\rightleftharpoons}} LR^*$$

where $L$ is generally referred to as ligand concentration (since many drugs are small molecules) and $LR$ is analogous to the [drug–receptor complex]. $LR^*$ is the activated form, which results in the drug eliciting the response.

The last step is written to accommodate different modes of how $LR$ leads to a drug response. For example, the interaction of a subsequent ligand with the receptor may involve a conformation change of the receptor or simply lead to an additional response.

This model makes the following assumptions:

1. The drug molecule combines with the receptor molecule as a bimolecular association, and the resulting drug–receptor complex disassociates as a unimolecular entity.

2. The binding of the drug with the receptor is fully reversible.

3. The basic model assumes a single type of receptor binding site, with one binding site per receptor molecule. It is also assumed that a receptor with multiple sites may be modeled after this (Cox, 1990).

4. The occupancy of the drug molecule at one receptor site does not change the affinity of more drug molecules to complex at additional receptor sites.

Generally, each receptor has an equal affinity for its drug molecule. The model is not suitable for drugs with *allosteric binding* to receptors, in which the binding of one drug molecule to the receptor affects the binding of subsequent drug molecules, as in the case of oxygen molecules binding to iron in hemoglobin. As more receptors are occupied by drug molecules, a greater pharmacodynamic response is obtained until a maximum response is reached.

Based on the interaction of the drug with the receptor, a drug can be classified as an agonist, partial agonist, inverse agonist, or antagonist. An *agonist* is an agent that interacts with a receptor, producing effects similar to that of an endogenous ligand (eg, stimulation of the $\mu$ opioid receptor by morphine) (Yaksh and Wallace, 2011). An *antagonist* is an agent that blocks the effect of an agonist by binding to the receptor, thereby inhibiting the effect of an endogenous ligand or agonist (eg, atenolol, a blood pressure–lowering agent is a $\beta_1$ receptor antagonist) (Westfall and Westfall, 2011). A *partial agonist* is an agent that produces a response similar to an agonist but cannot reach a maximal response as that of an agonist (eg, buspirone, an anxiolytic agent is a partial agonist of 5-HT$_{1a}$ receptor) (O'Donnell and Shelton, 2011). An *inverse agonist* selectively binds to the inactive form of the receptor and shifts the conformational equilibrium towards the inactive state (eg, famotidine, a gastric acid production inhibitor

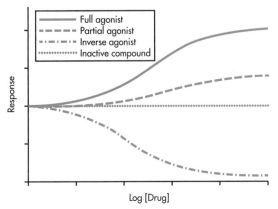

FIGURE 22-3 • Representation of different drug–receptor interactions. (Modified with permission from Brunton LL, Hilal-Dandan R, Knollmann BC: Goodman & Gilman's: The Pharmacological Basis of Therapeutics, 13th ed. New York, NY: McGraw Hill; 2018.)

is an inverse agonist of $H_2$ receptor) (Skidgel et al, 2011). The manner in which different drugs/ligands interact with the receptors can be represented graphically as shown in Fig. 22-3.

## RELATIONSHIP OF DOSE TO PHARMACOLOGIC RESPONSE

The onset, intensity, and duration of the pharmacologic effect depend on the dose and the PK of the drug. As the dose increases, the drug concentration at the receptor site increases, and the pharmacologic response increases up to a maxima. A plot of the pharmacologic response to dose on a linear scale

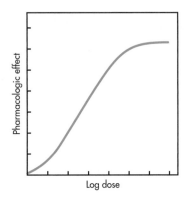

FIGURE 22-5 • A typical log dose versus pharmacologic response curve.

generally results in a hyperbolic curve with maximum response at the plateau (Fig. 22-4). The same data may be compressed and plotted on a log-linear scale and results in a sigmoid curve (Fig. 22-5).

For many drugs, the graph of the log dose–response curve shows a linear relationship at a dose range between 20% and 80% of the maximum response, which typically includes the therapeutic dose range for many drugs. For a drug that follows linear PK, the volume of distribution is constant; therefore, the pharmacologic response is also proportional to the log plasma drug concentration within a therapeutic range, as shown in Fig. 22-6.

Mathematically, the relationship in Fig. 22-6 may be expressed by the following equation, where $m$ is the slope, $e$ is an extrapolated intercept, and $E$ is the drug effect at drug concentration $C$:

$$E = m\log C + e \qquad (22.1)$$

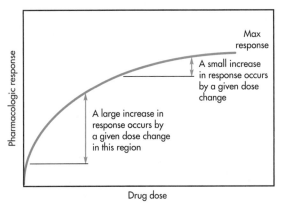

FIGURE 22-4 • A plot of pharmacologic response versus dose on a linear scale.

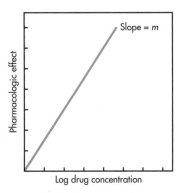

FIGURE 22-6 • Graph of log drug concentration versus pharmacologic response. Only the linear portion of the curve is shown.

Solving for log C yields

$$\log C = \frac{E - e}{m} \tag{22.2}$$

However, after an intravenous dose, the concentration of a drug in the body in a one-compartment open model is described as follows:

$$\log C = \log C_0 - \frac{kt}{2.3} \tag{22.3}$$

By substituting Equation 22.2 into Equation 22.3, we get Equation 21.4, where $E_0$ = effect at concentration $C_0$:

$$\frac{E - e}{m} = \frac{E_0 - e}{m} - \frac{kt}{2.3}$$

$$E = E_0 - \frac{kmt}{2.3} \tag{22.4}$$

The theoretical pharmacologic effect at any time after an intravenous dose of a drug may be calculated using Equation 22.4. Equation 22.4 predicts that the pharmacologic effect will decline linearly with time for a drug that follows a one-compartment model, with a linear log dose–pharmacologic response. From this equation, the pharmacologic effect declines with a slope of $k.m/2.3$. The decrease in pharmacologic effect is affected by both the elimination constant $k$ and the slope $m$. For a drug with a large $m$, the pharmacologic response declines rapidly, and multiple doses must be given at short intervals to maintain the pharmacologic effect.

The relationship between PK and pharmacologic response can be demonstrated by observing the percent depression of muscular activity after an IV dose of ± tubocurarine. The decline of pharmacologic effect is linear as a function of time (Fig. 22-7). For each dose and resulting pharmacologic response, the slope of each curve is the same. Because the values for each slope, which include $km$ (Equation 22.4), are the same, the sensitivity of the receptors for ± tubocurarine is assumed to be the same at each site of action. Note that a plot of the log concentration of drug versus time yields a straight line.

A second example of the pharmacologic effect declining linearly with time was observed with lysergic acid diethylamide (LSD) (Fig. 22-8). After an IV dose of the drug, log concentrations of drug

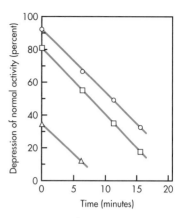

FIGURE 22-7 • Depression of normal muscle activity as a function of time after IV administration of 0.1–0.2 mg ± tubocurarine per kilogram to unanesthetized volunteers, presenting mean values of six experiments on five subjects. Circles represent head lift; squares, hand grip; and triangles, inspiratory flow. (Data from Johanson CE, Fischman MW. The pharmacology of cocaine related to its abuse, Pharmacol Rev. 1989 Mar;41(1):3–52.)

**A**

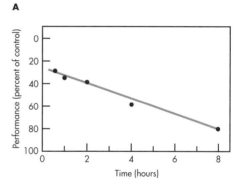

**B**

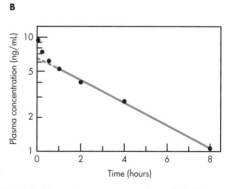

FIGURE 22-8 • Mean plasma concentrations of LSD (figure 22-8B) and performance test scores as a function of time (figure 22-8A) after IV administration of 2 μg LSD per kilogram to five normal human subjects. (Data from Aghajanian GK, Bing OH: Persistence of Lysergic Acid Diethylamide in the Plasma of Human Subjects, Clin Pharmacol Ther Sep-Oct 1964;5:611–614.)

decreased linearly with time except for a brief distribution period. Furthermore, the pharmacologic effect, as measured by the performance score of each subject, also declined linearly with time. Because the slope is governed in part by the elimination rate constant, the pharmacologic effect declines much more rapidly when the elimination rate constant is increased as a result of increased metabolism or renal excretion. Conversely, a longer pharmacologic response is experienced in patients when the drug has a longer half-life.

## RELATIONSHIP BETWEEN DOSE AND DURATION OF ACTIVITY ($t_{eff}$), SINGLE IV BOLUS INJECTION

The relationship between the duration of the pharmacologic effect and the dose can be inferred from Equation 22.3. After an intravenous dose, assuming a one-compartment model, the time needed for any drug to decline to a concentration $C$ is given by the following equation, assuming the drug takes effect immediately:

$$t = \frac{2.3(\log C_0 - \log C)}{k} \qquad (22.5)$$

Using $C_{eff}$ to represent the minimum effective drug concentration, the duration of drug action can be obtained as follows:

$$t_{eff} = \frac{2.3\left[\log\left(\dfrac{D_0}{V_D}\right) - \log C_{eff}\right]}{k} \qquad (22.6)$$

Some practical applications are suggested by this equation. For example, a doubling of the dose will not result in a doubling of the effective duration of pharmacologic action. On the other hand, a doubling of $t_{1/2}$ or a corresponding decrease in $k$ will result in a proportional increase in duration of action.

A clinical situation is often encountered in the treatment of infections in which $C_{eff}$ is the bactericidal concentration of the drug by prolonging its elimination $t_{1/2}$. Probenecid is a competitive inhibitor of organic anion transporter in the kidney and is used as a uricosuric agent in the treatment of chronic gout. Probenecid blocks the active secretion of penicillins and cephalosporins and has been used as an adjunct to enhance blood levels of these antibiotics (Cunningham et al, 1981). Probenecid can block the excretion of other drugs, such as methotrexate, thereby enhancing its toxicity.

## PRACTICE PROBLEM

The minimum effective concentration (MEC or $C_{eff}$) in plasma for an antibiotic is 0.1 $\mu g/mL$. The drug follows a one-compartment open model, has an apparent volume of distribution, $V_D$, of 10 L, and a first-order elimination rate constant of 1.0 h$^{-1}$.

**a.** What is the $t_{eff}$ after a single 100-mg IV bolus dose of this antibiotic?

**b.** What is the new $t_{eff}$ or $t'_{eff}$ for this drug if the dose were increased 10-fold, to 1000 mg?

### Solution

**a.** The $t_{eff}$ for a 100-mg dose is calculated as follows. Because $V_D = 10,000$ mL,

$$C_0 = \frac{100 \text{ mg}}{10,000 \text{ mL}} = 10 \ \mu g/mL$$

For a one-compartment-model IV dose, $C = C_0 e^{-kt}$. Then,

$$0.1 = 10e^{-(1.0)t_{eff}}$$
$$t_{eff} = 4.61 \text{ h}$$

**b.** The $t'_{eff}$ for a 1000-mg dose is calculated as follows (prime refers to a new dose). Because $V_D = 10,000$ mL,

$$C'_0 = \frac{1000 \text{ mg}}{10,000 \text{ mL}} = 100 \ \mu g/mL$$

and

$$C'_{eff} = C'_0 e^{-kt'_{eff}}$$
$$0.1 = 100e^{-(1.0)t'_{eff}}$$
$$t'_{eff} = 6.91 \text{ h}$$

The percent increase in $t_{eff}$ is therefore found as

$$\text{Percent increase in } t_{eff} = \frac{t'_{eff} - t_{eff}}{t_{eff}} \times 100$$

$$\text{Percent increase in } t_{\text{eff}} = \frac{6.91 - 4.61}{4.61} \times 100$$

Percent increase in $t_{\text{eff}} = 50\%$

This example shows that a 10-fold increase in the dose increases the duration of action of a drug ($t_{\text{eff}}$) by only 50%.

## EFFECT OF BOTH DOSE AND ELIMINATION HALF-LIFE ON THE DURATION OF ACTIVITY

After an IV bolus injection for a drug well characterized by a one-compartment model, a single equation can be derived to describe the relationship of dose ($D_0$) and the elimination half-life ($t_{1/2}$) on the effective time for therapeutic activity ($t_{\text{eff}}$). This expression is derived below:

$$\ln C_{\text{eff}} = \ln C_0 - kt_{\text{eff}}$$

Because $C_0 = D_0/V_D$,

$$\ln C_{\text{eff}} = \ln\left[\frac{D_0}{V_D}\right] - kt_{\text{eff}}$$

$$= \ln\left[\frac{D_0}{V_D}\right] - \ln C_{\text{eff}} \qquad (22.7)$$

$$= \frac{1}{k}\ln\left[\frac{\dfrac{D_0}{V_D}}{C_{\text{eff}}}\right]$$

Substituting $0.693/t_{1/2}$ for $k$,

$$= 1.44 t_{\frac{1}{2}}\ln\left(\frac{D_0}{V_D C_{\text{eff}}}\right) \qquad (22.8)$$

From Equation 22.8, an increase in $t_{1/2}$ will increase the $t_{\text{eff}}$ in direct proportion. However, an increase in the dose, $D_0$, does not increase the $t_{\text{eff}}$ in direct proportion. The effect of an increase in $V_D$ or $C_{\text{eff}}$ can be seen by using generated data. Only the positive solutions for Equation 21.8 are valid, although mathematically a negative $t_{\text{eff}}$ can be obtained by increasing $C_{\text{eff}}$ or $V_D$. The effect of changing dose on $t_{\text{eff}}$ is shown in Fig. 22-9 using data generated with Equation 21.8. A nonlinear increase in $t_{\text{eff}}$ is observed as dose increases.

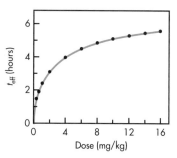

FIGURE 22-9 • Plot of $t_{\text{eff}}$ versus dose.

## EFFECT OF ELIMINATION HALF-LIFE ON DURATION OF ACTIVITY

Because elimination of drugs is due to the processes of excretion and metabolism, an alteration of any of these elimination processes will affect the $t_{1/2}$ of the drug. In certain disease states, pathophysiologic changes in hepatic or renal function will decrease the elimination of a drug, as observed by a prolonged $t_{1/2}$. This prolonged $t_{1/2}$ will lead to retention of the drug in the body, thereby increasing the duration of activity of the drug ($t_{\text{eff}}$) as well as increasing the possibility of drug toxicity.

As discussed, to improve antibiotic therapy with the penicillin and cephalosporin antibiotics, clinicians have intentionally prolonged the elimination of these drugs by giving a second drug, probenecid, which competitively inhibits renal excretion of the antibiotic. This approach to prolonging the duration of activity of antibiotics that are rapidly excreted through the kidney has been used successfully for a number of years. Similarly, Augmentin is a combination of amoxicillin and clavulanic acid; the latter is an inhibitor of $\beta$-lactamase. This $\beta$-lactamase is a bacterial enzyme that degrades penicillin-like drugs. The data in Table 22-2 illustrate how a change in the elimination $t_{1/2}$ will affect the $t_{\text{eff}}$ for a drug. For all doses, a 100% increase in the $t_{1/2}$ will result in a 100% increase in the $t_{\text{eff}}$. For example, for a drug whose $t_{1/2}$ is 0.75 hour and that is given at a dose of 2 mg/kg, the $t_{\text{eff}}$ is 3.24 hours. If the $t_{1/2}$ is increased to 1.5 hours, the $t_{\text{eff}}$ is increased to 6.48 hours, an increase of 100%. However, the effect of doubling the dose from 2 to 4 mg/kg (no change in elimination processes) will only increase the $t_{\text{eff}}$ to 3.98 hours, an increase of 22.8%. The effect of prolonging the elimination

**TABLE 22-2 •** Relationship between Elimination Half-Life and Duration of Activity

| Dose (mg/kg) | $t_{1/2} = 0.75$ h $t_{eff}$ (h) | $t_{1/2} = 1.5$ h $t_{eff}$ (h) |
|---|---|---|
| 2.0 | 3.24 | 6.48 |
| 3.0 | 3.67 | 7.35 |
| 4.0 | 3.98 | 7.97 |
| 5.0 | 4.22 | 8.45 |
| 6.0 | 4.42 | 8.84 |
| 7.0 | 4.59 | 9.18 |
| 8.0 | 4.73 | 9.47 |
| 9.0 | 4.86 | 9.72 |
| 10 | 4.97 | 9.95 |
| 11 | 5.08 | 10.2 |
| 12 | 5.17 | 10.3 |
| 13 | 5.26 | 10.5 |
| 14 | 5.34 | 10.7 |
| 15 | 5.41 | 10.8 |
| 16 | 5.48 | 11.0 |
| 17 | 5.55 | 11.1 |
| 18 | 5.61 | 11.2 |
| 19 | 5.67 | 11.3 |
| 20 | 5.72 | 11.4 |

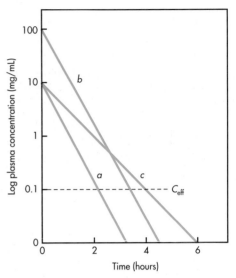

FIGURE 22-10 • Plasma level–time curves describing the relationship of both dose and elimination half-life on duration of drug action. $C_{eff}$ = effective concentration. Line $a$ = single 100 mg IV injection of drug; $k = 1.0$ h⁻¹. Line $b$ = single 1000 mg IV injection; $k = 1.0$ h⁻¹. Line $c$ = single 100 mg IV injection; $k = 0.5$ h⁻¹. $V_D$ is 10 L.

half-life has an extremely important effect on the treatment of infections, particularly in patients with high metabolism, or high clearance, of the antibiotic. Therefore, antibiotics must be dosed with full consideration of the effect of alteration of the $t_{1/2}$ on the $t_{eff}$. Consequently, a simple proportional increase in dose will leave the patient's blood concentration below the effective antibiotic level most of the time during drug therapy. The effect of a prolonged $t_{eff}$ is shown in lines $a$ and $c$ in Fig. 22-10, and the disproportionate increase in $t_{eff}$ as the dose is increased 10-fold is shown in lines $a$ and $b$.

## SUBSTANCE ABUSE POTENTIAL

The rate of drug absorption has been associated with the potential for substance abuse. Drugs taken by the oral route have the lowest abuse potential. For example, coca leaves containing cocaine alkaloid have been chewed by South American Indians for centuries (Johanson and Fischman, 1989). Cocaine abuse became a problem because of the availability of cocaine alkaloid ("crack" cocaine) and the use of other routes of drug administration (intravenous, intranasal, or smoking) that allow a very rapid rate of drug absorption and onset of action (Cone, 1995). Studies on diazepam (de Wit et al, 1993) and nicotine (Henningfield and Keenan, 1993) have shown that the rate of drug delivery correlates with the abuse liability of such drugs. Thus, the rate of drug absorption influences the abuse potential of these drugs. The route of drug administration that provides faster absorption and more rapid onset leads to greater abuse.

## DRUG TOLERANCE AND PHYSICAL DEPENDENCY

The study of drug tolerance and physical dependency is of particular interest in understanding the actions of abused drug substances, such as opiates and cocaine. *Drug tolerance* is a quantitative change in the sensitivity of the drug of the receptor site and is demonstrated by a decrease in PD effect after repeated exposure to the same drug. The degree of tolerance may vary greatly (Cox, 1990). Drug tolerance has been well described for organic nitrates, opioids, and other drugs. For example, the nitrates relax vascular smooth muscle and have been used for both acute angina (eg, nitroglycerin sublingual spray or transmucosal tablet) or angina prophylaxis (eg, nitroglycerin transdermal, oral controlled-release isosorbide dinitrate). Well-controlled clinical studies have shown that tolerance to the vascular and antianginal effects of nitrates may develop. For nitrate therapy, the use of a low nitrate or nitrate-free periods has been advocated as part of the therapeutic approach. The magnitude of drug tolerance is a function of both the dosage and the frequency of drug administration. Cross tolerance can occur for similar drugs that act on the same receptors. Tolerance does not develop uniformly to all the pharmacologic or toxic actions of the drug. For example, patients who show tolerance to the depressant activity of high doses of opiates will still exhibit "pinpoint" pupils and constipation.

The mechanism of drug tolerance may be due to (1) disposition or PK tolerance or (2) PD tolerance. PK tolerance is often due to enzyme induction (discussed in earlier chapters), in which the hepatic drug clearance increases with repeated drug exposure. PD tolerance is due to a cellular or receptor alteration in which the drug response is less than what is predicted in the patient given subsequent drug doses. Measurement of serum drug concentrations may differentiate between PK tolerance and PD tolerance.

Acute tolerance, or *tachyphylaxis*, which is the rapid development of tolerance, may occur due to a change in the sensitivity of the receptor or depletion of a cofactor after only a single or a few doses of the drug. Drugs that work indirectly by releasing norepinephrine may show tachyphylaxis. Drug tolerance should be differentiated from genetic factors which account for normal variability in the drug response.

*Physical dependency* is demonstrated by the appearance of withdrawal symptoms after cessation of the drug. Workers exposed to volatile organic nitrates in the workplace may initially develop headaches and dizziness followed by tolerance with continuous exposure. However, after leaving the workplace for a few days, the workers may demonstrate nitrate withdrawal symptoms. Factors that may affect drug dependency may include the dose or amount of drug used (intensity of drug effect), the duration of drug use (months, years, and peak use), and the total dose (amount of drug × duration). The appearance of withdrawal symptoms may be abruptly precipitated in opiate-dependent subjects by the administration of naloxone (Suboxone®), an opioid antagonist that has no agonist properties.

---

**FREQUENCY ASKED QUESTION**

▶ How does the rate of systemic drug absorption affect the abuse potential of drugs such as cocaine or heroin?

---

## HYPERSENSITIVITY AND ADVERSE RESPONSE

Many drug responses, such as hypersensitivity and allergic responses, are not fully explained by PD and PK. Some penicillin-sensitive patients may respond to threshold skin concentrations, but otherwise no dose–response relationship has been established. Skin eruption is a common symptom of drug allergy. Allergic reactions can occur at extremely low drug concentrations. Some urticaria episodes in patients have been traced to penicillin contamination in food or to penicillin contamination during dispensing or manufacturing of other drugs. A patient's allergic reactions are important data that must be recorded in the patient's profile along with other adverse reactions. Penicillin allergic reaction in the population is often detected by skin test with benzylpenicilloyl polylysine (PPL). The incidence of penicillin allergic reaction occurs in about 1%–10% of patients. The majority of these reactions are minor cutaneous reactions such as urticaria, angioedema, and pruritus. Serious allergic reactions such as anaphylaxis are rare, with an incidence of 0.021%–0.106% for penicillins (Lin, 1992). For cephalosporins, the incidence of anaphylactic reaction is less than 0.02%. Anaphylactic reaction for cefaclor was reported to be 0.001% in a postmarketing survey. There are emerging trends showing that there may be a difference between the original and the new generations of cephalosporins (Anne and Reisman 1995). Cross-sensitivity to similar chemical classes of drugs can occur.

Allergic reactions may be immediate or delayed and have been related to IgE mechanisms. In β-lactam (penicillin) drug allergy, immediate reactions occur in about 30 to 60 minutes, but either a delayed reaction or accelerated reaction may occur from 1 to 72 hours after administration. Anaphylactic reaction may occur in both groups. Although some early evidence of cross-hypersensitivity between penicillin and cephalosporin was observed, the incidence in patients sensitive to penicillin shows only a 2-fold increase in sensitivity to cephalosporin compared with that of the general population. The report rationalized that it is safe to administer cephalosporin to penicillin-sensitive patients and that the penicillin skin test is not useful in identifying patients who are allergic to cephalosporin, because of the low incidence of cross-reactivity (Anne and Reisman 1995). In practice, the clinician should evaluate the risk of drug allergy against the choice of alternative medication. Some earlier reports showed that cross-sensitivity between penicillin and cephalosporin was due to the presence of trace penicillin present in cephalosporin products.

## BIOLOGICAL MARKERS (BIOMARKERS)

As described previously, the interaction of the drug with the receptor results in a cascade of events ultimately leading to a PD response. The PD response measured could be a biomarker level, which could be linked to a clinical endpoint. This section provides an overview of biomarkers and surrogate endpoints and their application in drug development and clinical practice.

*Biomarkers* are a set of parameters that can be measured quantitatively to represent a healthy or a pathological process within the body. A biomarker could be a simple physical measurement like blood pressure or a biochemical endpoint such as blood glucose. Biomarkers can be applied to complex situations that involve genomic markers such as Taq1B polymorphism in the cholesteryl ester transfer protein (*CETP*) gene that code for cholesterol

ester transfer protein (Kuivenhoven et al, 1998), or the *HER2* (a tyrosine kinase that is a member of the epidermal growth factor receptor (EGFR) family) expression in metastatic breast cancer (Shak, 1999). Lesko and Atkinson (2001) have proposed a working definition of a biological marker, referring to a biological marker as a physical sign or laboratory measurement that occurs in association with a pathological process and that has putative diagnostic and/or prognostic utility.

Biomarkers can accelerate clinical drug development by fostering informed decision making, by bridging preclinical mechanistic studies and empirical clinical trials. Some examples, where use of biomarkers leads to accelerated drug development are described below. For example, the number of bone fractures is considered as a primary response variable for approving drugs to treat osteoporosis. Clinical trials are typically lengthy and hence very costly. To approve a different dosing regimen for drugs such as alendronate, which was approved based on number of fractures as the primary endpoint, the changes in the bone mineral density could be utilized as a biomarker for drug approval. Bone mineral density is relatively simpler and easier to measure and hence shorter and less costly clinical trials are required. For example, aminobisphosphonate, risedronate 5 mg once daily (Proctor and Gamble, 2000) was approved based on fracture as the endpoint. Subsequently, 35 mg once weekly and two 75-mg tablets monthly were approved based on changes in bone mineral density.

Along similar lines, if we assume that the progression of disease and treatment intervention is similar among adult and child populations, then drug approvals in the pediatric population can be based on PK studies (exposure) and/or biomarker data. For example, sotalol (a β-blocker) that was approved for ventricular tachycardia in adults using atrial fibrillation and flutter as endpoints was approved in the pediatric population based on a PK study and its effect on QTc and heart rate (Gobburu, 2009).

Besides bridging preclinical and clinical phases of development, biomarkers can be used as (1) a diagnostic tool to detect and diagnose disease conditions in patients (eg, elevated blood glucose levels are indicative of onset of diabetes mellitus), (2) as a tool for the staging of disease (eg, levels of prostate-specific antigen concentration in blood that is correlated to tumor growth and metastasis), (3) indicator of disease prognosis (anatomically measuring size of tumors), and (4) as a predictive and monitoring tool to assess the extent of clinical response to a therapeutic intervention (eg, measuring blood cholesterol as a means to assess cardiac disease or viral load used to assess the efficacy of an antiviral therapy) (Biomarkers Definitions Working Group, 2001).

A *surrogate endpoint* is a biomarker that is intended to substitute a clinically meaningful endpoint. Thus, a surrogate endpoint is expected to predict the presence or absence of clinical benefit or harm based on epidemiologic, therapeutic, pathophysiologic, or other forms of scientific evidence (Lesko and Atkinson, 2001). In a way, surrogate endpoints are a subset of biomarkers. However, not all biomarkers can achieve the status of a surrogate endpoint. A clinical endpoint relates to a clinically meaningful measure of how a patient feels, functions, or survives (Strimbu and Tavel, 2010). Blood pressure is a well-studied surrogate that correlates well with the cardiovascular health of the individual. Elevated blood pressure (also called hypertension) is known to be a direct cause of stroke, heart failure, renal failure, and accelerated coronary artery disease, and lowering blood pressure can lead to reduction in the rates of morbidity and mortality outcomes (Temple, 1999).

An example where a surrogate endpoint that has created immense interest is the CD4$^+$ count in the treatment of AIDS and HIV infections (Weiss and Mazade, 1990). The surrogate endpoints not only reduce the overall cost of the trial but also allow shorter follow-up periods than would be possible during clinical endpoint studies.

Among the successes of surrogate endpoints in predicting clinical outcomes, certain failures of perceived surrogate endpoints not predicting meaningful clinical outcomes have created doubts about whether surrogate markers should be the principal driver for making decisions for drug approvals (Colburn, 2000). To this context, one of many examples where surrogate endpoints have been proven to mislead clinical outcomes, posing greater threat to health and safety of thousands of patients, was in the Cardiac Arrhythmia Suppression Trial (CAST). In this trial, three antiarrhythmic drugs—flecainide, encainide, and moricizine—were compared to placebo treatment in patients with myocardial infarction who frequently experienced premature ventricular contractions where sudden death was considered a primary outcome. Although these drugs were successful in suppressing arrhythmias, they were responsible for increasing the risk of death from other causes (Echt et al, 1991). In this case, the surrogate endpoint "arrhythmia" was unable to capture the effect of the treatment on the true outcome, "death," of the treatment.

In the drug development process, the rationale of introducing a biomarker or surrogate endpoint should begin as early as possible, typically as a receptor- or enzyme-based high-throughput screening rationale during the preclinical phases. As newer technologies develop through genomics and proteomics, these existing biomarkers would evolve further as correct clinical targets get identified. The ability of a surrogate endpoint to predict clinical outcome is only as good as the intermediate bridge that is developed to link the surrogate to the clinical endpoint. If the mechanism of drug action to efficacy and toxicity are thoroughly studied, the surrogate endpoints would be predictive of clinical outcomes. Examples of biomarkers described in Table 22-3 that substitute for specific clinical endpoints may differ from one another in their predictive ability; nonetheless, their clinical utility cannot be underestimated.

---

### FREQUENTLY ASKED QUESTIONS

▶ What is a drug receptor?

▶ Explain why a drug that binds to a receptor may be an agonist, a partial agonist, or an antagonist?

▶ If we need to develop a drug where only 25% of maximal activation is needed to achieve therapeutic benefit, what type of agent among the four classes will you pick and why?

▶ What are the utilities of biomarkers besides being used as a bridging tool to link preclinical and clinical drug development?

**TABLE 22-3 •** Examples of Biomarkers/Surrogate Endpoints and Their Respective Clinical Endpoints

| Therapeutic Class | Biomarker/Surrogate | Clinical Endpoint |
|---|---|---|
| **Physiological Markers** | | |
| Antihypertensive drugs | Reduce blood pressure | Reduce stroke |
| Drugs for glaucoma | Reduce intraocular pressure | Preservation of vision |
| Drugs for Osteoporosis | Increase bone density | Reduce fracture rate |
| Antiarrhythmic drugs | Reduce arrhythmias | Increase survival |
| **Laboratory Markers** | | |
| Antibiotics | Negative culture | Clinical cure |
| Antiretroviral drugs | Increase CD4 counts and reduce viral RNA | Increase survival |
| Antidiabetic drugs | Reduce blood glucose | Reduce morbidity |
| Lipid-lowering drugs | Reduce cholesterol | Reduce coronary artery disease |
| Drugs for prostate cancer | Reduce prostate-specific antigen | Tumor response |

*Adapted with permission from Atkinson AJJ: Physiological and Laboratory Markers of Drug Effect. New York, NY: Academic Press; 2001.*

## TYPES OF PHARMACODYNAMIC RESPONSE

PD responses can be continuous, discrete (categorical), and time-to-event outcomes. Continuous PD responses can take any value in a range such as blood glucose levels, blood pressure readings, or enzyme levels. Categorical or discrete responses are either binary (eg, death or no death) or ordinal (eg, graded pain scores or counts over a time period, such as number of seizures in a month). Time-to-event outcomes constitute continuous measures of time but with censoring (eg, time to relapse or time until transplant). In this chapter, we will deal with continuous PD responses only.

### Components of PK–PD models

The use of mathematical modeling to link the PK of the drug to the time course of drug effects (PD) has evolved greatly since the pioneering work of Gerhard Levy in the mid-1960s (Levy 1964; Levy 1966). Today, PK–PD modeling is a scientific discipline in its own right, which characterizes the PK of a drug and relates PK to the PD. This PK–PD relationship is then applied for predictions of the response under new conditions (eg, new dose or dosing regimen). For any PK–PD model, the conceptual framework of the relationship is depicted in Fig. 22-11 (Jusko et al, 1995; Mager et al, 2003). The scheme describes that there may be at least four intermediary components between drug in plasma ($C_p$) and the measured response ($R$).

The first component of the PK–PD framework is the administration of the drug and the time course of drug in the relevant biological fluid (plasma, $C_p$). The drug is eliminated from the body depending on its disposition kinetics. The plasma drug concentration–time profile is typically represented by a PK model or function given as:

$$C_p = f(\theta_{PK}, X, t) \qquad (22.9)$$

The PK model or function can be thought of as a one-compartment model after an intravenous bolus administration, described as

$$C_p = \frac{\text{Dose}}{V_D} \cdot e^{-\frac{CL}{V_D} \cdot t} \qquad (22.10)$$

$\theta_{PK}$ denotes the fundamental PK parameters; namely, clearance ($CL$) and volume of distribution ($V_D$); $X$ refers to the subject variables such as dose or dosing regimen, and $t$ is the time. The drug

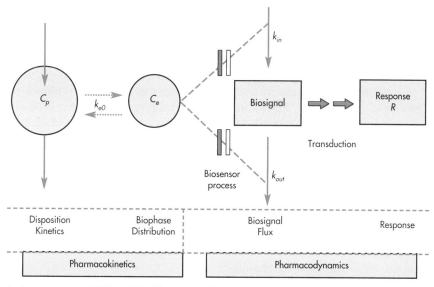

**FIGURE 22-11** • Basic components of PD models of drug action. (Reproduced with permission from Jusko WJ, Ko HC, Ebling WF. Convergence of direct and indirect pharmacodynamic response models, J Pharmacokinet Biopharm 1995 Feb;23(1):5–8.)

concentration in plasma then distributes to the site of action or the effect site, referred to as biophase drug concentration, $C_e$. The plasma drug concentration, $C_p$, can be tested, for example, to be proportional to the biophase concentration by linking it to the effect. Additionally, if it does not appear to be proportional or in equilibrium with the effect, then an effect compartment can be used, where $C_e$ would exist, and the distribution of the drug to the effect site could be governed by a very slow rate constant going in and a rate constant going out, called $k_{e0}$. The effect site or the biophase concentrations then serve as the driving function responsible for pharmacodynamic response, $R$, by influencing the production or degradation of the biosignal. The formation rate constant for the biosignal is denoted as $k_{in}$ and the degradation rate constant is denoted as $k_{out}$. Analogous to PK Equation 22.9 above, the time course of response, is described by a mathematical function as:

$$R = f(\theta_{PD}, C_p \text{ or } C_e, Z) \quad (22.11)$$

The mathematical function can be thought of as an equation linking the pharmacodynamic response to the drug concentrations. Here, $\theta_{PD}$ represents the fundamental pharmacodynamic parameters, namely maximum effect, $E_{max}$, and potency of the drug, $EC_{50}$, which is described in detail in later sections; $C_p$ and

$C_e$ are the concentrations of the drug in plasma or at the biophase, and $Z$ represents a vector of drug-independent system parameters. As seen from Fig. 22-11, the effect site concentrations affect formation or degradation of the biosignal via a biosensor process, and further undergo a transduction process to elicit the response. Thus, biosignal can be considered as a biomarker and is related to clinical endpoint or the response. Depending on the nature of the experiment, either only data on the biosignal are measured, or both biosignals, and the clinical outcome information may be available. In a typical situation, it might not be possible to capture all components of PK–PD framework; rather, the manifestation of the response will depend on which of the processes dominate the overall response. For example, there are three rate constants involved, namely $k_{e0}$ which controls the distribution of the drug concentration between plasma and the biophase, and $k_{in}$ and $k_{out}$, which are formation and degradation rate constants of the biosignal, and the role of these three rate constants may influence the type of the PK–PD relationship. When the biophase distribution represents a rate-limiting step (ie, $k_{e0}$) is slow compared to $k_{in}$ or $k_{out}$ for drugs in producing their response, a distributional delay or a link compartment model is used to explain the PK–PD relationship. The drug elicits a direct response but there is a delay in the response due to distributional delay in the drug to reach the biophase. Alternatively, if the distribution of the drug to effect site is very fast, then the process involving the formation or degradation of the biosignal may take over. Such instances occur when the drug acts via an indirect mechanism and the biosensor process (depicted in Fig. 22-11) may stimulate or inhibit the production or degradation of the biosignal. In such a case, an indirect response model is used to describe the PK–PD relationship. The biosensor process involves interaction between the drug and the pharmacological target and can be explained by the receptor theory.

In summary, the conceptual PK–PD framework is broadly applicable to various drugs with different mechanisms of action, and the final PK–PD model chosen should encompass the principles of pharmacology of the drug and the system. The various PD models described in this section are dealt with in detail, with examples in the following sections.

## Pharmacodynamic Models

PD models involve complex mechanisms that may not be easily simplified. Researchers have employed empirical, semi-mechanistic, or mechanistic models to explain the complex mechanisms of drug action. The predictive ability of empiric models might be limited under new scenarios such as new dose or dosing regimen. The understanding of drug response is greatly enhanced when PK modeling techniques are combined with clinical pharmacology, resulting in the development of mechanism-based PK–PD models. In this section, we will explore in detail different types of PD models with examples.

## Noncompartmental PK–PD Models

Under this approach, PK parameters like peak plasma drug concentrations ($C_{max}$), area under the curve (AUC), and half-life ($t_{1/2}$) are often correlated to PD parameters such as half maximal inhibitory concentration ($IC_{50}$). Such PK–PD relationship has been applied successfully among antimicrobials where the minimum inhibitory concentration (MIC) is often the PD parameter. The PK parameters $C_{max}$, AUC, and $t_{1/2}$ are considered because they are often influenced by the choice of drug or by the manner in which the antibiotics are administered

(route and dosing regimen). Large doses of antibiotics administered via intravenous route can produce high $C_{max}$, whereas a large AUC can be achieved by administering a large dose that has a relatively longer plasma half-life or by multiple dosing. A longer half-life drug will persist in the plasma for an extended period of time compared to a drug with shorter half-life. Thus, the manner by which these PK parameters relate to the MIC of the infecting pathogen becomes a key factor to the observed effect. Hence, the MIC is then designated to play an important role as a PD parameter. Usually, the PK parameters $C_{max}$ and AUC are divided by the MIC, yielding PK–PD indices—namely $C_{max}$/MIC and AUC/MIC (or AUIC)—whereas time over which drug concentrations remain above its MIC is another PK–PD index referred to as T>MIC. Better predictions of clinical efficacy using PK–PD indices can be sought if protein binding is adequately factored into these considerations, as the therapeutic effect of a drug is often produced by the free fraction of the drug rather than the total drug concentrations in plasma. The most relevant drug concentrations are the free drug concentrations at the site of action. Antibiotics that distribute into the interstitial fluid may have much lower tissue concentrations compared to plasma drug concentrations (Lorentzen et al, 1996). Figure 22-12 shows the three MIC-based PK–PD indices for a hypothetical antimicrobial drug.

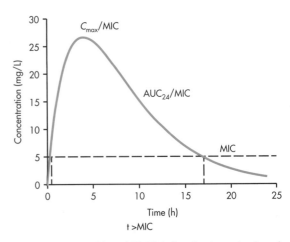

FIGURE 22-12 • MIC based PK–PD indices for the evaluation of a hypothetical anti-infective agent. MIC, minimum inhibitory concentrations; PD, pharmacodynamics; PK, pharmacokinetics.

Now let us understand what these indices really are and how they relate to the two distinct patterns associated with killing of antimicrobials (Craig, 2002); viz: (1) concentration-dependent and (2) time-dependent killing patterns.

*Concentration-dependent* killing pattern is associated with a *higher rate and extent* of killing with increasing concentrations of the antibiotic drug above the MIC of the pathogen. Hence, drugs that follow this pattern can maximize killing by maximizing their systemic drug exposure that is often represented by peak plasma drug concentration ($C_{max}$) and the extent of exposure (AUC). The $C_{max}$/MIC ratio relates to the efficacy of drugs that exhibit a concentration-dependent killing pattern. Figure 22-13 shows a plot of colony-forming units (CFUs) against three PK–PD indices: AUC/MIC ratio, $C_{max}$/MIC ratio, and time above MIC in a mouse infection model where an infection in the thigh due to *Streptococcus pneumoniae* was treated with temafloxacin (Craig, 2002). It was interesting to note that there was no correlation between CFU/thigh and the percentage of time the drug levels exceeded the MIC in the serum. However, an excellent relationship was evident between CFU/thigh and the AUC/MIC ratio followed by $C_{max}$/MIC. The AUC/MIC and $C_{max}$/MIC

ratios have been the PK–PD indices that often well correlate with the therapeutic efficacy of aminoglycoside and fluoroquinolone antimicrobials. Most often the AUC/MIC ratio shows a better correlation to efficacy compared to the $C_{max}$/MIC ratio. However, the latter index may be more relevant and thus is important where there is a significant risk of emergence of a resistant microbial subpopulation.

*Time-dependent* killing produces higher systemic concentrations beyond a threshold value or MIC, and does not cause a proportional increase in the killing rate of the microbes. In fact, the killing proceeds at a *zero-order rate* when systemic drug concentrations are above the MIC for its pathogen and under such conditions, a minimal correlation is expected between $C_{max}$/MIC and the pathogen survival rates. However, the PK–PD index that would most likely correlate to the killing would be the %T>MIC, which is the percentage of time within the dosing interval during which the systemic drug concentrations remain above the MIC of the drug for the pathogen. In contrast to aminoglycosides and fluoroquinolones, all β-lactam antibiotics and macrolides (Vogelman et al, 1988; Craig, 1995) follow a time-dependent bactericidal activity. To illustrate this killing pattern, Craig (1995) studied the activity

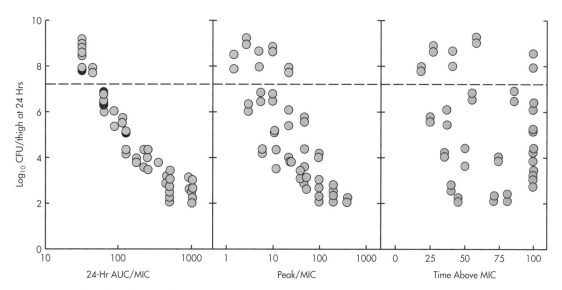

FIGURE 22-13 • Relationship between three PD parameters (24-h AUC/MIC ratio, $C_{max}$/MIC ratio and percentage of time that serum levels exceed above MIC) and the number of *S. pneumoniae* ATCC 10813 in the thighs of neutropenic mice after 24 h of therapy with temafloxacin. Each point represents one data for one mouse. The dotted line reflects the number of bacteria at the time of therapy initiation.

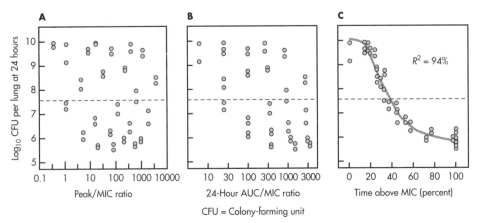

CFU = Colony-forming unit

**FIGURE 22-14** • Relationship between three PD parameters ($C_{max}$/MIC ratio, 24-h AUC/MIC ratio and percentage of time that serum levels exceed above MIC) and the number of *K. pneumoniae* ATCC 43816 in the lungs of neutropenic mice after 24 h of therapy with cefotaxime. Each point represents one mouse. Animals were infected by a 45-min aerosol given 14 h prior to therapy. The dotted line reflects the number of bacteria at the time of therapy initiation (7.5 $\log_{10}$ colony forming units (CFU)/lung. The $R^2$ value in (**C**) represents the percentage of variation in bacterial numbers than could be attributed to differences in time above MIC. (Reproduced with permission from Craig WA. Interrelationship between pharmacokinetics and pharmacodynamics in determining dosage regimens for broad-spectrum cephalosporins, Diagn Microbiol Infect Dis. 1995 May-Jun;22(1–2):89–96.)

of cefotaxime against the standard strain of *Klebsiella pneumoniae* in the lungs of a neutropenic mouse model. In this study, pairs of mice were treated with multiple-dose regimens that varied by the dose and the dosing interval (ie, a 500-mg single oral dose, 250 mg bid, 125 mg qid, and so on). Lungs were assessed for remaining CFUs after 24 h of therapy and the PK–PD indices $C_{max}$/MIC, AUC/MIC, and %T>MIC were determined for each dosing regimen. Figure 22-14 parts A and B showed a poor relationship between the CFU per lung and the $C_{max}$/MIC, AUC/MIC ratios. A highly significant correlation between the CFU remaining per lung and the duration of time that serum levels were above the MIC (%T>MIC) was evident. Thus, depending upon the type of antimicrobial, there would be one PK–PD index that would be highly correlated with its antimicrobial efficacy. It may be worth considering that percent time above MIC could be enhanced by dose fractionation such that the total daily dose remains constant. Table 22-4 illustrates some of the specific PK–PD indices that correlate with efficacy in the animal infection models for different class of antimicrobials.

### $E_{max}$ Drug-Concentration Effect Model

*Receptor occupancy theory* forms the basis of pharmacodynamic response evaluation and is routinely employed to describe concentration–effect/exposure–response relationship in drug discovery and development. The origins of the fundamental PD models can be derived using the receptor occupancy theory. The theory and derivation are described in detail as follows.

In general, as the drug is absorbed, one or more drug molecules may interact with a receptor to form

**TABLE 22-4** • PK–PD Indices Determining the efficacy for Different Antimicrobials

| PK–PD Index | Antimicrobial |
| --- | --- |
| % Time above MIC | Penicillins, cephalosporins, aztreonam, carbapenems, tribactams, macrolides, clindamycin, oxazolidinones, flucytosine, Vancomycin |
| Peak/MIC ratio | Aminoglycosides, fluoroquinolones, daptomycin, amphotericin B |
| AUC/MIC ratio | Aminoglycosides, fluoroquinolones, daptomycin, ketolides, Quinupristin/dalfopristin,* tetracyclines, fluconazole |

*Quinupristin and dalfopristin are approved for use as a combination product.

a complex that in turn elicits a pharmacodynamic response.

$$R + C \leftrightarrow RC \qquad (22.12)$$

The rate of change of the drug–receptor ($RC$) complex is given by the following equation:

$$\frac{d[RC]}{dt} = k_{on} \cdot (R_T - RC) \cdot C - k_{off} \cdot RC \qquad (22.13)$$

where $R_T$ is the maximum receptor density, $C$ is the concentration of the drug at the site of action, $k_{on}$ is the second-order association rate constant, and $k_{off}$ is the first-order dissociation rate constant. The term $(R_T - RC)$ represents the free receptors, $R$ available as the total number of receptors or the maximum receptor density can be written as $R_T = R + RC$. Under equilibrium conditions, ie, when $\frac{d[RC]}{dt} = 0$, the above equation becomes:

$$k_{on} \cdot (R_T - RC) \cdot C = k_{off} \cdot RC \qquad (22.14)$$

Upon further rearrangement, we get:

$$k_{on} \cdot R_T \cdot C = RC \cdot (k_{on} \cdot C + k_{off}) \qquad (22.15)$$

$$RC = \frac{k_{on} \cdot R_T \cdot C}{k_{off} + k_{on} \cdot C} \qquad (22.16)$$

$$RC = \frac{R_T \cdot C}{\frac{k_{off}}{k_{on}} + C} \qquad (22.17)$$

$$RC = \frac{R_T \cdot C}{K_D + C} \qquad (22.18)$$

where $K_D$ is the equilibrium dissociation constant $\left(\frac{k_{off}}{k_{on}}\right)$. Under the assumption that the magnitude of effect, $E$, is proportional to the $[RC]$ complex, the fraction of maximum possible effect, $E_{max}$, is equal to the fractional occupancy, $f_b = \frac{E}{E_{max}}$, of the receptor, which can be described as

$$f_b = \frac{E}{E_{max}} = \frac{[RC]}{R_T} \qquad (22.19)$$

Hence,

$$E = E_{max} \cdot \frac{\frac{R_T \cdot C}{K_D + C}}{R_T} \qquad (22.20)$$

$$E = \frac{E_{max} \cdot C}{k_D + C} \qquad (22.21)$$

Here, $K_D$ has the units of concentration and represents the concentration at which 50% of $E_{max}$ is achieved. Substituting $K_D = EC_{50}$ yields the classical $E_{max}$ concentration–effect relationship as below:

$$E = \frac{E_{max} \cdot C}{EC_{50} + C} \qquad (22.22)$$

$E_{max}$ refers to the maximum possible effect that can be produced by a drug and $EC_{50}$ is the sensitivity parameter or the potency parameter representing the drug concentration producing 50% of $E_{max}$. As the fundamental PK parameters of a drug are clearance ($CL$) and volume of distribution ($V_D$), $E_{max}$ and $EC_{50}$ are the fundamental PD parameters for a drug, and hence they define the pharmacodynamic properties of the drug. From Equation 22.22, it can be inferred that the typical effect–concentration relationship is curvilinear, as shown in Fig. 22-15 with parameters as $E_{max} = 100$ and $EC_{50} = 50\ \mu g/mL$.

The Hill equation, or the sigmoidal $E_{max}$ model, contains an additional parameter, typically represented as $\gamma$ and called the Hill coefficient. The sigmoidal $E_{max}$ model is shown in Equation 21.23.

$$E = \frac{E_{max} \cdot C^\gamma}{EC_{50}^\gamma + C^\gamma} \qquad (22.23)$$

The *Hill coefficient*, $\gamma$ (or the slope term) describes the steepness of the effect–concentration relationship. Some researchers also describe $\gamma$ as the

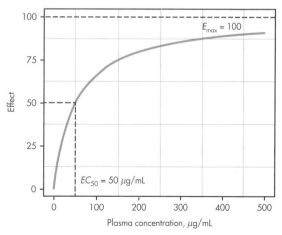

FIGURE 22-15 • The $E_{max}$ concentration–effect relationship. Fifty percent of the maximum effect is achieved at the $EC_{50}$ concentration.

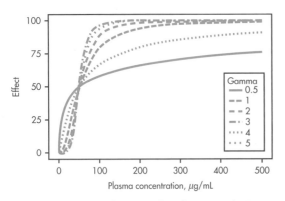

FIGURE 22-16 • Effect of varying Hill coefficients on the $E_{max}$ concentration–effect relationship.

number of drug molecules binding to a receptor. When more drug molecules bind (typically γ > 5) to the receptor, the effect–concentration relationship is very steep. Figure 22-16 shows the sigmoidal $E_{max}$ model for different Hill coefficient values. As seen from Fig. 22-16, values of γ less than or equal to unity have broader slopes, and as γ increases, the steepness of the relationship increases with values of γ > 4, signifying an all-or-none response. The utility of the Hill coefficient in model building is an empirical approach to provide improved model fit for the data. However, the value of the Hill coefficient potentially is from its real application in terms treatment adherence. For example, if a drug has a steep concentration effect relationship, then missing a dose can have greater impact on the response for a subject as compared to a drug for which the Hill coefficient is around unity. Examples of drugs where an $E_{max}$ model was used to describe the PK–PD relationships are discussed in detail in a later section of this chapter on direct effect models.

## Linear Concentration Effect Model

The linear concentration effect model is based on the assumption that the effect ($E$) is proportional to the drug concentration, typically the plasma drug concentration ($C$). This model can be derived from the $E_{max}$ model under the conditions that drug concentration ($C$) << $EC_{50}$, reducing Equation 22.23 to the following:

$$E = S \cdot C \qquad (22.24)$$

where mathematically $S$ is defined as the slope of linear concentration–effect relationship line (Holford and Sheiner, 1981). Pharmacodynamically, $S$ is the effect produced by one unit of drug concentration. This relationship can be observed visually in Fig. 22-15, when the concentration is << $EC_{50}$, the concentration–effect (C-E) follows approximately linear relationship. This model assumes that effect will continue to increase as the drug concentration is increased, although as we know there is always a maximal pharmacological effect ($E_{max}$) beyond which increasing drug concentrations does not yield further increase in the effect. Also, the C-E relationship is seldom linear over a broad range of drug concentrations. Thus, this simple model has limited application in PD modeling. Nonetheless, a specific PD effect where linear C-E model is utilized extensively is in evaluation of drug effects on cardiac repolarization (as measured by QT interval from an electrocardiogram) in humans (Garnett et al, 2008; Russell et al, 2008; Florian et al, 2011). Linear C-E model has been applied to describe the concentration–QTc relationship for moxifloxacin (Florian et al, 2011) as shown in Fig. 22-17, and also applied for modeling the concentration–QTc relationship for new drugs under development. The concentration–QTc relationship and analysis have played key role in the US FDA regulatory review of new drugs for pro-arrhythmic risk evaluation (Garnett et al, 2008).

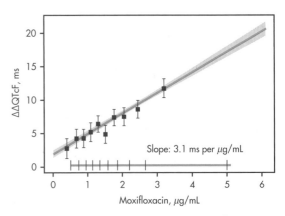

FIGURE 22-17 • ΔΔQTcF versus concentration predictions with 90% confidence interval (CI). Data points depict quantile means ± 90% CI. Decile ranges are displayed along with x-axis.

## Log-Linear Concentration–Effect Model

The log-linear model is based on the assumption that effect is proportional to the log of drug concentration and can be described as:

$$E = S \cdot \log C + E_0 \qquad (22.25)$$

where $S$ is same as that described for the linear concentration–effect model previously and $E_0$ is the baseline effect. This model is also a special case of $E_{max}$ model, as the log $C$ versus effect follow a nearly linear relationship between 20% and 80% of $E_{max}$ (Meibohm and Derendorf, 1997). The limitation of this model is that it cannot predict effect when drug concentrations are zero or the maximal effect ($E_{max}$). This model has been used to describe concentration–effect relationship for (1) synthesis rate of prothrombin complex activity in relation to warfarin plasma concentrations (Nagashima et al, 1969) and (2) propranolol concentration and reduction of exercise-induced tachycardia (Coltart and Hamer, 1970) (Fig. 22-18).

## Additive and Proportional Drug Effect Models

The fundamental $E_{max}$ model (Equation 22.22) or the linear effect model (Equation 22.24) signify that when the drug concentration is not present, then there is no effect. But there often exists a baseline response, which implies that even when the drug

is not present, there exists a baseline response. The effect of baseline can be additive or proportional to the drug effect, leading to additive or proportional drug response model.

### Additive Drug Effect Model

When a drug exhibits an additive drug effect, it implies that the drug response is independent of the baseline as represented by the equation below:

$$R(t) = R(0) + E \qquad (22.26)$$

where $R(t)$ is the drug response at time $t$, $R(0)$ is the response at baseline or time $= 0$ and $E$ represents the drug effect, which could be linear as in Equation 21.27, or $E_{max}$ type of relationship as shown in Equation 21.28 below:

Additive linear drug effect model: $R(t) = R(0) + S \cdot C$
$$\qquad (22.27)$$

Additive $E_{max}$ drug effect model: $R(t) = R(0) + \frac{E_{max} \cdot C}{EC_{50} + C}$
$$\qquad (22.28)$$

Here, $C$ is the plasma concentration at any time $t$. The interpretation of $E_{max}$ is the maximal drug effect that can be obtained and has the same units as the response. Based on the equations above, it can be inferred that there is a constant baseline response added to the drug effect. In this case, the drug effect is independent of the baseline response. The baseline response in mathematical terms can be considered similar to an intercept term. The additive drug effect for the linear and the $E_{max}$ drug effect model, where the slope is positive, is shown in Fig. 22-19. The slopes for the different baseline responses remain the same. Depending on whether it is a stimulatory (positive slope: $S > 0$ or $E_{max} > 0$) or an inhibitory effect (negative slope: $S < 0$ or $E_{max} < 0$), the graphs have an increasing or a decreasing trend with increasing concentrations.

## EXERCISE

*Using Excel, create the graph for a linear effect model with a slope of −0.3 at three different baseline values. Similarly, for $E_{max}$ model with negative $E_{max}$ value, inhibitory.*

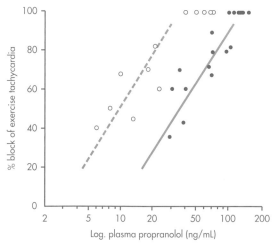

FIGURE 22-18 • Log plasma concentration/response relationship for orally administered (○) and intravenously administered (•) propranolol.

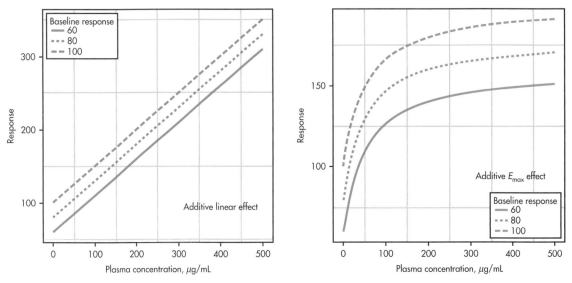

FIGURE 22-19 • Additive drug effect (linear and $E_{max}$) upon varying baseline values. For the linear effect model, $S = 0.5$ units was used. For the $E_{max}$ model, the drug effect parameters are $E_{max} = 100$ units and $EC_{50} = 50$ µg/mL.

**Application:** An example where an additive $E_{max}$ effect model is used to explain the PK–PD relationship of activated plasma thromboplastin time (aPTT) to argatroban concentrations (Madabushi et al, 2011). Argatroban is a synthetic thrombin inhibitor and is approved in the United States to be used for prophylaxis or as anticoagulant therapy for adult subjects with heparin-induced thrombocytopenia (HIT). Initially, there were no dosing recommendations for argatroban in pediatric subjects with HIT and dosing was often extrapolated from adult dose. Madabushi et al used PK (argatroban concentrations) and PD (aPTT) data from healthy adults and pediatric patients to derive dosing recommendations of argatroban in pediatric subjects with HIT. They used a direct additive $E_{max}$ model to describe the argatroban concentrations–aPTT relationship as shown below:

$$aPTT\ (t, \text{seconds}) = aPTT\ (t = 0, \text{seconds})$$

$$+ \frac{E_{max}(\text{seconds}) \cdot C}{EC_{50} + C} \quad (22.29)$$

The argatroban concentration producing 50% of maximal aPTT response ($EC_{50}$) was estimated as 959 ng/mL, the maximal aPTT response from baseline ($E_{max}$) was estimated as 84.4 seconds, and the baseline aPTT response is estimated at 32 seconds as evident in Fig. 22-20. The article also considered different subject specific factors, such as hepatic status, that might explain the variability seen in the data, which is beyond the scope of this chapter. The PK–PD relationship developed was used for simulations based on which pediatric dosing recommendations was derived and is currently available in argatroban label (http://www.accessdata.fda.gov/drugsatfda_docs/label/2014/020883s016lbl.pdf, accessed September 29, 2019, Section 8.4).

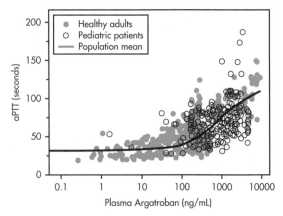

FIGURE 22-20 • Predicted Argatroban plasma concentration–aPTT relationship. Filled circles, healthy adults; open circles, pediatric patients.

## Proportional Drug Effect Model

As the name suggests, the response at any time depends proportionally on the baseline response. If the baseline response is higher, depending on whether we have stimulatory or inhibitory drug effect, a greater stimulation or inhibition can be expected. The general form of a proportional drug effect model is given as:

$$R(t) = R(0) \cdot (1 + E) \qquad (22.30)$$

where $R(t)$ is the drug response at time $t$, $R(0)$ is the response at baseline or time $= 0$, and $E$ represents the drug effect, which could be linear or $E_{max}$ type of relationship, as shown below:

Proportional linear drug effect model (stimulatory)

$$R(t) = R(0) \cdot (1 + S \cdot C) \qquad (22.31)$$

Proportional $E_{max}$ drug effect model (stimulatory)

$$R(t) = R(0) \cdot \left( 1 + \frac{S_{max} \cdot C}{SC_{50} + C} \right) \qquad (22.32)$$

Proportional $E_{max}$ drug effect model (inhibitory)

$$R(t) = R(0) \cdot \left( 1 - \frac{I_{max} \cdot C}{IC_{50} + C} \right) \qquad (22.33)$$

where $C$ is the plasma concentration of the drug at time $t$. However, the interpretation of $S_{max}$ or $I_{max}$ is different from that of an additive effect model. They represent fractional stimulation or inhibition from the baseline response, which may be considered as a proportional change (increase or decrease) of the response from baseline and hence a unit-less quantity. The drug concentrations at which 50% of $S_{max}$ or $I_{max}$ is obtained refers to $SC_{50}$ and $IC_{50}$, respectively, and have the units of concentration. The proportional drug effect for three different baseline values of a response is depicted in Fig. 22-20.

As seen in Fig. 22-21, the response is dependent on the baseline value, with a steeper decrease for the largest baseline as compared to small baseline. For both linear (proportional increase) and the inhibitory $I_{max}$ effect, for a baseline of 150 units, the decrease in response is much higher as compared to the baseline value of 60 units, but the fractional decrease from the baseline value is the same. For example, let us consider the graph on the right in Fig. 22-21, with the baseline value as 150 and 60. When baseline is 150 units, the response decreased to 95 units upon increase in drug concentrations, whereas when baseline was 60 units, the maximum inhibitory response in the presence of drug reaches 38 units. Thus, the absolute difference in the response is 55 units for higher baseline and 22 units for lower baseline, whereas the fractional decrease

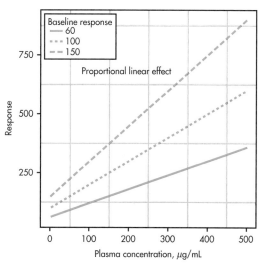

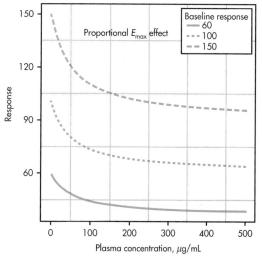

FIGURE 22-21 • Proportional drug effect (linear and $E_{max}$) model upon varying baseline values. For the linear effect, a proportional increase of 0.01 ($S = 0.01$) was used and for the $I_{max}$ effect model, the value of $I_{max} = 0.40$ (40% decrease from baseline).

in response $(I_{max})$ is $\frac{150-95}{150} = 0.37$ for the higher baseline and $\frac{60-38}{60} = 0.37$ for the lower baseline. Hence, the general expression for $I_{max} = \frac{R_0 - R_{min}}{R_0}$, where $R_0$ is the response at time, $t = 0$ or at baseline, and $R_{min}$ is the maximum inhibitory response.

The same argument can be applied when there is a stimulatory effect on the baseline. Typically, such a proportional drug effect model is employed for a drug wherever baseline response plays an important role (eg, blood pressure–lowering drugs).

The model descriptions so far have dealt with the different types of the drug concentration–effect relationships (eg, linear, $E_{max}$, additive drug effect, proportional drug effect). As described in Figure 22-11 (conceptual PK–PD model), the site at which the concentration–effect relationship drives the PD process leads to further PD models that are used for describing the different mechanisms by which the drug acts. For this section, the notation "$C_p$" is used to refer to plasma concentrations of the drug.

## Direct Effect Model

When the distribution of the drug to the site of action is very rapid and when the drug elicits the response by a direct mechanism (no biosensor process involved), then a model directly linking the concentration to the drug response can be used. Such a model is referred to as a *direct effect model*. The direct effect model could be linearly related to concentrations or via an $E_{max}$ model as shown in Fig. 22-22. The time course of plasma concentrations and the time course of effect will be in parallel to each other. The argatroban example discussed previously is an example of a direct effect where the argatroban

plasma concentrations were directly related to aPTT response via an $E_{max}$ model.

## Effect Compartment or Link model

Some drugs may produce a delayed pharmacologic response that may not directly parallel the time course of the plasma drug concentration. The maximum pharmacologic response produced by the drug may be observed after the plasma drug concentration has peaked. In such cases, the drug distribution to the site of action or biophase may represent a rate-limiting step for drugs to elicit the biological response. The delay could be caused due to convection transport and diffusion processes that deliver the drug to the site of action. To describe the delay in effect, Sheiner et al proposed a hypothetical effect compartment as a mathematical link between the time course of plasma concentrations and the PD effect (Sheiner et al, 1979). The effect compartment models account for this delay by representing it as an additional compartment between the plasma concentration and the effect defined by a first-order rate constant, $k_{e0}$, that dictates the disappearance of the effect. A slightly different model is shown in Fig. 22-23, where $k_{e0}$ is presented as a bidirectional clearance between the plasma and the theoretical effect compartment. The hypothetical effect site concentration is represented as $C_e$. The equilibrium rate constant, $k_{e0}$ accounts for the delay in the drug concentrations reaching the effect site or the biophase, and therefore the time course of concentration at the effect site mimic the time course of the pharmacodynamic effect. The effect compartment model is also called a distributional delay model or a link model, since the effect site concentrations now are linked to the PD effect.

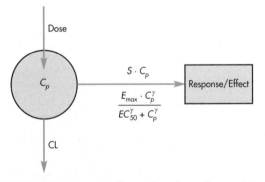

FIGURE 22-22 • Schematic diagram for a direct effect model.

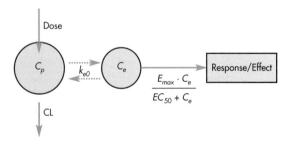

FIGURE 22-23 • Schematic diagram for effect compartment model.

One of the important assumptions in this model is that the amount of drug entering the hypothetical effect compartment is considered negligible and hence need not be reflected in the PK of the drug. The rate of change of drug concentration at the effect site is then given as:

$$\frac{dC_e}{dt} = k_{e0} \cdot (C_p - C_e) \qquad (22.34)$$

The effect site concentration, $C_e$, profile is governed by the plasma concentration, $C_p$, and the equilibration rate constant, $k_{e0}$. A large value of $k_{e0}$ versus the drug CL would imply that the effect site concentrations closely follow the plasma concentration profile and the effect compartment is rapidly equilibrating, whereas a smaller $k_{e0}$ value versus the CL would signify that the effect compartment equilibrates slowly with $C_e$ profile and hence the effect is delayed as compared to $C_p$. The effect is then linked to the effect site concentrations typically via a $E_{max}$ model as:

$$E = \frac{E_{max} \cdot C_e}{EC_{50} + C_e} \qquad (22.35)$$

Figure 22-24 depicts the $C_p$, $C_e$ and the response profile for a hypothetical drug with two different $k_{e0}$ values. As seen from the figure, the $C_e$ profile mimics

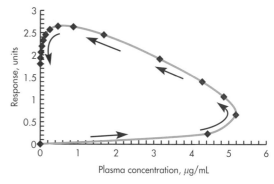

FIGURE 22-25 • Anti-clockwise loop (hysteresis) to describe the temporal difference between PK and PD.

the time course of PD and the delay between the PK and PD is accounted by the equilibration clearance $k_{e0}$. When there is a temporal difference between the PK and the PD, and when time-matched response and plasma concentrations are plotted, the plot depicts a *hysteresis* loop which is anticlockwise in nature as seen in Fig. 22-25. Another feature of the effect compartment models are though the peak effects will be delayed relative to plasma concentrations, the times at which peak $C_e$ occurs and hence the peak effect occurs is dose independent. Another type of time-dependent pharmacologic response

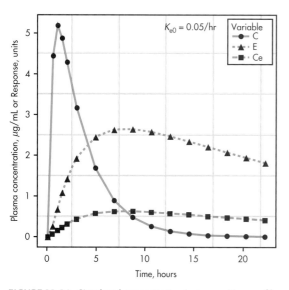

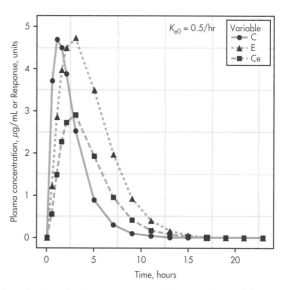

FIGURE 22-24 • Simulated concentration/response time profiles obtained using effect compartment model to describe the influence of $k_{e0}$: distributional delay rate constant. C, plasma concentration; $C_e$, concentrations at the hypothetical effect site; E, drug effect. Drug concentrations from a one-compartment model is used to derive the effect using the effect compartment model, with $E_{max} = 20$ units, $EC_{50} = 4 \, \mu g/mL$.

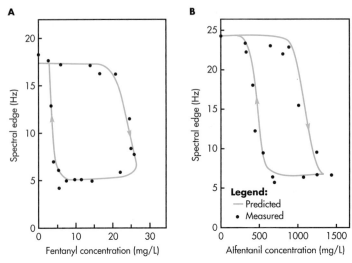

FIGURE 22-26 • Response of the EEG spectral edge to changing fentanyl (**A**) and alfentanil (**B**) serum concentrations. Plots are data from single patients after rapid drug infusion. Time is indicated by arrows. The clockwise loop (proteresis) indicates a significant time lag between blood and effect site. Spectral edge frequency (Hz) in the figure represents the depth of anesthesia.

may occur due to development of tolerance, induced metabolite deactivation, reduced response or translocation of receptors at the site of action. This type of time-dependent pharmacological response is characterized by a clockwise profile (called *proteresis*) when the pharmacological response is plotted versus the plasma drug concentration over time (Fig. 22-26). Drugs like fentanyl (lipid soluble, opioid anesthetic) and alfentanyl (an analog of fentanyl) display a *proteresis loop* apparently due to lipid partitioning effect of these drugs. Similarly, euphoria produced by cocaine also displayed a clockwise profile when responses were plotted versus plasma cocaine concentration (Fig. 22-27).

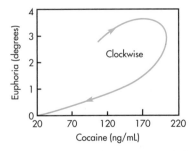

FIGURE 22-27 • Clockwise loop (*proteresis*) typical of tolerance is seen after intranasal administration of cocaine when related to degree of euphoria experienced in volunteers.

**Application:** An early example in which an effect compartment model is to describe the PK–PD relationship is to compare the PD effects of midazolam and diazepam using a surrogate measure for psychomotor performance (Mould et al, 1995). In the study, the PK and PD of midazolam and diazepam were compared after two intravenous infusions of 0.03 and 0.07 mg/kg of midazolam and 0.1 mg/kg and 0.2 mg/kg of diazepam on four occasions in healthy adults. The Digit Symbol Substitution Test (DSST), a neuropsychological test often used to study associative learning, was used as the pharmacodynamic response as it was thought to be a more sensitive measure for drug-induced changes in psychomotor performances than an electroencephalogram (EEG). Plasma concentrations of diazepam and midazolam, and DSST were measured at different times up to 180 minutes. The authors described the PK-DSST relationship using an effect compartment model with additive baseline effect, as there was a slight delay in the PD effect as compared the plasma concentrations of the drugs. The estimated distributional delay half-life $\left(t_{\frac{1}{2}} - k_{e0}\right)$ of midazolam was 3.2 minutes, and 1.2 minutes for diazepam. The use of effect compartment model was able to collapse the temporal difference between the PK and DSST as seen from the hysteresis plots in a representative subject (Figs. 22-28

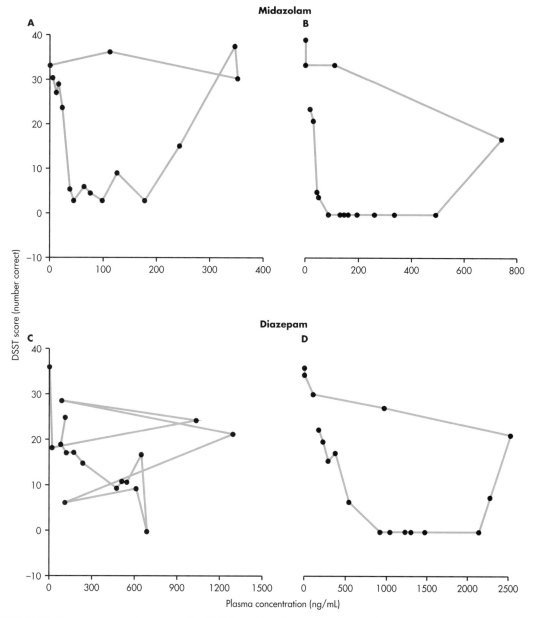

FIGURE 22-28 • Plasma concentration versus effect (DSST score) in subject 6 after 0.03 mg/kg midazolam (a), 0.07 mg/kg midazolam (b), 0.1 mg/kg diazepam (c), and 0.2 mg/kg diazepam (d).

and 22-29). Based on this analysis, the authors were able to confirm the fact that midazolam has a delayed onset of peak effect and the potency of midazolam was 6 times higher than that of diazepam. Moreover, the use of DSST as a surrogate measure instead of EEG was supported by this analysis.

### Indirect Response Models

When the pharmacological response is seen immediately in parallel to the plasma drug concentrations, pharmacodynamic models such a linear model, $E_{max}$ model or a sigmoid $E_{max}$ models are used to model PK–PD relationship. When there is a delay in the

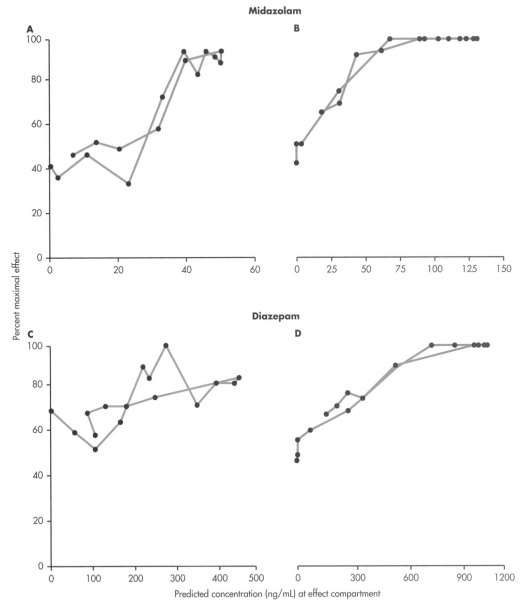

**FIGURE 22-29 •** Percent maximal effect versus predicted concentration at the effect site after determination of $K_{eo}$ and collapse of hysteresis loop in subject 6 after 0.03 mg/kg midazolam (a), 0.07 mg/kg midazolam (b), 0.1 mg/kg diazepam (c), and 0.2 mg/kg diazepam (d).

pharmacological response as compared to the drug concentrations, an *effect compartment* or the link model is used. The use of an effect compartment model is justified when the delay in the pharmacodynamic response can be attributed to the distribution of the drug to the effect site characterized by a hypothetical effect compartment. The equilibrium between the plasma and the effect site is characterized by the equilibration rate constant as described under "effect compartment or link model."

Many drugs, however, exhibit pharmacological response via an indirect mechanism. The drugs

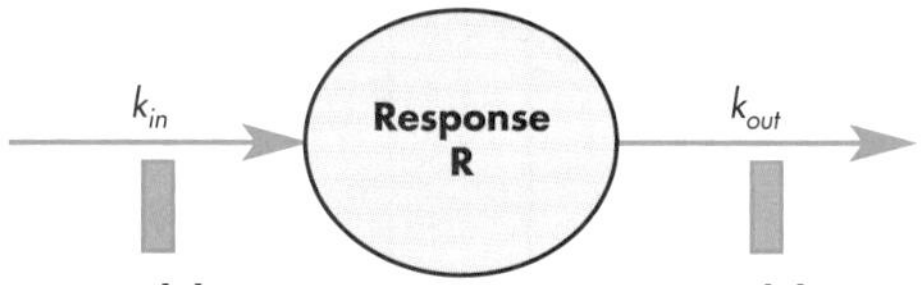


**Model I**

$$\frac{dR}{dt} = k_{in} \cdot \left(1 - \frac{I_{max} \cdot C_p}{IC_{50} + C_p}\right) - k_{out} \cdot R$$

**Model II**

$$\frac{dR}{dt} = k_{in} - k_{out} \cdot \left(1 - \frac{I_{max} \cdot C_p}{IC_{50} + C_p}\right) \cdot R$$

$$0 < I_{max} \leq 1$$

FIGURE 22-30 • Schematic diagram for basic indirect response Models I and II. In Model I, the drug inhibits the production of response. In Model II, the drug inhibits the degradation of the response.

might induce their effects not by direct interaction with the receptors, but rather the interaction with receptors might affect the production or degradation of an endogenous compound and the subsequent response is mediated by those substances. The earliest reference to a PK–PD model using an indirect mechanism of action for a drug was described for the anticoagulant effect of warfarin (Nagashima et al, 1969). A systematic modeling approach for characterizing diverse types of indirect response models in to four basic models was described by Sharma and Jusko (1996). The context where the use of an indirect response model may arise was briefly explained in the section on conceptual PK–PD framework. The characteristics of four basic indirect response models which are most commonly used are described in detail.

The four basic indirect response models arise when the factors controlling the input or production ($k_{in}$) of the response variable is either stimulated or inhibited, or the loss or degradation ($k_{out}$) of an endogenous compound or the response variable is either stimulated or inhibited. The rate of change of a response variable in the *absence of the drug* is given as

$$\frac{dR}{dt} = k_{in} - k_{out} \cdot R \tag{22.36}$$

where, $k_{in}$ represents the zero-order production rate constant of the response and $k_{out}$ represents the first-order degradation rate constant of the response variable. It is assumed that $k_{in}$ and $k_{out}$ fully account for the production and degradation of the response. In the presence of the drug, inhibition of $k_{in}$ or $k_{out}$ by the drug concentration gives rise to the Model I and Model II, and stimulation of $k_{in}$ or $k_{out}$ in the presence of drug leads to Model III and Model IV. Model I is the inhibition of $k_{in}$ and Model II is the inhibition of $k_{out}$ as shown in Fig. 22-30.

### *Inhibition of Production of Response, $k_{in}$ (Model I) and Inhibition of Degradation of Response, $k_{out}$ (Model II)*

The rate of change of response in model I is described as:

$$\frac{dR}{dt} = k_{in} \cdot (1 - E) - k_{out} \cdot R \tag{22.37}$$

and the rate of change of response in model II is explained by:

$$\frac{dR}{dt} = k_{in} - k_{out} \cdot (1 - E) \cdot R \tag{22.38}$$

where the inhibitory action of the drug is given by $E = \frac{I_{max} \cdot C_p}{IC_{50} + C_p}$. Here, $C_p$ represents the plasma concentration of the drug as a function of time, $I_{max}$ refers to the maximal fractional inhibition of production or degradation of the response by the drug and is always takes value between 0 and 1 ($0 < I_{max} \leq 1$), $IC_{50}$ is the plasma concentration producing 50% of the maximal inhibition achieved at the effect site. Since stationarity is assumed for all models, in the absence of drug at steady state, $\frac{dR}{dt} = 0$, hence

$$k_{in} = k_{out} \cdot R_0 \tag{22.39}$$

Thus, the response variable, *R*, begins at predetermined baseline value, $R_0$, changes with drug concentrations, and returns to the baseline value. This assumption further reduces the number of functional parameters in the models described above. When the plasma drug concentrations are very high, ie, at steady state ($C_p >> IC_{50}$), the value of $IC_{50}$ is insignificant and

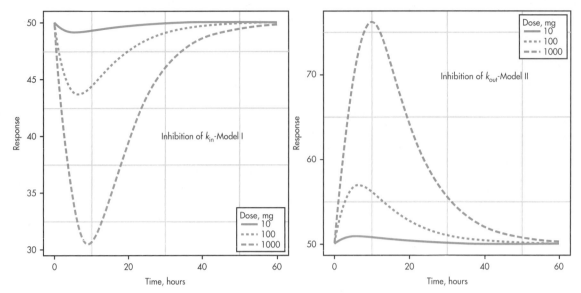

FIGURE 22-31 • Simulated response profiles for Model I and Model II. Three intravenous doses were used, and plasma concentrations follow a one-compartment model. The PD parameters used are $k_{in} = 5$ mg/hr; $k_{out} = 0.1$/hr $I_{max} = 5$; $IC_{50} = 10$ mg/L or $\mu$g/mL.

when $I_{max} = 1$, then the value of $E = 1$ ($C_p$ cancels out), and hence complete inhibition of production of the response variable occurs in Model I.

Later, when drug concentrations reduce to low values $C_p << IC_{50}$, the value of $E = 0$, and hence the production of the response variable will return to $k_{in}$ and the PD system returns to its baseline value, $R_o$. The same concept is applicable to inhibition of the $k_{out}$ model, wherein when the drug concentrations are much higher, there is complete blockade of degradation of the response variable and there is a build of response to its maximum and as concentrations decrease, the system returns to it baseline response. The response profiles for Model I and Model II at three different doses of the drug are shown in Fig. 22-31.

### Stimulation of Production of Response $k_{in}$ (Model III) and Stimulation of Degradation of Response $k_{out}$ (Model IV)

Model III and Model IV represent the stimulation of factors that control the production ($k_{in}$) and dissipation ($k_{out}$) of the drug response, respectively, as shown in Fig. 22-32.

The rate of change of drug response in Model III is given as:

$$\frac{dR}{dt} = k_{in} \cdot (1 + E) - k_{out} \cdot R \qquad (22.40)$$

whereas in Model IV, the differential equation corresponds to

$$\frac{dR}{dt} = k_{in} - k_{out} \cdot (1 + E) \cdot R \qquad (22.41)$$

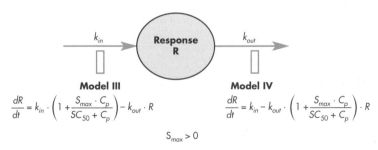

$$\text{Model III}$$
$$\frac{dR}{dt} = k_{in} \cdot \left(1 + \frac{S_{max} \cdot C_p}{SC_{50} + C_p}\right) - k_{out} \cdot R$$

$$\text{Model IV}$$
$$\frac{dR}{dt} = k_{in} - k_{out} \cdot \left(1 + \frac{S_{max} \cdot C_p}{SC_{50} + C_p}\right) \cdot R$$

$$S_{max} > 0$$

FIGURE 22-32 • Schematic diagram for basic indirect response Models III and IV. In Model III, the drug stimulates the production of response. In Model IV, the drug stimulates the degradation of the response.

Here, the drug effect, $E$, is described as $E = \frac{S_{max} \cdot C_p}{SC_{50} + C_p}$, providing a stimulatory effect for the factors controlling the response. $S_{max}$ refers to the maximal fractional stimulation of production or degradation of the response by the drug and it always has a value greater than 0 ($S_{max} > 0$), and $SC_{50}$ plasma concentration producing 50% of the maximal stimulation achieved at the effect site. As described in the inhibitory models, in the absence of drug, the drug response is at its baseline value as expressed in Equation 21.40. As drug concentrations becomes much higher ($C_p \gg SC_{50}$) there is maximal buildup of response (Model III) based on the value of $S_{max}$, and as drug concentrations decrease, the response returns to its baseline value. In the case of Model IV, the steady-state concentrations of the drug produce maximal stimulation of the loss of factors controlling the drug response. The response profiles for Model III and Model IV at three different doses of the drug are shown in Fig. 22-33.

In general, the characteristics of the four basic indirect response models can be summarized as follows:

1. There is a delay in the maximal PD response ($R_{max}$) as compared to the peak plasma concentrations of the drug ($C_{max}$), which is attributed to the indirect mechanism by which the drug acts.

2. The response time profiles show a slow decline or rise in the response variable to a maximum value ($R_{max}$) dictated by the steady-state concentrations of the drug followed by a gradual return to baseline conditions $\left(\frac{k_{in}}{k_{out}} \text{ or } R_0\right)$ as drug concentrations decline below $IC_{50}$ or $SC_{50}$ values.

3. Typically, the initial rate of decline or rise in the response profiles is governed by $k_{out}$, independent of dose. The gradual return to baseline after $R_{max}$ is reached is governed by both $k_{in}$ and the elimination rate constant of the drug $\left(k_{el} = \frac{CL}{V_D}\right)$.

4. The time to peak pharmacodynamic response ($t_{R_{max}}$) occurs at later times for larger doses owing to the increased duration of the plasma drug concentrations above $IC_{50}$ or $SC_{50}$ values.

Complete reviews of the basic properties of these models and the application of these models for different drugs are described in the literature (Jusko and Ko, 1994; Sharma and Jusko, 1998). Two applications of the indirect response models in the context of drug development are described here.

**Application:** Indirect response models have been used in the context of making decisions on dosing recommendations or selection of drug candidates early in the drug development process. A physiologic indirect response model was developed to

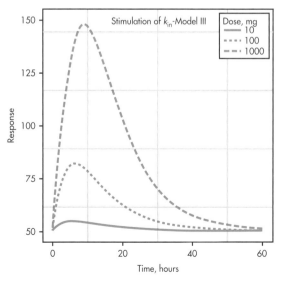
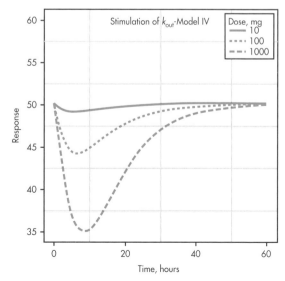

FIGURE 22-33 • Simulated response profiles for Model III and Model IV. Three intravenous doses were used, and plasma concentrations follow a one-compartment model. The PD parameters used are $k_{in} = 5$ mg/hr; $k_{out} = 0.1$/hr; $S_{max} = 5$; $SC_{50} = 10$ mg/L or µg/mL.

characterize the time course of the flare area (cm²) after oral administration of single ascending doses of mizolastine, a new $H_1$-receptor antagonist in healthy volunteers (Nieforth et al, 1996). The *in vivo* test in which histamine induced skin wheal and flare reactions is inhibited by $H_1$-receptor antagonist is considered a predictive test for demonstrating the clinical anti-allergic activity of investigative $H_1$-receptor antagonists. In this study, mizolastine was orally administered to healthy volunteers at four different doses (5, 10, 15, and 20 mg), including placebo. The pharmacodynamic response was measured in terms of histamine induced flare area (cm²) and wheal area (cm²) at different time points until 24 hours after administration of the mizolastine. A PK–PD model was developed to predict the mizolastine PD and further use the model for prediction purposes. The authors used an indirect response model to describe the flare area response over time considering inhibition of the production of histamine (Model I) in the presence of mizolastine concentrations as given below.

$$\frac{d\text{Flare}_{\text{area}}}{dt} = k_{\text{in}} \cdot \left(1 - \frac{I_{\text{max}} \cdot C}{IC_{50} + C}\right) - k_{\text{out}} \cdot \text{Flare}_{\text{area}} \quad (21.42)$$

where $C$ refers to the plasma mizolastine concentrations, $\text{Flare}_{\text{area}}$ refers to the area of the histamine induced flare on the skin, $I_{\text{max}}$ is the maximum fractional inhibition $(k_{\text{in}})$ of production of histamine response indicated by area of flare, $IC_{50}$ is the plasma concentration of mizolastine producing 50% of the $I_{\text{max}}$, and $k_{\text{out}}$ is the first-order rate constant for the flare disappearance. The PK–PD model provided adequate fit of the data, as seen in Fig. 22-34. As seen in Fig. 22-34, there is a dose-dependent inhibition in the flare area with inhibition sustained at higher doses, which is indicative of the indirect mechanism of action of the drug. The authors reported 92% maximal inhibition $(I_{\text{max}})$ of flare area by the drug with 50% of the maximal inhibition $(IC_{50})$ obtained at 21 ng/mL of mizolastine.

Another application of an indirect response model is in deciding the dosing regimen for abatacept, a recombinant soluble fusion protein, used in the treatment of rheumatoid arthritis (RA) (Roy et al, 2007). The pharmacodynamic response to abatacept was measured in terms of a biomarker, interleukin-6

(IL-6), as abatacept causes reduction of IL-6 levels, and increased IL-6 levels are indicated in RA disease pathology. The authors utilized data from Phase II and Phase III studies of abatacept (at doses 2 mg/kg and 10 mg/kg) to characterize the abatacept–IL-6 suppression relationship and to predict IL-6 suppressions at different doses not studied in clinical studies by clinical trial simulations. An indirect response model where there is stimulation of IL-6 degradation (Model IV) was used to describe the abatacept–IL-6 relationship as shown below

$$\frac{dC_{\text{IL6}}}{dt} = k_{\text{in}} - k_{\text{out}} \cdot \left(1 + \frac{S_{\text{max}} \cdot C_{\text{p}}}{SC_{50} + C_{\text{p}}}\right) \cdot C_{\text{IL6}} \quad (22.43)$$

where $C_{\text{IL6}}$ represents serum IL-6 concentrations. The developed PK–PD model adequately described the IL-6 data, and further simulations using the model at doses unstudied in the clinical studies revealed that the studied 10 mg/kg doses produced increased suppression over 2 mg/kg dose (Fig. 22-35), but doses higher than 10 mg/kg did not offer any additional therapeutic benefit and hence the PK–PD analysis and simulations supported the recommended abatacept doses studied in the clinical trials.

---

### FREQUENTLY ASKED QUESTIONS

▶ Explain why the log-linear model cannot be used to determine effect when concentration is zero. Describe which simple model could be used in such situation.

▶ Explain why doubling the dose of a drug may not double the pharmacodynamic effect of the drug.

▶ What is meant by a hysteresis loop? Why do some drugs follow a clockwise loop (hysteresis) and others follow a counterclockwise loop (proteresis)?

▶ When is an effect compartment model used? How does the effect compartment differ from pharmacokinetic compartmental model, such as the central compartment and the peripheral (tissue) compartment?

---

### Systems Pharmacodynamic Models

The field of PK–PD modeling has made tremendous progress over the last two decades, in progressing

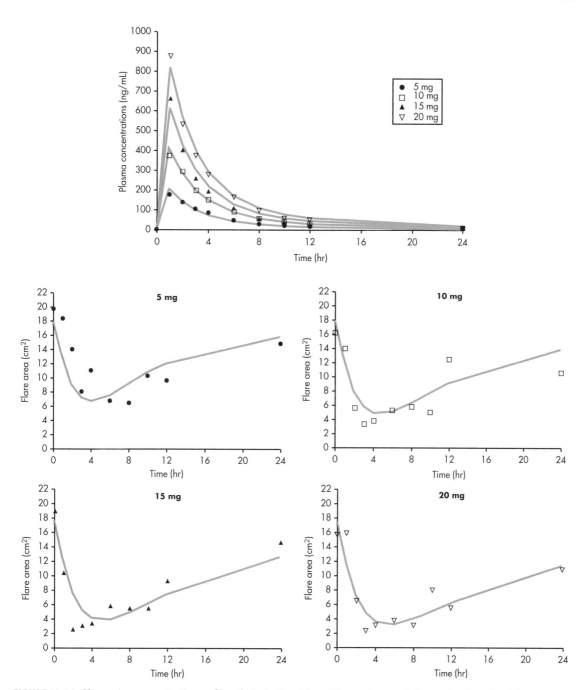

**FIGURE 22-34** • Plasma time concentration profiles of mizolastine at four different doses and observed and predicted flare area–time course profiles after oral administration of 5, 10, 15, and 20 mg of mizolastine. An indirect response model with inhibition of production of response (Model I) was used to predict the flare area responses.

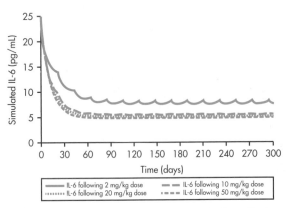

FIGURE 22-35 • Simulated average serum interleukin-6 (IL-6) concentrations versus time by abatacept dose. Simulated median IL-6 concentrations over time for 2 mg/kg abatacept (solid line), 10 mg/kg abatacept (long dashed line), 20 mg/kg abatacept (intermediate dashed line), and 50 mg/kg abatacept (short dashed line).

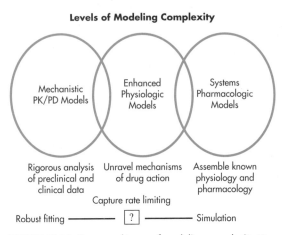

FIGURE 22-36 • Range and types of modeling complexity at three modeling levels of quantitative and systems pharmacology (QSP).

from empirical PK–PD models to mechanism-based PK–PD models. Although mechanistic PK–PD modeling incorporates drug–receptor interaction and/or physiology, these models still focus on the specific subsystem of physiology which is impacted by the drug. Systems PD models aim to incorporate all known and understood biological processes that control body events into the model (Jusko, 2013). These models capture a multitude of processes via mathematical equations, incorporating homeostasis as well as feedback mechanisms that are hallmarks of a complex biological system. Thus, systems pharmacology models represent probably the most complex models in the area of PK–PD modeling. The greatest advantage of systems models is that they can be used to assess the impact of perturbing one process on the overall biological system under consideration. The challenge that remains with the systems model includes a multitude of mathematical equations, functions, and parameter values for each step of the biological process. In the interim, models that are more mature than the mechanism-based PK–PD model but somewhat less than the complete systems pharmacology models are being employed, as depicted by the following Fig. 22-36.

This hybrid approach was utilized by Earp et al's, 2008 PK–PD model for dexamethasone effects in rat model of collagen-induced arthritis as shown in Fig. 22-37.

## PK–PD Models and Their Role in Drug Approval and Labeling

The impact of PK–PD modeling in regulatory decision-making has increased. The US FDA has been utilizing PK–PD modeling and simulation for drug approval as well as labeling related decisions (Bhattaram et al, 2005, 2007). To illustrate the role of PK–PD in regulatory decision making and approval, two examples from approved drugs are described through two cases.

### Case 1: Nesiritide

Case 1 demonstrates how PK–PD modeling and simulation can be applied to learn from an existing set of clinical trials results and design future clinical trials with greater probability of success, which in this example resulted in the approval of a drug by the FDA (Bhattaram et al, 2005). Nesiritide (Natrecor®), a recombinant human brain natriuretic peptide was being developed for the treatment of acute decompensated congestive heart failure (CHF). The new drug application (NDA) for nesiritide was rejected after review by the FDA in April 1999 on the basis that at a given dose, (1) the desired maximal effect (change in pulmonary capillary wedge pressure [PCWP], which is used to diagnose the severity of left ventricular failure) was not achieved instantaneously and (2) the PCWP could not be achieved without the undesired effect of hypotension. The FDA

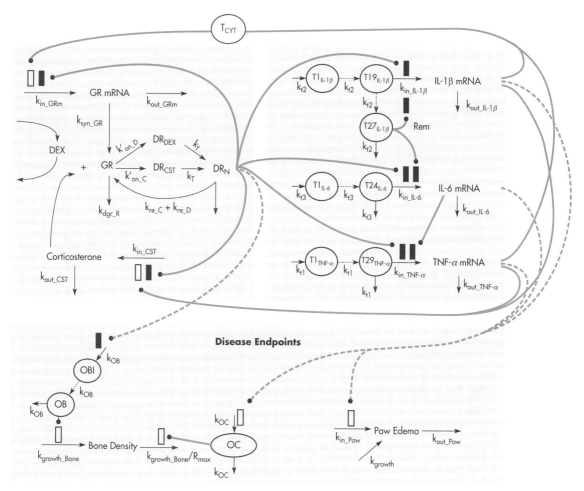

**FIGURE 22-37** • Model schematic for corticosteroid and cytokine inter-regulation during arthritis progression. Lines with arrows indicate conversion to or turnover of the indicated responses. Lines ending in closed circles indicate an effect is being exerted by the connected factors.

recommended the sponsor to optimize the nesiritide dosing regimen that would result in instantaneous effect on PCWP (benefit) and minimize hypotension (risk). As part of the regulatory review, nesiritide exposure–response data were modeled to develop a PK–PD model. The PK–PD model was then applied to evaluate different dosing regimens via simulations. The analysis suggested that a loading dose followed by a maintenance infusion should result in faster onset of desired action. Additionally, the simulations suggested that the lower infusion rates might result in smaller effect on the undesired side effect of hypotension. The analysis indicated that a loading bolus dose of 2 µg/kg with a maintenance dose of

0.01 µg/min/kg infusion could provide optimal risk–benefit profile. The sponsor investigated this PK–PD simulation-based modeling dosing regimen in an actual clinical trial for management of acute CHF and submitted the results for supporting a modified dosing regimen (Publication Committee, 2002). The modeled and actual results are shown in Fig. 22-38. The drug was subsequently approved by the FDA for treatment of acute CHF in May 2001.

### Case 2: Micafungin

This example focuses on how the US FDA as a regulatory authority recommended approval for a particular dosage for micafungin, a semisynthetic

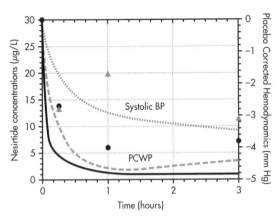

FIGURE 22-38 • Typical time course of nesiritide plasma concentrations (——), and the effects on the PCWP (• indicates observed; - - - - indicates model predicted) and systolic blood pressure (systolic BP; ▲ indicates observed; ..... indicates model predicted) after a 2-mg/kg bolus followed by a fixed-dose infusion of 0.01 mg/kg/min. Data for the initial 3 hours are shown here.

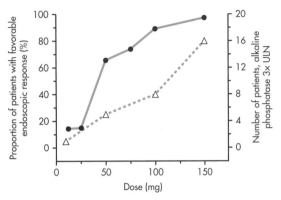

FIGURE 22-39 • Benefit–risk plot for micafungin. The solid line represents the proportion of patients with endoscopic response increased with dose. The dotted like represents incidence of elevations in alkaline phosphatase levels (> 3 × ULN) with dose.

lipopeptide formulated as an intravenous infusion for the treatment of esophageal candidiasis (Bhattaram et al, 2007). The review involved dose optimization by quantifying the exposure–response relationship by performing a benefit-to-risk assessment over a dynamic range of doses. Micafungin is an antifungal agent that belongs to the echinocandin class of compounds. The proposed dosage for treatment of esophageal candidiasis was 150 mg given every 24 hours for a period of 2 to 3 weeks (FUJISAWA, 2005). During the review, a thorough assessment of the dose to the clinical effectiveness was performed from two available Phase II trials and a registration study where the endoscopic response rate (proportion of patients that were cleared of the infection at the end of the therapy) was the primary

endpoint. A clinical response endpoint was considered a secondary parameter for effectiveness. Biochemical markers like alkaline phosphatase, serum glutamic oxaloacetic transaminase (SGOT), serum glutamic pyruvic transaminases (SGPT), and total bilirubin were assessed for a relationship between enzymatic elevations to the dose of antifungal agent. It was observed that both 100- and 150-mg doses of micafungin were able to achieve a maximal response as the primary endpoint (Fig. 22-39). Interestingly, patients that were treated with higher dose (150 mg) had a 15% lower relapse compared to the lower dose that was associated with a much lower of clinical cure rate. Of all biochemical markers, the alkaline phosphatase was correlated to the entire dynamic range of dose studied (12.5 to 150 mg). These elevations in the liver enzymes were transient and returned to normal levels upon discontinuation of the treatment.

## CHAPTER SUMMARY

Both agonist and antagonist drug effects can be quantitatively simulated by PK–PD models. The most common models are $E_{max}$ models mechanistically based on drug–receptor theory. Although most drug responses are complex, pharmacologic response versus log dose–type plots have been shown to follow a sigmoid type of curve (S-curve), with maximum response peaking when all receptors

become saturated. *In vitro* screening preparations are useful to study $EC_{50}$, potency, and mechanism of a drug. However, pharmacologic response in a patient is generally far more complicated. Physiologically based PD models must consider how the drug is delivered to the active site and the effect of various drug disposition processes, as well as plasma and tissue drug binding. In addition, pharmacogenomics of the drug and disease processes must be considered in the model. Appropriately developed PK–PD models may be applied to predict onset, intensity, and duration of action of a drug. Toxicokinetics may also be applied to explain the side effects or drug–drug interactions.

The progress of a disease or its response to a therapeutic agent is often accompanied by biologic changes (markers or biomarkers) that are observable and/or measurable. Biomarkers may be selected and validated to monitor the course of drug response in the body. Biomarkers should be mechanistically based and fulfill several clinically relevant criteria in order to be useful as potential clinical endpoints. Biomarkers together with PK–PD could be a very useful tool in expediting drug development, and many reviews and discussions are available about this application.

## LEARNING QUESTIONS

1. On the basis of the graph in Fig. 22-40, answer "true" or "false" to statements (a) through (e) and state the reason for each answer.

   a. The plasma drug concentration is more related to the pharmacodynamic effect of the drug compared to the dose of the drug.

   b. The pharmacologic response is directly proportional to the log plasma drug concentration.

   c. The volume of distribution is not changed by uremia.

   d. The drug is exclusively eliminated by hepatic biotransformation.

   e. The receptor sensitivity is unchanged in the uremic patient.

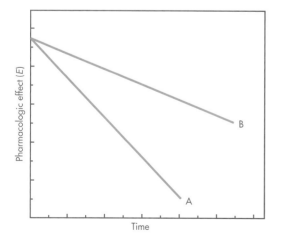

FIGURE 22-40 • Graph of pharmacologic response E as a function of time for the same drug in patients with normal (A) and uremic (B) function, respectively.

2. How would you define a response and an effect? Identify whether the following is a pharmacodynamic response or a pharmacodynamic effect:

   a. Change from baseline in HbA1c at the end of 26 weeks

   b. Blood histamine levels

   c. Number of sleep awakenings at week 4

   d. Percent reduction in seizures at end of 8 weeks

   e. Measure of body weight at the end of 52 weeks

3. What is the difference between a partial and an inverse agonist? Name a drug with its therapeutic class that behaves like a (a) partial agonist (b) inverse agonist?

4. What is the difference between biomarkers and surrogate endpoints? Give an example.

5. Explain why subsequent equal doses of a drug do not produce the same pharmacodynamic effect as the first dose of a drug.

   a. Provide an explanation based on pharmacokinetic considerations.

   b. Provide an explanation based on pharmacodynamic considerations.

6. How are the parameters AUC and $t_{eff}$ used in pharmacodynamic models?

7. What class of drug tends to have a lag time between the plasma and the effect compartment?

8. Name an example of a pharmacodynamic response that does not follow a drug dose–response profile.

9. What is AUIC with regard to an antibiotic?

10. What is the difference between $IC_{50}$ and $EC_{50}$? Are the values reproducible from one lab to another?

11. $K_i$ refers to the equilibrium dissociation constant of a ligand determined in inhibition studies. The $K_i$ for a given ligand is typically determined in a competitive radioligand binding study by measuring the inhibition of the binding of a reference radioligand by the inhibiting ligand of under equilibrium conditions. Why?

12. What is the dissociation constant $K$ in the following interaction between a drug ligand $L$ and a drug receptor $R$?

$$L + R \underset{k_{-1}}{\overset{k_{+1}}{\rightleftharpoons}} LR$$

$$P_{LR} = \frac{|L|}{|L| + K}$$

where $K$ is expressed as $k_{-1}/k_{+1}$ and $P_{LR}$ is the proportion of receptor occupied by $L$.

How many binding sites are assumed in the above model?

13. Which one of the following would you select as a biomarker for a type II diabetic patient? State the reasons that support your selection.

a. Blood sugar level

b. Blood insulin level

c. HbA1C

14. What are the three types of pharmacodynamic responses? Give an example for each type of PD response that will help to differentiate between them.

15. Explain the principal difference between concentration-dependent and time-dependent killing patterns associated with the use of antibiotics. What PK–PD index would be most appropriate to predict the therapeutic efficacy of antibiotics associated with respect to these two killing patterns?

16. For an investigative antibiotic under early discovery, series of efficacy studies in a mouse thigh infection model were conducted. The following are results for three PK–PD indices of AUC/MIC ratio, $C_{max}$/MIC ratio, and % time above MIC. Analyze these results and determine what PK–PD index is best correlated to the log CFU reduction. Explain why you picked the particular PK–PD index.

| AUC/MIC ratio | Log (CFU) reduction | $C_{max}$/MIC ratio | Log (CFU) reduction | (%) Time above MIC | Log (CFU) reduction |
|---|---|---|---|---|---|
| 31 | 8.9 | 1.4 | 7.8 | 18 | 7.7 |
| 32 | 8.4 | 2.6 | 8.8 | 25 | 5.7 |
| 40 | 7.5 | 2.7 | 9.1 | 27 | 8.8 |
| 61 | 6.7 | 4.7 | 8.6 | 35 | 3.9 |
| 64 | 5.9 | 4.9 | 7.9 | 35 | 4.2 |
| 88 | 5.8 | 5.7 | 6.8 | 36 | 5.3 |
| 93 | 5.3 | 9.4 | 6.7 | 37 | 6.0 |
| 108 | 5.6 | 9.7 | 6.4 | 39 | 2.7 |
| 122 | 5.0 | 10.8 | 5.0 | 41 | 8.6 |
| 125 | 4.2 | 11.1 | 3.5 | 45 | 2.2 |
| 168 | 3.7 | 12.6 | 4.3 | 50 | 4.3 |
| 172 | 3.9 | 20.3 | 6.0 | 55 | 6.8 |
| 210 | 4.2 | 21.4 | 7.6 | 58 | 8.9 |

| AUC/MIC ratio | Log (CFU) reduction | C$_{max}$/MIC ratio | Log (CFU) reduction | (%) Time above MIC | Log (CFU) reduction |
|---|---|---|---|---|---|
| 226 | 3.4 | 34.3 | 3.0 | 71 | 2.2 |
| 250 | 4.2 | 37.2 | 3.3 | 75 | 4.1 |
| 328 | 3.6 | 44.3 | 5.7 | 75 | 3.8 |
| 488 | 3.5 | 47.8 | 5.4 | 81 | 2.0 |
| 488 | 2.3 | 50.7 | 3.0 | 85 | 6.5 |
| 500 | 3.1 | 91.8 | 4.0 | 99 | 8.8 |
| 841 | 2.5 | 97.6 | 1.9 | 99 | 2.5 |
| 862 | 3.2 | 99.1 | 3.9 | 99 | 3.8 |
| 952 | 2.6 | 183.5 | 2.7 | 100 | 3.0 |
| 975 | 2.0 | 190.5 | 2.5 | 100 | 3.1 |
| 975 | 2.8 | 383.6 | 2.2 | 100 | 3.2 |
| 1025 | 2.2 | 398 | 1.9 | 100 | 3.5 |

Hint: Plot each PK–PD index against log CFU reduction.

17. The below graph shows a concentration–effect relationship for three hypothetical drugs. Assuming all drugs produce a maximum effect of five units, determine $EC_{50}$ for each drug $X$, $Y$, and $Z$. What does $EC_{50}$ signify?

expression for $S_{max}$, the fractional stimulation from baseline. (*Hint:* Use the same approach as for $I_{max}$, but in the opposite direction.)

19. Based on the graphs below, identify what kind of a PK–PD relationship can be assumed for this hypothetical drug.

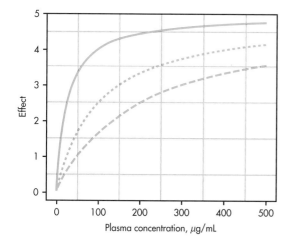

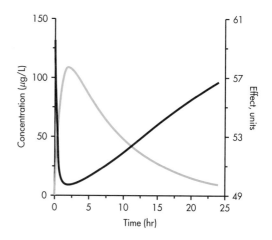

18. Assume a drug exhibits a proportional drug effect which is stimulatory in nature. Derive the

20. Hysteresis: What is the rationale for observing hysteresis in drug therapeutics?

## ANSWERS

### Frequently Asked Questions

*How does the rate of systemic drug absorption affect the abuse potential of drugs such as cocaine or heroin?*

■ A drug administered via a non-intravenous route such as oral, intranasal, or inhalation (smoking) undergoes absorption process. Post absorption, the drug enters systemic circulation (blood/plasma). If the rate of absorption ($k^a$) of a drug is faster via one route of administration over another route, higher levels of drug will be achieved quickly ($t_{max}$) for the route with faster absorption rate. Therefore, route with rapid rate of absorption will result in faster onset of action, which for drugs with abuse potential results in greater abuse.

*What is a drug receptor?*

■ Receptors can be defined as the cellular proteins that interact with endogenous ligands to elicit a physiological response thereby regulating cellular function(s).

*Explain why a drug that binds to a receptor may be an agonist, a partial agonist, or an antagonist?*

■ A drug may be defined as a chemical substance, which on introduction into the body at a relevant dose can elicit a physiological action after interacting with a receptor. As described in drug-receptor interaction section, if the drug mimics actions similar to the endogenous ligand, it is called an agonist. An antagonist can be classified as a drug that blocks the effect of an endogenous ligand by competitively binding to the given receptor. If a drug binds and activates a given receptor and produces a weak effect relative to that of a full agonist, it is classified as a partial agonist. As drug by definition produces a pharmacological effect, it will fall into one of these categories.

*If we need to develop a drug where only 25% of maximal activation is needed to achieve therapeutic benefit, what type of agent among the four classes will you pick and why?*

■ We will pick a partial agonist from the four classes (depicted in Figure 21-3) as partial agonist acts like an agonist but cannot reach the maximal response of a full agonist.

*What are the other utilities of biomarkers besides being used as a bridging tool to link preclinical and clinical drug development?*

■ Role of biomarkers in drug discovery and development is increasing day by day. In addition to serving as a bridging tool between preclinical and clinical drug development, biomarkers can be used as a diagnostic tool to detect and diagnose disease conditions such as elevated blood glucose levels for onset of diabetes mellitus, as a tool for the staging of disease such as levels of prostate-specific antigen concentration in blood to correlate tumor growth and metastasis, indicator of disease prognosis (anatomically measuring size of tumors), and as a predictive/monitoring tool to assess clinical response to a therapeutic intervention, a common example being blood cholesterol levels to assess cardiac disease.

*Explain why the log-linear model cannot be used to determine effect when concentration is zero? Describe which simple model could be used in such situation?*

■ The log-linear model is of the form: When the concentration is zero, logarithm of zero does not exist. Thus, when concentrations are zero, the concentration effect cannot be obtained. The effect will be same as the baseline effect. In such situations, a linear-concentration effect model could be used.

*Explain why doubling the dose of a drug may not double the pharmacodynamic effect of the drug.*

■ The scenario explained above could happen when relationship of the dose (or concentration)-response relationship follows an $E_{max}$ relationship, where the effect reaches a plateau after some dose (or concentration). Once the plateauing effect is reached, any additional increase in the dose will not affect the pharmacodynamic effect.

*What is meant by a hysteresis loop? Why do some drugs follow a clockwise hysteresis loop and other drugs follow a counterclockwise hysteresis loop?*

- When there is a temporal difference between the plasma drug concentration and the pharmacodynamic effect, ie, the maximum drug effect occurs later than the time of maximum plasma concentration, the effect vs plasma concentration graph depicts the profile as a loop, which is referred to as hysteresis loop. The hysteresis loop is anticlockwise in nature when the mechanism is delayed drug effect. However, if underlying mechanism is tolerance development, then the effect vs plasma concentration graph shows a clockwise loop.

*When is an effect compartment model used? How does the effect compartment differ from pharmacokinetic compartmental model, such as the central compartment and the peripheral (tissue) compartment?*

- When the drug effects are temporally delayed as compared to time course of the plasma concentration, the rate-limiting step in eliciting the drug effect could be due to distribution of the drug to the site of action. To describe the biodistributional delay mathematically, a hypothetical compartment is considered, which is referred to as the effect compartment model. The effect compartmental model is not typically applicable when there is an indirect mechanism involved in the elicitation of the drug response/effect. The central and peripheral compartments used in the pharmacokinetic model are a representation of how the drug distributes within the body based on its physicochemical properties and does not consider the drug effect. A one-compartment pharmacokinetic model (Central compartment only) indicates that the drug is instantaneously distributed within the body and

hence mathematically represented using only the central compartment. A two-compartment model (central+peripheral compartment) indicates a distinct distribution phase for the drug explaining that the drug does not instantaneously distribute rather the drug takes time to distribute to different tissues apart from the plasma.

## Learning Questions

1. **a. True.** Drug concentration is more precise because an identical dose may result in different plasma drug concentrations in different subjects due to individual differences in pharmacokinetics.

   **b. True.** The kinetic relationship between drug response and drug concentration is such that the response is proportional to log concentration of the drug.

   **c. True.** The data show that after IV bolus dose, the response begins at the same point, indicating that the initial plasma drug concentration is the same. In uremic patients, the volume of distribution may be affected by changes in protein binding and electrolyte levels, which may range from little or no effect to strongly affecting the $V_d$.

   **d. False.** The drug is likely to be excreted through the kidney since the slope (elimination) is reduced in uremic patients.

   **e. True.** Assuming that the volume of distribution is unchanged, the starting pharmacologic response should be the same if the receptor sensitivity is unchanged. In a few cases, receptor sensitivity to the drug can be altered in uremic patients. For example, the effect of digoxin will be more intense if the serum potassium level is depleted.

2. **a.** effect

   **b.** response

   **c.** response

   **d.** effect

   **e.** response

3. A partial agonist is an agent that produces a response similar to an agonist but cannot reach a maximal response as that of an agonist. However, an inverse agonist selectively binds to the inactive form of the receptor and shifts the conformational equilibrium towards the inactive state. An example of a partial agonist is buspirone (anxiolytic agent) and famotidine ($H_2$ receptor blocker) being an inverse agonist.

5. **a.** Pharmacokinetic considerations: Subsequent doses induce the hepatic drug metabolizing enzymes (auto-induction), thereby decreasing the elimination half-life, resulting in lower steady-state drug concentrations.

   **b.** Pharmacodynamic considerations: The patient develops tolerance to the drug, resulting in the need for a higher dose to produce the same effect.

7. CNS drugs

8. An allergic response to a drug may be unpredictable and does not generally follow a dose–response relationship.

9. AUC/MIC or AUIC is a pharmacokinetic parameter incorporating MIC together in order to provide better prediction of antibiotic response (cure percent). An example is ciprofloxacin. AUIC is a good predictor of percent cure in infection treated at various dose regimens.

10. In functional studies, the antagonist $IC_{50}$ is most useful if the concentration of the agonist is below maximal. Higher concentrations of the agonist will increase the $IC_{50}$ of the competitive antagonist well above its equilibrium dissociation constant. Even with low agonist concentrations, the $IC_{50}$ from functional studies, like an agonist $EC_{50}$ or maximal response, is dependent on the conditions of the experiment (tissue, receptor expression, type of measurement, etc).

14. Continuous, categorical, and time to event responses are the three types of responses. Blood pressure measurement is an example of continuous response. Mild, moderate, and severe status of an adverse event like diarrhea is an example of a discrete response. Time until relapse is an example of a time-to-event outcome. Here time to relapse is a continuous response, but not all patients would have relapse. Hence, patients who do not have relapse are censored, hence the distinction from continuous response.

17. $EC_{50}$ signifies the concentration of the drug at which 50% of $E_{max}$ (maximum effect is achieved or also referred to as the potency of the drug. Smaller the $EC_{50}$ value, more potent is the drug. For X (solid line), $E_{max}$ is approx.: 5 units, $EC_{50}$ approximately 25 $\mu g/ml$. This can be obtained by eyeballing the concentration corresponding to an effect of 2.5 units. For Y (short dotted line): $EC_{50}$: approx. 100 $\mu g/ml$; For Z (long dotted line): approximately 250 $\mu g/ml$.

19. The maximal drug concentrations are achieved at about 2.5 hrs and the corresponding PD response occurs at the same time indicating that the drug-effect relationship can be explained by a direct effect model.

20. Hysteresis occurs when there is time lag between the concentration and the corresponding effect. It could be manifested when there is a distributional delay of the drug reaching the effect site, or it could be based on the mechanism of action of the drug. Typically, hysteresis plots are observed when the maximum effect occurs later than the maximum concentrations.

## REFERENCES

Anne S, Reisman RE: Risk of administering cephalosporin antibiotics to patients with histories of penicillin allergy. *Ann Allergy Asthma Immunol* 74(2): 167-170, 1995.

Atkinson AJJ: *Physiological and Laboratory Markers of Drug Effect.* New York, Academic Press, 2001.

Bhattaram VA, Bonapace C, Chilukuri DM, et al: Impact of pharmacometric reviews on new drug approval and labeling decisions--a survey of 31 new drug applications submitted between 2005 and 2006. *Clin Pharmacol Ther* 81(2): 213-221, 2007.

Bhattaram VA, Booth BP, Ramchandani RP, et al: Impact of pharmacometrics on drug approval and labeling decisions: a survey of 42 new drug applications. *AAPS J* 7(3):E503–512, 2005.

Biomarkers Definitions Working Group: Biomarkers and surrogate endpoints: Preferred definitions and conceptual framework. *Clin Pharmacol Ther* **69**(3): 89-95, 2001.

Blumenthal DK, Garrison JC: Pharmacodynamics: Molecular mechanisms of drug action. In Brunton LL (ed). *The Pharmacological Basis of Therapeutics*. McGraw Hill, 2011, pp 41–72.

Clark AJ: The reaction between acetyl choline and muscle cells: Part II. *J Physiol* **64**(2):123–143, 1927.

Colburn WA: Optimizing the use of biomarkers, surrogate endpoints, and clinical endpoints for more efficient drug development. *J Clin Pharmacol* **40**(12 Pt 2):1419–1427, 2000.

Coltart DJ, Hamer J: A comparison of the effects of propranolol and practolol on the exercise tolerance in angina pectoris. *Br J Pharmacol* **40**(1):147P–148P, 1970.

Cone EJ: Pharmacokinetics and pharmacodynamics of cocaine. *J Anal Toxicol* **19**(6):459–478, 1995.

Cunningham RF, Israili ZH, Dayton PG: Clinical pharmacokinetics of probenecid. *Clin Pharmacokinet* **6**:135–151, 1981.

Cox BM: *Drug Tolerance and physical Dependence*, in Principles of Drug Action-The Basis of Pharmacology, (Pratt WB and Taylor, editors) Churchill Livingstone, NY, 3rd edition, Chapter 10, pp 639–690, 1990.

Craig WA: Interrelationship between pharmacokinetics and pharmacodynamics in determining dosage regimens for broad-spectrum cephalosporins. *Diagn Microbiol Infect Dis* **22**(1-2):89–96, 1995.

Craig WA: Pharmacodynamics of antimicrobials: General concepts and applications. *Antimicrobial Pharmacodynamics in Theory and Clinical Practice*. In Nightingale CH, Murakawa T, Ambrose PG (eds). New York, Marcel Dekker. **28**:1–22, 2002.

de Wit H, Dudish S, Ambre J: Subjective and behavioral effects of diazepam depend on its rate of onset. *Psychopharmacology (Berl)* **112**(2-3):324–330, 1993.

Derendorf H, Lesko LJ, Chaikin P, et al: Pharmacokinetic/pharmacodynamic modeling in drug research and development. *J Clin Pharmacol* **40**(12 Pt 2):1399–1418, 2000.

Echt DS, Liebson PR, Mitchell LB, et al: Mortality and morbidity in patients receiving encainide, flecainide, or placebo. The Cardiac Arrhythmia Suppression Trial. *New Engl J Med* **324**(12):781–788, 1991.

Florian JA, Tornoe CW, Brundage R, Parekh A, Garnett CE: Population pharmacokinetic and concentration--QTc models for moxifloxacin: Pooled analysis of 20 thorough QT studies. *J Clin Pharmacol* **51**(8):1152–1162, 2011.

FUJISAWA: Mycamine Prescribing label. FDA, 2005.

Garnett CE, Beasley N, Bhattaram VA, et al: Concentration-QT relationships play a key role in the evaluation of proarrhythmic risk during regulatory review. *J Clin Pharmacol* **48**(1):13–18, 2008.

Gobburu JV: Biomarkers in clinical drug development. *Clin Pharmacol Ther* **86**(1):26–27, 2009.

Gobburu JV, Marroum PJ: Utilisation of pharmacokinetic-pharmacodynamic modelling and simulation in regulatory decision-making. *Clin Pharmacokinet* **40**(12):883–892, 2001.

Henningfield JE, Keenan RM: Nicotine delivery kinetics and abuse liability. *J Consult Clin Psychol* **61**(5):743–750, 1993.

Holford NH, Sheiner LB: Understanding the dose-effect relationship: Clinical application of pharmacokinetic-pharmacodynamic models. *Clin Pharmacokinet* **6**(6):429–453, 1981.

J. C. Earp, D. C. Dubois, D. S. Molano, N. A. Pyszczynski, R. R. Almon and W. J. Jusko (2008). Modeling corticosteroid effects in a rat model of rheumatoid arthritis II: mechanistic pharmacodynamic model for dexamethasone effects in Lewis rats with collagen-induced arthritis. *J Pharmacol Exp Ther* **326**(2):546–554, 2008.

Johanson CE, Fischman MW: The pharmacology of cocaine related to its abuse. *Pharmacol Rev* **41**(1): 3–52, 1989.

Jusko WJ: Moving from basic toward systems pharmacodynamic models. *J Pharm Sci* **102**(9):2930–2940, 2013.

Jusko WJ, Ko HC: Physiologic indirect response models characterize diverse types of pharmacodynamic effects. *Clin Pharmacol Ther* **56**(4):406–419, 1994.

Jusko WJ, Ko HC, Ebling WF: Convergence of direct and indirect pharmacodynamic response models. *J Pharmacokinet Biopharm* **23**(1):5–8; discussion 9–10, 1995.

Katzung BG, Masters SB, Trevor AJ: Drug receptors and pharmacodynamics. In *Basic and Clinical Pharmacology*. McGraw-Hill, 2011, pp 15–35.

Kimko H, Pinheiro J: Model-based clinical drug development in the past, present and future: A commentary. *Br J Clin Pharmacol* **79**(1):108–116, 2015.

Kuivenhoven JA, Jukema JW, Zwinderman AH, et al: The role of a common variant of the cholesteryl ester transfer protein gene in the progression of coronary atherosclerosis. The Regression Growth Evaluation Statin Study Group. *N Engl J Med* **338**(2):86–93, 1998.

Lesko LJ, Atkinson AJ Jr: Use of biomarkers and surrogate endpoints in drug development and regulatory decision making: Criteria, validation, strategies. *Annu Rev Pharmacol Toxicol* **41**:347–366, 2001.

Levy G: Relationship between elimination rate of drugs and rate of decline of their pharmacologic effects. *J Pharm Sci* **53**: 342–343, 1964.

Levy G: Kinetics of pharmacologic effects. *Clin Pharmacol Ther* **7**(3):362–372, 1966.

Lin RY: A perspective on penicillin allergy. *Arch Intern Med* **152**(5):930–937, 1992.

Lorentzen H, Kallehave F, Kolmos HJ, Knigge U, Bulow J, Gottrup F: Gentamicin concentrations in human subcutaneous tissue. *Antimicrob Agents Chemother* **40**(8):1785–1789, 1996.

Madabushi R, Cox DS, Hossain M, et al: Pharmacokinetic and pharmacodynamic basis for effective argatroban dosing in pediatrics. *J Clin Pharmacol* **51**(1):19–28, 2011.

Mager DE, Wyska E, Jusko WJ: Diversity of mechanism-based pharmacodynamic models. *Drug Metab Dispos* **31**(5): 510–518, 2003.

Meibohm B, Derendorf H: Basic concepts of pharmacokinetic/pharmacodynamic (PK/PD) modelling. *Int J Clin Pharmacol Ther* **35**(10):401–413, 1997.

Moroney AC: PharmD Drug–Receptor Interactions. In *The MERCK Manual of Diagnosis and Therapy*. Whitehouse Station, NJ, Merck Sharp & Dohme, 2011.

Mould DR, DeFeo TM, Reele S, et al: Simultaneous modeling of the pharmacokinetics and pharmacodynamics of midazolam and diazepam. *Clin Pharmacol Ther* **58**(1):35–43, 1995.

Nagashima R, O'Reilly RA, Levy G: Kinetics of pharmacologic effects in man: The anticoagulant action of warfarin. *Clin Pharmacol Ther* **10**(1):22–35, 1969.

Neubig RR, Spedding M, Kenakin T, Christopoulos A: International Union of Pharmacology Committee on Receptor and C: Drug International Union of Pharmacology Committee on Receptor Nomenclature and Drug Classification. XXXVIII. Update on terms and symbols in quantitative pharmacology. *Pharmacol Rev* **55**(4):597–606, 2003.

Nieforth KA, Nadeau R, Patel IH, Mould D: Use of an indirect pharmacodynamic stimulation model of MX protein induction to compare in vivo activity of interferon alfa-2a and a polyethylene glycol-modified derivative in healthy subjects. *Clin Pharmacol Ther* **59**(6):636–646, 1996.

O'Donnell JM, Shelton RC: Drug therapy of depression and anxiety disorders. In Brunton LL (ed). *The Pharmacological Basis of Therapeutics*. McGraw Hill, 2011, pp 397–415.

Peck CC, Barr WH, Benet LZ, et al: Opportunities for integration of pharmacokinetics, pharmacodynamics, and toxicokinetics in rational drug development. *J Clin Pharmacol* **34**(2):111–119, 1994.

Proctor and Gamble: Risedronate prescribing label, 2000.

Publication Committee for the, V. I. Intravenous nesiritide vs nitroglycerin for treatment of decompensated congestive heart failure: a randomized controlled trial. *JAMA* **287**(12):1531–1540, 2002.

Roy A, Mould DR, Wang XF, Tay L, Raymond R, Pfister M: Modeling and simulation of abatacept exposure and interleukin-6 response in support of recommended doses for rheumatoid arthritis. *J Clin Pharmacol* **47**(11):1408–1420, 2007.

Russell T, Riley SP, Cook JA, Lalonde RL: A perspective on the use of concentration-QT modeling in drug development. *J Clin Pharmacol* **48**(1):9–12, 2008.

Shak S. Overview of the trastuzumab (Herceptin) anti-HER2 monoclonal antibody clinical program in HER2-overexpressing metastatic breast cancer. Herceptin Multinational Investigator Study Group. *Semin Oncol* **26**(4 Suppl 12):71–77, 1999.

Sharma A, Jusko WJ: Characterization of four basic models of indirect pharmacodynamic responses. *J Pharmacokinet Biopharm* **24**(6):611–635, 1996.

Sharma A, Jusko WJ: Characteristics of indirect pharmacodynamic models and applications to clinical drug responses. *Br J Clin Pharmacol* **45**(3):229–239, 1998.

Sheiner LB, Stanski DR, Vozeh S, Miller RD, Ham J: Simultaneous modeling of pharmacokinetics and pharmacodynamics: Application to d-tubocurarine. *Clin Pharmacol Ther* **25**(3):358–371, 1979.

Sheiner LB, Steimer JL: Pharmacokinetic/pharmacodynamic modeling in drug development. *Annu Rev Pharmacol Toxicol* **40**:67–95, 2000.

Skidgel RA, Kaplan AP, Erdös EG: Histamine, bradykinin, and their antagonists. In Brunton LL (ed). *The Pharmacological Basis of Therapeutics*. McGraw Hill, 2011, pp 911–935.

Strimbu K, Tavel JA: What are biomarkers? *Curr Opin HIV AIDS* **5**(6):463–466, 2010.

Temple R: Are surrogate markers adequate to assess cardiovascular disease drugs? *JAMA* **282**(8):790–795, 1999.

Vogelman B, Gudmundsson S, Leggett J, Turnidge J, Ebert S, Craig WA: Correlation of antimicrobial pharmacokinetic parameters with therapeutic efficacy in an animal model. *J Infect Dis* **158**(4):831–847, 1988.

Weiss R, Mazade L: *Surrogate Endpoints in Evaluating the Effectiveness of Drugs Against HIV Infection and AIDS*. Institute of Medicine, Washington DC: National Academy Press, 1990.

Westfall TC, Westfall DP: Adrenergic agonists and antagonists. In Brunton LL (ed). *The Pharmacological Basis of Therapeutics*. McGraw Hill, 2011, pp 275–333.

Yaksh TL, Wallace MS: Opioids, analgesia, and pain management. In Brunton LL (ed). *The Pharmacological Basis of Therapeutics*. McGraw Hill, 2011, pp 481–526.

# 23

# Application of Pharmacokinetics to Clinical Situations

Dana R. Bowers and Vincent H. Tam

## CHAPTER OBJECTIVES

- Define Medication Therapy Management (MTM) and explain how MTM can improve the success of drug therapy.

- Explain what "critical-dose drugs" are and name an example.

- Define therapeutic drug monitoring and explain which drugs should be monitored through a therapeutic drug monitoring service.

- Calculate a drug dosage regimen in an individual patient for optimal drug therapy for a drug that has complete pharmacokinetic information and for a drug that has incomplete pharmacokinetic information.

- Explain the relationship of changing the dose and/or the dosing interval on the $C_{max(ss)}$, $C_{min(ss)}$, and $C_{av(ss)}$.

- Define drug–drug interactions and the mechanisms of drug–drug interactions, and provide examples.

- Define population pharmacokinetics and explain how population pharmacokinetics enables the estimate of pharmacokinetic parameters from relatively sparse data obtained from study subjects.

The success of drug therapy is highly dependent on the choice of the drug, the drug product, and the design of the dosage regimen. The choice of the drug is generally made by the physician after careful patient diagnosis and physical assessment. The choice of the drug product (eg, immediate release versus modified release) and dosage regimen is based on the patient's individual characteristics and known pharmacokinetics of the drug, as discussed in earlier chapters. Ideally, the dosage regimen is designed to achieve a desired drug concentration at a receptor site to produce an optimal therapeutic response with minimum adverse effects. Individual variations in pharmacokinetics and pharmacodynamics make the design of dosage regimens difficult. Therefore, the application of pharmacokinetics to dosage regimen design must be coordinated with proper clinical evaluation of the patient. For certain critical-dose drugs, monitoring both the patient and drug regimen is even more important for proper efficacy.

## MEDICATION THERAPY MANAGEMENT

*Medication Therapy Management* (MTM) was officially recognized by the United States Congress in the Medicare Prescription Drug, Improvement, and Modernization Act of 2003.[1] The objective of this act is to improve the quality, effectiveness, and efficiency of healthcare delivery, including prescription drugs. An MTM program is developed in cooperation with pharmacists and physicians to optimize therapeutic outcomes through improved medication use. MTM provides consultative, educational, and monitoring services to patients to obtain

---

[1]https://www.cms.gov/Medicare/Prescription-Drug-Coverage/PrescriptionDrugCovContra/MTM.html.

better therapeutic outcomes from medications by the enhanced understanding of medication therapy, improved compliance, control of costs, and prevention of adverse events and drug interactions. MTM programs have been developed for specific practice areas such as elderly care, diabetes, and asthma (Barnett et al, 2009).

## INDIVIDUALIZATION OF DRUG DOSAGE REGIMENS

Not all drugs require rigid individualization of the dosage regimen. Many drugs have a large margin of safety (ie, exhibit a wide therapeutic window), and strict individualization of the dose is unnecessary. For a number of drugs generally recognized as safe (GRAS) and effective, the US Food and Drug Administration (FDA) has approved an *over-the-counter* (OTC) classification for drugs that the public may buy without prescription. In addition, many prescription drugs, such as ibuprofen, loratadine, omeprazole, naproxen, nicotine patches, and others, that were originally prescription drugs have been approved by the FDA and other regulatory agencies for OTC status. These OTC drugs and certain prescription drugs, when taken as directed, are generally safe and effective for the labeled indications without medical supervision. For drugs that are relatively safe and have a broad safety-dose range, such as the penicillins, cephalosporins, and tetracyclines, the antibiotic dosage is not dose titrated precisely but is based rather on the clinical judgment of the physician to maintain an effective plasma antibiotic concentration above a minimum inhibitory concentration. Individualization of the dosage regimen is very important for drugs with a narrow therapeutic window (also known as *critical-dose drugs* and *narrow therapeutic index* [NTI] drugs), such as digoxin, aminoglycosides, antiarrhythmics, anticoagulants, anticonvulsants, and some antiasthmatics, such as theophylline. Critical-dose drugs are defined as those drugs where comparatively small differences in dose or concentration lead to dose- and concentration-dependent, serious therapeutic failures and/or serious adverse drug reactions. These adverse reactions may be persistent, irreversible, slowly reversible life threatening, or could result in inpatient hospitalization or prolongation of existing hospitalization, persistent or significant disability or incapacity, or death. Adverse reactions that require significant medical intervention to prevent one of these outcomes are also considered to be serious (Alloway et al, 2000; Guidance for Industry, 2018).

The objective of the dosage regimen design is to produce a safe plasma drug concentration that does not exceed the minimum toxic concentration or fall below a critical minimum drug concentration below which the drug is not effective. For this reason, the dose of these drugs is carefully individualized to avoid plasma drug concentration fluctuations due to intersubject variation in drug absorption, distribution, or elimination processes. For drugs such as phenytoin, a critical-dose drug that follows nonlinear pharmacokinetics at therapeutic plasma drug concentrations, a small change in the dose may cause a huge increase in the therapeutic response and possible adverse effects.

## THERAPEUTIC DRUG MONITORING

Many nonsteroidal anti-inflammatory drugs (NSAIDs) such as ibuprofen, and calcium channel-blocking agents, such as nifedipine, have a wide therapeutic range and do not need therapeutic drug monitoring. In addition, OTC drugs such as various cough and cold remedies, analgesics, and other products are also generally safe when used as directed. Therapeutic monitoring of plasma drug concentrations is valuable only if a relationship exists between the plasma drug concentration and the desired clinical effect or between the plasma drug concentration and an adverse effect. For those drugs in which plasma drug concentration and clinical effect are not directly related, other pharmacodynamic or "surrogate" parameters may be monitored. For example, clotting time may be measured directly in patients on warfarin anticoagulant therapy. Glucose concentrations are often monitored in diabetic patients using insulin products. Asthmatic patients may use the bronchodilator, albuterol taken by inhalation via a metered-dose inhaler. For these patients, forced expiratory volume ($FEV_1$) may be used as a measure of drug efficacy. In cancer chemotherapy, dose adjustment for individual patients may depend more on the severity of side effects and the patient's ability to tolerate the drug. For some drugs that have large inter- and intrasubject variability, clinical judgment and experience with the drug are needed to dose the patient properly.

The therapeutic range for a drug is an approximation of the average plasma drug concentrations that are safe and efficacious in most patients. When using published therapeutic drug concentration ranges, such as those in Table 23-1, the clinician must realize that the therapeutic range is essentially a probability concept and should never be considered as absolute values (Evans et al, 1992; Schumacher, 1995). For example, the accepted therapeutic range for theophylline is 10–20 $\mu$g/mL. Some patients may exhibit signs of theophylline intoxication such as central nervous system excitation and insomnia at serum drug concentrations below 20 $\mu$g/mL (Fig. 23-1), whereas other patients may show drug efficacy at serum drug concentrations below 10 $\mu$g/mL.

In administering potent drugs to patients, the physician must maintain the plasma drug level within a narrow range of therapeutic concentrations (see Table 23-1). Various pharmacokinetic methods

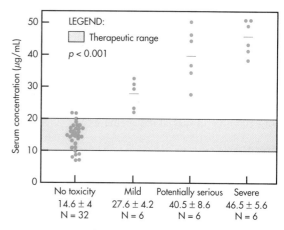

FIGURE 23-1 • Correlation between the frequency and severity of adverse effects and plasma concentration of theophylline (mean ± SD) in 50 adult patients. Mild symptoms of toxicity included nausea, vomiting, headache, and insomnia. A potentially serious effect was sinus tachycardia, and severe toxicity was defined as the occurrence of life-threatening cardiac arrhythmias and seizures. (Adapted with permission from Hendeles L, Weinberger M. Avoidance of adverse effects during chronic therapy with theophylline, Eur J Respir Dis Suppl. 1980;109:103-119.)

(or nomograms) may be used to calculate the initial dose or dosage regimen. Usually, the initial dosage regimen is calculated based on body weight or body surface after a careful consideration of the known pharmacokinetics of the drug, the pathophysiologic condition of the patient, and the patient's drug history including nonprescription drugs and nutraceuticals.

Because of interpatient variability in drug absorption, distribution, and elimination as well as changing pathophysiologic conditions in the patient, *therapeutic drug monitoring* (TDM) or clinical pharmacokinetic (laboratory) services (CPKS) have been established in many hospitals to evaluate the response of the patient to the recommended dosage regimen. The improvement in the clinical effectiveness of the drug by TDM may decrease the cost of medical care by preventing untoward adverse drug effects. The functions of a TDM service are listed below.

- Select drug.
- Design dosage regimen.
- Evaluate patient response.
- Determine need for measuring serum drug concentrations.

## TABLE 23-1 • Therapeutic Range for Commonly Monitored Drugs

| | |
|---|---|
| Amikacin | 20–30 $\mu$g/mL |
| Carbamazepine | 4–12 $\mu$g/mL |
| Digoxin | 1–2 ng/mL |
| Gentamicin | 5–10 $\mu$g/mL |
| Lidocaine | 1–5 $\mu$g/mL |
| Lithium | 0.6–1.2 mEq/L |
| Phenytoin | 10–20 $\mu$g/mL |
| Procainamide | 4–10 $\mu$g/mL |
| Quinidine | 1–4 $\mu$g/mL |
| Theophylline | 10–20 $\mu$g/mL |
| Tobramycin | 5–10 $\mu$g/mL |
| Valproic acid | 50–100 $\mu$g/mL |
| Vancomycin | 20–40 $\mu$g/mL |

*Reproduced with permission from Schumacher GE: Therapeutic Drug Monitoring. Norwalk, CT: Appleton & Lange; 1995.*

- Recommend an assay and/or assay for drug concentration in biological fluids.
- Perform pharmacokinetic evaluation of drug concentrations.
- Readjust dosage regimen, if necessary.
- Monitor serum drug concentrations.
- Recommend special requirements.

## Drug Selection

The choice of drug and drug therapy is usually made by the physician. However, many practitioners consult with the clinical pharmacist in drug product selection and dosage regimen design. Increasingly, clinical pharmacists in hospitals and nursing care facilities are closely involved in prescribing, monitoring, and substituting medications as part of a total MTM program. The choice of drug and the drug product is made not only on the basis of therapeutic consideration but also based on cost and therapeutic equivalency.

Hospitals and various prescription reimbursement plans have a drug formulary.[2] Pharmacokinetics and pharmacodynamics are part of the overall considerations in the selection of a drug for inclusion in the drug formulary. An Institutional Pharmacy and Therapeutic Committee (IPTC) periodically reviews clinical efficacy data on new drug products for inclusion in the formulary and on older products for removal from the formulary. Drugs with similar therapeutic indications may differ in dose and pharmacokinetics. The pharmacist may choose one drug over another based on therapeutic, adverse effect, pharmacokinetic (dosing convenience), and cost considerations. Other factors include patient-specific information such as medical history, pathophysiologic states, concurrent drug therapy, known allergies, drug sensitivities, and drug interactions; all are important considerations in drug selection (Table 23-2). As discussed in Chapter 21, the use of pharmacogenetic data may become another tool in assisting in drug selection for the patient.

---

[2]A drug formulary contains a list of prescription drug products that will be reimbursed fully or partially by the prescription plan provider. Drug products not listed in the formulary may be reimbursed if specially requested by the physician.

**TABLE 23-2 • Factors Associated with Variability in Drug Response**

| Patent Factors | Drug Factors |
|---|---|
| Age | Bioavailability and biopharmaceutics |
| Weight | Pharmacokinetics (including absorption, distribution, and elimination) |
| Pathophysiology | Drug interactions |
| Nutritional status | Receptor sensitivity |
| Genetic variability/ Gender | Rapid or slow metabolism |

## Dosage Regimen Design

The main objective of designing an appropriate dosage regimen for the patient is to provide a drug dose and dosing interval that achieve a *target* drug concentration at the receptor site. Once the proper drug is selected for the patient, a number of factors must be considered when designing a therapeutic dosage regimen. Usually, the manufacturer's dosing recommendations in the package insert will provide guidance on the initial starting dose and dosing interval in the typical patient population. These recommendations are based upon clinical trials performed during and after drug development. The package insert containing the FDA-approved label suggests an average dose and dosage regimen for the "average" patient who was enrolled in these studies. Genetic variation, drug interactions, or physiologic conditions such as disease or pregnancy may change the pharmacokinetics and/or pharmacodynamics of a drug, therefore requiring dosing regimen individualization. First, the known pharmacokinetics of the drug, including its absorption, distribution, and elimination profile, are considered in the patient who is to be treated. Some patients may have unusual metabolism (eg, fast or slow metabolizers) that will affect bioavailability after oral administration (due to first pass) and the elimination half-life after systemic drug absorption. Second, the physiology of the patient—their age, weight, gender, and nutritional status—will affect the disposition of the drug and should be considered. Third, any pathophysiologic conditions, such as renal dysfunction, hepatic disease, or congestive heart failure, may change the normal pharmacokinetic profile of the drug, and the dose must be carefully adjusted. Fourth, the effect of long-term exposure to the medication in the patient must be considered, including the possibility of drug abuse by the patient. In addition, personal lifestyle factors, such as cigarette and/or marijuana smoking, alcohol abuse, and obesity, are other issues that are known to alter the pharmacokinetics of drugs. Lastly, lack of patient compliance (ie, patient noncompliance) in taking the medication can also be a problem in achieving effective therapeutic outcomes.

An optimal dosing design can greatly improve the safety and efficacy of the drug, including reduced side effects and a decrease in frequency of TDM and its associated costs. For some drugs, TDM will be necessary because of the unpredictable nature of their pharmacodynamics and pharmacokinetics. Changes in drug or drug dose may be required after careful patient assessment by the pharmacist, including changes in the drug's pharmacokinetics, drug tolerance, cross-sensitivity, or history of unusual reactions to related drugs. The pharmacist must develop competency and experience in clinical pharmacology and therapeutics in addition to the necessary pharmacokinetic skills. Several mathematical approaches to dosage regimen design are given in later sections of this chapter and in Chapter 25.

Dosage regimen guidelines obtained from the literature and from approved product labeling are often based upon average patient response. However, substantial individual variation to drug response can occur. The design of the dosage regimen must be based upon clinical assessment of the patient. Labeling for recently approved drugs provides information for dosing in patients with renal and/or hepatic disease. Frequently, drug dose adjustment of another coadministered drug may be necessary due to drug–drug interactions. For example, an elderly patient who is on haloperidol (Haldol®) may require a reduction of his usual morphine dose. With many new drugs, pharmacogenetic information is also available and should be considered for dosing individual patients. For example, the extents of drug resistance are important considerations during dosage regimen design in cancer and anti-infective chemotherapy.

## Pharmacokinetics of the Drug

Various popular drug references list pharmacokinetic parameters such as clearance, bioavailability, and elimination half-life. The values for these pharmacokinetic parameters are often obtained from small clinical studies. Therefore, it is difficult to determine whether these reported pharmacokinetic parameters are reflected in the general population or in a specific patient group. Differences in study design, patient population, and data analysis may lead to conflicting values for the same pharmacokinetic parameters. For example, values for the apparent volume of distribution and clearance can be estimated by different methods, as discussed in previous chapters.

Ideally, the effective target drug concentration and the therapeutic window for the drug should be obtained. When using the target drug concentration in the development of a dosage regimen, the clinical pharmacist should know whether the reported target drug concentration represents an average steady-state drug concentration, a peak drug concentration, or a trough concentration.

## Drug Dosage Form (Drug Product)

The dosage form of the drug will affect drug bioavailability and the rate of absorption and thus the subsequent pharmacodynamics of the drug in the patient (see also Chapter 7). The choice of drug dosage form may be based on the desired route of drug administration, the desired onset and duration of the clinical response, cost, and patient compliance. For example, an extended-release drug product instead of an immediate-release drug product may provide a longer duration of action and better patient compliance. An orally disintegrating tablet (ODT) may be easier for the patient who has difficulty in swallowing a conventional tablet. Patients with profuse vomiting may prefer the use of a transdermal delivery system rather than an oral drug product. Available dosage forms and strengths are usually listed under the *How Supplied* section in the package insert.

## Patient Compliance

Factors that may affect patient compliance include the cost of the medication, complicated instructions, multiple daily doses, difficulty in swallowing, type of dosage form, and adverse drug reactions. The patient who is in an institution may have different issues compared to an ambulatory patient. Patient compliance in institutions is maintained by the healthcare personnel who provide/administer the medication on schedule. Ambulatory patients must remember to take the medication as prescribed to obtain the optimum clinical effect of the drug. It is very important that the prescriber or clinical pharmacist consider the patient's lifestyle and personal needs when developing a drug dosage regimen. The FDA-approved labeling in the package insert contains *Patient Counseling Information* to improve patient compliance. There are also sections on *Information for Patients* and *Medication Guide*.

### Evaluation of Patient's Response

After the drug and drug products are chosen and the patient receives the initial dosage regimen, the practitioner should evaluate the patient's clinical response. If the patient is not responding to drug therapy as expected, then the drug and dosage regimen should be reviewed. The dosage regimen should be reviewed for adequacy, accuracy, and patient compliance with the drug therapy. In many situations, sound clinical judgment may preclude the need for measuring serum drug concentrations.

### Measurement of Drug Concentrations

Before biological samples are taken from the patient, the need to determine drug concentrations should be assessed by the practitioner. In some cases, adverse events may not be related to a specific systemic drug concentrations and will preclude the patient from using the prescribed drug. For example, allergy or mild nausea may not be dose related. Plasma, serum, saliva, urine, and occasionally tissue drug concentrations may be measured for (1) therapeutic drug monitoring to improve drug therapy, (2) drug abuse screening, and (3) toxicology evaluation such as poisoning and drug overdose. Examples of common drugs that may be measured are listed in Table 23-3. In addition, many prescription medications (eg, opiates, benzodiazepines, NSAIDs, anabolic steroids) and nonprescription drugs (eg, dextromethorphan, NSAIDs) can also be abused. Analyses have been used for measurement of the presence of abused drugs in blood, urine, saliva, hair, and breath (alcohol).

A major assumption often made is that systemic drug concentrations relate to the therapeutic and/or toxic effects of the drug. For many drugs, clinical studies have demonstrated a therapeutically effective range of systemic concentrations. Knowledge of the systemic drug concentration may clarify why a patient is not responding to the drug therapy or is experiencing an adverse effect. For example, it may help recognize medication adherence issues.

The timing of the blood sample and the number of blood samples to be taken from the patient must be considered. In many cases, a single blood sample gives insufficient information. Occasionally, more than one blood sample is needed to clarify the adequacy of the dosage regimen. When ordering systemic drug concentrations to be measured, a single drug concentration may not yield useful information unless other factors are considered. For example, the dosage regimen of the drug should be known, including the dose and the dosage interval, the route of drug administration, the time of sampling (peak, trough, or steady state), and the type of drug product (eg, immediate-release or extended-release drug product).

In practice, trough systemic concentrations ($C_{trough}$) are easier to obtain than peak or $C_{av(ss)}$ samples under a multiple-dose regimen. In addition, there are limitations in terms of the number of blood samples that may be taken, total volume of blood needed for the assay, and time to perform the drug analysis. Schumacher (1985) has suggested that blood sampling times for TDM should be taken during the postdistributive phase for loading and maintenance doses, but at steady state for maintenance doses. After distribution equilibrium has been achieved, the plasma drug concentration during the postdistributive phase is better correlated with the tissue concentration and, presumably, the drug concentration at the site of action. In some cases, the clinical pharmacist may want an early-time sample that approximates the peak drug level, whereas a blood sample taken at three or four elimination half-lives during multiple dosing will approximate the steady-state drug concentration. The practitioner who orders the measurement of systemic concentrations should also consider the cost of the assays, the risks and discomfort for the patient, and the utility of the information gained.

**TABLE 23-3 • Drugs Commonly Measured in Serum, Plasma, or Other Tissues**

| Therapeutic Drug Monitoring | Drug Abuse Screen | Drug Overdose or Poisoning |
|---|---|---|
| *Anticonvulsants* | *Alcohol* | *Alcohol* |
| Carbamazepine, phenytoin, valproic acid, primidone | Cotinine | Ethyl alcohol, methanol |
| *Antibiotics* | *Anabolic steroids* | *Opiates* |
| Aminoglycosides (gentamicin), vancomycin | *Opiates* | Heroin, morphine, codeine derivatives, methadone, buprenorphine |
| | Heroin, morphine, codeine derivatives, methadone, buprenorphine | *Stimulants* |
| *Cardiovascular agents:* Digoxin, lidocaine, procainamide, quinidine | *Stimulants:* Cocaine, amphetamine, methamphetamine | Cocaine, amphetamine, methamphetamine, pseudoephedrine |
| *Immunosupressants:* Cyclosporine, tacrolimus, sirolimus | *Cannabinoids:* Marijuana, hashish | *Hallucinogens and related drugs* These drugs are subject to overdose and/or poisoning |
| *Antipsychotics:* Clozapine | | *Other drugs:* Barbiturates, benzodiazepines, tricyclics |
| *Other drugs:* Lithium, theophylline | *Hallucinogens and related drugs:* Phencyclidine, PCP, ketamine, MDMA (ecstasy, 3,4-methylenedioxy-N-methylamphetamine) | *Inhalants:* Nitrous oxide, paint thinners, solvents |
| *Hormonal drugs:* TSH, thyroxin, estrogens | *Other drugs:* Barbiturates, benzodiazepines, various hypnotics and sedatives | *Heavy metals:* Lead, mercury, arsenic, chromium |
| | | *Various nonprescription medications such as acetaminophen* |

Nicotine from tobacco is often included in some drug abuse literature but is not usually part of a drug abuse screen.

## Assay for Drug

Drug analyses are usually performed either by a clinical chemistry laboratory or by a clinical pharmacokinetics laboratory. A variety of analytical techniques are available for drug measurement, such as high-pressure liquid chromatography coupled with mass spectrometry, immunoassay, and other methods. The methods used by the analytic laboratory may depend on such factors as the physicochemical characteristics of the drug, target drug concentration, amount (volume) and nature of the biologic specimen (serum, urine, saliva), available instrumentation, cost for each assay, and analytical skills of the laboratory personnel. The laboratory should have a standard operating procedure for each drug analysis method and follow good laboratory practices. Moreover, analytical methods used for the assay of drugs in serum or plasma should be validated with respect to specificity, linearity, sensitivity, precision, accuracy, stability, and ruggedness. The times to perform the assays and receive the results are important factors that should be considered if the clinician needs this information to make a quick therapeutic decision.

### Specificity

Chromatographic evidence is generally required to demonstrate that the analytical method is specific for detection of the drug and other analytes, such as an active metabolite. The method should demonstrate that there is no interference between the drug and its metabolites and endogenous or exogenous substances such as other drugs that the patient may have taken. In addition, the internal standard should be resolved completely and also demonstrate no interference with other compounds. Immunoassays depend on an antibody and antigen (usually the drug to be measured) reaction. The antibody should be specific for the drug analyte but may instead also cross-react with drugs that have similar structures, including related compounds (endogenous or exogenous chemicals) and metabolites of the drug. Colorimetric and spectrophotometric assays are usually less specific. Interference from other materials may overestimate the results.

### Sensitivity

Sensitivity is the minimum detectable level or concentration of drug in serum that may be approximated as the lowest drug concentration that is two to three times the background noise. A *minimum quantifiable level* or *minimum detectable limit* is a statistical method for the determination of the precision of the lower level of quantitation.

### Linearity and Dynamic Range

Dynamic range refers to the relationship between the drug concentration and the instrument response (or signal) used to measure the drug. Many assays show a linear drug concentration–instrument response relationship. Immunoassays generally have a nonlinear dynamic range. High serum drug concentrations, above the dynamic range of the instrument response, must be diluted before assay. The dynamic range is determined by using serum samples that have known (standard) drug concentrations (including a blank serum sample or zero drug concentration). Extrapolation of the assay results above or below the measured standard drug concentrations are usually inaccurate; therefore, samples should be re-analyzed after dilution. If extrapolated results are used, they should be labeled accordingly, as the uncertainty related to them will be larger than the concentrations that directly come from the validated assay.

### Precision

Precision is a measurement of the variability or reproducibility of the data. Precision measurements are obtained by replication of various drug concentrations and by replication of standard concentration curves prepared separately on different days. A suitable statistical measurement of the dispersion of the data, such as standard deviation or coefficient of variation, is then performed.

### Accuracy

Accuracy refers to the difference between the average assay values and the true or known drug concentrations. Control (known) drug serum concentrations should be prepared by an independent technician using such techniques to minimize any error in their preparation. These samples, including a "zero" drug concentration, are assayed by the technician assigned to the study along with a suitable standard drug concentration curve.

### Stability

Standard drug concentrations should be maintained under the same storage conditions as the unknown serum samples and assayed periodically. The stability study should continue for at least the same length of time as the patient samples are to be stored. Freeze–thaw stability studies are performed to determine the effect of thawing and refreezing on the stability of the drug in the sample. On occasion, a previously frozen biologic sample must be thawed and reassayed if the first assay result is uncertain.

Plasma samples obtained from subjects on a drug study are usually assayed along with a minimum of three standard processed serum samples containing known standard drug concentrations and a minimum of three control plasma samples whose concentrations are unknown to the analyst. These control plasma samples are randomly distributed in each day's run. Control samples are replicated in duplicate to evaluate both within-day and between-day precision. The concentration of drug in each sample is based on each day's processed standard curve.

### Ruggedness

Ruggedness is the degree of reproducibility of the test results obtained by the analysis of the same samples by different analytical laboratories or by different instruments. The determination of ruggedness measures the reproducibility of the results under normal operational conditions from laboratory to laboratory, instrument to instrument, and analyst to analyst.

Because each method for drug assay may have differences in sensitivity, precision, and specificity, the clinical pharmacokineticist should be aware of which drug assay method the laboratory used.

## Pharmacokinetic Evaluation

After the serum or plasma drug concentrations are measured, the clinical pharmacokineticist must evaluate the data. Many laboratories report total drug (free plus bound drug) concentrations in the serum. The pharmacokineticist should be aware of the usual therapeutic range of serum drug concentrations from the literature. However, the literature may not indicate whether the reported values were trough, peak serum, or average drug levels. Moreover, the methodology for the drug assay used in the analytical laboratory may be different in terms of accuracy, specificity, and precision.

The assay results from the analytical laboratory may show that the patient's serum drug levels are higher, lower, or similar to the expected serum levels. The pharmacokineticist should evaluate these results while considering the patient and the patient's pathophysiologic condition. Table 23-4 lists a number of factors the pharmacokineticist should consider when interpreting serum drug concentration. Often, additional data, such as a high serum creatinine and high blood urea nitrogen, may help verify that an observed high serum drug concentration in a patient is due to lower renal drug clearance because of compromised kidney function. In another scenario, a complaint by the patient of overstimulation and insomnia might corroborate the laboratory's finding of higher-than-anticipated serum concentrations of theophylline. Therefore, the clinician or pharmacokineticist should evaluate the data using sound clinical judgment and observation. The therapeutic decision should not be based solely on serum drug concentrations.

## Dosage Adjustment

From the serum drug concentration data and patient observations, the clinician or pharmacokineticist may recommend an adjustment in the dosage regimen. Ideally, the new dosage regimen should be

### TABLE 23-4 • Pharmacokinetic Evaluation of Serum Drug Concentrations

| Serum Concentrations Lower Than Anticipated |
| --- |
| Patient compliance |
| Error in dosage regimen |
| Wrong drug product (controlled release instead of immediate release) |
| Poor bioavailability |
| Rapid elimination (efficient metabolizer) |
| Reduced plasma–protein binding |
| Enlarged apparent volume of distribution |
| Steady state not reached |
| Timing of blood sample |
| Improving renal/hepatic function |
| Drug interaction due to upregulation of enzyme or autoinduction |
| Changing hepatic blood flow |

| Serum Concentrations Higher Than Anticipated |
| --- |
| Patient compliance |
| Error in dosage regimen |
| Wrong drug product (immediate release instead of controlled release) |
| Rapid bioavailability |
| Smaller-than-anticipated apparent volume of distribution |
| Slow elimination (poor metabolizer) |
| Increased plasma–protein binding |
| Deteriorating renal/hepatic function |
| Drug interaction due to inhibition of elimination |

| Serum Concentration Correct but Patient Does Not Respond to Therapy |
| --- |
| Altered receptor sensitivity (eg, tolerance) |
| Drug interaction at receptor site |
| Changing hepatic blood flow |

calculated using the pharmacokinetic parameters derived from the *patient's* serum drug concentrations. Although there may not be enough data for a complete pharmacokinetic profile, the pharmacokineticist should still be able to derive a new dosage regimen based on the available data and the pharmacokinetic parameters in the literature that are based on average population data.

## Monitoring Serum Drug Concentrations

In many cases, the patient's pathophysiology may be unstable, either improving or deteriorating further. For example, proper therapy for congestive heart failure will improve cardiac output and renal perfusion, thereby increasing renal drug clearance. Therefore, continuous monitoring of serum drug concentrations is necessary to ensure proper drug therapy for the patient. When deciding to monitor serum concentrations, it is important to consider its distribution in the body. For example, azithromycin achieves high tissue concentrations, and therefore it would make more sense to monitor tissue concentrations rather than serum concentrations.

Commercial assays may not be available for all medications; therefore, acute pharmacologic response can be monitored in lieu of actual serum drug concentration. For example, prothrombin time might be useful for monitoring anticoagulant therapy and blood pressure monitoring for antihypertensive agents.

## Special Recommendations

At times, the patient may not be responding to drug therapy because of other factors. For example, the patient may not be following instructions for taking the medication (patient noncompliance). The patient may be taking the drug after a meal instead of before, or may not be adhering to a special diet (eg, low-salt diet). Therefore, the patient may need special instructions that are simple and easy to follow. It may be necessary to discontinue the drug and prescribe another drug from the same therapeutic class.

### FREQUENTLY ASKED QUESTIONS

▶ Can therapeutic drug monitoring be performed without taking blood samples?

▶ What are the major considerations in therapeutic drug monitoring?

## CLINICAL EXAMPLE

### Dosage and Administration of Lanoxin® (Digoxin) Tablets, USP

In the package insert, dosing information is available under *Dosage and Administration*. In addition, the section under *Clinical Pharmacology* provides valuable information for therapeutic considerations such as:

- Mechanism of action
- Pharmacodynamics
- Pharmacokinetics

Lanoxin (digoxin) is one of the cardiac (or digitalis) glycosides indicated for the treatment of congestive heart failure and atrial fibrillation. According to the approved label[3] for Lanoxin, the recommended dosages of digoxin may require considerable modification because of individual sensitivity of the patient to the drug, the presence of associated conditions, or the use of concurrent medications. In selecting a dose of digoxin, the following factors must be considered:

1. The body weight of the patient. Doses should be calculated based upon lean (ie, ideal) body weight.

2. The patient's renal function, preferably evaluated on the basis of estimated creatinine clearance.

3. The patient's age. Infants and children require different doses of digoxin than adults. Also, advanced age may be indicative of diminished renal function even in patients with normal serum creatinine concentration (ie, below 1.5 mg/dL).

4. Concomitant disease states, concurrent medications, or other factors likely to alter the pharmacokinetic or pharmacodynamic profile of digoxin.

### Serum Digoxin Concentrations

In general, the dose of digoxin used should be determined based on clinical grounds. However, measurement of serum digoxin concentrations can be helpful to the clinician in determining the adequacy of digoxin therapy and in assigning certain probabilities to the likelihood of digoxin intoxication.

[3]Lanoxin (digoxin) tablets, NDA 20405/SUPPL-15, Food and Drug Administration, Revised February 2019.

About two-thirds of adults considered adequately digitalized (without evidence of toxicity) have serum digoxin concentrations ranging from 0.8 to 2.0 ng/mL; lower serum trough concentrations of 0.5–1 ng/mL may be appropriate in some adult patients. About two-thirds of adult patients with clinical toxicity have serum digoxin concentrations greater than 2.0 ng/mL. Since one-third of patients with clinical toxicity have concentrations less than 2.0 ng/mL, values below 2.0 ng/mL do not rule out the possibility that a certain sign or symptom would be related to digoxin therapy. Rarely, there are patients who are unable to tolerate digoxin at serum concentrations below 0.8 ng/mL. Consequently, the serum concentration of digoxin should always be interpreted in the overall clinical context, and an isolated measurement should not be used alone as the basis for increasing or decreasing the dose of the drug.

To allow adequate time for equilibration of digoxin between serum and tissue, sampling of serum concentrations should be done just before the next scheduled dose of the drug (trough level). If this is not possible, sampling should be done at least 6–8 hours after the last dose, regardless of the route of administration or the formulation used. On a once-daily dosing schedule, the concentration of digoxin will be 10%–25% lower when sampled at 24 versus 8 hours, depending upon the patient's renal function. On a twice-daily dosing schedule, there will be only minor differences in serum digoxin concentrations whether sampling is done at 8 or 12 hours after a dose.

If a discrepancy exists between the reported serum concentration and the observed clinical response, the clinician should consider the following possibilities:

1. Analytical problems in the assay procedure.
2. Inappropriate serum sampling time.
3. Administration of a digitalis glycoside other than digoxin.
4. Conditions causing an alteration in the sensitivity of the patient to digoxin.
5. Serum digoxin concentration may decrease acutely during periods of exercise without any associated change in clinical efficacy due to increased binding of digoxin to skeletal muscle.

An important statement in the approved label for Lanoxin is the following, which is in bold for emphasis: "**It cannot be overemphasized that both the adult and pediatric dosage guidelines provided are based upon average patient response and substantial individual variation can be expected. Accordingly, ultimate dosage selection must be based upon clinical assessment of the patient.**"

### Adverse Events and Therapeutic Monitoring

An *adverse drug reaction*, also called a *side effect* or *adverse event* (AE), is any undesirable experience associated with the use of a medicine in a patient. AEs can range from mild to severe. Serious AEs are those that can cause disability, are life threatening, result in hospitalization or death, or cause birth defects.[4] Some AEs are expected and are documented in the literature and in the approved labeling for the drug. Other AEs may be unexpected. The severity of these AEs and whether the AE is related to the patient's drug therapy should be considered. The FDA maintains safety information and an AE reporting program (MedWatch) that provides important and timely medical product information to healthcare professionals, including information on prescription and over-the-counter drugs, biologics, medical devices, and special nutritional products.

It is sometimes difficult to determine whether the AE in the patient is related to the drug, due to progression of the disease or other pathology, or due to some unknown source. There are several approaches to determining whether the observed AE is due to the drug:

1. Check that the correct drug product and dose was ordered and given to the patient.
2. Verify that the onset of the AE was after the drug was taken and not before.
3. Determine the time interval between the beginning of drug treatment and the onset of the event.

---

[4]FDA Consumer Health Information, August 11, 2019 (http://www.fda.gov/downloads/ForConsumers/ConsumerUpdates/ucm107976.pdf).

4. Discontinue the drug and monitor the patient's status, looking for improvement.

5. Rechallenge or restart the drug, if appropriate, and monitor for recurrence of the AE.

For some drugs, there may be an AE due to the initial exposure to the drug. However, the patient may become desensitized to the AE after longer drug treatment or drug dose titration. The clinician should be familiar with the drug and relevant literature concerning AEs. Generally, the manufacturer of the drug can also be a resource to consult.

## CLINICAL EXAMPLE

### Serum Vancomycin Concentrations

Vancomycin is a glycopeptide antibiotic commonly used in the treatment of serious gram-positive infections. Nephrotoxicity is often cited as an adverse effect, especially when high dose therapy is used for

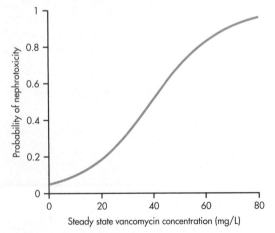

**FIGURE 23-2** • Correlation between the probability of nephrotoxicity and steady state serum vancomycin concentration. (Data from Ingram et al, 2008; Spapen et al, 2011; Norton K et al, 2014.)

a prolonged duration. The feasibility of using vancomycin as a continuous infusion has been examined recently in a variety of settings (eg, in intensive care units and as outpatient parenteral therapy) (Spapen et al, 2011; Norton et al, 2014).

Regardless of the clinical setting, the likelihood of nephrotoxicity was found to be significantly higher if the steady-state vancomycin trough concentrations ($C_{trough}$) were >25–32 $\mu$g/mL (Fig. 23-2) (Ingram et al, 2008). Unless there is a compelling clinical reason to do otherwise, it would be prudent to adjust dosing and maintain serum vancomycin trough concentrations to below 25 $\mu$g/mL.

## DESIGN OF DOSAGE REGIMENS

Several methods may be used to design a dosage regimen. Generally, the initial dosage of the drug is estimated using average population pharmacokinetic parameters obtained from the literature and modified according to the patient's known diagnosis, pathophysiology, demographics, allergy, and any other known factor that might affect the patient's response to the dosage regimen.

After initiation of drug therapy, the patient is then monitored for the therapeutic response by clinical and physical assessment. After evaluation of the patient, adjustment of the dosage regimen may be needed. If necessary, measurement of plasma drug concentrations may be used to obtain the patient's individual pharmacokinetic parameters from which the data are used to modify the dosage regimen. Further TDM in the patient may be needed.

Various clinical pharmacokinetic software programs are available for dosage regimen calculations. The dosing strategies are based generally on pharmacokinetic calculations that were previously performed manually. Computer automation and pharmacokinetic software packages improve the accuracy of the calculation, make the calculations "easier," and have an added advantage of maintaining proper documentation (see Chapter 19). However, the use of these software programs should not replace good clinical judgment.

• The package insert is a useful source for dose regimen. The section *Use in Specific Populations* provides information that may apply to individual patients.

- Pregnancy
- Labor and delivery
- Nursing mothers
- Pediatric use
- Geriatric use
- Hepatic impairment
- Renal impairment
- Gender effect

## Individualized Dosage Regimens

The most accurate approach to dosage regimen design is to calculate the dose based on the pharmacokinetics of the drug in the individual patient. This approach is not feasible for calculation of the initial dose. However, once the patient has been medicated, the readjustment of the dose may be calculated using pharmacokinetic parameters derived from measurement of the systemic drug levels from the patient after the initial dose. Most dosing programs record the patient's age and weight and calculate the individual dose based on creatinine clearance and lean body weight.

## Dosage Regimens Based on Population Averages

The method most often used to calculate a dosage regimen is based on average pharmacokinetic parameters obtained from clinical studies published in the drug literature. This method may be based on a fixed or an adaptive model (Mawer, 1976; Greenblatt, 1979).

The *fixed model* assumes that population average pharmacokinetic parameters may be used directly to calculate a dosage regimen for the patient, without any alteration. Usually, pharmacokinetic parameters such as absorption rate constant $k_a$, bioavailability factor $F$, apparent volume of distribution $V_D$, and elimination rate constant $k$ are assumed to remain constant. Most often the drug is assumed to follow the pharmacokinetics of a one-compartment model. When a multiple-dose regimen is designed, multiple-dosage equations based on the principle of superposition (see Chapter 17) are used to evaluate the dose. The practitioner may use the usual dosage suggested by the literature and then make a small adjustment of the dosage based on the patient's weight and/or age.

The *adaptive model* for dosage regimen calculation uses patient variables such as weight, age, sex, body surface area, and known patient pathophysiology, such as renal disease, as well as the known population average pharmacokinetic parameters of the drug. In this case, calculation of the dosage regimen takes into consideration any changing pathophysiology of the patient and attempts to adapt or modify the dosage regimen according to the needs of the patient. In some cases, pharmacogenetic data may be helpful in determining dosing. For example, clopidogrel (Plavix) has a black box warning cautioning use in patients who have slow CYP2D6 metabolism and who will therefore have slower activation of the prodrug to the active metabolite. However, an appropriate dose regimen has not been established for these patients. The adaptive model generally assumes that pharmacokinetic parameters such as drug clearance do not change from one dose to the next. However, some adaptive models allow for continuously adaptive change with time in order to simulate more closely the changing process of drug disposition in the patient, especially during a disease state (Whiting et al, 1991).

## Dosage Regimens Based on Partial Pharmacokinetic Parameters

For many old drugs, the entire pharmacokinetic profile of the drug is unknown or unavailable. Therefore, the pharmacokineticist needs to make some assumptions in order to calculate the dosage regimen in the absence of pharmacokinetic data in animals or humans. For example, a common assumption is to let the bioavailability factor $F$ equal 1% or 100%. Thus, if the drug is less than fully absorbed systemically, the patient will be undermedicated rather than overmedicated. Some of these assumptions will depend on the safety, efficacy, and therapeutic range of the drug. The use of population pharmacokinetics (discussed later in this chapter) employs average patient population characteristics and only a few serum drug concentrations from the patient. Population pharmacokinetic approaches to TDM have increased with the increased availability of computerized databases and the development of statistical tools for the analysis of observational data (Schumacher, 1985).

## Nomograms and Tabulations in Dosage Regimen Designs

For ease of calculation of dosage regimens, many clinicians rely on nomograms to calculate the proper dosage regimen for their patients. The use of a nomogram may give a quick dosage regimen adjustment for patients with characteristics requiring adjustments, such as age, body weight, and physiologic state. In general, the nomogram of a drug is based on population pharmacokinetic data collected and analyzed using a specific pharmacokinetic model. In order to keep the dosage regimen calculation simple, complicated equations are often solved and the results displayed diagrammatically on special scaled axes or as a table to produce a simple dose recommendation based on patient information. Some nomograms make use of certain physiologic parameters, such as serum creatinine concentrations, to help modify the dosage regimen according to renal function (see Chapter 25).

Pharmaceutical manufacturers provide dosage recommendations in the approved label for many marketed drugs in the form of a table or as a nomogram. These are general guidelines to aid the clinician in establishing an initial dosage regimen for patients. The tables may include loading and maintenance doses that are modified for the demographics of the patient (eg, age, weight) and for certain disease states (eg, renal insufficiency).

For drugs with a narrow therapeutic range, such as theophylline, a guide for monitoring serum drug concentrations is given. Another example is the aminoglycoside antibiotic, tobramycin sulfate USP (Nebcin, Eli Lilly), which is eliminated primarily by renal clearance. Thus, the dosage of tobramycin sulfate should be reduced in almost direct proportion to a reduction in creatinine clearance (see Chapter 25). The manufacturer provides a nomogram for estimating the percent of the normal dose of tobramycin sulfate assuming the serum creatinine level (mg/100 mL) has been obtained.

## Empirical Dosage Regimens

In many cases, the physician selects a dosage regimen for the patient without using any pharmacokinetic variables. In such a situation, the physician makes the decision based on empirical clinical data, personal experience, and clinical observations. The physician characterizes the patient as representative of a similar well-studied clinical population that has used the drug successfully.

## CONVERSION FROM INTRAVENOUS INFUSION TO ORAL DOSING

After the patient's dosing is controlled by intravenous infusion, it is often desirable to continue to medicate the patient with the same drug using the oral route of administration. When intravenous infusion is stopped, the serum drug concentration decreases according to first-order elimination kinetics for drugs displaying linear pharmacokinetic characteristics (see Chapters 6, 14, and 15). For oral drug products that display linear pharmacokinetics, the time to reach steady state will depend on the terminal first-order rate constant for the drug. For drugs having faster absorption than elimination, the terminal rate constant is the elimination one. For drugs having slower absorption than elimination (most extended-release or long-acting formulations), the terminal rate constant will be the absorption one. Therefore, if the patient starts the dosage regimen with the oral drug product at the same time as the intravenous infusion is stopped, then the exponential decline of serum levels from the intravenous infusion should be matched by the exponential increase in serum drug levels from the oral drug product.

The conversion from intravenous infusion to an oral medication is very common in infectious diseases, where severely infected patients must begin with intravenous therapy and then can be converted to oral medication once the infection is under control. Theophylline is usually given orally; however, intravenous therapy can be used at the beginning of treatment if, as in the case of infected patients, the oral bioavailability of the drug is thought to be compromised or if immediate bronchodilation is needed. Computer simulation for the conversion of intravenous theophylline (aminophylline) therapy to oral controlled-release theophylline demonstrated that oral therapy should be started at the same time as intravenous infusion is stopped (Iafrate et al, 1982). With this method, minimal fluctuations are observed between the peak and trough serum theophylline levels. Moreover, giving the first oral dose when intravenous infusion is stopped may make it easier for the nursing staff or patient to comply with the dosage regimen. The following method may be used to calculate an appropriate oral dosage regimen for a patient whose condition has been stabilized by an intravenous drug infusion, where $F$ is the bioavailability of the formulation (in the case of theophylline, $F$ represents the salt form of the drug) and $D_0/\tau$ is the dosing rate:

$$C_{av(ss)} = \frac{D_0 \cdot F}{\tau \cdot CL} \qquad (23.1)$$

$$\frac{D_0}{\tau} = \frac{C_{av(ss)} \cdot CL}{F} \qquad (23.2)$$

Note that this method assumes that the steady-state plasma drug concentration, $C_{ss}$, after intravenous infusion is identical to the desired $C_{av(ss)}$ after multiple oral doses of the drug.

## EXAMPLE ▷ ▷ ▷

An adult male asthmatic patient (age 55 years, 78 kg) has been maintained on an intravenous infusion of aminophylline at a rate of 34 mg/h. The steady-state theophylline drug concentration was 12 $\mu$g/mL and total body clearance was calculated as 3.0 L/h. Calculate an appropriate oral dosage regimen of theophylline for this patient.

### Solution
Aminophylline is a soluble salt of theophylline and contains 85% theophylline ($S = 0.85$). Theophylline is 100% bioavailable ($F = 1$) after an oral dose. The dose rate, $D_0/\tau$ (34 mg/h), was calculated on the basis of aminophylline dosing. The patient, however, will be given theophylline orally. To convert to oral theophylline, $S$ and $F$ should be considered.

$$\text{Theophylline dose rate} = \frac{SFD_0}{\tau} = \frac{0.85 \cdot 1 \cdot 34}{1} = 28.9 \text{ mg/h}$$

The theophylline dose rate of 28.9 mg/h must be converted to a reasonable schedule for the patient with a consideration of the various commercially available theophylline drug products. Therefore, the total daily dose is 28.9 mg/h · 24 h or 693.6 mg/d. Possible theophylline dosage schedules might be 700 mg/d, 350 mg every 12 hours, or 175 mg every 6 hours. Each of these dosage regimens would achieve the same $C_{av(ss)}$ but different $C_{max(ss)}$ and $C_{min(ss)}$, which should be calculated. The dose of 350 mg every 12 hours could be given in sustained-release form to minimize the fluctuations between peaks and throughs (ie, peaks will be lower, and troughs will be higher).

## DETERMINATION OF DOSE

The calculation of the starting dose of a drug and dosing interval is based on the objective of delivering a desirable (target) therapeutic level of the drug in the body. For many drugs, the desirable therapeutic drug levels and pharmacokinetic parameters are available in the literature. However, the literature in some cases may not yield complete drug information, or some of the information available may be equivocal. Therefore, the pharmacokineticist must make certain necessary assumptions in accordance with the best pharmacokinetic information available.

For a drug that is given in multiple doses for an extended period of time, the dosage regimen is usually calculated to maintain the average steady-state systemic level within the therapeutic range. The dose can be calculated through re-arrangement of Equation 23.1, which expresses $C_{av(ss)}$ in terms of dose ($D_0$), dosing interval ($\tau$), and clearance ($CL$). $F$ is the fraction of drug absorbed, which is equal to 1 for drugs administered intravenously.

## PRACTICE PROBLEMS

1. Pharmacokinetic data for clindamycin are as follows (DeHaan et al, 1972):

   $$CL = 10.8 \text{ L/h}; \ t_{1/2} = 2.81 \text{ h}; \ Vd = 43.9 \text{ L}$$

   What is the steady-state concentration of the drug after 150 mg of the drug is given orally every 6 hours for a week? (Assume the drug is 100% bioavailable.)

## Solution

The steady state concentration of a drug exhibiting linear pharmacokinetics is equal to dividing the bioavailable dose per hour $((F \times D_0)/\tau)$ administered by the clearance $(CL)$. Using Equation 23.1:

$$C_{av(ss)} = \frac{D_0 \cdot F}{\tau \cdot CL} = \frac{150 \cdot 1}{6 \cdot 10.8} = 2.3 \text{ mg/L}$$

2. Aminoglycosides such as gentamicin and tobramycin distribute in extracellular fluid volume (0.3 L/kg), are well described with a one-compartment model, and have an elimination half-life in a patient with normal renal function of 2.15 hours.

   What would be the daily AUC obtained at steady state for a patient with normal renal function receiving 5 mg/kg every 24 hours?

## Solution

$$CL = \frac{\ln(2)}{t_{1/2}} \cdot V_D = \frac{0.693}{2.15\text{h}} \cdot (0.3) = 0.097 \, L/(\text{h.kg})$$

$$C_{av(ss)} = \frac{D_0 \cdot F}{\tau \cdot CL}$$

$$C_{av(ss)} = \frac{5}{24 \cdot 0.097} = 2.148 \text{ mg/L}$$

$$AUCss = Cav(ss) x \ 24 = 51.5 \text{ mg.h/L}$$

## EFFECT OF CHANGING DOSE AND DOSING INTERVAL ON $C_{MAX(SS)}$, $C_{MIN(SS)}$, AND $C_{AV(SS)}$

During intravenous infusion, $C_{ss}$ may be used to monitor the steady-state serum concentrations. In contrast, when considering TDM of serum concentrations after the initiation of a multiple-dosage regimen, the trough serum drug concentrations or $C_{min(ss)}$ may be used to validate the dosage regimen. The blood sample withdrawn just prior to the administration of the next dose represents $C_{min(ss)}$. To obtain $C_{max(ss)}$, the blood sample must be withdrawn exactly at the time for peak absorption, or closely spaced blood samples must be taken and the plasma drug concentrations graphed. In practice, an approximate

time for maximum drug absorption is estimated and a blood sample is withdrawn. Because of differences in rates of drug absorption, $C_{max(ss)}$ measured in this manner is only an approximation of the true $C_{max(ss)}$.

The $C_{av(ss)}$ is used most often in dosage calculation. The advantage of using $C_{av(ss)}$ as an indicator for deciding therapeutic blood level is that $C_{av(ss)}$ is determined on a set of points and generally fluctuates less than either $C_{max(ss)}$ or $C_{min(ss)}$. Moreover, when the dosing interval is changed, the dose may be increased proportionally, to keep $C_{av(ss)}$ constant. This approach works well for some drugs. For example, if the drug diazepam is given either 10 mg TID (three times a day) or 15 mg BID (twice daily), the same $C_{av(ss)}$ is obtained, as shown by Equation 23.1. In fact, if the daily dose is the same, the $C_{av(ss)}$ should be the same (as long as clearance is linear). However, when monitoring serum drug concentrations, $C_{av(ss)}$ cannot be measured directly but may be obtained from AUC/$\tau$ during multiple-dosage regimens. As discussed in Chapter 17, the $C_{av(ss)}$ is not the arithmetic average of $C_{max(ss)}$ and $C_{min(ss)}$ because serum concentrations decline exponentially.

The dosing interval must be selected while considering the elimination half-life of the drug; otherwise, the patient may suffer the toxic effect of a high $C_{max(ss)}$ or subtherapeutic effects of a low $C_{min(ss)}$ even if the $C_{av(ss)}$ is kept constant. For example, using the same example of diazepam, the same $C_{av(ss)}$ is achieved at 10 mg TID or 60 mg every other day. Obviously, the $C_{max(ss)}$ of the latter dose regimen would produce a $C_{max(ss)}$ several times larger than that achieved with 10-mg-TID dose regimen. In general, if a drug has a relatively wide therapeutic index and a relatively long elimination half-life, then flexibility exists in changing the dose or dosing interval, $\tau$, using $C_{av(ss)}$ as an indicator. When the drug has a narrow therapeutic index, $C_{max(ss)}$ and $C_{min(ss)}$ must be monitored to ensure safety and efficacy.

As the dose or dosage intervals change proportionately, the $C_{av(ss)}$ may be the same but the steady-state peak, $C_{max(ss)}$, and trough, $C_{min(ss)}$, drug levels will change. $C_{max(ss)}$ is influenced by the dose and the dosage interval. An increase in the dose given at a longer dosage interval will cause an increase in $C_{max(ss)}$ and a decrease in $C_{min(ss)}$. In certain cases, $C_{max(ss)}$ may be very close or above the minimum toxic drug concentration (MTC). In other cases, the $C_{\min(ss)}$ may be lower than the minimum effective drug concentration (MEC). In this latter case, the low $C_{\min(ss)}$ may be subtherapeutic and dangerous for the patient, depending on the mechanism of action of the drug and the relationship between concentrations and effect.

## DETERMINATION OF FREQUENCY OF DRUG ADMINISTRATION

The drug dose is often related to the frequency of drug administration. The more frequently a drug is administered, the smaller the dose is needed to obtain the same $C_{av(ss)}$. Thus, a dose of 250 mg every 3 hours can be changed to 500 mg every 6 hours without affecting the average steady-state plasma concentration of the drug. However, as the dosing intervals get longer, the dose required to maintain the average plasma drug concentration gets correspondingly larger.

In general, the dosing interval for most drugs is determined by the terminal half-life and the relationship between concentrations and effect. Drugs such as the penicillins, which have relatively low toxicity, may be given at intervals much longer than their elimination half-lives without any toxicity problems. Drugs having a narrow therapeutic range, such as digoxin and phenytoin, must be given relatively frequently to minimize excessive "peak-and-trough" fluctuations in blood levels. For example, the common maintenance schedule for digoxin is 0.25 mg/d and the elimination half-life of digoxin is 1.7 days. In contrast, penicillin G may be given at 250 mg every 6 hours, while its elimination half-life is 0.75 hour. Penicillin can be given at a dosage interval equal to 8 times its elimination half-life, whereas digoxin is given at a dosing interval only 0.59 times its elimination half-life. The toxic plasma concentration of penicillin G is over 100 times greater than its effective concentration, whereas digoxin has an effective concentration of 1–2 ng/mL and a toxicity level of 3 ng/mL. The toxic concentration of digoxin is only 1.5 times effective concentration. Therefore, a drug with a large therapeutic index (ie, a large margin of safety) can be given in large doses and at an interval equals to many times its terminal half-life.

## DETERMINATION OF BOTH DOSE AND DOSAGE INTERVAL

Both the dose and the dosing interval should be considered in the dosage regimen calculations. For intravenous multiple-dosage regimens, and assuming a one-compartment linear pharmacokinetic model, the ratio of $C_{\max(ss)}/C_{\min(ss)}$ may be expressed by

$$\frac{C_{\max(ss)}}{C_{\min(ss)}} = \frac{C_0/(1-e^{-k\tau})}{C_0 e^{-k\tau}(1-e^{-k\tau})} \qquad (23.3)$$

which can be simplified to

$$\frac{C_{\max(ss)}}{C_{\min(ss)}} = \frac{1}{e^{-k\tau}} \qquad (23.4)$$

From Equation 23.4, a maximum dosage interval, $\tau$, may be calculated that will maintain the serum concentration between desired $C_{\min(ss)}$ and $C_{\max(ss)}$. After the dosage interval is calculated, then a dose may be calculated.

### PRACTICE PROBLEM

The elimination half-life of an antibiotic is 3 hours with an apparent volume of distribution equivalent to 20% of body weight. The usual therapeutic range for this antibiotic is between 5 and 15 $\mu$g/mL. Adverse toxicity for this drug is often observed at serum concentrations greater than 20 $\mu$g/mL. Calculate a dosage regimen (multiple intravenous doses) that will just maintain the serum drug concentration between 5 and 15 $\mu$g/mL.

#### Solution

From Equation 23.4, determine the maximum possible dosage interval $\tau$.

$$\frac{15 \ \mu\text{g/mL}}{5 \ \mu\text{g/mL}} = \frac{1}{e^{-(0.693/3)\tau}}$$

$$e^{-0.231\tau} = 0.333$$

Take the natural logarithm (ln) on both sides of the equation.

$$-0.231\tau = -1.10$$

$$\tau = 4.76 \ \text{h}$$

Then determine the dose required to produce $C_{max(ss)}$ from Equation 23.5 after substitution of $C_0 = D_0/V_D$:

$$C_{max(ss)} = \frac{D_0/V_D}{1 - e^{-k\tau}} \tag{23.5}$$

Solve for dose, $D_0$, letting $V_D = 200$ mL/kg (20% body weight).

$$15 = \frac{D_0/200}{1 - e^{-(0.231)(4.76)}}$$

$$D_0 = 2 \text{ mg/kg}$$

To check this dose for therapeutic effectiveness, calculate $C_{min(ss)}$ and $C_{av(ss)}$.

$$C_{min(ss)} = \frac{(D_0/V_D)e^{-k\tau}}{1 - e^{-k\tau}} = \frac{(2000/200)e^{-(0.231)(4.76)}}{1 - e^{-(0.231)(4.76)}}$$

$$C_{min(ss)} = 4.99 \ \mu\text{g/mL}$$

As a further check on the dosage regimen, calculate $C_{av(ss)}$.

$$C_{av(ss)} = \frac{D_0}{V_D k\tau} = \frac{2000}{(200)(0.231)(4.76)}$$

$$C_{av(ss)} = 9.09 \ \mu\text{g/mL}$$

By calculation, the dose of this antibiotic should be 2 mg/kg every 4.76 hours to maintain the serum drug concentration between 5 and 15 $\mu$g/mL.

In practice, rather than a dosage interval of 4.76 hours, the dosage regimen and the dosage interval should be made as convenient as possible for the patient, and the size of the dose should take into account the commercially available drug formulation. Therefore, the dosage regimen should be recalculated to have a convenient value (below the maximum possible dosage interval) and the dose adjusted accordingly.

## DETERMINATION OF ROUTE OF ADMINISTRATION

Selection of the proper route of administration is an important consideration in drug therapy. The rate of drug absorption and the duration of action are influenced by the route of drug administration.

However, the use of certain routes of administration is precluded by physiologic and safety considerations. For example, intra-arterial and intrathecal drug injections are less safe than other routes of drug administration and are used only when absolutely necessary. Drugs that are unstable in the gastrointestinal tract, such as proteins, or drugs that undergo complete first-pass metabolism, are not suitable for oral administration. For example, insulin is a protein that is degraded in the gastrointestinal tract by proteolytic enzymes. Drugs such as xylocaine and nitroglycerin are not suitable for oral administration because of complete first-pass effect. These drugs must therefore be given by an alternate route of administration.

Intravenous administration is the fastest and most reliable way of delivering a drug into the circulatory system. Drugs administered by intravenous bolus are delivered to the plasma immediately, and the entire dose is immediately subject to elimination. Consequently, more frequent drug administration is required. Drugs administered extravascularly must be absorbed into the bloodstream, and because of the absorption process, the total dose will take a longer time to disappear completely from the body. The frequency of administration can be lessened by using routes of administration that give a sustained and slower rate of drug absorption.

Certain drugs are not suitable for administration intramuscularly because of erratic drug release, pain, or local irritation. After being injected into the muscle mass, the drug must reach the circulatory system or other body fluid to become bioavailable. The anatomic site of drug deposition following intramuscular injection will affect the rate of drug absorption. A drug injected into the deltoid muscle may be more rapidly absorbed than a drug injected similarly into the gluteus maximus, because there is better blood flow in the former. In general, the method of drug administration that provides the most consistent and greatest bioavailability should be used to ensure maximum therapeutic effect. The various routes of drug administration can be classified as either *extravascular* or *intravascular* and are listed in Table 23-5.

Precipitation of an insoluble drug at the injection site may result in slower absorption, incomplete bioavailability, and/or a delayed response. For example,

**TABLE 23-5 • Common Routes of Drug Administration**

| Parenteral | Extravascular |
|---|---|
| Intravascular | Enteral |
|    Intravenous injection (IV bolus) |    Buccal |
|    Intravenous infusion (IV drip) |    Sublingual |
|    Intra-arterial injection |    Oral |
|    Intramuscular injection |    Rectal |
| Intradermal injection | Inhalation |
| Subcutaneous injection | Transdermal |
| Intrathecal injection | |

a dose of 50 mg of chlordiazepoxide (Librium) is more quickly absorbed after oral administration than after intramuscular injection. Some drugs, such as haloperidol decanoate, are oil-soluble products that release very slowly after intramuscular injection.

## DOSING IN SPECIFIC POPULATIONS

Pharmacokinetics of a drug may be altered in special populations, such as the elderly, infants, obese patients, and patients with renal or hepatic disease. Elderly patients may have several different pathophysiologic conditions that require multiple drug therapy, which increases the likelihood for a drug interaction. Infants and children have different dosing requirements than adults. Dosing of drugs in this population requires a thorough consideration of the differences in the pharmacokinetics and pharmacology of a specific drug in the preterm newborn infant, newborn infant, infant, young child, older child, adolescent, and adult. Unfortunately, the pharmacokinetics and pharmacodynamics of most drugs are not well known in children under 12 years of age. Obesity often is defined by *body mass index*. For some drugs, dosing is based on ideal body weight. Chapter 24 provides more detailed information on this topic.

## PHARMACOKINETICS OF DRUG INTERACTIONS

A *drug interaction* generally refers to a modification of the expected drug response in the patient as a result of exposure of the patient to another drug or substance. Some unintentional drug interactions produce adverse reactions in the patient, whereas some drug interactions may be intentional, to provide an improved therapeutic response or to decrease adverse drug effects. Drug interactions may include drug–drug interactions, food–drug interactions, or chemical–drug interactions, such as the interaction of a drug with alcohol or tobacco. A listing of food interactions is given in Chapter 4. A drug–laboratory test interaction pertains to an alteration in a diagnostic clinical laboratory test result because of the drug.

Drug interactions may cause an alteration in the pharmacokinetics of the drug due to an interaction in drug absorption, distribution, or elimination (Tables 23-6 and 23-7). Drug interactions can also be pharmacodynamic interactions at the receptor site in which the competing drug potentiates or antagonizes the action of the first drug. Pharmaceutical drug interaction occurs when physical and/or chemical incompatibilities arise during extemporaneous pharmaceutical compounding. Pharmaceutical drug interactions, such as drug–excipient interactions, are considered during the development and manufacture of new and generic drug products.

The risk of a drug interaction increases with multiple drug therapy, multiple prescribers, poor patient compliance, and patient risk factors, such as predisposing illness (diabetes, hypertension, etc) or advancing age. Multiple drug therapy has become routine in most acute and chronic care settings. Elderly patients and patients with various predisposing illnesses tend to be a population using multiple drug therapy. A recent student survey found an average of 8–12 drugs per patient used in a group of hospital patients.

An important source of drug interactions is the combination of herbal remedies (sometimes referred to as *nutraceuticals* or dietary supplements) with drug therapy. Although many herbal products are safe when taken alone, many drug–herbal interactions have been reported (Izzo and Ernst, 2009). For example, St. John's wort is an inducer of CYP3A enzymes, which are involved in the metabolism of many drugs. St. John's wort reduces, for example, the plasma drug concentrations of indinavir, a protease inhibitor used to treat HIV infection and AIDS.

Screening for drug interactions is generally performed whenever multiple drug products are

## TABLE 23-6 • Sources of Drug Interactions

| Type of Drug Interaction | Source | Example |
|---|---|---|
| Pharmacokinetic | Absorption | Drug interactions can affect the rate and the extent of systemic drug absorption (bioavailability) from the absorption site, resulting in increased or decreased drug bioavailability. |
| | Distribution | Drug distribution may be altered by displacement of the drug from plasma protein or other binding sites due to competition for the same binding site. |
| | Hepatic elimination | Drugs that share the same drug-metabolizing enzymes have a potential for a drug interaction. |
| | Renal clearance | Drugs that compete for active renal secretion may decrease renal clearance of the first drug. Probenecid blocks the active renal secretion of penicillin drugs. |
| Pharmacodynamic | Drug receptor site | Pharmacodynamic drug interactions at the receptor site in which the competing drug potentiates or antagonizes the action of the first drug. |
| Pharmaceutical compounding | Pharmaceutical interactions are caused by a chemical or physical incompatibility when two or more drugs are mixed together | An IV solution of aminophylline has an alkaline pH and should not be mixed with such drugs as epinephrine which decompose in an alkaline pH. |

## TABLE 23-7 • Pharmacokinetic Drug Interactions

| Drug Interaction | Examples (Precipitant Drugs) | Effect (Object Drugs) |
|---|---|---|
| **Bioavailability** | | |
| Complexation/chelation | Calcium, magnesium, or aluminum and iron salts | Tetracycline complexes with divalent cations, causing a decreased bioavailability |
| Adsorption binding/ionic interaction | Cholestyramine resin (anion exchange resin binding) | Decreased bioavailability of thyroxine, and digoxin; binds anionic drugs and reduces absorption. Some antacid may cause HCl salt to precipitate out in stomach. |
| Adsorption | Antacids (adsorption) Charcoal, antidiarrheals | Decreased bioavailability of antibiotics. Decreased bioavailability of many drugs. |
| Increased GI motility | Laxatives, cathartics | Increases GI motility, decreases bioavailability for drugs which are absorbed slowly; may also affect the bioavailability of drugs from controlled-release products. |
| Decreased GI motility | Anticholinergic agents | Propantheline decreases the gastric emptying of acetaminophen (APAP), delaying APAP absorption from the small intestine. |
| Alteration of gastric pH | H-2 blockers, antacids | Both H-2 blockers and antacids increase gastric pH; the dissolution of ketoconazole is reduced, causing decreased drug absorption. |
| Alteration of intestinal flora | Antibiotics (eg, tetracyclines, penicillin) | Digoxin has better bioavailability after erythromycin; erythromycin administration reduces bacterial inactivation of digoxin. |
| Inhibition of drug metabolism in intestinal cells | Monoamine oxidase inhibitors (MAO-I) (eg, tranylcypromine, phenelzine) | Hypertensive crisis may occur in patients treated with MAO-I and foods containing tyramine. |

## TABLE 23-7 • Pharmacokinetic Drug Interactions (*Continued*)

| Drug Interaction | Examples (Precipitant Drugs) | Effect (Object Drugs) |
|---|---|---|
| **Distribution** | | |
| Protein binding | Warfarin–phenylbutazone Phenytoin–valproic acid | Displacement of warfarin from binding. Displacement of phenytoin from binding. |
| **Hepatic Elimination** | | |
| Enzyme induction | Smoking (polycyclic aromatic hydrocarbons) Barbiturates | Smoking increases theophylline clearance. Phenobarbital increases the metabolism of warfarin. |
| Enzyme inhibition Mixed-function oxidase | Cimetidine | Decreased theophylline, diazepam metabolism. |
| | Fluvoxamine | Diazepam $t_{1/2}$ longer. |
| | Quinidine | Decreased nifedipine metabolism. |
| | Fluconazole | Increased levels of phenytoin, warfarin. |
| Other enzymes | Monoamine oxidase inhibitors, MAO-I (eg, pargyline, tranylcypromine) | Serious hypertensive crisis may occur following ingestion of foods with a high content of tyramine or other pressor substances (eg, cheddar cheese, red wines). |
| Inhibition of biliary secretion | Verapamil | Decreased biliary secretion of digoxin causing increased digoxin levels. |
| **Renal Clearance** | | |
| Glomerular filtration rate (GFR) and renal blood flow | Methylxanthines (eg, caffeine, theobromine) | Increased renal blood flow and GFR will decrease time for reabsorption of various drugs, leading to more rapid urinary drug excretion. |
| Active tubular secretion | Probenecid | Probenecid blocks the active tubular secretion of penicillin and some cephalosporin antibiotics. |
| Tubular reabsorption and urine pH | Antacids, sodium bicarbonate | Alkalinization of the urine increases the reabsorption of amphetamine and decreases its clearance. |
| | | Alkalinization of urine pH increases the ionization of salicylates, decreases reabsorption, and increases its clearance. |
| **Diet** | | |
| Charcoal hamburgers | Theophylline Terfenadine, cyclosporin | Increased elimination half-life of theophylline decreases due to increased metabolism. Blood levels of terfenadine and cyclosporine increase due to decreased metabolism. |
| Grapefruit juice | Lovastatin, simvastatin, nifedipine | Grapefruit juice is a moderate CYP3A inhibitor and increases plasma drug concentrations. |
| Alcohol (ethanol) | Acetaminophen | Possible hepatotoxicity. |
| Alcohol (ethanol) | | May increase or decrease absorption of many drugs. |
| **Environmental** | | |
| Smoking | Theophylline | Cigarette smoke contains aromatic hydrocarbons that induce cytochrome isozymes involved in metabolism of theophylline, thereby shortening the elimination $t_{1/2}$. |
| **Pharmacodynamic** | | |
| Alcohol (ethanol) | Antihistamines, opioids | Increased drowsiness. |
| Reye's syndrome | Aspirin | Aspirin in children exposed to certain viral infections such as influenza B virus leads to Reye's syndrome. |

dispensed to the patient. However, the pharmacist should ask the patient when dispensing any medication whether the patient is taking OTC drugs, herbal supplements, or contraceptive drugs. Some patients do not realize that these products may interact with their drug therapy. There are many computer programs that will "flag" a potential drug interaction. However, the pharmacist needs to determine the clinical significance of the interaction and whether there is an alternate drug or alternate dosage regimen design that will prevent the drug interaction. The clinical significance of a potential drug interaction should be documented in the literature. The likelihood of a drug interaction may be classified as an established drug interaction, probable drug interaction, possible drug interaction, or unlikely drug interaction. The dose and the duration of therapy, the onset (rapid, delayed), the severity (major, minor) of the potential interaction, and extrapolation to related drugs should also be considered.

Preferably, drugs that interact should be avoided or doses of each drug should be given sufficiently far apart so that the interaction is minimized. In situations involving two drugs of choice that may interact, dose adjustment based on pharmacokinetic and therapeutic considerations of one or both of the drugs may be necessary. Dose adjustment may be based on clearance or elimination half-life of the drug. Assessment of the patient's renal function, such as serum creatinine concentration, and liver function indicators, such as alkaline phosphatase, alanine aminotransferase, aspartate aminotransferase, or other markers of hepatic metabolism (see Chapter 25), should be undertaken. In general, if the therapeutic response is predictable from serum drug concentration, dosing at regular intervals may be based on a steady-state concentration equation such as Equation 23.1. When the elimination half-life is lengthened by drug interaction, the dosing interval may be extended or the dose reduced according to Equation 23.1. Some examples of pharmacokinetic drug interactions are listed in Table 23-7. A more complete discussion of pharmacologic and therapeutic drug interactions of drugs is available in standard textbooks on clinical pharmacology.

Many drugs affect the CYP superfamily of hemoprotein enzymes (formerly called "cytochrome P450 enzymes") that catalyze drug biotransformation

(see also Chapter 21). Dr. David A. Flockhart, Indiana University School of Medicine, has compiled an excellent website that lists various drugs that may be substrates or inhibitors of these enzymes (https://drug-interactions.medicine.iu.edu/Main-Table.aspx). Some examples of substrates of CYPs are:

| CYP1A2 | Amitriptyline, fluvoxamine, theophylline |
|--------|-------------------------------------------|
| CYP2B6 | Cyclophosphamide |
| CYP2C9 | Ibuprofen, fluoxetine, tolbutamide, amitriptyline |
| CYP2C19 | Omeprazole, S-mephenytoin, amitriptyline |
| CYP2D6 | Propranolol, amitriptyline, fluoxetine, paroxetine |
| CYP2E1 | Halothane, ethanol |
| CYP3As | Erythromycin, clarithromycin, midazolam, diazepam, cyclosporine |

Many calcium channel blockers, macrolides, and protease inhibitors are substrates of CYP3A enzymes. An enzyme substrate may competitively interfere with other substrates' metabolism if coadministered. Drug inducers of CYPs may also result in drug interactions by accelerating the rate of drug metabolism. When an unusually high plasma level is observed as a result of coadministration of a second drug, pharmacists should check whether the two drugs share a common CYP metabolic pathway. New substrates are still being discovered. For example, many proton pump inhibitors are substrates of CYP2C19, and many calcium channel blockers are CYP3A substrates. It is important to assess the clinical significance with the prescriber before alarming the patient. It is also important to suggest an alternative drug therapy to the prescriber if a clinically significant drug interaction is likely to be occurring.

Some examples of pharmacokinetic drug interactions are discussed in more detail below and in Chapter 21. Many side effects occur as a result of impaired or induced (enhanced) drug metabolism. Changes in pharmacokinetics due to impaired drug metabolism should be evaluated quantitatively. For example, acetaminophen is an OTC drug that has been used safely for decades, but incidences of severe hepatic toxicity leading to coma have occurred in some subjects with impaired liver function because of chronic alcohol use. Drugs that have reactive intermediates, active metabolites, and/or metabolites with a longer half-life than the parent drug need to be considered carefully if there is a potential for a drug interaction. A polar metabolite may also distribute to a smaller fluid volume, leading to high concentration in some tissues. Drug interactions involving metabolism may be temporal, observed as a delayed effect. Temporal drug interactions are more difficult to detect in a clinical situation.

## INHIBITION OF DRUG METABOLISM, MONOAMINE OXIDASE (MAO), DRUG METABOLISM, DRUG ABSORPTION, AND BILIARY EXCRETION

### Inhibition of Drug Metabolism

Numerous clinical instances of severe adverse reactions as a result of drug interactions involving a change in the rate of drug metabolism have been reported. Knowledge of pharmacokinetics allows the clinical pharmacist to evaluate the clinical significance of the drug interaction. Pharmacokinetic models help determine the need for dose reduction or discontinuing a drug. In assessing the situation, the pathophysiology of the patient and the effect of chronic therapy on drug disposition in the patient must be considered. In some patients with traumatic injury or severe cardiovascular disease, blood flow may be impaired, resulting in delayed drug absorption and distribution. Potent drugs such as morphine, midazolam, lidocaine, sodium thiopental, and fentanyl can result in serious adverse reactions if the kinetics of multiple dosing are not carefully assessed.

## EXAMPLES ▷ ▷ ▷

1. *Fluvoxamine doubles the half-life of diazepam.* The effect of fluvoxamine on the pharmacokinetics of diazepam was investigated in healthy volunteers (Perucca et al, 1994). Concurrent fluvoxamine intake increased mean peak plasma diazepam concentrations from 108 to 143 ng/mL, and oral diazepam clearance was reduced from 0.40 to 0.14 mL/min/kg. The half-life of diazepam increased from

51 to 118 hours. The area under the plasma concentration–time curve for the diazepam metabolite *N*-desmethyldiazepam was also significantly increased during fluvoxamine treatment. These data suggest that fluvoxamine inhibits the biotransformation of diazepam and its active *N*-demethylated metabolite.

In this example, the dosing interval, $\tau$, may be increased twofold to account for the doubling of elimination half-life to keep average steady-state concentration unchanged based on Equation 23.1. The rationale for this recommendation may be demonstrated by sketching a diagram showing how the steady-state plasma drug level of diazepam differs after taking 10 mg orally twice a day with or without taking fluvoxamine for a week.

$$C_{av(ss)} = \frac{D_0 \cdot F}{\tau \cdot CL}$$

2. *Quinidine inhibits the metabolism of nifedipine and other calcium channel-blocking agents.* Quinidine coadministration significantly inhibited the aromatization of nifedipine to its major first-pass pyridine metabolite and prolonged the elimination half-life by about 40% (Schellens et al, 1991). Quinidine and nifedipine are both metabolized by CYP3A enzymes which explains this interaction. Other calcium channel antagonists may also be affected by a similar interaction. What could be a potential problem if two drugs metabolized by the same enzyme are coadministered?

3. *Theophylline clearance is decreased by cimetidine.* Controlled studies have shown that cimetidine can decrease theophylline plasma clearance by 20%–40% (apparently by inhibiting demethylation) (Loi et al, 1997). Prolongation of half-life by as much as 70% was found in some patients. Elevated theophylline plasma concentrations with toxicity may lead to nausea, vomiting, cardiovascular instability, and even seizure. What could happen to an asthmatic patient whose meals are high in protein and low in carbohydrate, and who takes Tagamet 400 mg BID? (*Hint:* Check the effect of food on theophylline, below.)

4. *Interferon-β reduces metabolism of theophylline.* Theophylline pharmacokinetics was also examined before and after interferon treatment (Okuno et al, 1993). Interferon-β treatment reduced the activities of both O-dealkylases by 47%. The total body clearance of theophylline was also decreased (from 0.76 to 0.56 mL/kg/min) and its elimination half-life was increased (from 8.4 to 11.7 hours; $p < 0.05$). This study provided the first direct evidence that interferon-β can depress the activity of drug-metabolizing enzymes in the human liver. What percent of steady-state theophylline plasma concentration would be changed by the interaction? (Use Equation 23.1.)

5. *Torsades de pointes interaction.* A life-threatening ventricular arrhythmia associated with prolongation of the QT interval, known as torsades de pointes, caused the removal of the antihistamine terfenadine (Seldane) from the market because of drug interactions with cisapride, astemizole, and ketoconazole. Clinical symptoms of torsades de pointes include dizziness, syncope, irregular heartbeat, and sudden death. The active metabolite of terfenadine is not cardiac toxic and is now marked as fexofenadine (Allegra), a nonsedative antihistamine.

6. *Cimetidine and diazepam interaction.* The administration of 800 mg of cimetidine daily for 1 week increased the steady-state plasma diazepam and nordiazepam concentrations due to a cimetidine-induced impairment in microsomal oxidation of diazepam and nordiazepam. The concurrent administration of cimetidine caused a decrease in total metabolic clearance of diazepam and its metabolite, nordiazepam (Lima et al, 1991). How would the following pharmacokinetic parameters of diazepam be affected by the coadministration of cimetidine?

   a. Area under the curve in the dose interval ($AUC_{0-24\,h}$)
   b. Maximum plasma concentration ($C_{max}$)
   c. Time to peak concentration ($t_{max}$)
   d. Elimination rate constant ($k_{el}$)
   e. Total body clearance ($CL_T$)

## Inhibition of MAO

Nonhepatic enzymes can be involved in drug interactions. For example, drug interactions have been reported for patients taking the antibacterial drug linezolid (Zyvox) who are concurrently taking certain psychiatric medications that work through the serotonin system of the brain (serotonergic psychiatric medications). Linezolid is a reversible monoamine oxidase inhibitor (MAOI). Serotonergic psychiatric medications may include antidepressant drugs such as citalopram, paroxetine, fluoxetine, sertraline, and others that affect the serotonergic pathway in the brain. MAOIs, such as phenelzine and isocarboxazid, are also contraindicated. Although the exact mechanism of this drug interaction is unknown, linezolid inhibits the action of monoamine oxidase A—an enzyme responsible for breaking down serotonin in the brain. It is believed that when linezolid is given to patients taking serotonergic psychiatric medications, high levels of serotonin can build up in the brain, causing toxicity. This is referred to as *serotonin syndrome.* Its signs and symptoms include mental changes (confusion, hyperactivity, memory problems), muscle twitching, excessive sweating, shivering or shaking, diarrhea, trouble with coordination, and/or fever. A complete list is posted on the FDA website, http://www.fda.gov/Drugs/DrugSafety/ucm265305.htm (accessed August 12, 2019).

## Induction of Drug Metabolism

CYP enzymes are often involved in the metabolic oxidation of many drugs (see Chapter 21). Many drugs can stimulate the production of hepatic enzymes. Therapeutic doses of phenobarbital and other barbiturates accelerate the metabolism of coumarin anticoagulants such as warfarin and substantially reduce the hypoprothrombinemic effect. Fatal hemorrhagic episodes can result when phenobarbital is withdrawn and warfarin dosage maintained at its previous level. Other drugs known to induce drug metabolism include carbamazepine, rifampin, valproic acid, and phenytoin. Enzymatic stimulation can shorten the elimination half-life of the affected drug. For example, phenobarbital can result in lower levels of dexamethasone in asthmatic patients taking both drugs. St. John's wort, a herbal supplement, also induces CYP3A enzymes and is known to reduce plasma drug concentrations of digoxin, indinavir, and other drugs.

### Inhibition of Drug Absorption

Various drugs and dietary supplements can decrease the absorption of drugs from the gastrointestinal tract. Antacids containing magnesium and aluminum hydroxide often interfere with absorption of many drugs. Coadministration of magnesium and aluminum hydroxide caused a decrease in plasma levels of pefloxacin. This drug interaction is caused by the formation of chelate complexes and is possibly also due to adsorption of the quinolone to aluminum hydroxide gel. Pefloxacin should be given at least 2 hours before the antacid to ensure sufficient therapeutic efficacy of the quinolone.

Sucralfate is an aluminum glycopyranoside complex that is not absorbed but retards the oral absorption of ciprofloxacin. Sucralfate is used in the local treatment of ulcers. Cholestyramine is an anion-exchange resin that binds bile acid and many drugs in the gastrointestinal tract. Cholestyramine can bind digitoxin in the gastrointestinal tract and shortens the elimination half-life of digitoxin by approximately 30%–40%. Absorption of thyroxine may be reduced by 50% when it is administered closely with cholestyramine.

### Inhibition of Biliary Excretion

The interaction between digoxin and verapamil (Hedman et al, 1991) was studied in six patients (mean age 61 ± 5 years) with chronic atrial fibrillation. The effects of adding verapamil (240 mg/d) on steady-state plasma concentrations of digoxin were studied. Verapamil induced a 44% increase in steady-state plasma concentrations of digoxin. The biliary clearance of digoxin was determined by a duodenal perfusion technique. The biliary clearance of digoxin decreased by 43%, from 187 ± 89 to 101 ± 55 mL/min, whereas the renal clearance was not significantly different (153 ± 31 versus 173 ± 51 mL/min).

## ALTERED RENAL REABSORPTION DUE TO CHANGING URINARY PH

The normal adult urinary pH ranges from 4.8 to 7.5 but can increase due to chronic antacid use. This change in urinary pH affects the ionization

and reabsorption of weak electrolyte drugs (see Chapter 6). An increased ionization of salicylate due to an increase in urine pH reduces salicylate reabsorption in the renal tubule, resulting in increased renal excretion. Magnesium aluminum hydroxide gel (Maalox), 120 mL/d for 6 days, decreased serum salicylate levels from 19.8 to 15.8 mg/dL in six subjects who had achieved a control serum salicylate level of 0.10 mg/dL with the equivalent of 3.76 g/d aspirin (Hansten and Hayton, 1980). Single doses of magnesium aluminum hydroxide gel did not alter urine pH significantly. Five milliliters of Titralac (calcium carbonate with glycine) 4 times a day or magnesium hydroxide for 7 days also increased urinary pH. In general, drugs with $pk_a$ values within the urinary pH range are affected the most. Basic drugs tend to have longer half-lives when urinary pH is increased, especially near its $pk_a$.

## PRACTICAL FOCUS

Some drugs can change urinary pH and thereby affect the rate of excretion of weak electrolyte drugs in the urine. Which of the following treatments would be most likely to decrease the elimination $t_{1/2}$ of aspirin? Explain the rationale for your answer.

1. Calcium carbonate PO
2. Sodium carbonate PO
3. Intravenous sodium bicarbonate

## EFFECT OF FOOD ON DRUG DISPOSITION

### Diet–Theophylline Interaction

Theophylline disposition is influenced by diet. A protein-rich diet will increase theophylline clearance. Average theophylline half-lives in subjects on a low-carbohydrate, high-protein diet increased from 5.2 to 7.6 hours when subjects were changed to a high-carbohydrate, low-protein diet. A diet of charcoal-broiled beef, which contains polycyclic aromatic hydrocarbons from the charcoal, resulted in a decrease in theophylline half-life of up to 42% when compared to a control non-charcoal-broiled-beef diet. Irregular intake of vitamin K may modify the anticoagulant effect of warfarin. Many foods, especially green, leafy vegetables such as broccoli and spinach, contain high concentrations of vitamin K. In one study, warfarin therapy was interfered with inpatients receiving vitamin K, broccoli, or spinach daily for 1 week (Pedersen et al, 1991).

### Grapefruit–Drug Interactions

The ingredients in a common food product, grapefruit juice, taken in usual dietary quantities, can significantly inhibit CYP3A and P-Glycoprotein activity in the gut wall (Ducharme et al, 1995; Spence, 1997). For example, grapefruit juice increases average felodipine levels about 3-fold, increases cyclosporine levels, and increases the levels of terfenadine, a common antihistamine. In the case of terfenadine, Spence (1997) reported the death of a 29-year-old man who had been taking terfenadine and drinking grapefruit juice 2–3 times per week. Death was attributed to terfenadine toxicity.

## ADVERSE VIRAL DRUG INTERACTIONS

Recent findings have suggested that some interactions between viruses and drugs may predispose individuals to specific disease outcomes (Haverkos et al, 1991). For example, Reye's syndrome has been observed in children who had been taking aspirin and were concurrently exposed to certain viruses, including influenza B virus and varicella zoster virus. The mechanism by which salicylates and certain viruses interact is not clear. However, the publication of this interaction has led to the prevention of morbidity and mortality due to this complex interaction (Haverkos et al, 1991).

## POPULATION PHARMACOKINETICS

Population pharmacokinetics (PopPK) is the study of variability in plasma drug concentrations between and within patient populations receiving therapeutic doses of a drug. Traditional pharmacokinetic studies are usually performed on healthy volunteers or highly selected patients, and the average behavior of a group (ie, the mean plasma concentration–time profile) is the main focus of interest. PopPK examines the relationship of the demographic, genetic, pathophysiological, environmental, and other

drug-related factors that contribute to the variability observed in safety and efficacy of the drug. The PopPK approach encompasses some of the following features (FDA Guidance for Industry, 1999):

- The collection of relevant pharmacokinetic information in patients who are representative of the target population to be treated with the drug
- The identification and measurement of variability during drug development and evaluation
- The explanation of variability by identifying factors of demographic, pathophysiological, environmental, or concomitant drug-related origin that may influence the pharmacokinetic behavior of a drug
- The quantitative estimation of the magnitude of the unexplained variability in the patient population

The resolution of the issues causing variability in patients allows for the development of an optimum dosing strategy for a population, subgroup, or individual patient. The importance of developing optimum dosing strategies has led to an increase in the use of PopPK approaches in new drug development.

### Introduction to Bayesian Theory

Bayesian theory can be applied in PopPK analyses when few analytical samples are measured. The different types of PopPK analyses and software packages are detailed in Chapters 11, 19, and 20, therefore this chapter will briefly discuss Bayesian theory, as it is important to understand in clinical practice when receiving the results of a Bayesian analysis.

Bayesian theory was originally developed to improve forecast accuracy by combining subjective prediction with improvement from newly collected data. In the diagnosis of disease, the physician may make a preliminary diagnosis based on symptoms and physical examination. Later, the results of laboratory tests are received. The clinician then makes a new diagnostic forecast based on both sets of information. Bayesian theory provides a method to weigh the prior information (eg, physical diagnosis) and new information (eg, results from laboratory tests) to estimate a new probability for predicting the disease.

In developing a drug dosage regimen, we assess the patient's medical history and then use average or population pharmacokinetic parameters appropriate for the patient's condition to calculate the initial dose. After the initial dose, plasma or serum drug concentrations are obtained from the patient that provide new information to assess the adequacy of the dosage. The dosing approach of combining old information with new involves a "feedback" process and is to some degree inherent in many dosing methods involving some parameter readjustment when new serum drug concentrations become known. The advantage of the Bayesian approach is the improvement in estimating the patient's pharmacokinetic parameters based on Bayesian probability versus an ordinary least-squares–based program. The method is particularly useful when only a few blood samples are available.

Because of inter- and intrasubject variability, the pharmacokinetic parameters of an individual patient must be estimated from limited data in the presence of unknown random error (assays, etc), known covariates and variables such as clearance, weight, and disease factor, etc, and possible structural (kinetic model) error. From the knowledge of mean population pharmacokinetic parameters and their variability, Bayesian methods often employ a special *weighted least-squares* approach and allow improved estimation of patient pharmacokinetic parameters when there is a lot of variation in data.

## EXAMPLE ▷ ▷ ▷

After diagnosing a patient, the physician gave the patient a probability of 0.4 of having a disease. The physician then ordered a clinical laboratory test. A positive laboratory test value had a probability of 0.8 of positively identifying the disease in patients with the disease (true positive) and a probability of 0.1 of positive identification of the disease in subjects without the disease (false positive). From the prior information (physician's diagnosis) and current patient-specific data (laboratory test), what is the posterior probability of the patient having the disease using the Bayesian method?

### Solution

Prior probability of having the disease (positive) = 0.4

Prior probability of not having the disease (negative) = 1 − 0.4 = 0.6

Ratio of disease positive to disease negative = 0.4/0.6 = 2/3, or the physician's evaluation shows a 2/3 chance for the presence of the disease

The probability of the patient actually having the disease can be better evaluated by including the laboratory findings. For this same patient, the probability of a positive laboratory test of 0.8 for the detection of disease in positive patients (with disease) and the probability of 0.1 in negative patients (without disease) are equal to a ratio of 0.8/0.1 or 8/1. This ratio is known as the *likelihood ratio*. Combining with the prior probability of 2/3, the posterior probability ratio is

Posterior probability ratio = (2/3) (8/1) = 16/3

Posterior probability = 16/(16 + 3) = 84.2%

Thus, the laboratory test that estimates the likelihood ratio and the preliminary diagnostic evaluation are both used in determining the posterior probability. The results of this calculation show that with a positive diagnosis by the physician and a positive value for the laboratory test, the probability that the patient actually has the disease is 84.2%.

Bayesian probability theory when applied to dosing of a drug involves a given pharmacokinetic parameter ($P$) and plasma or serum drug concentration (C), as shown in Equation 23.6. The probability of a patient with a given pharmacokinetic parameter $P$, taking into account the measured concentration, is Prob($P$/C):

$$\text{Prob}(P/C) = \frac{\text{Prob}(P) \cdot \text{Prob}(C/P)}{\text{Prob}(C)} \quad (23.6)$$

where Prob($P$) = the probability of the patient's parameter within the assumed population distribution, Prob(C/$P$) = the probability of measured concentration within the population, and Prob(C) = the unconditional probability of the observed concentration.

## EXAMPLE  ▷ ▷ ▷

Theophylline has a therapeutic window of 10–20 $\mu$g/mL. Serum theophylline concentrations above 20 $\mu$g/mL produce mild side effects, such as nausea and insomnia; more serious side effects, such as sinus tachycardia, may occur at drug concentrations above 40 $\mu$g/mL; at serum concentrations above 45 $\mu$g/mL, cardiac arrhythmia and seizure may occur (see Fig. 23-1). However, the probability of some side effect occurring is by no means certain. Side effects are not determined solely by plasma concentration, as other known or unknown variables (called covariates) may affect the side effect outcome. Some patients have initial side effects of nausea and restlessness (even at very low drug concentrations) that later disappear when therapy is continued. The clinician should therefore assess the probability of side effects in the patient, order a blood sample for serum theophylline determination, and then estimate a combined (or posterior) probability for side effects in the patient.

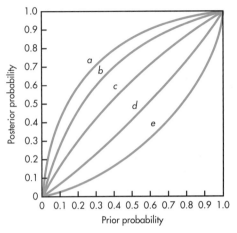

**FIGURE 23-3** • Conditional probability curves relating prior probability of toxicity to posterior probability of toxicity of STC, theophylline serum concentrations: (*a*) 27–28.9, (*b*) 23–24.9, (*c*) 19–20.9, (*d*) 15–16.9, and (*e*) 11–12.9 (all STC in $\mu$g/mL). (Reproduced with permission from Schumacher GE, Barr JT. Applying decision analysis in therapeutic drug monitoring: using decision trees to interpret serum theophylline concentrations, Clin Pharm. 1986 Apr;5(4):325–333.)

The decision process is illustrated graphically in Fig. 23-3. The probability of initial (prior) estimation of side effects is plotted on the *x* axis, and the final (posterior) probability of side effects is plotted on the *y* axis for various serum theophylline concentrations. For example, a patient was placed on theophylline and the physician estimated the chance of side effects to be 40%, but therapeutic drug monitoring showed a theophylline level of 27 $\mu$g/mL. A vertical line of prior probability at 0.4 intersects curve *a* at about 0.78, or 78%. Hence, the Bayesian probability of having side effects is 78% taking both the laboratory and physician assessments into consideration. The curves (*a–e* in Fig. 23-3) for various theophylline concentrations are called *conditional probability curves*. Bayesian theory does not replace clinical judgment, but it provides a quantitative tool for incorporating subjective judgment (human) with objective (laboratory assay) in making risk decisions. When complex decisions involving several variables are involved, this objective tool can be very useful.

Bayesian probability is used to improve forecasting in medicine. One example is its use in the diagnosis of healed myocardial infarction from a 12-lead electrocardiogram by artificial neural networks using the Bayesian concept. Bayesian results were comparable to those of an experienced electrocardiographer (Heden et al, 1996). In pharmacokinetics, Bayesian theory is applied to "feed-forward neural networks" for gentamicin concentration predictions (Smith and Brier, 1996). Bayesian parameter estimations were most frequently used for drugs with narrow therapeutic ranges, such as the aminoglycosides, cyclosporin, digoxin, anticonvulsants (especially phenytoin), lithium, and theophylline. The technique has now been extended to cytotoxic drugs, factor VIII, and warfarin. Bayesian methods have also been used to limit the number of samples required in more conventional pharmacokinetic studies with new drugs (Thomson and Whiting, 1992). The main disadvantage of Bayesian methods is the subjective selection of prior probability.

### Analysis of Population Pharmacokinetic Data

Traditional pharmacokinetic studies involve taking multiple blood samples periodically over time in a few individual patients, and characterizing basic pharmacokinetic parameters such as $k$, $V_D$, and $CL$;

because the studies are generally well designed, there are fewer parameters than data points (ie, to allow the identifiability of the parameters), and the parameters are efficiently estimated even with simple noncompartmental methods. Traditional pharmacokinetic parameter estimation is very accurate, provided that enough samples can be taken for the individual patient. The disadvantage is that only a few relatively homogeneous healthy subjects are included in the majority of pharmacokinetic studies, from which dosing in different patients must be projected.

In the clinical setting, patients are usually less homogeneous; patients vary in sex, age, and body weight; they may have concomitant disease and may be receiving multiple drug treatments. Even the diet, lifestyle, ethnicity, and geographic location can differ from a selected group of "normal" subjects. Further, it is often not possible to take multiple samples from the same subject, and therefore no data are available to reflect intrasubject variability, so that iterative procedures for finding the maximum likelihood estimate can be complex and unpredictable due to incomplete or missing data. However, the vital information needed about the pharmacokinetics of drugs in patients at different stages of their disease with various therapies can only be obtained from the same population, or from a collection of pooled blood samples. The advantages of population pharmacokinetic analysis using pooled data were reviewed by Sheiner and Ludden (1992) and included a summary of population pharmacokinetics for dozens of drugs. Pharmacokinetic analysis of pooled data of plasma drug concentration from a large group of subjects may reveal much information about the disposition of a drug in a population. Unlike data from an individual subject collected over time, inter- and intrasubject variations must be considered. Both pharmacokinetic and nonpharmacokinetic factors, such as age, weight, sex, and creatinine concentration, should be examined in the model to determine the relevance to the estimation of pharmacokinetic parameters.

One example involving analysis of population plasma concentration data involved the drug procainamide. The drug clearance of an individual in a group may be assumed to be affected by several factors (Whiting et al, 1986). These factors include body weight, creatinine clearance, and a clearance factor $P_1$ described in the following equation:

$$CL_{drug\,j} = P_1 + P_2\,(C_{creatinine\,j}) + P_3(weight_j) + \eta_{CLj}\quad(23.7)$$

where $\eta_{CLj}$ is the intersubject error of clearance and its variance is $\omega^2_{CLj}$.

In another mixed-effect model involving the analysis of lidocaine and mexiletine, Vozeh et al (1984) tested age, sex, time on drug therapy, and congestive heart failure (CHF) for effects on drug clearance. The effects of CHF and weight on $V_D$ were also examined. The test statistic, DELS (*difference extended least-squares*), was significant for CHF and moderately significant for weight on lidocaine clearance.

Population pharmacokinetics may be analyzed from various clinical sites. The information content is better when sampling is strategically designed. Proper sampling can yield valuable information about the distribution of pharmacokinetic parameters in a population. Pooled clinical drug concentrations taken from hospital patients are generally not well controlled and are much harder to analyze. A mixed-effect model can yield valuable information about various demographic and pathophysiologic factors that may influence drug disposition in the patient population.

## Decision Analysis Involving Diagnostic Tests

Diagnostic tests may be performed to determine the presence or absence of a disease. A scheme for the predictability of a disease by a diagnostic test is shown in Table 23-8. A true positive, represented by *a*, indicates that the laboratory test correctly predicted the disease, whereas a false positive, represented by *b*, shows that the laboratory test incorrectly predicted that the patient had the disease when, in fact, the patient did not have the disease. In contrast, a true negative, represented by *d*, correctly gave a negative test in patients without the disease, whereas a false negative, represented by *c*, incorrectly gave a negative test when, in fact, the patient did have the disease.

## CLINICAL EXAMPLE 1

A new diagnostic test for HIV+/AIDS was developed and tested in 5772 intravenous drug users. The results of this study are tabulated in Table 23-9. From

**TABLE 23-8** • Errors in Decision Predictability

| Decision | Diagnostic Test Result | | Totals |
| --- | --- | --- | --- |
| | Disease Present | Disease Absent | |
| Accept disease | Test positive | Test positive | |
| Present | (True positive) $a$ | (False positive) $b$ | $a + b$ |
| Reject disease | Test negative | Test negative | |
| Present | (False negative) $c$ | (True negative) $d$ | $c + d$ |
| Totals | $a + c$ | $b + d$ | $a + b + c + d$ |

the results in Table 23-9, a total of 2863 subjects had a positive diagnostic test for HIV+/AIDS and 2909 subjects had a negative diagnostic test for HIV+/AIDS. Further tests on these subjects showed that 2967 subjects actually had HIV+/AIDS, although 211 of these subjects had negative diagnostic test results. Moreover, 107 subjects who had a positive diagnostic test result did not, in fact, have HIV+/AIDS after further tests were made.

1. The *positive predictability* of the test is the likelihood that the test will correctly predict the disease if the test is positive and is estimated as

$$\text{Positive predictability} = \frac{a}{a+b} = \frac{2756}{2863} = 0.963 = 96.3\%$$

2. The *negative predictability* of the test is the likelihood that the patient will not have the disease if the test is negative and is estimated as

$$\text{Negative predictability} = \frac{d}{c+d} = \frac{2698}{2909} = 0.927 = 92.7\%$$

3. The *total predictability* of the test is the likelihood that the patient will be predicted correctly and is estimated as

$$\text{Total predictability} = \frac{a+d}{a+b+c+d} = \frac{2756+2698}{5772} = 0.945 = 94.5\%$$

4. The *sensitivity* of the test is the likelihood that a test result will be positive in a patient with the disease and is estimated as

$$\text{Sensitivity} = \frac{a}{a+c} = \frac{2756}{2967} = 0.929 = 92.9\%$$

5. The *specificity* of the test is the likelihood that a test result will be negative in a patient without the disease and is estimated as

$$\text{Specificity} = \frac{d}{b+d} = \frac{2698}{2805} = 0.962 = 96.2\%$$

Analysis of the results in Table 23-9 shows that a positive result from the new test for HIV+/AIDS will only predict the disease correctly 94.5% of the time. Therefore, the clinician must use other measures to

**TABLE 23-9** • Results of HIV+/AIDS Test

| Decision | Diagnostic Test Result | | Totals |
| --- | --- | --- | --- |
| | Disease Present | Disease Absent | |
| | 2756 | 107 | 2863 |
| Reject HIV+/AIDS present | 211 | 2698 | 2909 |
| Totals | 2967 | 2805 | 5772 |

predict whether the patient has the disease. These other measures may include physical diagnosis of the patient, other laboratory tests, normal incidence of the disease in the patient population (in this case, intravenous drug users), and the experience of the clinician. Each test has different predictive values.

## CLINICAL EXAMPLE 2

An area-under-concentration time curve to minimum inhibitory concentration (AUC/MIC) ratio of ≥400 is recognized as the most appropriate pharmacokinetic/pharmacodynamic (PK/PD) target for vancomycin. Since many clinicians find manual calculation time consuming, an AUC/MIC approach to vancomycin dosing has not been routinely incorporated into practice but rather measurement of serum trough concentrations as a surrogate marker of the AUC. Recently, newer studies have been able to demonstrate successful application of Bayesian methods to vancomycin dosing (Fuchs et al, 2013; Neely et al, 2014; Pai et al, 2014; Heil et al, 2018). These methods have been able to determine precise and consistent AUC values using either vancomycin peaks, troughs or both (Pai et al, 2014; Heil et al, 2018). One method uses a Bayesian approach with the principles previously described (see "Introduction to Bayesian Theory" section). The patient has a $C_{max}$ collected 1 hour after the end of the infusion and a trough concentration. This information is then input into a software program that calculates the AUC. The dose will then be adjusted to maintain an AUC/MIC between 400 and 600 (Pai et al, 2014; Heil et al, 2018). This current PK/PD target is recommended in clinical practice guidelines in order to maximize efficacy and minimize the likelihood of nephrotoxicity (Rybak et al, 2020). It is also recommended to use a $MIC_{BMD90}$ of 1 mg/L, as this reflects most MICs encountered in clinical practice (Rybak et al, 2020).

Another method is to use an equation-based method. This could be used by institutions without access to Bayesian software or used to create an institution-specific spreadsheet. This approach requires two levels: a $C_{max}$ ("peak"), measured 1 hour after the end of the infusion, and a $C_{min}$ ("trough"), usually measured 30 min before the next dose. These two levels are then used to calculate a patient-specific $k_{el}$ assuming a one-compartment model. Once a $k_{el}$

is determined, the next steps are to back-extrapolate and calculate the concentration at the end of the infusion ($C_{eoi'}$) and then forward-extrapolate the concentration for the true trough, at the end of the dosing interval. This approach is illustrated using the equation below (Pai et al, 2014):

$$AUC_{0-t} = t' \cdot \frac{C_{eoi'} + C_{trough}}{2} + \frac{C_{eoi'} - C_{trough}}{k_{el}}$$

Where $t'$ = given infusion time, $C_{eoi'}$ = calculated value for end of infusion, $C_{trough}$ = calculated value for "true" trough, $k_{el}$ = elimination rate constant.

The above equation will estimate the AUC over the dosing interval ($AUC_{0-12}$ for a dose given every 12 hours) assuming a one-compartment model. The $AUC_{0-24}$ is the sum of the AUC of identical doses and intervals in 24 hours. For example, to calculate the $AUC_{0-24}$ of a dose administered every 12 hours, the $AUC_{0-12}$ will have to be multiplied by 2. This equation method will underestimate the AUC if the pharmacokinetics of the drug is not well described by a one-compartment model, as it does not account for the distribution phase and the concentration increase is not linear at the end of the infusion (Pai et al, 2014). For vancomycin, a drug known to be described by a two-compartment model, a Bayesian approach using a two-compartment model would be the recommended method (Pai et al, 2014; Heil et al, 2018; Rybak et al, 2020).

## PRACTICE PROBLEM

A 65-year-old female is started on vancomycin for bacterial meningitis. She weighs 60 kg and her estimated creatinine clearance is 60 mL/min. She is started on a dose of vancomycin 1000 mg intravenous every 12 hours. She has a $C_{max}$ drawn 1 hour after the end of a 1-hour infusion, and it is 32 μg/mL. Her $C_{min}$ drawn 30 min before her next dose is 13 μg/mL. Assuming a $MIC_{BMD90}$ of 1 mg/L, a $V_D$ of 0.65 L/kg, and a one-compartment model, calculate the $AUC_{0-24}$ for this patient.

### Solution

$C_1$ = 32 μg/mL drawn at 2 hours after start of infusion

$C_2$ = 13 μg/mL drawn at 11.5 hours after start of infusion

$\Delta t = 11.5 - 2 = 9.5$ hours

$V_D = 0.65$ L/kg $\times$ 60 kg $= 39$ L

Dose $= 1000$ mg

$\tau = 12$ hours

$t' = 1$ hour

1. Solve for $k_{el} = \dfrac{\ln(C_1/C_2)}{\Delta t} = \dfrac{\ln(32/13)}{9.5\ \text{h}} = 0.09$

2. Solve for $C_{eoi'} = \dfrac{\text{dose}/V_D\ (e^{-kt'})}{(1-e^{-k\tau})} = \dfrac{1000/39\ (e^{-0.09 \cdot 1})}{(1-e^{-0.09 \cdot 12})} = 34.5\ \mu\text{g/mL}$

3. Solve for $C_t = C_{eoi'} \cdot e^{-kt} = 34.5\ \mu\text{g/mL} \cdot e^{-0.09 \cdot 11.5} = 12.3\ \mu\text{g/mL}$

4. Calculate $\text{AUC}_{0-12} = t' \cdot \dfrac{C_{eoi'} + C_{trough}}{2} + \dfrac{C_{eoi'} - C_{trough}}{k_{el}} = 260\ \text{h} \cdot \text{mg/L}$

5. Calculate $\text{AUC}_{0-24} = \text{AUC}_{0-12} \cdot 2 = 520\ \text{h} \cdot \text{mg/L}$

Clinical interpretation: This dose estimates an AUC/MIC of 400–600 which is within our desired range for efficacy and acceptable likelihood of nephrotoxicity.

## REGIONAL PHARMACOKINETICS

Pharmacokinetics is the study of the time course of drug concentrations in the body. It is based generally on the time course of drug concentrations in systemic blood sampled from either a vein or an artery. This general approach is useful as long as the drug concentrations in the tissues of the body are well reflected by drug concentrations in the blood. Clinically, the blood drug concentration may not be proportional to the drug concentration in tissues. For example, after intravenous bolus administration, the distributive phase is attributed to temporally different changes in mixing and redistribution of drug in organs such as the lung, heart, and kidney (Upton, 1990). The time course for the pharmacodynamics of the drug may have no relationship to the time course for the drug concentrations in the blood. The pharmacodynamics of the drug may be related to local tissue drug levels and the status of homeostatic physiologic functions. After an intravenous bolus dose, Upton (1990) reported that lignocaine (lidocaine) rapidly accumulates in the spleen and kidney but is slowly sequestered into fat. More than 30 minutes were needed before the target-site (heart and brain) drug levels established equilibrium with drug concentrations in the blood. These *regional equilibrium factors* are often masked in conventional pharmacokinetic models that assume rapid drug equilibrium.

*Regional pharmacokinetics* is the study of pharmacokinetics within a given tissue region. The tissue region is defined as an anatomic area of the body between specified afferent and efferent blood vessels. For example, the myocardium includes the region perfused by the coronary arterial (afferent) and the coronary sinus (efferent) blood vessels. The selection of a region bounded by its network of blood vessel is based on the movement of drug between the blood vessels and the interstitial and intracellular spaces of the region. The conventional pharmacokinetic approach for calculating systemic clearance and volume of distribution tends to average various drug distributions together such that the local perturbations are neglected. Regional pharmacokinetics (see Mather, 2001; Chapter 18) supplement systemic pharmacokinetics when inadequate information is provided by conventional pharmacokinetics.

Various homeostatic physiologic functions may be responsible for the nonequilibrium of drug concentrations between local tissue regions and the blood. For example, most cells have an electrochemical difference across the cell membrane consisting of a membrane potential of negative 70 mV inside the membrane relative to the outside. Moreover, regional differences in pH normally exist within a cell. For example, the pH within the lysosome is between 4 and 5, which could allow a basic drug to accumulate within the lysosome with a concentration gradient of 400-fold to 160,000-fold over the blood. Other explanations for regional drug concentration differences have been reviewed by Upton (1990), who also considers that dynamic processes may be more important than equilibrium processes in affecting dynamic response. Thus, regional pharmacokinetics is another approach in applying pharmacokinetics to pharmacodynamics and clinical effect.

### FREQUENTLY ASKED QUESTIONS

▶ What is meant by population pharmacokinetics? What advantages does population pharmacokinetics have over classical pharmacokinetics?

▶ Why is it possible to estimate individual pharmacokinetic parameters with just a few data points using the Bayesian method?

▶ Why is pharmacokinetics important in studying drug interactions?

## CHAPTER SUMMARY

Successful drug therapy involves the selection of the drug, the drug product, and the development of a dosage regimen that meets the needs of the patient. Often, drug dosage regimens are based on average population pharmacokinetics. Ideally, the dosage regimen can be developed for the individual patient by taking into consideration the patient's demographics, genetics, pathophysiology, environmental issues, possible drug–drug interactions, known variability in drug response, and other drug-related issues. The development of MTM and therapeutic drug monitoring services can improve patient compliance and the success of drug therapy. Drug dosage regimens may be calculated in an individual patient based on complete or incomplete pharmacokinetic information. Changes in the dose and/or in the dosing interval can affect the $C_{max(ss)}$, $C_{min(ss)}$, and $C_{av(ss)}$. Furthermore, pharmacokinetics of a drug may be altered in special populations (eg, the elderly, infants, obese patients, and patients with renal or

hepatic disease) and/or by interaction with concomitant medication. A drug interaction generally refers to a modification of the expected drug response in the patient as a result of exposure of the patient to another drug or substance. Drug–drug interactions may cause an alteration in the pharmacokinetics of the drug due to an interaction in drug absorption, distribution, or elimination. Bayesian analyses are useful in clinical practice as they allow clinicians and researchers to find the pharmacokinetic parameters of a drug in a given patient using very few pharmacokinetic samples. In order for clinicians to use Bayesian analyses, knowledge about the population pharmacokinetics of a drug is necessary. PopPK is the study of variability in plasma drug concentrations between and within patient populations receiving therapeutic doses of a drug and enables the estimate of pharmacokinetic parameters from relatively sparse data obtained from study subjects.

## LEARNING QUESTIONS

1. Why is it harder to titrate patients with a drug whose elimination half-life is 36 hours compared to a drug whose elimination is 6 hours?

2. Penicillin G has a volume of distribution of 42 L/1.73 m² and an elimination rate constant of 1.034 h⁻¹. Calculate the maximum peak concentration ($C_{max}$) that would be produced if the drug was given intravenously at a rate of 250 mg every 6 hours for a week.

3. Dicloxacillin has an elimination half-life of 42 minutes and a volume of distribution of 20 L. Dicloxacillin is 97% protein bound. What would be the steady-state free concentration of dicloxacillin if the drug was given intravenously at a rate of 250 mg every 6 hours?

4. The maintenance dose of digoxin was reported to be 0.5 mg/day for a 60-kg patient with normal renal function. The half-life of digoxin is

0.95 days and the volume of distribution is 306 L. The bioavailability of the digoxin tablet is 0.56.

   a. Calculate the steady-state concentration of digoxin.

   b. Determine whether the patient is adequately dosed (effective serum digoxin concentration is 1–2 ng/mL).

   c. What is the steady-state concentration if the patient is dosed with the elixir instead of the tablet? (Assume the elixir to be 100% bioavailable.)

5. An antibiotic has an elimination half-life of 2 hours and an apparent volume of distribution of 200 mL/kg. The minimum effective serum concentration is 2 μg/mL and the minimum toxic serum concentration is 16 μg/mL. A physician ordered a dosage regimen of this antibiotic

to be given at 250 mg every 8 hours by repetitive intravenous bolus injections.

a. Comment on the appropriateness of this dosage regimen for an adult male patient (23 years, 80 kg) whose creatinine clearance is 122 mL/min.

b. Would you suggest an alternative dosage regimen for this patient? Give your reasons and suggest an alternative dosage regimen.

6. A potent drug with a narrow therapeutic index is ordered for a patient. After making rounds, the attending physician observes that the patient is not responding to drug therapy and orders a single plasma-level measurement. Comment briefly on the value of measuring the drug concentration in a single blood sample and on the usefulness of the information that may be gained.

7. Calculate an oral dosage regimen for a cardiotonic drug for an adult male (63 years old, 68 kg) with normal renal function. The elimination half-life for this drug is 30 hours and its apparent volume of distribution is 4 L/kg. The drug is 80% bioavailable when given orally, and the suggested therapeutic serum concentrations for this drug range from 0.001 to 0.002 $\mu g/mL$.

a. This cardiotonic drug is commercially supplied as 0.075-mg, 0.15-mg, and 0.30-mg white, scored, compressed tablets. Using these readily available tablets, what dose would you recommend for this patient?

b. Are there any advantages for this patient to give smaller doses more frequently compared to a higher dosage less frequently? Any disadvantages?

c. Is there a rationale for preparing a controlled-release product of this drug?

8. The dose of sulfisoxazole (Gantrisin, Roche) recommended for an adult female patient (age 26 years, 63 kg) with a urinary tract infection was 1.5 g every 4 hours. The drug is 85% bound to serum proteins. The elimination half-life of this drug is 6 hours and the apparent volume of distribution is 1.3 L/kg. Sulfisoxazole is 100% bioavailable. Calculate the steady-state plasma concentration of sulfisoxazole in this patient.

9. An antibiotic is to be given to an adult male patient (75 kg, 58 years of age) by intravenous infusion. The elimination half-life for this drug is 8 hours and the apparent volume of distribution is 1.5 L/kg. The drug is supplied in 30-mL ampules at a concentration of 15 mg/mL. The desired steady-state serum concentration for this antibiotic is 20 mg/mL. What infusion rate ($R$) would you suggest for this patient?

10. Nomograms are frequently used in lieu of pharmacokinetic calculations to determine an appropriate drug dosage regimen for a patient. Discuss the advantages and disadvantages of using nomograms to calculate a drug dosage regimen.

11. Based on the following pharmacokinetic data for drugs A, B, and C: **(a)** Which drug takes the longest time to reach steady state? **(b)** Which drug would achieve the highest steady-state drug concentration? **(c)** Which drug has the largest apparent volume of distribution?

| | Drug A | Drug B | Drug C |
|---|---|---|---|
| Rate of infusion (mg/h) | 10 | 20 | 15 |
| $k_{el}$ (h$^{-1}$) | | 0.5 | 0.1 | 0.05 |
| CL (L/h) | | 5 | 20 | 5 |

12. The effect of repetitive administration of phenytoin (PHT) on the single-dose pharmacokinetics of primidone (PRM) was investigated by Sato et al (1992) in three healthy male subjects. The peak concentration of unchanged PRM was achieved at 12 and 8 hours after the administration of PRM in the absence and the presence of PHT, respectively. The elimination half-life of PRM was decreased from 19.4 ± 2.2 (mean ± SE) to 10.2 ± 5.1 hours ($p < 0.05$), and the total body clearance was increased from 24.6 ± 3.1 to 45.1 ± 5.1 mL/h/kg ($p < 0.01$) in the presence of PHT. No significant change was observed for the apparent volume of distribution between the two treatments. Based on pharmacokinetics of the two drugs, what are the possible reasons for phenytoin to reduce primidone elimination half-life and increase its renal clearance?

13. Itraconazole (Sporanox, Janssen) is a lipoph-
    ilic drug with extensive lipid distribution. The
    drug levels in fatty tissue and organs contain
    2–20 times the drug levels in the plasma. Little or
    no drug was found in the saliva and in the cere-
    brospinal fluid, and the half-life is 64 ± 32 hours.
    The drug is 99.8% bound. How do (a) plasma
    drug–protein binding, (b) tissue drug distribu-
    tion, and (c) lipid tissue partitioning contribute
    to the long elimination half-life for itraconazole?

14. JL (29-year-old man, 180 kg) received oral oflox-
    acin 400 mg twice a day for presumed bronchi-
    tis due to *Streptococcus pneumoniae*. His other
    medications were 400 mg cimetidine, orally,
    3 times a day and 400 mg metronidazole, as
    directed. JL was still having a fever of 100.1°C a
    day after taking the quinolone antibiotic. Com-
    ment on any appropriate action.

## ANSWERS

### Frequently Asked Questions

*Can therapeutic drug monitoring be performed with-
out taking blood samples?*

- TDM may be performed by sampling other biologic fluids, such as saliva or, when available, tissue or ear fluids. However, the sample must be
  correlated to blood or special tissue level. Urinary
  drug concentrations generally are not reliable.
  Saliva is considered an ultrafiltrate of plasma and
  does not contain significant albumin. Saliva drug
  concentrations represent free plasma drug levels
  and have been used with limited success to monitor some drugs.
- Pharmacodynamic endpoints such as prothrombin clotting time for warfarin, blood glucose
  concentrations for antidiabetic drugs, blood pressure for antihypertensive drugs, and other clinical
  observations are useful indications that the drug
  is dosed correctly.

*What are the major considerations in therapeutic drug
monitoring?*

- The major considerations in TDM include the
  pathophysiology of the patient, the blood sample
  collection, and the data analysis. Clinical assessment of patient history, drug interaction, and
  demographic factors are all part of a successful
  program for TDM.

*What is meant by population pharmacokinetics?
What advantages does population pharmacokinetics
have over classical pharmacokinetics?*

- Most pharmacokinetic models require well-
  controlled studies in which many blood samples
  are taken from each subject and the pharmacokinetic parameters estimated. In patient care situations, only a limited number of blood samples
  is collected, which does not allow for the complete determination of the drug's pharmacokinetic profile in the individual patient. However,
  the data from blood samples taken from a large
  demographic sector are more reflective of the disease states and pharmacogenetics of the patients
  treated. Population pharmacokinetics allow data
  from previous patients to be used in addition
  to the limited blood sample from the individual
  patient. The type of information obtained is less
  constrained and is sometimes dependent on the
  model and algorithm used for analysis. However,
  many successful examples have been reported in
  the literature.

*Why is it possible to estimate individual pharmacoki-
netic parameters with just a few data points using the
Bayesian method?*

- With the Bayesian approach, the estimates of
  patient parameters are constrained more nar-
  rowly, to allow easier parameter estimation based
  on information provided from the population.
  The information is then combined with one or
  more serum concentrations from the patient to
  obtain a set of final patient parameters (generally
  $CL$ and $V_D$). When no serum sample is taken, the
  Bayesian approach is reduced to an *a priori* model
  using only population parameters.

*Why is pharmacokinetics important in studying drug interactions?*

■ Pharmacokinetics provides a means of studying whether an unusual drug action is related to pharmacokinetic factors, such as drug disposition, distribution, or binding, or is related to pharmacodynamic interaction, such as a difference in receptor sensitivity, drug tolerance, or some other reason. Many drug interactions involving enzyme inhibition, stimulation, and protein binding were discovered as a result of pharmacokinetic, pharmacogenetic, and pharmacodynamic investigations.

*Why are drugs that demonstrate high intrasubject variability generally safer than critical-dose drugs?*

■ Drug safety is more closely linked to the therapeutic window of a drug. Despite great variability in drug handling due to physiological or disease changes of a patient, a drug could still be well tolerated if the therapeutic window is wide enough.

*What type of drugs should be monitored?*

■ Drugs with a narrow therapeutic window (where comparatively small differences in dose or concentration lead to serious therapeutic failures and/or serious adverse drug reactions) should be closely monitored.

*How does one determine whether an adverse event is drug related?*

■ The determination is usually composed of several factors: prior knowledge/experience with the drug, temporal relationship between drug administration and adverse effect onset, dechallenge with an antagonist, rechallenge with repeat exposure(s), availability of objective evidence (eg, elevated plasma drug concentration or abnormal laboratory test value), and plausible alternative explanations.

## Learning Questions

1. Steady-state drug concentrations are achieved in approximately five half-lives. For a drug with a half-life of 36 hours, steady-state drug concentrations are achieved in approximately 180 hours

(or 7.5 days). Thus, dose adjustment in patients is difficult for drugs with very long half-lives. In contrast, steady-state drug concentrations are achieved in approximately 20–30 hours (or 1 day) for drugs whose half-lives are 4–6 hours.

2. $C_{\max(ss)} = \dfrac{D_0/V_D}{1-e^{-k\tau}} = \dfrac{250,000/42,000}{1-e^{-6 \cdot 1.034}} = \dfrac{5.95}{0.998} = 5.96 \,\mu g/mL$

At steady state, the peak concentration of penicillin G will be 5.96 $\mu g/mL$.

3. $CL = \dfrac{\ln(2)}{t_{1/2}} \cdot V_D = \dfrac{0.693}{0.7\text{ h}} \cdot 20,000\text{ mL} = 19,804\text{ mL/h}$

$C_{\mathrm{av(ss)}} = \dfrac{D_0 \cdot F}{\tau \cdot CL} = \dfrac{250,000\,\mu g \cdot (1-0.97)}{6\text{ h} \cdot 19,804\text{ mL/h}} = 0.063\,\mu g/mL$

Free drug concentration at steady state 0.063 $\mu g/mL$.

4. **a.** $CL = \dfrac{\ln(2)}{t_{1/2}} \cdot V_D = \dfrac{0.693}{0.95\text{ days}} \cdot 306,000\text{ mL} = 223,218.95\text{ mL/day}$

$C_{\mathrm{av(ss)}} = \dfrac{D_0 \cdot F}{\tau \cdot CL} = \dfrac{500,000\text{ ng} \cdot 0.56}{1 \cdot 223,218.95\text{ mL/day}} = 1.25\text{ ng/mL}$

**b.** The patient is adequately dosed.

**c.** $F = 1$; using the above equation, the $C_{\mathrm{av(ss)}}$ is 2.2 ng/mL; although still effective, the $C_{\mathrm{av(ss)}}$ will be closer to the toxic serum concentration of 3 ng/mL.

5. The $CL_{CR}$ for this patient shows normal kidney function.

$t_{1/2} = 2\text{h}$

$k_{el} = \dfrac{0.693}{2\text{ h}} = 0.347\text{ h}^{-1}$

$V_D = 0.2\text{ L/kg} \cdot 80\text{ kg} = 16\text{ L}$

**a.** $C_{\max(ss)} = \dfrac{D_0/V_D}{1-e^{-k\tau}} = \dfrac{250/16}{1-e^{-(0.3465)(8)}} = 16.68\text{ mg/L}$

$C_{\min(ss)} = C_{\max(ss)} \cdot e^{-k\tau} = C_{\max(ss)} \cdot e^{-(0.3465)(8)} = 1.04\text{ mg/L}$

The dosage regimen of 250 mg every 8 hours gives a $C_{\max(ss)}$ above 16 mg/L and a $C_{\min(ss)}$ below 2 mg/L. Therefore, this dosage regimen is not correct.

**b.** Several trials might be necessary to obtain a more optimal dosing regimen. One approach is to change the dosage interval, $\tau$, to 6 hours and to calculate the dose, $D_0$:

$D_0 = C_{\max(ss)} \cdot V_D \cdot (1-e^{-k\tau}) = 16 \cdot 16 \cdot (1-e^{-(0.3465)(6)}) = 224\text{ mg}$

$$C_{min(ss)} = C_{max(ss)} \cdot e^{-k\tau} = 16 \cdot e^{-(0.3465)(6)} = 2 \text{ mg/L}$$

A dose of 224 mg given every 6 hours should achieve the desired drug concentrations.

7. Assume desired $C_{av(ss)} = 0.0015 \ \mu g/mL$ and $\tau = 24$ h

$$CL = \frac{\ln(2)}{t_{1/2}} \cdot V_D = \frac{0.693}{30 \text{ h}} \cdot (4 \text{ L} \cdot 68 \text{ kg}) = 6.283 \text{ L/h}$$

$$D_0 = \frac{C_{av(ss)} \cdot \tau \cdot CL}{F} = \frac{0.0015 \ \mu g/mL \cdot 24 \cdot 6.283 \text{ L/h}}{0.80} = 0.283 \text{ mg}$$

Give 0.283 mg every 24 hours.

a. For a dosage regimen of one 0.30-mg tablet daily

$$C_{av(ss)} = \frac{D_0 \cdot F}{\tau \cdot CL} = \frac{0.30 \text{ mg} \cdot 0.80}{24 \cdot 6.283 \text{ L/h}} = 0.0016 \ \mu g/mL$$

which is within the therapeutic window.

b. A dosage regimen of 0.15 mg every 12 hours would provide smaller fluctuations between $C_{max(ss)}$ and $C_{min(ss)}$ compared to a dosage regimen of 0.30 mg every 24 hours.

c. There is no rationale for a controlled-release drug product because of the long elimination half-life of 30 hours inherent in the drug.

8. $CL = \dfrac{\ln(2)}{t_{1/2}} \cdot V_D = \dfrac{0.693}{6 \text{ h}} \cdot (1.3 \text{ L} \cdot 63 \text{ kg}) = 9.46 \text{ L/h}$

$$C_{av(ss)} = \frac{D_0 \cdot F}{\tau \cdot CL} = \frac{1,500 \text{ mg} \cdot 1}{4 \cdot 9.46 \text{ L/h}} = 39.6 \ \mu g/mL$$

9. $k_{el} = \dfrac{\ln(2)}{t_{1/2}} = \dfrac{0.693}{8 \text{ h}} = 0.866 \text{ h}^{-1}$

$V_D = 1.5 \text{ L/kg} \cdot 75 \text{ kg} = 112.5 \text{ L}$

$CL = V_D \cdot k_{el} = 0.866 \text{ h}^{-1} \cdot 112.5 \text{ L} = 9.74 \text{ L/h}$

$C_{ss} = 20 \ \mu g/mL$

$$R = \frac{C_{av(ss)} \cdot CL}{F} = \frac{20 \ \mu g/mL \cdot 9.74 \text{ L/h}}{1} = 194.8 \text{ mg/h}$$

10. Advantages: logistic convenience, feasible for a large patient load. Disadvantages: dosing not individualized based on patient-specific pharmacokinetics (ie, empiric dosing adjustment), considerable efforts to develop a new nomogram, established nomograms may not be applicable to other institutions / patient cohorts.

11. (a) Drug C – it has the longest half-life; (b) Drug C – it has greatest rate of infusion/$CL$ ratio; (c) Drug B – it has greatest $CL/k$ ratio

12. Phenytoin is an inducer of CYP3A4. Administration of phenytoin would increase the metabolism of primidone, resulting in a shorter elimination half-life. With a greater amount of metabolites (cleared renally) formed, the renal clearance of primidone could also be increased.

13. In all cases, limited itraconazole is available for metabolism: (a) high protein binding limits free drug available; (b) extensive drug distribution in peripheral organs limits drug availability systemically; (c) preferential drug accumulation in fatty tissue limits drug availability systemically.

14. The patient is morbidly obese. The use of a standard ofloxacin dose may not be adequate to achieve effective concentrations at the site of infection. If the patient is not responding to therapy as expected, a higher dose should be considered with close monitoring for adverse effects (preferably with TDM guidance if available).

## REFERENCES

Alloway R, Barr WH, Flagstad M, et al: Substitution of critical dose drugs: Issues, analysis, and decision making. Washington, DC, American Pharmaceutical Association, 2000.

Barnett M, Frank J, Wehring H, et al: Analysis of pharmacist-provided medication therapy management (MTM) services in community pharmacies over 7 years. *J Manag Care Pharm* **15**(1):18–31, 2009.

DeHaan RM, Metzler CM, Schellenberg D, et al: Pharmacokinetic study of clindamycin hydrochloride in humans. *Int J Clin Pharmacol Biopharm* **6**:105–119, 1972.

Ducharme MP, Warbasse LH, Edwards DJ. Disposition of intravenous and oral cyclosporine following administration with grapefruit juice. *Clin Pharmacol Ther* **57**:485–491, 1995.

Evans WE, Schentag JJ, Jusko WJ: *Applied Pharmacokinetics. Principles of Therapeutic Drug Monitoring.* San Francisco, Applied Therapeutics, 1992.

FDA Guidance for Industry: Population Pharmacokinetics, 1999.

Fuchs A, Csajka C, Thoma Y, et al: Benchmarking therapeutic drug monitoring 1390 software: A review of available computer tools. *Clin Pharmacokinet* **52**(1):9–22, 2013.

Greenblatt DJ: Predicting steady state serum concentration of drugs. *Annu Rev Pharmacol Toxicol* **19**:347–356, 1979.

Guidance Document: Comparative Bioavailability Standards: Formulations Used for Systemic Effects, Minister of Health, Therapeutic Products Directorate (TPD), 2018.

Hansten PD, Hayton WI: Effect of antacid and ascorbic acid on serum salicylate concentration. *J Clin Pharmacol* **20**:326–331, 1980.

Haverkos HW, Amsel Z, Drotman DP: Adverse virus–drug interactions. *Rev Infect Dis* **13**:697–704, 1991.

Heden B, Ohlsson M, Rittner R, et al: Agreement between artificial neural networks and experienced electrocardiographer on electrocardiographic diagnosis of healed myocardial infarction. *J Am Coll Cardiol* **28**(4):1012–1016, 1996.

Hedman A, Angelin B, Arvidsson A, et al: Digoxin–verapamil interaction: Reduction of biliary but not renal digoxin clearance in humans. *Clin Pharmacol Ther* **49**(3):256–262, 1991.

Heil EL, Claeys KC, Mynatt RP, et al: Making the change to area under the curve-based 1386 vancomycin dosing. *Am J Health Syst Pharm* **75**(24):1986–1995, 2018.

Hendeles L, Weinberger M: Avoidance of adverse effects during chronic therapy with theophylline. *Drug Intell Clin Pharm* **14**:523, 1980.

Iafrate RP, Glotz VP, Robinson JD, Lupkiewicz SM: Computer simulated conversion from intravenous to sustained-release oral theophylline drug. *Intell Clin Pharm* **16**:19–25, 1982.

Ingram PR, Lye DC, Tambyah PA, et al: Risk factors for nephrotoxicity associated with continuous vancomycin infusion in outpatient parenteral antibiotic therapy. *J Antimicrob Chemother* **62**:168–71, 2008.

Izzo AA, Ernst E: Interactions between herbal medicines and prescribed drugs: An updated systematic review. *Drugs* **69**(13):1777–1798, 2009.

Lima DR, Santos RM, Werneck E, Andrade GN: Effect of orally administered misoprostol and cimetidine on the steady-state pharmacokinetics of diazepam and nordiazepam in human volunteers. *Eur J Drug Metab Pharmacokinet* **16**(3):61–70, 1991.

Loi CM, Parker BM, Cusack BJ: Aging and drug interactions. III. Individual and combined effects of cimetidine and cimetidine and ciprofloxacin on theophylline metabolism in healthy male and female nonsmokers. *J Pharmacol Exp Ther* **280**(2):627–637, 1997.

Mather LE: Anatomical-physiological approaches in pharmacokinetics and pharmacodynamics. *Clin Pharmacokinet* **40**:707–722, 2001.

Mawer GE: Computer assisted prescribing of drugs. *Clin Pharmacokinet* **1**:67–78, 1976.

Medicare Prescription Drug, Improvement, and Modernization Act of 2003 (/www.fda.gov/ohrms/dockets/dockets/04s0170/04s-0170-bkg0001-108s1013.pdf).

Neely MN, Young G, Jones B, et al. Are vancomycin concentrations adequate for optimal dosing? *Antimicrob Agents Chemother* **58**(1):309–16, 2014.

Norton K, Ingram PR, Heath CH, Manning L: Risk factors for nephrotoxicity in patients receiving outpatient continuous infusions of vancomycin in an Australian tertiary hospital. *J Antimicrob Chemother* **69**:805–8, 2014.

Okuno H, Takasu M, Kano H, Seki T, Shiozaki Y, Inoue K: Depression of drug metabolizing activity in the human liver by interferon-beta. *Hepatology* **17**(1):65–69, 1993.

Pai MP, Neely M, Rodvold KA, Lodise TP. Innovative approaches to optimizing the delivery of 1381 vancomycin in individual patients. *Adv Drug Deliv Rev* **77**:50-7, 2014.

Pedersen FM, Hamberg O, Hess K, Ovesen L: The effect of dietary vitamin K on warfarin-induced anticoagulation. *J Intern Med* **229**:517–20, 1991.

Perucca E, Gatti G, Cipolla G, et al: Inhibition of diazepam metabolism by fluvoxamine: A pharmacokinetic study in normal volunteers. *Clin Pharmacol Ther* **56**(5):471–476, 1994.

Rybak MJ, Le J, Lodise TP et al. Therapeutic monitoring of vancomycin for serious methicillin-resistant Staphylococcus aureus: A revised consensus guideline and review of the American Society of Health-System Pharmacists, the Infectious Diseases Society of America, the Pediatric Infectious Diseases Society and the Society of Infectious Diseases Pharmacists. *Am J Health Syst Pharm* **77**(11):835–864, 2020.

Sato J, Sekizawa Y, Yoshida A, et al: Single-dose kinetics of primidone in human subjects: Effect of phenytoin on formation and elimination of active metabolites of primidone, phenobarbital and phenylethylmalonamide. *J Pharmacobiodyn* **15**(9):467–472, 1992.

Schellens JH, Ghabrial H, van-der-Wart HH, Bakker EN, Wilkinson GR, Breimer DD: Differential effects of quinidine on the disposition of nifedipine, sparteine, and mephenytoin in humans. *Clin Pharmacol Ther* **50**(5 pt 1):520–528, 1991.

Schumacher GE: Choosing optimal sampling times for therapeutic drug monitoring. *Clin Pharm* **4**:84–92, 1985.

Schumacher GE: *Therapeutic Drug Monitoring*. Norwalk, CT, Appleton & Lange, 1995.

Schumacher GE, Barr JT: Applying decision analysis in therapeutic drug monitoring: Using decision trees to interpret serum theophylline concentrations. *Clin Pharm* **5**:325–333, 1986.

Sheiner LB, Ludden TM: Population pharmacokinetics/dynamics. *Annu Rev Pharmacol Toxicol* **32**:185–209, 1992.

Smith BP, Brier ME: Statistical approach to neural network model building for gentamicin peak predictions. *J Pharm Sci* **85**(1):65–69, 1996.

Spapen HD, Janssen van Doorn K, Diltoer M, et al: Retrospective evaluation of possible renal toxicity associated with continuous infusion of vancomycin in critically ill patients. *Ann Intensive Care* **1**:26, 2011.

Spence JD: Drug interactions with grapefruit: Whose responsibility is it to warn the public? *Clin Pharmacol Ther* **61**:395–400, 1997.

Thomson AH, Whiting B: Bayesian parameter estimation and population pharmacokinetics. *Clin Pharmacokinet* **22**(6):447–467, 1992.

Upton RN: Regional pharmacokinetics, I. Physiological and physicochemical basis. *Biopharm Drug Disp* **11**:647–662, 1990.

Vozeh S, Wenk M, Follath F: Experience with NONMEM: Analysis of serum concentration data in patients treated with mexiletine and lidocaine. *Drug Metab Rev* **15**:305–315, 1984.

Whiting B, Kelman AW, Grevel J: Population pharmacokinetics: Theory and clinical application. *Clin Pharmacokinet* **11**: 387–401, 1986.

Whiting B, Niven AA, Kelman AW, Thomson AH: A Bayesian kinetic control strategy for cyclosporin in renal transplantation. In D'Argenio DZ (ed). *Advanced Methods of Pharmacokinetic and Pharmacodynamic Systems Analysis.* New York, Plenum, 1991.

# BIBLIOGRAPHY

Abernethy DR, Azarnoff DL: Pharmacokinetic investigations in elderly patients. Clinical and ethical considerations. *Clin Pharmacokinet* **19**:89–93, 1990.

Abernethy DR, Greenblatt DJ, Divoll M, et al: Alterations in drug distribution and clearance due to obesity. *J Pharmacol Exp Ther* **217**:681–685, 1981.

Anderson KE: Influences of diet and nutrition on clinical pharmacokinetics. *Clin Pharmacokinet* **14**:325–346, 1988.

Aranda JV, Stern L: Clinical aspects of developmental pharmacology and toxicology. *Pharmacol Ther* **20**:1–51, 1983.

Atkinson AJ, Daniels CE, Dedrick RL, Grudzinskas CV, Markey SP: *Principles of Clinical Pharmacology.* New York, Academic, 2001.

Bartelink IH, Rademaker CMA, Schobben AFAM, van den Anker JN: Guidelines on paediatric dosing on the basis of developmental physiology and pharmacokinetic considerations. *Clin Pharmacokinet* **45**(11):1077–1097, 2006.

Beal SL: *NONMEM Users Guide VII: Conditional Estimation Methods.* San Francisco, NONMEM Project Group, University of California, San Francisco, 1992.

Benet LZ (ed): *The Effect of Disease States on Drug Pharmacokinetics.* Washington, DC, American Pharmaceutical Association, 1976.

Benowitz NL, Meister W: Pharmacokinetics in patients with cardiac failure. *Clin Pharmacokinet* **1**:389–405, 1976.

Besunder JB, Reed MD, Blumer JL: Principles of drug biodisposition in the neonate: A critical evaluation of the pharmacokinetic–pharmacodynamic interface, Part I. *Clin Pharmacokinet* **14**:189–216, 1988.

Chiou WL, Gadalla MAF, Pang GW: Method for the rapid estimation of total body clearance and adjustment of dosage regimens in patients during a constant-rate infusion. *J Pharmacokinet Biopharm* **6**:135–151, 1978.

Chrystyn H, Ellis JW, Mulley BA, Peak MD: The accuracy and stability of Bayesian theophylline predictions. *Ther Drug Monit* **10**:299–303, 1988.

Clinical Symposium on Drugs and the Unborn Child. *Clin Pharmacol Ther* **14**:621–770, 1973.

Crooks J, O'Malley K, Stevenson IH: Pharmacokinetics in the elderly. *Clin Pharmacokinet* **1**:280–296, 1976.

Crouthamel WG: The effect of congestive heart failure on quinidine pharmacokinetics. *Am Heart J* **90**:335, 1975.

DeVane CL, Jusko WJ: Dosage regimen design. *Pharmacol Ther* **17**:143–163, 1982.

Dimascio A, Shader RI: Drug administration schedules. *Am J Psychiatry* **126**:6, 1969.

Friis-Hansen B: Body-water compartments in children: Changes during growth and related changes in body composition. *Pediatrics* **28**:169–181, 1961.

Giacoia GP, Gorodisher R: Pharmacologic principles in neonatal drug therapy. *Clin Perinatol* **2**:125–138, 1975.

Gillis AM, Kates R: Clinical pharmacokinetics of the newer anti-arrhythmic agents. *Clin Pharmacokinet* **9**:375–403, 1984.

Godley PJ, Black JT, Frohna PA, Garrelts JC: Comparison of a Bayesian program with three microcomputer programs for predicting gentamicin concentrations. *Ther Drug Monit* **10**:287–291, 1988.

Gomeni R, Pineau G, Mentre F: Population kinetics and conditional assessment of the optimal dosage regimen using the P-pharm software package. *Cancer Res* **14**:2321–2326, 1994.

Grasela TH, Sheiner LB: Population pharmacokinetics of procainamide from routine clinical data. *Clin Pharmacokinet* **9**:545, 1984.

Gross G, Perrier CV: Intrahepatic portosystemic shunting in cirrhotic patients. *N Engl J Med* **293**:1046, 1975.

Harnes HT, Shiu G, Shah VP: Validation of bioanalytical methods. *Pharm Res* **8**:421–426, 1991.

Holloway DA: Drug problems in the geriatric patient. *Drug Intell Clin Pharm* **8**:632–642, 1974.

Jaehde U, Sorgel F, Stephan U, Schunack W: Effect of an antacid containing magnesium and aluminum on absorption, metabolism, and mechanism of renal elimination of pefloxacin in humans. *Antimicrob Agents Chemother* **38**(5):1129–1133, 1994.

Jensen EH: Current concepts for the validation of compendial assays. *Pharm Forum* March–April:1241–1245, 1986.

Jusko WJ: Pharmacokinetic principles in pediatric pharmacology. *Pediatr Clin N Am* **19**:81–100, 1972.

Kamimori GH, Somani SM, Kawlton, et al: The effects of obesity and exercise on the pharmacokinetics of caffeine in lean and obese volunteers. *Eur J Clin Pharmacol* **31**:595–600, 1987.

Klotz U, Avant GR, Hoyumpa A, et al: The effects of age and liver disease on the disposition and elimination of diazepam in adult man. *J Clin Invest* **55**:347, 1975.

Krasner J, Giacoia GP, Yaffe SJ: Drug–protein binding in the newborn infant. *Ann NY State Acad Sci* **226**:102–114, 1973.

Kristensen M, Hansen JM, Kampmann J, et al: Drug elimination and renal function. *Int J Clin Pharmacol Biopharm* **14**:307–308, 1974.

Latini R, Bonati M, Tognoni G: Clinical role of blood levels. *Ther Drug Monit* **2**:3–9, 1980.

Latini R, Maggioni AP, Cavalli A: Therapeutic drug monitoring of antiarrhythmic drugs. Rationale and current status. *Clin Pharmacokinet* **18**:91–103, 1990.

Lehmann K, Merten K: Die Elimination von Lithium in Abhängigkeit vom Lebensalten bei Gesunden und Niereninsuffizienten. *Int J Clin Pharmacol Biopharm* **10**:292–298, 1974.

Levy G (ed): *Clinical Pharmacokinetics: A Symposium.* Washington, DC, American Pharmaceutical Association, 1974.

Ludden TM: Population pharmacokinetics. *J Clin Pharmacol* **28**:1059–1063, 1988.

Matzke GR, St Peter WL: Clinical pharmacokinetics 1990. *Clin Pharmacokinet* **18**:1–19, 1990.

Maxwell GM: Paediatric drug dosing. Body weight versus surface area. *Drugs* **37**:113–115, 1989.

Meister W, Benowitz NL, Melmon KL, Benet LZ: Influence of cardiac failure on the pharmacokinetics of digoxin. *Clin Pharmacol Ther* **23**:122, 1978.

Mentre F, Pineau, Gomeni R: Population kinetics and conditional assessment of the optimal dosage regimen using the P-Pharm software package. *Anticancer Res* **14**:2321–2326, 1994.

Morley PC, Strand LM: Critical reflections on therapeutic drug monitoring. *J Pharm Pract* **2**:327–334, 1989.

Morselli PL: Clinical pharmacokinetics in neonates. *Clin Pharmacokinet* **1**:81–98, 1976.

Mungall DR: *Applied Clinical Pharmacokinetics.* New York, Raven, 1983.

Neal EA, Meffin PJ, Gregory PB, Blaschke TF: Enhanced bioavailability and decreased clearance of analgesics in patients with cirrhosis. *Gastroenterology* **77**:96, 1979.

Niebergall PJ, Sugita ET, Schnaare RL: Potential dangers of common drug dosing regimens. *Am J Hosp Pharm* **31**:53–58, 1974.

Rane A, Sjoquist F: Drug metabolism in the human fetus and newborn infant. *Pediatr Clin N Am* **19**:37–49, 1972.

Rane A, Wilson JT: Clinical pharmacokinetics in infants and children. *Clin Pharmacokinet* **1**:2–24, 1976.

Richey DP, Bender DA: Pharmacokinetic consequences of aging. *Annu Rev Pharmacol Toxicol* **17**:49–65, 1977.

Roberts J, Tumer N: Age and diet effects on drug action. *Pharmacol Ther* **37**:111–149, 1988.

Rowland M, Tozer TN: *Clinical Pharmacokinetics Concepts and Applications.* Philadelphia, Lea & Febiger, 1980.

Schumacher GE, Barr JT: Pharmacokinetics in drug therapy. Bayesian approaches in pharmacokinetic decision making. *Clin Pharm* **3**:525–530, 1984.

Schumacher GE, Barr JT: Making serum drug levels more meaningful. *Ther Drug Monit* **11**:580–584, 1989.

Schumacher GE, Griener JC: Using pharmacokinetics in drug therapy II. Rapid estimates of dosage regimens and blood levels without knowledge of pharmacokinetic variables. *Am J Hosp Pharm* **35**:454–459, 1978.

Sheiner LB, Benet LZ: Premarketing observational studies of population pharmacokinetics of new drugs. *Clin Pharmacol Ther* **35**:481–487, 1985.

Sheiner LB, Rosenberg B, Marathe V: Estimation of population characteristics of pharmacokinetic parameters from routine clinical data. *J Pharmacokinet Biopharm* **9**:445–479, 1977.

Shirkey HC: Dosage (dosology). In Shirkey HC (ed). *Pediatric Therapy.* St. Louis, Mosby, 1975, pp 19–33.

Spector R, Park GD, Johnson GF, Vessell ES: Therapeutic drug monitoring. *Clin Pharmacol Ther* **43**:345–353, 1988.

Thompson PD, Melmon KL, Richardson JA, et al: Lidocaine pharmacokinetics in advanced heart failure, liver disease, and renal failure in humans. *Ann Intern Med* **78**:499–508, 1973.

Thomson AH: Bayesian feedback methods for optimizing therapy. *Clin Neuropharmacol* **15**(suppl 1, part A):245A–246A, 1992.

Uematsu T, Hirayama H, Nagashima S, et al: Prediction of individual dosage requirements for lignocaine. A validation study for Bayesian forecasting in Japanese patients. *Ther Drug Monit* **11**:25–31, 1989.

Vestel RE: Drug use in the elderly: A review of problems and special considerations. *Drugs* **16**:358–382, 1978.

Vonesh EF, Carter RL: Mixed-effects nonlinear regression for unbalanced repeated measures. *Biometrics* **48**:1–17, 1992.

Williams RW, Benet LZ: Drug pharmacokinetics in cardiac and hepatic disease. *Annu Rev Pharmacol Toxicol* **20**:289, 1980.

Winter ME: *Basic Clinical Pharmacokinetics.* San Francisco, Applied Therapeutics, 1980.

Yuen GJ, Beal SL, Peck CC: Predicting phenytoin dosages using Bayesian feedback. A comparison with other methods. *Ther Drug Monit* **5**:437–441, 1983.

# 24

# Application of Pharmacokinetics and Pharmacodynamics to Aging, Obese, and Pediatric Patients

Brian R. Overholser, Michael B. Kays, and Kevin M. Sowinski*

## CHAPTER OBJECTIVES

- Describe the age-related physiological changes to the gastrointestinal tract in older adults and pediatric patients.

- Describe the effects of age on drug absorption in older adults and pediatric patients.

- Describe the effects of age on drug metabolism and disposition in older adults, pediatric patients, and obese patients.

- Provide examples of pharmacodynamic changes in older adults and pediatric patients.

- Describe the pharmacokinetics and pharmacodynamics changes in obese patients.

- Describe the global prevalence of obesity and the impact of obesity on the health of an individual.

- Classify obesity based on body mass index.

- List the classification of the pediatric age categories.

- Explain the differences in volume distribution in obese versus non-obese patients.

- Describe the differences in renal elimination between obese and non-obese patients.

- Apply pharmacokinetic principles for drug dosing in obese patients.

- Calculate different body weight descriptors and estimate creatinine clearance for obese patients.

## INTRODUCTION

To ensure safe and effective therapy for special populations, an understanding of the pharmacokinetics and pharmacodynamics in those patients is essential. Earlier in the book the impact of disease states, such as renal disease or hepatic disease, on pharmacokinetics and pharmacodynamics was discussed. The focus of this chapter is to discuss the impact that special populations have on pharmacokinetics and pharmacodynamics. The populations that are discussed in this chapter are age (pediatric and older adults) and obese patients. There are additional populations that may be impacted, such as sex differences in pharmacokinetics and pharmacodynamics, but these are not addressed in this chapter. Finally, additional alterations in pharmacokinetics may occur due to renal impairment, hepatic impairment, pregnancy, various pathophysiologic conditions, and are discussed elsewhere.

## APPLICATION OF PHARMACOKINETICS TO OLDER ADULTS

### Introduction

Aging is a complex and multifactorial process that includes functional deficits of multiple organs and tissue. The gradual decline in system function impacts the pharmacokinetics and pharmacodynamics of many drugs. However, the actual impact on drug therapy is often difficult to predict since system function often declines at varying rates with age. Given the difficulty to predict, patients are often stratified into subgroups to make drug, dosing, and frequency decisions (eg, 65–75; 75–85; and ≥85 years). Adding even more complexity, older patients usually have more disease burden and thus take multiple drug therapies. In fact, persons aged 65 and older are the most medicated group of patients and receive the highest proportion of prescription drugs. Therefore, elderly patients with a chronological age of 65 years and over have increased likelihood for underlying diseases, drug interactions, and adverse drug events (Hilmer and Gnjidic, 2009).

The age group of 65 and over is the fastest growing segment of the population in many developed countries, including the United States. In 2030, the projected number of people in the United States aged 65 and over will outnumber children for the first time in U.S. history (U.S. Census Bureau, 2018). This is an added obstacle to healthcare delivery since there has been a historical underrepresentation of older individuals in clinical trials in many therapeutic areas, including cancer, dementia, epilepsy, incontinence, transplantation, and cardiovascular disease. This underrepresentation phenomenon is also common to pharmacokinetic and pharmacodynamic trials (Chien and Ho, 2011; Mangoni et al, 2013). Understanding the effect of aging on pharmacokinetics and pharmacodynamics is important since it can help maximize the therapeutic effects and minimize the adverse effects of medications for better care of older patients.

## Effects of Age on Pharmacokinetics in Older Adults

Almost all drugs can be affected by a patient's underlying disease states or other conditions that may change their pharmacokinetic or pharmacodynamic profiles. This adds complexity to making drug therapy and dosing predictions in aging patients, since multiple disease states are more frequent than in the younger population. Of course, any prediction about pharmacokinetics in the elderly should include an assessment of comorbidities and drug interactions in addition to the changes that occur with age. The following section describes changes in the absorption, distribution, metabolism, and excretion of drugs that occurs with age alone and not due to common disease states in the elderly.

### Drug Absorption

**Gastrointestinal.** Aging results in many physiological changes in the gastrointestinal tract such as increased gastric pH, delayed gastric emptying, decreased splanchnic blood flow, decreased absorption surface, and decreased gastrointestinal motility. Thus, it can be expected that there will be some absorption changes likely to occur with many drugs with aging. For example, theoretically drugs that are dependent on ionization for absorption may have altered absorption profiles. However, there are not many actual clinical examples of how these physiological changes with age alter the absorption profiles of drugs (Schwartz, 2007; Klotz, 2009). While oral absorption changes can be expected in the elderly, they may reflect the rate of absorption more than the overall extent of drug absorption. Thus, the overall implications of gastrointestinal absorption changes with aging are not of clinical significance for most drugs.

**Transdermal.** The transdermal route provides benefit to elderly patients who are often taking multiple drugs to help maintain constant and effective plasma drug concentrations. Transdermal absorption requires drugs to penetrate multiple layers of skin that have known composition changes that occur with age. The compositional changes include thinning of the dermis with decreased structural integrity. Indeed, older adults have an increased sensitivity to transdermal fentanyl than younger subjects (Holdsworth et al, 1994). This, of course, could be a combination of pharmacodynamic sensitivity in addition to altered absorption. Thus, like gastrointestinal absorption, there are not many examples of clinically relevant differences in the absorption of drugs from transdermal delivery systems between young and old individuals (Kaestli et al, 2008).

**Subcutaneous/Intramuscular.** Subcutaneous and intramuscular drug absorption occurs through the vascular capillaries and lymphatic channels. Molecular size primarily determines the passage across the capillary endothelium. Smaller molecules chiefly pass through the capillary pathway, whereas larger molecules (eg, polypeptides) enter the blood via the lymphatic pathway. The skin blood supply and lymphatic drainage change with age (Ryan, 2004). Thus, subcutaneous and intramuscular absorption of drugs may be affected with aging but there are few studies directly assessing the impact of aging. The effects of subcutaneously administered fast-acting insulin generally have a more rapid onset and shorter duration of action in the elderly, but this may be due to a combination of pharmacokinetic and pharmacodynamic differences. Additionally, the intramuscular absorption of two small molecules, diazepam and midazolam, does not appear to alter with older age (Divoll et al, 1983; Holazo et al, 1988). More research is necessary to better understand how age-related changes may affect subcutaneous or intramuscular drug absorption.

**Pulmonary.** Like many of the vital organs, lung anatomy and physiology has been extensively studied and is known to change with age. Older individuals show a decrease of the alveolar surface, reduced lung elasticity, a decrease of the alveolar capillary volume combined with a decline of the ventilation/perfusion ratio, a decrease of the pulmonary diffusion capacity for carbon monoxide, and an increase of the pulmonary residual volume (Siekmeier and Scheuch, 2008). These altered functions that occur with advancing age have been demonstrated to affect the pharmacokinetics of inhaled drugs (Siekmeier and Scheuch, 2008). For example, the concentrations of isoflurane and sevoflurane (inhalation anesthetic drugs) necessary to maintain adequate depth of anesthesia are decreased in older age (Matsuura et al, 2009).

Not all inhaled drugs have demonstrated altered pharmacokinetic profiles in the elderly. For example, absorption was comparable among young (18–45 years of age) and older (over 65 years) patients with type 2 diabetes following a single inhalation of insulin. However, the older patients had an attenuated glucose reduction effect, again demonstrating that pharmacodynamic differences exist (Henry et al, 2003). Overall, there has been very little research for the pharmacokinetic and pharmacodynamic characteristics of newer inhaled drugs in older patients, and the effects of lung aging and with comorbidities are not well described. This is particularly important in patients over 85 years of age, where almost no data are available but physiological changes are expected to alter absorption.

*Drug Distribution*

Changes in body composition progress with chronological aging. A notable change relevant to the distribution of drugs is a decreasing ratio of muscle to fat tissue content. This lower ratio is due to the combination of a decreased lean body mass with a redistribution of body fat with aging. The decrease in lean body mass includes a decrease in total body water. For example, the total body water for an 80-year old is 10%–20% lower than a 20-year old (Vestal, 1997; Beaufrere and Morio, 2000). Thus, the distribution volume of hydrophilic drugs such as digoxin, theophylline, and aminoglycosides decrease with aging (Shi and Klotz, 2011). In contrast, body fat is 18%–36% higher in men and 33%–45% higher in women (Vestal, 1997; Beaufrere and Morio, 2000). This increase in body fat may provide partial explanation for the increase in volume of distribution for lipophilic drugs such as benzodiazepines (Greenblatt et al, 1991). Given the changes in distribution, hydrophilic drugs will generally have lower volumes of distribution and therefore higher peak plasma concentrations in the elderly, whereas lipophilic drugs will generally have an increased volume of distribution and decreased overall exposure in the elderly.

In addition to a lowering of the lean-to-fat tissue ratio, elderly patients generally weigh less than younger patients. Thus, an important body composition change that should not be overlooked is a decrease in total body weight. This influences the doses of drugs, which are generally lower in older patients as compared to younger patients to achieve similar effects. Thus, weight-based loading regimens should be considered (Schwartz, 2007).

The protein binding of drugs in both plasma and tissue can also impact a drug's volume of distribution. Albumin and α1-acid glycoprotein are the major drug binding proteins in plasma. In general, blood albumin concentrations are about 10% lower, whereas α1-acid glycoprotein concentrations are higher in older people (McLean and Le Couteur, 2004). These changes in plasma proteins may not be due to aging itself but to pathophysiological states that occur more commonly in older patients. In general, these changes do not necessitate any adjustments in dosing regimens (Benet and Hoener 2002).

*Hepatic and Extrahepatic Drug Metabolism*

Phase I drug metabolism is primarily catalyzed by CYP enzymes. The key drug-metabolizing enzymes of this superfamily are CYP3A, CYP2D6, CYP2C9, CYP2C19, CYP1A2, CYP2B6, and CYP2E1. The human liver, gastrointestinal tract, kidneys, lung, and skin contain quantitatively important amounts of CYP enzymes for drug metabolism. However, the vast majority of drug metabolism occurs via the liver. The content and activity of various CYP enzymes, as assessed from liver microsomal preparations, does not decline with advancing age from 10–85 years (Parkinson et al, 2004). Overall, CYP activity from liver microsomal preparations is variable but not significantly different between the age group of 20–60 years and the age group of 60 years and greater (Parkinson et al, 2004).

The hepatic drug clearance of drugs primarily eliminated via CYP metabolism is therefore expected to be mostly unchanged or modestly decreased in the elderly. It should be noted that these data usually originate from individuals under 75 years of age and are generally in good health. However, another study of older patients and nursing home residents demonstrated a decrease in the oral clearance of the CYP3A substrate atorvastatin (Schwartz and Verotta, 2009). This decrease could have been due to an increased bioavailability and decreased liver clearance via CYP3A, or altered drug transport. Nonetheless, age is a significant factor in predicting the concentrations of atorvastatin for patients up to 86 years of age (DeGorter et al, 2013). These observations are consistent with early pharmacokinetic studies that demonstrated that the elderly have increased exposure of atorvastatin, and a dose reduction should be considered (Gibson et al, 1996).

In general, the reduction of drug metabolism with advancing age appears modest, certainly for patients less than 75 years of age. Phase II drug metabolism including glucuronidation, sulfation, and acetylation does not appear to change with age (Benedetti et al, 2007). Changes in extrahepatic drug metabolism such as pulmonary metabolism that occur with age are unknown. In addition to enzymatic function changes, the liver has a reduced blood flow. A reduction in blood flow would theoretically involve a reduction in clearance of high-extraction-ratio drugs, but there is a lack of studied examples (McLean and Le Couteur, 2004).

## Drug Excretion

Renal clearance is the most consistent and predictable age-related change that alters the pharmacokinetics of drugs. Renal function, including renal blood flow, glomerular filtration rate (GFR), and active renal tubular secretory processes, all decline with increasing age. Mean inulin clearance, used as a measure of GFR, decreased from 122.8 to 65.3 mL/min/1.73 m$^2$ between 20 and 90 years of age in 70 men (Davies and Shock, 1950). Renal tubular reabsorption also decreases, at least measured as glucose reabsorption, and appears to parallel the decline in GFR (Miller et al, 1952).

Serum creatinine concentration is a common endogenous glomerular filtration marker in clinical practice. Creatinine is predominantly produced from creatine and phosphocreatine in skeletal muscle (Sandilands et al, 2013). As mentioned, lean muscle mass declines with age at a rate of about 1% a year after 30 years of age (Morley et al, 2010). Creatinine is freely filtered at the glomerulus and is not reabsorbed, but up to 15% is actively secreted by the tubules (Traynor et al, 2006). For renally impaired patients, the age-associated decrease in creatinine production may significantly blunt an increase of serum creatinine concentration despite a marked decrease in the GFR and creatinine clearance. This is particularly an issue with small women or in malnourished individuals whose creatinine production is well below normal (Perrone et al, 1992). Thus, serum creatinine concentration alone may lead to serious errors in assessing the severity of renal disease in the older population. A retrospective medical record review study showed that serum creatinine concentration is an inadequate screening test for renal failure in older patients (Swedko et al, 2003).

A direct measure of GFR is the best overall indicator of renal function but it is cumbersome to collect urine for extended period of time (24 hours) and is more prone to error of measurement. Furthermore, the diurnal variation in GFR and day-to-day variation in creatinine excretion may also contribute to the errors for GFR measurements with timed urine collection. Additionally, since GFR is estimated during drug development using calculated creatinine clearance equations, they are often more useful than measured GFR for drug therapy adjustments. Thus, despite limitations, serum creatinine is the most common estimate of GFR through the following two formulas to estimate creatinine clearance:

The Cockcroft–Gault (CG) equation for creatinine clearance as GFR estimate (Cockcroft and Gault, 1976):

$$cl_{cr}(mL/min) = \frac{(140 - age\ in\ years) \times (weight\ in\ kg)}{72 \times (serum\ creatinine\ in\ mg/dL)}$$

$$(24.1)$$

For women, the $Cl_{cr}$ estimate should be reduced by 15%.

The Modification of Diet in Renal Disease (MDRD) equation for GFR estimate (Levey et al, 2006):

GFR (mL/min/1.73 m$^2$)

$= 175 \times$ (standardized serum creatinine)$^{-1.154}$

$\times$ (age)$^{-0.203} \times$ (0.742 if female)

$\times$ (1.212 if African American)        $(24.2)$

The CG equation-estimated creatinine clearance predicts a linear decrease with age that is steeper than the nonlinear decline predicted via the MDRD equation. Either one of these equations gives a reasonable estimate for dosing drugs that are predominantly renal cleared. The merits and limitations of the CG versus MDRD equation to estimate renal function exist but are beyond the scope of this chapter (Spruill et al, 2009; Stevens and Levey, 2009; Nyman et al, 2011). The major disadvantage of the MDRD equation is the limited information available on dosage adjustments, as many of the age-adjusted recommendations in prescribing information have been based on the CG equation. It should be noted that neither the CG nor MDRD equations were derived from a large proportion of people over the age of 70 years when they were introduced. This lack of information may be the greatest limitation of either equation, but it is important to note that despite having been proposed in 1976 from a limited number of patients, the CG equation is to this day the most commonly used and useful equation to relate estimated renal function and the clearance of drugs. No other more recent formula has been shown to be significantly better in the last 40 years.

The clearance of drugs that are primarily eliminated via glomerular filtration (eg, aminoglycoside antibiotics, lithium, and digoxin) decreases with age in parallel with the decline in measured or calculated creatinine clearance (Cusack et al, 1979; Ljungberg and Nilsson-Ehle, 1987; Sproule et al, 2000). The renal clearance of drugs undergoing active renal tubular secretion also decreases with aging. For example, the decrease in renal tubular secretion of cimetidine parallels the decrease in creatinine clearance in older patients (Drayer et al, 1982).

### Age-Related Changes in Transporters

Transporters such as P-glycoprotein, organic anion transporting peptide, organic cation transporter, and organic anion transporter are involved in drug absorption, distribution, metabolism, and excretion. The potential age-related changes in expression and function of drug transporters and subsequent effect on pharmacokinetics is largely unknown. However, data are emerging that change in the blood–brain barrier, including alterations in transporter expression, may increase the brain exposure of drugs in elderly patients (Pan and Nicolazzo, 2018). P-glycoprotein is one of the better characterized drug transporters at the blood–brain barrier. There are conflicting data on the impact of advancing age on P-glycoprotein activity and expression (Mangoni, 2007). For example, an *ex vivo* uptake study of MDR1-encoded P-glycoprotein in leukocytes from healthy older and frail older participants as well as healthy young participants showed that aging and frailty had minor impact on this validated cellular P-glycoprotein model (Brenner and Klotz, 2004). However, a positron emission tomography study showed that older participants have significantly reduced P-glycoprotein function in the internal capsule and corona radiata white matter and in orbitofrontal regions (Bartels et al, 2009). Further studies are needed to address the potential for P-glycoprotein decline in elderly patients and the impact on drug therapy and response.

### Effects of Age on Pharmacodynamics in Older Adults

Limited information exists for age-related changes in pharmacodynamics. Factors such as pharmacogenetic polymorphisms, nutrition, concomitant medications, smoking, and drinking habits can influence the disposition and action of drugs in older patients. Another confounding factor for drug disposition and action in older patients can be frailty (Shi and Klotz, 2011; Sitar, 2012). While there has not been a uniform definition of frailty in research studies, it has been associated with higher inflammatory markers such as C-reactive protein, interleukin-6, or tumor necrosis factor-alpha (Clegg et al, 2013).

In general, elderly and particularly frail patients are more sensitive to drug effects, but this is likely due to a combination of pathophysiology, drug interactions, and aging. In fact, there are examples where elderly patients have reduced sensitivity to drug action. Thus, it is often difficult to differentiate chronological age versus biological age or physiological effects versus pathological effects in studies assessing pharmacodynamic changes with aging. Additionally, the oldest study cohort of research studies include only those participants who survived to reach that age, and these participants may be unique regarding the variable of interest (Bowie and Slattum, 2007; Trifiro and Spina, 2011). In general, interindividual variability is prominent, which is usually due not only to the influence of age-related physiological changes but also to the impact of comorbidities and drug interactions (Shi and Klotz, 2011). These limitations hinder the generalizability of results for the pharmacodynamic studies to the entire older population. With those limitations noted, the following are examples to illustrate the effect of aging on the pharmacodynamics of specific therapeutic areas.

### Drugs That Act on the Central Nervous Systems

**Benzodiazepines.** Changes in pharmacodynamics rather than pharmacokinetics with increasing age may explain the well-described altered response to benzodiazepines in the elderly. Many studies document a greater sensitivity to the clinical action of benzodiazepines in older people, which is not attributable to the differences in plasma concentrations, half-life, or apparent volume of distribution of drugs. For example, diazepam, flurazepam, midazolam, and triazolam show age-related increase in sensitivity to cognitive and sedative effects in the absence of significant pharmacokinetic changes (Castleden et al, 1977; Greenblatt et al, 1981; Kanto et al, 1981;

Swift et al, 1985; Albrecht et al, 1999; Greenblatt et al, 2004). The exact mechanisms responsible for the increased sensitivity to benzodiazepines with aging are unknown despite considerable efforts to define such a mechanism. Notably, there are no significant age-related differences in GABA receptor binding properties or GABA receptor numbers, both in animal models (Bickford and Breiderick, 2000) and in humans (Sundman et al, 1997).

**Psychotropic Drugs.** The function of different neurotransmitters in dopaminergic, serotonergic, and cholinergic systems may be influenced by the aging process itself. Additionally, the psychopathology of psychiatric disorders, including schizophrenia, depression, or dementia can be altered by the aging process (Meltzer, 1999). Thus, the effects of psychotropic drugs in the older patients may differ between patients with and without these mental diseases.

### Drugs with Anticholinergic Effects

An estimated one-third to more than half of the most commonly prescribed medications for older patients have anticholinergic effects (Tune et al, 1992; Chew et al, 2008). These anticholinergic effects have been linked with cognitive impairment in older patients, and attempts have been made to deprescribe drugs with these properties (Cancelli et al, 2008). Drugs with sedative adverse effects are also of concern for older patients, since these sedative effects can cause falls and bone fractures (Leipzig et al, 1999; Ensrud et al, 2002), which may further cause older patients to lose independence.

### Drugs That Act on the Cardiovascular System

**β-adrenergic Receptors.** The sensitivity to drugs that act on the β-adrenergic receptors declines with age. A reduced response to both agonists and antagonists of the $\beta_1$- and $\beta_2$-adrenergic receptors has been reported (Vestal et al, 1979; Scott et al, 1995). These age-related changes may not be attributed to reduced β–receptor density or affinity alone but may at least partially be due to impaired signal transduction (Landmann et al, 1981; Doyle et al, 1982). β-adrenergic receptors are largely coupled with G proteins, including Gs, which in turn are linked to adenylate cyclase. Age-associated decreases in β-adrenergic receptors related Gs activity in human heart tissue has been reported (White et al, 1994). A downregulation of β-adrenergic receptors may also explain why higher systemic drug concentrations are necessary with increasing age to reach desired effects (Scarpace et al, 1991). Reduced β-adrenergic receptor sensitivity does not imply the absence of safety issues for β-adrenergic receptors agonists or antagonists in older patients. Thus, the risk–benefit ratio for the treatment of β-adrenergic receptor modulators needs careful evaluation because higher doses may be more effective but with safety concerns (Dobre et al, 2007).

**Warfarin.** Evidence exists of a greater inhibition of synthesis of vitamin K-dependent clotting factors at similar plasma warfarin concentrations for older versus younger patients. However, the exact mechanism of this age-related change in sensitivity is unknown. Age is one of the strongest predictors of the anticoagulant effects of warfarin (Miao et al, 2007; Schwartz, 2007).

**QT Prolonging Drugs.** The arrhythmogenic potential of antipsychotic and antidepressant drugs, which may lead to QTc interval prolongation as well as polymorphic ventricular tachycardia, torsade de pointes, and sudden cardiac death, is significantly higher in older patients with preexisting cardiovascular disease or who are treated with concomitant QTc-prolonging drugs (Vieweg et al, 2009).

### Clinical Examples of Concomitant Medication in Older Patients

The following two examples have been modified from Mallet and colleagues (Mallet et al, 2007). Example 1 illustrates an older patient with the potential for multiple drug interactions. Example 2 illustrates an older patient's prescribing cascade due to drug adverse effects.

## EXAMPLE 1 ▷ ▷ ▷

An 82-year-old man was hospitalized for general deterioration. His medical history included renal transplant 18 years ago, type 2 diabetes mellitus, atrial fibrillation, heart failure, and early Alzheimer dementia. He was taking cyclosporine, prednisone, warfarin, digoxin, furosemide, levothyroxine, losartan, glyburide, donepezil,

lactulose, calcium carbonate, vitamin D, and ginkgo biloba. A week before admission, clarithromycin was started to treat bronchitis.

Assessment of Drug Therapy:

- Potential drug–drug interactions:
  - Clarithromycin + warfarin: Clarithromycin is a CYP3A inhibitor. Warfarin is a CYP3A substrate. This combination has risk of increased warfarin exposure and anticoagulant effect.
  - Clarithromycin + cyclosporine: Clarithromycin is a CYP3A inhibitor. Cyclosporine is a CYP3A substrate. This combination has risk of increased cyclosporine exposure and nephrotoxicity.
  - Calcium carbonate + levothyroxine: Decreased absorption of levothyroxine.
  - Ginkgo biloba + warfarin: Increased risk of hemorrhage.
- Potential drug–disease interactions:
  - Prednisone in patients with heart failure may cause fluid and electrolyte disturbances.
  - Prednisone in diabetic patients increase requirements for insulin or oral hypoglycemic agents.

Therapeutic plan: Management of drug interactions in older patients often requires a team effort, and communication is pivotal to achieve this goal. Several clinicians may take care of this patient, such as nephrologist, endocrinologist, cardiologist, neurologist, geriatrician, and family practice physician to prescribe medications. The pharmacist is likely to have access to this patient's most complete medication records and may help the following:

- Communicate with clarithromycin's prescriber for the potential interaction between clarithromycin and cyclosporine as well as warfarin. Azithromycin or another antibiotic should be considered to minimize the potential for drug interactions with cyclosporine and warfarin.
- Communicate with the patient or caregiver to take calcium carbonate and levothyroxine at least 4 hours apart to prevent the potential of calcium carbonate interfering with the absorption of levothyroxine.

- Communicate with the nurse or caregiver to watch for signs of worsening heart failure such as shortness of breath and fluid retention as well as signs of fall from hypotension or hypoglycemia for further evaluation.

## EXAMPLE 2 ▷ ▷ ▷

A 75-year-old man was taking paroxetine and haloperidol for the treatment of psychotic depression. His primary care physician sent him for a neurological consult of his new-onset tremors. The neurologist started him with carbidopa and levodopa for probable Parkinson disease. He was eventually hospitalized after several recurrent falls. The initial assessment attributed his falls to worsening instability secondary to suboptimally treated Parkinson disease. Thus, his carbidopa and levodopa dose was increased. Risperidone was prescribed for nighttime agitated behavior (haloperidol was discontinued). He was still taking paroxetine.

Assessment of Drug Therapy: Paroxetine and haloperidol can prompt extrapyramidal adverse effects which may be the underlying cause of the tremors. Moreover, these two drugs are CYP2D6 substrates and inhibitors with potential risk to increase exposure resulting in an increased risk of extrapyramidal symptoms. The nighttime agitation may have been a result of the central nervous system adverse effects secondary to increased doses of carbidopa and levodopa and subsequent risperidone prescription. Risperidone is also a CYP2D6 substrate and inhibitor with potential to prompt extrapyramidal adverse effects.

Therapeutic plan for this 75-year-old patient:

- Communicate with the neurologist that the patient is taking paroxetine and haloperidol for the treatment of psychotic depression, which may cause the extrapyramidal adverse effects and tremors.
- Communicate with the neurologist that discontinuation or dose reductions of carbidopa and levodopa may be considered as potential underlying cause for nighttime agitation, prompting drug therapy changes that increase the risk for extrapyramidal symptoms.
- Communicate with the primary care physician that dose reduction for paroxetine and haloperidol may be necessary for this patient.
- Communicate with the nurse or caregiver for mouth, dental, and bowel hygiene to watch for potential anticholinergic adverse effects with paroxetine.

### Summary

Careful consideration of drug therapy is essential to take care of older patients, who usually have comorbidities and concurrently take multiple medications. Knowledge of the effect of age on pharmacokinetics and pharmacodynamics will help maximize the therapeutic effects and minimize the adverse effects of drugs. This is particularly important, since people 65 years of age and older are the fastest growing demographic in the United States.

Oral absorption of drugs is not significantly altered with advancing age despite well-characterized physiological changes in the gastrointestinal tract. Plasma albumin concentration decreases about 10% with advancing age, whereas plasma $\alpha_1$-acid glycoprotein concentration increases due to comorbidities. These may alter drug distribution but do not necessitate dosage adjustments under most circumstances. Phase I or degradative process of drug metabolism modestly decrease and on occasion may require dose adjustments, whereas Phase II or synthetic process of drug metabolism do not appear to change with advancing age. In general, the overall decrease in drug metabolism due to advancing age is modest. Renal drug clearance is the most consistent and predictable age-related change in pharmacokinetics.

Age-related changes in pharmacodynamics are more difficult to study than age-related changes in pharmacokinetics. In general, older patients have increased sensitivity to drugs that act in the central nervous system. Based on the limited knowledge of the impact of aging on pharmacokinetic and pharmacodynamic properties, it is difficult to make definitive dosage recommendations for older patients. The complex interactions among comorbidity, polypharmacy, changes in pharmacodynamic sensitivity, and relatively modest pharmacokinetic changes in the older patients warrant the dosing recommendation to follow the conventional wisdom of "start low and go slow" (Shi and Klotz, 2011).

## APPLICATION OF PHARMACOKINETICS TO THE OBESE PATIENT

### Introduction

Obesity is defined by excess body fat and is recognized as a global health problem by the World Health Organization (WHO), as obesity rates have more than doubled worldwide since 1980 (World Health Organization, 2019). In addition, several leading medical associations have classified obesity as a disease (Jensen et al, 2014). Classification of obesity is most commonly based on body mass index (BMI), which is calculated as actual body weight in kilograms divided by height in meters squared. The international weight classification of the WHO and the United States National Institutes of Health define overweight, obesity, and morbid (or extreme) obesity as a BMI of 25–29.99 kg/m$^2$, 30–30.99 kg/m$^2$, and ≥40 kg/m$^2$, respectively (Table 24-1) (World Health Organization, 2000). Some authors have added definitions for super obesity (BMI ≥ 50 kg/m$^2$) and super-super obesity (BMI ≥ 60 kg/m$^2$), but these definitions are not used by the WHO (Janson and Thursky, 2012) (Table 24-1).

### TABLE 24-1 • Classification of Obesity Based on BMI

| Classification | BMI (kg/m$^2$) |
| --- | --- |
| Underweight | < 18.5 |
| Normal body weight | 18.5 – < 25 |
| Overweight | 25– < 30 |
| Obese | ≥ 30 |
| Obese (obesity class I) | 30– < 35 |
| Severely obese (obesity class II) | 35– < 40 |
| Morbidly obese (obesity class III) | ≥ 40 |

In 2016, more than 1.9 billion adults worldwide were overweight, and over 650 million of these adults were obese. These numbers represent 39% and 13% of the world's population, respectively (World Health Organization, 2019). In 2015–2016, 39.6% of adults in the United States were obese, and the prevalence of obesity was higher in women compared to men (41.1% vs. 37.9%) (Hales et al, 2018). During this time period, the prevalence of morbid obesity was 7.7% overall, with 5.6% of men and 9.7% of women being classified as morbidly obese (Hales et al, 2018). The prevalence of obesity and morbid obesity varies by sex and race/Hispanic origins with the highest prevalence observed in non-Hispanic black women and the lowest prevalence observed in non-Hispanic Asian men and women (Flegal et al, 2016).

Nearly all physiologic functions of the body are adversely affected by obesity, and excess body fat increases the risk of death and major comorbidities. Medical care costs related to obesity are staggering, and much of the cost is associated with obesity-related chronic conditions, including diabetes mellitus, renal disease, cardiovascular disease, cancer, and musculoskeletal disorders. The prevalence of infections, including postoperative and hospital-acquired infections, is also higher in obese patients. Adipose tissue plays an active role in immunity and the inflammatory process by producing various pro- and anti-inflammatory mediators, leading to a chronic low-grade inflammatory state of adipose tissue and increased susceptibility to infection (Wellen and Hotamisligil, 2003; Falagas and Kompoti, 2006). Obesity is a significant risk factor for antibiotic treatment failure and has been identified as an independent risk factor for mortality in patients hospitalized in an intensive care unit (Bercault et al, 2004; Longo et al, 2013).

### Body Weight Descriptors

Although BMI is used to classify obesity and increases with total body weight (TBW), it is a poor metric for drug dosing because BMI cannot differentiate adipose tissue from muscle mass. However, many adults with increased BMI encountered in clinical practice have increased total body fat. A number of body size descriptors have been developed and utilized by clinicians for dosage

**TABLE 24-2 •** Body Weight Descriptors and Related Equations

| Weight Descriptor | Equation | Reference |
|---|---|---|
| Body mass index (BMI), kg/m² | TBW/[Height (m) × Height (m)] | (World Health Organization, 2000) |
| Body surface area (BSA), m² | √[(Height (cm) × Weight)/3600] | (Mosteller, 1987) |
| Total body weight (TBW), kg | Measured body weight | |
| Ideal body weight (IBW), kg | Male: 50 + 2.3 × [Height (inches) − 60] | |
| | Female: 45.5 + 2.3 × [Height (inches) − 60] | |
| Adjusted body weight (AdjBW), kg | IBW + [CF × (TBW − IBW)] | (Bauer et al, 1983) |
| Lean body weight (LBW), kg | Male: (9270 × TBW)/[6680 + (216 × BMI)] | (Janmahasatian et al, 2005) |
| | Female: (9270 × TBW)/[8780 + (244 × BMI)] | |

*CF, correction factor (usually 0.3 or 0.4).*

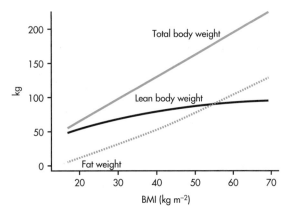

FIGURE 24-1 • Relationship of total body weight, fat weight, and lean body weight to body mass index (BMI) in a standard height male. (Lean body weight and fat weight were derived from the equations of Janmahasatian et al.)

calculations in obese patients (Table 24-2). Ideal body weight (IBW) was associated with the lowest mortality derived from data relating body size to mortality (Pai and Paloucek, 2000). Thus, IBW was originally developed for insurance purposes, not for drug dosing. Clinically, a patient may be considered obese and morbidly obese when their TBW is 125%–190% and >195% of their IBW, respectively (Pai and Bearden, 2007).

Lean body weight (LBW) describes body weight of all "non-fat" body components, including muscle, bone, vascular organs, and extracellular fluid (ECF) and is more representative of fat-free mass (Smit et al, 2018). LBW increases in obesity but in a nonlinear manner with TBW (Fig. 24-1) (Ingrande and Lemmens, 2010). Some clinicians may use the terms IBW and LBW interchangeably; however, these two terms are not synonymous. IBW is only a function

of sex and height. Therefore, all patients of the same sex and height will have the same IBW regardless of body composition. Obese patients tend to have greater lean body mass than non-obese patients based on sex and height (Janmahasatian et al, 2005; Falagas and Karageorgopoulos, 2010). For example, a male patient who is 72 inches tall weighing 75 kg will have the same IBW as a male patient who is 72 inches tall weighing 150 kg (IBW 77.6 kg). However, LBW is 41% higher in the patient weighing 150 kg. Clinical pharmacokinetic studies have demonstrated the difference in body size description between IBW and LBW in obese patients (Chung et al, 2015; Chung et al, 2017a).

Adjusted body weight (AdjBW) is the sum of the IBW and a proportion of adipose tissue as calculated by the difference between TBW and IBW. A correction factor, usually 0.3 or 0.4, is frequently utilized to estimate drug distribution into the excess adipose tissue. AdjBW using a correction factor of 0.4 is frequently utilized when dosing aminoglycoside antibiotics in obesity, although the actual correction factor may range from 0.38–0.58 for this drug class (Janson and Thursky, 2012). It is a common practice to calculate AdjBW as an estimate of lean body mass. However, as mentioned previously, the relationship between LBW and TBW is nonlinear where the relationship between AdjBW and TBW is linear and will overestimate lean body mass. One study found LBW a better normalized volume of distribution for tobramycin and gentamicin across a wide range of body weights (Pai et al, 2011).

## Pharmacokinetic Changes in Obesity

### Absorption

Although many drugs are administered orally, data are limited on the effect of obesity on pharmacokinetics following oral administration. Despite faster gastric emptying time, increased gut permeability, and increased splanchnic blood flow in obese patients, no differences in bioavailability or rate of oral absorption were found for trazodone, cyclosporine, dexfenfluramine, moxifloxacin, and propranolol between obese and non-obese subjects, although there was a trend toward higher bioavailability for propranolol in obese subjects (Knibbe et al, 2015; Smit et al, 2018). One study compared the oral bioavailability of metformin between patients who underwent gastric bypass surgery and their sex- and BMI-matched (non-surgery) cohorts. A 50% increase in bioavailability was observed in the surgery group despite no differences in age, weight, and BMI between the two groups (Padwal et al, 2011). Another study compared oral atorvastatin exposure in 12 patients before and after gastric bypass surgery in the same patients. Gastric bypass surgery had variable effects on individual systemic exposures, ranging from a 3-fold decrease to a 2-fold increase in area under the serum concentration–time curve (AUC) (Skottheim et al, 2009). In another study, the pharmacokinetics of intravenous and oral linezolid were compared before and 3 months after gastric bypass surgery. Oral bioavailability was 114% before and after gastric bypass surgery. TBW decreased by 25%, but the mean $AUC_{0-\infty}$ increased from 41.6 mg*h/L before surgery to 98.9 mg*h/L after surgery (Hamilton et al, 2013). In addition to being present in hepatocytes, CYP3A4 enzymes are also present in the gut wall. In one study, the bioavailability of midazolam was higher in obese patients, which was hypothesized to be due to reduced gut CYP3A4 activity (Brill et al, 2012).

### Distribution

Drug distribution, measured as volume of distribution (V), depends on the physicochemical properties of the drug, physiologic changes secondary to obesity,

and perhaps severity of the patient's illness (eg, sepsis/septic shock). Physiochemical drug properties include molecular weight, lipid solubility, protein binding, and degree of ionization. Obesity is associated with increased adipose tissue mass, lean body mass, plasma volume, cardiac output, and splanchnic blood flow along with decreased tissue perfusion and changes in plasma proteins as compared to non-obese individuals (Jain et al, 2011; Knibbe et al, 2015). Hydrophilic drugs do not distribute well into adipose tissue; however, V of hydrophilic drugs may be increased in obesity since adipose tissue is approximately 30% water, and obese patients have increased lean body mass and plasma volume. For lipophilic drugs, V is generally increased in obesity; however, the pharmacokinetics of highly lipophilic drugs in obesity are not predictable, and lipophilicity alone does not predict changes in V. Other variables, such as protein binding, binding in adipose and lean tissues, and blood flow to adipose tissues, play an important role in drug distribution (Falagas and Karageorgopoulos, 2010).

Assessment of the absolute V (uncorrected for weight) and the weight-normalized V (eg, V/TBW) may provide information regarding drug distribution into excess body weight. If estimates for V/TBW are similar between obese and non-obese individuals, the drug exhibits marked uptake into adipose tissue. However, there are exceptions to this rule. Cyclosporine is highly lipophilic, but the V was 295 L (4.54 L/kg) in non-obese patients and 229 L (2.55 L/kg) in obese patients (Flechner et al, 1989). Propofol and digoxin are both highly lipophilic, but the V for these drugs is not increased in obesity (Smit et al, 2018). Conversely, if the absolute V of the drug is increased but the V/TBW is significantly lower in obesity, the drug exhibits incomplete distribution into excess body weight (Hanley et al, 2010). In general, β-lactam antibiotics are considered to be hydrophilic drugs. Piperacillin/tazobactam is a β-lactam/β-lactamase inhibitor combination that has been studied in obese and non-obese patients. The absolute V of piperacillin was significantly higher in obese patients, but V/TBW was significantly higher in the non-obese patients (Chung et al, 2015). The absolute V of meropenem, a carbapenem antibiotic, was not significantly different between non-obese, obese, and morbidly obese patients; however, its V/TBW was 0.47 L/kg, 0.31 L/kg, and 0.21 L/kg in non-obese, obese, and morbidly obese patients (Chung et al, 2017a). Vancomycin, a glycopeptide antibiotic, is also hydrophilic, and previous studies have shown increased V in obese patients. However, the weight-normalized V (in L/kg) is different when adjusting for different body weights. Vancomycin V in obesity has been reported to be 0.26–0.52 L/kg using TBW, 0.76 L/kg using AdjBW, and 0.68–0.89 L/kg using IBW (Ducharme et al, 1994; Grace, 2012; Adane et al, 2015).

Albumin and total protein concentrations are not altered in obesity compared to lean subjects. However, $\alpha_1$-acid glycoprotein can be elevated in morbid obesity (Smit et al, 2018). Previous studies have shown that unbound concentrations of alprazolam, cefazolin, daptomycin, lorazepam, midazolam, oxazepam, propranolol, and triazolam are not significantly altered in obesity (Smit et al, 2018).

Tissue penetration is an important consideration in obesity, especially for antibiotics that may be used for surgical prophylaxis or to treat bacterial skin infections. Cefazolin is commonly used in both of these situations, and a study demonstrated significantly lower interstitial fluid concentrations in the subcutaneous tissue in morbidly obese patients (Brill et al, 2014). As a result, higher doses and/or increased dosing frequency may be needed.

Pathophysiologic changes are also observed in obese patients who are critically ill and hospitalized in an intensive care unit (ICU). A study evaluated the population pharmacokinetics of doripenem in obese patients who were hospitalized on a general medical ward and in the ICU. Volume of the central compartment ($V_C$) was associated with both TBW and ICU residence, and ICU patients had significantly increased $V_C$ when compared to obese, non-ICU patients (Chung et al, 2017b).

### Metabolism

A majority of obese patients have fatty infiltration in the liver (Machado et al, 2006), resulting in nonalcoholic fatty liver disease (NAFLD) with steatosis or steatohepatitis (NASH). Therefore, Phase I and II enzyme activities in obesity may be affected by the fatty infiltration of the liver and its associated changes.

**Phase I Metabolism.** It has been reported that CYP3A4 metabolic activity was reduced in the obese patients, either significantly, as for triazolam and carbamazepine, or not significantly, as for midazolam and cyclosporine (Brill et al, 2012), when compared to the non-obese patients. The weight-normalized oral clearances were invariably lower in the obese patients. Various studies have shown consistent and significant increases in the clearance of CYP2E1 substrates in obese patients, including chlorzoxazone, enflurane, sevoflurane, and halothane (Brill et al, 2012). These data suggest an increased CYP2E1 activity in obesity. When normalized for body weight, clearance values of these drugs are approximately equal between obese and non-obese individuals, suggesting CYP2E1 activity increases with body weight. CYP2E1 mediates the metabolism of fatty acids, ketones, and ethanol. Chronic exposure to these substrates in large amounts induces CYP2E1, leading to free-radical formation, lipid peroxidation, and liver injury (Buechler and Weiss, 2011). Studies on dexfenfluramine and nebivolol showed a trend toward increased CYP2D6 activity in the obese patients (Brill et al, 2012). However, its activity may also vary based on its genetic polymorphisms (May, 1994; van den Anker, 2010). Studies on caffeine and theophylline showed a trend toward higher clearances in the obese group, indicating a slight increase in CYP1A2 activity in obese patients (Brill et al, 2012). Studies with glimepiride and ibuprofen showed a small but significantly increased CYP2C9 activity in obese patients (Abernethy and Greenblatt, 1985a; Shukla et al, 2004), and studies on glipizide and phenytoin showed an insignificant increase in the obese group (Abernethy and Greenblatt, 1985b, Jaber et al, 1996). When normalized for body weight, lower enzyme activity of CYP2C9 was associated with the obese group. CYP2C19 activity is largely dependent on genetic polymorphisms. Diazepam clearance was higher in the obese group with no difference in desmethyl diazepam clearance between obese and non-obese subjects. When normalized for body weight, clearance was slightly decreased in obese subjects for both compounds (Brill et al, 2012).

Studies comparing xanthine oxidase activities using caffeine (Chiney et al, 2011) and mercaptopurine (Balis, 1986) in obese versus non-obese children showed significantly increased enzyme activity in the obese group.

**Phase II Metabolism.** Uridine diphosphate glucuronosyltransferase (UGT) enzymes catalyze the conjugation of endogenous substances and exogenous compounds and are involved in approximately 50% of the Phase II metabolism of drugs. Since the liver is the main organ for UGT enzymatic activities, liver disease or an increased size of the liver, as seen in obese patients, may correlate with UGT activities. Studies have shown a significantly increased clearance in obese subjects for medications metabolized via this pathway, including acetaminophen, oxazepam, and lorazepam (Abernethy et al, 1983; Brill et al, 2012). With the exception of oxazepam, the weight-normalized clearance values were either the same or slightly lower in the obese group. Besides UGT, other Phase II metabolic processes include *N*-acetyl-, methyl, glutathione, and sulfate conjugation of substrates. Procainamide, which is metabolized via *N*-acetylation, showed an increased plasma clearance in the obese group, but the difference was not statistically significant (Christoff et al, 1983). The weight-normalized clearance for procainamide was lower in the obese group. A study with busulfan, which is metabolized via glutathione S-transferase, showed a significantly increased *CL/F* in the obese group while the weight-normalized clearance was significantly lower in the obese group (Gibbs et al, 1999).

Obesity is associated with absolute increases in cardiac output and blood volume, as compared to non-obese subjects. Yet the effect of obesity on liver blood flow has not been fully determined, partly because NAFLD increases fat deposition in the liver, resulting in sinusoidal narrowing and altered morphology of the liver (Smit et al, 2018). Drugs with high-extraction ratio, such as propofol, sufentanil, and paclitaxel, could potentially serve as markers of liver blood flow because they are rapidly metabolized and sensitive to changes in the blood flow of the liver, and less sensitive to changes in enzyme activities. Studies of these drugs showed higher clearances in the obese subjects. However, studies on propranolol, a drug with high-extraction ratio but less clearance rate, showed variable results (Brill et al, 2012).

*Drug Excretion*

Many drugs are eliminated through the kidney via glomerular filtration, tubular secretion, and tubular reabsorption. The size of the kidney, renal blood flow, and urine flow rate may influence the function of the kidney. The relationship between obesity and kidney function is complex. In general, obesity is associated with enhanced renal function but is also an important factor in the development of chronic kidney disease. Studies comparing clearance of drugs that are primarily eliminated by glomerular filtration have shown a significantly higher clearance in the obese group for vancomycin (Bauer et al, 1998), daptomycin (Dvorchik and Damphousse, 2005), and enoxaparin (Barras et al, 2009). Studies for carboplatin (Sparreboom et al, 2007) and dalteparin (Yee and Duffull, 2000) showed higher clearances in the obese group, but not statistically significant as compared to the non-obese group. A significantly higher tubular secretion in the obese group was reported for procainamide, ciprofloxacin, and cisplatin (Christoff et al, 1983; Allard et al, 1993; Sparreboom et al, 2007). Studies for topotecan and digoxin (Abernethy et al, 1981; Sparreboom et al, 2007) showed a trend toward higher tubular secretion in the obese group, but the differences were not statistically significant. It appears that tubular reabsorption of lithium was significantly lower in the obese group as compared with the non-obese group (Reiss et al, 1994). In this study, the renal clearance of lithium was significantly increased in the obese patients while the glomerular filtration rates were not different between obese and non-obese groups.

## Dosing Considerations in the Obese Patients

Studies for various drugs have been conducted to evaluate appropriate dosing regimens for obese patients. It is not possible to list all the studies and dosing recommendations in this text. However, based on the findings from the pharmacokinetic studies, principles of drug dosing for obese patients may be adopted to calculate loading and maintenance doses. The loading dose is calculated using a target desired concentration multiplied by a volume of distribution. For drugs that are well described by multicompartment models and for which the loading dose is given acutely in one dose, the volume of distribution that is used is generally $V_C$ to avoid achieving maximum systemic concentrations that will be above the desired target. For drugs that are best described by a one-compartment model or are assumed to follow one compartment pharmacokinetics (eg, aminoglycosides, vancomycin), $V_{ss}$ should be utilized to calculate the loading dose. For some drugs, the relationship between weight and the volume of distribution is known, and that weight, whether it is TBW, IBW, or AdjBW, should be used. If the relationship is not known, the weight to use to estimate the volume of distribution and therefore the loading dose will depend on how the drug is distributed into lean and adipose tissues. If the drug is primarily distributed into lean mass, IBW may be used to calculate the loading dose. In contrast, if the drug is largely distributed into adipose tissues, TBW may be used to calculate the loading dose. Lastly, if the drug distributes into lean body mass and a proportion of adipose tissue, AdjBW may be used to calculate the loading dose.

The maintenance dose depends on drug clearance ($CL$). For renally eliminated drugs, the most common method for estimating drug $CL$ is to estimate the glomerular filtration rate (GFR) by calculating creatinine clearance ($CL_{cr}$) using the patient's serum creatinine ($S_{cr}$). Clearance of endogenous creatinine in serum is dependent on GFR and renal tubular secretion. Production of endogenous creatinine is affected by diet and muscle mass. The most commonly used equations to calculate $CL_{cr}$ are the CG equation (Cockcroft and Gault, 1976) and the Modification of Diet in Renal Disease (MDRD) equation (Levey et al, 2006).

One of the primary challenges when using the CG equation (Equation 24.1) in obesity is determining which body weight to incorporate into the equation. The CG equation was developed using TBW to predict creatinine clearance, but there were no obese or morbidly obese patients in the study. Several studies have evaluated the effects of different body weight descriptors on the accuracy and bias of the CG equation. Two studies recommend using AdjBW calculated using a correction factor of 0.3 or 0.4 to estimate $CL_{cr}$ in obese patients (Wilhelm and Kale-Pradhan, 2011; Winter et al, 2012). However, the primary utility of AdjBW in pharmacokinetics is to account for drug distribution into excess body weight, not to

estimate lean body mass in an obese patient. In a study with 31 obese patients (TBW 143–178 kg; BMI 44.3–54.8 kg/m²), the median (interquartile range) 24-hour measured $CL_{cr}$ was 84 mL/min (70–122 mL/min). However, estimated $CL_{cr}$ using the CG equation was 207 mL/min (157–230 mL/min) using TBW and 147 mL/min (109–155 mL/min) using AdjBW (Adane et al, 2015). Thus, using a more accurate estimate of lean body mass may better predict creatinine clearance. In clinical practice, however, the creatinine clearance obtained by the CG equation is not used per se to determine the patient's true creatinine clearance or GFR, but instead to adjust the dosing regimen of a drug using the relationship identified between the CG and drug clearance in studies. Such relationship is presented in the official product monograph and approved label dosing instructions, and TBW is always used in the CG equation. Obese patients may be included in these studies, but usually the number of morbidly obese patients is small. It is therefore unknown for patients with BMI > 40 kg/m² if drug $CL$ will continue to correlate better with TBW or with another body weight descriptor, such as LBW.

Some investigators have argued that LBW provides better estimates of $CL_{cr}$ in obese patients and should be used in the CG equation instead of TBW (Demirovic et al, 2009; Pai, 2010). In a study evaluating GFR determined by inulin clearance, GFR was 42% higher in the obese group (BMI > 30 kg/m²) compared to the lean group (BMI < 25 kg/m²). When normalized for TBW, GFR was 36% lower in the obese group, suggesting that excess adipose tissue does not contribute entirely to increased GFR. When normalized for LBW, there was no difference in GFR between obese and lean subjects, suggesting preference of LBW over TBW for estimating GFR (Fig. 24-2) (Janmahasatian et al, 2008). However, a recent population pharmacokinetic study of vancomycin in 346 patients (TBW 70–294 kg; BMI 30.1–85.7 kg/m²), in whom the authors referred to as "super obese," did not identify a relationship between vancomycin $CL$ and $CL_{cr}$ estimated using the CG equation and any of the different body weight descriptors (TBW, IBW, AdjBW, LBW). Instead, vancomycin $CL$ was better associated with a specific fitted formula using age, $S_{cr}$, sex, and TBW allometrically scaled to an exponent of 0.75 (Crass et al, 2018).

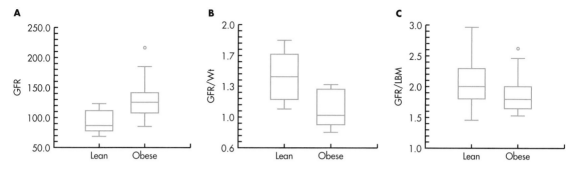

FIGURE 24-2 • Box plots of glomerular filtration rate (GFR) for lean and obese subjects. In all figures, there were 11 observations of GFR from lean subjects (9 from the original lean patients and 2 from patients who were obese and became lean after surgery) and 13 observations from obese subjects (8 from obese patients presurgery and 6 from the same cohort 12 months after surgery). (a) Non-normalized GFR ($P = 0.003$, repeated measures analysis of variance comparing lean with obese). (b) GFR normalized to total body weight ($P = 0.002$, repeated measures analysis of variance comparing lean with obese). (c) GFR normalized to lean body mass (LBM) ($P = 0.27$, repeated measures analysis of variance comparing lean with obese; power is approximately 0.65 to show 25% difference assuming same variability).

The MDRD equation (Equation 24.2) estimates GFR based on a normalized body surface area of 1.73 m². Unfortunately, this equation has been shown to significantly underestimate $CL_{cr}$ in obese patients (Demirovic et al, 2009), which may lead to inadequate dosing and undesirable patient outcomes. In addition, conversion of the MDRD estimate of GFR to a non-normalized body surface area overestimates GFR in obese patients (Pai, 2010). Applying these pharmacokinetic principles and using modified weight strategies may help improve initial drug dosing in the obese patient. However, due to limitations with published pharmacokinetic studies in obesity and substantial interindividual variations within the obese population, it may be prudent to determine the measured 24-hour $CL_{cr}$ and incorporate individualized therapeutic drug monitoring, especially for drugs with a narrow therapeutic index.

## Clinical Examples on Estimating Creatinine Clearance in Obesity

## EXAMPLE 3 ▷ ▷ ▷

A 47-year-old male, SR, was admitted to the hospital with sepsis and positive blood cultures for methicillin-resistant *Staphylococcus aureus*. His height is 72 inches, and his weight is 240 kg. His serum creatinine is 1.55 mg/dL. The primary medical team consults the infectious diseases service, and they recommend starting SR on vancomycin.

Discussion (use equations in Table 24-2):

- First, calculate BMI for SR:
  TBW = 240 kg
  Height= 72 inches × 2.54 cm/inch, which is 182.9 cm or 1.829 m
  BMI = 240/(1.829 × 1.829) = 71.7 kg/m²
  He is morbidly obese according to the obesity classification based on BMI (Table 24-1).
- Calculate the patient's IBW, AdjBW, and LBW:
  IBW = 50 + 2.3 × [72 inches – 60] = 77.6 kg
  AdjBW = 77.6 + [0.4 × (240 – 77.6)] = 142.6 kg
  LBW = (9270 × 240)/[6680 + (216 × 71.7)]
  = 100.3 kg
- Calculate $CL_{cr}$ (mL/min) using the CG equation for TBW, IBW, AdjBW, and LBW:
  $CL_{cr}$ (mL/min) = [(140 – 47) × 240]/(72 × 1.55)
  = 200 mL/min
  $CL_{cr}$ (mL/min) = [(140 – 47) × 77.6]/(72 × 1.55)
  = 65 mL/min
  $CL_{cr}$ (mL/min) = [(140 – 47) × 142.6]/(72 × 1.55)
  = 119 mL/min
  $CL_{cr}$ (mL/min) = [(140 – 47) × (100.3)]/(72 × 1.55)
  = 84 mL/min

Using TBW and AdjBW overestimate $CL_{cr}$ and may result in supratherapeutic dosing since these body weights are not likely good estimates of the patient's lean body mass. IBW underestimates $Cl_{cr}$ because it does not account for the increase in lean body mass in a patient who is morbidly obese. Thus, it is recommended to incorporate LBW into the CG equation to estimate $Cl_{cr}$ in patients who are morbidly obese.

# EXAMPLE 4 ▷ ▷ ▷

A 45-year-old female was admitted to the hospital with chief complaints of shortness of breath, wheezing, chills, and fever. Past medical history included hypertension, arthritis, and asthma. The patient's height and weight are 64 inches and 130 kg, respectively, and her serum creatinine is 0.9 mg/dL.

Discussion:

- Calculate BMI as in Example 1:
  TBW in kilograms = 130 kg
  Height in centimeters (cm) = 64 inches × 2.54 cm/inch =162.6 cm or 1.626 m
  BMI = 130/(1.626 × 1.626) = 49.2 kg/m²
  She is morbidly obese according to the obesity classification based on BMI (Table 24-1).
- Calculate the patient's IBW, AdjBW, and LBW:
  IBW = 45.5 + 2.3 × [64 inches – 60] = 54.7 kg
  AdjBW = 54.7 + [0.4 × (130 – 54.7)] = 84.8 kg
  LBW = (9270 × 130)/[8780 + (244 × 49.2)] = 58 kg
- Calculate $Cl_{cr}$ (mL/min) using the CG equation for TBW, IBW, AdjBW, and LBW:
  $Cl_{cr}$ (mL/min) = [[(140 – 45) × (130)]/(72 × 0.9)] × 0.85 = 162 mL/min
  $Cl_{cr}$ (mL/min) = [[(140 – 45) × (54.7)]/(72 × 0.9)] × 0.85 = 68 mL/min
  $Cl_{cr}$ (mL/min) = [[(140 – 45) × (84.8)]/(72 × 0.9)] × 0.85 = 106 mL/min
  $Cl_{cr}$ (mL/min) = [[(140 – 45) × (58)]/(72 × 0.9)] × 0.85 = 72 mL/min

Although the patient is morbidly obese, her LBW is only slightly larger than her IBW. In this patient, estimating $Cl_{cr}$ using IBW and LBW result in similar rates. Once again, using TBW and AdjBW to estimate $Cl_{cr}$ in this patient will likely overestimate $Cl_{cr}$ and lead to supratherapeutic dosing recommendations.

## Summary

Our understanding of obesity and its implications continue to improve as more research has been devoted to this area. However, the complexity of physiological changes in obesity combined with obesity-related comorbidities frequently encountered in the obese population may render interpretation of available pharmacokinetic studies challenging. More studies are needed on the bioavailability of drugs in the obese population, as well as specific studies on drug distribution, metabolism, and elimination in obesity.

For Phase I metabolism, CYP3A4 activity was consistently lower while CYP2E1 and xanthine oxidase activities were consistently higher in obesity. Other Phase I metabolism enzymes showed trends toward higher activities in obesity, but the results were not conclusive. For Phase II metabolism, UGT-mediated drug clearances were significantly higher in the obese group. Liver blood flow may be increased in obesity, but the number of the drugs studied is relatively small, and the weight difference between obese and non-obese groups was limited in these studies. As a note, the weight-normalized clearance values may provide information on quantitative differences for drug clearance.

Renal clearance is increased in obese patients due to increased glomerular filtration and tubular secretion. The impact of obesity on tubular reabsorption is currently inconclusive due to limited data. Weight-normalized clearances for many drugs studied for renal elimination showed similar or lower values in the obese group as compared to the non-obese group.

In terms of drug dosing, even with the same BMI, individual obese patients may present with unique body composition and fat distribution. Thus, drug dosing for the obese patients continues to be empiric and individualized. Presently, in an effort to ensure optimal therapeutic outcomes for drug therapies in obesity, we need to keep abreast with published pharmacokinetic data, apply the information to patients prudently, and provide individualized therapeutic drug monitoring as indicated.

## APPLICATION OF PHARMACOKINETICS TO PEDIATRIC PATIENTS

### Pediatric Age Subpopulations

Pediatric patients are not small adults, nor do they belong to a homogeneous population, as their anatomical development and physiological functions vary depending on their age subpopulations. Therefore, the pharmacokinetic characteristics of medications may differ in adults and among the pediatric subpopulations. The pediatric subpopulations are illustrated in Table 24-3, with the age ranges defined in the Food and Drug Administration (FDA) Guidance for Industry (FDA, 2014). The upper age limits used to define the pediatric subpopulations vary among sources (Murphy and American Society of Health-System Pharmacists, 2017; FDA, 1997; Williams et al, 2012; Hardin et al, 2017) as shown in Table 24-3 as an example of different classifications used.

### Inadequate Guidance in Dosing Recommendation for Pediatric Patients

Pediatric patients have different dosing requirements from those for adults, although information for pediatric dosing is generally lacking. Most (75%) drugs are marketed without specific pediatric dosing recommendations. In December 1994, the FDA required drug manufacturers to determine whether existing data were sufficient to support information on pediatric use for drug labeling purposes and implemented a plan to encourage the voluntary collection of pediatric data. The FDA Modernization Act authorized a pediatric exclusivity with an additional 6 months of patent protection for manufacturers who conducted pediatric clinical trials (FDA, 1997). As a consequence, the pediatric studies resulted in 805 drugs labeled for pediatric use in 2003–2019, with the inclusion of new indications and enhanced pediatric safety information for pediatric population (FDA, 2019); this progress also includes studies conducted in neonates and labeling and indications changes or additions. Overall, these studies reveal significant new information regarding dosing and pharmacokinetic differences between children and adults (Burton, 2006).

When information is not available to allow for the determination of pediatric doses, empirical dose adjustment methods are often used. Dosage normalization has been proposed by some based on the child's age or body weight from adult drug dosages (eg, Young's rule and Clark's rule, respectively) (Kearns et al, 2003). Dosage based on body surface area may have an advantage of avoiding bias due to unusual body weight because both the height and the weight of the patient are considered.

## TABLE 24-3 • Age Ranges of Pediatric Subpopulations

| Age Terminology | Murphy (Murphy and American Society of Health-System Pharmacists, 2017) | FDA (FDA, 2014) | Williams (Williams et al, 2012) |
|---|---|---|---|
| Neonate | Birth to 4 weeks | Birth to 1 month | Birth to 27 days |
| Preterm | Gestational age < 37 wks | Gestational age < 37 wks | Before full gestational period |
| Full term | Gestational age 39–40 wks | | |
| Post term | Gestational age ≥ 38 wks | | |
| Infant | 1 month to < 12 months | > 1 month to 2 years | 28 days–12 mo (Infant) 13 mo–2 years (Toddler) |
| Child | 1 to 12 years | > 2 to 12 years | 2–5 yrs (Early) 6–11 yrs (Middle) |
| Adolescent | 13 to 18 years | >12 to 16–21 years | 12–18 yrs (Early) 19–21 yrs (Late) |
| Pediatric | Birth to 18 years | Birth to 16–21 years | Birth to 21 years |

These equations and/or principles are often inadequate in describing the range of doses required from birth through adulthood and are inadequate to reflect the developmental and physiological differences that lead to pharmacokinetic consequences across the pediatric subpopulations, as well as between pediatric and adult patients. Therefore, pediatric subjects should not be considered as simply "small adults" in the aspect of pharmacokinetics.

## Impact of Pediatrics on the Pharmacokinetics of Drugs

The rational, effective, and safe use of drugs in pediatric patients requires a thorough understanding of the differences in developmental pharmacology, pharmacokinetics, and pharmacodynamics of specific drugs, in pediatric subpopulations, as well as between pediatric and adult patients. The following section highlights the potential impact on pharmacokinetics based on ADME principles. A summary of these changes is highlighted in Table 24-4.

### Absorption

The physiological variables for oral absorption, such as gastric pH, gastric emptying time, intestinal transit time, and biliary function, vary among neonates, infants, and children. In newborns, the gastric pH is elevated (>4), and gastric emptying and intestinal transit are faster and irregular with immature biliary function (Murphy and American Society of Health-System Pharmacists, 2017). In infants, the gastric pH is lower (2–4) with increasing emptying and transit time, but biliary function is near the adult pattern. As a consequence, the higher pH in newborns and infants may result in higher bioavailability of acid-labile drugs, such as penicillin G, ampicillin, and nafcillin, but lower bioavailability of weak acids, such as phenobarbital that may require higher relative doses as compared to those for children and adults (Kearns et al, 2003). The impact of gastric emptying time on the rate of absorption in neonates and infants has not been extensively studied, although it has been suggested that processes have fully matured by 4 months of age (Kearns et al, 2003). Neonates have difficulty

| TABLE 24-4 • Trends in the Determinants of Developmental Pharmacokinetics from Neonates to Adolescents | | | | |
|---|---|---|---|---|
| | **Neonate** | **Infant** | **Child** | **Adolescent** |
| Absorption | | | | |
| Gastric pH | ↑↑ | ↑ | ↑ | ↔ |
| GI transit time | ↓↓ | ↓ | ↔ | ↔ |
| Biliary function | ↓ | ~↔ | ↔ | ↔ |
| Distribution | | | | |
| Total water/ECF | ↑ | ↑ | ↓~↔ | ↔ |
| Total body fat | ↓ | ↓ | ↑ by 1–10 mo | ↔ |
| Plasma protein | ↓ | ↓~↔ | ↔ | ↔ |
| Metabolism | | | | |
| CYP enzymes | ↓↓ | ↓~↔ by 1 yr | ↑ | ↔ |
| Phase II enzymes | ↓ | ↓ | ↔ | ↔ |
| Excretion | | | | |
| Glomerular filtration | ↓ | ↔ | ↔ | ↔ |
| Tubular secretion | ↓ | ~↔ | ↔ | ↔ |

absorbing fat-soluble vitamins compared to infants and children due to their immature biliary function (Heubi et al, 1982).

### Drug Distribution

Age-related changes or differences in factors such as plasma and tissue protein concentration, body composition, blood flow, permeability, and acid–base balance are important for drug distribution. Of these factors, changes in (a) body composition (body fat and total body water and extracellular water) and (b) plasma protein concentration, are major factors exerting important effects on drug distribution in pediatric patients (Murphy and American Society of Health-System Pharmacists, 2017).

The total body water is relatively high, constituting ~80% of total body weight in neonates and infants up to the first 6–12 months of life, compared to about 60% in children and adults. The extracellular water is relatively high in neonates, ~45%, and approaching the adult value of ~25% in adults during the first year of life. The total body fat is lower in neonates and infants, peaks at 1 year, then decreases gradually to adult value. As a result, the apparent volume of distribution of hydrophilic drugs is age dependent, as illustrated in Table 24-5 with the well-documented case of gentamicin (Shevchuk and Taylor, 1990; Semchuk et al, 1995) but not lipophilic drugs, such as diazepam, where a smaller apparent

volume of distribution may be observed. Therefore, hydrophilic drugs may have reduced plasma concentrations due to increased apparent volume of distribution when dosed on a weight basis, lower plasma concentrations for hydrophilic drugs are expected in neonates and young infants.

The relative concentrations of circulating drug-binding proteins, such as albumin and α-acid glycoprotein, are lower in the neonates and infants up to 1 year of age. The changes in these proteins may impact the unbound fraction and distribution of highly protein-bound drugs. In neonates and young infants, the unbound fraction of phenytoin is higher, leading to elevated free phenytoin concentrations. This may lead to misinterpretation of total phenytoin concentrations which are typically measured clinically (Burton, 2006). Micafungin unbound fraction has also been observed to be higher in neonates than adults (Yanni et al, 2011). The presence of fetal albumin and the increased concentrations of bilirubin and free fatty acids are also important issues in neonates. Both these factors, albeit via different mechanisms, lead to increased unbound fractions of drugs that are bound to albumin (Kearns et al, 2003; Allegaert et al, 2008).

The ontogeny of drug transporters has recently been reviewed by the Pediatric Transporter Working Group; interested readers are encouraged to seek additional information (Brouwer et al, 2015). As reviewed, there has been little research regarding the impact of drug transporters on pharmacokinetics in pediatrics or the impact that these alterations in pharmacokinetics may have on therapeutic outcomes or toxicity.

### Hepatic and Extrahepatic Drug Metabolism

The developmental differences in drug-metabolizing enzymes and transporters are still inadequately characterized, although it is clear that there are marked changes in the expression and function in Phase I drug-metabolizing enzymes (Murphy and American Society of Health-System Pharmacists, 2017; Allegaert et al, 2008).

**Phase I Metabolism.** The traditional view is that there is a delayed maturation of CYP enzymes in newborns that changes markedly and increases throughout the first year to adult levels. Thereafter,

### TABLE 24-5 • Age-Dependent Apparent Volumes of Distribution of Gentamicin and Diazepam

| Age | $V$ (L/kg) | |
| --- | --- | --- |
| | Gentamicin | Diazepam |
| <34 weeks postnatal | 0.67 | |
| 34–48 weeks postnatal | 0.52 | 1.3–2.6 |
| 1–4.9 years | 0.38 | |
| 5–9.9 years | 0.33 | |
| 10–16 years | 0.31 | |
| Adults | 0.30 | 1.6–3.2 |

in early childhood and through the onset of puberty, its activity exceeds that seen in adults, before declining to adult levels (Leeder and Kearns, 1997). This pattern for CYP enzyme development contributes to the variability in drug pharmacokinetics in pediatric subpopulations. It should be noted that this is an oversimplification of the process and that not all CYP enzymes nor individuals share this development profile. While an extensive description of the distinct patterns that exist for different enzymes is beyond the scope of this chapter section, the following will briefly review some important CYP enzymes. A study of the development of CYP Phase I drug-metabolizing enzymes identified three distinct groups: (1) fetal expression (CYP3A7 and 4A1); (2) early neonatal expression (CYP2D6 and 2E1) and (3) late neonatal expression (CYP3A4, 2C19, 2C9, and 1A2). At birth, activity of enzymes of CYPs 1A2, 2E1, 3A4, 2D6, 2C9, and 2C19 are all reduced, as compared with that of adult activities (Murphy and American Society of Health-System Pharmacists, 2017; Kearns et al, 2003; Lu and Rosenbaum, 2014).

CYP2D6 is very low to absent in the fetus, with uniform presence as early as 1–2 weeks postnatal age. Increased activity throughout infancy, until the age of ~3–5 years when activity is similar to adults. CYP2C9 and 2C19 are not observed in the fetal liver, with low activity in the first 1–2 weeks of life, with adult activity achieved reached at 6 months and continued increased activity at 3–4 years of age, before returning to adult levels during puberty. CYP1A2 has very little fetal activity, with adult activity reached at ~4 months and may exceed adult activity during early childhood before returning to adult activity during puberty. CYP3A7 is the predominant isozyme in the fetus and shortly peaks at birth and declines rapidly thereafter (Kearns et al, 2003). It is detectable as early as 2 months' gestation, declines after birth, and is undetectable by ~1 year of age. CYP3A7 has lower metabolic capacity than other CYP3A enzymes. CYP3A4 has lower fetal activity than adults and increases throughout infancy until 1–4 years of age, when it decreases to adult levels.

Significant impacts of the age-dependent development of Phase I enzymes on the pharmacokinetics of many drugs have been documented. The hepatic metabolism of carbamazepine (substrate of CYP3A4) is increased in infants and children

as compared to neonates and adults (Korinthenberg et al, 1994). Phenytoin (substrate of CYP2C9 and CYP2C19) concentrations were markedly increased in preterm infants, than term first-week-of-life infants- and term second-week-of-life infants (Loughnan et al, 1977; Besunder et al, 1988a, b; Kearns et al, 2003;). With diazepam (substrate of CYP2C19), the age-dependent changes in oxidative metabolism result in the shortest half-life in children, 7–37 hours, as compared to those of 25–100 hours in neonates and infants- and 20–50 hours in adults (Kearns et al, 2003).

Clinical observations are consistent with the notion that hepatic metabolism is age dependent in pediatric patients. Hepatic metabolism in children of 3–10 years of age may be greater than that of adults. The greater hepatic clearance in this subpopulation remains significant even after the correction for the age-dependent liver weight (Murry et al, 1995). Therefore, the doses required for this subpopulation of children are often higher on a pure body weight basis as compared to adolescents and adults.

**Phase II Metabolism.** The understanding of the age-related development of Phase II conjugation metabolism is less well characterized than Phase I. Like Phase I metabolism, there is a unique pattern observed for each of the different Phase II enzymes. Among the Phase II drug-metabolizing enzymes, glucuronosyltransferase (UGT) has markedly reduced activity in neonates and early infants but approaches adult level by early childhood (6–18 months). Glucuronidation of acetaminophen (primarily UGT1A6, and to a lesser extent UGT1A9) is decreased in neonates and children 3–10 years of age, compared to adults (Murphy and American Society of Health-System Pharmacists, 2017; Kearns et al, 2003; Burton, 2006). N-acetyl transferase (NAT2) has reduced activity in neonates, and activity increases in infants and children until 1–3 years of age, when adult activity is attained (Murphy and American Society of Health-System Pharmacists; Burton, 2006). Methyltransferase in children has increased activities, 50% higher than that in adults (Burton, 2006).

*Excretion*

The rates of glomerular filtration, tubular secretion, and tubular reabsorption are slower at birth, but rapidly rise to adult levels in 8–12 months of age (van den Anker et al, 1995; van den Anker, 2010). Therefore, drugs that are primarily excreted in the urine unchanged (eg, high fraction excreted in urine unchanged) require an extension of dosing intervals to accommodate the slower drug renal clearance. Numerous drugs have been studied and required interval and/or dosage adjustment. A common example of drugs requiring dosage adjustment is aminoglycoside antibiotics, drugs that have a narrow therapeutic index. In term newborns, the dosing interval of aminoglycosides is typically 24 hours, compared to 36–48 hours for preterm newborns (Schwartz et al, 1987; Brion et al, 1991; Kearns et al, 2003).

In summary, the understanding of differences in developmental changes and their impacts on the pharmacokinetics of medications is essential to interpret observations correctly and to recommend rational modification in dosing regimen for safe and effective therapy. Antiretroviral therapy, used for HIV-infected pediatric patients, provides an example of how pharmacokinetics of drugs may differ within a drug class and across the pediatric subpopulation. The oral absorption of antiretrovirals is affected by the presence of food in the gastrointestinal tracts of infants. For example, the bioavailability of nelfinavir (a weak acid) in newborns and infants <2 years of age is lower than that in older children, due to the food effect, higher gastric pH, or both (Hirt et al, 2006). Decreased albumin concentrations in newborns and neonates cause increases in the unbound fraction of highly protein-bound drugs, such as enfuvirtide (>90% bound) that result in increased efficacy and toxicity. The current cocktail regimen with fixed-dose combinations of antiretrovirals for adults cannot be extrapolated to the pediatric population, because the varied metabolic changes among the pediatric subpopulations may result in subtherapeutic concentrations of one agent in young children, such as nevirapine (metabolized by CYP3A4 and CYP2B6), but overdosing of another agent, such as lamivudine of high $f_e = 0.7$ (eliminated by GFR and active tubular secretion) in neonates (Ellis et al, 2007).

## Age-Dependent Pharmacodynamics

In contrast to the current understanding of ontogeny and pharmacokinetics, much less information is available for the developmental impacts on drug actions (Holford, 2010). Several developmental age–dependent differences in treatment responses are recognized (van den Anker et al, 2018). These include a higher incidence of valproic acid–induced hepatotoxicity, a higher incidence of paradoxical excitement associated with antihistamines, a higher incidence of acute dystonic reactions associated with dopamine antagonists, and greater lansoprazole antisecretory effects. Whether these are true pharmacodynamic differences, due to pharmacokinetic differences, or some combination of the two is not known. Developmental pharmacodynamics has recently been reviewed (van den Anker et al, 2018), and suggests that human *in vivo* studies show that developmental pharmacodynamics differences exist for numerous drugs when studied in animals and humans. Currently available data in humans suggest that children are more sensitive to the effects of immunosuppressants due to differences that exist in the developing immune system. Increased sensitivity to warfarin due to decreased concentrations of vitamin K–dependent clotting factors has been observed. Finally, several studies have suggested that children are more susceptible to paradoxical seizure occurrence due to the increased excitatory $GABA_A$ receptor density. Additional study is required and several researchers (Burton, 2006; Holford, 2010; van den Anker et al, 2018) have called for more intense study of the developmental aspects of pharmacodynamics.

## Clinical Example of Rational Dosing in Pediatric Patients

Busulfan is a bifunctional alkylating agent used for the preparative regimen before blood, bone marrow, or stem cell transplantation. Before the FDA approval of IV Busulfex˚ in 1999 for parenteral administration, patients had to receive 35 tablets q6h around the clock for 4 days (total 16 doses). Moreover, the drug triggered vomiting and resulted in erratic systemic exposure, as assessed by AUC. However, the grafting success depends on reaching a target AUC of 900–1500 $\mu$Mol•min, and adverse effects are observed when AUC is >1500 $\mu$Mol•min. Therefore, dosing busulfan precisely and effectively is challenging in adults, and even more so in pediatric patients.

With the availability of IV busulfan, the age-dependent clearance is characterized based on five body-weight strata from <9 kg to >34 kg for 55 pediatric patients 0.3–17.2 years old with 20 subjects younger than 4 years old. The population clearance (*CL*) in children is 3.96 L/h (Vassal et al, 2008), whereas that of adults is ~ 2.5 L/h (Nguyen et al, 2006). Busulfan *CL* varied among the subjects, with the greatest value for subjects of 9- to 16-kg body weight, and reducing to approach the adult value at a weight >34 kg. With the specifically derived *CL*, rational doses can be derived for individual subsets of pediatric patients, based on the following relationship

Total dose (mg/kg) = *CL* (L/h/kg) × (Target AUC)

The dose levels adjusted are 1, 1.2, 1.1, and 0.95 mg/kg for patients with body weights of <9, 9–16, 16–23, and 23–34 kg, respectively, higher than the dose of 0.8 mg/kg for adults. The resulting busulfan AUCs were all within the therapeutic range of 900–1500 $\mu$Mol•min. The example shown here is not meant to illustrate how to dose busulfan, but instead illustrates that with the concept of combining pharmacokinetics (*CL*) and response (therapeutic range of the AUC that predicts positive outcomes) we can make rational dosing choices.

## Approaches to Study Pharmacokinetics and Pharmacodynamics in Pediatrics

Awareness has grown about the developmental pharmacokinetics of medications, resulting from physiological and pharmacological differences observed across the entire pediatric age range, and between pediatric and adult populations. With the legislative incentive from the FDA and Pediatric Research Equity Act and the European Union, an increasing number of studies on pediatric pharmacokinetics and pharmacodynamics were conducted in both academic and industrial settings.

In general, clinical pediatric pharmacokinetic data are scarce and often do not cover the entire pediatric age range. In addition, the study enrollment is small, and the number of observations is limited due to constraints in the blood volume and frequency of blood sampling. Advances have been made to overcome some of these constraints (Knibbe et al, 2011).

Several approaches have been described in an attempt to more efficiently study pharmacokinetics

and pharmacodynamics of drugs in pediatric population, allometric scaling (Knibbe et al, 2011; Wang et al, 2014), and pharmacokinetic–pharmacodynamic (PK/PD) modeling (Holford, 2010; Leong et al, 2012; Himebauch and Zuppa, 2014).

In performing allometric scaling, the pharmacokinetic parameters of clearance (*CL*) and volume of distributions ($V_c$, $V_p$, or $V_{ss}$) of pediatric subjects are often predicted by scaling down from adult values with fixed exponent values of 0.75 for *CL* and of 1 for *Vs*. The allometric exponent for scaling *CL* has been recognized to vary with ages in subpopulations of pediatric population (Wang et al, 2014). Current allometric scaling approach may be of value for scaling from adults to adolescents and perhaps children, while it is inadequate for scaling from adults to neonates, or between pediatric subpopulations (Wang et al, 2014).

Pediatric pharmacokinetic and pharmacodynamic modeling and simulation have been increasingly employed in pediatric drug development, as well as in FDA regulatory review and decision making (Leong et al, 2012). The PK/PD modeling is most commonly implemented in pediatric drug development for first-time-in-pediatrics dose selection, which is a critical milestone and decision point in pediatric drug development (Edginton, 2011).

Holford reviews some of these concepts in which rational dosing in pediatrics is reviewed, named the target concentration approach. The approach is intuitive and links pharmacokinetics and pharmacodynamics, through four steps: (1) choosing the target effect, (2) using pharmacodynamic parameters ($E_{max}$ and $EC_{50}$) to predict the target concentration, (3) using apparent volume of distribution to choose loading dose, and (4) using clearance to predict the maintenance dose rate (Holford, 2010).

## Summary

Pediatric patients consist of four subpopulation groups: neonates, infants, children, and adolescents. The pharmacokinetics of drugs in pediatric patients are distinct from those of adult subjects, as well as among the pediatric subpopulations. Therefore, a thorough understanding of their developmental and physiological differences and the resulting impact on pharmacokinetics and pharmacodynamics is essential to design safe and effective therapy.

Drug absorption in neonates and infants may differ from that of children and adolescents, due to high gastric pH, short gastric emptying time and intestinal transit time, and immature biliary function. Drug distribution is impacted by the composition of total body water and total body fat and plasma protein concentrations. Drug clearance may be altered by changes in Phase I- and II-mediated metabolism and renal clearance. The current understanding of age-related pharmacodynamic variation in pediatrics is still limited and requires more studies. Over the past two decades, there have been an increasing number of studies on pediatric pharmacokinetics and pharmacodynamics performed in both academic and industrial settings. Emerging approaches of pharmacokinetic and pharmacodynamic modeling have been gaining acceptance in rational clinical trial design, trial execution, and data analysis. It is anticipated that more useful PK/PD information will be generated in the next few decades, to further facilitate safe and effective drug therapy in pediatric patients.

## LEARNING QUESTIONS

1. Which of the following is the most appropriate choice that describes a physiological change with aging?

   a. Increased transporter activity

   b. Increased hepatic blood flow

   c. Increased renal function

   d. Increased muscle as a percentage of total body mass

   e. Decrease in total body water

2. Which of the following is the most appropriate to describe age-associated changes that can affect pharmacokinetics in older patients?

   a. Changes in gastrointestinal function that reduces the extent of drug absorption

   b. Increase in total body water that lower peak concentrations of hydrophilic drugs

   c. Decrease in body fat that increases peak concentrations of hydrophilic drugs

   d. Decrease in serum albumin concentrations to increase volume of distribution

   e. Decrease in creatinine clearance to increase renal clearance

3. Which of the following statements regarding renal function and pharmacokinetics in older patients is most accurate?

   a. Decreased muscle mass is a reason for the normal or low serum creatinine concentrations in older patients even in the presence of decreased renal function.

   b. Renal tubular secretion does not change with aging.

   c. Renal function estimations that are based on serum creatine concentrations are identical between older men and women.

   d. Glomerular function is more accurately estimated in older patients.

   e. Gentamicin can be used safely in older patients with serum creatinine concentrations of 1.7 mg/dL.

4. Which of the following is the most appropriate to describe age-associated changes that can affect pharmacodynamics in older patients?

   a. Increased sensitivity to $\beta_1$–adrenergic receptor agonism

   b. Increased sensitivity to $\beta_2$–adrenergic receptor antagonism

   c. Increased sensitivity to anticholinergic effects of drugs

   d. Decreased sensitivity to drugs that prolong the QT interval

   e. Decreased sensitivity to benzodiazepines

5. Which of the following age-related changes is the most likely to cause a clinically significant adverse drug effect?

   a. Increased gastrointestinal transit time

   b. Increased P-glycoprotein function

   c. Increased Phase II drug metabolism

   d. Increased permeability at the blood–brain barrier

   e. Changes in plasma protein binding

6. Which of the following answers is correct for this patient's body mass index (BMI)?

   a. 39.3

   b. 46.7

   c. 52.1

   d. 59.3

   e. 64.7

7. If this patient has a serum creatinine of 1.4 mg/dL, calculate her estimated creatinine clearance in mL/min using lean body weight (LBW) in the Cockcroft–Gault equation.

   a. 40 mL/min

   b. 55 mL/min

   c. 70 mL/min

   d. 82 mL/min

   e. 127 mL/min

8. Which of the following CYP450 isoenzymes has reduced activity in obese patients?

   a. CYP3A4

   b. CYP2E1

   c. CYP2C9

   d. CYP2D6

   e. Xanthine oxidase

9. Which of the following statements most accurately reflects the physiological changes commonly occurred with obesity?

   a. Glomerular filtration is usually increased in obese patients.

   b. Tubular reabsorption is usually increased in obese patients.

   c. Tubular secretion is usually decreased in obese patients.

   d. The activity of uridine diphosphate glucuronosyltransferase is usually decreased in obese patients.

   e. The size of the kidney is usually smaller in obese patients.

10. Which of the following statements most accurately reflects an appropriate drug dosing strategy for the obese patients?

    a. The TBW should always be used to calculate the loading dose for obese patients.

    b. The IBW should always be used to calculate the loading dose for obese patients.

    c. The TBW should always be used to calculate the maintenance dose for obese patients.

    d. The IBW should always be used to calculate the maintenance dose for obese patients.

    e. Apply pharmacokinetic principles using modified weight strategies combined with therapeutic drug monitoring.

11. List the subpopulations that belong to the pediatric population.

12. Temozolomide is an alkylating agent, indicated for the management of pediatric brain tumors. When used for the treatment of refractory anaplastic astrocytoma, the recommended treatment is to give oral doses of 200 mg/m$^2$/day for 5 days and to repeat every 28 days. The bioavailability of temozolomide is 0.98 on an empty stomach and 0.6 when the drug is given with a fatty meal. The $CL$ and $t_{1/2}$ of temozolomide are 100 mL/min/m$^2$ and 1.8 hours, respectively. The available capsule strengths are 5, 20, 100, and 250 mg. CB is a 15-month-old patient of 7-kg body weight (0.3 m$^2$). (a) What is the $CL$ of temozolomide in CB? (b) Recommend a regimen for CB; which $F$ is to be used? (c) Predict the $C_{ss,ave}$.

13. WS, an 8-year-old, 25-kg male, is receiving a 250-mg capsule of valproic acid (VA) q12h for the treatment of seizures. The $CL$s of VA are 13 mL/kg/h for children and 8 mL/kg/h for adults. The $V$ and $F$ of VA are 0.14 L/kg and 1, respectively. The therapeutic plasma VA concentration range is 50–100 mg/L. The toxicity may be observed when plasma concentrations are >200 mg/L. WS has normal hepatic and renal function. (a) Predict the steady state trough concentration ($C_{ss,min}$) for WS, and (b) comment on the adequacy of his current regimen, using a one-compartment intravenous bolus model.

# ANSWERS

## Learning Questions

1. **e.**
2. **e.**
3. **a.**
4. **c.**
5. **d.**
6. **c.**
7. **b.**
8. **a.**
9. **a.**
10. **e.**
11. Children, Infants, Adolescents, Neonates
12. **(a)** $CL = (100 \text{ mL/min/m}^2)(0.3 \text{ m}^2)$
    $\qquad = 30 \text{ mL/min}$
    $\qquad = [30 (60)/1000] \text{ L/h} = 1.8 \text{ L/h}$

    The $CL$ in the infant is significantly lower than that of 10.3 L/h in adults with 1.73 m² of body surface area.

    **(b)** $D/\tau = (200 \text{ mg/m}^2/\text{day})(0.3 \text{ m}^2)$
    $\qquad = 60 \text{ mg/day} = 60 \text{ mg/24 hours}$
    $\qquad = 20 \text{ mg/8 hours}$

    The dose will be given with 3 × 20-mg capsules or in divided doses per day.

    **(c)** $C_{ss,ave} = [F\,D]/[CL \cdot \tau]$

    **Which *F* is to be used?**

    $F = \mathbf{0.6}$ (not 0.98) is used to predict the $C_{ss,ave}$, because infants are fed regularly; therefore, the medication is NOT given to the infant with empty stomach, and infant formula is rich in the fat content.

    $C_{ss,ave} = [F\,D]/[CL \cdot \tau]$
    $\qquad = [(0.6)(60 \text{ mg})]/[(1.8 \text{ L/h})(24 \text{ h})]$
    $\qquad = 0.83 \text{ mg/L}$

    The $C_{ss,ave}$ will be overestimated by 1.6 times as 1.36 mg/L, if an incorrect $F$ (0.98) is selected.

13. **(a)** The one-compartment IV bolus model can be used to estimate the concentration,

because VA is rapidly (with very high $k_a$) and completely absorbed.

For the one-compartment IV bolus model,

$C_{ss,max} = C_0/(1 - e^{-k \cdot \tau})$

$C_{ss,min} = C_{ss,max}\, e^{-k \cdot \tau}$
$\qquad = C_0\, e^{-k\tau}/(1 - e^{-k \cdot \tau})$
$\qquad = [(D/V)e^{-k\tau}]/(1 - e^{-k \cdot \tau})$

$\qquad D = 250 \text{ mg} \quad \tau = 12 \text{ h}$
$\qquad V = (0.14 \text{ L/kg})(25 \text{ kg}) = 3.5 \text{ L}$
$\qquad k = CL/V$

**What is the *CL* for AH?**

$CL = (13 \text{ mL/kg/h})(25 \text{ kg})$
$\qquad = 325 \text{ mL/h} = 0.325 \text{ L/h}$
$\qquad k = CL/V = (0.325 \text{ L/h})/3.5 \text{ L}$
$\qquad = 0.093 \text{ h}^{-1}$

$C_{ss,min} = [(D/V)\, e^{-k \cdot \tau}]/(1 - e^{-k \cdot \tau})$
$\qquad = [(250 \text{ mg})/(3.5 \text{ L})][e^{-(0.093)(12)}]/$
$\qquad\quad [1 - e^{-(0.093)(12)}]$
$\qquad = (71.43 \text{ mg/L})(0.328)/(0.672)$
$\qquad = 34.8 \text{ mg/L} \sim 35 \text{ mg/L}$

**(b)** The $C_{ss,min}$ is *below* the therapeutic range of 50–100 mg/L. The current regimen is required to be modified.

**Discussion: If *CL* of 8 mg/kg/h for adults is misused,**

$CL = (\mathbf{8} \text{ mL/kg/h})(25 \text{ kg})$
$\qquad = 200 \text{ mL/h} = \mathbf{0.20} \text{ L/h}$
$\qquad k = CL/V = (\mathbf{0.20} \text{ L/h})/3.5 \text{ L}$
$\qquad = \mathbf{0.057} \text{ h}^{-1}$

$C_{ss,min} = [(D/V)\, e^{-k \cdot \tau}]/(1 - e^{-k \cdot \tau})$
$\qquad = [(250 \text{ mg})/(3.5 \text{ L})][e^{-(0.057)(12)}]/$
$\qquad\quad [1 - e^{-(0.057)(12)}]$
$\qquad = (71.43 \text{ mg/L})(\mathbf{0.505})/(\mathbf{0.495})$
$\qquad = 72.8 \text{ mg/L} \sim \mathbf{73} \text{ mg/L}$

(overestimated for ~ 2 times)

The comment on the regimen will then be mistakenly made as adequate, because the overestimated trough concentration of 73 mg/L is within the therapeutic range of 50–100 mg/L.

$$\frac{\tau_1}{\tau_2} = \frac{(t_{1/2})_1}{(t_{1/2})_2}$$

$$t_{1/2} = 0.5\,h$$

$$\tau_2 = \frac{4 \times 3.2}{0.5} = 25.6\,h$$

Therefore, this infant may be given the following dose:

$$Dose = 4\,mg/kg\,[11\,lb/(2.2\,lb/kg)]$$

$$= 20\,mg\,every\,24\,h$$

Alternatively, 10 mg every 12 hours would achieve the same $C_{ss,ave}$.

## REFERENCES

Abernethy DR, Greenblatt DJ: Ibuprofen disposition in obese individuals. *Arthritis Rheum* **28**(10):1117–1121, 1985a.

Abernethy DR, Greenblatt DJ: Phenytoin disposition in obesity. Determination of loading dose. *Arch Neurol* **42**(5):468–471, 1985b.

Abernethy DR, Greenblatt DJ, Divoll M, Shader RI: Enhanced glucuronide conjugation of drugs in obesity: Studies of lorazepam, oxazepam, and acetaminophen. *J Lab Clin Med* **101**(6):873–880, 1983.

Abernethy DR, Greenblatt DJ, Smith TW: Digoxin disposition in obesity: Clinical pharmacokinetic investigation. *Am Heart J* **102**(4):740–744, 1981.

Adane ED, Herald M, Koura F: Pharmacokinetics of vancomycin in extremely obese patients with suspected or confirmed *Staphylococcus aureus* infections. *Pharmacotherapy* **35**(2):127–139, 2015.

Albrecht S, Ihmsen H, Hering W, et al: The effect of age on the pharmacokinetics and pharmacodynamics of midazolam. *Clin Pharmacol Ther* **65**(6):630–639, 1999.

Allard S, Kinzig M, Boivin G, Sorgel F, LeBel M: Intravenous ciprofloxacin disposition in obesity. *Clin Pharmacol Ther* **54**(4):368–373, 1993.

Allegaert K, Rayyan M, Vanhaesebrouck S, Naulaers G: Developmental pharmacokinetics in neonates. *Expert Rev Clin Pharmacol* **1**(3):415–428, 2008.

Balis FM: Pharmacokinetic drug interactions of commonly used anticancer drugs. *Clin Pharmacokinet* **11**(3):223–235, 1986.

Barras MA, Duffull SB, Atherton JJ, Green B: Modelling the occurrence and severity of enoxaparin-induced bleeding and bruising events. *Br J Clin Pharmacol* **68**(5):700–711, 2009.

Bartels AL, Kortekaas R, Bart J, et al: Blood-brain barrier P-glycoprotein function decreases in specific brain regions with aging: A possible role in progressive neurodegeneration. *Neurobiol Aging* **30**(11):1818–1824, 2009.

Bauer LA, Black DJ, Lill JS. Vancomycin dosing in morbidly obese patients. *Eur J Clin Pharmacol* **8**: 621–625, 1998.

Bauer LA, Edwards WA, Dellinger EP, Simonowitz DA: Influence of weight on aminoglycoside pharmacokinetics in normal weight and morbidly obese patients. *Eur J Clin Pharmacol* **24**(5):643–647, 1983.

Beaufrere B, Morio B: Fat and protein redistribution with aging: Metabolic considerations. *Eur J Clin Nutr* **54**(Suppl 3):S48–53, 2000.

Benedetti MS, Whomsley R, Canning M: Drug metabolism in the paediatric population and in the elderly. *Drug Discov Today* **12**(15-16):599–610, 2007.

Benet LZ, Hoener BA: Changes in plasma protein binding have little clinical relevance. *Clin Pharmacol Ther* **71**(3):115–121, 2002.

Bercault N, Boulain T, Kuteifan K, Wolf M, Runge I, Fleury JC: Obesity-related excess mortality rate in an adult intensive care unit: A risk-adjusted matched cohort study. *Crit Care Med* **32**(4):998–1003, 2004.

Besunder JB, Reed MD, Blumer JL: Principles of drug biodisposition in the neonate. A critical evaluation of the pharmacokinetic-pharmacodynamic interface (Part I). *Clin Pharmacokinet* **14**(4):189–216, 1988a.

Besunder JB, Reed MD, Blumer JL: Principles of drug biodisposition in the neonate. A critical evaluation of the pharmacokinetic-pharmacodynamic interface (Part II). *Clin Pharmacokinet* **14**(5):261–286, 1988b.

Bickford PC, Breiderick L: Benzodiazepine modulation of GABAergic responses is intact in the cerebellum of aged F344 rats. *Neurosci Lett* **291**(3):187–190, 2000.

Bowie MW, Slattum PW: Pharmacodynamics in older adults: A review. *Am J Geriatr Pharmacother* **5**(3):263–303, 2007.

Brenner SS, Klotz U: P-glycoprotein function in the elderly. *Eur J Clin Pharmacol* **60**(2):97–102, 2004.

Brill MJ, Diepstraten J, van Rongen A, van Kralingen S, van den Anker JN, Knibbe CA: Impact of obesity on drug metabolism and elimination in adults and children. *Clin Pharmacokinet* **51**(5):277–304, 2012.

Brill MJ, Houwink AP, Schmidt S, et al: Reduced subcutaneous tissue distribution of cefazolin in morbidly obese versus non-obese patients determined using clinical microdialysis. *J Antimicrob Chemother* **69**(3):715–723, 2014.

Brion LP, Fleischman AR, Schwartz GJ: Gentamicin interval in newborn infants as determined by renal function and postconceptional age. *Pediatr Nephrol* **5**(6):675–679, 1991.

Brouwer KL, Aleksunes LM, Brandys B, et al: Human ontogeny of drug transporters: Review and recommendations of the Pediatric Transporter Working Group. *Clin Pharmacol Ther* **98**(3):266–287, 2015.

Buechler C, Weiss TS: Does hepatic steatosis affect drug metabolizing enzymes in the liver? *Curr Drug Metab* **12**(1):24–34, 2011.

Burton ME: *Applied Pharmacokinetics and Pharmacodynamics: Principles of Therapeutic Drug Monitoring.* Baltimore, Lippincott Williams & Wilkins, 2006.

Cancelli I, Gigli GL, Piani A, et al: Drugs with anticholinergic properties as a risk factor for cognitive impairment in elderly people: A population-based study. *J Clin Psychopharmacol* **28**(6):654–659, 2008.

Castleden CM, George CF, Marcer D, Hallett C: Increased sensitivity to nitrazepam in old age. *Br Med J* **1**(6052):10–12, 1977.

Chew ML, Mulsant BH, Pollock BG, et al: Anticholinergic activity of 107 medications commonly used by older adults. *J Am Geriatr Soc* **56**(7):1333–1341, 2008.

Chien JY, Ho RJ: Drug delivery trends in clinical trials and translational medicine: Evaluation of pharmacokinetic properties in special populations. *J Pharm Sci* **100**(1):53–58, 2011.

Chiney MS, Schwarzenberg SJ, Johnson LA: Altered xanthine oxidase and N-acetyltransferase activity in obese children. *Br J Clin Pharmacol* **72**(1):109–115, 2011.

Christoff PB, Conti DR, Naylor C, Jusko WJ: Procainamide disposition in obesity. *Drug Intell Clin Pharm* **17**(7-8):516–522, 1983.

Chung EK, Cheatham SC, Fleming MR, Healy DP, Kays MB: Population pharmacokinetics and pharmacodynamics of meropenem in nonobese, obese, and morbidly obese patients. *J Clin Pharmacol* **57**(3):356–368, 2017a.

Chung EK, Cheatham SC, Fleming MR, Healy DP, Shea KM, Kays MB: Population pharmacokinetics and pharmacodynamics of piperacillin and tazobactam administered by prolonged infusion in obese and nonobese patients. *J Clin Pharmacol* **55**(8):899–908, 2015.

Chung EK, Fleming MR, Cheatham SC, Kays MB: Population pharmacokinetics and pharmacodynamics of doripenem in obese, hospitalized patients. *Ann Pharmacother* **51**(3):209–218, 2017b.

Clegg A, Young J, Iliffe S, Rikkert MO, Rockwood K: Frailty in elderly people. *Lancet* **381**(9868):752–762, 2013.

Cockcroft DW, Gault MH: Prediction of creatinine clearance from serum creatinine. *Nephron* **16**(1):31–41, 1976.

Crass RL, Dunn R, Hong J, Krop LC, Pai MP: Dosing vancomycin in the super obese: Less is more. *J Antimicrob Chemother* **73**(11):3081–3086, 2018.

Cusack B, Kelly J, O'Malley K, Noel J, Lavan J, Horgan J: Digoxin in the elderly: Pharmacokinetic consequences of old age. *Clin Pharmacol Ther* **25**(6):772–776, 1979.

Davies DF, Shock NW: Age changes in glomerular filtration rate, effective renal plasma flow, and tubular excretory capacity in adult males. *J Clin Invest* **29**(5):496–507, 1950.

DeGorter MK, Tirona RG, Schwarz UI, et al: Clinical and pharmacogenetic predictors of circulating atorvastatin and rosuvastatin concentrations in routine clinical care. *Circ Cardiovasc Genet* **6**(4):400–408, 2013.

Demirovic JA, Pai AB, Pai MP: Estimation of creatinine clearance in morbidly obese patients. *Am J Health Syst Pharm* **66**(7):642–648, 2009.

Divoll M, Greenblatt DJ, Ochs HR, Shader RI: Absolute bioavailability of oral and intramuscular diazepam: Effects of age and sex. *Anesth Analg* **62**(1):1–8, 1983.

Dobre D, Haaijer-Ruskamp FM, Voors AA, van Veldhuisen DJ: beta-Adrenoceptor antagonists in elderly patients with heart failure: A critical review of their efficacy and tolerability. *Drugs Aging* **24**(12):1031–1044, 2007.

Doyle V, O'Malley K, Kelly JG: Human lymphocyte beta-adrenoceptor density in relation to age and hypertension. *J Cardiovasc Pharmacol* **4**(5):738–740, 1982.

Drayer DE, Romankiewicz J, Lorenzo B, Reidenberg MM: Age and renal clearance of cimetidine. *Clin Pharmacol Ther* **31**(1):45–50, 1982.

Ducharme MP, Slaughter RL, Edwards DJ: Vancomycin pharmacokinetics in a patient population: Effect of age, gender, and body weight. *Ther Drug Monit* **16**(5):513–518, 1994.

Dvorchik BH, Damphousse D: The pharmacokinetics of daptomycin in moderately obese, morbidly obese, and matched nonobese subjects. *J Clin Pharmacol* **45**(1):48–56, 2005.

Edginton AN: Knowledge-driven approaches for the guidance of first-in-children dosing. *Paediatr Anaesth* **21**(3):206–213, 2011.

Ellis JC, L'Homme, Ewings FM, et al: Nevirapine concentrations in HIV-infected children treated with divided fixed-dose combination antiretroviral tablets in Malawi and Zambia. *Antivir Ther* **12**(2):253–260, 2007.

Ensrud KE, Blackwell TL, Mangione CM, et al: Central nervous system-active medications and risk for falls in older women. *J Am Geriatr Soc* **50**(10):1629–1637, 2002.

Falagas ME, Karageorgopoulos DE: Adjustment of dosing of antimicrobial agents for bodyweight in adults. *Lancet* **375**(9710):248–251, 2010.

Falagas ME, Kompoti M: Obesity and infection. *Lancet Infect Dis* **6**(7):438–446, 2006.

FDA: Qualifying for Pediatric Exclusivity Under Section 505A of the Federal Food, Drug, and Cosmetic Act: Frequently Asked Questions on Pediatric Exclusivity (505A). 1997. Retrieved September 30, 2019, from https://www.fda.gov/drugs/development-resources/qualifying-pediatric-exclusivity-under-section-505a-federal-food-drug-and-cosmetic-act-frequently.

FDA: Premarket Assessment of Pediatric Medical Devices, Guidance for Industry and FDA Staff. 2014. Retrieved September 30, 2019, from https://www.fda.gov/regulatory-information/search-fda-guidance-documents/premarket-assessment-pediatric-medical-devices.

FDA: New Pediatric Labeling Information Database. 2019. Retrieved September 30, 2019, from https://www.accessdata.fda.gov/scripts/sda/sdNavigation.cfm?sd=labelingdatabase.

Flechner SM, Kolbeinsson ME, Tam J, Lum B: The impact of body weight on cyclosporine pharmacokinetics in renal transplant recipients. *Transplantation* **47**(5):806–810, 1989.

Flegal KM, Kruszon-Moran D, Carroll MD, Fryar CD, Ogden CL: Trends in obesity among adults in the United States, 2005 to 2014. *JAMA* **315**(21):2284–2291, 2016.

Gibbs JP, Gooley T, Corneau B, Murray G, et al: The impact of obesity and disease on busulfan oral clearance in adults. *Blood* **93**(12):4436–4440, 1999.

Gibson DM, Bron NJ, Richens A, Hounslow NJ, Sedman AJ, Whitfield LR: Effect of age and gender on pharmacokinetics of atorvastatin in humans. *J Clin Pharmacol* **36**(3):242–246, 1996.

Grace E: Altered vancomycin pharmacokinetics in obese and morbidly obese patients: What we have learned over the past 30 years. *J Antimicrob Chemother* **67**(6):1305–1310, 2012.

Greenblatt DJ, Divoll M, Harmatz JS, MacLaughlin DS, Shader RI: Kinetics and clinical effects of flurazepam in young and elderly noninsomniacs. *Clin Pharmacol Ther* **30**(4):475–486, 1981.

Greenblatt DJ, Harmatz JS, Shader RI: Clinical pharmacokinetics of anxiolytics and hypnotics in the elderly. Therapeutic considerations (Part I). *Clin Pharmacokinet* **21**(3):165–177, 1991.

Greenblatt DJ, Harmatz JS, von Moltke LL, Wright CE, Shader RI: Age and gender effects on the pharmacokinetics and pharmacodynamics of triazolam, a cytochrome P450 3A substrate. *Clin Pharmacol Ther* **76**(5):467–479, 2004.

Hales CM, Fryar CD, Carroll MD, Freedman DS, Ogden CL: Trends in obesity and severe obesity prevalence in US youth and adults by sex and age, 2007-2008 to 2015-2016. *JAMA* **319**(16):1723–1725, 2018.

Hamilton R, Thai XC, Ameri D, Pai MP: Oral bioavailability of linezolid before and after Roux-en-Y gastric bypass surgery: Is dose modification necessary in obese subjects? *J Antimicrob Chemother* **68**(3):666–673, 2013.

Hanley MJ, Abernethy DR, Greenblatt DJ: Effect of obesity on the pharmacokinetics of drugs in humans. *Clin Pharmacokinet* **49**(2):71–87, 2010.

Hardin AP, Hackell JM, Committee On P, Ambulatory M: Age limit of pediatrics. *Pediatrics* **140**(3), 2017.

Henry RR, Mudaliar S, Chu N, et al: Young and elderly type 2 diabetic patients inhaling insulin with the AERx insulin diabetes management system: A pharmacokinetic and pharmacodynamic comparison. *J Clin Pharmacol* **43**(11):1228–1234, 2003.

Heubi JE, Balistreri WF, Suchy FJ: Bile salt metabolism in the first year of life. *J Lab Clin Med* **100**(1):127–136, 1982.

Hilmer SN, Gnjidic D: The effects of polypharmacy in older adults. *Clin Pharmacol Ther* **85**(1):86–88, 2009.

Himebauch AS, Zuppa A: Methods for pharmacokinetic analysis in young children. *Expert Opin Drug Metab Toxicol* **10**(4):497–509, 2014.

Hirt D, Urien S, Jullien V, et al: Age-related effects on nelfinavir and M8 pharmacokinetics: A population study with 182 children. *Antimicrob Agents Chemother* **50**(3):910–916, 2006.

Holazo AA, Winkler MB, Patel IH: Effects of age, gender and oral contraceptives on intramuscular midazolam pharmacokinetics. *J Clin Pharmacol* **28**(11):1040–1045, 1988.

Holdsworth M, Forman WB, Killilea TA, et al: Transdermal fentanyl disposition in elderly subjects. *Gerontology* **40**(1):32–37, 1994.

Holford N: Dosing in children. *Clin Pharmacol Ther* **87**(3): 367–370, 2010.

Ingrande J, Lemmens HJ: Dose adjustment of anaesthetics in the morbidly obese. *Br J Anaesth* **105**(1): i16–23, 2010.

Jaber LA, Ducharme MP, Halapy H: The effects of obesity on the pharmacokinetics and pharmacodynamics of glipizide in patients with non-insulin-dependent diabetes mellitus. *Ther Drug Monit* **18**(1):6–13, 1996.

Jain R, Chung SM, Jain L, et al: Implications of obesity for drug therapy: Limitations and challenges. *Clin Pharmacol Ther* **90**(1):77–89, 2011.

Janmahasatian S, Duffull SB, Ash S, Ward LC, Byrne NM, Green B: Quantification of lean bodyweight. *Clin Pharmacokinet* **44**(10):1051–1065, 2005.

Janmahasatian S, Duffull SB, Chagnac A, Kirkpatrick CM and Green B: Lean body mass normalizes the effect of obesity on renal function. *Br J Clin Pharmacol* **65**(6): 964–965, 2008.

Janson B, Thursky K: Dosing of antibiotics in obesity. *Curr Opin Infect Dis* **25**(6):634–649, 2012.

Jensen MD, Ryan DH, Apovian CM, et al: 2013 AHA/ACC/TOS guideline for the management of overweight and obesity in adults: A report of the American College of Cardiology/ American Heart Association Task Force on Practice Guidelines and The Obesity Society. *J Am Coll Cardiol* **63**(25 Pt B): 2985–3023, 2014.

Kaestli LZ, Wasilewski-Rasca AF, Bonnabry P, Vogt-Ferrier N: Use of transdermal drug formulations in the elderly. *Drugs Aging* **25**(4):269–280, 2008.

Kanto J, Kangas L, Aaltonen L, Hilke H: Effect of age on the pharmacokinetics and sedative of flunitrazepam. *Int J Clin Pharmacol Ther Toxicol* **19**(9):400–404, 1981.

Kearns GL, Abdel-Rahman SM, Alander SW, Blowey DL, Leeder JS, Kauffman RE: Developmental pharmacology--drug disposition, action, and therapy in infants and children. *N Engl J Med* **349**(12):1157–1167, 2003.

Klotz U: Pharmacokinetics and drug metabolism in the elderly. *Drug Metab Rev* **41**(2):67–76, 2009.

Knibbe CA, Brill MJ, van Rongen A, Diepstraten J, van der Graaf PH, Danhof M: Drug disposition in obesity: Toward evidence-based dosing. *Annu Rev Pharmacol Toxicol* **55**:149–167, 2015.

Knibbe CA, Krekels EH, Danhof M: Advances in paediatric pharmacokinetics. *Expert Opin Drug Metab Toxicol* **7**(1):1–8, 2011.

Korinthenberg R, Haug C, Hannak D: The metabolization of carbamazepine to CBZ-10,11-epoxide in children from the newborn age to adolescence. *Neuropediatrics* **25**(4):214–216, 1994.

Landmann R, Bittiger H, Buhler FR: High affinity beta-2-adrenergic receptors in mononuclear leucocytes: Similar density in young and old normal subjects. *Life Sci* **29**(17):1761–1771, 1981.

Leeder JS, Kearns, GL: Pharmacogenetics in pediatrics. Implications for practice. *Pediatr Clin North Am* **44**(1):55–77, 1997.

Leipzig RM, Cumming RG, Tinetti ME: Drugs and falls in older people: A systematic review and meta-analysis: II. Cardiac and analgesic drugs. *J Am Geriatr Soc* **47**(1):40–50, 1999.

Leong R, Vieira ML, Zhao P, et al: Regulatory experience with physiologically based pharmacokinetic modeling for pediatric drug trials. *Clin Pharmacol Ther* **91**(5):926–931, 2012.

Levey AS, Coresh J, Greene T, et al: Using standardized serum creatinine values in the modification of diet in renal disease study equation for estimating glomerular filtration rate. *Ann Intern Med* **145**(4):247–254, 2006.

Ljungberg B, Nilsson-Ehle I: Pharmacokinetics of antimicrobial agents in the elderly. *Rev Infect Dis* **9**(2):250–264, 1987.

Longo C, Bartlett G, Macgibbon B, Mayo N, Rosenberg E, Nadeau L, Daskalopoulou SS: The effect of obesity on antibiotic treatment failure: A historical cohort study. *Pharmacoepidemiol Drug Saf* **22**(9):970–976, 2013.

Loughnan PM, Greenwald A, Purton WW, Aranda JV, Watters G, Neims AH: Pharmacokinetic observations of phenytoin disposition in the newborn and young infant. *Arch Dis Child* **52**(4):302–309, 1977.

Lu H, Rosenbaum S: Developmental pharmacokinetics in pediatric populations. *J Pediatr Pharmacol Ther* **19**(4):262–276, 2014.

Machado M, Marques-Vidal P, Cortez-Pinto H: Hepatic histology in obese patients undergoing bariatric surgery. *J Hepatol* **45**(4):600–606, 2006.

Mallet L, Spinewine A, Huang A: The challenge of managing drug interactions in elderly people. *Lancet* **370**(9582):185–191, 2007.

Mangoni AA: The impact of advancing age on P-glycoprotein expression and activity: Current knowledge and future directions. *Expert Opin Drug Metab Toxicol* **3**(3):315–320, 2007.

Mangoni AA, Jansen PA, Jackson SH: Under-representation of older adults in pharmacokinetic and pharmacodynamic studies: A solvable problem? *Expert Rev Clin Pharmacol* **6**(1): 35–39, 2013.

Matsuura T, Oda Y, Tanaka K, Mori T, Nishikawa K, Asada A: Advance of age decreases the minimum alveolar concentrations of isoflurane and sevoflurane for maintaining bispectral index below 50. *Br J Anaesth* **102**(3):331–335, 2009.

May DG: Genetic differences in drug disposition. *J Clin Pharmacol* **34**(9):881–897, 1994.

McLean AJ, Le Couteur DG: Aging biology and geriatric clinical pharmacology. *Pharmacol Rev* **56**(2):163–184, 2004.

Meltzer CC: Neuropharmacology and receptor studies in the elderly. *J Geriatr Psychiatry Neurol* **12**(3):137–149, 1999.

Miao L, Yang J, Huang C, Shen Z: Contribution of age, body weight, and CYP2C9 and VKORC1 genotype to the anticoagulant response to warfarin: Proposal for a new dosing regimen in Chinese patients. *Eur J Clin Pharmacol* **63**(12):1135–1141, 2007.

Miller JH, Mc DR, Shock NW: Age changes in the maximal rate of renal tubular reabsorption of glucose. *J Gerontol* **7**(2): 196–200, 1952.

Morley JE, Argiles JM, Evans WJ, et al: Nutritional recommendations for the management of sarcopenia. *J Am Med Dir Assoc* **11**(6):391–396, 2010.

Mosteller RD: Simplified calculation of body-surface area. *N Engl J Med* **317**(17):1098, 1987.

Murphy JE e. *Clinical Pharmacokinetics.* American Society of Health-System Pharmacists. Bethesda, MD, 2017.

Murry DJ, Crom WR, Reddick WE, Bhargava R, Evans WE: Liver volume as a determinant of drug clearance in children and adolescents. *Drug Metab Dispos* **23**(10):1110–1116, 1995.

Nguyen L, Leger F, Lennon S, Puozzo C: Intravenous busulfan in adults prior to haematopoietic stem cell transplantation: A population pharmacokinetic study. *Cancer Chemother Pharmacol* **57**(2):191–198, 2006.

Nyman HA, Dowling TC, Hudson JQ, Peter WL, Joy MS Nolin TD: Comparative evaluation of the Cockcroft-Gault Equation and the Modification of Diet in Renal Disease (MDRD) study equation for drug dosing: An opinion of the Nephrology Practice and Research Network of the American College of Clinical Pharmacy. *Pharmacotherapy* **31**(11):1130–1144, 2011.

Padwal RS, Gabr RQ, Sharma AM, et al: Effect of gastric bypass surgery on the absorption and bioavailability of metformin. *Diabetes Care* **34**(6):1295–1300, 2011.

Pai MP: Estimating the glomerular filtration rate in obese adult patients for drug dosing. *Adv Chronic Kidney Dis* **17**(5): e53–62, 2010.

Pai MP, Bearden DT: Antimicrobial dosing considerations in obese adult patients. *Pharmacotherapy* **27**(8):1081–1091, 2007.

Pai MP, Nafziger AN, Bertino JS Jr: Simplified estimation of aminoglycoside pharmacokinetics in underweight and obese adult patients. *Antimicrob Agents Chemother* **55**(9): 4006–4011, 2011.

Pai MP, Paloucek FP: The origin of the "ideal" body weight equations. *Ann Pharmacother* **34**(9):1066–1069, 2000.

Pan Y, Nicolazzo JA: Impact of aging, Alzheimer's disease and Parkinson's disease on the blood-brain barrier transport of therapeutics. *Adv Drug Deliv Rev* **135**:62–74, 2018.

Parkinson A, Mudra DR, Johnson C, Dwyer A, Carroll KM: The effects of gender, age, ethnicity, and liver cirrhosis on cytochrome P450 enzyme activity in human liver microsomes and inducibility in cultured human hepatocytes. *Toxicol Appl Pharmacol* **199**(3):193–209, 2004.

Perrone RD, Madias NE, Levey AS: Serum creatinine as an index of renal function: New insights into old concepts. *Clin Chem* **38**(10):1933–1953, 1992.

Reiss RA, Haas CE, Karki SD, Gumbiner B, Welle SL, Carson SW: Lithium pharmacokinetics in the obese. *Clin Pharmacol Ther* **55**(4):392–398, 1994.

Ryan T: The ageing of the blood supply and the lymphatic drainage of the skin. *Micron* **35**(3):161–171, 2004.

Sandilands EA, Dhaun N, Dear JW, Webb DJ: Measurement of renal function in patients with chronic kidney disease. *Br J Clin Pharmacol* **76**(4):504–515, 2013.

Scarpace P J, Tumer N, Mader SL: Beta-adrenergic function in aging. Basic mechanisms and clinical implications. *Drugs Aging* **1**(2):116–129, 1991.

Schwartz GJ, Brion LP, Spitzer A: The use of plasma creatinine concentration for estimating glomerular filtration rate in infants, children, and adolescents. *Pediatr Clin North Am* **34**(3):571–590, 1987.

Schwartz JB: The current state of knowledge on age, sex, and their interactions on clinical pharmacology. *Clin Pharmacol Ther* **82**(1):87–96, 2007.

Schwartz JB, Verotta D: Population analyses of atorvastatin clearance in patients living in the community and in nursing homes. *Clin Pharmacol Ther* **86**(5):497–502, 2009.

Scott PJ, Meredith PA, Kelman AW, Hughes DM, Reid JL: The effects of age on the pharmacokinetics and pharmacodynamics of cardiovascular drugs: Application of concentration-effect modeling. 2. Acebutolol. *Am J Ther* **2**(8):537–540, 1995.

Semchuk W, Shevchuk YM, Sankaran K, Wallace SM: Prospective, randomized, controlled evaluation of a gentamicin loading dose in neonates. *Biol Neonate* **67**(1):13–20, 1995.

Shevchuk YM, Taylor DM: Aminoglycoside volume of distribution in pediatric patients. *DICP* **24**(3):273–276, 1990.

Shi S, Klotz U: Age-related changes in pharmacokinetics. *Curr Drug Metab* **12**(7):601–610, 2011.

Shukla UA, Chi EM, Lehr KH: Glimepiride pharmacokinetics in obese versus non-obese diabetic patients. *Ann Pharmacother* **38**(1):30–35, 2004.

Siekmeier R, Scheuch G: Inhaled insulin--does it become reality? J Physiol Pharmacol **59 Suppl 6**:81–113, 2008.

Sitar DS: Clinical pharmacology confounders in older adults. *Expert Rev Clin Pharmacol* **5**(4):397–402, 2012.

Skottheim IB, Stormark K, Christensen H, et al: Significantly altered systemic exposure to atorvastatin acid following gastric bypass surgery in morbidly obese patients. *Clin Pharmacol Ther* **86**(3):311–318, 2009.

Smit C, De Hoogd S, Bruggemann RJM, Knibbe CAJ: Obesity and drug pharmacology: A review of the influence of obesity on pharmacokinetic and pharmacodynamic parameters. *Expert Opin Drug Metab Toxicol* **14**(3):275–285, 2018.

Sparreboom A, Wolff AC, Mathijssen RH, et al: Evaluation of alternate size descriptors for dose calculation of anticancer drugs in the obese. *J Clin Oncol* **25**(30):4707–4713, 2007.

Sproule BA, Hardy BG, Shulman KI: Differential pharmacokinetics of lithium in elderly patients. *Drugs Aging* **16**(3):165–177, 2000.

Spruill WJ, Wade WE, Cobb HH 3rd: Continuing the use of the Cockcroft-Gault equation for drug dosing in patients with impaired renal function. *Clin Pharmacol Ther* **86**(5):468–470, 2009.

Stevens LA, Levey AS: Use of the MDRD study equation to estimate kidney function for drug dosing. *Clin Pharmacol Ther* **86**(5):465–467, 2009.

Sundman I, Allard P, Eriksson A, Marcusson J: GABA uptake sites in frontal cortex from suicide victims and in aging. *Neuropsychobiology* **35**(1):11–15, 1997.

Swedko PJ, Clark HD, Paramsothy K, Akbari A: Serum creatinine is an inadequate screening test for renal failure in elderly patients. *Arch Intern Med* **163**(3):356–360, 2003.

Swift CG, Ewen JM, Clarke P, Stevenson IH: Responsiveness to oral diazepam in the elderly: Relationship to total and free plasma concentrations. *Br J Clin Pharmacol* **20**(2):111–118, 1985.

Traynor J, Mactier R, Geddes CC, Fox JG: How to measure renal function in clinical practice. *BMJ* **333**(7571):733–737, 2006.

Trifiro G, Spina E: Age-related changes in pharmacodynamics: Focus on drugs acting on central nervous and cardiovascular systems. *Curr Drug Metab* **12**(7):611–620, 2011.

Tune L, Carr S, Hoag E, Cooper T: Anticholinergic effects of drugs commonly prescribed for the elderly: Potential means for assessing risk of delirium. *Am J Psychiatry* **149**(10):1393–1394, 1992.

U.S. Census Bureau: Older People Projected to Outnumber Children for First Time in U.S. History. U. S. C. Bureau. 2018. https://www.census.gov/newsroom/press-releases/2018/cb18-41-population-projections.html.

van den Anker J, Reed MD, Allegaert K, Kearns GL: Developmental changes in pharmacokinetics and pharmacodynamics. *J Clin Pharmacol* **58**(Suppl 10):S10–S25, 2018.

van den Anker JN: Developmental pharmacology. *Dev Disabil Res Rev* **16**(3):233–238, 2010.

van den Anker JN, Schoemaker RC, Hop WC, et al: Ceftazidime pharmacokinetics in preterm infants: Effects of renal function and gestational age. *Clin Pharmacol Ther* **58**(6):650–659, 1995.

Vassal G, Michel G, Esperou H, et al: Prospective validation of a novel IV busulfan fixed dosing for paediatric patients to improve therapeutic AUC targeting without drug monitoring. *Cancer Chemother Pharmacol* **61**(1):113–123, 2008.

Vestal RE: Aging and pharmacology. *Cancer* **80**(7):1302–1310, 1997.

Vestal RE, Wood AJ, Shand DG: Reduced beta-adrenoceptor sensitivity in the elderly. *Clin Pharmacol Ther* **26**(2):181–186, 1979.

Vieweg WV, Wood MA, Fernandez A, Beatty-Brooks M, Hasnain M, Pandurangi AK: Proarrhythmic risk with antipsychotic and antidepressant drugs: Implications in the elderly. *Drugs Aging* **26**(12):997–1012, 2009.

Wang C, Allegaert K, Peeters MY, Tibboel D, Danhof M, Knibbe CA: The allometric exponent for scaling clearance varies with age: A study on seven propofol datasets ranging from preterm neonates to adults. *Br J Clin Pharmacol* **77**(1):149–159, 2014.

Wellen KE, Hotamisligil GS: Obesity-induced inflammatory changes in adipose tissue. *J Clin Invest* **112**(12):1785–1788, 2003.

White M, Roden R, Minobe W, et al: Age-related changes in beta-adrenergic neuroeffector systems in the human heart. *Circulation* **90**(3):1225–1238, 1994.

Wilhelm SM, Kale-Pradhan PB: Estimating creatinine clearance: A meta-analysis. *Pharmacotherapy* **31**(7):658–664, 2011.

Williams K, Thomson D, Seto I, et al: Standard 6: Age groups for pediatric trials. *Pediatrics* **129**(Suppl 3):S153–S160, 2012.

Winter MA, Guhr KN, Berg GM: Impact of various body weights and serum creatinine concentrations on the bias and accuracy of the Cockcroft-Gault equation. *Pharmacotherapy* **32**(7):604–612, 2012.

World Health Organization: *Obesity: Preventing and Managing the Global Epidemic.* Geneva, CH, 2000.

World Health Organization: Obesity and overweight fact sheet. 2019. Retrieved September 30, 2019, from https://www.who.int/news-room/fact-sheets/detail/obesity-and-overweight.

Yanni SB, Smith PB, Benjamin DK Jr, Augustijns PF, Thakker DR, Annaert PP: Higher clearance of micafungin in neonates compared with adults: Role of age-dependent micafungin serum binding. *Biopharm Drug Dispos* **32**(4):222–232, 2011.

Yee JY, Duffull SB: The effect of body weight on dalteparin pharmacokinetics. A preliminary study. *Eur J Clin Pharmacol* **56**(4):293–297, 2000.

# 25 Dose Adjustment in Renal and Hepatic Diseases

Yuen Yi Hon* and Murray P. Ducharme

## CHAPTER OBJECTIVES

- List the common causes of chronic kidney disease (CKD) and describe how CKD affects drug elimination.

- Compare the advantages and disadvantages of the use of drugs or endogenous substances as markers for the measurement of renal function.

- Describe the relationships between creatinine clearance, serum creatinine concentration, and glomerular filtration rate (GFR).

- Explain and contrast the methods of Cockcroft–Gault and Modification of Diet in Renal Disease (MDRD) for the calculation of creatinine clearance and for adjusting dosing regimens with a patient's estimated renal function.

- List the causes for fluctuating serum creatinine concentrations in the body.

- Calculate the dose for a drug in a patient with renal disease.

- Describe quantitatively using equations how renal or hepatic disease can alter the disposition of a drug.

- Describe hemoperfusion and the limitations of its use.

- Distinguish between hemodialysis and peritoneal dialysis and calculate dose adjustments of a drug in patients undergoing dialysis.

- Describe the principle of the fraction of drug excreted unchanged ($f_e$) method and how it is applied to adjust doses in renal disease.

- Describe the effects of hepatic disease on the pharmacokinetics of a drug.

- List the reasons why dose adjustment in patients with hepatic impairment is more difficult than dose adjustment in patients with renal disease.

- Explain how liver function tests relate to drug absorption and disposition.

- List the pharmacokinetic properties of a drug for which dose adjustment would not be required in patients with renal or hepatic impairment.

## RENAL IMPAIRMENT

Chronic kidney disease (CKD) is a worldwide public health problem affecting more than 50 million people, and more than 1 million are receiving kidney replacement therapy (Levey et al, 2009). The kidney is an important organ in regulating body fluids, electrolyte balance, removal of metabolic waste, and drug excretion from the body. Impairment or degeneration of kidney function affects the pharmacokinetics of drugs. Some of the more common causes of kidney failure include disease, injury, and drug intoxication. Table 25-1 lists some of the conditions that may lead to chronic or acute renal failure. Acute diseases or trauma to the kidney can cause *uremia*, in which glomerular filtration is impaired or reduced, leading to accumulation of excessive fluid and blood nitrogenous products in the body. Uremia generally reduces

---

*Disclaimer: The contents of this article reflect the views of the author and should not be construed to represent the US Food and Drug Administration (FDA)'s views or policies. No official support or endorsement by the FDA is intended or should be inferred.

**TABLE 25-1 •** Common Causes of Kidney Failure

| | |
|---|---|
| Pyelonephritis | Inflammation and deterioration of the pyelonephrons due to infection, antigens, or other idiopathic causes. |
| Hypertension | Chronic overloading of the kidney with fluid and electrolytes may lead to kidney insufficiency. |
| Diabetes mellitus | The disturbance of sugar metabolism and acid–base balance may lead to or predispose a patient to degenerative renal disease. |
| Nephrotoxic drugs/metals | Certain drugs taken chronically may cause irreversible kidney damage—eg, the aminoglycosides, phenacetin, and heavy metals, such as mercury and lead. |
| Hypovolemia | Any condition that causes a reduction in renal blood flow will eventually lead to renal ischemia and damage. |
| Neophroallergens | Certain compounds may produce an immune type of sensitivity reaction with nephritic syndrome—eg, quartan malaria nephrotoxic serum. |

glomerular filtration and/or active secretion, which leads to a decrease in renal drug excretion resulting in a longer elimination half-life of the administered drug.

In addition to changing renal elimination directly, uremia can affect drug pharmacokinetics in unexpected ways. For example, declining renal function leads to disturbances in electrolyte and fluid balance, resulting in physiologic and metabolic changes that may alter the pharmacokinetics and pharmacodynamics of a drug. Pharmacokinetic processes such as drug distribution (including both the volume of distribution and protein binding) and elimination (including both biotransformation and renal excretion) may also be altered by renal impairment. Both therapeutic and toxic responses may be altered as a result of changes in drug sensitivity at the receptor site. Overall, uremic patients have special dosing considerations to account for such pharmacokinetic and pharmacodynamic alterations.

## PHARMACOKINETIC CONSIDERATIONS

Patients with renal impairment may exhibit pharmacokinetic changes in bioavailability, volume of distribution, and clearance. The oral bioavailability of a drug in severe uremia may be decreased as a result of disease-related changes in gastrointestinal motility and pH that are caused by nausea, vomiting, and diarrhea. Mesenteric blood flow may also be altered. However, the oral bioavailability of a drug such as propranolol (which has a high first-pass effect) may

be increased in patients with renal impairment as a result of the decrease in first-pass hepatic metabolism (Bianchetti et al, 1978).

The apparent volume of distribution depends largely on drug–protein binding in plasma or tissues and total body water. Renal impairment may alter the distribution of the drug as a result of changes in fluid balance, drug–protein binding, or other factors that may cause changes in the apparent volume of distribution (see Chapter 5). The plasma protein binding of weak acidic drugs in uremic patients is decreased, whereas the protein binding of weak basic drugs is less affected. A decrease in drug–protein binding results in a larger fraction of free drug and an increase in the volume of distribution. However, the net elimination half-life is generally increased as a result of the dominant effect of reduced glomerular filtration. Protein binding of the drug may be further compromised due to the accumulation of metabolites of the drug and various biochemical metabolites, such as free fatty acids and urea, which may compete for the protein-binding sites for the active drug.

Total body clearance of drugs in uremic patients is also reduced by either a decrease in the glomerular filtration rate (GFR) and possibly active tubular secretion or a reduced hepatic clearance resulting from a decrease in intrinsic hepatic clearance.

In clinical practice, estimation of the appropriate drug dosage regimen in patients with impaired renal function is based on an estimate of the remaining renal function of the patient and a prediction of the total body clearance. A complete pharmacokinetic

**TABLE 25-2 •** Common Assumptions in Dosing Renally-Impaired Patients

| Assumption | Comment |
|---|---|
| Creatinine clearance accurately measures the degree of renal impairment | Creatinine clearance estimates may be biased. Renal impairment should also be verified by physical diagnosis and other clinical tests. |
| Drug follows dose-independent pharmacokinetics | Pharmacokinetics should not be dose dependent (nonlinear). |
| Nonrenal drug elimination remains constant | Renal disease may also affect the liver and cause a change in nonrenal drug elimination (drug metabolism). |
| Drug absorption remains constant | Unchanged drug absorption from gastrointestinal tract. |
| Drug clearance, $CL_U$, declines linearly with creatinine clearance, $CL_{CR}$ | Normal drug clearance may include active secretion and passive filtration and may not decline linearly. |
| Unaltered drug–protein binding | Drug–protein binding may be altered due to accumulation of urea, nitrogenous wastes, and drug metabolites. |
| Target drug concentration remains constant | Changes in electrolyte composition such as potassium may affect response to the effect of digoxin. Accumulation of active metabolites may cause more intense pharmacodynamic response compared to parent drug alone. |

analysis of the drug in the uremic patient may not be possible. Moreover, the patient's uremic condition may not be stable and may be changing too rapidly for pharmacokinetic analysis. Each of the approaches for the calculation of a dosage regimen has certain assumptions and limitations that must be carefully assessed by the clinician before any approach is taken. Dosing guidelines for individual drugs in patients with renal impairment may be found in various reference books, such as the *Physicians' Desk Reference*, and in the medical literature (Bennett 1988, 1990; St. Peter et al, 1992). Most newly approved drugs now contain dosing instructions for CKD patients.

## GENERAL APPROACHES FOR DOSE ADJUSTMENT IN RENAL DISEASE

Several approaches are available for estimating the appropriate dosage regimen for a patient with renal impairment. Each of these approaches has similar assumptions, as listed in Table 25-2. Most of these methods assume that the required therapeutic plasma drug concentration in patients with renal impairment is similar to that required in patients with normal renal function. Patients with renal impairment are maintained on the same $C_{av}^{\infty}$ after multiple oral doses or multiple IV bolus injections. For IV infusions, the same $C_{ss}$ is maintained. ($C_{ss}$ is the same as $C_{av}^{\infty}$ after the plasma drug concentration reaches steady state.)

The design of dosage regimens for uremic patients is based on the pharmacokinetic changes that have occurred as a result of the uremic condition. Generally, drugs in patients with uremia or kidney impairment have prolonged elimination half-lives and a change in the apparent volume of distribution. In less severe uremic conditions, there may be neither edema nor a significant change in the apparent volume of distribution. Consequently, the methods for dose adjustment in uremic patients are based on an accurate estimation of the drug clearance in these patients.

Several specific clinical approaches for the calculation of drug clearance based on monitoring kidney function are presented later in this chapter.

### Dose Adjustment Based on Drug Clearance and Elimination Rate Constants

Methods based on drug clearance try to maintain the desired mean concentration at steady state ($C_{av(ss)}$) after multiple oral doses or multiple IV bolus injections as total body clearance, $CL$ changes. As seen in previous chapters, $C_{av(ss)}$ is obtained by dividing the dosing rate by the $CL$. With oral administration, the equation is therefore:

$$C_{av(ss)} = (Do/\tau)/(CL/F) \text{ or } F \cdot Do/(CL \cdot \tau) \qquad (25.1)$$

As we have seen in Chapter 15, the clearance in a given patient can be calculated via different approaches, namely via the noncompartmental method when a lot of concentrations are taken after a dose, or via fitting using a compartmental model especially when less samples are available. It can also be "estimated" using a nomogram that is based on the renal function of the patient with renal impairment. These nomograms are proposed after a population pharmacokinetic analysis has been conducted and the clearance of a drug is related to clinical covariates such as the creatinine clearance ($CL_{CR}$), weight, and/or age, to name a few. More details on this will follow in this chapter.

The renal clearance and the renal elimination rate constants are decreased in a patient with renal impairment. The largest the overall contribution of the renal clearance or renal elimination rate constant to the overall clearance and elimination rate constant, and the greater the decrease in renal function will affect the dose to administer in order to reach the same exposure, as we have seen in Chapter 15.

Renal impairment does not typically affect protein binding and therefore the volume of distribution of drugs until it becomes very severe. Consequently, the calculated elimination rate constant can be used in a given patient to calculate what is the dose to administer in order to reach a target exposure.

## Practical Example:

The official monograph and product label states that a drug is thought to be 70% eliminated renally but does not provide dosing information in patients with renal impairment. The monograph does state that the oral clearance in a patient with normal renal function is 10 L/h, its elimination half-life is 6 h, and that the recommended dosing regimen to administer is 300 mg per day. What may be the dosing regimen to administer in a patient that has 50% of its renal function (eg, creatinine clearance of 50 mL/min)?

## Solutions:

- The expected AUC at steady state over a dosing interval in a patient with normal renal function can be calculated to be:
  - $CL/F = \text{Dose}/AUC_{inf}$
  - Therefore, $AUC_{\infty}$ or $AUC_{\tau(ss)} = \text{DOSE}/(CL/F)$, $= 300/10 = 30$ mg.h/L
- The expected renal and non-renal clearance and the expected renal and non-renal elimination rate constant in a patient with normal renal function can be calculated to be:
  - $CL_R = 0.7 \cdot CL = 7$ L/h, therefore the $CL_{NR} = 10 - 7 = 3$ L/h
  - $K_R = 0.7 \cdot K = 0.7 \cdot 0.693/6 = 0.08085$ h$^{-1}$
  - Therefore, the $K_{NR} = 0.3 \cdot 0.693/6$ $= 0.03465$ h$^{-1}$
- Our patient has a 50% decrease in renal function, so its renal clearance and its renal elimination rate constant can both be expected to be half of their normal value:
  - $CL_R = 0.5 \cdot 7 = 3.5$ L/h
  - $K_R = 0.5 \cdot 0.08085 = 0.040425$ h$^{-1}$
- Because the nonrenal component of both the clearance and elimination rate constant are unchanged, the overall clearance and elimination half-life can be estimated to be:
  - $CL = CL_R + CL_{NR} = 3.5 + 3 = 6.5$ L/h instead of the normal value of 10 L/h
  - $K = K_R + K_{NR} = 0.040425 + 0.03465$ $= 0.075$ h$^{-1}$
  - $t_{1/2} = 0.693/0.075 = 9.24$ h instead of the normal value of 6 h
- The dose to administer in our patient in order to reach the same target $AUC_{\tau(ss)}$ of 30 $\mu$g·h/L (0.03 mg·h/L) is therefore:
  - Dose $= CL/F \times AUC_{\tau(ss)} = 30 \times 6.5 = 195$ or ~200 mg PO per day
- $C_{max}$ at steady state will be slightly decreased (because the volume of distribution should not be affected by the change in renal function), and with an elimination half-life 50% longer we can also anticipate that the $C_{min(ss)}$ will be slightly increased.

**FREQUENTLY ASKED QUESTIONS**

▶ How does renal impairment affect the pharmacokinetics of a drug that is primarily eliminated by hepatic clearance?

▶ What are the main factors that influence drug dosing in renal disease?

## MEASUREMENT OF THE KIDNEY'S GLOMERULAR FILTRATION RATE

The GFR is important clinically to estimate for two main reasons. First, it will provide an estimation of the patient's filtration capability of the kidney for its treating physician. To this end, it is important for the estimation to be as accurate and precise as possible, and not be influenced, for example, by secretion or reabsorption. The second reason for which we estimate the GFR has more to do with estimating the overall renal function than the GFR per se, because it is to adjust drug dosing regimens based on the overall renal function, not just the GFR, because drugs are often reabsorbed and secreted in addition to being filtered. In this circumstance, drug dosing regimens are adjusted because of the correlation that exists between the renal clearance and the estimate of the renal function, for example, the calculated creatinine clearance using the Cockcroft–Gault method. The renal drug clearance will be correlated with the GFR estimate. Here it is no so important to have an accurate and precise estimation of the true GFR. It is better instead to have an estimate of the overall renal function so that a better correlation exist with the drug's renal clearance. These two reasons for using creatinine clearances are therefore fundamentally different. In this chapter, we will focus on the second reason, because what is important is a predictor of the overall renal function to estimate a drug's overall renal clearance, and not to estimate the GFR more precisely.

Several drugs and endogenous substances have been used as markers to measure the GFR in a given patient. These markers are carried to the kidney by the blood via the renal artery and are filtered at the glomerulus. Several criteria are necessary to use a drug as a marker to measure the GFR:

1. The drug must be freely filtered at the glomerulus.
2. The drug must neither be reabsorbed nor actively secreted by the renal tubules.

3. The drug should not be metabolized.
4. The drug should not bind significantly to plasma proteins.
5. The drug should neither have an effect on the filtration rate nor alter renal function.
6. The drug should be nontoxic.
7. The drug may be infused in a sufficient dose to permit simple and accurate quantitation in plasma and in urine.

Therefore, the rate at which these drug markers are filtered from the blood into the urine per unit of time reflects the GFR of the kidney. Changes in GFR reflect changes in kidney function that may be diminished in uremic conditions.

*Inulin*, a fructose polysaccharide, fulfills most of the criteria listed above and is therefore used as a standard reference for the measurement of GFR. In practice, however, the use of inulin involves a time-consuming procedure in which inulin is given by intravenous infusion until a constant steady-state plasma level is obtained. Clearance of inulin may then be measured by the rate of infusion divided by the steady-state plasma inulin concentration. Although this procedure gives an accurate value for GFR, inulin clearance is not used frequently in clinical practice.

The clearance of creatinine is used most extensively as a measurement of GFR. *Creatinine* is an endogenous substance formed from creatine phosphate during muscle metabolism. Creatinine production varies with age, weight, and gender of the individual. In humans, creatinine is filtered mainly at the glomerulus, with no tubular reabsorption. However, a small amount of creatinine may be actively secreted by the renal tubules, and the values of GFR obtained by the creatinine clearance tend to be higher than GFR measured by inulin clearance. Because of that, using creatinine clearance as an overall measure of renal function, and not just GFR, may be better for predicting a patient's drug's clearance in renal impairment conditions. Creatinine clearance tends to decrease in the elderly patient. As mentioned in Chapter 24, the physiologic changes due to aging may necessitate special considerations in administering drugs to the elderly.

Measurement of *blood urea nitrogen* (BUN) is a commonly used clinical diagnostic laboratory test for renal disease. Urea is the end product of protein catabolism and is excreted through the kidney. Normal

BUN levels range from 10 to 20 mg/dL. Higher BUN levels generally indicate the presence of renal disease. However, other factors, such as excessive protein intake, reduced renal blood flow, hemorrhagic shock, or gastric bleeding, may affect increased BUN levels. The renal clearance of urea is by glomerular filtration and partial reabsorption in the renal tubules. Therefore, the renal clearance of urea is less than creatinine or inulin clearance and does not give a quantitative measure of kidney function.

## SERUM CREATININE CONCENTRATION AND CREATININE CLEARANCE

Under normal circumstances, creatinine production is roughly equal to creatinine excretion, so the serum creatinine level remains constant. In a patient with reduced glomerular filtration, serum creatinine will accumulate in accordance with the degree of loss of glomerular filtration in the kidney. The serum creatinine concentration alone is frequently used to determine creatinine clearance, $CL_{CR}$. Creatinine clearance from the serum creatinine concentration is a rapid and convenient way to monitor kidney function.

*Creatinine clearance* may be defined as the volume of plasma cleared of creatinine per unit time. Creatinine clearance can be calculated directly in a given patient by dividing the rate of urinary excretion of creatinine by the patient's serum creatinine concentration. The approach is similar to that used in the determination of drug clearance. In practice, the serum creatinine concentration is determined at the midpoint of the urinary collection period and the rate of urinary excretion of creatinine is measured for the entire day (24 hours) to obtain a reliable excretion rate. This is called the "midpoint" clearance method and has been presented in Chapter 15:

$$CL_{CR} = \text{Rate of urinary excretion of creatinine}/S_{creat} \text{ at midpoint} \quad (25.2)$$

$$CL = (Cu \cdot Vu)/(S_{creat} \cdot 1440)$$

where $S_{creat}$ is the serum creatinine concentration (mg/dL) taken at the 12th hour or at the midpoint of the urine collection period, $Vu$ is the volume of urine excreted (mL) in 24 hours, and $C_u$ is the

concentration of creatinine in urine (mg/mL). The units for $CL_{CR}$ are in mL/min.

Creatinine is eliminated primarily by glomerular filtration. A small fraction of creatinine also is eliminated by active secretion and some nonrenal elimination. Therefore, $CL_{CR}$ values obtained from creatinine measurements overestimate the actual GFR.

Creatinine clearance has been normalized both to body surface area, using 1.73 m² as the average, and to body weight for a 70-kg adult male. Creatinine distributes into total body water.

Creatinine clearance values must be considered carefully in special populations such as elderly, obese, and emaciated patients. In elderly and emaciated patients, muscle mass may have declined, thus lowering the production of creatinine. However, serum creatinine concentration values may appear to be in the normal range because of lower renal creatinine excretion. Thus, the calculation of creatinine clearance from serum creatinine may give an inaccurate estimation of the renal function. For obese patients, generally defined as patients more than 20% over *ideal body weight* (IBW), estimation of creatinine clearance based on *total body weight* (TBW) may exaggerate the $CL_{CR}$ values. Women with normal kidney function have smaller creatinine clearance values than men, which are approximately 80%–85% of those in men with normal kidney function.

Several empirical equations have been used to estimate lean body weight (LBW) based on the patient's height and actual (total) body weight (see Chapter 24). The following equations have been used to estimate LBW in renally impaired patients in order to propose adjustments in aminoglycosides dosing (Devine, 1974):

LBW (males) = 50 kg

+ 2.3 kg for each inch over 5 ft

LBW (females) = 45.5 kg

+ 2.3 kg for each inch over 5 ft

$$(25.3)$$

For the purpose of dose adjustment in renal patients, normal creatinine clearance is generally assumed to be between 100 and 125 mL/min for a healthy adult subject of typical body weight (72 kg):

$CL_{CR} = 108.8 \pm 13.5$ mL/min for an adult female and $CL_{CR} = 124.5 \pm 9.7$ mL/min for an adult male (Diem and Lentner, 1973). Creatinine clearance is affected by diet and salt intake. As a convenient approximation and to simplify calculations, the normal creatinine clearance is often assumed by clinicians to be approximately 100 mL/min.

---

**FREQUENTLY ASKED QUESTIONS**

▶ Why is creatinine clearance used in renal disease?

▶ What patient-specific factors influence the accuracy of $CL_{CR}$ estimates?

▶ How is $CL_{CR}$ determined?

---

### Calculation of Creatinine Clearance from Serum Creatinine Concentration

The problems of obtaining a complete 24-hour urine collection from a patient, the time necessary for urine collection, and the analysis time preclude a direct estimation of creatinine clearance. This is not that clinically relevant, regardless, as the calculated creatinine clearance is not a good estimation of the GFR for reasons mentioned previously, and for adjusting drug dosing regimen the "estimated" creatinine clearance obtained from a nomogram is more appropriate because this is what is used in official product monographs and labels to correlate with drug's clearances and therefore doses. Several nomogram methods have been proposed for the calculation of creatinine clearance from the serum creatinine concentration. The more accurate methods are based on the patient's age, height, weight, and gender. These methods have been developed in patients with intact liver function and no abnormal muscle disease, such as hypertrophy or dystrophy, and most methods also assume a stable creatinine clearance. The typical units for reporting $CL_{CR}$ are mL/min.

### Adults

The proposed nomogram of Cockcroft and Gault (1976) shown in Equation 25.4 is arguably the most used to estimate creatinine clearances from serum creatinine concentrations. This method considers both the age and the weight of the patient. For males:

$$CL_{CR} = (140 - \text{Age (years)} \cdot \text{Actual Body Weight (kg)}/(72 \cdot S_{creat})) \quad (25.4)$$

For females, the use of 85% of the $CL_{CR}$ value obtained in males, and as originally proposed by Cockcroft and Gault has been consistently use with good results (Stevens et al, 2006).

Other methods have been proposed prior to the Cockcroft–Gault equation; namely, the nomogram method of Siersback-Nielsen et al (1971), Kampmann et al (1974) as shown in Fig. 25-1, and the method proposed by Jelliffe RW (1973), but in both clinical and regulatory practice (to relate drug's clearances with estimates of renal function), the Cockcroft–Gault method is by far the one that has been and still is the most used.

### Children

There are a number of methods for calculation of creatinine clearance in children, based on body length

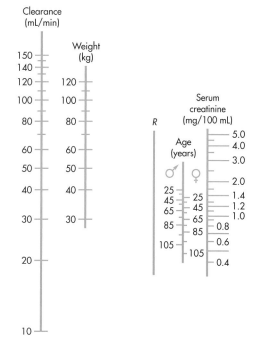

FIGURE 25-1 • Nomogram for evaluation of endogenous creatinine clearance. To use the nomogram, connect the patient's weight on the second line from the left with the patient's age on the fourth line with a ruler. Note the point of intersection on *R* and keep the ruler there. Turn the right part of the ruler to the appropriate serum creatinine value and the left side will indicate the clearance in mL/min. (Reproduced with permission from Siersbaek-Nielsen K, Hansen JM, Kampmann J, et al: Rapid evaluation of creatinine clearance, *Lancet.* 1971 May 29; **1**(7709):1133-1134.)

and serum creatinine concentration. Equation 25.5 is a method developed by Schwartz et al (1976):

$$CL_{CR} = \frac{0.55 \times \text{body length (cm)}}{S_{creat}} \qquad (25.5)$$

where $CL_{CR}$ is given in mL/min/1.73 m$^2$ and $S_{creat}$ is the serum creatinine value in American units (mg/dL). The value 0.55 represents a factor used for children aged 1–12 years.

Another method for calculating creatinine clearance in children uses the nomogram of Traub and Johnson (1980) as shown in Fig. 25-2. This nomogram is based on observations from 81 children aged 6–12 years and requires the patient's height and serum creatinine concentration.

## PRACTICE PROBLEMS

1. What is the creatinine clearance for a 25-year-old male patient with a $S_{creat}$ of 1 mg/dL and a body weight of 80 kg?

**Solution**

- Using the nomogram (see Fig. 25-1), join the points at 25 years (male) and 80 kg with a ruler—let the line intersect line $R$. Connect the intersection point at line $R$ with the creatinine concentration point of 1 mg/dL, and extend the line to intersect the "clearance line." The extended line will intersect the clearance line at 110 mL/min, giving the creatinine clearance for the patient.
- Using the Cockcroft–Gault (C&G) equation, the $CL_{CR}$ is $(140 - 25) \cdot (80/(72 \cdot 1))$ which is 128 mL/min.

2. What is the creatinine clearance for a 25-year-old male patient with a $S_{creat}$ of 1 mg/dL? The patient is 5 ft, 4 in. in height and weighs 103 kg. Use ideal body weight in the calculation.

**Solution**

$$\text{LBW (males)} = 50 \text{ kg} + (2.3 \cdot 4) = 59.2 \text{ kg}$$

Using the C&G method (Equation 25.4), the $CL_{CR}$ can be calculated.

$$CL_{CR} = \frac{(140 - 25) \cdot (59.2 \text{ kg})}{72(1)} = 94.6 \text{ mL/min}$$

The serum creatinine methods for the estimation of the creatinine clearance assume stabilized kidney function and a steady-state serum creatinine concentration. In acute renal failure and in other situations in which kidney function is changing, the serum creatinine may not represent steady-state conditions. If $C_{CR}$ is measured daily and the $C_{CR}$ value is constant, then the serum creatinine concentration is probably at steady state. If the $C_{CR}$ values are changing daily, then kidney function is changing.

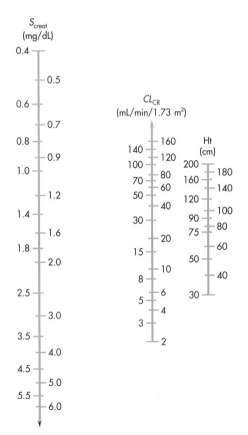

FIGURE 25-2 • Nomogram for rapid evaluation of endogenous creatinine clearance ($CL_{CR}$) in pediatric patients (aged 6–12 years). To predict $CL_{CR}$, connect the child's $S_{creat}$ (serum creatinine) and HT (height) with a ruler and read the $CL_{CR}$ where the ruler intersects the center line. (Reproduced with permission from Traub SL, Johnson CE. Comparison of methods of estimating creatinine clearance in children, Am J Hosp Pharm. 1980 Feb; 37(2):195–201.)

**TABLE 25-3 •** Classification of Renal Function Based on Estimated GFR (eGFR) or Estimated Creatinine Clearance ($CL_{CR}$)

| Stage | Description[†] | eGFR[‡] (mL/min/1.73m²) | $CL_{CR}$[*][§] (mL/min) |
|-------|------------|------------------------|------------------------|
| 1 | Normal GFR | ≥90 | ≥90 |
| 2 | Mild decrease in GFR | 60–89 | 60–89 |
| 3 | Moderate decrease in GFR | 30–59 | 30–59 |
| 4 | Severe decrease in GFR | 15–29 | 15–29 |
| 5 | End-stage renal disease | <15 Not on dialysis | <15 Not on dialysis |
|   |   | Requiring dialysis | Requiring dialysis |

[*]*In some situations, collection of 24-hour urine samples for measurement of creatinine clearance, or measurement of clearance of an exogenous filtration marker, may provide better estimates of GFR than the prediction equations. The situations include determination of GFR for patients in the following scenarios: undergoing kidney replacement therapy; acute renal failure; extremes of age, body size, or muscle mass; conditions of severe malnutrition or obesity; disease of skeletal muscle; or on a vegetarian diet.*

[†]*Stages of renal impairment are based on K/DOQI Clinical Practice Guidelines for chronic kidney disease (CKD) from the National Kidney Foundation in 2002; GFR: glomerular filtration rate.*

[‡]*eGFR: estimate of GFR based on an MDRD equation.*

[§]*$CL_{CR}$: estimated creatinine clearance based on the Cockcroft–Gault equation.*

Although the C&G method for estimating $CL_{CR}$ has some biases, this method has gained general acceptance for the determination of renal impairment (Spinler et al, 1998;  Hailmeskel et al, 1999; Schneider et al, 2003) and is routinely used in the renal impairment studies that are conducted before any new drug product is approved for marketing. A suggested representation of patients with various degrees of renal impairment based on creatinine clearance is shown in Table 25-3 and can also be found in the FDA draft guidance on pharmacokinetics in patients with impaired renal function (FDA Guidance for Industry, 2010).

The practice problems show that, depending on the formula used, the calculated $CL_{CR}$ can vary considerably. Consequently, unless a clinically significant change in the creatinine clearance occurs, dosage adjustment may not be needed. According to St. Peter et al (1992), dose adjustment of many antibiotics is necessary only when the GFR, as measured by $CL_{CR}$, is less than 50 mL/min. But in contrast, for drugs with narrow therapeutic range such as the aminoglycosides and vancomycin, dose adjustment is individualized according to each patient's own $CL_{CR}$. The need to adjust dosing regimens based on renal function will therefore depend on the following combination of factors: the percentage of the overall clearance that is renally based, and the relationship between concentrations and efficacy as well as the relationship between concentrations and side effects (eg, whether the drug has a "narrow" or "wide" therapeutic range).

### Estimated Glomerular Filtration Rate using Modification of Diet in Renal Disease Formula or using the Chronic Kidney Disease–Epidemiology Collaboration Equations

We have seen that various approaches for the estimation of GFR from serum creatinine have been published (Levey et al, 1999, 2009; FDA Guidance for Industry, 2010). The Modification of Diet in Renal Disease (MDRD) equation is a simple and effective method that is more and more utilized, and is considered to be a better estimator of the GFR than the C&G creatinine clearance equation. An example of the MDRD equation is presented below (future modifications are possible),

$$\text{eGFR (mL/min/1.73 m}^2) = 175 \cdot (C_{CR})^{-1.154}$$
$$\times \text{(age)}^{-0.203} \cdot (0.742 \text{ if female})$$
$$\times (1.212 \text{ if African American}) \qquad (25.6)$$

where estimated glomerular filtration rate (eGFR) is the abbreviation for the estimated GFR using that equation.

The MDRD equation does not require weight or height measurements and the results are normalized to 1.73 m² body surface area, which is an accepted average adult surface area.

The Chronic Kidney Disease–Epidemiology Collaboration (CKD-EPI) reviewed various approaches for GFR measurements based on serum creatinine concentration and other factors (Levey et al, 2009). Based on the same four variables as the MDRD equation, the CKD-EPI equation uses a two-slope "spline" to model the relationship between estimated GFR and serum creatinine, and a different relationship for age, sex, and race. In the validation data set, the CKD-EPI equation performed better than the MDRD equation, with less bias (median difference between measured and estimated GFR of 2.5 versus 5.5 mL/min/1.73 m²) especially at higher GFR ($p < .001$ for all subsequent comparisons). The CKD-EPI equation was reported as being more accurate than the MDRD equation for estimating GFR (Levey et al, 2009). No comparison between the CKD-EPI and the C&G methods was made in that research.

While the MDRD and CKD-EPI equations are considered to be more accurate than the C&G method to predict GFR, they give an estimate that is normalized to a body surface area of 1.73 m², which is not directly useful when adjusting dosing regimens based on renal function. Doses of drugs are not normalized to 1.73 m², so the correct dose to administer to a patient for a given target AUC can only be calculated with the specific clearance of that patient, not with a normalized clearance for a body surface area of 1.73 m². In this regard, the C&G method for estimating renal function and creating correlations with clearances in patients with diverse degrees of renal function is more directly useful. To this end, and while the MDRD equation is being more considered within drug development, most studies relating drug's clearances with renal function that have been and are submitted to regulatory agencies before approval and marketing have used the Cockcroft–Gault equation. Regardless of the method used however, the official product monograph and label will state directly how to adjust a drug's dosing regimen with a patient's estimated renal function and with which formula (eg, MDRD or C&G).

## Comparison of Methods for the Measurement of GFR

The estimate of GFR based on serum creatinine concentration is widely used, even though serum creatinine concentrations are known to fluctuate with disease state and patient conditions such as age, gender, and endogenous factors that affect creatinine synthesis and elimination (Table 25-4). These estimation methods are referred to as creatinine-based methods in the clinical literature (Stevens et al, 2006; Levey et al, 2009). Two creatinine-based methods that have been extensively studied and widely applied are the Cockcroft–Gault and the MDRD study equations. The Cockcroft–Gault has a longer history of use but the original equation was based on fewer subjects. The MDRD method is a more recent method based on more subjects with application better defined for certain groups of patients. For example, the relationship of serum creatinine

**TABLE 25-4 • Factors Affecting Creatinine Generation**

| Factor | Effect on Serum Creatinine |
|---|---|
| Aging | Decreased |
| Female sex | Decreased |
| Race or ethnic group | |
| Black | Increased |
| Hispanic | Decreased |
| Asian | Decreased |
| Body habitus | |
| Muscular | Increased |
| Amputation | Decreased |
| Obesity | No change |
| Chronic illness | |
| Malnutrition, inflammation, deconditioning (eg, cancer, severe cardiovascular disease, hospitalized patients) | Decreased |
| Neuromuscular diseases | Decreased |
| Diet | |
| Vegetarian diet | Decreased |
| Ingestion of cooked meat | Increased |

Reproduced with permission from Stevens LA, Coresh J, Greene T, et al: Assessing kidney function—measured and estimated glomerular filtration rate, N Engl J Med. 2006 Jun 8;354(23):2473-2483.

concentration and GFR may be different between subjects with diabetic nephropathy and those without real renal disease. Some reports indicated that the MDRD method is less biased for obese and diabetic patients, whereas other studies do not find a difference between the two methods.

The Cockcroft–Gault formula was developed with data from 249 men with measured $CL_{CR}$ ranging from 30 to 130 mL/min. The equation as already presented in (25.4) is

$$CL_{CR} = ((140 - age) \cdot weight)/(72 \cdot S_{creat}) \cdot 0.85 \text{ (for female subjects)}$$

where weight referred to the patient's actual body weight in kg, and age and $S_{creat}$ are in years of age and American units (mg/dL), respectively.

The C&G formula systematically overestimates the GFR because of the tubular secretion of creatinine. So, this may be a benefit when correlating renal clearance and clearance of drugs that are secreted with this estimation of $CL_{CR}$, but it certainly is not when a true estimation of GFR is needed by a clinician. On the positive side, the $CL_{CR}$ estimate obtained by the method is not normalized for a body surface area of 1.73 m², so it is a more appropriate covariate to use to correlate a patient's clearance with its administered dose and measured systemic exposure.

The MDRD study equation was initially developed in 1999 with the use of data from 1628 patients with CKD. Its estimated GFR is adjusted for body-surface area. The estimating equation is

$$GFR \text{ (mL/min/1.73 m}^2) = 186 \cdot (C_{CR})^{-1.154} \cdot (age)^{-0.203} \cdot 0.742$$
(if the subject is female).

This equation was revised in 2005 for use with a standardized serum creatinine assay that yields serum creatinine values that are 5% lower.

$$\begin{aligned} GFR \text{ (mL/min/1.73 m}^2) &= 175 \\ &\times (\text{standardized } C_{CR})^{-1.154} \cdot (age)^{-0.203} \\ &\times 0.742 \text{ (if the subject is female) or} \\ &\times 1.212 \text{ (if the subject is black)} \end{aligned} \quad (25.8)$$

In the MDRD study population, 91% of the GFR estimates were within 30% of the measured values, and this approach was more accurate than the use of the C&G equation. The C&G equation was reported to be less accurate than the MDRD study equation in older and obese people. Both methods are less accurate in healthy subjects.

While the MDRD method will provide a more accurate GFR estimate, renal drug clearance as mentioned previously is not entirely governed by GFR. Reabsorption and secretion are also important for many drugs. In patients with CKD, the following recommendations are good practices that physicians and pharmacists should be aware of (Munar and Singh, 2007):

1. Assess the use of OTC and herbal medicine to ensure proper indication, and avoid medications with toxic metabolites, or use the least nephrotoxic agents.

2. Use alternative medications if potential drug interactions exist.

3. Use caution for drugs with active metabolites that can exaggerate pharmacologic effects in patients with renal impairment.

4. Adjust dosages of drugs cleared renally based on the patient's kidney function (calculated as $CL_{CR}$ or eGFR); determine initial dosages using published guidelines and adjust based on patient response or monitoring if appropriate.

## DOSE ADJUSTMENT IN PATIENTS WITH RENAL IMPAIRMENT

Dose adjustment for drugs in renally impaired patients should be made in accordance with changes in pharmacodynamics and pharmacokinetics of the drug in the individual patient. Whether renal impairment will alter the pharmacokinetics of the drug enough to justify dosage adjustment is an important consideration. For many drugs that are eliminated primarily by metabolism and/or biliary secretion (80% or more), renal impairment may not alter the pharmacokinetics sufficiently to warrant dosage adjustment.

Active metabolites of the drug may also be formed and must be considered for additional pharmacologic effects when adjusting dose. The classical example is procainamide, which is almost exclusively metabolized and not eliminated unchanged in the urine. Procainamide dosing regimens would therefore not need to be adjusted in renal failure if it was not for its main metabolite, N-acetylprocainamide (NAPA) which is pharmacologically active (it is a Class III, while its parent drug, procainamide, is a class Ia antiarrhythmic agent) and will accumulate in patients with renal impairment. For some drugs, the free drug concentrations may need to be considered due to decreased or altered protein binding in uremia. Combination products that contain two or more active drugs in a fixed-dose combination may be differentially affected by decreased renal function and thus, from a general point of view, combination drug products are more challenging to administer in patients with renal impairment.

The following methods may be used to estimate initial and maintenance dose regimens. After initiating the dosage, the clinician should continue to monitor the pharmacodynamics and pharmacokinetics of the drug. They should also evaluate the patient's renal function, which may be changing over time.

### Basis for Dose Adjustment in Renal Impairment

The loading drug dose is based on the apparent central volume of distribution of the drug. Moderate or mild renal impairment does not normally impair protein binding significantly, and therefore the volume of distribution, but severe impairment can. Patients with severe renal impairment may have lower concentrations of proteins in blood and the proteins like albumin may be of "lesser quality," affecting the percentage of free drug within the systemic circulation. It is thought, however, that this should not be clinically relevant if drugs are 80% or less bound to plasma proteins (FDA Guidance for Industry, 2010).

The maintenance dose is always based on the clearance of the drug in the patient for a given target systemic exposure as seen in this equation for clearance already presented in Chapter 15:

$$AUC_\infty \text{ or } AUC\tau_{(ss)} = Dose/CL/F \quad (25.9)$$

In patients with renal impairment, the rate of renal drug excretion decreases, leading to a decrease in renal and therefore overall clearance. Most methods for dose adjustment assume that the nonrenal drug clearance is unchanged, which is a reasonable assumption to make until severe renal impairment

is seen and where hepatorenal syndrome can occur. The fraction of normal renal function remaining in the patient with renal impairment is simply estimated from the fraction of normal $CL_{CR}$ that is observed in that patient. The total clearance in the renally impaired patient is therefore obtained by adding their estimated renal clearance to the typical nonrenal clearance. The dosage regimen may then be developed by (1) decreasing the maintenance dose, (2) increasing the dosage interval, or (3) changing both maintenance dose and dosage interval.

Although total body clearance is the accurate parameter to relate the overall dose to administer per day (or per week or month), the change in the elimination half-life of the drug will be used to decide if the dosing interval has to be adjusted.

### Nomograms

Nomograms are charts available for use in estimating dosage regimens in patients with renal impairment (Tozer, 1974; Chennavasin and Brater, 1981; Bjornsson, 1986). The nomograms may be based on serum creatinine concentrations, patient data (height, weight, age, gender), and the pharmacokinetics of the drug. As discussed by Chennavasin and Brater (1981), each nomogram has errors in its assumptions and drug database. Nomograms are not as useful clinically as they once were, simply because drugs that have been approved for market commercialization in the last 30 years have been obligated to be studied in renal impaired patients. Clear tables for dosing are therefore included in product labels and monographs, and can also be found in small clinical books such as those introduced originally by William Bennet and called "Bennet tables." We will discuss this in the next section.

Most nomogram methods for dose adjustment in renal disease assume that nonrenal elimination of the drug is not affected by renal impairment and that the remaining renal excretion rate constant in the renally impaired patient is proportional to the product of a constant and of the $CL_{CR}$:

$$k = k_{NR} + \alpha \cdot CL_{CR} \quad (25.10)$$

where $k_{NR}$ is the nonrenal elimination rate constant and $\alpha$ is a constant relating a clearance to a rate constant, so in the case of a drug well characterized by a

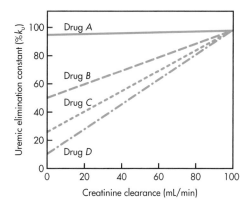

FIGURE 25-3 • Relationship between creatinine clearance and the drug elimination rate constant.

respectively. A $CL_{CR}$ of $\geq 80$ mL/min is considered an adequate GFR in subjects with normal renal function. The patient elimination rate constant ($k$) is the sum of the nonrenal elimination rate constant and the renal elimination rate constant, which is decreased due to renal impairment. If the patient has complete renal shutdown (ie, $CL_{CR} = 0$ mL/min), then the intercept on the $y$ axis represents the percent of drug elimination due to nonrenal drug elimination routes. Drug $D$, which is excreted 90% unchanged in the urine, has the steepest slope (equivalent to $\alpha$ in Equation 25.14) and is most affected by small changes in $CL_{CR}$. In contrast, drug $A$, which is excreted only 5% unchanged in the urine (ie, 95% eliminated by nonrenal routes), is least affected by a decrease in $CL_{CR}$.

The nomogram method of Welling and Craig (1976) provides an estimate of the ratio of the patient's elimination rate constant ($k$) to the normal elimination rate constant ($k_N$) on the basis of $CL_{CR}$ (Fig. 25-4). For this method, Welling and Craig (1976) provided a list of drugs grouped according to the amount of drug excreted unchanged in the urine (Table 25-5). From the $k/k_N$ ratio, the dose to

one-compartment model it would be $\alpha = 1/V_D$, and it can then be used for the construction of a nomogram. Figure 25-3 shows a graphical representation of Equation 25.10 for four different drugs, each with a different renal excretion rate constant. The fractions of drug excreted unchanged in the urine ($f_e$) for drugs $A$, $B$, $C$, and $D$ are 5%, 50%, 75%, and 90%,

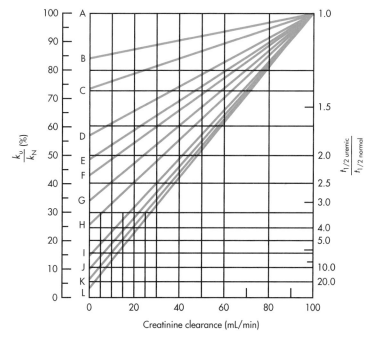

FIGURE 25-4 • This nomograph describes the changes in the percentage of normal elimination rate constant (left ordinate) and the consequent geometric increase in elimination half-life (right ordinate) as a function of creatinine clearance. The drugs associated with the individual slopes are given in Table 25-5. (Reproduced with permission from Benet LZ: The Effects of Disease States on Drug Pharmacokinetics. Washington, DC: American Pharmaceutical Association; 1976.)

## TABLE 25-5 • Elimination Rate Constants for Various Drugs*

| Group | Drug | $k_N$ (h$^{-1}$) | $k_{nr}$ (h$^{-1}$) | $k_{nr}/k_N$% |
|---|---|---|---|---|
| A | Minocycline | 0.04 | 0.04 | 100.0 |
| | Rifampicin | 0.25 | 0.25 | 100.0 |
| | Lidocaine | 0.39 | 0.36 | 92.3 |
| | Digitoxin | 0.114 | 0.10 | 87.7 |
| B | Doxycycline | 0.037 | 0.031 | 83.8 |
| | Chlortetracycline | 0.12 | 0.095 | 79.2 |
| C | Clindamycin | 0.16 | 0.12 | 75.0 |
| | Chloramphenicol | 0.26 | 0.19 | 73.1 |
| | Propranolol | 0.22 | 0.16 | 72.8 |
| | Erythromycin | 0.39 | 0.28 | 71.8 |
| D | Trimethoprim | 0.054 | 0.031 | 57.4 |
| | Isoniazid (fast) | 0.53 | 0.30 | 56.6 |
| | Isoniazid (slow) | 0.23 | 0.13 | 56.5 |
| E | Dicloxacillin | 1.20 | 0.60 | 50.0 |
| | Sulfadiazine | 0.069 | 0.032 | 46.4 |
| | Sulfamethoxazole | 0.084 | 0.037 | 44.0 |
| F | Nafcillin | 1.26 | 0.54 | 42.8 |
| | Chlorpropamide | 0.020 | 0.008 | 40.0 |
| | Lincomycin | 0.15 | 0.06 | 40.0 |
| G | Colistimethate | 0.154 | 0.054 | 35.1 |
| | Oxacillin | 1.73 | 0.58 | 33.6 |
| | Digoxin | 0.021 | 0.007 | 33.3 |
| H | Tetracycline | 0.120 | 0.033 | 27.5 |
| | Cloxacillin | 1.21 | 0.31 | 25.6 |
| | Oxytetracycline | 0.075 | 0.014 | 18.7 |
| I | Amoxicillin | 0.70 | 0.10 | 14.3 |
| | Methicillin | 1.40 | 0.19 | 13.6 |
| J | Ticarcillin | 0.58 | 0.066 | 11.4 |
| | Penicillin G | 1.24 | 0.13 | 10.5 |
| | Ampicillin | 0.53 | 0.05 | 9.4 |
| | Carbenicillin | 0.55 | 0.05 | 9.1 |
| K | Cefazolin | 0.32 | 0.02 | 6.2 |
| | Cephaloridine | 0.51 | 0.03 | 5.9 |
| | Cephalothin | 1.20 | 0.06 | 5.0 |
| | Gentamicin | 0.30 | 0.015 | 5.0 |
| L | Flucytosine | 0.18 | 0.007 | 3.9 |
| | Kanamycin | 0.28 | 0.01 | 3.6 |
| | Vancomycin | 0.12 | 0.004 | 3.3 |
| | Tobramycin | 0.32 | 0.010 | 3.1 |
| | Cephalexin | 1.54 | 0.032 | 2.1 |

*$k_N$ = patients with normal renal function, $k_{nr}$ = patients with severe renal impairment, $k_{nr}/k_N$% = percent of normal elimination in severe renal impairment. Reproduced with permission from Benet LZ: The Effects of Disease States on Drug Pharmacokinetics. Washington, DC: American Pharmaceutical Association; 1976.

administer to a patient with renal impairment can be estimated according to Equation 25.11:

$$\text{DOSE} = k/k_N \cdot \text{DOSE}_N \qquad (25.11)$$

When the dosage interval $\tau$ is kept constant, the patient's dose is always a smaller fraction of the normal dose. Instead of reducing the dose for the renally impaired patient, the usual dose is kept constant and the dosage interval $\tau$ is prolonged according to the following equation:

$$\tau = k_N/k \cdot \tau_N \qquad (25.12)$$

where $\tau$ is the dosage interval for the renally impaired patient while $\tau_N$ is the dosage interval for the dose in patients with normal renal function.

These nomogram methods are not really used nowadays, as they propose to either alter the dose or the dosing interval, when in reality the optimum dosing regimen to administer to a renally impaired patient may be one that uses a combination of dose and interval adjustments. We will see this in the following section.

## Tables for Adjusting Drug Dosage Regimens

William Bennet was instrumental in creating tables for dosing of drugs in patients with renal impairment. The tables that were proposed influenced regulatory guidances and how companies needed to study drug dosing regimen in renally impaired patients.

An example of drug dosing table in renal impairment for a recently approved product, Fetroja® (cefiderocol, a new cephalosporin approved in the United States in 2019), presented in Table 25-6,

shows how these tables are now part of every new drug label and monograph.

The recommendation in terms of dose and therapeutic interval adjustment that are presented in these tables and in approved drug product's label and monograph should be based on the relationship between exposure, safety, and efficacy.

- The simplest example is for a drug product where efficacy and safety would only correlate with AUC. For that product only, the dose would need to be adjusted and the therapeutic interval would stay constant. In that particular case, the overall exposure would be the same at steady state ($\text{AUC}_{t(ss)}$), but the $C_{max(ss)}$ would be slightly lower and the $C_{min(ss)}$ would be slightly higher.
- Should the efficacy not only relate to AUC but also to $C_{max}$ and $C_{min}$, such as the case for an antibiotic agent, then the dosing interval will be adjusted primarily instead of the dose, so that both $C_{max(ss)}$, $\text{AUC}_{t(ss)}$, and $C_{min(ss)}$ would stay as close to their intended normal exposure as much as possible.

The following steps explain how to relate the pharmacokinetics of a drug with changing renal function, and how to decide whether to adjust primarily the dose or the dosing interval of a drug in a patient with impaired renal function.

1. Calculation of the overall dose to administer at every dosing interval in order to reach the same exposure (AUC):
   - Until only severe renal impairment is seen, only the renal clearance of a drug

## TABLE 25-6 • Example of Drug Dosing for Patients in Renal Impairment as Presented in a Drug Approved Monograph or Label (2019 Recommendations for Fetroja® Shionogi Inc., 2019 Presented)

| Estimated Creatinine (CLcr)* | Dose | Frequency | Infusion Time |
|---|---|---|---|
| Patients with CLcr 30 to 59 mL/min | 1.5 grams | Every 8 hours | 3 hours |
| Patients with CLcr 15 to 29 mL/min | 1 gram | Every 8 hours | 3 hours |
| ESRD Patients (CLcr less than 15 mL/min) with or without HD† | 0.75 grams | Every 12 hours | 3 hours |

*CLcr = creatinine clearance estimated by Cockcroft--Gault equation.
†Cefiderocol is removed by hemodialysis (HD); thus, complete hemodialysis (HD) at the latest possible time before the start of cefiderocol dosing.
ESRD = end-stage renal disease; HD = hemodialysis.

will be affected. The non-renal clearance (most of the time hepatic) will remain constant. As clearances are additive,

$$CL = CL_R + CL_{NR} \qquad (25.13)$$

and

$$CL_R = f_e \cdot CL \qquad (25.14)$$

The renal clearance will correlate with the estimated $CL_{CR}$ (eg, using the C&G equation)

$$CL_R = a \cdot CL_{CR} \qquad (25.15)$$

The overall clearance can be correlated with the C&G equation:

$$CL = CL_{NR} + a \cdot CL_{CR} \qquad (25.16)$$

where $CL_{NR}$ can be estimated from a drug product monograph that specifies what the normal $CL$ and the $f_e$ is by rearranging Equations 25.13 and 25.14 to:

$$CL_{NR} = CL \cdot (1 - f_e) \qquad (25.17)$$

Table 25-7 lists various drugs with their $f_e$ values and elimination half-lives.

The dose to administer over the normal therapeutic interval in order to reach the exact same exposure at steady state is therefore:

$$DOSE = AUC_{t(ss)} \cdot (CL_{NR} + a \cdot CL_{CR}) \qquad (25.18)$$

Or using the normal dose ($DOSE_N$) that is associated with the targeted AUC and 100 mL/min as a "normal" creatinine clearance:

$$DOSE = DOSE_N \cdot \frac{(CL_{NR} + a \cdot CL_{CR})}{(CL_{NR} + a \cdot 100)} \qquad (25.19)$$

2. Calculation of the impact of renal impairment on the half-life:

Assuming a one-compartment model, where $CL = k_{el} \cdot V_{ss}$, and assuming that the degree of renal impairment in a patient does not affect the $V_{ss}$, the change in the therapeutic interval will be dictated by the change in the $k_{el}$ and corresponding half-life:

$$CL = CL_N \times \frac{(CL_{NR} + a \cdot CL_{CR})}{(CL_{NR} + a \cdot 100)} \qquad (25.20)$$

And because $CL = k_{el} \cdot V_{ss}$, then:

$$k_{el} = k_{elN} \times (k_{NR} + a \cdot CL_{CR})/(k_{NR} + a \cdot 100) \qquad (25.21)$$

$$\text{And } t_{1/2} = 0.693/k_{el} \qquad (25.22)$$

where $CL_N$ and $k_{elN}$ represents the normal expected $CL$ and $k_{el}$ in a normal patient (N) with normal renal function ($CL_{CR}$ of 100 mL/min).

3. Estimation of the impact on $C_{max(ss)}$ and $C_{min(ss)}$

The exact predicted $C_{max(ss)}$ and $C_{min(ss)}$ can be obtained using a multicompartment model and for any type of administration by conducting simple simulations with a compartmental pharmacokinetic tool such as ADAPT 5® or NONMEM® (see Chapter 20). In the absence of easy access to a computer, the impact on $C_{max(ss)}$ and $C_{min(ss)}$ can simply be rounded off by assuming a one-compartment model and assuming that the absorption process will not be affected by renal impairment.

We have seen in Chapter 12 that the degree of accumulation will be dependent on the relationship between the therapeutic interval and the terminal half-life:

$$AR = 1/(1 - \exp(-k_{el} \cdot \tau)) \qquad (25.23)$$

A patient with renal impairment will present the same exact first $C_{max}$ when given the same dose as a normal patient, assuming as presented before that the volume of distribution and the absorption process are unaffected. The $C_{max(ss)}$ will, however, be different for a patient with renal impairment receiving the same dose over the same dosing interval, because the AR will be different.

$$C_{max(ss)} = C_{max(SD)} \cdot AR \qquad (25.24)$$

Because $AR = 1/(1 - \exp(-k_{el} \cdot \tau))$

Then $C_{max(ss)} = C_{max(SD)}/(1 - \exp(-k_{el} \cdot \tau)) \qquad (25.25)$

In order to reach a similar $C_{max(ss)}$ for a patient with renal impairment, the therapeutic interval will need to be changed to:

$$\tau = k_{el(N)} \times \tau_{(N)}/k_{el} \qquad (25.26)$$

where $k_{el(N)}$ and $\tau_{(N)}$ are the $k_{el}$ and $\tau$ expected in a patient with normal renal function.

## TABLE 25-7 • Fraction of Drug Excreted Unchanged ($f_e$) and Elimination Half-Life Values

| Drug | $f_e$ | $t_{1/2\ normal}$ (h)* | Drug | $f_e$ | $t_{1/2\ normal}$ (h)* |
|------|-------|------------------------|------|-------|------------------------|
| Acebutolol | 0.44 ± 0.11 | 2.7 ± 0.4 | Chlorthalidone | 0.65 ± 0.09 | 44 ± 10 |
| Acetaminophen | 0.03 ± 0.01 | 2.0 ± 0.4 | Cimetidine | 0.77 ± 0.06 | 2.1 ± 1.1 |
| Acetohexamide | 0.4 | 1.3 | Clindamycin | 0.09–0.14 | 2.7 ± 0.4 |
| Active metabolite | | 16–30 | Clofibrate | 0.11–0.32 | 13 ± 3 |
| Allopurinol | 0.1 | 2–8 | Clonidine | 0.62 ± 0.11 | 8.5 ± 2.0 |
| Alprenolol | 0.005 | 3.1 ± 1.2 | Colistin | 0.9 | 3 |
| Amantadine | 0.85 | 10 | Cyclophosphamide | 0.3 | 5 |
| Amikacin | 0.98 | 2.3 ± 0.4 | Cytarabine | 0.1 | 2 |
| Amiloride | 0.5 | 8 ± 2 | Dapsone | 0.1 | 20 |
| Amoxicillin | 0.52 ± 0.15 | 1.0 ± 0.1 | Dicloxacillin | 0.60 ± 0.07 | 0.7 ± 0.07 |
| Amphetamine | 0.4–0.45 | 12 | Digitoxin | 0.33 ± 0.15 | 166 ± 65 |
| Amphotericin B | 0.03 | 360 | Digoxin | 0.72 ± 0.09 | 42 ± 19 |
| Ampicillin | 0.90 ± 0.08 | 1.3 ± 0.2 | Disopyramide | 0.55 ± 0.06 | 7.8 ± 1.6 |
| Atenolol | 0.85 | 6.3 ± 1.8 | Doxycycline | 0.40 ± 0.04 | 20 ± 4 |
| Azlocillin | 0.6 | 1.0 | Erythromycin | 0.15 | 1.1–3.5 |
| Bacampicillin | 0.88 | 0.9 | Ethambutol | 0.79 ± 0.03 | 3.1 ± 0.4 |
| Baclofen | 0.75 | 3–4 | Ethosuximide | 0.19 | 33 ± 6 |
| Bleomycin | 0.55 | 1.5–8.9 | Flucytosine | 0.63–0.84 | 5.3 ± 0.7 |
| Bretylium | 0.8 ± 0.1 | 4–17 | Flunitrazepam | 0.01 | 15 ± 5 |
| Bumetanide | 0.33 | 3.5 | Furosemide | 0.74 ± 0.07 | 0.85 ± 0.17 |
| Carbenicillin | 0.82 ± 0.09 | 1.1 ± 0.2 | Gentamicin | 0.98 | 2–3 |
| Cefalothin | 0.52 | 0.6 ± 0.3 | Griseofulvin | 0 | 15 |
| Cefamandole | 0.96 ± 0.03 | 0.77 | Hydralazine | 0.12–0.14 | 2.2–2.6 |
| Cefazolin | 0.80 ± 0.13 | 1.8 ± 0.4 | Hydrochlorothiazide | 0.95 | 2.5 ± 0.2 |
| Cefoperazone | 0.2–0.3 | 2.0 | Indomethacin | 0.15 ± 0.08 | 2.6–11.2 |
| Cefotaxime | 0.5–0.6 | 1–1.5 | Isoniazid | | |
| Cefoxitin | 0.88 ± 0.08 | 0.7 ± 0.13 | Rapid acetylators | 0.07 ± 0.02 | 1.1 ± 0.2 |
| Cefuroxime | 0.92 | 1.1 | Slow acetylators | 0.29 ± 0.05 | 3.0 ± 0.8 |
| Cephalexin | 0.96 | 0.9 ± 0.18 | Isosorbide dinitrate | 0.05 | 0.5 |
| Chloramphenicol | 0.05 | 2.7 ± 0.8 | Kanamycin | 0.9 | 2.1 ± 0.2 |
| Chlorphentermine | 0.2 | 120 | Lidocaine | 0.02 ± 0.01 | 1.8 ± 0.4 |
| Chlorpropamide | 0.2 | 36 | Lincomycin | 0.6 | 5 |

*(Continued)*

**TABLE 25-7 • Fraction of Drug Excreted Unchanged ($f_e$) and Elimination Half-Life Values (*Continued*)**

| Drug | $f_e$ | $t_{1/2\,normal}$ (h)* | Drug | $f_e$ | $t_{1/2\,normal}$ (h)* |
|---|---|---|---|---|---|
| Lithium | 0.95 ± 0.15 | 22 ± 8 | Primidone | 0.42 ± 0.15 | 8.0 ± 4.8 |
| Lorazepam | 0.01 | 14 ± 5 | Procainamide | 0.67 ± 0.08 | 2.9 ± 0.6 |
| Meperidine | 0.04–0.22 | 3.2 ± 0.8 | Propranolol | 0.005 | 3.9 ± 0.4 |
| Methadone | 0.2 | 22 | Quinidine | 0.18 ± 0.05 | 6.2 ± 1.8 |
| Methicillin | 0.88 ± 0.17 | 0.85 ± 0.23 | Rifampin | 0.16 ± 0.04 | 2.1 ± 0.3 |
| Methotrexate | 0.94 | 8.4 | Salicylic acid | 0.2 | 3 |
| Methyldopa | 0.63 ± 0.10 | 1.8 ± 0.2 | Sisomicin | 0.98 | 2.8 |
| Metronidazole | 0.25 | 8.2 | Sotalol | 0.6 | 6.5–13 |
| Mexiletine | 0.1 | 12 | Streptomycin | 0.96 | 2.8 |
| Mezlocillin | 0.75 | 0.8 | Sulfinpyrazone | 0.45 | 2.3 |
| Minocycline | 0.1 ± 0.02 | 18 ± 4 | Sulfisoxazole | 0.53 ± 0.09 | 5.9 ± 0.9 |
| Minoxidil | 0.1 | 4 | Tetracycline | 0.48 | 9.9 ± 1.5 |
| Moxalactam | 0.82–0.96 | 2.5–3.0 | Thiamphenicol | 0.9 | 3 |
| Nadolol | 0.73 ± 0.04 | 16 ± 2 | Thiazinamium | 0.41 | |
| Nafcillin | 0.27 ± 0.05 | 0.9–1.0 | Theophylline | 0.08 | 9 ± 2.1 |
| Nalidixic acid | 0.2 | 1.0 | Ticarcillin | 0.86 | 1.2 |
| Neostigmine | 0.67 | 1.3 ± 0.8 | Timolol | 0.2 | 3–5 |
| Netilmicin | 0.98 | 2.2 | Tobramycin | 0.98 | 2.2 ± 0.1 |
| Nitrazepam | 0.01 | 29 ± 7 | Tocainide | 0.20–0.70 (0.40 mean) | 1.6–3 |
| Nitrofuraniton | 0.5 | 0.3 | | | |
| Nomifensine | 0.15–0.22 | 3.0 ± 1.0 | Tolbutamide | 0 | 5.9 ± 1.4 |
| Oxacillin | 0.75 | 0.5 | Triamterene | 0.04 ± 0.01 | 2.8 ± 0.9 |
| Oxprenolol | 0.05 | 1.5 | Trimethoprim | 0.53 ± 0.02 | 11 ± 1.4 |
| Pancuronium | 0.5 | 3.0 | Tubocurarine | 0.43 ± 0.08 | 2 ± 1.1 |
| Pentazocine | 0.2 | 2.5 | Valproic acid | 0.02 ± 0.02 | 16 ± 3 |
| Phenobarbital | 0.2 ± 0.05 | 86 ± 7 | Vancomycin | 0.97 | 5–6 |
| Pindolol | 0.41 | 3.4 ± 0.2 | Warfarin | 0 | 37 ± 15 |
| Pivampicillin | 0.9 | 0.9 | | | |
| Polymyxin B | 0.88 | 4.5 | | | |
| Prazosin | 0.01 | 2.9 ± 0.8 | | | |

*Half-life is a derived parameter that changes as a function of both clearance and volume of distribution. It is independent of body size, because it is a function of these two parameters (CL, $V_D$), each of which is proportional to body size. It is important to consider that half-life is the time to eliminate 50% of the "drug" from the body (plasma), not the time in which 50% of the effect is lost.

Data from Chennavasin and Brater, 1981; Dettli, 1976; Gilman et al, 1980.

Once the $C_{max(ss)}$ has been calculated for a given patient, then the $C_{min(ss)}$ can be calculated assuming a monoexponential decline as follows:

$$C_{min(ss)} = C_{max(ss)} \cdot \exp(-k_{el} \cdot \tau) \qquad (25.27)$$

## PRACTICE PROBLEM

Assuming that the maintenance dose of gentamicin in a bacterial infected patient with normal renal function (100 mL/min) is 140 mg every 12 hours, calculate the maintenance dose to administer to a similar patient in terms of age, gender, and body weight, except for a $CL_{CR}$ of 50 mL/min. Assume that for gentamicin the $CL = 0.0216 + 0.0648 \cdot CL_{CR}$, that the volume of distribution is 21 L (0.3 L/kg), that it is well characterized by a one-compartment model, and that the minimum inhibitory concentration (MIC) of the bacteria causing the infection is 0.5 mg/L.

### Solution

1. A simple solution adjusting only the dose, keeping the same dosing interval.

   We can use Equation 25.19:

   $$DOSE = DOSE_N \times \frac{(CL_{NR} + a \cdot CL_{CR})}{(CL_{NR} + a \cdot 100)}$$

   Therefore, the dose to administer over the same dosing interval would be:

   $$DOSE = 140 \times \left( \frac{0.2216 + 0.0648 \cdot 50}{0.2216 + 0.0648 \cdot 100} \right) = 70 \text{ mg}$$

   The problems with this approach are that despite having the same $AUC_{t(ss)}$, this regimen will be associated with a much lower $C_{max}$ (half) and a much higher $C_{min}$, which in the case of aminoglycosides will lead to renal and ear toxicity.

2. A slightly more complicated solution taking also $C_{max}$ and $C_{min}$ into account.

   Let's calculate the pharmacokinetic parameters first for the "normal" patient.

   $$C_{max(SD)} = DOSE/V_C = 140/21 = 6.67 \text{ mg/L}$$

   $$CL = 0.0216 + 0.0648 \cdot CL_{CR} = 0.0216 + 0.0648 \cdot 100$$
   $$= 6.50 \text{ L/h}$$

$$k_{el} = CL/V_C = 6.50/21 = 0.3096 \text{ h}^{-1}$$

$$C_{max(ss)} = C_{max(SD)}/(1 - \exp(-k_{el} \cdot \tau))$$
$$= 6.67/(1 - \exp(-0.3096 \cdot 12)) = 6.84 \text{ mg/L}$$

$$C_{min(ss)} = C_{max(ss)} \cdot \exp(-k_{el} \cdot \tau) = 6.84 \cdot \exp(-0.3096 \cdot 12)$$
$$= 0.166 \text{ mg/L}$$

The patient with impaired renal function will not have a different volume of distribution than the "normal" patient, so his first $C_{max}$ will be approximately the same, but his accumulation ratio will not be the same. So, his pharmacokinetic parameters associated with the same dosage and therapeutic intervals would be:

$$C_{max}(SD) = 6.67 \text{ mg/L}$$

$$CL = 0.0216 + 0.0648 \cdot CL_{CR} = 0.0216 + 0.0648 \cdot$$
$$50 = 3.262 \text{ L/h}$$

$$k_{el} = CL/V_C = 3.262/21 = 0.1553 \text{ h}^{-1}$$

$$C_{max(ss)} = C_{max(SD)}/(1 - \exp(-k_{el} \cdot \tau))$$
$$= 6.67/(1 - \exp(-0.1553 \cdot 12)) = 7.895 \text{ mg/L}$$

$$C_{min(ss)} = C_{max(ss)} \cdot \exp(-k_{el} \cdot \tau) = 7.895 \cdot \exp(-0.1553 \cdot 12)$$
$$= 1.225 \text{ mg/L}$$

Let's calculate what the dosing interval would need to be in order to get the same AR:

$$\tau = k_{el(N)} \times \tau_{(N)}/k_{el} = 0.3096 \cdot 12/0.1553 = 23.92 \text{ mg/L}$$

In order for us to have similar AR in our patient with renal impairment, the therapeutic interval would need to be extended to 24 hours. The $C_{max(ss)}$ and $C_{min(ss)}$ would therefore be:

$$C_{max(ss)} = C_{max(SD)}/(1 - \exp(-k_{el} \cdot \tau))$$
$$= 6.67/(1 - \exp(-0.1553 \cdot 24)) = 6.83 \text{ mg/L}$$

$$C_{min(ss)} = C_{max(ss)} \cdot \exp(-k_{el} \cdot \tau)$$
$$= (6.83 \cdot \exp(-0.1553 \cdot 24)) = 0.164 \text{ mg/L}$$

## PRACTICE PROBLEM

What is the dose to administer, keeping the same dosing interval, for a drug that is 75% excreted unchanged through the kidney in a patient with a creatinine clearance of 20 mL/min?

## Solution

Assuming no change in the $CL_{NR}$, the $CL_R$ will be directly affected by the change in the $CL_{CR}$ (versus a normal value of 100 mL/min) such that it will only be 20% of its normal value. The overall clearance will therefore be the following fraction of its normal value ($CL_N$):

$$CL/CL_N = 0.25 + 20/100 = 0.45 \text{ or } 45\%$$

Because $CL = DOSE/AUC$, the proportion of the normal dose ($DOSE_N$) to administer to this patient in order to reach the exact same $AUC_{t(ss)}$ will be 45%.

Table 25-8 provides some calculated dose adjustments for drugs eliminated to various degrees by renal excretion in different stages of renal failure.

### Limitations of Dose Adjustment Methods in Patients with Renal Impairment

All of the methods mentioned previously have similar limitations (see Table 25-2). For example, the drug must follow linear pharmacokinetics, and the

---

### FREQUENTLY ASKED QUESTIONS

▶ What are the advantages and disadvantages of using a nomogram such as the C&G using serum creatinine concentrations for the estimation of renal function?

▶ What is the most accurate approach for the estimation of glomerular filtration rate?

▶ Why does each method based on serum creatinine concentrations for dosage adjustment in renal impairment give somewhat different values?

▶ What are some of the PK/PD considerations that one needs to consider when adjusting a dosing regimen in a renally impaired patient?

---

non-renal clearance and/or the volume of distribution of the drug must remain relatively constant. If there is a change in an active metabolite formation or elimination, then both parent and active metabolites must be considered when adjusting a dosage regimen for patients with renal disease, because potential side effects may result from an increase in the half-life of the parent drug and/or an accumulation of the active metabolites, as we have seen previously with procainamide and its active metabolite NAPA. Similarly, Bodenham et al (1988) have shown that although lorazepam pharmacokinetics were not significantly altered in patients with chronic renal failure, the clearance of lorazepam glucuronide, a major metabolite, was reduced significantly. Therefore, there are potential sedative side effects in the renally impaired patient as a result of the longer metabolite half-life. Bodenham and coworkers (1988) also cited literature references to potentiation of sedative and analgesic drug effects in renal, liver, and other multisystem disease states.

Another assumption in the use of these methods is that pharmacologic response is unchanged in the renal impaired patient. This assumption may be unrealistic for drugs that act differently in the disease state, and possible changes in pharmacodynamic effects in patients with renal and other diseases must be considered. For example, the pharmacologic response with digoxin is dependent on the potassium level in the body, and potassium level in the renally impaired patients may be rather different from that of the normal individual. In a patient undergoing dialysis, loss of potassium may increase the potential for toxic effects of the drug digoxin. In addition, neuromuscular-blocking drugs may be potentiated or antagonized by changes in potassium, phosphate, and hydrogen ion concentration brought

---

## TABLE 25-8 • Dosage Adjustment in Patients with Renal Impairment

| Fraction of Drug Excreted Unchanged ($k_R/k_N$) or $f_e$ | Percent of Normal Dose | | | |
|---|---|---|---|---|
| | 50% Normal $CL_{CR}$ | 25% Normal $CL_{CR}$ | 10% Normal $CL_{CR}$ | 0% Normal $CL_{CR}$ |
| 0.25 | 87 | 81 | 77 | 75 |
| 0.50 | 75 | 62 | 55 | 50 |
| 0.75 | 62 | 44 | 32 | 25 |
| 0.90 | 55 | 32 | 19 | 10 |

about by uremic states, and morphine potentiation has been reported in hypocalcemic states.

For many drugs, studies have shown that the incidence of adverse effects is increased in renally impaired patients. It is often impossible in these studies to distinguish whether the increase in adverse effect is due to a pharmacokinetic change and/or a pharmacodynamic change in the receptor sensitivity to the drug. Serum creatinine concentration may not rise for some time until $CL_{CR}$ has fallen significantly, thereby adding to the uncertainty of any method that depends on serum $CL_{CR}$ for dose adjustment in unstable renal disease. In any event, these observations point out the fact that dose adjustment must be regarded as a preliminary estimation to be followed with further adjustments in accordance with the observed clinical response.

## EXTRACORPOREAL REMOVAL OF DRUGS

Patients with *end-stage renal disease* (ESRD) and those who have become intoxicated with a drug as a result of drug overdose require supportive treatment to remove the accumulated drug and its metabolites. Several methods are available for the extracorporeal removal of drugs, including hemoperfusion, hemofiltration, and dialysis. The objective of these methods is to rapidly remove the undesirable drugs and metabolites from the body without disturbing the fluid and electrolyte balance in the patient.

Patients with impaired renal function may be taking other medication concurrently. For these patients, dosage adjustment may be needed to replace drug loss during extracorporeal drug and metabolite removal.

### Dialysis

*Dialysis* is an artificial process in which the accumulation of drugs or waste metabolites is removed by diffusion from the body into the dialysis fluid. Two common dialysis treatments are *peritoneal dialysis* and *hemodialysis*. The principle underlying both processes is that as the patient's blood or fluid is equilibrated with the dialysis fluid across a dialysis membrane, waste metabolites from the patient's blood or fluid diffuse into the dialysis fluid and are

removed. The dialysate is balanced with electrolytes and with respect to osmotic pressure. The dialysate contains water, dextrose, electrolytes (potassium, sodium, chloride, bicarbonate, acetate, calcium, etc), and other elements similar to normal body fluids without the toxins.

### Peritoneal Dialysis

Peritoneal dialysis uses the peritoneal membrane in the abdomen as the filter. The peritoneum consists of visceral and parietal components. The peritoneum membrane provides a large natural surface area for diffusion of approximately 1–2 m² in adults; it is permeable to solutes of molecular weights ≤ 30,000 Da (*Merck Manual*, 1996–1997). However, only a small portion of the total splanchnic blood flow (70 mL/min out of 1200 mL/min at rest) comes into contact with the peritoneum and gets dialyzed. Placement of a peritoneal catheter is surgically simpler than hemodialysis and does not require vascular surgery and heparinization. The dialysis fluid is pumped into the peritoneal cavity, where waste metabolites in the body fluid are discharged rapidly. The dialysate is drained and fresh dialysate is reinstilled and then drained periodically. Peritoneal dialysis is also more amenable to self-treatment. However, slower drug clearance rates are obtained with peritoneal dialysis compared to hemodialysis, and thus longer dialysis time is required.

*Continuous ambulatory peritoneal dialysis* (CAPD) is the most common form of peritoneal dialysis. Many diabetic patients become uremic as a result of lack of control of their disease. About 2 L of dialysis fluid is instilled into the peritoneal cavity of the patient through a surgically placed resident catheter. The objective is to remove accumulated urea and other metabolic waste in the body. The catheter is sealed and the patient is able to continue in an ambulatory mode. Every 4–6 hours, the fluid is emptied from the peritoneal cavity and replaced with fresh dialysis fluid. The technique uses about 2 L of dialysis fluid; it does not require a dialysis machine and can be performed at home.

### Hemodialysis

Hemodialysis uses a dialysis machine and filters blood through an artificial membrane. Hemodialysis requires access to the blood vessels to allow the blood to flow to the dialysis machine and back to the body. For temporary access, a shunt is created in the arm, with one tube inserted into an artery and another tube inserted into a vein. The tubes are joined above the skin. For permanent access to the blood vessels, an arteriovenous fistula or graft is created by a surgical procedure to allow access to the artery and vein. Patients who are on chronic hemodialysis treatment need to be aware of the need for infection control of the surgical site of the fistula. At the start of the hemodialysis procedure, an arterial needle allows the blood to flow to the dialysis machine, and blood is returned to the patient to the venous side. Heparin is used to prevent blood clotting during the dialysis period.

During hemodialysis, the blood flows through the dialysis machine, where the waste material is removed from the blood by diffusion through an artificial membrane before the blood is returned to the body. Hemodialysis is a much more effective method of drug removal and is preferred in situations when rapid removal of the drug from the body is important, as in overdose or poisoning. In practice, hemodialysis is most often used for patients with end-stage renal failure. Early dialysis is appropriate for patients with acute renal failure in whom resumption of renal function can be expected and in patients who are to be renally transplanted. Other patients may be placed on dialysis according to clinical judgment concerning the patient's quality of life and risk/benefit ratio (Carpenter and Lazarus, 1994).

Dialysis is usually required 2 or 3 times per week (eg, Mon/Wed/Fri, or Tue/Thur/Sat, or Tue/Thur), with each treatment period lasting for 2–4 hours. The time required for dialysis depends on the amount of residual renal function in the patient, any complicating illness (eg, diabetes mellitus), the size and weight of the patient, including muscle mass, and the efficiency of the dialysis process (eg, 2 hours for "high-flux" dialysis and 4 hours for regular dialysis). Dosing of drugs in patients receiving hemodialysis is affected greatly by the frequency and type of dialysis machine used and by the physicochemical and pharmacokinetic properties of the drug. Factors that affect drug removal in hemodialysis are listed in Table 25-9. These factors are carefully considered before hemodialysis is used for drug removal.

## TABLE 25-9 • Factors Affecting Dialyzability of Drugs

| Physicochemical and Pharmacokinetic Properties of the Drug | |
|---|---|
| Water solubility | Insoluble or fat-soluble drugs are not dialyzed—eg, glutethimide, which is very water insoluble. |
| Protein binding | Tightly bound drugs are not dialyzed because dialysis is a passive process of diffusion—eg, propranolol is 94% bound. |
| Molecular weight | Only molecules with molecular weights of less than 500 are easily dialyzed—eg, vancomycin is poorly dialyzed and has a molecular weight of 1800. |
| Drugs with large volumes of distribution | Drugs widely distributed are dialyzed more slowly because the rate-limiting factor is the volume of blood entering the machine—eg, for digoxin, $V_D = 250$–$300$ L. Drugs concentrated in the tissues are usually difficult to remove by dialysis. |
| **Characteristics of the Dialysis Machine** | |
| Blood flow rate | Higher blood flows give higher clearance rates. |
| Dialysate | Composition of the dialysate and flow rate. |
| Dialysis membrane | Permeability characteristics and surface area. |
| Transmembrane pressure | Ultrafiltration increases with increase in transmembrane pressure. |
| Duration and frequency of dialysis | |

In hemodialysis, blood is pumped to the dialyzer by a roller pump at a rate of 300–450 mL/min. The drug and metabolites diffuse from the blood through the semipermeable membrane. In addition, hydrostatic pressure also forces the drug molecules into the dialysate by ultrafiltration. The composition of the dialysate is similar to plasma but may be altered according to the needs of the patient. Many dialysis machines use a hollow fiber or capillary dialyzer in which the semipermeable membrane is made into fine capillaries, of which thousands are packed into bundles with blood flowing through the capillaries and the dialysate circulating outside the capillaries. The permeability characteristics of the membrane and the membrane surface area are determinants of drug diffusion and ultrafiltration.

Hemodialysis will remove drugs that are "free" from protein binding directly from the central volume of distribution. Drugs that are well described by a one-compartment model, that distribute mostly in extracellular fluid volume, that do not have a high molecular weight, and that are minimally bound to plasma proteins such as the aminoglycosides are removed approximately 40% during a 4-hour dialysis session, and therefore have a dialysis elimination rate constant ($K_D$) of about 0.1 h$^{-1}$ during hemodialysis.

In contrast, drugs that have a higher molecular weight and are described by a two-compartment model, such as vancomycin, are not appreciably removed by a normal 4-hour dialysis session, but a "high-flux" analysis will remove some vancomycin. The efficacy of hemodialysis membranes for the removal of vancomycin by hemodialysis has been reviewed by De Hart (1996). Vancomycin is an antibiotic effective against most gram-positive organisms such as *Staphylococcus aureus*, which may be responsible for vascular access infections in patients undergoing dialysis. In De Hart's study, vancomycin hemodialysis in patients was compared using a cuprophan membrane or a cellulose acetate and polyacrylonitrile membrane. The cellulose acetate and polyacrylonitrile membrane are considered a "high-flux" filter. Serum vancomycin concentrations decreased only 6.3% after dialysis when using the cuprophan membrane, whereas the serum drug concentration decreased 13.6%–19.4% after dialysis with the cellulose acetate and polyacrylonitrile

membrane. It is estimated clinically that patients on vancomycin receiving high-flux hemodialysis should either receive their dose after dialysis, or they should receive a 250–500 mg supplemental dose after dialysis to compensate for the loss of drug.

In dialysis involving patients receiving drugs for therapy, the rate at which a given drug is removed depends on the flow rate of blood to the dialysis machine and the performance of the dialysis machine. The term *dialysance* is used to describe the process of drug removal from the dialysis machine. Dialysance is a clearance term similar in meaning to renal clearance, and it describes the amount of blood completely cleared of drugs (in mL/min). Dialysance is defined by the following equation for calculating the clearance of the drug through the dialysis machine ($CL_{DIAL}$):

$$CL_{DIAL} = Q\,(C_a - C_v)/C_a \qquad (25.28)$$

where $C_a$ = drug concentrations in arterial blood (blood entering dialysis machine), $C_v$ = drug concentration in venous blood (blood leaving kidney machine), and $Q$ = rate of blood flow to the kidney machine.

## PRACTICE PROBLEM

Assume the flow rate of blood to the dialysis machine is 350 mL/min. By chemical analysis, the concentrations of drug entering and leaving the machine are 30 and 12 $\mu$g/mL, respectively. What is the dialysis clearance?

### Solution

The rate of drug removal is equal to the volume of blood passed through the machine divided by the arterial difference in blood drug concentrations before and after dialysis. Thus,

Rate of drug removal = 350 mL/min · (30 − 12) $\mu$g/mL
= 6300 $\mu$g/min

Since clearance is equal to the rate of drug removal divided by the arterial concentration of drug,

$$CL_{DIAL} = (6300/30) = 210 \text{ mL/min}$$

Alternatively, using Equation 25.28,

$$CL_{DIAL} = 350 \cdot (30 - 12)/30 = 210 \text{ mL/min}$$

These calculations show that the two terms are the same. In practice, dialysance has to be measured experimentally by determining $C_a$, $C_v$, and $Q$. In dosing of drugs for patients who are on continuous dialysis, the average plasma drug concentration of a patient will be given by:

$$C_{av(ss)} = F \cdot \text{DOSE}/((CL_{DIAL} + CL) \cdot \tau) \quad (25.29)$$

where $F$ represents the fraction of the dose that is bioavailable, $CL$ is the total body drug clearance of the patient, $C_{av(ss)}$ is the average steady-state plasma drug concentration, and $\tau$ is the dosing interval.

In practice, if $CL_{DIAL}$ is 30% or more of the $CL$, then adjustments are usually made for the amount of drug lost during dialysis.

The elimination half-life, $t_{1/2}$, for the drug in the patient off dialysis is related to the remaining total body clearance, $CL_t$, and the volume of distribution, $V_D$, assuming a one-compartment model as shown below.

$$t_{1/2} = 0.693 \cdot V_D/CL \quad (25.30)$$

Drugs that are easily dialyzed will have a high dialysis clearance, $CL_{DIAL}$, and the elimination half-life, $t_{1/2}$, will be shorter in a patient on dialysis.

$$t_{1/2} = 0.693 \cdot V_D/(CL + CL_{DIAL}) \quad (25.31)$$

$$k_{ON} = (CL + CL_{DIAL})/V_D \quad (25.32)$$

where $k_{ON}$ is the first-order elimination half-life of the drug in the patient while on dialysis.

The *fraction of drug lost* due to elimination and dialysis may be estimated from Equation 25.33.

$$\text{Fraction of drug lost} = 1 - \exp(-k_{ON} \cdot t) \quad (25.33)$$

Equation 25.33 is based on first-order drug elimination and the substitution of $t$ hours for the dialysis period.

Several hypothetical examples illustrating the use of Equation 25.33 have been developed by Gambertoglio (1984). These are given in Table 25-10.

In Table 25-10, the fraction of drug lost during a 4-hour dialysis period for phenobarbital and salicylic acid is reported to be 0.30 and 0.50, respectively, whereas for digoxin and phenytoin- it is only 0.07 and 0.04, respectively. Both phenobarbital and salicylic acid are easily dialyzed because of their smaller volumes of distribution, small molecular weights, and aqueous solubility. These are drugs that are well described by a one-compartment model, and the hemodialysis removes drugs that are present in the central volume of distribution. In contrast, digoxin has a large volume of distribution and is well characterized by a two-compartment model, and phenytoin is highly bound to plasma proteins, making these drugs difficult to dialyze. Thus, dialysis is not very useful for treating digoxin intoxication, but is useful for salicylate overdose.

**TABLE 25-10** • Predicted Effects of Hemodialysis on Drug Half-Life and Removal in the Overdose Setting

| Drug | $V_D$ (L) | $CL$ (mL/min) | $CL_{DIAL}$ (mL/min) | $t_{1/2\,off}$ (h) | $t_{1/2\,on}$ (h) | FL[*] |
|------|-----------|---------------|----------------------|--------------------|-------------------|-------|
| Digoxin[†] | 560 | 150 | 20 | 43 | 38 | 0.07 |
| Digoxin[‡] | 300 | 40 | 20 | 86 | 58 | 0.05 |
| Ethchlorvynol | 300 | 35 | 60 | 99 | 36 | 0.07 |
| Phenobarbital | 50 | 5 | 70 | 115 | 8 | 0.30 |
| Phenytoin | 100 | 5 | 10 | 231 | 77 | 0.04 |
| Salicylic acid | 40 | 20 | 100 | 23 | 4 | 0.51 |

[*]FL = fraction lost during a dialysis period of 4 hours.
[†]Parameters for a patient with normal renal function.
[‡]Parameters for a patient with no renal function.
Reproduced with permission from Benet LZ, Massoud N, Gambertoglio JG: Pharmacokinetic Basis of Drug Treatment. New York, NY: Raven; 1984.

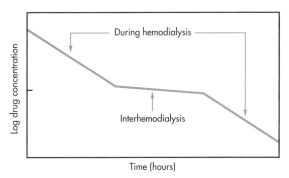

FIGURE 25-5 • Effect of dialysis on drug elimination.

An example of the effect of hemodialysis on drug elimination is shown in Fig. 25-5. During the interdialysis period, the patient's total body clearance is very low and the drug concentration declines slowly. In this example, the drug has an elimination $t_{1/2}$ of 48 hours during the interdialysis period. When the patient is placed on dialysis, the drug clearance (sum of the total body clearance and the dialysis clearance) removes the drug more rapidly.

## CLINICAL EXAMPLE

The aminoglycoside antibiotics, such as gentamicin and tobramycin, are eliminated primarily by the renal route, and their pharmacokinetics is well described by a one-compartment model. Dosing of these aminoglycosides is adjusted according to the residual renal function in the patient as estimated by creatinine clearance. During hemodialysis or peritoneal dialysis, the elimination half-lives for these antibiotics are significantly decreased. After dialysis, the aminoglycoside concentrations may be below the therapeutic range, and the patient may need to be given another dose of the aminoglycoside antibiotic.

Using the nomogram presented earlier relating creatinine clearance and the aminoglycoside clearance, a $V_D$ of 0.3 L/kg, and an elimination rate constant while on dialysis of 0.1 h$^{-1}$ ($k_{DIAL}$), address the following case study:

An adult male (73 years old, 65 kg) with diabetes mellitus receives 4-hour hemodialysis sessions three times a week (Mon/Wed/Fri). His residual creatinine clearance is approximately 2.5 mL/min. The attending physician wants to start a regimen of

gentamicin, an aminoglycoside antibiotic, in order to "synergize" the bactericidal activity of nafcillin 1 g IV q6h against a systemic infection of *S. aureus*. Today is Tuesday and the patient had his last hemodialysis session 24 hours earlier (Monday).

Assuming that peak levels of 3–5 mg/L are all that is necessary to synergize the activity of nafcillin against *S. aureus*, propose a dosing regimen of gentamicin that would be effective while associated with $C_{min}$ levels of less than 1 mg/L to avoid ototoxicity.

### Solution
The pharmacokinetic parameters for gentamicin based on population averages (nomograms) off dialysis in this patient may be:

$$V_D = 0.3 \text{ L/kg} = 0.3 \cdot 65 = 19.5 \text{ L}$$

$$CL = 0.0216 + 0.0648 \cdot CL_{CR} = 0.0216 + 0.0648 \cdot 2.5$$
$$= 0.1836 \text{ L/h}$$

$$k = CL/V_D = 0.1836/19.5 = 0.009415 \text{ h}^{-1}$$

$$t_{1/2} = 0.693/k = 73.6 \text{ h}$$

The elimination rate constant and clearance due to the dialysis may be:

$$k_{DIAL} = 0.1 \text{ h}^{-1}$$

$$CL_{DIAL} = k_{DIAL} \cdot V_D = 0.1 \cdot 19.5 = 1.95 \text{ L/h}$$

The pharmacokinetic parameters while on dialysis may therefore be:

$$CL_{ON} = CL + CL_{DIAL} = 1.95 + 0.1836 = 2.1336 \text{ L/h}$$

$V_D$ is unaffected at 19.5 L

$$k_{ON} = k + k_{DIAL} = 0.009415 + 0.1 = 0.109415 \text{ h}^{-1}$$

$$t_{1/2ON} = 0.693/k_{ON} = 6.33 \text{ h}$$

The patient can be started on a 60-mg dose of gentamicin, and this dose will be associated with a first $C_{max}$ of:

$$C_{max} = \text{Dose}/V_D = 60/19.5 = 3.08 \text{ mg/L}$$

In 24 hours (Wednesday, just before hemodialysis) the remaining systemic concentrations will be:

$$C = C_{max} \cdot \exp(-k \cdot t) = 3.08 \cdot \exp(-0.009415 \cdot 24)$$
$$= 2.45 \text{ mg/L}$$

After the 4-hour dialysis session (Wednesday), the remaining concentrations will be:

$$C = 3.27 \cdot \exp(-k_{ON} \cdot 4) = 1.58 \text{ mg/L}$$

This level is still significant and the concentrations should drop further (<1 mg/L) before another dose is given. The concentration before and after the next dialysis session will be (Friday):

Pre-dialysis: $C = 1.58 \cdot \exp(-k \cdot (48 - 4))$
$= 1.58 \cdot \exp(-0.009415 \cdot 44) = 1.05 \text{ mg/L}$

Post-dialysis: $C = 1.05 \cdot \exp(-k_{ON} \cdot 4)$
$= 1.05 \cdot \exp(-0.109415 \cdot 4) = 0.66 \text{ mg/L}$

Administering aminoglycosides in renally impaired patients is tricky, as concentrations stay above 1 mg/L for a very long time, and so these administrations can lead to ototoxicity (nephrotoxicity is obviously not a concern in this already renally impaired patient). Aminoglycosides should be given one dose at a time, and concentrations should be obtained to verify that the predictions are accurate. If they are and the predicted concentration of 0.66 mg/L is verified, a supplemental dose of 60 mg can then be given if the patient still needs the nafcillin treatment to be synergized; otherwise it can be stopped.

Assuming that the infection is still severe, and the gentamicin synergism is still desired, in order to reach a peak of approximately 3 mg, the following dose can be given post hemodialysis on the Friday:

$$C = \text{DOSE}/V_D + 0.66$$

Therefore, DOSE $= (3 - 0.66) \cdot 19.5 = 45.63 \sim 50 \text{ mg}$

The new $C_{max}$ after a 50-mg dose will therefore be:

$$C_{max} = 0.66 + 50/19.5 = 3.224 \text{ mg/L}$$

The remaining concentration the following Monday before dialysis will therefore be:

$$C = 3.224 \cdot \exp(-0.009415 \cdot (72 - 4)) = 1.70 \text{ mg/L}$$

After the 4-hour dialysis session, the remaining concentration may therefore be:

$$C = 1.70 \cdot \exp(-k_{ON} \cdot 4) = 1.10 \text{ mg/L}$$

## Hemoperfusion

*Hemoperfusion* is the process of removing drug by passing the blood from the patient through an adsorbent material and back to the patient. Hemoperfusion is a useful procedure for rapid drug removal in accidental poisoning and drug overdose. Because the drug molecules in the blood are in direct contact with the adsorbent material, any molecule that has great affinity for the adsorbent material will be removed. The two main adsorbents used in hemoperfusion include (1) activated charcoal, which adsorbs both polar and nonpolar drug, and (2) AmberLite resins. AmberLite resins, such as AmberLite XAD-2 and AmberLite XAD-4, are available as insoluble polymeric beads, with each bead containing an agglomerate of cross-linked polystyrene microspheres. The AmberLite resins have a greater affinity for nonpolar organic molecules than activated charcoal. The important factors for drug removal by hemoperfusion include affinity of the drug for the adsorbent, surface area of the adsorbent, absorptive capacity of the adsorbent, rate of blood flow through the adsorbent, and the equilibration rate of the drug from the peripheral tissue into the blood.

## Hemofiltration

An alternative to hemodialysis and hemoperfusion is hemofiltration. *Hemofiltration* is a process by which fluids, electrolytes, and small-molecular-weight substances are removed from the blood by means of low-pressure flow through hollow artificial fibers or flat-plate membranes (Bickley, 1988). Because fluid is also filtered out of the plasma during hemofiltration, replacement fluid is administered to the patient for volume replacement. Hemofiltration is a slow, continuous filtration process that removes nonprotein-bound small molecules (<10,000 Da) from the blood by convective mass transport. The clearance of the drug depends on the sieving coefficient and ultrafiltration rate. Hemofiltration provides a creatinine clearance of approximately 10 mL/min (Bickley, 1988) and may have limited use for drugs that are widely distributed in the body. A major problem with this method is the formation of blood clots within the hollow filter fibers.

## Continuous Renal Replacement Therapy

Because of the initial loss of fluid that results during hemofiltration, intermittent hemofiltration results in concentration of red blood cells in the resulting reduced plasma volume. Therefore, blood becomes more viscous with a high hematocrit and high colloid osmotic pressure at the distal end of the hemofilter. *Predilution* may be used to circumvent this problem, but this method is rarely used because of cost and inefficiency.

*Continuous replacement therapy* allows ongoing removal of fluid and toxins by relying on a patient's own blood pressure to pump blood through a filter. The continuous filtration is better tolerated by patients than intermittent therapy and provides optimal control of circulating volumes and ongoing toxin removal. Because continuous replacement therapies are hemofiltration methods, replacement fluid must be administered to the patient to replace fluid lost to the hemofiltrate, though the volume of fluid removed can be easily controlled compared to intermittent hemofiltration. Heparin infusions are also provided for anticoagulation.

*Continuous renal replacement therapy* (CRRT) includes *continuous veno-venous hemofiltration* (CVVH) and *continuous arteriovenous hemofiltration* (CAVH). In CAVH, blood passes through a hemofilter that is placed between a cannulated femoral artery and vein. A dialysis filter may be added to CAVH to improve small-molecule clearance. Circulating dialysate on the outside of the filters allows more efficient toxin removal. However, this method is inefficient (10–15 mL filtered per minute) and complex and is not widely used in comparison to CVVH.

CVVH provides a hemofilter that is placed between cannulated femoral, subclavian, or internal jugular veins. Rather than relying on arterial pressure to filter blood, a pump can be used to provide filtration rates greater than 100 mL/min. Like CAVH, a dialysis filter may be added to CVVH to improve clearance of small molecules.

As with other extracorporeal removal systems, hemofiltration methods can alter drug pharmacokinetics. A study by Hansen et al (2001) showed that acute renal failure patients on CVVH demonstrated a 50% decrease in clearance of levofloxacin. However, because of the large volume and moderate renal clearance of fluoroquinolones, levofloxacin does not require dosing adjustment.

## Drug Removal during Continuous Renal Replacement Therapy

During CAVH, solutes are removed by convection. The efficiency of the removal of drugs is related to the *sieving coefficient S*, which reflects the solute removal ability during hemofiltration and is equal to the ratio of solute concentration in the ultrafiltrate to the solute concentration in the retentate. When $S = 1$, the solute passes freely through the membrane. When $S = 0$, the solute is retained in the plasma. The $S$ is constant and independent of blood flow; therefore,

$$CL_{CAVH} = S \cdot rate_{UF} \qquad (25.34)$$

where rate$_{uf}$ is the ultrafiltration rate. The concentration of drug in the ultrafiltrate is also equal to the unbound drug concentration in the plasma. So, the amount of drug removed during CAVH is

$$\text{Amount removed per time unit} = C_p \cdot \alpha \cdot rate_{uf} \quad (25.35)$$

where $\alpha$ = the unbound fraction.

---

**FREQUENTLY ASKED QUESTION**

▶ Which pharmacokinetic properties of a drug would predict a greater or lesser rate of elimination in a patient undergoing hemo dialysis?

---

## EFFECT OF HEPATIC DISEASE ON PHARMACOKINETICS

Hepatic disease can alter drug pharmacokinetics, including its bioavailability and disposition as well as sometimes its pharmacodynamics, including efficacy and safety. Hepatic disease may include common hepatic diseases, such as alcoholic liver disease (cirrhosis) and chronic infections with hepatitis viruses B and C, and less common diseases, such as acute hepatitis D or E, primary biliary cirrhosis, primary sclerosing cholangitis, and $\alpha_1$-antitrypsin deficiency (FDA Guidance for Industry, 2003). In addition, drug-induced hepatotoxicity is the leading cause of acute liver failure in the United States (Chang and Schiano, 2007).

Drugs are often metabolized by one or more enzymes located in cellular membranes in different parts of the liver. Drugs and metabolites may also be excreted by biliary secretion. Hepatic disease may lead to drug accumulation, failure to form an active or inactive metabolite, increased bioavailability after oral administration, and other effects including possible alteration in drug–protein binding. Liver disease may also alter kidney function, which can lead to accumulation of a drug and its metabolites even when the liver is not primarily responsible for elimination.

The major difficulty in estimating hepatic clearance in patients with hepatic disease is the complexity and stratification of the liver enzyme systems. In contrast, creatinine clearance has been used successfully to measure kidney function and correlates very well with the renal clearance of drugs. Clinical laboratory tests measure only a limited number of liver functions. Some clinical laboratory tests, such as the *aspartate aminotransferase* (AST) and *alanine aminotransferases* (ALT), are common serum enzyme tests that detect liver cell damage rather than liver function. Other laboratory tests, such as serum bilirubin, are used to measure biliary obstruction or interference with bile flow. Presently, no single test accurately assesses the total liver function. Usually, a series of clinical laboratory tests are used in clinical practice to detect the presence of liver disease, distinguish among different types of liver disorders, gauge the extent of known liver damage, and follow the response to treatment. A few tests have been used to relate the severity of hepatic impairment to predicted changes in the pharmacokinetic profile of a drug (FDA Guidance for Industry, 2003). Examples of these tests include the ability of the liver to eliminate marker drugs such as antipyrine, indocyanine green, monoethylglycine-xylidide, and galactose. Furthermore, endogenous substrates, such as albumin or bilirubin, or a functional measure, such as prothrombin time, have been used for the evaluation of liver impairment. As we will see later, the main method currently used to classify the impact of hepatic function on a drug's clearance is a classification that was not originally built for that task, the Child–Pugh classification method. The Child–Pugh score is a composite ordinal score consisting of three laboratory-based biomarkers (serum albumin levels, serum bilirubin levels, and prothrombin time) and two clinically assessed variables (presence/degree of ascites and presence/degree of hepatic encephalopathy).

## Dosage Considerations in Hepatic Disease

Several physiologic and pharmacokinetic factors are relevant in considering dosage of a drug in patients with hepatic disease (Table 25-11). Chronic disease or tissue injury may change the accessibility of some enzymes as a result of redirection or detour of hepatic blood circulation. Liver disease affects the quantitative and qualitative synthesis of albumin, globulins, and other circulating plasma proteins that subsequently affect plasma drug–protein binding and distribution (see Chapter 5). As mentioned, most liver function tests indicate only that the liver has been damaged; they do not assess the function of the CYP enzymes or intrinsic clearance by the liver.

Unlike estimates of GFR (ie, creatinine clearance calculated by the Cockcroft–Gault equation or eGFR by MDRD equation), currently there is no readily available measure of hepatic function that can be applied to calculate appropriate doses. Information that may help guide dosing in patients with hepatic impairment is usually obtained by conducting PK/PD assessments based on hepatic function as determined by the Child–Pugh classification during drug development in clinical studies and may be available in the product labeling. If no recommendations for dosage adjustment based on Child–Pugh score are available in the labeling, the use of the drugs in patients with hepatic impairment should take into consideration pharmacokinetic characteristics and therapeutic index of the drugs, and the severity of hepatic dysfunction of the patients. Careful monitoring of the patients is warranted in some situations. For instance, drugs with flow-dependent clearance should be avoided if possible in patients with liver failure. When necessary, doses of these drugs may need to be reduced to as low as one-tenth of the conventional dose for an orally administered agent. Starting therapy with low doses and monitoring response or plasma levels provides the best opportunity for safe and efficacious treatment.

If some of the efflux proteins that normally protect the body against drug accumulation are reduced or not functioning, this could potentially cause hepatic drug injury as drug concentration begins

**TABLE 25-11** • Considerations in Dosing Patients with Hepatic Impairment

| Item | Comments |
|---|---|
| Nature and severity of liver disease | Not all liver diseases affect the pharmacokinetics of the drugs to the same extent. |
| Drug elimination | Drugs eliminated by the liver >20% are less likely to be affected by liver disease. Drugs that are eliminated mainly via renal route will be least affected by liver disease. |
| Route of drug administration | Oral drug bioavailability may be increased by liver disease due to decreased first-pass effects. |
| Protein binding | Drug–protein binding may be altered due to alteration in hepatic synthesis of albumin. |
| Hepatic blood flow | Drugs with flow-dependent hepatic clearance will be more affected by change in hepatic blood flow. |
| Intrinsic clearance | Metabolism of drugs with high intrinsic clearance may be impaired. |
| Biliary obstruction | Biliary excretion of some drugs and metabolites, particularly glucuronide metabolites, may be impaired. |
| Pharmacodynamic changes | Tissue sensitivity to drug may be altered. |
| Therapeutic range | Drugs with a wide therapeutic range will be less affected by moderate hepatic impairment. |

to increase. Compounds that form glucuronide, sulfate, glutathione (GSH), and other substrates that are involved in phase II metabolism (see Chapter 6) may be depleted during hepatic impairment, potentially interrupting the normal path of drug metabolism. Indeed, even albumin or alpha-1-acid glycoprotein (AAG) concentrations can be altered in hepatic impairment and affect drug distribution or drug disposition in many unpredictable ways that can affect drug safety.

### Fraction of Drug Metabolized

Drug elimination in the body may be divided into (1) fraction of drug excreted unchanged in the urine, $f_e$, and (2) fraction of drug metabolized, $f_m$. The latter is usually estimated from $1 - f_e$; alternatively, the fraction of drug metabolized may be estimated after IV administration from the ratio of $CL_H/CL$ should hepatic clearance $(CL_H)$ be known. Knowing the fraction of drug eliminated by the liver allows estimation of total body clearance when hepatic clearance is reduced. Drugs with low $f_e$ values (or conversely, drugs with a higher fraction of metabolized drug)

are more affected by a change in liver function due to hepatic disease.

$$CL_H = CL \cdot (1 - f_e) \qquad (25.36)$$

Equation 25.36 assumes that drug metabolism occurs only in the liver and that the unchanged drug is excreted in the urine. If there is no enzyme saturation and a drug exhibits linear kinetics, dosing adjustment may be based on residual hepatic function in patients with hepatic disease as shown in the following example.

### PRACTICE PROBLEM

The hepatic clearance of a drug in a patient is reduced by 50% due to chronic viral hepatitis. How is the total body clearance of the drug affected? What should be the new dose of the drug for the patient? Assume that the drug is only metabolized and transported in the liver, and that renal drug clearance $(f_e = 0.4)$ and plasma drug–protein binding are not altered.

## Solution

$$CL = CL_H + CL_R \text{ and } CL_R = f_e \cdot CL$$

so $CL_R = 0.4 \cdot CL$ and $CL_H = 0.6 \cdot CL$ in a normal patient

In a patient with 50% less hepatic function, the $CL_H$ will be equal to $0.3 \cdot CL$, and the total clearance will therefore equal $0.4 + 0.3 = 0.7$ or 70% of the normal clearance.

Because Dose $= CL \cdot AUC$, the dose will have to be decreased by 30% to reach the same overall systemic exposure (AUC).

An example of a correlation established between actual residual liver function (as assessed by measuring galactose blood concentration one hour after galactose administration) and hepatic clearance was reported for cefoperazone (Hu et al, 1995) and other drugs in patients with cirrhosis. The method should be applied only to drugs that have linear pharmacokinetics or low protein binding, or that are non-restrictively eliminated (ie, drugs whose hepatic clearance is flow-limited and have extraction ratios > 0.7).

Many variables can complicate dose correction when drug–protein binding profoundly affects distribution, elimination, and penetration of the drug to the active site. For drugs with restrictive elimination (ie, drugs whose hepatic clearance is limited by protein binding and have extraction ratios < 0.3), the fraction of free drug must be used to correct the change in free drug concentration and the change in free drug clearance. In some cases, the increase in free drug may be partly offset by a larger volume of distribution as a result of decrease in protein binding, leading to no or minimal change in pharmacokinetic and/or pharmacodynamic response.

## Active Drug and the Metabolite

For many drugs, both the drug and the metabolite contribute to the overall therapeutic response of the patient to the drug. The concentration of both the drug and the metabolite in the body should be known. When the pharmacokinetic parameters of the metabolite and the drug are similar, the overall activity of the drug can become more or less potent as a result of a change in liver function; that is, (1) when the drug is more potent than the metabolite,

the overall pharmacologic activity will increase in the hepatic-impaired patient because the parent drug concentration will be higher, and (2) when the drug is less potent than the metabolite, the overall pharmacologic activity in the hepatic patient will decrease because less of the active metabolite is formed.

Changes in pharmacologic activity due to hepatic disease may be much more complex when both the pharmacokinetic parameters and the pharmacodynamics of the drug change as a result of the disease process. In such cases, the overall pharmacodynamic response may be greatly modified, making it necessary to monitor the response change with the aid of a pharmacodynamic model (see Chapters 11 and 22). For example, a decrease in pharmacodynamic effect has been observed for the diuretic furosemide in patients with cirrhosis (Keller et al, 1981; Villeneuve et al, 1986). The reduced pharmacodynamic effect was caused by a decrease in renal clearance of unchanged furosemide, which changes in proportion to the reduction in the GFR as well as a decrease in maximum rate of sodium excretion that was proportionally greater than the reduction in creatinine clearance (Villeneuve et al, 1986).

## Hepatic Blood Flow and Intrinsic Clearance

Blood flow changes can occur in patients with chronic liver disease (often due to viral hepatitis or chronic alcohol use). In some patients with severe liver cirrhosis, fibrosis of liver tissue may occur, resulting in intra- or extrahepatic shunt. Hepatic arterial-venous shunts may lead to reduced fraction of drug extracted (see Chapter 15) and an increase in the bioavailability of drug. In other patients, resistance to blood flow may be increased as a result of tissue damage and fibrosis, causing a reduction in intrinsic hepatic clearance.

The following equation from the well-stirred hepatic model may be applied to estimate hepatic clearance of a drug after assessing changes in blood flow and intrinsic clearance ($CL_{int}$):

$$CL_H = Q_H \cdot f_u \cdot CL_{int(u)}/(Q_H + f_u \cdot CL_{int(u)}) \qquad (25.37)$$

Alternatively, when both $Q_H$ and the hepatic extraction ratio, $E_H$, are both known in the patient, $CL_H$ may also be estimated:

$$CL_H = Q_H \cdot E_H \qquad (25.38)$$

Unlike changes in renal disease, in which serum creatinine concentration may be used to monitor relatively small changes in renal function such as GFR, there are no pharmacodynamic markers known that enables one to monitor changes in hepatic function. The only classification that is used commonly is the Child–Pugh, and we will see that it provides only three different levels of hepatic function (normal, moderate, and severe).

## Pathophysiologic Assessment

In practice, patient information about changes in hepatic blood flow may not be available. Special electromagnetic (Nuxmalo et al, 1978) or ultrasound techniques are required to measure blood flow and are not routinely available. The clinician/pharmacist may have to make an empirical estimate of the blood flow change after examining the patient and reviewing the available liver function tests.

Various approaches have been used to assess hepatic impairment. The *Child–Pugh* (or Child–Turcotte–Pugh) score assesses the overall hepatic impairment as normal/mild, moderate, or severe (Figg et al, 1995). The score employs five clinical measures of liver disease, including total bilirubin, serum albumin, international normalized ratio (INR), ascites, and hepatic encephalopathy (Tables 25-12 and 25-13). Different publications use different measures. Some older references substitute prothrombin time (PT) prolongation for INR.

### TABLE 25-12 • Child–Pugh Classification of Severity of Liver Disease

| Parameter | Points Assigned | | |
|---|---|---|---|
| | 1 | 2 | 3 |
| Ascites | Absent | Slight | Moderate |
| Bilirubin, mg/dL | ≤ 2 | 2–3 | >3 |
| Albumin, g/dL | >3.5 | 2.8–3.5 | <2.8 |
| Prothrombin time | | | |
| Seconds over control | 1–3 | 4–6 | >6 |
| INR | <1.8 | 1.8–2.3 | >2.3 |
| Encephalopathy | None | Grade 1–2 | Grade 3–4 |

*Data from Trey C, Burns DG, Saunders SJ. Treatment of hepatic coma by exchange blood transfusion, N Engl J Med. 1966 Mar 3;274(9):473–481.*

### TABLE 25-13 • Severity Classification Schemes for Liver Disease

| | Child–Turcotte Classification | | |
|---|---|---|---|
| | Grade A | Grade B | Grade C |
| Bilirubin (mg/dL) | <2.0 | 2.0–3.0 | >3.0 |
| Albumin (g/dL) | >3.5 | 3.0–3.5 | <3.0 |
| Ascites | None | Easily controlled | Poorly controlled |
| Neurological disorder | None | Minimal | Advanced |
| Nutrition | Excellent | Good | Poor |

*Data from Evans WE, Schewtag, J, Jusko, J: Applied Pharmacokinetics—Principles of Therapeutic Drug Monitoring. Baltimore, MD: Lippincott Williams & Wilkins; 1992.*

The original classification used nutrition, which was later replaced by PT prolongation. The model for end-stage liver disease (MELD) is a scoring system for assessing the severity of chronic liver disease based on mortality after liver surgery (Cholongitas et al, 2005; Kamath and Kim, 2007). While neither of these approaches for assessing hepatic disease and hepatic impairment provides a measurement that can be used quantitatively for determining dose adjustments, the Child–Pugh classification has been used in evaluating drug PK/PD in clinical studies and to inform dosing in patients with hepatic impairment.

While chronic hepatic disease is more likely to change the metabolism of a drug (Howden et al, 1989), acute hepatitis due to hepatotoxin or viral inflammation is often associated with marginal or less severe changes in metabolic drug clearance (Farrell et al, 1978). The clinician should make an assessment based on acceptable risk criteria on a case-by-case basis.

In general, basic pharmacokinetics treats the body globally and more readily applies to dosing estimation. However, drug clearance based on individual eliminating organs is more informative and provides more insight into the pharmacokinetic changes in the disease process. While the hepatic blood flow model (see Chapter 15) is useful for predicting changes in hepatic clearance resulting from alterations in hepatic blood flow, $Q_a$ and $Q_v$, extrahepatic changes can also influence pharmacokinetics

**TABLE 25-14 •** Drugs with Significantly Decreased Metabolism in Chronic Liver Disease

| | |
|---|---|
| Antipyrine | Caffeine |
| Cefoperazone | Chlordiazepoxide |
| Chloramphenicol | Diazepam |
| Erythromycin | Hexobarbital |
| Metronidazole | Lidocaine |
| Meperidine | Metoprolol |
| Pentazocine | Propranolol |
| Tocainide | Theophylline |
| Verapamil | Promazine |

*Data from Howden et al (1989), Williams (1983), and Hu et al. (1995).*

in hepatic-impaired patients. Global changes in distribution may occur outside the liver. Extrahepatic metabolism and other hemodynamic changes may also occur and can be accounted for more completely by monitoring total body clearance of the drug using basic pharmacokinetics. For example, lack of local change in hepatic drug clearance should not be prematurely interpreted as "no change" in overall drug clearance. Reduced albumin and AAG, for example, may change the volume of distribution of the drug and therefore alter total body clearance on a global basis.

Chronic liver disease has been shown to decrease the metabolism of many drugs, as shown in Table 25-14. However, the amount of decrease in metabolism is difficult to assess.

## EXAMPLE ▷ ▷ ▷

After IV bolus administration of 1 g of cefoperazone to normal and chronic hepatitis patients, urinary excretion of cefoperazone was significantly increased in cirrhosis patients, from 23.95% ± 5.06% for normal patients to 51.09% ± 11.50% in cirrhosis patients (Hu et al, 1995). Explain **(a)** why there is a change in the percent of unchanged cefoperazone excreted in the urine of patients with cirrhosis, and **(b)** suggest a quantitative test to monitor the hepatic elimination of cefoperazone. (*Hint:* Consult Hu et al, 1994.)

## Liver Function Tests and Hepatic Metabolic Markers

Drug markers used to measure residual hepatic function may correlate well with hepatic clearance of one drug but correlate poorly with another substrate metabolized by a different CYP enzyme. Some useful endogenous markers of hepatic function are listed below:

1. *Aminotransferase* (normal ALT: male, 10–55 U/L; female, 7–30 U/L; normal AST: male, 10–40 U/L; female, 9–25 U/L): Aminotransferases are enzymes found in many tissues that include serum aspartate aminotransferase (AST, formerly SGOT) and alanine aminotransferase (ALT, formerly SGPT). ALT is liver specific, but AST is found in liver and many other tissues, including cardiac and skeletal muscles. Leakage of aminotransferases into the plasma is used as an indicator for many types of hepatic disease and hepatitis. The AST/ALT ratio is used in differential diagnosis. In acute liver injury, AST/ALT is ≤1, whereas in alcoholic hepatitis the AST/ALT >2.

2. *Alkaline phosphatase* (normal: male, 45–115 U/L; female, 30–100 U/L): Like aminotransferase, alkaline phosphatase (AP) is normally present in many tissues, and it is also present on the canalicular domain of the hepatocyte plasma membrane. Plasma AP may be elevated in hepatic disease because of increased AP production and released into the serum. In cholestasis, or bile flow obstruction, AP release is facilitated by bile acid solubilization of the membranes. Marked AP elevations may indicate hepatic tumors or biliary obstruction in the liver, or disease in other tissues such as bone, placenta, or intestine.

3. *Bilirubin* (normal total = 0–1.0 mg/dL: direct = 0–0.4 mg/dL): Bilirubin consists of both a water-soluble, conjugated, "direct" fraction and a lipid-soluble, unconjugated, "indirect" fraction. The unconjugated form is bound to albumin and is therefore not filtered by the kidney. Since impaired biliary excretion results in increases in conjugated (filtered) bilirubin, hepatobiliary disease can result in increases in urinary bilirubin. Unconjugated hyperbilirubinemia results from either increased bilirubin production or

defects in hepatic uptake or conjugation. Conjugated hyperbilirubinemia results from defects in hepatic excretion.

4. *Prothrombin time* (PT; normal, 11.2–13.2 s): With the exception of Factor VIII, all coagulation factors are synthesized by the liver. Therefore, hepatic disease can alter coagulation. Decreases in PT (the rate of conversion of prothrombin to thrombin) are suggestive of acute or chronic liver failure or biliary obstruction. Vitamin K is also important in coagulation, so Vitamin K deficiency can also decrease PT.

## EXAMPLE ▷ ▷ ▷

Paclitaxel, an anticancer agent for solid tumors and leukemia, has extensive tissue distribution, high plasma protein binding (approximately 90%–95%), and variable systemic clearance. Average paclitaxel clearance ranges from 87 to 503 mL/min/m$^2$ (5.2–30.2 L/h/m$^2$), with minimal renal excretion (10%) of the parent drug (Sonnichsen and Relling, 1994). Paclitaxel is extensively metabolized by the liver to three primary metabolites. CYP2C8 and CYP3A enzymes appear to be involved in hepatic metabolism of paclitaxel. What are the precautions in administering paclitaxel to patients with liver disease?

### Solution

Although paclitaxel has first-order pharmacokinetics at normal doses, its elimination may be saturable in some patients with genetically reduced intrinsic clearance due to reduced CYP3A or CYP2C8 activity. The clinical importance of saturable elimination will be greatest when large dosages are infused over a shorter period of time. In these situations, achievable plasma concentrations are likely to cause saturation of binding. Thus, small changes in dosage or infusion duration may result in disproportionately large alterations in paclitaxel systemic exposure, potentially influencing patient response and toxicity.

## Hepatic Impairment and Dose Adjustment

Hepatic impairment may not sufficiently alter the pharmacokinetics of some drugs to require dosage adjustment. Drugs that have the following properties are less likely to need dosage adjustment in patients with hepatic impairment (FDA Guidance for Industry, 2003):

- The drug is excreted entirely via renal routes of elimination with no involvement of the liver.
- The drug is metabolized in the liver to a small extent (<20%), and the therapeutic range of the drug is wide, so that modest impairment of hepatic clearance will not lead to toxicity of the drug directly or by increasing its interaction with other drugs.
- The drug is gaseous or volatile, and the drug and its active metabolites are primarily eliminated via the lungs.

For each drug case, the clinician needs to assess the degree of hepatic impairment and consider the known pharmacokinetics and pharmacodynamics of the drug. For example, Mallikaarjun et al (2008) studied the effects of hepatic or renal impairment on the pharmacokinetics of aripiprazole (Abilify), an atypical antipsychotic used to treat schizophrenia. These investigators concluded that there were no meaningful differences in aripiprazole pharmacokinetics between groups of subjects with normal hepatic or renal function and those with either hepatic or renal impairment. Thus, dose adjustment of the aripiprazole does not appear to be required in populations with hepatic or renal impairment.

In contrast, Muirhead et al (2002) studied the effects of age and renal and hepatic impairments on the pharmacokinetics, tolerability, and safety of sildenafil (Viagra), a drug used to treat erectile dysfunction. They observed significant differences in $C_{max}$ and AUC between the young and the elderly subjects for both the parent drug and the metabolite. In addition, the hepatic impairment study demonstrated that pharmacokinetics of sildenafil was altered in subjects with chronic stable cirrhosis, as shown by a 46% reduction in $CL/F$ and a 47% increase in $C_{max}$ compared with subjects with normal hepatic function. Sildenafil pharmacokinetics was affected by age and by renal and hepatic impairments, suggesting that a lower starting dose of 25 mg should be considered for patients with severely compromised renal or hepatic function.

---

**FREQUENTLY ASKED QUESTIONS**

▶ Why do changes in drug–protein binding affect dose adjustment in patients with renal and/or hepatic disease?

▶ Which pharmacokinetic properties of a drug are more likely to be affected by renal disease or liver hepatotoxicity?

▶ Can you quantitatively predict the change in the pharmacokinetics of a drug that normally has high hepatic clearance in a patient with hepatic impairment? Explain.

---

## CHAPTER SUMMARY

The kidney and liver are important organs involved in regulating body fluids, electrolyte balance, removal of metabolic waste, and drug excretion from the body. Impairment of kidney or liver function affects the pharmacokinetics of drugs as well as safety and efficacy. Renal function may be assessed by several methods. Creatinine clearance calculated by using the serum concentration of endogenous creatinine is used most often to measure GFR. Creatinine clearance values must be considered carefully in special populations such as elderly, obese, and emaciated patients. The Cockcroft–Gault method is frequently used to estimate creatinine clearance from serum creatinine concentration. Dose adjustment in renal disease is based on the fraction of drug that is really excreted and generally assumes that nonrenal drug elimination remains constant. Different approaches for dose adjustment in renal disease give somewhat different values. Patients with ESRD and other patients without kidney function require supportive treatment such as dialysis to remove the

accumulated drug and its metabolites. The objective of these dialysis methods is to rapidly remove the undesirable drugs and metabolites from the body without disturbing the fluid and electrolyte balance in the patient. Dosage adjustment may be needed to replace drug loss during extracorporeal drug and metabolite removal. The major difficulty in estimating hepatic clearance in patients with hepatic disease is the complexity and stratification of the liver enzyme systems. Presently, no single test accurately assesses the total liver function. Various approaches such as the Child–Pugh (or Child–Turcotte–Pugh) score have been used diagnostically to assess hepatic impairment. Hepatic impairment may not sufficiently alter the pharmacokinetics of some drugs to require dosage adjustment. Physicians and/or pharmacists must understand the pharmacokinetic and pharmacodynamic properties of each drug in patients with hepatic and/or renal impairment for proper dose adjustment.

---

## LEARNING QUESTIONS

1. The normal dosing schedule for a patient on tetracycline is 250 mg PO (by mouth) every 6 hours. Suggest a dosage regimen for this patient when laboratory analysis shows that his renal function has deteriorated from a $CL_{CR}$ of 90 mL/min to a $CL_{CR}$ of 20 mL/min.

2. A patient receiving antibiotic treatment is on dialysis. The flow rate of serum into the kidney machine is 50 mL/min. Assays show that the concentration of drug entering the machine is 5 $\mu$g/mL and the concentration of drug in the serum leaving the machine is 2.5 $\mu$g/mL. The drug clearance for this patient is 10 mL/min. To what extent should the dose be increased if the average concentration of the antibiotic is to be maintained?

3. A patient excreted 0.9 L of urine in 24 hours, with a urinary creatinine concentration of 0.5 mg/mL, and an associated mid-point serum creatinine of 2.2 mg/dL. What is the *measured* creatinine clearance in that patient? How would you adjust the dose of a drug that is eliminated unchanged in the urine at 50% and normally given at 100 mg every 6 hours in a "normal" patient having a GFR of 100 mL/min?

4. A patient is to receive 1000 mg of ceftriaxone for the treatment of a respiratory infection every 12 hours. The patient has a creatinine clearance of 20 mL/min. Should the dosing regimen be modified? According to the approved drug label, ceftriaxone is 33% to 67% eliminated unchanged in the urine.

5. Calculate the creatinine clearance for a woman (38 years old, 62 kg) whose serum creatinine is 1.8 mg/dL using the nomogram method of Cockcroft–Gault.

6. Would you adjust the normal dose of piperacillin (4g IV every 4 hours), an antibiotic that has a reported $k_R$ of 0.413 h$^{-1}$ and a $k_{NR}$ of 0.165 h$^{-1}$ for the patient in Question 5? If so, why?

7. What assumptions are usually made when adjusting a dosage regimen according to the creatinine clearance in a patient with renal failure?

8. A patient suffers from a systemic infection of *E. Coli* for which gentamicin will be needed.

   a. Using the nomogram proposed for dosing gentamicin and tobramycin using a one-compartment model in the chapter (ie, $CL = 0.0216 + 0.0648 \times CL_{creat}$, and $V = 0.3$ L/kg), propose an initial dosing regimen to achieve an $AUC_{\tau(ss)}$ 24 h of 50 mg h/L for a 70-year-old male patient of 72 kg and having a serum creatinine of 1 mg/dL.

   b. The first maximum concentration after the end of a 30-minute infusion comes back at 12 mg/L and a concentration 12 hours after dosing is 1.5. Understanding that the MIC for the *E. coli* of this patient came back at 0.5 mg/L, that the post-antibiotic effect is expected to last for a maximum of 6 hours, that the safe maximum peak concentration can be up to 20 mg/L while the $C_{min}$ should be as low as possible and lower than 1 mg/L to avoid oto and nephrotoxicity, state whether the dosing regimen will need to be adjusted or not after this first dose (reference: Ducharme MP. Chapter 45: Principes d'utilisation des antibiotiques. In: Calop J (ed). Pharmacie Clinique et Therapeutique. Paris: Masson. 2008.)

9. A single intravenous bolus injection (1 g) of an antibiotic was given to a male anephric patient (age 68 years, 75 kg). During the next 48 hours, the elimination half-life of the antibiotic was 16 hours. The patient was then placed on hemodialysis for 8 hours and the elimination half-life was reduced to 4 hours.

   a. How much drug was eliminated by the end of the dialysis period? Calculate the elimination rate of the patient and what is due to the dialysis.

   b. Assuming the apparent volume of distribution of this antibiotic is 0.5 L/kg, what was the plasma drug concentration just before and just after dialysis?

10. After assessment of the renal impairment condition of a patient, the drug dosage regimen may be adjusted by one of two methods: **(a)** by keeping the dose constant and prolonging the dosage interval, τ, or **(b)** by decreasing the dose and maintaining the dosage interval constant. Discuss the advantages and disadvantages of adjusting the dosage regimen using either method.

## ANSWERS

**Frequently Asked Questions**

*How does renal impairment affect the pharmacokinetics of a drug that is primarily eliminated by hepatic clearance?*

■ For simplicity purposes and for adjusting dosing regimens of drugs in patients with renal-impairment, we often assume that intestinal and liver metabolism and transport of drugs are unaffected. While this is a reasonable assumption to make in mild-to-moderate renal impairment, patients with severe renal impairment often display an associated decrease in intestinal and liver metabolism, which may be due to several factors, including the degree of uremia, the presence of several circulating toxins, as well as a potential reduced gene expression for CYP enzymes, for example (*Ladda MA, Goralski KB. The Effects of CKD on Cytochrome P450-Mediated Drug Metabolism. Adv Chronic Kidney Dis. 2016 Mar;23(2):67-75. doi: 10.1053/j.ackd.2015.10.002. PMID: 26979145.*).

*What are the main factors that influence drug dosing in renal disease?*

■ The main factor influencing drug dosing in renal disease is the alteration in the renal clearance of the drug. We typically do not consider that any significant change in the non-renal clearance of drug and in protein binding (affecting the volume of distribution) will occur until severe renal impairment is seen. Therefore, for at least mild-to-moderate renal impairment, the decrease in the overall clearance of the drug that is due to a lesser renal clearance will affect the daily dose to administer (as $CL/F = \text{DOSE}/AUC_{inf}$), and the therapeutic interval may also have to be enlarged (as $CL/F = k_{10} \times V_c/F$, where $V_c/F$ is expected to stay unchanged, so changes in $CL/F$ due to reduced $CL_R$ will decrease $k_{10}$).

*Why is creatinine clearance used in renal disease?*

■ The creatinine clearance is used medically to estimate what the glomerular filtration rate (GFR) may be in a patient. The measured creatinine clearance is the preferred method for this, although because creatinine is also known to be secreted in addition to being filtered, the measured creatinine clearance is known to overestimate the true GFR.

*What patient-specific factors influence the accuracy of $CL_{CR}$ estimates?*

■ Diet and salt intake will affect creatinine clearance.

*How is $CL_{CR}$ determined?*

■ The measured $CL_{CR}$ is typically calculated using the "mid-point clearance formula." It is usually calculated by measuring the clearance of creatinine over a 24-hour period.

*What are the advantages and disadvantages of using a nomogram such as the C&G using serum creatinine concentrations for the estimation of renal function?*

■ The advantages of the C&G method are that it is simple, it enables a quick estimation of renal function, and it provides a sound basis for adjusting dosing regimens of drugs because it is the most commonly used method in approved drug labels. The disadvantages of the method are that it is not always accurate enough as a measure of the glomerular filtration rate (GFR) because serum creatinine can be affected by diet, exercise, drug-lab interactions, and because creatinine is secreted in addition to being filtered.

*What is the most accurate approach for the estimation of glomerular filtration rate?*

■ Inulin clearance, through its actual calculations using plasma concentration measurements after constant intravenous infusion, is an accurate approach for the estimation of GFR, as inulin is only filtered. Creatinine clearance using the mid-point method and 24-hour urinary excretion measurements is often used, because it is practically simpler. The resulting GFR will however be overestimated because creatinine is secreted in addition to being filtered.

*Why does each method based on serum creatinine concentrations for dosage adjustment in renal impairment give somewhat different values?*

■ Each proposed method is a nomogram that was developed statistically based on a specific patient population. A nomogram provides only a mean or median value for a population based on the clinical covariates specified in the formula (eg, with the C&G method, based on age, actual body weight, and gender). They are therefore not meant to be exact methods, and their prediction will be associated with a certain degree of uncertainty.

*What are some of the PK/PD considerations that one needs to consider when adjusting a dosing regimen in a renally impaired patient?*

■ When efficacy and safety only relate with the overall systemic exposure ($AUC_{\tau(ss)}$), the dosing regimen of a drug product in a patient with renal impairment can be adjusted simply by modifying the daily dose to administer, as Dose = $CL/F \times AUC_{\tau(ss)}$. Should efficacy and safety also relate to $C_{max}$ and $C_{min}$, such as with antiviral and anti-infective agents, the dosing interval will also have to be adjusted.

*Which pharmacokinetic properties of a drug would predict a greater or lesser rate of elimination in a patient undergoing hemodialysis?*

■ Hemodialysis removes drugs that are polar, are well described by a one-compartment model, and that exist mostly in an unbound form in the systemic circulation. The properties of a drug that would predict a greater rate of elimination are therefore those associated with a one-compartment model (ie, small volume of distribution, short elimination half-life), and when the drug is not much bound to plasma proteins. In contrast, drugs that are associated with a long elimination half-life and a large volume of distribution (indicative of multi-compartment pharmacokinetics), and those that are highly bound to plasma proteins will have their rate of elimination less affected by hemodialysis as they will not be removed easily.

*Why do changes in drug–protein binding affect dose adjustment in patients with renal and/or hepatic disease?*

■ Only free drug is filtered by the kidney and metabolized in the liver. In addition, only the free drug concentrations relate to efficacy and safety. Changes in protein-binding will therefore affect dose adjustments in patients with renal and/or hepatic disease.

*Which pharmacokinetic properties of a drug are more likely to be affected by renal disease or liver hepatotoxicity?*

■ Among main PK parameters (bioavailability, clearance, volume of distribution, and elimination half-life), and unless it is severe, renal disease only affects the renal component of the total body clearance without affecting bioavailability and volumes of distribution. The elimination half-life is therefore affected as well, as clearance changes while the volume of distribution does not.

■ Hepatic disease results in more complex changes, as protein binding, metabolism, and transport are all affected. In severe hepatic disease, renal impairment can also be seen (hepatorenal syndrome). Protein binding changes will affect the volume of distribution of drugs, while decrease in enzymatic and transporter activity will affect bioavailability and clearance. Because free drug exposure relates to safety and efficacy, it is important to follow free drug concentrations in patients with liver disease.

*Can you quantitatively predict the change in the pharmacokinetics of a drug that normally has high hepatic clearance in a patient with hepatic impairment? Explain.*

■ A quantitative prediction of the changes in the pharmacokinetics of any drug using the 'well-stirred" model can be made. Although it provides only an approximation, as it is not exact like $CL/F = \text{DOSE}/AUC_{\tau(ss)}$, the formulas of the well-stirred model have been proven to be reasonable compared to those of more complicated models such as the parallel tube or the sinusoidal parallel tube models for predicting the results of drug–drug interaction studies. Using these formulas, assumed changes in free drug fraction ($f_u$) and enzymatic activity ($CL_{int(u)}$), depending on the level of hepatic impairment that is seen in a patient using the Child-Pugh classification, for example, can be set to predict what any pharmacokinetic parameter value may be.

## Learning Questions

1. Tetracycline is reported to be eliminated unchanged in the urine ($f_e$) between 30% and 50% of the dose based on approved FDA drug labels. Assuming the dosing regimen of 250 mg every 6 hours was optimized for this patient, and therefore that the exposure was ideal when the $CL_{CR}$ was 90 mL/min, the impact of the decrease in $CL_{CR}$ to 20 mL/min will only be in the $CL_R$ and not in the $CL_{NR}$. Therefore:

> $CL/F = \text{DOSE} / AUC$ with the dose being 1 g per day originally (250 mg q. 6 hours). The change in $CL/F$ will have to be exactly reflected by a change in the daily dosage, as we will want to keep AUC exactly the same.
>
> Where $CL = CL_{NR} + CL_R$ and where $CL_R = f_e \times CL$
>
> Therefore, the $CL_R$ is now 20/90 (22.22%) of what it was before. As the $CL_R$ accounts

for 30% to 55% of the total clearance, and the $CL_{NR}$ should be unchanged, the new $CL$ should range between these two estimates:

- If $f_e$ = 30%, $(0.7+0.3\times 0.2222) = 0.7666$ or 76.66% of what it was.
- If $f_e$=55%, $(0.45+0.55\times0.2222) = 0.5722$ or 57.22% of what it was.

The total daily dose to administer to get the same overall exposure should therefore range between 766 and 572 mg per day. Tetracycline is available in immediate formulations of 250 mg and 500 mg strengths, and so therefore the dosing regimen of 250 mg q. 6 hours (1000 mg per day) could be changed to a dosing regimen of 250 mg q. 8 hours (750 mg per day).

2. This patient is on dialysis and can be assumed to have no renal component to its clearance left. So in this patient, the $CL$ of 10 mL/min (or more appropriately 0.6 L/h) reflects the $CL_{NR}$.

When the patient is off dialysis, the $CL \sim CL_{NR}$, while when it is on dialysis, the $CL \sim CL_{DIAL} + CL_{NR}$.

The assay results show that the drug is removed at 50% through a flow rate of 50 mL/min, so the $CL_{DIAL}$ is $(50 \times 60/1000) \times 0.5 = 1.5$ L/h

So the $CL$ will be 0.6 L/h when off dialysis, while it will be 2.1 L/h (ie, 0.6 + 1.5), an increase of 3.5-fold.

Should the drug be given by a constant infusion, then the dosing rate of infusion of the drug would have to be increased by 3.5-fold only while on dialysis, so that the $C_{ss}$ would not be affected.

If the drug is given once a day, and the dialysis is only occurring two or three times a week for a few hour sessions, the drug product should therefore be given once a day at the time when dialysis stops, not before it starts. For example, if dialysis occurs between 8 and 12h00, then the drug product could be administered every day at 12h00. It would not serve any purpose to administer the drug just before the dialysis sessions, as it would be completely removed by dialysis and the remaining exposure for the rest of the day would then be too small.

3. The $CL_{creat}$ in this patient can be calculated using the mid-point $CL$ formula, where $CL = U \times V/P$, where U represents the urine creatinine concentration, V the urinary volume, and P the mid-point systemic concentration.

$CL_{creat} = 0.9$ L $\times$ 500 mg/L / 22 mg/L = 20.45 L/24 h or 14.2 mL/min

The $CL_R$ of the drug is therefore 14.2% of what it should be, while the $CL_{NR}$ should stay unchanged. The overall $CL$ will therefore be $0.5 + 0.5 \times 0.142 = 0.571$ or 57% of what we would expect in a "normal" patient. The daily dose therefore needs to be 57% of the normal daily dose in order to reach the same daily systemic exposure. The dosing regimen can therefore be changed to 100 mg every 12 hours instead of 100 mg every 6 hours.

4. The $CL_R$ of the drug is therefore 20% of what it should be ($CL_{creat}$ of 20 mL/min instead of 100), while the $CL_{NR}$ should stay unchanged. Assuming a mean fe of 50% (range of 33% to 67%), the overall $CL$ will therefore be $0.5 + 0.5\times0.2 = 0.6$ or 60% of what we would expect in a "normal" patient. The daily dose therefore needs to be 60% of the normal daily dose in order to reach the same daily systemic exposure. The dosing regimen can therefore be changed from 1000 mg every 24 hours instead of 1000 mg every 12 hours.

5. $CL_{creat}$(C&G) = $(140 - AGE) \times$ ABW/$(72 \times S_{creat})$ $\times 0.85 = 41.5$ mL/min

6. Yes, of course we would need to adjust the dosing regimen in order to ensure that this patient receives a safe and effective dosing regimen.

This patient has a renal function that is approximately 41.5% from the expected normal one (ie, $CL_{creat}$ of 41.5 versus 100 mL/min). The $CL_R$ will therefore be 41.5% of what it should be, while the $CL_{NR}$ can be expected to be similar. The volume of distribution should not be affected, so all differences that are seen in $k_R$ will be reflected in $CL_R$.

Therefore, the $CL_R$ of the drug will be 41.5% of what it should be, while the $CL_{NR}$ should stay unchanged. The $f_e$ can be calculated to be $k_R/(k_R + k_{NR}) = 0.413/(0.165 + 0.413) = 0.715$ or 71.5%. The overall $CL$ will therefore be 0.285 + 0.715 $\times$ (41.5/100) = 0.58 or 58% of what we would expect in a "normal" patient. The daily dose therefore needs to be 58% of the normal daily dose in order to reach the same daily systemic exposure (14 g per day instead of 24 g per day). The dosing regimen can therefore be changed to 3500 mg every 6 hours instead of 4000 mg every 4 hours.

7. The usual assumptions that are made are that protein binding and therefore volumes of distribution are not affected, and that the non-renal clearance is also not affected.

8. a) The predicted population parameters for this patient based on the nomogram are:

   - Volume of distribution, $V = 0.3 \times 72 = 21.6$ L
   - Creatinine clearance, $CL_{CREAT} = (140 - 70) \times 72/72 \times 1 = 70$ mL/min
   - Clearance, $CL = CL_{NR} + CL_R = 0.0216 + 0.0648 \times CL_{creat} = 4.56$ L/h
   - Elimination half-life, $T_{1/2} = 0.693/(CL/V) = 0.693/(4.56/21.6) = 3.28$ h
   - Dose to administer per day to achieve an $AUC_{0-24(ss)}$ of: DOSE $= AUC \times CL = 50 \times 4.56 = 228$ mg. The dose can therefore be rounded to 220 mg for ease of dosing.

   b) Using a one-compartment model, the PK parameters in this patient can now be calculated:

$$k = (\ln(C1) - \ln(C2))/(t2 - t1)$$
$$= (\ln(12) - \ln(1.5))/(12 - 0.5) = 0.180 \text{ h}^{-1}$$
$$t_{1/2} = 0.693/k = 0.693/0.180 = 3.83$$

The $C_{max}$ is seen at the end of infusion, so it was 12 mg/L, while the $C_{min}$ will be just before the 2nd dose, so 23.5 hours later. Therefore, $C_{min} = C_{max} \times \exp(-k \times t) = 12 \times \exp(-0.18 \times 23.5) = 0.175$ mg/L

The time at which the MIC (0.5 mg/L) will have been reached from this minimum concentration (0.175) will be: $t2 - t1 = (\ln(C1) - \ln(C2))/k = (\ln(0.5) - \ln(0.175))/0.18 = 5.83$ hours.

No changes are therefore necessary. The peak concentration is more than 10 to 20 times above the MIC, ensuring maximum bactericidal activity, the $C_{min}$ concentration is well below 1 for safety purposes, and the post-antibiotic effect of 6 hours is not overcome.

9. a. The hemodialysis occurred over 8 hours, and the elimination half-life while on it was 4 hours. Therefore two elimination half-lives occurred while on hemodialysis, and consequently, 75% of the drug was removed during that time.

   An anephric patient is a patient that does not have any significant urinary output. So the $CL_R$ or $k_R$, of that patient is essentially zero. The half-life of 16 hours is therefore due to the $CL_{NR}$, or $k_{NR}$.

$$k_{NR} = 0.693/16 = 0.043 \text{ h}^{-1}$$

   While on dialysis, $k = 0.693/4 = 0.173$ h$^{-1}$ and $k = k_{NR} + k_{DIAL}$, so $k_{DIAL} = 0.173 - 0.043 = 0.13$ h$^{-1}$.

   b. The volume of distribution is 0.5 L/kg or $0.5 \times 75 = 37.5$ L. The concentration at the end of the bolus injection should therefore have been 1000/37.5 = 26.67 mg/L

   The concentration 48 hours later, which is 3 times the elimination half-life of 16 hours should therefore have been 87.5% lower, so $26.67 \times 0.125 = 3.33$ mg/L

   After dialysis, when 75% of the drug remaining should have been further eliminated, the concentrations should be $3.33 \times 0.25 = 0.83$ mg/L

10. a. By keeping the dose constant and prolonging the dosage interval, the AUC over the dosing interval (or the $C_{avg}$) will be unchanged (but the new dosing interval will be longer) while the $C_{max}$ and $C_{min}$ will be little affected. But the new dosing interval will be longer. So in some circumstances, should the dosing interval span multiple days, then the Daily AUC may be much higher one day than the next. For example, should the dosing interval have to be every 48 hours, instead of being 24 hours or less in a normal patient, then it will mean that the AUC will have to be higher than normal for the first 24 hours and much less than normal over the remaining 24 hours. This may not be the right thing to do for some drugs.

    b. By decreasing the dose and maintaining the dosage interval constant, the $C_{max}$ will be lower (as the dose is lower), the $C_{min}$ will be higher, but the AUC over the dosing interval will be unchanged. Having a lower $C_{max}$ and higher $C_{min}$ may not be the right thing to do for some drugs.

Each method therefore has to be considered, and the most appropriate one based on the relationship between the PK and PD of the drug will have to be selected.

## REFERENCES

Bennett WM: Guide to drug dosage in renal failure. *Clin Pharmacokinet* **15**:326–354, 1988.

Bennett WM: Guide to drug dosage in renal failure. In Holford N (ed). *Clinical Pharmacokinetics Drug Data Handbook*. New York, Adis, 1990.

Bianchetti G, Graziani G, Brancaccio D, et al: Pharmacokinetics and effects of propranolol in terminal uremic patients and in patients undergoing regular dialysis treatment. *Clin Pharmacokinet* **1**:373–384, 1978.

Bickley SK: Drug dosing during continuous arteriovenous hemofiltration. *Clin Pharm* **7**:198–206, 1988.

Bjornsson TD: Nomogram for drug dosage adjustment in patients with renal failure. *Clin Pharmacokinet* **11**:164–170, 1986.

Bodenham A, Shelly MP, Park GR: The altered pharmacokinetics and pharmacodynamics of drugs commonly used in critically ill patients. *Clin Pharmacokinet* **14**:347–373, 1988.

Brouwer KBR, Dukes GE, Powell JR: Influence of liver function on drug disposition. In Evans WE, Schewtag, J, Jusko, J (eds). *Applied Pharmacokinetics—Principles of Therapeutic Drug Monitoring*. Baltimore, MD, Lippincott Williams & Wilkins, 1992, Chap 6.

Carpenter CB, Lazarus JM: Dialysis and transplantation in the treatment of renal failure. In Isselbacher KJ, et al (eds). *Harrison's Principles of Internal Medicine*. New York, McGraw-Hill, 1994, Chap 238.

Chennavasin P, Brater DC: Nomograms for drug use in renal disease. *Clin Pharmacokinet* **6**:193–215, 1981.

Cholongitas E, Papatheodoridis GV, Vangeli M, et al: Systematic review: The model for end-stage liver disease—Should it replace Child-Pugh's classification for assessing prognosis in cirrhosis? *Aliment Pharmacol Ther* **22**(11):1079–1089, 2005.

Cockcroft DW, Gault MH: Prediction of creatinine clearance from serum creatinine. *Nephron* **16**:31–41, 1976.

De Hart RM: Vancomycin removal via newer hemodialysis membranes. *Hosp Pharm* **31**:1467–1477, 1996.

Dettli L: Drug dosage in renal disease, *Clin Pharmacokinet* **1**(2):126–34, 1976.

Devine BJ: Gentamicin therapy. *DICP* **8**:650–655, 1974.

Diem K, Lentner C (eds): *Scientific Tables*, 7th ed. New York, Geigy Pharmaceuticals, 1973.

Farrell GC, Cooksley WG, Hart P, et al: Drug metabolism in liver disease. Identification of patients with impaired hepatic drug metabolism. *Gastroenterology* **75**:580, 1978.

FDA Guidance for Industry: Pharmacokinetics in patients with impaired hepatic function: Study design, data analysis, and impact on dosing and labeling, FDA, Center for Drug Evaluation and Research (CDER), May 2003.

FDA Guidance for Industry: Pharmacokinetics in patients with impaired renal function—Study design, data analysis, and impact on dosing and labeling, Draft Guidance, FDA, Center for Drug Evaluation and Research (CDER), March 2010.

Gambertoglio JG: Effects of renal disease: Altered pharmacokinetics. In Benet LZ, Massoud N, Gambertoglio JG (eds). *Pharmacokinetic Basis of Drug Treatment*. New York, Raven, 1984.

Gilman AG, et al: *Pharmacological Basis of Therapeutics*, MacMillan, New York, 1980.

Hailmeskel B, Lakew D, Yohannes L, Wutoh AK, Namanny M: Creatinine clearance estimation in elderly patients using the Cockcroft and Gault equation with ideal, actual, adjusted or no body weight. *Consult Pharm* **14**:72–75, 1999.

Hansen E, Bucher M, Jakob W, Lemberger P: Pharmacokinetics of levofloxacin during continuous veno-venous hemofiltration. *Intensive Care Med* **27**:371–375, 2001.

Howden CW, Birnie GG, Brodie MJ: Drug metabolism in liver disease. *Pharmacol Ther* **40**:439, 1989.

Hu OY, Tang HS, Chang CL: The influence of chronic lobular hepatitis on pharmacokinetics of cefoperazone: A novel galactose single-point method as a measure of residual liver function. *Biopharm Drug Dispos* **15**(7):563–576, 1994.

Hu OY, Tang HS, Chang CL: Novel galactose single point method as a measure of residual liver function: Example of cefoperazone kinetics in patients with liver cirrhosis. *J Clin Pharmacol* **35**(3):250–258, 1995.

Jelliffe RW. Creatinine clearance: Bedside estimate. *Ann Intern Med* **79**:604–605, 1973.

Kamath PS, Kim WR: The model for end-stage liver disease (MELD). *Hepatology* **45**(3):797–805, 2007.

Kampmann J, Siersback-Nielsen K, Kristensen M: Rapid evaluation of creatinine clearance. *Acta Med Scand* **196**(6):517–520, 1974.

Keller E, Hoppe-Seyler G, Mumm R, Schollmeyer P: Influence of hepatic cirrhosis and end-stage renal disease on pharmacokinetics and pharmacodynamics of furosemide. *Eur J Clin Pharmacol* **20**(1):27–33, 1981.

Levey AS, Bosch JP, Lewis JB, Greene T, Rogers N, Roth D: A more accurate method to estimate glomerular filtration rate from serum creatinine: A new prediction equation, Modification of Diet in Renal Disease Study Group. *Ann Intern Med* **130**(6):461–470, 1999.

Levey AS, Stevens LA, Schmid CH, et al: A new equation to estimate glomerular filtration rate. *Ann Intern Med* **150**(9): 604–612, 2009.

Mallikaarjun S, Shoaf SE, Boulton DW, Bramer SL: Effects of hepatic or renal impairment on the pharmacokinetics of aripiprazole. *Clin Pharmacokinet* **47**(8):533–542, 2008.

*Merck Manual*. Merck, Whitehouse Station, NJ, 1996–1997.

Muirhead GJ, Wilner K, Colburn W, Haug-Pihale G, Rouviex B: The effects of age and renal and hepatic impairment on the pharmacokinetics of sildenafil. *Br J Clin Pharmacol* 53(suppl 1):21S–30S, 2002.

Munar M, Singh H: Drug dosing adjustments in patients with chronic kidney disease. *American Fam Physician* 75(10): 1489–1496, 2007.

Nuxmalo JL, Teranaka M, Schenk WG, Jr Hepatic blood flow measurement. *Arch Surg* 113:169, 1978.

*Physicians' Desk Reference*. Montvale, NJ, Medical Economics (published annually).

Schneider V, Henschel V, Tadjalli-Mehr K, Mansmann U, Haefeli WE: Impact of serum creatinine measurement error on dose adjustment in renal failure. *Clin Pharmacol Ther* 74:458–467, 2003.

Schwartz GV, Haycock GB, Edelmann CM, Spitzer A: A simple estimate of glomerular filtration rate in children derived from body length and plasma creatinine. *Pediatrics* 58:259–263, 1976.

Siersback-Nielsen K, Hansen JM, Kampmann J, Kirstensen M: Rapid evaluation of creatinine clearance. *Lancet* **i**:1133–1134, 1971.

Sonnichsen DS, Relling MV: Clinical pharmacokinetics of paclitaxel. *Clin Pharmacokinet* 27(4):256–269, 1994.

Spinler SA, Nawarskas JJ, Boyce EG, Connors JE, Charland SL, Goldfarb S: Predictive performance of ten equations for estimating creatinine clearance in cardiac patients. *Ann Pharmacother* 32:1275–1283, 1998.

Stevens LA, Coresh J, Greene T, Levey AS: Assessing kidney function: Measured and estimated glomerular filtration rate. *N Eng J Med* 354(23):2473–2483, 2006.

St. Peter WL, Redic-Kill KA, Halstenson CE: Clinical pharmacokinetics of antibiotics in patients with impaired renal function. *Clin Pharmacokinet* 22:169–210, 1992.

Tozer TN: Nomogram for modification of dosage regimen in patients with chronic renal function impairment. *J Pharmacokinet Biopharm* 2:13–28, 1974.

Traub SL, Johnson CE: Comparison methods of estimating creatinine clearance in children. *Am J Hosp Pharm* 37:195–201, 1980.

Trey C, Burns DG, Saunders SJ: Treatment of hepatic coma by exchange blood transfusion. *N Engl J Med* 274:473–448, 1966.

Villeneuve JP, Verbeeck RK, Wilkinson GR, Branch RA: Furosemide kinetics and dynamics in cirrhosis. *Clin Pharmacol Ther* 40(1):14–20, 1986.

Welling PG, Craig WA: Pharmacokinetics in disease states modifying renal function. In Benet LZ (ed). *The Effects of Disease States on Drug Pharmacokinetics*. Washington, DC, American Pharmaceutical Association, 1976.

Williams RL: Drug administration in hepatic disease. *N Engl J Med* 309:1616, 1983.

## BIBLIOGRAPHY

Benet L: *The Effect of Disease States on Drug Pharmacokinetics*. Washington, DC, American Pharmaceutical Association, 1976.

Bennett WM, Singer I: Drug prescribing in renal failure: Dosing guidelines for adults—An update. *Am J Kidney Dis* 3:155–193, 1983.

Bjornsson TD: Use of serum creatinine concentration to determine renal function. *Clin Pharmacokinet* 4:200–222, 1979.

Bjornsson TD, Cocchetto DM, McGowan FX, et al: Nomogram for estimating creatinine clearance. *Clin Pharmacokinet* 8:365–399, 1983.

Brater DC: *Drug Use in Renal Disease*. Boston, AIDS Health Science Press, 1983.

Brater DC: Treatment of renal disorders and the influence of renal function on drug disposition. In Melmon KL, Morrelli HF, Hoffman BB, Nierenberg DW (eds). *Clinical Pharmacology—Basis Principles in Therapeutics*, 3rd ed. New York, McGraw-Hill, 1992, Chap 11.

Brenner BM (ed): *Brenner and Rector's The Kidney*, 8th ed. New York, Elsevier, 2007.

Chang CY, Schiano TD: Drug hepatotoxicity. *Aliment Pharmacol Ther* 25:1135–1151, 2007.

Chennavasin P, Brater DC: Nomograms for drug use in renal disease. *Clin Pharmacokinet* 6:193–214, 1981.

Child C, Turcotte J: The liver and portal hypertension. In Child CI (ed). *Surgery and Portal Hypertension*. Philadelphia, WB Saunders, 1964, pp 50–58.

Craig BD, Chennavasin P: Effects of renal disease: Pharmacokinetic considerations. In Benet LZ (eds). *Pharmacokinetic Basis of Drug Treatment*. New York, Raven, 1984.

Cutler RE, Forland SC, St. John PG, et al: Extracorporeal removal of drugs and poisons by hemodialysis and hemoperfusion. *Annu Rev Pharmacol Toxicol* 27:169–191, 1987.

Dettli L: Elimination kinetics and dosage adjustment of drugs in patients with kidney disease. In Grobecker H, et al (eds). *Progress in Pharmacology*, Vol 1. New York, Gustav Fischer Verlag, 1977.

Fabre J, Balant L: Renal failure, drug pharmacokinetics and drug action. *Clin Pharmacokinet* 1:99–120, 1976.

*Facts and Comparisons*: St. Louis, MO, Walter Kluwer Health, (updated monthly), 1992.

FDA Guidance for Industry: Pharmacokinetics in patients with impaired renal function—Study design, data analysis and impact on dosing and labeling, 1998.

Feldman M: Biochemical liver tests. In Feldman M, Friedman LS, Sleisenger MH, et al (eds). *Gastrointestinal and Liver Disease*, 7th ed. New York, Elsevier, 2002, pp 1227–1231.

Figg WD, Dukes GE, Lesesne HR, et al: Comparison of quantitative methods to assess hepatic function: Pugh's classification, indocyanine green, antipyrine, and dextromethorphan. *Pharmacotherapy* 15:693–700, 1995.

Ford M: *Clinical Toxicology*. Philadelphia, Saunders, 2001, pp 43–48.

Gibaldi M: Drug distribution in renal failure. *Am J Med* 62:471–474, 1977.

Gibson TP, Nelson HA: Drug kinetics and artificial kidneys. *Clin Pharmacokinet* 2:403–426, 1977.

Giusti DL, Hayton WL: Dosage regimen adjustments in renal impairment. *Drug Intell Clin Pharm* 7:382–387, 1973.

Hallynck TH, Soeph HH, Thomis VA, et al: Should clearance be normalized to body surface or lean body mass? *Br J Clin Pharm* **11**:523–526, 1981.

Jellife RW: Estimation of creatinine clearance when urine cannot be collected. *Lancet* **1**:975–976, 1971.

Jellife RW: Estimation of creatinine clearance in patients with unstable renal function, without a urine specimen. *Am J Nephrol* **22**:320–324, 2002.

Jellife RW, Jellife SM: A computer program for estimation of creatinine clearance from unstable serum creatinine concentration. *Math Biosci* **14**:17–24, 1972.

Kampmann JP, Hansen JM: Glomerular filtration rate and creatinine clearance. *Br J Clin Pharmacol* **12**:7–14, 1981.

Lee CC, Marbury TC: Drug therapy in patients undergoing haemodialysis. Clinical pharmacokinetic considerations. *Clin Pharmacokinet* **9**:42–66, 1984.

LeSher DA: Considerations in the use of drugs in patients with renal failure. *J Clin Pharmacol* **16**:570, 1976.

Levy G: Pharmacokinetics in renal disease. *Am J Med* **62**:461–465, 1977.

Lott RS, Hayton WL: Estimation of creatinine clearance from serum creatinine concentration: A review. *Drug Intell Clin Pharm* **12**:140–150, 1978.

Maher JF: Principle of dialysis and dialysis of drugs. *Am J Med* **62**:475–481, 1977.

Paton TW, Cornish WR, Manuel MA, Hardy BG: Drug therapy in patients undergoing peritoneal dialysis. Clinical pharmacokinetic considerations. *Clin Pharmacokinet* **10**:404–426, 1985.

Ratz A, Ewandrowski K: Normal reference laboratory values. *N Engl J Med* **339**:1063–1071, 1998.

Rhodes PJ, Rhodes RS, McClelland GH, et al: Evaluation of eight methods for estimating creatinine clearance in man. *Clin Pharm* **6**:399–406, 1987.

Rosenberg J, Benowitz NL, Pond S: Pharmacokinetics of drug overdosage. *Clin Pharmacokinet* **6**:161–192, 1981.

Schumacher GE: Practical pharmacokinetic techniques for drug consultation and evaluation, II: A perspective on the renal impaired patient. *Am J Hosp Pharm* **30**:824–830, 1973.

Traub SL: Creatinine and creatinine clearance. *Hosp Pharm* **13**:715–722, 1978.

Watanabe AS: Pharmacokinetic aspects of the dialysis of drugs. *Drug Intell Clin Pharm* **11**:407–416, 1977.

Watkins PB, Hamilton TA, Annesley TM, Ellis CN, Kolars JC, Voorhees JJ: The erythromycin breath test as a predictor of cyclosporine blood levels. *Clin Pharmacol Ther* **48**:120–129, 1990.

# PART V

Biopharmaceutics and
Pharmacokinetics in
Drug Product Development

# 26

# Biopharmaceutical Aspects of the Active Pharmaceutical Ingredient and Pharmaceutical Equivalence

Changquan Calvin Sun, Andrew B.C. Yu, and Leon Shargel

## CHAPTER OBJECTIVES

- Define active pharmaceutical ingredient[1] (API) and drug product (finished dosage form).

- Define pharmaceutical equivalence (PE) and therapeutic equivalence (TE).

- Describe the physical and biopharmaceutical properties of API that are important in the design and performance of drug products.

- Describe the main methods used to test PE of the API or the dosage form (drug product).

- Explain the relationship of PE, bioequivalence (BE), and TE.

- Explain whether a generic drug product that is not an exact PE can be TE.

- Explain why a generic drug product with identical PE may not lead to equivalent pharmacokinetic and pharmacodynamic performance.

- Define complex drug products and explain the problems for establishing pharmaceutical equivalence for these products.

---

[1]The active pharmaceutical ingredient (API) is also referred to as the drug substance. Both drug substance and API will be used interchangeably in this chapter.

## INTRODUCTION

In order to bring a new drug to the United States market, a company must submit a new drug application (NDA) to the FDA for review and approval. Regulatory approval is based on evidence that establishes the safety and efficacy of the new drug product through one or more clinical trials (FDA, cited June 5, 2014). The development of a new drug, from discovery to entering the market, is a lengthy and expensive process. These clinical studies are typically performed by a large pharmaceutical company known as the innovator company. The innovator company patents the new drug and gives it a brand name. The brand drug product is available from only one manufacturer until patent expiration. These drug products are also known as single-source drugs, which are marketed at a high price, a practice that allows the company to recover the costs in development and to make a profit. Patents are critical for encouraging innovation that is needed for developing new drugs to effectively treat diseases. Once the patent expires, other companies can manufacture and market generic versions of the brand drug product after gaining approval for marketing by a regulatory agency through an Abbreviated New Drug Application (ANDA) process, which presents a substantially lower barrier than the NDA process (Fig. 26-1). At that point, the drug becomes a multisource drug, provided the generic drug products contain the same active pharmaceutical ingredient (API) in the same dosage form and given by the same route of administration (Chapters 8 and 29). Through market competition, the price of a multisource drug is lower than the single-source brand drug (Cook, et al 1998). This makes the drug more affordable to the general public. The competition of generic drug products reduces global healthcare costs and motivates brand name companies to sustain their business through more innovations. Generic drug products are especially important

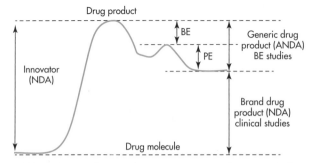

FIGURE 26-1 • Illustration of the different barriers that must be overcome to gain the approval of a new drug product through either New Drug Application (NDA) or Abbreviated New Drug Application (ANDA) approval processes. BE = bioequivalence, PE = pharmaceutical equivalence.

for countries where innovator drug products are not available. Therefore, a balance must be reached to both encourage innovation by brand name companies and curb costs in drug purchasing through generic drug competition.

The safety and efficacy of a generic drug product is established by demonstrating that the generic drug product is a *therapeutic equivalent* (TE) to the branded or innovator drug product (Chapters 8 and 29). Under the current United States ANDA process for approval of generic drug products, TE of a generic drug product is assumed if the following conditions are met:

- They are approved as safe and effective.
- They are pharmaceutical equivalents.
- They are bioequivalent (BE) in that (a) they do not present a known or potential bioequivalence problem, and they meet an acceptable *in vitro* standard, or (b) if they do present such a known or potential problem, they are shown to meet an appropriate bioequivalence standard.
- They are adequately labeled.
- They are manufactured in compliance with Current Good Manufacturing Practice regulations.

Among the list of criteria, the requirements of pharmaceutically equivalent (PE) and BE to the innovator drug product are most crucial for a generic drug product to be considered as being therapeutically equivalent (TE) to the innovator drug product (Fig. 26-2) (FDA Guidance for Industry, 2003). The substitution of innovator drug products with TE generic drug products by a pharmacist is allowed

without the permission of the prescriber. The FDA believes that products classified as TE can be substituted with the full expectation that the substituted product will produce the same clinical effect and safety profile as the prescribed product.

Although the cost-saving advantage of generic substitution is obvious, the absence of direct clinical studies in patients leads to a lingering concern about efficacy of generic drug products. Patients often ask, "Are they [generic drugs] really as safe and efficacious as the innovator drug products?" To answer this question, the concepts of PE and BE must be carefully examined.[2,3]

---

**FREQUENTLY ASKED QUESTIONS**

▶ If two APIs are pharmaceutical equivalents, can we assume that these two APIs are also identical?

▶ Can drug products that are not pharmaceutical equivalents be bioequivalent in patients?

---

### Pharmaceutical Equivalents

FDA defines *pharmaceutical equivalents* as drug products in identical dosage forms and route(s) of administration that contain identical amounts of the identical active drug ingredient, ie, the same salt or ester of the same therapeutic moiety, or, in the case

---

[2] As noted in Chapters 8 and 29, the currently marketed brand drug product may not have the identical formulation as the original formulation used in the safety and efficacy studies in patients. Brand and generic manufacturers may make changes in the formulation after approval.

[3] Additional definitions appear in Chapter 8.

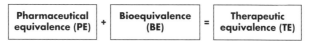

FIGURE 26-2 • Relationship between pharmaceutical equivalence, bioequivalence, and therapeutic equivalence in the current regulatory framework.

of modified-release dosage forms that require a reservoir or overage or such forms as prefilled syringes where the residual volume may vary, that deliver identical amounts of the active drug ingredient over the identical dosing period; do not necessarily contain the same inactive ingredients; and meet the identical compendial or other applicable standard of identity, strength, quality, and purity, including potency and, where applicable, content uniformity, disintegration times, and/or dissolution rates. They may differ in characteristics such as shape, scoring configuration, release mechanisms, packaging, excipients (including colors, flavors, preservatives), expiration date/time, and, within certain limits, labeling (see Approved Drug Products with Therapeutic Equivalence Evaluations, or Orange Book).

Pharmaceutical equivalence is used to compare the active pharmaceutical ingredient and the finished dosage form of a reference drug product (usually the brand) to a test drug product (eg, a proposed generic drug product). In the United States, pharmaceutical equivalents are not identical[4] and may have certain allowable differences. In contrast, Health Canada (HC) and the European Medicines Agency (EMA) demand identicality. For example, IV iron formulations of iron dextran, iron gluconate, and iron sucrose can be submitted to the FDA as an ANDA even though the API of the proposed generic may not be identical to that of the reference product. In contrast, these formulations will not be accepted at this time as generic submissions by HC and EMA.

### Pharmaceutical Equivalence of the Active Pharmaceutical Ingredient

The therapeutic moiety or active pharmaceutical ingredient (API) must be the same salt or ester and meet compendial standards (eg, USP-NF) for identity, strength, quality, purity, and potency. Salts such as tetracycline hydrochloride and tetracycline phosphate are not considered identical since different salts have different ionization constants and different aqueous solubility. Different salt forms may have different dissolution rates. Many prodrugs are esters of the active drug (eg, tetracycline stearate). Different esters of the same active drug are not pharmaceutical equivalents since esters have different aqueous solubility and hydrolyze at different rates. The stability of esters is also a problem. Various issues in establishing pharmaceutical equivalence of the API are listed in Table 26-1.

### Pharmaceutical Equivalence of the Drug Product

A *drug product* is a finished dosage form (eg, tablet, capsule, solution) that contains the active drug ingredient, generally, but not necessarily, in association with inactive ingredients (Code of Federal Regulations, §320.1 Title 21). Same or equivalent drug product formulations mean that the formulation of the generic drug product submitted for FDA approval may have minor differences in composition or method of manufacture from the approved brand formulation (ie, Reference Listed Drug Product; Chapters 8 and 29) but are similar enough to be relevant to the FDA's determination of bioequivalence.

For generic drug products to be pharmaceutical equivalents, they must be identical dosage forms that contain identical amounts of the chemically identical API. Pharmaceutical equivalents deliver identical amounts of the API over the identical dosing period. APIs must meet the identical compendial (eg, USP-NF) or other applicable standards on potency, content uniformity, disintegration times, and dissolution rates where applicable (CFR Part 320, 2013).

Pharmaceutically equivalent drug products may contain different inactive ingredients, or excipients; for example, colorant, flavor, and preservative. They may contain different amounts of impurities within an allowable range. This flexibility in compositions of the drug product sometimes, though rarely, leads

---

[4] The terms "identical" and "same" are often used interchangeably.

## TABLE 26-1 • Issues in Establishing Pharmaceutical Equivalence (PE) of the API

| Active Pharmaceutical Ingredient (API) | Comments |
| --- | --- |
| Particle size | Particle size differences can lead to differences in dissolution rates and differences in bulk density. In solution, the API is PE. However, particle size is important in suspensions and can cause a problem in dissolution. In suspensions, PE can be problematic. |
| Polymorph | Different crystalline forms and also amorphous API may have different dissolution rates. However, in solution the API is PE. In the case of an IV solution made with an API containing a polymorphic form impurity, after initial solubilization, the API may precipitate out during its product cycle. Long-term stability of this solution may be a problem. |
| Hydrate/Anhydrous | Although differences in the water of hydration, in solution the API is PE. There may be dissolution rate different between different hydrates and anhydrous forms of the API. Different water contents in hydrates and anhydrous forms affect API potency. |
| Impurities | PE may be synthesized using different synthetic pathways, leading to differences in impurities. Different purification methods can also lead to residual solvents and different impurities that need to be qualified depending on whether these are above or below threshold level. |
| Stability | Crystal defects as a result of different methods of synthesis and purification may affect the shelf life of the drug substance. Amorphous forms often degrade more rapidly for many APIs.<br><br>Thus, stability is a PE issue, which may lead to a change in efficacy of the API due to more rapid decomposition. |
| Racemic/Chirality | Racemic APIs may be PE if the ratio of isomers is the same in both products. However, the racemate (R,S) omeprazole (Prilosec) is not a PE to its single efficacious isomer esomeprazole (Nexium), the S-isomer of omeprazole, since different isomers may have different pharmacokinetic and pharmacodynamic activity. |
| Biotechnology-derived drugs | Biotechnology-derived products include protein and peptide products. Currently, it is not technically possible to ensure identicality for most of these products. Therefore, PE cannot be established between two APIs. Follow-on products are thereby termed "biosimilars" as they can be established to be similar in terms of PE and pharmacokinetic and pharmacodynamic activity. Additionally, differences may lead to immunogenicity problems. |

to undesirable consequences on the therapeutic performance, as discussed later. In addition, pharmaceutically equivalent drug products may differ in characteristics, such as shape, release mechanism, scoring (for tablets), packaging, and even labeling to some extent.

Strictly speaking, only identical drug products are truly BE and TE. However, in practice, two drug products are generally viewed as BE under the current FDA policies when they do not significantly differ in the rate and extent of the API (or its active moiety) reaching the site of drug action when administered at the same molar dose and under similar conditions in an appropriately designed study (see Chapter 29). If the rate of API released from a product is purposely modified, such as certain extended-release dosage forms, but the change in rate does not significantly affect the clinical performance, they may still be considered as BE, provided such change is reflected in the labeling and it does not affect the effective drug concentration in body on chronic use. Some of the issues concerning pharmaceutical equivalence of the drug product are listed in Table 26-2.

**TABLE 26-2 •** Issues in Establishing Pharmaceutical Equivalence of the Drug Product

| Dosage Form (Drug Product) | Comments |
|---|---|
| Drug product delivery system | Transdermal systems and oral ER drug products may have different drug delivery systems but are considered PE to their respective brand drug product provided they meet the additional requirements for therapeutic equivalence. |
| Size, shape, and other physical attributes of generic tablets and capsules | Differences in physical characteristics (eg, size and shape of the tablet or capsule) are not strictly a PE issue but may affect patient compliance and acceptability of medication regimens, could lead to medication errors, and could have different GI transit times. |
| Excipients | Generic and brand drug products may have different excipients and still be considered PE provided they meet the requirements for therapeutic equivalence. |
| Sterile solutions | The ingredients in many sterile drug solutions (eg, ophthalmic solutions) must be the same, both qualitatively and quantitatively. |
| Overage | Overage is generally disallowed unless justified by data. Transdermal products using a reservoir system may have an overage to maintain the desired bioavailability. |
| Liposomes and emulsions | Liposomes and emulsions are dispersed systems with two or more liquid phases, generally composed of lipid and aqueous phases. PE is difficult to establish for these drug products. For example, there may be differences in drug concentration in the lipid phase and in the aqueous phase. |
| Inhalation products | Different designs in inhalation devices may deliver drugs with different particle size, plume geometry, etc, which may produce different clinical efficacy. Certain inhalation products may be considered PE provided they meet the requirements for therapeutic equivalence. |
| Manufacturing process | The manufacturing process can affect drug product performance. For example, an increase in compaction may produce a harder tablet that disintegrates more slowly, thereby releasing the drug more slowly (see also Chapter 27). |

## Drug Master Files[5]

Drug substances are usually chemically synthesized from starting materials or extracted from natural sources including plants or microorganisms. The synthetic or isolation process is proprietary in nature and is documented confidentially in a drug master file (DMF). A DMF is a submission to the FDA that may be used to provide confidential detailed information about facilities, processes, or articles used in the manufacturing, processing, packaging, and storing of one or more human drugs. There are five types of DMFs:

- Type I: Manufacturing Site, Facilities, Operating Procedures, and Personnel

- Type II: Drug Substance, Drug Substance Intermediate, and Material Used in Their Preparation, or Drug Product
- Type III: Packaging Material
- Type IV: Excipient, Colorant, Flavor, Essence, or Material Used in Their Preparation
- Type V: FDA Accepted Reference Information

The drug substance or API is referred to as Type II DMF. The details of the DMF are not necessarily known to a drug product manufacturer although the specification of the API is generally known and meets compendial standards. An API manufacturer may sell the same API to multiple generic manufacturers. The ANDA submission refers to the DMF. The DMF summarizes all significant steps in the manufacturing and controls of the drug intermediate or substance. Each additive must be identified and

---

[5]Drug Master Files: Guidelines https://www.fda.gov/drugs/guidances-drugs/drug-master-files-guidelines

characterized by its method of manufacture, release specifications, and testing methods.

A recent FDA Guidance for Industry: Good ANDA Submission Practices, draft January 2018, highlights common, recurring deficiencies that may lead to a delay in the approval of an ANDA. Among the deficiencies that are highlighted include the characterization of the API and the drug product.

## PHARMACEUTICAL ALTERNATIVES

Drug products that contain the same therapeutic moiety or its precursor but differ in dosage form, API amount, or chemical structure (different salt forms, prodrugs, complexes, etc) are considered *pharmaceutical alternatives* by the FDA as long as they meet applicable standards. Tablet products containing different chemical form of an API—for example, a prodrug or a different salt—are pharmaceutical alternatives regardless of whether the molar dose is the same. In addition, the route of administration should be the same for two products to qualify as pharmaceutical alternatives. For example, an IV injectable drug product cannot be a pharmaceutical alternative to an oral tablet. Pharmaceutical alternatives may or may not be a pharmacokinetic or therapeutic equivalent with the innovator drug product. US FDA considers capsules and tablets containing the same API—for example, quinidine sulfate 200-mg tablets versus quinidine sulfate 200-mg capsules—as pharmaceutical alternatives even if the products have equivalent bioavailability. In the European Union, an immediate-release (IR) capsule may be considered as a pharmaceutical equivalent to an IR tablet containing the same API, but not in Canada and the United States.

Although pharmaceutical alternatives are not pharmaceutical equivalents, pharmaceutical alternatives have been used to provide a similar clinical endpoint. For example, naproxen capsules (220 mg) and naproxen tablets (220 mg) are different dosage forms but are often clinically interchanged to provide the same therapeutic objective. In this case, some patients might find a capsule easier to swallow than a tablet. Amoxicillin and ampicillin are two different antibiotic drugs but may be prescribed for the same therapeutic indications.

### Stability-Related Therapeutic Nonequivalence

True solutions of drug are considered pharmaceutical equivalents, provided that different excipients, if present, do not affect their pharmacokinetic characteristics (eg, different amounts of sorbitol or mannitol are known to affect the pharmacokinetics (PK) of some APIs). Intravenous drug solutions are BE because their bioavailability is 100% by the nature of their route of administration. It should be noted that the FDA may demand that excipients are qualitatively and quantitatively the same.[6] However, these drug products may have different stability. Instability can significantly impact therapeutic performance of a drug product that is otherwise pharmaceutically equivalent to the innovator products.

### Clinical Example of Non-United States Approved Generic Drug Product

Cefuroxime is an antimicrobial prophylaxis that is given as a single-dose IV injection in patients prior to undergoing coronary artery bypass grafting surgery (Mastoraki et al, 2008). When a brand name drug product is used, a single dose of 3 g of cefuroxime prior to surgery generally achieves and maintains serum levels sufficient to prevent infections during the surgery. Occasionally, a 0.75 g dose is administered 12 hours after the surgery to prevent infection. However, when a generic cefuroxime IV solution was used to substitute the brand drug for cost saving, an increased frequency of post-surgical infections occurred (Fujimura et al, 2011). Some patients had to be admitted to the surgical intensive care unit. When the brand name drug product was again used, new cases of severe postoperative infection stopped. When the generic drug product was reintroduced, higher incidence of postoperative infections again occurred. Subsequent investigation confirmed that,

---

[6]For drug products, such as sterile solutions, topical ointments, and other products, the FDA considers formulation Q1/Q2 sameness, ie, the test and reference listed drug product (RLD) are qualitatively and quantitatively the same. In addition, FDA may consider Q3 similarity, ie, the physicochemical properties of test and RLD products are similar.

although both drug products were chemically identical, the generic product hydrolyzed very quickly to render it less effective by the time it is administered (Fujimura et al, 2011). Although reasons that caused the poor stability in the generic product were not given, it is likely that the differences in formulation and/or manufacturing process were responsible. It should be clarified that no such case study has been reported for FDA, or HC, or European approved generic version of cefuroxime.

## Excipients and Impurities-Related Therapeutic Nonequivalence

Drugs are rarely administered alone. Various excipients, such as binder, solubilizer, stabilizer, preservatives, lubricant, diluents, and colorants, are added to make the final drug product. Sometimes, impurities and contaminants are present in the drug product. Unfortunately, the focus of quality control has traditionally been placed on the analysis of drug in the product. The recent safety problem with heparin due to the contamination by over-sulfated chondroitin sulfate, an impurity that is structurally similar to heparin, alerted the scientific community that impurities must also be considered to ensure pharmaceutical equivalence and therapeutic equivalence (Dodd and Besag, 2009; Vesga et al, 2010; FDA, 1999).

Although less dramatically, impurities are contained in drugs and excipients, and degradation can occur during manufacturing and storage. Interaction between drug and excipients may also have a negative impact on the safety and efficacy of a drug product. Interactions between drug and excipients should be considered when evaluating whether or not a follow-on and/or generic drug product is therapeutically equivalent to the reference drug product. In addition, some adverse reactions may not be evident in a single-dose BE study but may show up during chronic use of the drug. Hence, impurities in the drug and excipients must be controlled to avoid unintended problems in safety and efficacy of generic drug products. The absence of some critical functional excipients or the inappropriate amounts of them in a drug product may lead to poor efficacy even if the drug itself is of high quality (Zuluaga et al, 2010).

The potential problems mentioned above are true for both innovator and generic drug products. However, compared to generic products, the innovator drug products usually undergo fewer or less significant changes in the formulation, quality of drug and excipients, or manufacturing process when compared to the materials used in the Phase III clinical studies. In that case, the potential problems related to excipients and impurities are less of a concern for the clinical performance of innovator drug products.

## PRACTICE PROBLEM

A generic manufacturer wants to make an amoxicillin suspension, 250 mg/5 mL with identical excipients as in the brand product. The generic manufacturer purchased the API from a drug supplier who imported various grades of amoxicillin trihydrate from different countries. The supplier reported that the amoxicillin trihydrate drug substance is a pharmaceutical equivalent to the innovator's API. A consultant stated further that the proposed product has the same chemical formula, antibacterial activity, potency, and excipients as in the innovator's drug product. The generic drug product will be marketed in a similar package. A bioequivalence study was performed comparing the proposed generic drug product to the brand drug product. The rate and extent of the generic product was found to (Chapters 8 and 29) be within the required BE requirements (Chapter 29). After submission to the FDA, the product was rejected by the FDA's Office of Generic Drugs. Based on your understanding of the PE definition, what could be the possible reasons for the FDA not approving this product? (Consult Tables 26-1 and 26-2 about the potential issues with PE, TE, and BE.)

### Solution

The definition of pharmaceutical equivalence provides for a number of attributes that are possible sources for failure in PE. Product performance criteria for these drug products as described in the Code of Federal Regulations (CFR) must also be met.

PEs are drug products in identical dosage forms that contain identical amounts of the identical active drug ingredient and meet the identical compendial or other applicable standard of identity, strength, quality, and purity, including potency and, where applicable, content uniformity, disintegration times, and/or dissolution rates.

### Possible Sources of Pharmaceutical Inequivalence

1. Stability is affected by various factors such as residual solvent, reagents, and byproducts (impurities) that are the results of different methods of chemical synthesis and purification.

2. Drug substance suppliers may use different starting materials during synthesis. The starting materials may also have different impurities, depending on the method of crystallization method used for purification. Generally, impurity profiles are synthetic route dependent, and may not always be detected using the same analytical method as the innovator.

3. The stability may not be detected with the BA/BE test. However, the FDA requires clinical samples to be retained, and it is possible that the retained samples may fail stability specifications later. In addition, content uniformity may be a quality issue for failure under the definition of PE.

   *Comment 1:* The CFR states that the purity and identity criteria must be met. Although the CFR does not directly refer to the impurity profile and all the detailed drug substance properties, the comprehensive statements clearly state that the drug substance that ends up in the drug product must perform as intended.

   *Comment 2:* A change in particle size, or crystallinity, during product manufacturing can result in batch-to-batch or within-batch variability failure. When this occurs, even an objective BE study will not preclude regulatory rejection or product failure. Another important issue is the *content uniformity* in the context of the drug substance and the product in a multidrug source environment. The statistical nature of this is the recognition of an adequate design for sampling, and the relevance of quality-by-design (QbD) (see Chapter 27), which when properly implemented, minimizes the need for more testing of factors that affect PE.

4. A low level of an unsuspicious trace solvent may change the crystal form, solid-state stability of a drug substance.

5. Byproducts in a drug substance from starting materials may cause PE issues that affect quality. In some cases, toxicity or even carcinogenicity issues must be considered when different drug sources are used. It is important to note that as progress occurs, more efficient synthetic methods may be discovered for the API. The synthetic process may be quite different. Even though a higher yield may be achieved, the impurity profile should be also acceptable. Compendial standards such as the European Pharmacopeia or USP-NF are helpful, but additional evaluation may be needed. Some of this information may be in the DMF provided by the drug substance supplier.

6. Chirality is important, as the same chemical formula may be structurally different, resulting in different solubility and/or activity. Note the reference to "identical active drug ingredients" in the definition. Therefore, *d*-Thyroxine and *l*-Thyroxine will not be considered as PE, nor will *d,l*-Thyroxine.

### Polymorphic Form-Related Therapeutic Nonequivalence

For poorly soluble drugs, a change in polymorph form may impact bioavailability. The FDA does not consider polymorphism in the definition of pharmaceutical equivalence. Hence, two products are considered pharmaceutically equivalent even when different polymorphs are used. Since some polymorphs are patented, generic manufacturers will use a different polymorph than the brand name product. In this case, the potential phase change of the polymorph during manufacture and storage will need to be carefully evaluated and controlled. The potential impact due to polymorph form differences can be masked by appropriate formulation design. In some cases, even differences in drug crystal morphology may lead to different bioavailability (Modi et al, 2013). These factors should be evaluated in the design of generic drug product to ensure bioequivalence and therapeutic equivalence.

## Particle Size–Related Therapeutic Nonequivalence

Content uniformity is a challenge for low-dose tablet drug products for both generic and brand drug product manufacturers. A tablet containing 5 mg or less of the API may represent only 5% or less of a tablet weighing a total of 100 mg. In this case, 95% or more of the tablet weight is due to excipients. The high ratio of excipients to drug can produce problems of excipient–drug interactions (Fathima et al, 2011) and content uniformity. Unintended particle size variations have an impact on content uniformity in tablet products, especially when the manufacturer uses a direct compression tableting process (Rohrs et al, 2006). The batch of generic tablets that is used in studies for ANDA submission must meet the content uniformity requirement and demonstrate BE with the brand name product. Subsequent batches of the generic or brand tablets may fail to meet the content uniformity requirement, and clinical outcomes unexpectedly vary. In that case, drug product substitution may occasionally cause unintended problems in therapeutic performance. The problem of content uniformity can be minimized by stringent quality control.

Variations in particle size can also potentially impact bioavailability of poorly soluble drugs. Smaller drug particles correspond to larger surface area and more rapid dissolution leading to potentially higher bioavailability (Jounela et al, 1975). Therefore, adequate particle size control is needed to maintain consistent clinical performance.

## Bioequivalence of Drugs with Multiple Indications

Brand drug products may be approved for several clinical indications. Although a generic drug product may be therapeutically equivalent to a brand name for the exact same indications, it may not be approved for all of the indications. The demonstration of therapeutic equivalence in one population of patients plus the "bioequivalency" to the brand in healthy volunteers is strong evidence suggesting that the generic drug is TE for the other approved clinical indications. Theoretically a definitive answer can only be attained through a clinical study for each indication, because different characteristics of the drug may be critical for successful clinical outcomes in different patient populations. For example, a drug may dissolve quickly and get absorbed completely in one patient population with a normal pH environment in their GI tract. Hence, variation in particle size and formulation does not affect bioavailability. However, the bioavailability of the same two drug products in the same cancer patients may be very different because of the much slower dissolution of the drug in their GI tract, which has a higher pH. This is a topic of active research (Yue et al, 2015; Cristofoletti et al, 2017).

## CHANGES TO AN APPROVED NDA OR ANDA

After the approval of a new drug product or generic drug product, the manufacturer may make a change to the marketed product (FDA Guidance for Industry, April 2004). These changes may include changes in the API, changes in the manufacturing process, change in the formulation, scale-up or an increase in the batch size of the drug product, change in the manufacturing site, and change in the container closure system. In many cases, the manufacturer may make multiple changes to the drug product. For any of these changes, it is important to assess whether the change has a potential to have an adverse effect on the identity, strength, quality, purity, or potency of a drug product as these factors may relate to the safety or effectiveness of the drug product. The FDA must be notified whenever a manufacturer makes a change to an approved product. The reporting requirements for a change are listed in Table 26-3. The manufacturer must assess the effects of the change before distributing a drug product made with a manufacturing change. Significant change will trigger the need for a BE study comparing the previous formulation to the new one to show that the new formulation behaves clinically in the same manner.

## Formulation and Manufacturing Process Changes

After FDA approval, generic and brand drug product manufacturers may make changes in the formulation and/or the manufacturing process. In addition, the manufacturer might change equipment and/or the site of manufacture for the product. Due to

## TABLE 26-3 • Changes to an Approved NDA or ANDA

| Change | Definition | FDA Reporting Requirement | Example |
|---|---|---|---|
| Major change | A change that has a substantial potential to have an adverse effect on the identity, strength, quality, purity, or potency of a drug product as these factors may relate to the safety or effectiveness of the drug product | *Prior Approval Supplement*—requires the submission of a supplement and approval by the FDA prior to distribution of the drug product; may require a BE study | A move to a different manufacturing site for the manufacturer of an ER capsule |
| Moderate change | A change that has a moderate potential to have an adverse effect on the identity, strength, quality, purity, or potency of the drug product as these factors may relate to the safety or effectiveness of the drug product | (1) *Supplement—Changes Being Effected in 30 Days*—requires the submission of a supplement to FDA at least 30 days before the distribution of the drug product made using the change<br><br>(2) *Supplement—Changes Being Effected*—moderate changes for which distribution can occur when FDA receives the supplement | A change in the manufacturing process for an IR tablet |
| Minor change | A change that has minimal potential to have an adverse effect on the identity, strength, quality, purity, or potency of the drug product as these factors may relate to the safety or effectiveness of the drug product | *Annual report*—The applicant must describe minor changes in its next annual report | A change in an existing code imprint for a dosage form. For example, changing from a numeric to alphanumeric code |

*Data from Guidance for Industry Changes to an Approved NDA or ANDA. U.S. Department of Health and Human Services. Food and Drug Administration. Center for Drug Evaluation and Research (CDER), April 2004.*

post-approval changes, the current reference drug products and the approved generic drug product equivalent may not have the same formulation and manufacturing process as those of the original formulations used in clinical trials that established their efficacy and safety. Changes to the formulation, suppliers of excipients, manufacturing process, or manufacturing site may be necessary in order to manufacture the drug product at large scale after the approval. The FDA requires the manufacturer to demonstrate that drug product performance is not affected by these scale-up and post-approval changes (SUPAC) (FDA, 1995, 1997). If the changes in the formulation and manufacturing process for a brand name or generic drug product are more than allowed by FDA under the SUPAC guidances (considered a major change), a BE study is required (Table 26-3). The differences between currently marketed brand, generic drug products and the drug product used in the clinical trials are likely due to different formulations and different manufacturing processes. Hence, a BE study for both brand and generic drug products after a major post-approval change (SUPAC) is required.

### FREQUENTLY ASKED QUESTIONS

▶ Why do drug manufacturers make changes to an approved drug product that is currently on the market?

▶ Should a bioequivalence study be performed every time a drug manufacturer makes a change in the formulation of the drug product?

▶ Where can we find a list of United States products with therapeutic equivalence and a discussion of evaluation criteria?

## SIZE, SHAPE, AND OTHER PHYSICAL ATTRIBUTES OF GENERIC TABLETS AND CAPSULES

Generic formulations are required to be PE and TE to the corresponding brand drug product. There has been an increasing concern that differences in physical characteristics (eg, size and shape of the tablet or capsule) may affect patient compliance and acceptability of medication regimens or could lead to medication errors (FDA, 2015). For example, difficulty in swallowing tablets or capsules can be a problem for many individuals and may lead to a variety of adverse events and patient noncompliance with treatment regimens. In addition to possible swallowing difficulty, larger tablets and capsules have been shown to prolong esophageal transit time. This can lead to disintegration of the product in the esophagus and/or cause injury to the esophagus, resulting in pain and localized esophagitis and the potential for serious sequelae, including ulceration. Studies in humans have also suggested that oval tablets may be easier to swallow and have faster esophageal transit times than round tablets of the same weight. The weight of the tablet or capsule also may affect transit time, with heavier tablets or capsules having faster transit times compared to similarly sized lighter tablets or capsules. Surface area, disintegration time, and propensity for swelling when swallowed are additional parameters that can influence esophageal transit time and have the potential to affect the performance of the drug product for its intended use. Consequently, these physical attributes should also be considered for generic drug products intended to be swallowed intact.

> **FREQUENTLY ASKED QUESTION**
>
> ▶ How would the shape or size of an oral drug product affect compliance in an elderly patient?

## HOW PREVALENT IS THE THERAPEUTIC NONEQUIVALENCE OF A GENERIC PRODUCT?

FDA-approved generic drug products are TEs and PEs for which BE has, most of the time, been demonstrated. Once approved, the generic drug product is expected to have the same clinical effect and safety profile when administered to patients under the conditions specified in the labeling.

This assumption of similar clinical effect by the generic and brand drug products is generally true and is rarely challenged. However, the possibility of failures by generic or follow-on products by the innovator should not be overlooked. Therefore, it is prudent to ask the question: "How often is a generic drug product not therapeutically equivalent to a brand product?" While basic principles have been laid to ensure quality of approved generic products, situations can arise where generic products are not TE. The FDA constantly monitors safety and performance of approved drug products, both innovator and generic, and pulls problematic products off the market and investigates the causes. Once the science underlying an issue or problem is understood, the FDA updates relevant regulations to avoid similar problems.

In one United States example, a generic lansoprazole delayed-release orally disintegrating tablet unexpectedly clogged and blocked oral syringes and feeding tubes. In some cases, patients needed to seek emergency medical assistance. The problems with the generic lansoprazole tablet were traced to several differences in the generic product, including the use of more insoluble excipients, slower disintegration, and larger granular size, and higher tendency to stick to the inner wall of tubes. The generic drug manufacturer voluntarily withdrew the product from distribution. FDA subsequently made recommendations for generic product evaluation to address these issues and updated guidance for products with feeding tube administration. In another United States example, Bupropion XL 300-mg tablets by one generic manufacturer was not therapeutically equivalent to the brand name Wellbutrin XL 300-mg tablets. This generic Bupropion XL 300-mg tablet was approved based on BE studies comparing the 150-mg strength of the products to Wellbutrin XL 150 mg, which was then extrapolated on the "way-up" to the 300-mg product with dissolution studies only. Since then, the approach of extrapolating to a higher dose product to establish BE with dissolution studies only is viewed with extreme caution by regulators and may not be acceptable.

Cases of therapeutic equivalence failure of generic drug products approved by regulatory agencies outside the United States have been reported in the literature. One example of nontherapeutic equivalence was for an IV vancomycin solution. A non-FDA-approved generic IV vancomycin product failed to treat a liver transplant patient against infection in Colombia. However, switching to the brand name product led to a speedy recovery by the patient (Rodriguez et al, 2010). Had this case been non-life-threatening, the apparent different bactericidal activities between the generic and innovator products may have been ignored. A patient who requires longer treatment may be attributed to differential individual response to a therapy. The physician may simply switch to a different kind of antibiotics. Unfortunately, a death of the patient caused by ineffective drug therapy may be simply attributed to the severity of the disease, since a death is not an unexpected outcome (Rodriguez et al, 2010). Either scenario will conceal the problem in the antibiotic failure.

For drugs with narrow therapeutic indices, such as some antiepileptic drugs, concerns about therapeutic nonequivalence were raised in the United States by many and for a long time (Crawford et al, 2006; Andermann et al, 2007). However, a recent study using "generic-brittle" patients under clinical use conditions found a generic lamotrigine tablet was BE to the brand tablet, Lamictal (Ting et al, 2015). That study supports the soundness of the FDA BE standards. The issues observed with switching to generic products have even been attributed by some to be likely caused by quality issues of individual products that can face both brand name and generic products (Ting et al, 2015). The American Epilepsy Society subsequently issued a position statement in 2016, where substituting a brand drug with a BE FDA-approved generic product is supported in principle. Other concerns on therapeutic nonequivalence of generic products have been discussed (Dettelbach, 1986; Lamy 1986). Those have prompted tightened regulations to ensure quality of generic drug products.

Both brand and generic drug product manufacturers make changes in the formulation and manufacturing process. Some drug product manufacturers use a contract manufacturing organization (CMO) to manufacture the drug product. Internationally, brand name drug products containing the same active drug may not use the same formulation and manufacturing process as those used in the United States. Consequently, these drug products may not meet FDA BE criteria. For this reason, FDA implements a post-market surveillance program and performs post-market research to guide regulatory actions for ensuring the safety of generic drug products.

## THE FUTURE OF PHARMACEUTICAL EQUIVALENCE AND THERAPEUTIC EQUIVALENCE

Considering the potential therapeutic nonequivalence of generic drug products, suggestions have been made to require clinical evaluations on clinical efficacy of generic products with a randomized double-blind comparative study for each major indication (Fujimura et al, 2011). However, clinical trial comparisons are very expensive, often have very little discriminatory potential (eg, much less than a typical PK "BE" study), and their requirement would effectively stifle the competition for bringing down the cost of prescription drugs.

A reason for the documented failures in therapeutic equivalence of generic products, although very few, may be the empirical nature of drug product development. In absence of a clear understanding of the relationship among structure, property, and performance (Sun, 2009), each product by a different manufacturer can be potentially very different in terms of formulation compositions and manufacturing processes. Some may argue that a successful BE study may not assure the therapeutic equivalence. Having recognized the challenge, the way forward would be for the scientific community, pharmaceutical companies, and drug regulatory agencies (DRAs) worldwide to work together to advance the science that enables the design of high-quality and stable drug products in a consistent way. In the short term, DRAs have appropriately tightened the BE requirement, at least for types of products with known TE problems, to minimize the occurrence of drug therapy failure due to substandard generic drug products. In his 1986 editorial, Dr. Dettelbach stated, "However, until we institute a system of evaluating generic drugs in patients, in whom therapeutic and pharmacodynamic (PD) differences can be of critical importance, we may be playing a dangerous game" (Dettelbach, 1986). This concern has been continuously addressed by regulators and scientists worldwide through the development of science for the design and manufacture of high-quality generic drugs products.

## COMPLEX DRUG PRODUCTS

Complex drug products are products that contain various combinations of drugs for which it is very difficult to determine PE and BE (Table 26-4). Unlike simple APIs that are small molecules with well-defined chemical structures, complex APIs contain heterogeneous mixtures of small molecules or biotechnology-derived macromolecules that have complicated structures. These complex APIs are difficult to characterize by commonly used analytical methods. Formulations of complex drug products, such as liposomes, drug-impregnated stents, etc are also difficult to characterize.

The demonstration of pharmaceutical equivalence of complex drug products requires the development and validation of special analytical methods and *in vitro* methods. Manufacturers who want to develop complex drug products are encouraged to meet with the FDA to determine the most appropriate methodology needed for developing a therapeutically equivalent drug product.

### Clinical Example: Bioequivalence of Fluticasone Propionate Nasal Spray

Fluticasone propionate nasal spray (Flonase) is used for the management of the nasal symptoms of perennial non-allergic rhinitis. Fluticasone propionate nasal spray contains an aqueous suspension of fluticasone propionate for topical administration to the nasal mucosa by means of a metering, atomizing spray pump. Several issues must be considered in establishing pharmaceutical equivalence and bioequivalence of this product. Some of the major issues include (1) the particle size of the suspension and

**TABLE 26-4 • Complex Drug Products**

| Complex Drug Product | Comments | Examples |
|---|---|---|
| Complex active ingredients | Complex mixtures of APIs, polymeric compounds, peptides | Glatiramer acetate, iron dextran |
| Complex formulations | Liposomes, suspensions, emulsions, gels | Doxorubicin liposomal injection |
| Complex routes of delivery | Locally acting such as dermatologic, nasal, and ophthalmologic drugs | Estradiol vaginal cream USP |
| Complex dosage forms | Extended release injectables and implantables, transdermals, metered dose inhalers | PLGA microspheres |
| Complex drug-device combinations | Meter dose inhalers, medicated stents, transdermal therapeutic systems | Azelastine hydrochloride and fluticasone propionate nasal spray |

Other products where complexity or uncertainty would benefit from early scientific engagement

*Data from Jiang X: Introduction to Complex Products and FDA Considerations Demonstrating Equivalence of Generic Complex Drug Substances and Formulations, Workshop, 2017.*

dissolution rate of the API, (2) the droplet size, spray geometry, and plume geometry of the spray when the spray pump is actuated, and (3) demonstration of BE for a locally active product. Due to the complexity of this product, FDA requires both *in vivo* and *in vitro* studies. The *in vitro* studies quantitatively characterize the API, the formulation, and drug delivery by the metered dose spray. The *in vivo* studies require a BE study and clinical efficacy study comparisons (FDA Draft Guidance on Fluticasone Propionate, Recommended Sept 2015).

### FREQUENTLY ASKED QUESTION

▶ What considerations are needed to establish pharmaceutical equivalence of complex drug-device combinations?

## BIOSIMILAR DRUG PRODUCTS

The Biologics Price Competition and Innovation Act of 2009 (BPCI Act) amended the Public Health Service Act (PHS Act) and other statutes to create an abbreviated licensure pathway in Section 351(k) of the PHS Act for biological products shown to be biosimilar to, or interchangeable with, an FDA-licensed biological reference product. Biological products can present challenges given the scientific and technical complexities that are associated with the larger and typically more complex structure of biological products and the processes by which such products are manufactured. Most biological products are produced in a living system such as a microorganism, or plant or animal cells, whereas small-molecule drugs are typically manufactured through chemical synthesis (FDA Guidance for Industry, 2012a, 2012b).

*Biosimilar* or *biosimilarity* means that the biological product is highly similar to the reference product notwithstanding minor differences in clinically inactive components, and there are no clinically meaningful differences between the biological product and the reference product in terms of the safety, purity, and potency of the product.

*Interchangeable biosimilar drug products* include the following (FDA, 2019):

- The biological product is biosimilar to the reference product.
- It can be expected to produce the same clinical result as the reference product in any given patient.
- For a product administered more than once, the safety and reduced efficacy risks of alternating or switching are not greater than with repeated use of the reference product.

Due to the complexity of these products, regulatory agencies such as the FDA, EMA, or HC consider the totality of the evidence provided by a sponsor to support a demonstration of biosimilarity and recommend that sponsors use a stepwise approach in their development of biosimilar products. Evidence demonstrating biosimilarity can include a comparison of the proposed product and the reference product with respect to structure, function, animal toxicity, human PK and PD, clinical immunogenicity, and clinical safety and effectiveness. The complete biosimilar development program will be considered as well as the manufacturing process.

## HISTORICAL PERSPECTIVE

In the last decade, many FDA guidances were developed to guide the control and manufacturing of API that impact PE issues. Many of the guidances were withdrawn with the adoption of the International Conference on Harmonisation (ICH) quality guidances by the European Union, Japan, and the United States. The quality (Q) guidance for API (referred to as drug substance in ICH) is well discussed in the preamble for Q3A, which fully discusses API issues in the developed world: impurities, byproducts, enantiomers, crystallinity, and other quality attributes. The issue of degradation impurities that may still form due to processing in the formulated product is discussed in Q3B (drug product guidance). A series of Q Guidances (www.ich.org) are easily available. As the QbD and progress evolve, the regulations of drug source supply will be updated accordingly. Revision of compendial and compliance policy notification as well as CFR announcements should be frequently consulted—for example, Compliance Policy Guide Sec. 420.300, Changes in Compendial Specifications and New Drug Application Supplements; Withdrawal of Guidance. https://www.federalregister.gov/articles/2012/08/30/2012-21415/compliance-policy-guide-sec-420300-changes-in-compendial-specifications-and-new-drug-application

A pharmacist should recognize that even a compendial grade drug source, when manufactured by a new process, may potentially form new degradation impurities that are not controlled under the drug substance guidance. Therefore, the ICH Guidance ICH Q3A (2006) advises in the preamble that regardless of new or old molecules, any impurities above defined thresholds must be identified; additionally, total impurities must be reported. If impurities are relatively high with respect to dose, they must be qualified (ie, determined by toxicity studies to be within safe level). Consequently, most generic manufacturers tend to use historically known manufacturing methods without introducing new or unknown impurities.

## CHAPTER SUMMARY

Pharmaceutical equivalence (PE), along with bio-equivalence (BE), is important for establishing therapeutic equivalence (TE) between the reference product and generic and follow-on drug products. Both the active pharmaceutical ingredient (API) and finished dosage form must be PE. PE is also important for post-approval changes in both brand and generic drug products. The determination of PE depends upon the physical and chemical properties of the API as well as the design and manufacture of the finished dosage form (drug product). For the API, different synthetic pathways and purification steps can lead to physical and chemical differences, including particle size, degree of hydration, crystalline form, impurities, and stability. The drug product can differ in characteristics, such as shape, scoring configuration, release mechanisms, packaging, and excipients (including colors, flavors, and preservatives). PE is more difficult to establish for complex APIs, complex drug products, or multiple APIs within the drug product (eg, combination drug product). Biotechnology-derived drugs, such as proteins and polypeptides, that are proposed for biosimilar drug products have additional issues with respect to structure, function, animal toxicity, human PK and PD, clinical immunogenicity, and clinical safety and effectiveness. Complex drug products are products that contain various combinations of drugs that are very difficult to determine PE and BE.

## LEARNING QUESTIONS

1. The Reference Listed Drug marketed by a brand drug company has a patent on the crystalline form of the API. A generic drug manufacturer wants to make a therapeutic equivalent of the brand drug product using an amorphous form of the API. Will the generic manufacturer be able to meet the requirements for PE and TE with the amorphous form of the API?

2. Why is it more difficult to determine PE for biosimilars, such as erythropoietin injection (Procrit) compared to small molecules, such as atorvastatin calcium tablets (Lipitor)?

3. Explain why a generic drug product can be a PE but not identical to the brand drug product.

4. For a generic drug product to be "pharmaceutical equivalent" to the innovator drug (or reference drug product), which of the following is true? Explain your answer.

   a. API in the generic product must be identical to the API in the reference drug product.

   b. It is desirable but not necessary for API to be identical in the generic and reference drug products.

   c. Many APIs used in generic products are referenced by drug master files and meet compendial standards. For these APIs, generic products are always pharmaceutically equivalent to the brand name drug.

5. Under what circumstances is particle size distribution of API critical for the product performance?

6. Can a generic drug product containing a different polymorph of an API be pharmaceutically equivalent to an innovator drug product? How about if a different salt or cocrystal is used in the generic drug product?

7. The drug miconazole may contain benzyl chloride–related impurity/intermediate that may be potentially genotoxic as reported in the literature. This API is supplied by various suppliers with DMFs available. How would a generic manufacturer planning to market a miconazole vaginal cream ensure that the API purchased is safe? Does supplier-designated "EP or USP-NF" grade necessarily ensure that PE is met?

## ANSWERS

### Frequently Asked Questions

*If two APIs are pharmaceutical equivalents, can we assume that these two APIs are also identical?*

■ No. The API can differ in particle size, crystal structure, hydrate, impurities, and/or stability (see Table 26-1.)

*Can drug products that are not pharmaceutical equivalents be bioequivalent in patients?*

■ Yes. Capsules and tablets containing the same API can be bioequivalent. However, in the United States, capsules and tablets are pharmaceutical alternatives. Extended-release tablets or capsules that have different drug release processes can be bioequivalent in vivo. Tablets containing either the API or a salt of the API can be bioequivalent when absorption is not dissolution limited.

*Why do drug manufacturers make changes to an approved drug product that is currently on the market?*

■ There are many reasons that a manufacturer makes a change in the formulation. For example, changed physical properties of API, due to the use of a more economical API synthesis process, necessitate a change in the formulation to assure the same performance of drug product. A manufacturer may want to enlarge the units manufactured (scale-up), use new manufacturing equipment, and/or change the manufacturing site.

*Should a bioequivalence study be performed every time a drug manufacturer makes a change in the formulation of the drug product?*

■ If the change in formulation is minor, such as removal of the color, and the manufacturer can show the likelihood that the change would not affect the bioequivalence of the formulation after the minor change, no bioequivalence study would be needed.

*Where can we find a list of United States products with therapeutic equivalence and a discussion of evaluation criteria?*

■ The publication Approved Drug Products with Therapeutic Equivalence Evaluations (the List, commonly known as the Orange Book. http://www.fda.gov/Drugs/DevelopmentApprovalProcess/ucm079068.htm). A discussion of PE, TE, and other terms are found in the preface.

*How would the shape or size of an oral drug product affect compliance in an elderly patient?*

■ Certain shape, size, or color may discourage the patient from swallowing the tablet. For many patients, tablets containing a 1000 mg of active drug can be difficult to swallow.

### Learning Questions

1. A crystalline form of the API is a more rigid structure compared to the amorphous form of the API. Dissolution rates may be different for the amorphous form of the API compared to the crystalline form of the API. However, the generic manufacturer may develop a formulation with the amorphous form that has a similar in vitro dissolution rate as the brand and is bioequivalent to the brand, in vivo. Therefore, the generic manufacturer will be able to meet the requirements for pharmaceutical equivalence, bioequivalence, and therapeutic equivalence with the amorphous form of the API.

2. Procrit® (epoetin alfa) is a 165-amino acid erythropoiesis-stimulating glycoprotein manufactured by recombinant DNA technology and has a molecular weight of approximately 30,400. Lipitor® (atorvastatin calcium) is chemically synthesized and has a molecular weight of 1209.42. Large biotechnology derived molecules are difficult to characterize and may have impurities that are difficult to identify compared to small synthetic molecules.

3. FDA determines whether a generic drug product and the API are pharmaceutical equivalent to the Brand drug product and API. FDA allows for small differences in the API including particle sized, crystalline form, and hydrate versus anhydrous. In addition, the generic drug product may have different excipients, different colors, and different shapes compared to the Brand drug product. In the manufacturer of Brand and generic drug products, there are slight deviations from one batch to another, so that each manufactured batch is not identical to each other but must meet specifications agreed upon by the FDA.

4. The answer is b. *It is desirable but not necessary for API to be identical in the generic and reference drug products.* As explained in answer #3 above, FDA determines what minor differences may be in the generic API compared to the brand API and still be considered a pharmaceutical equivalent.

5. Two APIs may have the same mean particle size but a different particle size distribution. If the particle size distribution has many small size particles, then the API may dissolve more quickly and be absorbed more quickly. In contrast, if the particle size distribution has many large size particles, then the API may dissolve more slowly and be absorbed more slowly.

6. Different polymorphs of the same API can be pharmaceutical equivalents. Different salts or cocrystals of the same API have different physicochemical properties, such as solubility, and are not considered as pharmaceutical equivalents. Different salts or cocrystals of the same API may be pharmaceutical alternatives.

## REFERENCES

Andermann F, Duh MS, Gosselin A, Paradis PE: Compulsory generic switching of antiepileptic drugs: High switchback rates to branded compounds compared with other drug classes. *Epilepsia* 48:464–469, 2007.

Approved Drug Products with Therapeutic Equivalence Evaluations (the list, commonly known as the Orange Book), http://www.fda.gov/Drugs/DevelopmentApprovalProcess/ucm079068.htm

CFR Part 320: Bioavailability and Bioequivalence Requirements. Title 21—Food and Drugs, Chapter I: Food and Drug Administration, Department of Health and Human Services, Subchapter D—Drugs for Human Use, 2013. [Cited June 29, 2014] Available from http://www.accessdata.fda.gov/scripts/cdrh/cfdocs/cfcfr/cfrsearch.cfm?cfrpart=320.

Cook A, Acton JP, Schwartz E: How increased competition from generic drugs has affected prices and returns in the pharmaceutical industry. Congressional Budget Office, Washington, DC, 1998 (http://www.cbo.gov/ftpdocs/6xx/doc655/pharm.pdf1-75).

Crawford P, et al: Are there potential problems with generic substitution of antiepileptic drugs? A review of issues. *Seizure* 15(3):165–176, 2006.

Cristofoletti R, Patel N, Dressman JB: Assessment of bioequivalence of weak base formulations under various dosing conditions using physiologically based pharmacokinetic simulations in virtual populations. Case examples: Ketoconazole and Posaconazole. *J Pharm Sci* 106:560–569, 2017.

Dettelbach HR: A time to speak out on bioequivalence and therapeutic equivalence. *J Clin Pharmacol* 26(5):307–308, 1986.

Dodd S, Besag FMC: Editorial [Lessons from contaminated heparin]. *Curr Drug Saf* 4(1):1–1, 2009.

Fathima N, Mamatha T, Qureshi HK, Anitha N, Rao JV: Drug-excipient interaction and its importance in dosage form development. *J Appl Pharm Sci* 01(06):66–67; 2011 (www.japsonline.com).

FDA: Immediate Release Solid Oral Dosage Forms Scale-Up and Postapproval Changes: Chemistry, Manufacturing, and Controls, In Vitro Dissolution Testing, and In Vivo Bioequivalence Documentation. FDA, US Department of Health and Human Services, Center for Drug Evaluation and Research, Editor, 1995.

FDA: SUPAC-MR: Modified Release Solid Oral Dosage Forms Scale-Up and Postapproval Changes: Chemistry, Manufacturing, and Controls; In Vitro Dissolution Testing and In Vivo Bioequivalence Documentation. FDA, US Department of Health and Human Services, Center for Drug Evaluation and Research, Editor, 1997.

FDA: How Drugs are Developed and Approved. [Cited June 5, 2014] Available from http://www.fda.gov/Drugs/DevelopmentApprovalProcess/HowDrugsareDevelopedandApproved/default.htm.

FDA Guidance for Industry: Bioavailability and Bioequivalence Studies for Orally Administered Drug Products—General Considerations. FDA, US Department of Health and Human Services, Center for Drug Evaluation and Research, Editor, 2003.

FDA Guidance for Industry: Changes to an Approved NDA or ANDA, April 2004.

FDA Guidance for Industry ANDAs: Impurities in Drug Substances, November 1999.

FDA Guidance for Industry: Biosimilars: Questions and Answers Regarding Implementation of the Biologics Price Competition and Innovation Act of 2009, Draft Guidance, February 2012a.

FDA Draft Guidance on Fluticasone Propionate, Recommended Sept 2015

FDA Guidance for Industry: Scientific Considerations in Demonstrating Biosimilarity to a Reference Product, Draft Guidance, February 2012b.

FDA Guidance for Industry: Considerations in Demonstrating Interchangeability with a Reference Product, May 2019.

FDA Guidance for Industry: Size, Shape, and Other Physical Attributes of Generic Tablets and Capsules, December 2015.

FDA Guidance for Industry: Good ANDA Submission Practices FDA Guidance for Industry, Draft, January 2018 (https://www.fda.gov/media/110689/download)

Fujimura S, et al: Antibacterial effects of brand-name teicoplanin and generic products against clinical isolates of methicillin-resistant *Staphylococcus aureus*. *J Infect Chemother* 17(1):30–33, 2011.

ICH Guidance, Q3A, www.ICH.org. ICH Harmonised Tripartite Guideline—Impurities In New Drug Substances, Q3A(R2), Current Step 4 Version Dated October 25, 2006.

Jiang X: Introduction to Complex Products and FDA Considerations Demonstrating Equivalence of Generic Complex Drug Substances and Formulations, Workshop, 2017 (https://sbiaevents.com/complex-generics-2018/).

Jounela AJ, Pentikäinen PJ, Sothmann A: Effect of particle size on the bioavailability of digoxin. *Eur J Clin Pharmacol* **8**(5):365–370, 1975.

Lamy PP: Generic equivalents: Issues and concerns. *J Clin Pharmacol* **26**(5):309–316, 1986.

Mastoraki E, et al: Incidence of postoperative infections in patients undergoing coronary artery bypass grafting surgery receiving antimicrobial prophylaxis with original and generic cefuroxime. *J Infect* **56**(1):35–39, 2008.

Modi SR, et al: Impact of crystal habit on biopharmaceutical performance of celecoxib. *Cryst. Growth Des* **13**:2824–2832, 2013.

Rodriguez CA, et al: Potential therapeutic failure of generic vancomycin in a liver transplant patient with MRSA peritonitis and bacteremia. *J Infect* **59**(4):277–280, 2009.

Rodriguez C, et al: In vitro and in vivo comparison of the antistaphylococcal efficacy of generic products and the innovator of oxacillin. *BMC Infect Dis* **10**(1):153, 2010.

Rohrs BR, et al: Particle size limits to meet USP content uniformity criteria for tablets and capsules. *J Pharm Sci* **95**(5):1049–1059, 2006.

Sun CC: Materials science tetrahedron—A useful tool for pharmaceutical research and development. *J Pharm Sci* **98**:1671–1687, 2009.

Ting TY, Jiang W, Lionberger R, et al: Generic lamotrigine versus brand-name Lamictal bioequivalence in patients with epilepsy: A field test of the FDA bioequivalence standard. *Epilepsia* **56**:1415-1424, 2015.

Vesga O, et al: Generic vancomycin products fail in vivo despite being pharmaceutical equivalents of the innovator. *Antimicrob Agents Chemother* **54**(8):3271–3279, 2010.

Yue CS, Benvenga S, Scarsi C, Loprete L, Ducharme MP: When bioequivalence in healthy volunteers may not translate to bioequivalence in patients: differential effects of increased gastric pH on the pharmacokinetics of levothyroxine capsules and tablets. *J Pharm Pharm Sci* **18**:844–855, 2015.

Zuluaga AF, et al: Determination of therapeutic equivalence of generic products of gentamicin in the neutropenic mouse thigh infection model. *PLoS ONE* **5**(5):e10744, 2010.

# 27

# Rational Drug Product Development, Quality, and Performance

Trupti Dixit, and Leon Shargel

## CHAPTER OBJECTIVES

- Describe the types of safety and efficacy risks that may occur after taking a drug product and various means for preventing these risks.

- List the major reasons that a drug product might be recalled due to quality defects.

- Understand how biopharmaceutics risk assessment road map (BioRAM) can lead to rational drug product development.

- Differentiate between drug product quality and drug product performance.

- Differentiate between quality control (QC) and quality assurance (QA).

- Explain how quality by design (QbD) ensures the development and manufacture of a drug product that will deliver consistent quality and performance.

- Define quality target product profile (QTPP) and explain how QTPP is different from conventional quality product criteria.

- Describe the quality principles underlying basis for the development, manufacture, and QA of the drug product throughout its life cycle.

- Describe how product specifications relate to drug product quality and the relevance to QA of the drug product through QbD.

- Define critical quality attributes and how these attributes relate to clinical safety and efficacy.

- Explain how postapproval changes in a drug product may affect drug quality and performance.

Biopharmaceutics is the study of the relationship between physicochemical properties of the drug, the dosage form (drug product) in which the drug is given and the route of administration on the rate and extent of systemic absorption. As such, the design (development and mechanism of delivery) of drug product and its quality have a big impact on the safety and efficacy of the drug. In this chapter, we explore the impact of drug product formulation on its safety/efficacy (biopharmaceutics) and the ways of assuring the quality and performance of the product throughout the life cycle of the drug.

## RISKS FROM MEDICINES

Side effects from the use of drugs are the major cause of drug-related injuries, adverse events, and deaths. The FDA (FDA, 2005, 2007) has summarized various types of safety and efficacy risks from medicines (Fig. 27-1). Side effects are observed in clinical trials or postmarketing surveillance and result in listing of adverse events in the drug's labeling. Some side effects are avoidable, and others are unavoidable. Avoidable side effects may include known drug–drug or drug–food interactions, contraindications, improper compliance, etc. In many cases, drug therapy requires an individualized drug treatment plan and careful patient monitoring. Known side effects occur with the best medical practice and even when the drug is used appropriately. Examples include nausea from antibiotics or bone marrow suppression from chemotherapy. Medication errors include wrong drug, wrong dose, or incorrect drug administration. Some side effects are unavoidable. These uncertainties include unexpected adverse events, side effects due to long-term therapy, and unstudied uses and unstudied populations. For example, a rare adverse event occurring in fewer than 1 in 10,000 persons would not be identified

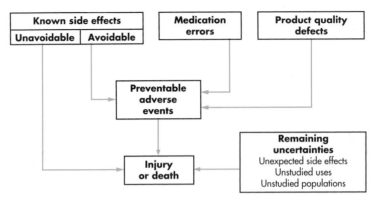

FIGURE 27-1 • Safety and efficacy risks from medicines. (Reproduced with permission from FDA: CDER Report to the Nation: 2005.)

in normal premarket testing. Chapters 21, 22, and 23 discuss how pharmacogenetics, pharmacokinetics, pharmacodynamics, and clinical considerations may improve drug efficacy and safety in many instances. The understanding of the biopharmaceutical properties of a drug helps the development of drug products with minimum side effects and maximum efficacy. For example, modified extended-release drug products formulations are formulated to decrease nausea caused by peak levels of drugs, or avoiding degradation in the stomach to increase the drug available for absorption in the intestines, etc. Once the drug is designed to minimize the side effects, pharmaceutical scientists focus on building quality by design in the drug product. *Drug product performance* relates to how the drug is presented to the body and is measured by release/dissolution and absorption parameters that impact bioavailability. *In vitro* drug product performance is evaluated using dissolution methods, whereas *in vivo* drug product performance uses bioavailability studies. These studies are dependent, as stated above, on how the drug is presented to the body (delivery system), and its pharmacokinetic and pharmacodynamic properties. *Drug product quality* is recognized and defined in the International Conference on Harmonisation (ICH), as the suitability of either a drug substance or drug product for its intended use. This term includes attributes such as identity, strength, and purity. An appropriately designed drug product is assured to provide the intended benefit to the patient through consistent quality of product measured by its key

attributes (ie, identity, strength, purity) as well as certain critical performance characteristics. Each batch of products is tested for these key attributes as defined in its specifications prior to release and distribution. However, occasionally there may be incidences of drug product defects observed either during release or on distribution. These quality defects are an important source of risk that affects drug product performance and can affect patient safety and therapeutic efficacy if not detected prior to consumption. Product quality is impacted by the quality of raw materials (excipients), the manufacturing process of the drug product, and storage and distribution controls.[1] This chapter will focus on how biopharmaceutical consideration can help design the right product, how quality can be built in by design, and how once a quality product is made, its quality can be assured throughout the life of the product. Successful development requires close collaboration between different pharmaceutical disciplines (pre-clinical, clinical, CMC) and regulatory authorities. A risk-based approach at each development stage demonstrating the scientific understanding of how formulation and manufacturing process factors affect product quality and performance will help regulatory agencies in the drug approval process. Understanding drug product quality and risks

---

[1]Pharmaceutical manufacturers are required to follow current Good Manufacturing Practices (cGMP) to ensure that the drug products are made consistently with high quality.

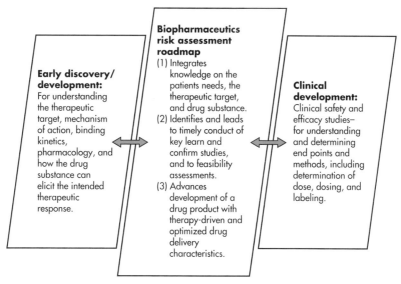

FIGURE 27-2 • Biopharmaceutics risk assessment roadmap as a connecting and translational tool for improving and enhancing product quality. (Reproduced with permission from Selen A, Dickinson PA, Müllertz A, et al: The biopharmaceutics risk assessment roadmap for optimizing clinical drug product performance, J Pharm Sci. 2014 Nov;103(11):3377–3397.)

of product quality defects that may affect drug product performance will help drive assurance of safer drugs for patients.

## Biopharmaceutics and Drug Product Development

Applying a patient-centric approach to drug development results in better drug development and assuring the benefits of intended therapy for patients. Understanding the impact of physicochemical characteristics of the drug, the mechanism of action *in vivo*, and the need for presenting the drug in a specific manner (input rate, maximum exposure, prolonged presence at site of action, etc) allows for rational development of drug product with maximum benefit. Figure 27-2 depicts how early discovery, the biopharmaceutics risk assessment roadmap (BioRAM), and clinical development are interlinked, and that the drug product development should be an iterative process.

### Quality Target Product Profile

Following a systems approach as outlined in BioRAM papers results in more efficient and effective drug product development. The drug product development process should ideally begin with the development of a *quality target product profile* (QTPP). ICH defines QTPP as a prospective summary of the quality characteristics of a drug product that ideally will be achieved to ensure the desired quality, taking into account safety and efficacy. The target product profile (TPP) is focused on safety and efficacy characteristics of the product. The Q in QTPP includes quality aspects that are needed to help meet the TPP. It is important to note that although both TPP and QTPP are predefined, some elements of QTPP are expected to be refined (rather targets that get better defined) as more information is gathered throughout development.

The key elements to be defined in the QTPP includes dosage form, strength, route of administration, intended patient population (adults, pediatric), frequency of administration, pharmacokinetic parameters desired, stability, quality attributes, container closure systems, and any alternate means of administration if available. Of these elements, some targets such as dose, type of dosage form (immediate versus modified), and quality attributes may evolve as more information becomes available based on clinical studies, *in vitro* modeling, and better understanding of risk/benefit.

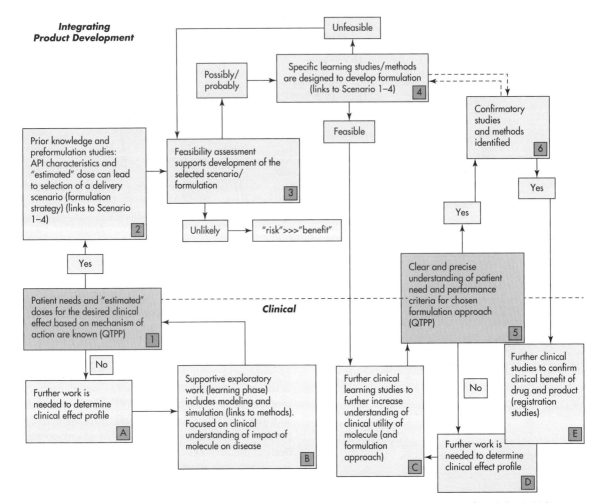

**FIGURE 27-3 •** The Biopharmaceutics Risk Assessment Roadmap (BioRAM). (Reproduced with permission from Selen A, Dickinson PA, Müllertz A, et al: The biopharmaceutics risk assessment roadmap for optimizing clinical drug product performance, J Pharm Sci. 2014 Nov;103(11):3377–3397.)

The integrated systems approach that can be applied to drug development is described in Fig. 27-3. Figure 27-3 shows how formulation development based on physicochemical characteristics of the drug substance and *in vitro* modeling can be done in parallel with clinical development. Integration of knowledge gained from both could lead to better drug development. The key at each step is to conduct a risk assessment and evaluate the information gained against the desired QTPP. The scheme in Fig. 27-3 illustrates various steps that are aligned with the integrated approach, beginning with mechanistic knowledge that leads to product definition; understanding the challenges based on drug substance characteristics

and expected *in vivo* performance could then lead to an optimized approach for developing the product.

The different steps involved in developing the optimized formulation can be outlined as follows:

1. Understanding the molecular mechanistic target (including temporal aspects) for the intended therapeutic outcome

2. Developing an appropriate drug delivery approach, taking into account patient needs

3. Assessing physicochemical and biopharmaceutic characteristics of the drug substance

4. Identifying the pharmacokinetic (PK)/pharmacodynamic (PD) profiles or the PD effect leading

to characterization of the target input profile (such as *in vitro* and *in vivo* dissolution/release profiles)

5. Developing a suitable formulation approach

6. Developing robust and reliable assessment tools to support each of these steps

## RISK ASSESSMENT

*Risk assessment* is a valuable science-based process used in quality risk management that can aid in identifying which material attributes and process parameters potentially have an effect on product *critical quality attributes* (CQAs). Risk assessment is typically initiated early in the pharmaceutical development process and is repeated as more information becomes available and greater knowledge is obtained. Risk assessment tools can be used to identify and rank parameters (eg, process, equipment, input materials) with potential to have an impact on product quality, based on prior knowledge and initial experimental data. Once the significant parameters are identified, they can be further studied to achieve a higher level of process understanding.

## DRUG PRODUCT QUALITY AND DRUG PRODUCT PERFORMANCE

*Drug product quality* relates to the biopharmaceutic and physicochemical properties of the drug substance and the drug product to the *in vivo* performance of the drug. The performance of each drug product must be consistent and predictable to assure both clinical efficacy and safety. Drug product attributes and performance are critical factors that influence product quality (Table 27-1) and are measured for each batch prior to acceptable release. Each component of the drug product and the method of manufacture contribute to quality. Quality must be built into the product during research, development, and production. Quality is maintained by implementing systems and procedures that are followed during the development and manufacture of the drug product. There are several regulatory guidance such as ICH Q8, Q9, Q10, Q11 that provide the framework for quality by design/quality expectations and risk assessment tools.

**TABLE 27-1 • Drug Product Quality and Performance Attributes**

Product quality
  Chemistry, manufacturing, and controls
  Microbiology
  Information that pertains to the identity, strength, quality, purity, and potency of the drug product
  Validation of manufacturing process and identification of critical quality attributes
Product performance
  *In vivo*
    Bioavailability and bioequivalence
  *In vitro*
    Drug release/dissolution

### Drug Recalls and Withdrawals

The FDA coordinates drug recall information and prepares health hazard evaluations to determine the risk to public health from products being recalled. The FDA classifies recall actions in accordance with the level of risk. The FDA and the manufacturer develop recall strategies based on the potential health hazard and other factors, including distribution patterns and market availability. The FDA also determines the need for public warnings and assists the recalling firm with public notification. Table 27-2 lists some of the major reasons for drug recalls.

As can be seen from the categories of recall, many recalls can be avoided if GMPs are followed and if the product is developed appropriately such that the formulation is robust, the process is well developed, and the quality is assured.

For convenience, drug product quality is listed in Table 27-3 separately from drug product performance. However, drug product quality must be maintained since drug product quality impacts directly on drug product performance.

## PHARMACEUTICAL DEVELOPMENT

Pharmaceutical development must design a quality drug product (*quality by design* [QbD]) using a manufacturing process that provides consistent drug product performance within the well-defined design space and achieves the desired therapeutic objective. The product development program is

**TABLE 27-2 • Top 20 Categories for Drug Recalls—2018**

| Sr. No. | Category | Number of Recalls |
|---|---|---|
| 1 | Violation of cGMP | 238 |
| 2 | Lack of sterility assurance | 171 |
| 3 | Lack of processing controls | 79 |
| 4 | Microbial contamination of non-sterile product | 49 |
| 5 | Out of specification | 26 |
| 6 | Marketed without an approved NDA/ANDA | 25 |
| 7 | Labeling issues | 24 |
| 8 | Presence of particulate matter | 22 |
| 9 | Subpotent drug | 13 |
| 10 | Defective delivery system | 12 |
| 11 | Non-sterility | 8 |
| 12 | Superpotent drug | 8 |
| 13 | Presence of foreign substance | 6 |
| 14 | Stability data does not support expiry | 6 |
| 15 | Defective container | 4 |
| 16 | Presence of foreign tablets/capsules | 4 |
| 17 | Temperature abuse | 3 |
| 18 | Incorrect product formulation | 2 |
| 19 | Presence of precipitate | 1 |
| 20 | Product mix-up | 1 |

Reproduced with permission from Pharma Times Now, Feb 2018; Top 20 Reasons for Drug Recalls in USA - Review of 2018 Data.

based on a sound understanding of the mechanistic activity of the drug substance and its optimal delivery to achieve the desired therapeutic outcome. The integration of biopharmaceutics and QbD optimizes drug product development and performance, which has been described by a biopharmaceutics risk assessment roadmap (Fig. 27-3) (Selen et al, 2014). The systematic product and process development should allow for developing a well-understood design space where the variability in quality of raw materials and the potential interaction/interdependency within the formulation and process is studied.

This manufacturing process is carefully designed using scientific principles throughout and integrating assurance of product quality into the design of the manufacturing process (quality assurance [QA]). Information gained from pharmaceutical development studies leads to identification of factors that impact CQAs which directly impact the performance of the drug product and hence its efficacy. The development of manufacturing process helps define critical material attributes (CMAs) and critical process parameters (CPPs), which directly impact the CQAs and thus support the establishment of the design space (see below), specifications, and manufacturing controls that ensure that each batch of the drug product will be produced with the same quality and performance. The advantage of a well-designed scientific study is that the interdependency of the components (quality of the drug substance, excipients, and their potential interactions) and process (manufacturing) is well understood. The quality of materials used can thus be controlled within the acceptable ranges (via specifications) and a process can be developed to accommodate those variations in quality to still produce a drug product of acceptable quality and performance. The information is also the basis for quality risk management. Changes in formulation and manufacturing processes during development and life cycle management after market approval provide additional knowledge and further support the manufacture of the drug product. Every step that affects CQA, CMAs, and CPP drug manufacture must also be tested to demonstrate that the desired physical and functional outcomes are achieved (process validation). Once the manufacturing process developed on scientific principles and thorough knowledge of interactions between components has been validated, every single lot produced by this method is assured to meet the desired specifications (quality control [QC]), which are directly related to the performance of the drug product.

**FREQUENTLY ASKED QUESTIONS**

▶ Explain how to "build in" drug quality to ensure that "the performance of a drug product will be predictable to assure clinical efficacy and safety."

▶ What do you use as a reference in evaluating performance of a new product in a quality system?

## TABLE 27-3 • Approaches to Pharmaceutical Development

| Aspect | Minimal Approaches | Enhanced, Quality-by-Design Approaches |
|---|---|---|
| Overall pharmaceutical development | • Mainly empirical<br>• Developmental research often conducted one variable at a time | • Systematic, relating mechanistic understanding of material attributes and process parameters to drug product CQAs<br>• Multivariate experiments to understand product and process<br>• Establishment of design space<br>• Process analytical technology (PAT) tools utilized |
| Manufacturing process | • Fixed<br>• Validation primarily based on initial full-scale batches<br>• Focus on optimization and reproducibility | • Adjustable within design space<br>• Life cycle approach to validation and ideally, continuous process verification<br>• Focus on control strategy and robustness<br>• Use of statistical process control methods |
| Process controls | • In-process tests primarily for go/no-go decisions<br>• Off-line analysis | • PAT tools utilized with appropriate feed forward and feedback controls<br>• Process operations tracked and trended to support continual improvement efforts postapproval |
| Product specifications | • Primary means of control<br>• Based on batch data available at the time of registration | • Part of the overall quality control strategy<br>• Based on desired product performance with relevant supportive data |
| Control strategy | • Drug product quality controlled primarily by intermediates (in-process materials) and end-product testing | • Drug product quality ensured by risk-based control strategy for well-understood product and process<br>• Quality controls shifted upstream, with the possibility of real-time release testing or reduced end-product testing |
| Life cycle management | • Reactive (ie, problem-solving and corrective action) | • Preventive action<br>• Continual improvement facilitated |

Reproduced with permission from FDA Guidance for Industry: Q8(R2) Pharmaceutical Development. U.S. Department of Health and Human Services. Food and Drug Administration Center for Drug Evaluation and Research (CDER). Center for Biologics Evaluation and Research (CBER), November 2009.

## Quality Risks in Drug Products

Although drug products are developed and manufactured using scientific considerations, specific knowledge gained during development, and adhering to GMPs, there may still be instances where quality risks are observed in marketed products. These risks related to drug product quality and performance can impact patient medication. Most serious side effects of drugs are recognized and are described in the approved product label to prevent serious injury. Quality risks are rarely very serious. Mostly, quality risks compromise the intended effect of medicine or produce unintended adverse reactions. These quality risks are in the form of damaged products (broken tablets, compromised packaging, etc) that could lead to some potential performance impact such as lower dose, or perhaps more degraded product (example from damaged protective packaging). By testing drug product quality of each lot, these effects are minimized. With evolving technology, better development techniques, such as QbD and risk assessment tools, the need for end product testing has also been minimized with emphasis on quality of design instead of testing in quality

Quality risks may be tracked by following all operation steps involved from drug product development throughout the manufacturing process, distribution, and patient utilization of the drug product. Key operations in manufacturing and pharmaceutical development are listed in the many FDA references along with quality controls essential for proper operation of those steps (http://www.fda.gov/Drugs/GuidanceComplianceRegulatoryInformation/Guidances/ucm065005.htm).

Quality documents are important to ensure FDA compliance, which inspects manufacturing facilities and its operation. The development pharmaceutics section can uncover product risks that are often an extension of poor formulation or poor product design. Modern design concepts involve identifying risk sources (variate) that take into account the frequency of occurrence and components (unit process) of the overall operation. The overall process involves many materials and operations. Hence a QbD approach is often multivariate by necessity. An understanding of risk involves some probability and statistics. QbD is very much rooted in statistics. However, an understanding of the basic material science and interplay of functional components should always override the tools and mathematics that are used to implement them. These tools should be viewed as an aid to discover or add more choices to manufacturing through QbD. The risks from drug product quality are sometimes described as *product drug quality defects*. Some of the quality elements important during product development are listed in Table 27-4.

## Quality by Design

A major principle that drives manufacturing process development is QbD. QbD is a systematic, scientific, risk-based, holistic, and proactive approach to pharmaceutical development that begins with predefined objectives and emphasizes the understanding of product and processes and process control. Product and process performance characteristics are scientifically designed to meet specific objectives (Cogdill and Drennen, 2008; Yu, 2008, 2015). To achieve QbD objectives, product and process characteristics important to desired performance must be derived from a combination of prior knowledge

**TABLE 27-4 •** Quality Elements of Pharmaceutical Development and Quality by Design

- Define quality target product quality profile.
- Design and develop formulations and manufacturing processes to ensure predefined product quality.
- Identify critical quality attributes (CQA), process parameters (CPP), and sources of variability that are critical to quality from the perspective of patients, and then translate them into the attributes that the drug product should possess.
- Perform a risk assessment linking material attributes (CMAs) and CPPs to drug product CQAs.
- Identify a design space for critical processing variables and formulation variables that impact *in vivo* product performance.
- Establish how the critical process parameters can be varied to consistently produce a drug product with the desired characteristics.
- Establish the relationships between formulation and manufacturing process variables (including drug substance and excipient attributes and process parameters); identify desired product characteristics and sources of variability.
- Implement a flexible and robust manufacturing process that can adapt and produce a consistent product over time.
- Develop process analytical technology (PAT) to integrate systems during drug product manufacture that provides continuous real-time quality assurance.
- Control manufacturing processes to produce consistent quality over time.
- Apply product life cycle management and continual improvement.

and experimental assessment during product development. Quality cannot be tested in drug products. Quality should be built into the design and confirmed by testing. With a greater understanding of the drug product and its manufacturing process, regulatory agencies are working with pharmaceutical manufacturers to use systematic approaches to drug product development that will achieve product quality and the desired drug product performance (FDA Guidance for Industry, 2009). The elements of QbD are listed in Table 27-4.

*Quality target product profile* (QTPP) is a prospective summary of the quality characteristics of a drug product that ideally will be achieved to ensure the desired quality, taking into account safety and efficacy of the drug product. As part of the quality system, the concept QTPP was introduced in QbD. QTPP summarizes all the important product attributes that are targeted and designed by the manufacturer during design and manufacturing. QTPP helps to maintain the quality throughout the life cycle of the product.

The following steps are informative in understanding various aspects of the overall scheme and its relevance:

1. QTPP-driven specifications: Desired product characteristics.

2. BioRAM (see Fig. 27-3): Development with clinical relevance and input.

3. Advancing and leveraging science and technology including mechanistic understanding, *in silico* tools, statistical evaluations use of biomarkers, QbD studies: Rationale drug development.

4. Knowledge sharing and collaborations based on multidimensional collaborations and shared database: Ensuring efficient and effective development.

By the use of an integrated approach to QbD using biopharmaceutic principles, drug products can be manufactured with the assurance that product quality and performance will be maintained throughout its life cycle.

## Quality (by) Design Critical Quality Attributes and Critical Process Parameters

In process development, the most important processes and component properties should be identified in the manufacturing process. A CQA is a physical, chemical, biological, or microbiological property or characteristic that needs to be controlled (directly or indirectly) to ensure product quality. The pharmaceutical manufacturer should identify CPPs and sources of variability that ensure the quality of the finished dosage form. The CQAs should be based on clinical relevance. Thus, the manufacturer of the drug product designs and develops the formulations and manufacturing processes to ensure a predefined quality.

## Design Space

The interaction between critical processes and materials should also be studied to optimize manufacturing processes. A *design space* is defined for critical processing variables and formulation variables that impact *in vivo* product performance. There may be several variables that affect the product variability *in vitro*. It is important to identify which of these variables are actually relevant to drug product performance *in vivo*. ICH defines design space in Q8 as follows:

- The multidimensional combination and interaction of input variables (eg, material attributes) and process parameters that have been demonstrated to provide assurance of quality.

- Working within the design space is not considered a change. Movement out of the design space is considered to be a change and would normally initiate a regulatory post-approval change process.

- Design space is proposed by the applicant and is subject to regulatory assessment and approval.

Design space is the geometrical region suitable for quality manufacturing when two or more process/material variables are plotted in a two-dimensional or higher-dimensional space to show the combined effects of the relevant processing variables during manufacturing. Some of these processing variables may or may not be critical to drug product performance. Thus, the manufacturer knows which process variable is critical and must have stricter control.

## Process Analytical Technology

Like design space, *process analytical technology* (PAT) also uses critical processes and materials to improve the quality of the product, but in PAT the emphasis is on monitoring these variables in a timely manner. PAT is intended to support innovation and efficiency in pharmaceutical development, manufacturing, and QA (FDA Guidance for Industry, September 2004). Conventional pharmaceutical manufacturing is generally accomplished using batch processing with laboratory testing conducted on samples collected during the manufacturing process and after the drug product is made (finished dosage form). These laboratory tests are used to evaluate the quality of the drug product (see quality control and quality assurance below). Newer methods based on science and engineering principles now exist for improving pharmaceutical development, manufacturing, and QA starting earlier in the development timeline through innovation in product and process development, analysis, and control.

PAT uses an integrated systems approach to regulating pharmaceutical product quality. PAT assesses mitigating risks related to poor product and process quality, and then monitors and controls them. PAT is characterized by the following:

- Product quality and performance are ensured through the design of effective and efficient manufacturing processes.
- Product and process specifications are based on a mechanistic understanding of how formulation and process factors affect product performance.
- Continuous real-time QA.
- Relevant regulatory policies and procedures are tailored to accommodate the most current level of scientific knowledge.
- Risk-based regulatory approaches recognize:
  - The scientific understanding of how formulation and manufacturing process factors affect product quality and performance.
  - The capability of process control strategies to prevent or mitigate the risk of producing a poor quality product.

PAT enhances manufacturing efficiencies by improving the manufacturing process through scientific innovation and with better communication between manufacturers and the regulatory agencies.

PAT may be considered a part of the overall QbD such that quality is built into the product during manufacture. An increased emphasis on building quality into drug products allows more focus to be placed on relevant multifactorial relationships among material, manufacturing process, environmental variables, and their effects on quality. This enhanced focus provides a basis for identifying and understanding the relationships among various critical formulation and process factors and for developing effective risk mitigation strategies (eg, product specifications, process controls, training). The data and information to help recognize these relationships can be leveraged through preformulation programs, development, and scale-up studies, as well as from improved analysis of manufacturing data collected over the life of a product.

The use of QbD principles for development, advances in overall manufacturing technology, and utilization of PAT techniques have led to development of continuous manufacturing (CM) concepts. This is a paradigm shift from the traditional batch manufacturing processes where each batch is distinct. CM is a seamless, fully integrated process applied for oral solid dosage (OSD) form production with real-time testing and monitoring at critical stages that allows for a high degree of control and QA. This results in reduced costs, better and faster product development, and more regulatory flexibility for manufacturing. The CM concept allows production of high-quality products with less resource utilization and enhanced safety. Several drugs listed in Table 27-5 are manufactured using CM. There is one company that switched the manufacturing of its product from batch to CM in 2016 because of the advantages of such a manufacturing concept in terms of quality as well as resources.

## TABLE 27.5 • First Adopters of Continuous Manufacturing

| Product | Manufacturer | Disease State | Date Approved |
|---------|--------------|---------------|---------------|
| Orkambi | Vertex | Cystic fibrosis | July 2015 |
| Prezista | J&J | HIV | April 2016 (switched from batch to continuous) |
| Verzenio | Eli Lilly | Breast cancer | September 2017 |
| Symdeko | Vertex | Cystic fibrosis | February 2018 |

# EXCIPIENT EFFECT ON DRUG PRODUCT PERFORMANCE

Drug products are finished dosage forms that contain the active pharmaceutical ingredient (API) along with suitable diluents and/or excipients. Excipients are generally considered inert in that they have no pharmacodynamic activity of their own. However, excipients have different functional purposes and influence the performance of the drug product (Shargel, 2010; Amidon et al, 2007). Compressed tablets may consist of the active ingredient, a diluent (filler), a binder, buffering agents, a disintegrating agent, and one or more lubricants. Approved FD&C and D&C dyes or lakes (dyes adsorbed onto insoluble aluminum hydroxide), flavors, and sweetening agents may also be present. These excipients provide various functional purposes such as improving compression, improving powder flow, stability of the active ingredient, and other properties (Table 27-6). For example, diluents such as lactose, starch, dibasic calcium phosphate, and microcrystalline cellulose are added where the quantity of active ingredient is small and/or difficult to compress. For highly insoluble drugs, solubilizing excipients are necessary to develop an acceptable drug product. Similarly, many drug delivery system functional excipients are the key for successfully delivering the drug to the site or releasing at a specific rate. For example, microspheres for delayed release, or some matrixes required for dermatological products.

The physical and chemical properties of the excipients, the physical and chemical properties of the API, and the manufacturing process all play a role in the performance of the finished dosage form. Each excipient must be evaluated to maintain consistent performance of the drug product throughout the product's life cycle. The quality of excipient may have an impact on the availability of the drug and hence the critical attributes of the excipients need to be understood and controlled.

## PRACTICAL FOCUS

### Bovine Spongiform Encephalopathy in Gelatin

Gelatin and other excipients may be produced from ruminant sources such as bones and hides obtained from cattle. In the early 1990s, the FDA became concerned about transmissible spongiform encephalopathies (TSEs) in animals and Creutzfeldt–Jakob disease in humans. In 1993, the FDA recommended against the use of materials from cattle that had resided in,

| **TABLE 27-6** • Common Excipients for Solid Oral Dosage Forms | | |
|---|---|---|
| Excipient | Function in Compressed Tablet | Possible Effect on Drug Product Performance |
| Microcrystalline cellulose, lactose, calcium carbonate | Diluent | Very low-dose drug (eg, 5 mg) may have high ratio of excipients to active drug, leading to a problem of homogeneous blending and possible interaction of drug with excipients. |
| Copovidone, starch, methylcellulose | Binder | Binders give adhesiveness to the powder blend and can affect tablet hardness. Harder tablets tend to disintegrate more slowly. |
| Magnesium stearate | Lubricant | Lubricants are hydrophobic; over-lubrication can slow dissolution of API. |
| Starch | Disintegrant | Disintegrant allows for more rapid fragmentation of tablet *in vivo*, reducing disintegration time and allowing for more rapid dissolution. |
| FD&C colors and lakes | Color | |
| Various | Coating | Coatings may have very little effect (film coat) or have rate-controlling effect on drug release and dissolution (eg, enteric coat). |

or originated from, countries in which *bovine spongiform encephalopathy* (BSE, or "mad cow disease") had occurred. The FDA organized a Transmissible Spongiform Encephalopathies Advisory Committee to help assess the safety of imported and domestic gelatin and gelatin by-products in FDA-regulated products with regard to the risk posed by BSE. The FDA published a guidance to industry concerning the sourcing and processing of gelatin used in pharmaceutical products to ensure the safety of gelatin as it relates to the potential risk posed by BSE (http://www.fda.gov/opacom/morechoices/industry/guidance/gelguide.htm). In some cases, such as the magnesium stearates, a vegetative source may be used to avoid the BSE/TSE concern.

## Gelatin Capsule Stability

Soft and hard gelatin capsules show a decrease in the dissolution rate as they age in simulated gastric fluid (SGF) with and without pepsin or in simulated intestinal fluid (SIF) without pancreatin. This has been attributed to pellicle formation. When the dissolution of aged or slower-releasing capsules was carried out in the presence of an enzyme (pepsin in SGF or pancreatin in SIF), a significant increase in dissolution was observed. In this setting, multiple dissolution media may be necessary to assess product quality adequately.

## Excipient Effects

Excipients can sometimes affect the rate and extent of drug absorption. In general, using excipients that are currently in FDA-approved immediate-release OSD forms within a suitable range will not affect the rate or extent of absorption of a highly soluble and highly permeable drug substance that is formulated in a rapidly dissolving immediate-release product.

Excessive use of lubricant should be avoided. When new excipients or atypically large amounts of commonly used excipients are included in an immediate-release solid dosage form, additional information documenting the absence of an impact on bioavailability of the drug may be requested by the FDA. Such information can be provided with a relative bioavailability study using a simple aqueous solution as the reference product. Large quantities of certain excipients, such as surfactants

(eg, polysorbate 80) and sweeteners (eg, mannitol or sorbitol), may be problematic.

### FREQUENTLY ASKED QUESTIONS

▶ How does a change in drug product quality change drug product performance?

▶ What is the difference between critical manufacturing attribute (CMA), critical product attribute (CPA), and critical quality attribute (CQA)?

▶ How can a pharmaceutical manufacturer ensure that a drug product has the same drug product performance before and after a change in the supplier of the active pharmaceutical ingredient or a change in the supplier of an excipient?

## Development of Age-Appropriate Formulations (Pediatric and Geriatric Populations)

It is recognized by the pharmaceutical scientists that special considerations are needed for developing pediatric formulations since children are not just mini-adults but have distinct physiological and metabolic differences that may have an impact on the pharmacokinetic parameters of the drug and hence its efficacy and or side effects. Traditionally, pediatric medication was just a dose adjustment of the adult dosage form without much effort spent on developing an age-appropriate formulation that the pediatric population could successfully ingest/tolerate. Examples of this could be too large a tablet to be chewed by younger children, or a non-taste-masked formulation that is not palatable to children and hence results in non-compliance. Often such dosage forms lead to non-optimized dose delivery; for example, if the tablet is too large, the caregivers may crush it for ease of administration, which in some cases may destroy the integrity of the dosage form resulting in suboptimal dosing. This is true for geriatric population as well, who may have difficulty in swallowing.

Another important issue is tolerance of certain excipients by the pediatric population. Examples of this include the use of propylene glycol, methyl and propylparaben, benzyl alcohol, etc. Screening and selection of excipients for pediatric formulations should be carefully conducted, since some of the excipients routinely used in the adult dosage forms are found to pose elevated toxicological risks for the children even if the doses are adjusted age-appropriately (Fabiano et al, 2011). A compilation of all nonclinical and human safety data should be assessed for inclusion of an excipient, and a risk-based justification of the excipient used needs to be presented.

## QUALITY CONTROL AND QUALITY ASSURANCE

An independent *quality assurance* (QA) unit is a vital part of drug development and manufacture. QA is responsible for ensuring that all the appropriate procedures have been followed and documented. QA provides a high probability that each dose or package of a drug product will have predictable characteristics and perform according to its labeled use. The *quality control* (QC) unit is responsible for all the testing, including in-process tests beginning with receipt of raw materials throughout production, finished product, packaging, and distribution.

Principles of QA include the following: (1) quality, safety, and effectiveness must be designed and built into the product; (2) quality cannot be inspected or tested into the finished product; and (3) each step of the manufacturing process must be controlled to maximize the probability that the finished product meets all quality and design specifications.

QA/QC has the responsibility and authority to approve or reject all components, drug product containers, closures, in-process materials, packaging material, labeling, and drug products, and has the authority to review production records to ensure that no errors have occurred or, if errors have occurred, that they have been fully investigated. QA/QC is responsible for approving or rejecting drug products manufactured, processed, packed, or held under contract by another company.

## PRACTICAL FOCUS

Tablet compression may affect drug product performance of either immediate-release or extended-release drug products even between products containing the same active drug. Metoprolol is a beta 1-selective (cardioselective) adrenoceptor blocking agent that is available as an immediate-release tablet

(metoprolol tartrate tablets, USP—Lopressor®) and an extended-release tablet (metoprolol succinate extended-release tablets—Toprol-XL®). Metoprolol is a highly soluble and highly permeable drug that meets the Biopharmaceutics Classification System, BCS 1 (Chapter 16). Metoprolol is rapidly and completely absorbed from the immediate-release tablet.

Compression makes the powder blend more compact and affects tablet hardness, especially when an inadequate amount of binder is added. Excessive compression may cause the tablet to disintegrate more slowly, resulting in a slower rate of dissolution and systemic drug absorption. Adequate use of binder and lubricant during product design obviates the need to use excessive force during compression/compaction.

The metoprolol succinate extended-release tablet (Toprol-XL®) is a multiple-unit system containing metoprolol succinate in a multitude of controlled-release pellets. Each pellet acts as a separate drug delivery unit and is designed to deliver metoprolol continuously over the dosage interval (Toprol-XL approved label). The controlled-release pellets are mixed with excipients and compressed into tablets. If the tablet is compressed too strongly, the high compression will not only increase tablet hardness but can also deform the controlled-release pellets. The deformed pellets lose their controlled-release characteristics and the active drug, metoprolol, dissolves more quickly, resulting in a faster-than-desired rate of systemic drug absorption. An inadequate amount of lubricant or glidant can also aggravate or damage pellets during compression.

## TYPES OF QUALITY RISK

Quality risks can be realized at various stages of development and manufacturing if proper controls and systems are not implemented to ensure acceptable quality. These can be seen right from the quality of materials including drug substance and excipients, developmental risks, and manufacturing risks as the main categories.

### Material (Components/Excipients)

It is critical that all the components that make up the drug product ultimately consumed by the patient are assured of quality and devoid of any risks that could impact the efficacy of the product. This can be done by implementing quality procedures as mandated by cGMP practices and having a well-defined vendor qualification and testing program. Periodic GMP audits to ensure that the vendor adheres to the quality procedures are necessary. This is most important for API manufacturer. The API is often sourced from different regions of the world and hence subjected to different quality standards. It is important to understand the quality of the API, the control of its starting materials, and the risks involved therein. At minimum, they should meet FDA expectations, but the supply chain and the probable risks involved due to sourcing, transportation, difference in standards, etc, should all be evaluated and assessed for potential risks to the quality of drug products as a good business practice as well.

API material properties include particle size, crystal forms, and compression characteristics. However, these properties may be reduced by the impact resulting from a poor API that has residual solvents (eg, chloroform, toluene), or solvents that may be classified as carcinogenic. With the adoption of recent FDA quality guidances, residual solvents are generally well controlled with generally recognized standards with FDA-approved products.

## Control of Starting Materials in API Synthesis

Sources of impurities such as heavy metals, solvents, and impurities are risks that may impact quality in subsequent steps in unknown ways. For example, metallic impurities, even if not harmful, may have an impact on the stability of some products, and a low level may alter the appearance of a product even if not harmful. Related impurities to an API may sometimes have pharmacologic properties of their own. The history or processes that precede starting materials is generally not documented. Starting materials may not be regulatory controlled or inspected. It is of particular importance to maintain a good quality practice by the vendor or supplier even though the starting materials are not strictly regulated. A chemical may be produced for chemical or industrial purposes. For example, urea is produced as fertilizer rather than for drug or excipient use.

The quality of excipients should also be monitored similarly, and the vendors should be qualified to ensure no unexpected changes during the life cycle of the product. Excipient quality may impact the physicochemical characteristics of the drug product that may sometimes be unacceptable. Having a well-understood supply chain and quality of excipients is important in maintaining drug product quality.

## Drug Development Quality Risks

These are risks to quality that occur due to inadequate development. If quality is not built in using sound scientific principles and development, testing in quality may become necessary and result in a poorly designed drug that may cause lot failures during manufacturing, or worse, recalls after being distributed. As an example, consider a tablet formulation that typically has a diluent, a binder, and a disintegrant. Choosing the wrong combination of these excipients may result in a tablet that is friable and soft, making it necessary to compensate by increasing the compression force to result in a harder tablet (and thus decrease friability) or increasing the binder level to maintain the tablet integrity. In this scenario, frequent testing for friability and hardness may be implemented to ensure the product exhibits suitable characteristics for handling (not soft to touch and friable). However, using the correct binder could result in a more robust formulation that will obviate the criticality of such a test. Too hard a tablet will make it brittle, and too much binder may increase the disintegration time. Appropriate development of this tablet formulation will typically evaluate the excipient compatibility, the different levels of excipients needed, and their impact on CQAs that will allow early selection of appropriate excipients at the right amounts, resulting in a robust formulation. A risk in QbD may be easily overlooked with an inadequate quality strategy. Too often, inadequate understanding of excipient functions or inclusion of suitable binders (eg, starch, macrocrystalline cellulose) results in an incorrect QbD strategy, such as testing friability and hardness at different hardness at appropriate levels instead of using a suitable binder or increasing the proportion of excipients. The proper inclusion of suitable ingredients may result in a product that is so robust that hardness has little or no effect on disintegration while still maintaining friability. A well-designed QbD study on such a product would do away with the need for extensive testing.

## Manufacturing Risks

Manufacturing includes API synthesis, Drug Product manufacturing, and final product packaging steps. API risks have been discussed in the previous chapter.

Control tests on the finished product are quality tests that are specified, including stability, dissolution, and other special product tests. It is important to consider whether the tests will have an impact on the performance of the product. Setting meaningful specifications which directly impact product performance and therefore efficacy is important. These should relate back to measurements of CQAs. It is therefore of utmost importance to ensure that CQAs have been identified accurately. This in turn relates to how CPPs are defined. Well-defined CQAs and CPPs lead to a robust formulation and manufacturing process that results in a product with consistent, well-defined quality and minimal postmarketing issues. Product developed using the concepts presented in Figs. 27-2 and 27-3 address these issues and lead to setting of meaningful specifications that provide QA throughout the life cycle of the product.

Protecting the finished product by ensuring appropriate packaging is important in maintaining quality throughout the life cycle of the product. For example, light-sensitive/moisture-sensitive drugs have specific packaging requirements that must be followed and accompanied with specific instructions for patients to follow after they open the package. Not adhering to these instructions may impact the quality of the product and hence efficacy in some cases.

---

### FREQUENTLY ASKED QUESTIONS

▶ Can a QbD strategy for testing hardness and disintegration replace the need for a full dissolution profile testing of all batches?

▶ Can a dissolution test of a tablet at the beginning and the end period of stability cycle replace dissolution testing every 3 or 6 months during the stability cycle?

▶ Is sterility testing of an injection product at the initial and the end of production batch adequate to justify the stability of a new product?

---

## Good Manufacturing Practices

*Good Manufacturing Practices* (GMPs) are FDA regulations that describe the methods, equipment, facilities, and controls required for producing human and veterinary products. GMPs define a quality system that manufacturers use to build quality into their products. For example, approved drug products developed and produced according to GMPs are considered safe, properly identified, of the correct strength, pure, and of high quality. The US regulations are called *current* Good Manufacturing Practices (cGMPs), to emphasize that the expectations are dynamic. These regulations are minimum requirements that may be exceeded by the manufacturer. GMPs help prevent inadvertent use or release of unacceptable drug products into manufacturing and distribution. GMP requirements include well-trained personnel and management, buildings and facilities, and written and approved standard operating procedures (SOPs), as listed in Table 27-7.

## Guidance for Industry

The FDA publishes guidances for the industry to provide recommendations to pharmaceutical manufacturers for the development and manufacture of drug substances and drug products (http://www.fda.gov/drugs/guidancecomplianceregulatoryinformation/guidances/ucm121568.htm). The International Conference on Harmonization of Technical Requirements for Registration of Pharmaceuticals for Human Use (ICH) is composed of the regulatory authorities of Europe, Japan, and the United States, and experts from the pharmaceutical industry. The ICH is interested in the global development and availability of new medicines while maintaining safeguards on quality, safety and efficacy, and regulatory obligations to protect public health (www.ich.org).

## Quality Standards

Public standards are necessary to ensure that drug substances and drug products have consistent and reproducible quality. The *United States Pharmacopeia* National Formulary (USP-NF, www.usp.org) is legally recognized by the US Food, Drug, and Cosmetic Act and sets public standards for drug products and drug substances. The USP-NF contains monographs for drug substances and drug

**TABLE 27-7** • Current Good Manufacturing Practice for Finished Pharmaceuticals

Subpart A—General Provisions
  Scope, definitions
Subpart B—Organization and Personnel
  Responsibilities of quality control unit, personnel qualifications, personnel responsibilities, consultants
Subpart C—Buildings and Facilities
  Design and construction features, lighting, ventilation, air filtration, air heating and cooling, plumbing, sewage and refuse, washing and toilet facilities, sanitation, maintenance
Subpart D—Equipment
  Equipment design, size, and location, equipment construction, equipment cleaning and maintenance, automatic, mechanical, and electronic equipment, filters
Subpart E—Control of Components and Drug Product Containers and Closures
  General requirements, receipt and storage of untested components, drug product containers and closures; testing and approval or rejection of components, drug product containers and closures; use of approved components, drug product containers and closures; retesting of approved components, drug product containers and closures, rejected components, drug product containers and closures, drug product containers and closures
Subpart F—Production and Process Controls
  Written procedures, deviations, change of components, calculation of yield, equipment identification, sampling and testing of in-process materials and drug products, time limitations on production, control of microbiological contamination, reprocessing
Subpart G—Packaging and Labeling Controls
  Materials examination and usage criteria, labeling issuance, packaging and labeling operations, tamper-resistant packaging requirements for over-the-counter human drug products, drug product inspection, expiration dating
Subpart H—Holding and Distribution
  Warehousing procedures, distribution procedures
Subpart I—Laboratory Controls
  General requirements, testing and release for distribution, stability testing, special testing requirements, reserve samples, laboratory animals, penicillin contamination
Subpart J—Records and Reports
  General requirements; equipment cleaning and use log; component, drug product, container, closure, and labeling records; master production and control records, batch production and control records, production record review, laboratory records, distribution, complaint files
Subpart K—Returned and Salvaged Drug Products
  Returned drug products, drug product salvaging

*Data from US Code of Federal Regulations (CFR), 21 CFR Part 211. U.S. Department of Health and Human Services. Food and Drug Administration.*

products that include standards for strength, quality, and purity. In addition, the USP-NF contains chapters that describe specific procedures that support the monographs. The tests in the monographs may provide *acceptance criteria*, that is, numerical limits, ranges, or other criteria for the test for the drug substance or drug product. An *impurity* is defined as any component of the drug substance that is not the entity defined as the drug substance. Drugs with a USP or NF designation that do not conform to the USP monograph may be considered adulterated. *Specifications* are the standards a drug product must meet to ensure conformance to predetermined

criteria for consistent and reproducible quality and performance.

The International Conference on Harmonization (ICH) has published several guidances to regulate drug substance and drug product manufacturing. The main approach is to promote "better understanding of manufacturing processes with quality (by) design." QbD improves the quality of the product and makes it easier for regulatory agencies to evaluate postapproval changes of a drug product. ICH Guidance Q8 describes pharmaceutical development, and ICH Guidance Q10 discusses pharmaceutical quality systems. Earlier guidances such as

ICH Q6A provide more specific details on setting acceptance criteria and test specifications for new drug substances and new drug products. The ICH Guidance Q6A has been recommended for adoption in the United States, the European Union, and Japan. These regulations will be applied to new drug substances and drug products.

## RISK MANAGEMENT

### Regulatory and Scientific Considerations

The FDA develops rational, science-based regulatory requirements for drug substances and finished drug products. The FDA establishes quality standards and acceptance criteria for each component used in the manufacture of a drug product. Each component must meet an appropriate quality and performance objective.

### Drug Manufacturing Requirements

Assurance of product quality is derived from careful attention to a number of factors, including selection of quality parts and materials, adequate product and process design, control of the process, and in-process and end-product testing. Because of the complexity of today's medical products, routine end-product testing alone often is not sufficient to ensure product quality. The *chemistry, manufacturing, and controls* (CMC) section of a drug application describes the composition, manufacture, and specifications of the drug substance and drug product (Table 27-8).

**TABLE 27-8** • Guidelines for the Format and Content of the Chemistry, Manufacturing, and Controls Section of an Application

Module 3: Quality
   3.1. Table of Contents of Module 3
   3.2. Body Of Data
   3.2. S Drug Substance
      3.2.S.1: General Information (Nomenclature, Structure, General Properties)
      3.2.S.2: Manufacture (Manufacturers, Description of Manufacturing Process and process controls, Control of materials, Control of Critical Steps and Intermediates, Process Validation and/or Evaluation, Manufacturing process development)
      3.2.S.3: Characterization (Elucidation of Structure and other characteristics), Impurities)
      3.2.S.4: Control of Drug Substance (Specification, analytical Procedures, Validation of Analytical Procedures, Batch Analyses, Justification of specifications
      3.2.S.5: Reference Standards or Materials
      3.2.S.6: Container Closure System
      3.2.S.7: Stability (Summary and Conclusions, Post-approval Stability Protocol and Stability Commitment, Stability data)
   3.2.P Drug Product
      3.2.P.1: Description and Composition of Drug Product
      3.2.P.2: Pharmaceutical Development (Components, Drug Product, Manufacturing Process Development, Manufacture, Container closure System, Microbiological Attributes, compatibility)
      3.2.P.3: Manufacture (Manufacturers, Batch Formula, Description of manufacturing process and process controls, Control of Critical Steps and Intermediates, Process Validation and/or Evaluation)
      3.2.P.4: Control of Excipients (Specifications, Analytical Procedures, Validation of Analytical Procedures, Justifications of Specifications, Excipients of human or Animal Origins, Novel Excipients)
      3.2.P.5: Control of Drug Product (Specification, Analytical Procedures, Validation of Analytical Procedures, Batch Analyses, Characterization of Impurities, Justification of specifications)
      3.2.P.6: Reference Standards or Materials
      3.2.P.7: Container Closure System
      3.2.P.8: Stability (Stability Summary and Conclusions, Post-Approval Stability Protocol and Commitment, Stability data)

*Data from FDA Guidance, 1999.*

## Process Validation

*Process validation* is the process for establishing documented evidence to provide a high degree of assurance that a specific process will consistently produce a product meeting its predetermined specifications and quality characteristics. Process validation is a key element in ensuring that these QA goals are met. Proof of validation is obtained through collection and evaluation of data, preferably beginning at the process development phase and continuing through the production phase.

The product's end use should be a determining factor in the development of product (and component) characteristics and specifications. All pertinent aspects of the product that may affect safety and effectiveness should be considered. These aspects include performance, reliability, and stability. Acceptable ranges or limits should be established for each characteristic to set up allowable variations. *Specifications* are the quality standards (ie, tests, analytical procedures, and acceptance criteria) that confirm the quality of drug substances, drug products, intermediates, raw material reagents, components, in-process material, container closure systems, and other materials used in the production of the drug substance or drug product. The standards or specifications that are critical to product quality are considered CMAs or CPPs.

Through careful design and validation of both the process and process controls, a manufacturer can establish with a high degree of confidence that all manufactured units from successive lots will be acceptable. Successfully validating a process may reduce the dependence on intensive in-process and finished product testing. In most cases, end-product testing plays a major role in ensuring that QA goals are met; that is, validation and end-product testing are not mutually exclusive.

## SCALE-UP AND POSTAPPROVAL CHANGES

A *postapproval change* is any change in a drug product after it has been approved for marketing by the FDA. Postapproval manufacturing changes may adversely impact drug product quality. Since safety and efficacy are established using clinical batches, the same level of quality must be ensured in the finished drug product released to the public. A change to a marketed drug product can be initiated for a number of reasons, including a revised market forecast, change in an API source, change in excipients, optimization of the manufacturing process, and upgrade of the packaging system. A change within a given parameter can have varied effects, depending on the type of product. For example, a change in the container closure/system of an OSD form may have little impact on an oral tablet dosage form unless the primary packaging component is critical to the shelf life of the finished product.

If a pharmaceutical manufacturer makes any change in the drug formulation, scales up the formulation to a larger batch size, or changes the process, equipment, or manufacturing site, the manufacturer should consider whether any of these changes will affect the identity, strength, purity, quality, safety, and efficacy of the approved drug product. Moreover, any changes in the raw material (ie, active pharmaceutical ingredient), excipients (including a change in grade or supplier), or packaging (including container closure system) should also be shown not to affect the quality of the drug product. The manufacturer should assess the effect of the change on the identity, strength (eg, assay, content uniformity), quality (eg, physical, chemical, and biological properties), purity (eg, impurities and degradation products), or potency (eg, biological activity, bioavailability, bioequivalence) of a product as they may relate to the safety or effectiveness of the product.

The FDA has published several Scale-Up and Postapproval Changes (SUPAC) guidances, including *Changes to an Approved NDA or ANDA* for the pharmaceutical industry. These guidances address the following issues:

- Components and composition of the drug product
- Manufacturing site change
- Scale-up of drug product
- Manufacturing equipment
- Manufacturing process
- Packaging
- Active pharmaceutical ingredient

These documents describe (1) the level of change, (2) recommended CMC tests for each level of change, (3) *in vitro* dissolution tests and/or

## TABLE 27-9 • FDA Definitions of Level of Changes That May Affect the Quality of an Approved Drug Product

| Change Level | Definition of Level |
|---|---|
| Level 1 | Changes that are unlikely to have any detectable impact on the formulation quality and performance. |
| Level 2 | Changes that could have a significant impact on formulation quality and performance. |
| Level 3 | Changes that are likely to have a significant impact on formulation quality and performance. |

bioequivalence tests for each level of change, and (4) documentation that should support the change. The level of change is classified as to the likelihood that a change in the drug product as listed above might affect the quality of the drug product. The levels of change as described by the FDA are listed in Table 27-9.

As noted in Table 27-9, a Level 1 change, which could be a small change in the excipient amount (eg, starch, lactose), would be unlikely to alter the quality or performance of the drug product, whereas a Level 3 change, which may be a qualitative or quantitative change in the excipients beyond an allowable range, particularly for drug products containing a narrow therapeutic window, might require an *in vivo* bioequivalence study to demonstrate that drug quality and performance were not altered by the change.

The SUPAC guidance is an early guidance that assesses changes in manufacturing and its effect on product quality. The basic concepts continue to be a useful guide, and in many respects, QbD extends its scope. With adequate QbD study, some changes in manufacturing may require only an annual report instead of a prior approval supplements for regulatory purposes. The ultimate question is whether the product quality will be assured to be equivalent or better, and meet with prior information described in the application with QbD data.

### Assessment of the Effects of the Change

Assessment of the effects of a change should include a determination that the drug substance intermediates,

drug substance, in-process materials, and/or drug product affected by the change conform to the approved specifications. *Acceptance criteria* are numerical limits, ranges, or other criteria for the tests described. *Conformance* to a specification means that the material, when tested according to the analytical procedures listed in the specification, will meet the listed acceptance criteria. Additional testing may be needed to confirm that the material affected by manufacturing changes continues to meet its specifications. The assessment may include, as appropriate, evaluation of any changes in the chemical, physical, microbiological, biological, bioavailability, and/or stability profiles. This additional assessment may involve testing of the postchange drug product itself or, if appropriate, the component directly affected by the change. The type of additional testing depends on the type of manufacturing change, the type of drug substance and/or drug product, and the effect of the change on the quality of the product. Examples of additional tests include:

- Evaluation of changes in the impurity or degradant profile
- Toxicology tests to qualify a new impurity or degradant or to qualify an impurity that is above a previously qualified level
- Evaluation of the hardness or friability of a tablet
- Assessment of the effect of a change on bioequivalence (may include multipoint and/or multimedia dissolution profiles and/or an *in vivo* bioequivalence study)
- Evaluation of extractables from new packaging components or moisture permeability of a new container closure system

### Equivalence

The manufacturer usually assesses the extent to which the manufacturing change has affected the identity, strength, quality, purity, or potency of the drug product by comparing test results from *pre-* and *postchange* material and then determining if the test results are equivalent. The drug product after any changes should be equivalent to the product made before the change. An exception to this general approach is that when bioequivalence should be redocumented for certain Abbreviated New

Drug Application (ANDA) postapproval changes, the comparator should be the reference listed drug. Equivalence does not necessarily mean identical. Equivalence may also relate to maintenance of a quality characteristic (eg, stability) rather than a single performance of a test.

### Critical Manufacturing Variables

*Critical manufacturing variables* (CMVs) include items in the formulation, process, equipment, materials, and methods for the drug product that can significantly affect *in vitro* dissolution. If possible, the manufacturer should determine whether there is a relationship between CMV, *in vitro* dissolution, and *in vivo* bioavailability.[2] The goal is to develop product specifications that will ensure bioequivalence of future batches prepared within limits of acceptable dissolution specifications. One approach to obtaining this relationship is to compare the bioavailability of test products with slowest and fastest dissolution characteristics to the bioavailability of the marketed drug product. Dissolution specifications for the drug product are then established so that future production batches do not fall outside the bioequivalence of the marketed drug product.

### Adverse Effects

Sometimes manufacturing changes have an adverse effect on the identity, strength, quality, purity, or potency of the drug product. For example, a type of process change could cause a new degradant to be formed that requires qualification and/or quantification. The manufacturer must show that the new degradant will not affect the safety or efficacy of the product. Changes in the qualitative or quantitative formulation, including inactive ingredients, are considered major changes and are likely to have a significant impact on formulation quality and performance. However, the deletion or reduction of an ingredient intended to affect only the color of a product is considered to be a minor change that is unlikely to affect the safety of the drug product.

---

[2]In vitro dissolution/drug release studies that relate to the in vivo drug bioavailability may be considered a drug product performance test.

### Postapproval Changes of Drug Substance

Manufacturing changes of the *active pharmaceutical ingredient* (API)—also known as the drug substance or bulk active—may change its quality attributes. These quality attributes include chemical purity, solid-state properties, and residual solvents. Chemical purity is dependent on the synthetic pathway and purification process. Solid-state properties include particle size, polymorphism, hydrate/solvate, and solubility. Small amounts of residual solvents such as dichloromethane may remain in the API after extraction and/or purification. Changes in the solid-state properties of the API may affect the manufacture of the dosage form or product performance. For example, a change in particle size may affect API bulk density and tablet hardness, whereas different polymorphs may affect API solubility and stability. Changes in particle size and/or polymorph may affect the drug's bioavailability *in vivo*. Moreover, the excipient(s) and vehicle functionality and possible pharmacologic properties may affect product quality and performance.

> **FREQUENTLY ASKED QUESTION**
>
> ▶ Does a change in the manufacturing process require FDA approval?

## PRACTICAL FOCUS

### Quantitative Change in Excipients

A manufacturer would like to increase the amount of starch by 2% (w/w) in an immediate-release drug product.

- Would you consider this change in an excipient to be a Level 1, 2, or 3 change? Why?

  The FDA has determined that small changes in certain excipients for immediate-release drug products may be considered Level 1 changes. Table 27-10 lists the changes in excipients, expressed as percentage (w/w) of the total formulation, less than or equal to the following percent ranges that are considered Level 1 changes. According to this table, a 2% increase in starch would be considered a Level 1 change.

  The total additive effect of all excipient changes should not be more than 5%. For example, in a drug product containing the active ingredient lactose,

## TABLE 27-10 • Level 1—Allowable Changes in Excipients

| Excipient | Percent Excipient (W/W) of Total Target Dosage Form Weight |
|---|---|
| Filler | ±5 |
| Disintegrant | ±3 |
|   Starch | ±1 |
|   Other | |
| Binder | ±0.5 |
| Lubricant | ±0.25 |
|   Calcium stearate | ±0.25 |
|   Magnesium stearate | ±1 |
|   Other | |
| Glidant | ±1 |
|   Talc | ±0.1 |
|   Other | |
| Film coat | ±1 |

*These percentages are based on the assumption that the drug substance in the product is formulated to 100% of label/potency.*
*Reproduced with permission from FDA Guidance: Immediate Release Solid Oral Dosage Forms: Scale-Up and Postapproval Changes. Center for Drug Evaluation and Research (CDER). November, 1995.*

microcrystalline cellulose, and magnesium stearate, the lactose and microcrystalline cellulose should not vary by more than an absolute total of 5% (eg, lactose increases 2.5% and microcrystalline cellulose decreases by 2.5%) relative to the target dosage form weight if it is to stay within the Level 1 range. The examples are for illustrations only and the latest official guidance should be consulted for current views.

It should be noted that a small change in the amount of excipients is less likely to affect the bioavailability of a highly soluble, highly permeable drug in an immediate-release drug product compared to a drug that has low solubility and low permeability.

### Changes in Batch Size (Scale-Up/Scale-Down)

For commercial reasons, a manufacturer may increase the batch size of a drug product from 100,000 units to 5 million units. Even though similar equipment and the same SOPs are used, there may be problems in manufacturing a very large batch. This problem is similar to a chef's problem of cooking the main entrée for two persons versus cooking the same entrée for a banquet of 200 persons using the same recipe. The FDA has generally considered that a change in batch size greater than 10-fold is a Level 2 change and requires the manufacturer to notify the FDA and provide documentation for all testing before marketing this product.

## PRODUCT QUALITY PROBLEMS

The FDA and industry are working together to establish a set of quality attributes and acceptance criteria for certain approved drug substances and drug products that would indicate less manufacturing risk. Table 27-11 summarizes some of the quality attributes for these products. However, all approved drug products must be manufactured under cGMPs.

Drug substances and drug products that have more quality risk are generally those products that are more complex to synthesize or manufacture. For example, biotechnology-derived drugs (eg, proteins) made by fermentation may have more quality risk than chemically synthesized small molecules. Extended-release and delayed-release drug products may also present a greater quality risk than an immediate-release drug product. Drug products that have a very small ratio of active drug substance to excipients are more difficult to blend uniformly and thus may have a greater quality risk. GMPs and control of the critical manufacturing operations help maintain the quality of the finished product. Complex operations can have consistent outcome quality as long as the manufacturer maintains control of the process and builds in quality during manufacturing operations.

## POSTMARKETING SURVEILLANCE

Pharmaceutical manufacturers are required to file periodic postmarket reports for an approved ANDA to the FDA through its *Postmarketing Surveillance Program*. The main component of the requirement is the reporting of adverse drug experiences. This

**TABLE 27-11** • Quality Attributes and Criteria for Certain Approved Drug Substances and Drug Products

| Drug Substances | | Drug Products | |
|---|---|---|---|
| **Attribute** | **Criteria** | **Attribute** | **Criteria** |
| Chemical structure | Well characterized | Dosage form | Oral (immediate release), simple solutions, others |
| Synthetic process | Simple process | | |
| Quality | No toxic impurities; adequate specifications | Manufacturing process Quality | Easy to manufacture (TBD) Adequate specifications |
| Physical properties | Polymorphic forms, particle size are well controlled | Biopharmaceutic Classification Systems | Highly permeable and highly soluble drugs |
| Stability | Stable drug substance | Stability | Stable drug product (TBD) |
| Manufacturing history | TBD | | |
| Others | TBD | Manufacturing history | TBD |
| | | Others | TBD |

TBD, to be defined.
Adapted with permission from Chui Y: Risk-Based CMC Review, An Update, Advisory Committee for Pharmaceutical Sciences Meeting, FDA, October 21, 2002.

is accomplished by reassessing drug risks based on data learned after the drug is marketed. In addition, labeling changes may occur after market approval. For example, a new adverse reaction discussed by postmarketing surveillance is required for both branded and generic drug products.

## GLOSSARY

**BioRAM:** The biopharmaceutics risk assessment roadmap (BioRAM) optimizes drug product development and performance by using therapy-driven target drug delivery profiles as a framework to achieve the desired therapeutic outcome.

**Continuous process verification:** An alternative approach to process validation in which manufacturing process performance is continuously monitored and evaluated.

**Critical Materials Attribute (CMA):** Attribute of the materials (excipients) that impacts drug product quality and/or performance.

**Critical Process parameter (CPP):** Process parameter that impacts the drug product quality and/or performance.

**Critical quality attribute (CQA):** A physical, chemical, biological, or microbiological property or characteristic that should be within an appropriate limit, range, or distribution to ensure the desired product quality.

**Design space:** The multidimensional combination and interaction of input variables (eg, material attributes) and process parameters that have been demonstrated to provide quality assurance. Working within the design space is not considered a change. Movement out of the design space is considered to be a change and would normally initiate a regulatory postapproval change process. Design space is proposed by the applicant and is subject to regulatory assessment and approval.

**Life cycle:** All phases in the life of a product from the initial development through marketing until the product's discontinuation.

**Process analytical technology (PAT):** A system for designing, analyzing, and controlling manufacturing through timely measurements (ie, during processing) of critical quality and performance attributes of raw and in-process materials and processes with the goal of ensuring final product quality.

**Quality:** The suitability of either a drug substance or a drug product for its intended use. This term includes such attributes as the identity, strength, and purity (from ICH Q6A specifications: test procedures and acceptance criteria for new drug substances and new drug products: chemical substances).

**Quality by design (QbD):** A systematic approach to development that begins with predefined objectives and emphasizes product and process understanding and process control, based on sound science and quality risk management.

**Quality target product profile (QTPP):** A prospective summary of the quality characteristics of a drug product that ideally will be achieved to ensure the desired quality, taking into account safety and efficacy of the drug product.

## CHAPTER SUMMARY

The pharmaceutical development process must design a quality drug product (QbD, quality by design) using a manufacturing process that provides consistent drug product performance and achieves the desired therapeutic objective. Drug product quality and drug product performance are important for patient safety and therapeutic efficacy. Drug product quality and drug product performance relate to the biopharmaceutic and physicochemical properties of the drug substance and the drug product and to the manufacturing process. The development of a drug product requires a systematic, scientific, risk-based, holistic, and proactive approach that begins with predefined objectives and emphasizes product and processes understanding and process control (QbD). Quality cannot be tested into drug products. Quality should be built in the design and confirmed by testing. Quality control (QC) and quality assurance (QA) help ensure that drug products are manufactured with quality and have consistent performance throughout their life cycle. Manufacturers must demonstrate that any changes in the formulation after FDA approval (SUPAC) does not alter drug product quality and performance compared to the initial formulation. Excipients that have no inherent pharmacodynamic activity may affect drug product performance. Drug products may be recalled due to deficiencies in drug product quality. Product quality defects are controlled through GMPs, monitoring, and surveillance. The QTPP approach is an approach commonly recommended for drug development. The need to "learn and confirm" is an important approach evaluating different quality systems balancing risk and need for progress.

## LEARNING QUESTIONS

1. Three batches of ibuprofen tablets, 200 mg, are manufactured by the same manufacturer using the same equipment. Each batch meets the same specifications. Does meeting specifications mean that each batch of drug product contains the identical amount of ibuprofen?

2. What should a manufacturer of a modified-release tablet consider when making a qualitative or quantitative change in an excipient?

3. Explain how a change in drug product quality may affect drug product performance. Provide at least three examples.

4. For solid oral drug products, a change in the concentration of which of the following excipients is more likely to influence the bioavailability of a drug? Why?

   Starch

   Magnesium stearate

   Microcrystalline cellulose

   Talc

   Lactose

5. How does the polymorphic form of the active drug substance influence the bioavailability of a drug? Can two different polymorphs of the same active drug substance have the same bioavailability?

## ANSWERS

### Learning Questions

1. Specifications provide a quantitative limit (acceptance criteria) to a test product (eg, the total drug content must be within ±5% or the amount of impurities in the drug substance must not be more than [NMT] 1%). Thus, one batch of nominally 200-mg ibuprofen tablets may contain an average content of 198 mg, whereas the average content for another batch of 200-mg ibuprofen tablets may have an average content of 202 mg. Both batches meet a specification of ±5% and would be considered to meet the label claim of 200 mg of ibuprofen per tablet.

2. The manufacturer must consider whether the excipient is critical or not critical to drug release. If the excipient (eg, starch) is not critical to drug release (ie, a non-release-controlling excipient), then small changes in the starch concentration, generally less than 3% of the total target dosage form weight, is unlikely to affect the formulation quality and performance. A qualitative change in the excipient may affect drug release and thus will have significant effect on the formulation performance.

## REFERENCES

Amidon GE, Peck GE, Block LH, et al: Proposed new USP general information chapter, excipient performance (1059). *Pharm Forum* **33**(6):1311–1323, 2007.

Chui Y: Risk-Based CMC Review, An Update. Advisory Committee for Pharmaceutical Sciences Meeting, FDA, October 21, 2002.

Cogdill RP, Drennen JK: Risk-based Quality by Design (QbD): A Taguchi perspective on the assessment of product quality, and the quantitative linkage of drug product parameters and clinical performance. *J Pharm Innov* **3**:23–29, 2008. DOI 10.1007/s12247-008-9025-3.

Fabiano, V, Mameli, C, Zuccotii, GV: Pediatric pharmacology: Remember the excipients. *Pharm Res* **63**(5):362–365, 2011.

FDA: CDER Report to the Nation: 2005.

FDA: CDER 2007 Update.

FDA Guidance: Immediate Release Solid Oral Dosage Forms: Scale-Up and Postapproval Changes, 1995.

FDA Guidance for Industry: Changes to an Approved NDA or ANDA, April 2004 http://www.fda.gov/drugs/guidancecompllanceregulatoryinformation/guidances/ucm121568.htm.

FDA Guidance for Industry: PAT—A Framework for Innovative Pharmaceutical Development, Manufacturing, and Quality Assurance, September 2004.

FDA Guidance for Industry: Q8(R1) Pharmaceutical Development, June 2009.

International Conference on Harmonisation (ICH) Guidances: http://www.ich.org.

Lionberger RL: FDA critical path initiatives: Opportunities for generic drug development. *AAPS J* **10**(1):103–109, 2008.

Sayeed, VA, Advisory Committee for Pharmaceutical Sciences: Risk-Based CMC Review. FDA, Oct 21, 2002.

Selen A: Office of New Drug Quality Assessment/CDER/FDA, 32nd Annual Midwest Biopharmaceutical Statistics Workshop, Ball State University, Muncie, Indiana, May 18–20, 2009.

Selen A, et al: The biopharmaceutics risk assessment roadmap for optimizing clinical drug product performance. *J Pharm Sci* **103**(11):3377–3397, 2014. Also published online in Wiley Online Library (wileyonlinelibrary.com). DOI 10.1002/jps.24162, August 22, 2014.

Shargel L: Drug product performance and interchangeability of multisource drug substances and drug products. *Pharm Forum* **35**:744–749, 2010.

US Code of Federal Regulations (CFR), 21 CFR Part 211. http://www.fda.gov/drugs/guidancecomplianceregulatoryinformation/guidances/ucm121568.htm. Accessed August 10, 2011.

Yu LX: Pharmaceutical quality by design: Product and process development, understanding, and control. *Pharm Res* **25**:781–791, 2008.

Yu LX: Regulatory Assessment of Pharmaceutical Quality for Generic Drugs. http://www.fda.gov/downloads/aboutfda/centersoffices/officeofmedicalproductsandtobacco/cder/ucm119204.pdf. Accessed June 10, 2015.

# BIBLIOGRAPHY

Buckley L, Salunke S, Thompson K, Baer G, Fegley D, Turner M: Challenges and strategies to facilitate formulation development of pediatric drug products: Safety qualification of excipients. *Int J Pharm* 2017. 536. 10.1016/j.ijpharm.2017.07.042.

International Conference on Harmonisation (ICH): http://www.fda.gov/Drugs/GuidanceComplianceRegulatoryInformation/Guidances/ucm065005.htm (source of regulatory documents for quality systems and QbD discussions).

Sood R: Question-Based Review—A Vision. 9-Jun-2014. http://www.fda.gov/downloads/aboutfda/centersoffices/officeofmedicalproductsandtobacco/cder/ucm410433.pdf. Accessed June 10, 2015.

Ternik R, Liu F, Bartlett J, et al: Assessment of swallowability and palatability of oral dosage forms in children: Report from an M-CERSI pediatric formulation workshop. *Int J Pharm*, 2017. 536. 10.1016/j.ijpharm.2017.08.088.

Yu LX, Amidon G, Khan MA, et al: Understanding pharmaceutical quality by design. *AAPS J* **6**(4):771–783, 2014.

# 28 FDA-Approved Novel Dosage Forms

Ziyaur Rahman, Naseem A. Charoo,
Mohammad T.H. Nutan, and Mansoor A. Khan

## CHAPTER OBJECTIVES

- Describe regulatory pathways for approval of new dosage forms of already approved drugs.

- Describe the regulatory pathway for approval of drug–device combination products

- Explain how dosage forms are printed using 3D printing technologies, advantages and disadvantages of the technologies.

- List various approaches employed in designing FDA approved abuse deterrent opioid formulations.

- Describe preformed and *in situ* methods for preparation of implants and discuss their release mechanism.

- Explain how microparticles/and microspheres differ from implants.

- Describe vaginal contraceptive rings, their primary application, and polymers used in their fabrication. Explain their differences with intrauterine devices.

- Describes various types of nanomedicines, ie, liposomes, nanocrystals, polymeric nanoparticles, micelles, nanoemulsion, microemulsion, nanotubes, and colloidal iron products, route of administration as presented in FDA approved nanomedicines.

- Explain how digital medicines are different from conventional medicines with discussion on the design of commercial products.

- Describe various types of drug-eluting stents, their design, and materials used in the fabrication of commonly used drugs.

- Explain the design of various types of transdermal systems, formulation components, and functions with FDA-approved transdermal products as examples.

- Describe advantages and disadvantages of nasal delivery systems, formulation components with function and examples, and different types of FDA-approved nasal delivery systems for topical and systemic drugs.

- Describe advantages of administering drugs by inhalation route, types of inhalation dosage forms, differences, and commercially available inhalation dosage forms.

## INTRODUCTION

Drug molecules have to be developed into a suitable dosage form for safe and effective administration. Before 1950, most of the approved dosage forms included conventional capsules, tablets, and liquid formulations. Dosage forms have undergone a radical transformation in the last six decades. The US Food and Drug Administration (FDA) approved the first extended-release formulation in 1952, which provided 12 hours of sustained release and was based on Spansule® technology. Since then, the FDA has approved a number of new and novel dosage forms, such as pressurized metered dose inhalers (pMDIs), transdermal patches, liposomes, microparticles, polymeric nanoparticles, digital dosage forms, drug–device combination products, etc, to improve the safety and efficacy of drugs and patient adherence.

The decision as to whether to develop a conventional dosage form or a novel formulation is made during the drug development phase and is determined by many factors, including physicochemical and biopharmaceutical properties of the drug candidate. The mode of delivery must ensure that the drug is safe and effective. For instance, poorly soluble and/or poorly permeable drug substances such as cyclosporine and tacrolimus, if formulated in conventional dosage forms such as tablets, capsules, or suspensions, would not produce the desired therapeutic response. Consequently, cyclosporine is commercially available as microemulsion and tacrolimus as an amorphous solid dispersion (Rahman et al 2014). By formulating cyclosporine and tacrolimus into new dosage forms, the therapeutic outcomes increased tremendously. Often, the development of new and novel dosage forms is guided purely by commercial reasons such as financial incentives, loss of sales due to generic competition, extend exclusivity period, and patents on conventional dosage forms, development of intellectual property assets, or meeting regulatory requirements. For example, the Best Pharmaceuticals for Children Act (BPCA) and Pediatric Research Equity Act (PREA) mandate that pediatric formulations of new drugs be developed to meet the needs of the diverse pediatric population. In turn, the sponsors are rewarded with incentives in terms of extended exclusivities and patent terms.

## REGULATORY PATHWAY FOR NEW, NOVEL, AND DRUG–DEVICE COMBINATION PRODUCTS

New drug application (NDA) is a regulatory pathway for FDA approval of new drug candidates. New dosage forms of already FDA-approved drugs also require submission of new NDA. Examples of new dosage forms are oral solutions and suspension formulations of already approved dosage forms for the pediatric population. Chewable, effervescent, sublingual, and orally disintegrating tablets, oral film, and granules are developed primarily for ease of administration in patients who have difficulty in swallowing. Dosage forms such as long-acting injectables or modified release formulations or combination products are novel formulations that decrease the dose with consequent reduction in adverse events and frequency of administration. Other novel dosage forms such as liposomes or polymeric nanoparticles deliver

drugs to specific organs or tissues by their targeting abilities, thereby making them more therapeutically useful to patients.

An NDA can be submitted under two regulatory pathways, 505(b)(1) or 505(b)(2). NDA of new drug molecules is submitted under 505(b)(1), which requires exhaustive data on safety and efficacy. On the other hand, NDA under 505(b)(2) regulatory pathway allows reliance on the data of an approved drug or from publicly available literature. In the 505(b)(2) pathway, the sponsor needs to conduct bridging studies, which could be pharmacokinetics, clinical, or both. Comparative bioavailability study is needed to demonstrate bioequivalence between new dosage forms of an approved drug if the route of administration is same as provided under 505(b)(2). For non-bioequivalent dosage forms, additional study(s) or justification may be required. If the route of administration and indications are different for the new dosage form, additional clinical studies are required to demonstrate safety and efficacy. For example, skin irritation, skin sensitivity, and adhesion studies are required for transdermal dosage forms of an orally administered drug, among other studies. The 505(b)(2) regulatory pathway is particularly valuable to pharmaceutical companies compared to 505(b)(1), owing to a higher FDA approval success rate, lower cost, accelerated development, and application may also qualify for 3, 5, or even 7 years of exclusivity.

New dosage forms also include drug–device combination products as defined in 21 CFR 3.2: (a) a product comprised of two or more regulated components, ie, drug/device, biologic/device, drug/biologic, or drug/device/biologic, that are physically, chemically, or otherwise combined or mixed and produced as a single entity; (b) two or more separate products packaged together in a single package or as a unit and comprised of drug and device products, device and biological products, or biological and drug products; (c) a drug, device, or biological product packaged separately that according to its investigational plan or proposed labeling is intended for use only with an approved individually specified drug, device, or biological product where both are required to achieve the intended use, indication, or effect and where upon approval of the proposed product the labeling of the approved product would need to be changed, eg, to reflect a change in intended use, dosage form, strength, route of administration, or significant change in dose; or (d) any investigational drug, device, or biological product packaged separately that according to its proposed labeling is for use only with another individually specified investigational drug, device, or biological product where both are required to achieve the intended use, indication, or effect. Examples of drug–device combination products are prefilled drug syringes, auto-injectors, metered dose inhalers, dry powder inhalers, transdermal systems, prefilled iontophoresis systems or microneedle "patches," drug pills embedded with sensors, drug-eluting stents, etc. Combining device with drug offers many advantages, such as more selective targeted therapy which cannot be easily achieved otherwise, improved safety and efficacy, reduced adverse events, and improved patient compliance. However, combining the drug with device raises many regulatory challenges due to the complex nature of the drug–device products, and additionally, components of the products are regulated by different centers of the FDA. While drugs are regulated by the Center for Drug Evaluation and Research (CDER), the devices are regulated by the Center for Devices and Radiological Health (CDRH). The FDA created the Office of Combination Products (OCP) in 2008 to streamline the assignment of drug–device combination submissions to specific centers. The primary mode of action (PMOA) of a drug–device combination product defines a regulatory approval pathway, ie, whether the PMOA is due to drug or device. OCP determines PMOA of a combination product and directs it to the relevant center for regulatory evaluation. Regulatory pathways for device approval are 510(k) and premarket approval. The FDA also established an intercenter agreement that establishes the lead center for review and oversight of certain categories of combination products (Bayarri 2015). In this chapter, new and novel dosage forms including drug–device combination products approved by the FDA are discussed.

## NEW AND NOVEL DOSAGE FORMS

### 3D Printed Dosage Forms

3D printing or additive manufacturing is a versatile manufacturing technology. It allows customized manufacturing of 3D objects without requiring mold or machining typical for a conventional manufacturing. 3D printing is widely used in prototyping, production, and proof-of-concept models in various industries including consumable goods, high tech, automotive, aerospace and defense, and education. 3D printing is a group of technologies, and more than two dozen printing methods have been reported in the literature. Each printing method is unique due to the technology it uses, raw material requirements, and characteristics of the printed object. In the first step of the printing process, a virtual object is created using CAD software, followed by digital slicing to generate a stereolithography (STL) file. STL file steers motors that control the position of the building device or 3D-disperser orifice. The object is formed of layer-by-layer deposition of a material (clay, metal or polymer, etc). The thickness of layer varies from 50 to 500 $\mu$m depending upon the 3D printing technology. Depending upon method of 3D printing, post-processing such as heating, drying, or UV curing may be required. Commonly reported 3D printing methods are fused deposition modeling, selective laser sintering, stereolithography, and binder jetting. The technology has the capability to fabricate complex dosage forms, which are very difficult to create using conventional pharmaceutical manufacturing. For instance, 3D printing technology makes it possible to fabricate dosage forms with complex designs and shapes, or having controlled release, hardness, high porosity, and quick dispersion features (Eigon et al 2017; Rahman et al 2018; Rahman et al 2019; Ventola 2014).

In the biomedical industry, 3D printing is mostly used in manufacturing of devices. The significance of 3D printing to the biomedical industry can be gauged by the number of devices approved by the FDA. So far, the FDA has approved over 100 medical devices by 3D printing (Columbus 2019; Jacobson 2018). On the other hand, only one drug product has received FDA approval, mainly due to the high cost of manufacturing, slow process, high wastage of raw material, non-availability of GMP compliant printers, challenges to monitoring the process, in-process controls, etc. Aprecia Pharmaceuticals received FDA approval of first and only commercially available 3D printed tablets (Spritam® levetiracetam, an antiepileptic drug) in 2015. The 3D printing method used was binder jetting; the manufacturer calls it ZipDose® technology (Fig. 28-1).

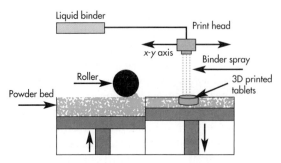

**FIGURE 28-1** • Binder jetting 3D printing process used in manufacturing Spritam® tablet.

The tablets disintegrate within a few seconds, which is similar to orally disintegrating tablets (ODT). However, the amount of drug substance in each dosage unit is much greater than 500 mg, which is the uppermost limit of most ODTs. Spritam tablets contain a high dose of 250–1250 mg of levetiracetam, which is difficult to formulate as an ODT using conventional pharmaceutical methods. The tablets are designed to melt or disintegrate, which is ideal for children or geriatric patients who may have difficulty in swallowing dosage forms. The technology imparts highly porous characteristics to the dosage form, causing it to disintegrate very rapidly (mean disintegration time is about 11 seconds in the mouth). Spritam contains conventional excipients, ie, colloidal silicon dioxide, glycerin, mannitol, microcrystalline cellulose, polysorbate 20, povidone, sucralose, butylated hydroxyanisole, and natural and artificial spearmint flavors.

## Abused Deterrent Products

Opioids such as oxycodone, hydrocodone, morphine, fentanyl, etc, are powerful analgesics. One of the adverse effects of opioids is euphoria, which is a highly sought-after effect by abusers. Opioid prescriptions are associated with abuse, misuse, overdose, addiction, and death due to their euphoric effects. They are abused by ingestion, snorting, smoking, and injection. The overuse and abuse of opioids can be traced back decades to before 1990, when physicians were criticized for undertreatment of pain. In the late 1990s, there was a paradigm shift about pain and its treatment. The pain was referred to as the fifth vital sign and physicians were encouraged to address and treat it. Coincidentally, the FDA approved an extended-release formulation of opioid (OxyContin®) for non-cancer pain in 1995. The current consumption

and mortality rate data reveal that abuse of prescription opioids has reached epidemic levels in the United States. Though the United States constitutes less than 5% of the world population, it consumes 75%–80% of global opioids. The National Institute of Drug Abuse (2019) estimates that every day about 130 people die in the United States due to opioids overdose. Besides morbidity and mortality issues, the opioid epidemic takes its toll on the economy. The cost of the epidemic to the economy is estimated to have topped $1 trillion from 2001 through 2017. The economic fallout from the epidemic of heroin and prescription opioid abuse is estimated to cost $500 billion from 2018 to 2020 alone (Mangan 2018). Considering the health and economic effects of opioid abuse, then-President Trump declared opioid addiction epidemic as "health emergency" in October 2017.

The FDA has taken many actions to address the epidemic of opioid abuse. One of these actions includes encouraging pharmaceutical companies to develop *abuse-deterrent formulations* (ADFs) of opioids. These formulations should meaningfully deter the abuser from abusing the products by various routes. ADFs are designed to be abuse deterrent rather than abuse resistant. Furthermore, the FDA does not use tamper-resistant terminology for these formulations, as this terminology is used in connection with packaging requirement of certain classes of drugs, devices, and cosmetics. The ADFs can be categorized based on the design as follows:

1. Physical/chemical barriers: This formulation design incorporates physical and/or, chemical barriers against abuse. A physical barrier imparts mechanical properties that resist chewing, crushing, cutting, grating, or grinding. The chemical barrier approach involves adding a gelling or swelling agent, which substantially decreases drug extraction in various solvents.

2. Agonist/antagonist combinations: These formulations contain both opioid agonists and antagonists. An antagonist does not release in patients. However, the abuser does not feel the euphoric effect of the opioid, which is blocked by the antagonist when the abuser tries to abuse the formulation.

3. Aversion: This formulation contains some averting agent which produces unpleasant effects if manipulated.

4. Delivery systems: Sustained-release depots and implants which are difficult to manipulate.

5. New molecular entities and prodrugs: New chemical entities with less brain penetration, and less euphoric effect than in currently available opioids or inactive as such but require enzymatic activation.

6. Combination of two or more approaches.

7. Novel approaches or technologies.

ADF products of morphine, oxycodone, and hydrocodone are available. OxyContin was reformulated as an ADF and received FDA approval in 2010. Since then, nine more ADF products have been approved (Table 28-1). Only one product is immediate-release and the rest are extended-release formulations. Currently, only three formulations are commercially available, as other products have been discontinued. However, the FDA has not approved a single generic version of ADF even though the exclusivity period of many of the approved products has expired a long time ago. The abuse deterrence of these approved products is based on physical and chemical, and agonist–antagonist approaches. A physical barrier increases the mechanical strength of tablets by a unique process, aided by the excipients or combination thereof, which resist mechanical manipulation by the abuser. These formulations are also referred to as crush resistant. Most of the crush-resistant formulations are based on polyethylene oxide (Polyox™) polymer. Polyox is a high molecular weight polyethylene glycol that has melting point of 62–67°C. Heating of Polyox tablets above their melting point leads to formation of a consolidated plastic structure due to melting, bridge formation, and fusion

## TABLE 28-1 • FDA-Approved Abuse Deterrent Formulations

| Brand Name | Opioids | Year of Approval | Company | Abuse Deterrent Design | Drug Release | Abuse-Deterrence Claim | Commercial Availability |
|---|---|---|---|---|---|---|---|
| OxyContin® | Oxycodone hydrochloride | 2010 | Purdue Pharma LP | Physical-chemical | Extended/long-acting | Intranasal injection | Yes |
| Hysingla™ ER | Hydrocodone bitartrate | 2014 | Purdue Pharma LP | Physical-chemical | Extended/long-acting | Oral Intranasal injection | Yes |
| MorphaBond ER™ | Morphine sulfate | 2015 | Daiichi Sankyo Inc | Physical-chemical | Extended/long-acting | Intranasal injection | Discontinue |
| Xtampza ER | Oxycodone | 2016 | Collegium Pharm Inc | Physical-chemical | Extended/long-acting | Intranasal injection | Yes |
| Arymo™ ER | Morphine sulfate | 2017 | Egalet | Physical-chemical | Extended/long-acting | Injection | Discontinue |
| Vantrela™ ER | Hydrocodone bitartrate | 2017 | Teva Branded Pharm | Physical-chemical | Extended/long-acting | Oral intranasal injection | Discontinue |
| RoxyBond™ | Oxycodone hydrochloride | 2017 | Inspiron Delivery | Physical-chemical | Immediate release | Intranasal injection | Discontinue |
| Embeda® | Morphine sulfate and naltrexone hydrochloride | 2014 | AlPharma Pharms | Agonist-antagonist | Extended/long-acting | Oral Intranasal | Discontinue |
| Targiniq™ ER | Oxycodone hydrochloride and naloxone hydrochloride | 2014 | Purdue Pharma LP | Agonist-antagonist | Extended/long-acting | Intranasal injection | Discontinue |
| Troxyca® ER | Oxycodone hydrochloride and naltrexone hydrochloride | 2016 | Pfizer Inc | Agonist-antagonist | Extended/long-acting | Oral Intranasal | Discontinue |

among particles (Rahman et al 2016; Xu et al; 2019). On the other hand, a chemical barrier approach is based on incorporating gelling agents in the formulation such as hydroxypropyl methyl cellulose, Polyox, alginic acid, sodium alginate, etc, which form a thick gel and resist drug extraction in commonly used solvents. Three out of the ten FDA-approved products are based on the agonist–antagonist design approach. The antagonist found in ADF products is either naloxone or naltrexone. Not all products have identical abuse deterrence claims. Some products claim abuse deterrence against multiple routes of abuse such as oral, intranasal, and injection routes, while other products claim abuse deterrence against only one route of abuse.

### Implants

Implantable drug delivery systems are used for both localized and systemic effects of drugs for an extended period of time, typically months to years. They offer many advantages over traditional oral or parenteral formulations, including achievement of therapeutic effects with low doses, potential adverse effects of therapy are minimized, patient compliance is increased, and they can be employed to administer drugs that are either not orally bioavailable or unstable in the gastrointestinal environment. Implants are of two types: preformed and *in-situ*. Preformed implants are pre-shaped implants available usually in cylindrical, circular disc, or octopus (Sinuva™) shapes (Fig. 28-2). The size of commercially available preformed cylindrical implants varies from 0.37 to 3 mm diameter with 3.5 to 35 mm length, depending upon the site of administration (Table 28-2). Implants are administered via subcutaneous, subdermal, intracranial, intravitreal, and ethmoid sinus regions. Cylinder-shaped implants are administered by 16–18 gauge syringes, with or without incision.

The commonly used manufacturing method employed for fabricating implants is melt extrusion. Both non-biodegradable and biodegradable polymers are used in their manufacture. Non-biodegradable polymers release drug primarily by passive diffusion; however, drug release behavior

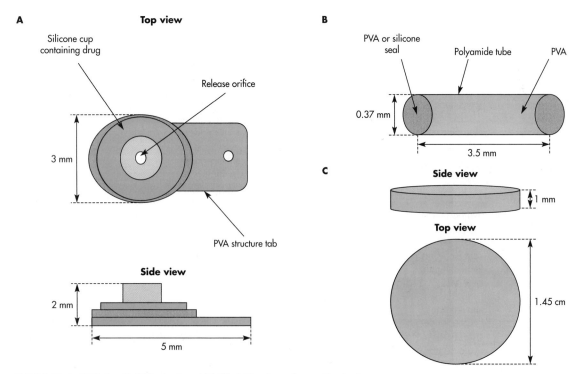

FIGURE 28-2 • (**A**) Retisert®; (**B**) Iluvien®; and (**C**) Gliadel® wafer preformed implants.

## TABLE 28-2 • FDA-Approved Preformed and *In-Situ* Implants

| Brand Name | Drug | Year of Approval | Company | Dimension | Polymer | Route of Administration | Duration |
|---|---|---|---|---|---|---|---|
| **Preformed implants** | | | | | | | |
| Zoladex® | Goserelin, 3.6 mg | 1989 | Tersera Therap LLC | 1 mm diameter Cylinder | Poly (DL-lactide-co-glycolide) | Subcutaneous | 28 days |
| Gliadel® Wafer | Carmustine | 1996 | Arbor Pharma LLC | 1.45 cm diameter × 1 mm thick | Copolymer, polifeprosan 20, consists of poly [bis (p-carboxyphenoxy)] propane and sebacic acid in a 20:80 molar ratio | Intracranial | 3 weeks |
| Retisert | Flurocinolone acetonide, 0.59 mg | 2004 | Bausch and Lomb | Tablets | Polyvinyl alcohol | Intravitreal | 30 months |
| Vantas | Histrelin acetonide, 50 mg | 2004 | Endo Pharm | 3 mm diameter × 35 mm length Cylinder | 2-hydroxyethyl methacrylate, 2-hydroxypropyl methacrylate, trimethylolpropane trimethacrylate, | Subcutaneous | 12 months |
| | Etonogestrel | 2006 | Organon USA Inc | 2 mm diameter × 4 mm length Cylinder | Ethylene vinyl acetate | Subdermal | Three years |
| Supprelin® LA | Histrelin acetonide | 2007 | Endo Pharm | 3 mm diameter × 35 mm length Cylinder | 2-hydroxyethyl methacrylate, 2-hydroxypropyl methacrylate, trimethylolpropane trimethacrylate | Subcutaneous | 12 months |
| Ozurdex™ | Dexamethasone | 2009 | Allergan | 0.46 mm in diameter × 6 mm length Cylinder | Poly (DL-lactide-co-glycolide) polymer | Intravitreal | 6 months |
| Iluvien® | Flurocinolone acetonide | 2014 | Alimera Sciences Inc | 0.37 mm diameter × 3.5 mm length Cylinder | Polyimide tube, polyvinyl alcohol, silicone adhesive | Intravitreal | 36 months |
| Probuphine® | Buprenorphine hydrochloride | 2016 | Braeburn Pharmaceuticals, Inc. | 2.5 mm diameter and 26 mm length Cylinder | Ethylene vinyl acetate | Subcutaneous | 6 months |
| Sinuva™ | Mometasone furoate | 2017 | Intersect ENT Inc | 34 mm expanded diameter and 20 length Octopus shape | Poly (DL-lactide-co-glycolide) | Ethmoid sinus | 90 days |
| Yutiq™ | Flurocinolone acetonide, 0.18 mg | 2018 | Eyepoint Pharms | 0.37 mm diameter × 3.5 mm length Cylinder | Polyimide tube, polyvinyl alcohol, silicone adhesive | Intravitreal | 36 months |

*(Continued)*

**TABLE 28-2** • FDA-Approved Preformed and *In-Situ* Implants (*Continued*)

| Brand Name | Drug | Year of Approval | Company | Dimension | Polymer | Route of Administration | Duration |
|---|---|---|---|---|---|---|---|
| **In-situ implants** | | | | | | | |
| Atridox® | Doxycycline hyclate | 1998 | Tolmar | — | Poly (DL-lactide-co-glycolide) Solvent - N-methyl pyrrolidone | Subgingival | 7 days |
| Eligard® | Leuprolide acetate | 2004 | Tolmar | — | Poly (DL-lactide-co-glycolide) Solvent - N-methyl pyrrolidone | Subcutaneous | 1–6 months |
| Perseris™ | Risperidone | 2018 | Indivior Inc | — | Poly (DL-lactide-co-glycolide) Solvent - N-methyl pyrrolidone. | Subcutaneous | Monthly |

may change depending on the physicochemical properties and concentration of drug, and polymer, design, and surface properties (Stewart 2018).

Based on the manufacturing process and modulation of drug release, non-biodegradable preformed implants are categorized into monolithic and reservoir type implants. In monolithic implants, drug is uniformly dispersed in the polymer. In reservoir implants, the drug reservoir is covered by permeable non-biodegradable polymer membrane. The membrane thickness and permeability of the drug through the membrane determine the release kinetics. Non-biodegradable implants have to be removed after the release period. Examples of non-biodegradable polymers are ethylene vinyl acetate, 2-hydroxyethyl methacrylate, 2-hydroxypropyl methacrylate, trimethylolpropane trimethacrylate, polyimide, silicone, etc. Biodegradable polymer–based preformed implants are fabricated from polylactide-co-glycolide (PLGA) polymer, which degrades into lactic and glycolic acids that are utilized by the body's metabolic cycles. Compared to non-biodegradable polymers, the drug release from biodegradable polymer is a very complex process, which involves a simultaneous process of diffusion, polymer degradation, and erosion. The other major difference is the duration of drug release, which is in months and not years as seen with non-biodegradable polymer–based implants (Table 28-2) (Stewart 2018).

*In-situ* implants are not only easy to manufacture but can be administered through small aperture size needles. *In-situ* implants are comprised of a low-viscosity solution of the polymer in which drug is either dissolved or dispersed prior to injection, depending upon the physicochemical properties of the drug. Once injected into the tissue, liquid solution of polymer solidifies into semi-solid or solid depot (Fig. 28-3). *In-situ* implants are typically based

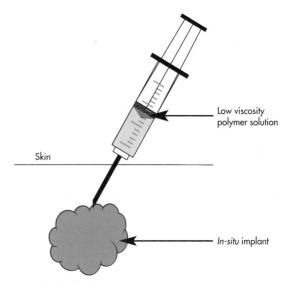

FIGURE 28-3 • Mechanism of *in-situ* implant formation.

on biodegradable polymer such as PLGA. A commonly used solvent to dissolve the polymer and disperse/dissolve drug is N-methyl pyrollidone (NMP). Once PLGA solution is injected, NMP dissipates into surrounding tissues, leaving behind the depot of polymer mass with the entrapped drug in it, which controls the duration of drug release (Fig. 28-3). Commercial *in-situ* implants are available in two prefilled syringes. One of the syringes contains a solution of PLGA in NMP and the other syringe contains the powder drug. The liquid polymer solution is added to the syringe containing powder drug to form solution or dispersion before injection. Compared to preformed implants, *in-situ* implants do not need to be removed after the drug release period. This feature greatly increases patient acceptance of *in-situ* implants over preformed implants (Kempe and Mader; 2012). The FDA has not yet approved any generic version of implant dosage forms due to their complex nature (Table 28-2).

## Microparticles/Microspheres

A needle gauge of 16–18 is needed to administer preformed implants, which induces fear and discomfort in some patients. Microparticles/microspheres represent a separate category of implants, which can be administered using smaller aperture size needles. Solvent evaporation, spray drying, and phase separation are common methods utilized in manufacturing of microspheres. PLGA is the most commonly used polymer to encapsulate the drug. Drug release occurs simultaneously by drug diffusion and polymer erosion processes. Duration of drug release varies widely from a few days to months and can be modulated by altering polymer composition, viscosity/molecular grade, and formulation composition. Commercially, PLGA is available in various lactate-to-glycolate content chain lengths ranging from 50:50 to 90:10. The rate of biodegradation and hence the duration of drug release is also determined by lactate content in the chain length. Higher the lactate content, longer it takes to degrade. Most commercially available microparticles/microspheres are available as dry powders except for Arestin® and Bydureon® Bcise™, which necessitate reconstitution in a liquid diluent before administration. The dry powder form prevents the premature release of drug

into the liquid vehicle. Diluent (liquid) component of the formulation contains buffering agent, osmotic agent, polymer, and surfactant. The most commonly used buffer system to prevent pH fluctuations is a phosphate and/or citrate buffer system. Osmotic agents like mannitol or 0.9% sodium chloride, surfactants (wetting agents) such as Poloxamer 188 or Polysorbate 20 or 80, and viscosity modifiers such as carboxymethylcellulose form integral parts of the diluent component. Arestin is available as cartridge containing dry powder which does not need reconstitution and is administered as such. Bydureon Bcise is available as a single-dose autoinjector containing powder suspension in a medium-chain triglycerides vehicle. Compared to *in-situ* implants, microparticles suffer from many drawbacks including a complex, time consuming, and expensive method of manufacturing, difficult administration procedure, incomplete dispersion, needle clogging, and administration of incomplete dose. Currently, ten microparticles/microspheres are available for clinical use; however, no generic formulation is available (Table 28-3).

## Vaginal Rings

Ideally, contraceptives should be highly effective, discreet, painless, and easy to use without a healthcare professional's assistance, reversible, and with no or minimal interference with daily life and bodily function. It should provide a constant release of the drug to avoid fluctuation in plasma drug concentration with no interference in drug absorption. Many of these criteria can be achieved by vaginal rings, also known as contraceptive vaginal rings (CVRs). Administration of contraceptives via vaginal ring offers many advantages, such as bypassing gastrointestinal absorption and first-pass effects, reduced possibility of elevated uterine concentration of hormones, and fluctuation in plasma concentration, increased bioavailability, reduction in dose, and improved patient compliance. The design of CVRs is based on combining two principles, slow diffusion of contraceptives (estrogen, progestin, or both) through biocompatible elastomeric polymers, and rapid absorption by the vaginal epithelium to distribute into systemic circulation. The vaginal epithelium is highly vascular in nature with low

## TABLE 28-3 • FDA-Approved Microparticles/Microspheres Dosage Forms

| Brand Name | Drug | Year of Approval | Company | Polymer | Route of Administration | Duration |
|---|---|---|---|---|---|---|
| Sandostatin® LAR Depot | Octreotide acetate | 1998 | Novartis | Poly (DL-lactide-co-glycolide) | Intramuscular | 4 weeks |
| Arestin® | Minocycline | 2001 | Orapharma | Poly (DL-lactide-co-glycolide) | Periodontal | 3 months |
| Risperdal Consta® | Risperidone | 2003 | Janssen Pharms | Poly (DL-lactide-co-glycolide) | Intramuscular | 4–6 weeks |
| Vivitrol | Naltrexone | 2006 | Alkermes | Poly (DL-lactide-co-glycolide) | Intramuscular | 4 weeks |
| Trelstar® | Triptorelin pamoate | 2010 | Allergan | Poly (DL-lactide-co-glycolide) | Intramuscular | 4–24 weeks |
| Lupaneta Pack | Leuprolide acetate | 2012 | Abbvie | Poly (DL-lactide-co-glycolide) | Intramuscular | 6 months |
| Signifor® LAR | Pasireotide pamoate | 2014 | Novartis Pharm Corp | Poly (DL-lactide-co-glycolide) | Intramuscular | 4 weeks |
| Bydureon® Bcise™ | Exenatide | 2017 | AstraZeneca | Poly (DL-lactide-co-glycolide) | Subcutaneous | 7 days |
| Triptodur | Triptorelin pamoate | 2017 | Arbor Pharm LLC | Poly (DL-lactide-co-glycolide) | Intramuscular | 24 weeks |
| Zilretta | Triamcinolone acetinide | 2017 | Flexion Therapeutics | Poly (DL-lactide-co-glycolide) | Intraarticular | — |

sensitivity to foreign bodies that favors the absorption of hormones into systemic circulation. Most CVRs provide an initial burst release of the drug due to release of surface drug deposited during storage. However, after the initial burst effect, drug release is near constant from the CVR to maintain steady-state plasma level of the drug. Unlike intrauterine devices (IUDs), the site of placement of the CVRs in the cavity is irrelevant. Any part of vaginal epithelium is equally capable of absorbing the drug, which makes it healthcare professional–free administration. It is the only long-acting contraceptive that is "user controlled," thus giving freedom to the user to initiate or discontinue its use. The ring is inserted by the patient and remains in place for the intended duration. The ring can be compressed into a linear shape and then placed deep in the cavity, where it regains its original shape. The dimensions of the ring are 54–56 mm outer diameter with 7.7–9 mm cross-sectional diameter. It is fabricated using non-biodegradable polymer, eg, ethylene vinyl acetate, copolymers, and silicone polymers in reservoir or monolithic type form. Duration of action is shorter compared to contraceptive implants or IUDs (Wieder and Pattimakiel 2010; Chen and Faundes 2010). The commercial CVRs are intended for 3 weeks' to 3 months' delivery of contraceptive hormones (Table 28-4). Four CVRs are available for clinical use, and the FDA has not yet approved a generic formulation (Fig. 28-4).

### Nanomedicines

Nanomedicines include dosage forms derived from nanotechnology. Physical, chemical, or biological properties of nanomaterials are different from conventionally scaled materials. Unlike conventional dosage forms, nanomedicines have a complex *in-vivo* transport mechanism, eg, opsonization and mononuclear phagocyte system, enhanced permeability retention effect, lymphatic transport, cellular recognition, internalization, enzymatic degradation, and physical modulations. Due to their unusual properties, nanomedicines have shown a great deal of promise in improving dissolution and bioavailability of poorly absorbed drugs, targeting drugs,

**TABLE 28-4 •** FDA-Approved Contraceptive Vaginal Rings

| Brand Name | Drug | Year of Approval | Company | Polymer | Dimension | Duration |
|---|---|---|---|---|---|---|
| Estring® | Estradiol | 1996 | Pharmacia and Upjohn | Silicone polymers | Outer diameter, 55 mm Cross-sectional diameter, 9 mm Core diameter, 2 mm | 3 months |
| Nuvaring® | Etonogestrel/ ethinyl estradiol | 2001 | Organon Sub Merck | Ethylene vinylacetate copolymers | Outer diameter, 54 mm Cross-sectional diameter, 4 mm | 3 weeks |
| Femring® | Estradiol acetate | 2003 | Millicent | Silicone polymers | Outer diameter, 56 mm Cross-sectional diameter, 7.6 mm Core diameter, 2 mm | 3 months |
| Annovera | Ethinyl estradiol/ Segesterone acetate | 2018 | TherapeuticsMD Inc | Silicone polymers | Outer diameter, 56 mm Cross-sectional diameter, 8.4 mm | 3 weeks |

and increased retention at diseased organ or tissue. Consequently, targeted drug delivery with polymeric nanoparticles and liposomes for cancer treatment is being widely explored. The FDA has approved a number of anticancer nanomedicines for delivering drugs directly to the disease site.

The FDA has not devised a separate regulatory framework for the review of nanomedicines. Rather, the FDA believes that the current regulatory framework is flexible and robust enough for safety and efficacy evaluation of nanomedicines. Moreover, the agency has issued guidelines to determine whether an FDA-regulated product involves application of nanotechnology. Two specific parameters applied to determine application of nanotechnology in medical product fabrication are: (1) whether a material or end product is engineered to have at least one external dimension, or an internal or surface structure, in the nanoscale range (approximately 1–100 nm); or (2) whether a material or end product is engineered to exhibit properties or phenomena, including physical or chemical properties or biological effects, which are attributable to its dimension(s), even if these dimensions fall outside the nanoscale range, up to 1 $\mu$m (1000 nm). It is to be noted that nanomedicines have to meet the same standards for quality, safety, and efficacy as for non-nanomaterial medicines. The FDA has approved various types of nanomedicines, including liposomes, nanocrystals, nanotubes, polymeric nanoparticles, micelles, nanoemulsions,

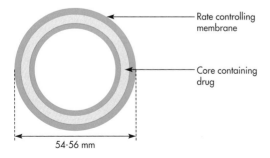

FIGURE 28-4 • Schematic presentation of contraceptive vaginal ring.

microemulsions, colloids, etc. Nanomedicines are considered complex drug products that explain why generic products of the majority of nanomedicines have not yet been approved, even though the FDA has issued products specific guidance document (Tyner et al 2017; Cruz et al 2013) (Table 28-5).

*Liposomes*: Liposomes are spherical-shaped vesicles of phospholipids. They consist of one or more layers of phospholipids with size varying from 30 nm to several micrometers (Fig. 28-5). Their properties differ significantly with lipid composition, surface charge, size, and method of preparation.

## TABLE 28-5 • FDA-Approved Nanomedicines

| Drug Product | Active Ingredient | Type of Nanomedicine | Indications | FDA Approval | Company | Generics |
|---|---|---|---|---|---|---|
| Abelcet® | Amphotericin B | Liposome lipid complex | Fungal infection | 1995 | Leadiant Biosci Inc | No |
| Doxil® | Doxorubicin | Stealth liposome | Ovarian cancer, AIDS related Kaposi's sarcoma, multiple myeloma | 1995 | Janssen Products | Yes |
| AmBisome® | Amphotericin | Liposome | Fungal infection | 1997 | Astellas | No |
| Depocyt | Cytarabine | Liposome | Lymphomatous meningitis | 1999 | Pacira Pharma | No |
| Curosurf® | Poractant alphs (Protein SP-B and SP-C) | Liposome | Respiratory surfactant | 1999 | Chiesi USA | No |
| Visudyne® | Verteporfin | Liposome | Subfoveal choroidal neovascularization | 2000 | Valeant | No |
| Marqibo® | Vincristine sulfate | Liposome | Acute lymphoblastic leukemia | 2012 | Talon Therapeutics | No |
| Onivyde® | Irinotecan hydrochloride | Liposome | Metastatic adenocarcinoma of pancreas | 2015 | Ipsen Inc | No |
| Vyxeos | Cytarabine and Daunorubicin | Liposome | Acute myeloid leukemia | 2017 | Celator Pharms | No |
| Emend® | Aprepitant | Nanocrystals | Antiemetic | 2003 | Merck | Yes |
| Tricor® | Fenofibrate | Nanocrystals | Primary hypercholesterolemia or mixed dyslipidemia | 2004 | Abbvie | Yes |
| Megace ES® | Megestrol acetate | Nanocrystals | Anorexia, cachexia in AIDS | 2005 | Endo Pharma | Yes |
| Abraxane® | Paclitaxel | Protein nanoparticles | Breast, lung, pancreatic cancers | 2005 | Abraxis Science | No |
| Taxotree® | Docetaxel | Micelles | Breast, prostrate, head and neck, and non-small cell lung cancers and gastric adenocarcinoma | 1996 | Sanofi Aventis | No |
| Cequa™ | Cyclosporine | Micellar | Dry eye | 2018 | Sun Pharma | No |
| Diprivan® | Propofol | Nanoemulsion | General anesthesia | 1989 | Fresenius Kabi USA | Yes |
| Restasis® | Cyclosporine | Nanoemulsion | Dry eye | 2002 | Allergan | No |
| Xelpros™ | Latanoprost | Nanoemulsion | Intraocular pressure | 2018 | Sun Pharma | No |
| Neoral® | Cyclosporine | Microemulsion | Immunosuppressant | 1995 | Novartis | Yes |
| Somatuline Depot | Lanreotide acetate | Nanotube | Acromegalis who have had an inadequate response to or cannot be treated with surgery and/or radiotherapy | 2007 | Ipsen Pharma | No |
| INFeD® | Iron dextran | Colloidal iron | Iron deficiency | 1974 | Allergan | No |
| Ferrlecit® | Sodium ferric gluconate complex | Colloidal iron | Iron deficiency anemia with chronic kidney disease | 1999 | Sanofi Aventis | Yes |
| Venofer® | Iron sucrose | Colloidal iron | Iron deficiency anemia with chronic kidney disease | 2000 | Luitpold | No |
| Feraheme® | Ferumoxytol | Colloidal iron | Iron deficiency anemia with chronic kidney disease | 2006 | AMAG Pharma | No |
| Injectafer® | Ferric carboxymaltose | Colloidal iron | Iron deficiency anemia with chronic kidney disease | 2013 | Luitpold Pharm | No |

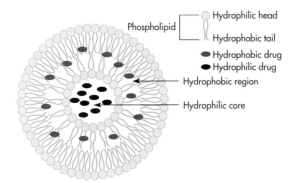

Phospholipid
- Hydrophilic head
- Hydrophobic tail
- Hydrophobic drug
- Hydrophilic drug
- Hydrophobic region
- Hydrophilic core

FIGURE 28-5 • Schematic presentation of liposome.

For example, liposomes of unsaturated phospholipids have high permeability but less stability characteristics. Conversely, liposomes of saturated phospholipids are rigid with less permeability and better stability (Akbarzadeh et al 2013). Commercially available liposomes contain both unsaturated as well as saturated phospholipids. The following phospholipids are present in commercial liposome nanomedicines: dimyristoylphosphatidylcholine, dimyristoylphosphatidylglycerol, dioleoylphosphatidylcholine, distearoylphosphatidylglycerol, distearoylphosphatidylcholine, dipalmitoylphosphatidylglycerol, dipalmitoylphosphatidylcholine, sphingomyelin, hydrogenated soy phosphatidylcholine, and N-(carbonyl-methoxypolyethylene glycol-2000)-1,2-distearoyl-sn-glycero-3-phosphoethanolamine sodium (MPEG-DSPE). Fluidity or rigidity of bilayers can be modulated by addition of cholesterol. Furthermore, surface properties can be modified for longer circulation times and targeted delivery of the drug (Doxil®). Doxil and Onivyde® contain MPEG-DSPE phospholipid, which prolongs circulation half-life by interfering with opsonization process. Liposomes are promising carriers for nanomedicines due to unique characteristics such as size and capability to encapsulate both hydrophilic and hydrophobic drugs. Currently, they are used for delivering single (Doxil) or two drugs (Vyxeos™) simultaneously. The first liposomal product was approved in 1995. Liposomes account for 30% of market share among nanomedicines (Bobo et al 2016; Kapoor et al 2017). A generic version of Doxil has been approved by FDA.

*Nanocrystals:* One of the challenges of polymeric nanocarrier–based systems (eg, polymeric nanoparticles) is limited drug loading. Drug loading can be increased by employing nanocrystals as delivery vehicles. The nanocrystals, also known as nanosuspensions, are solid crystalline particles with mean diameter <1 $\mu m$. Theoretically, high drug loading even up to 100% can be achieved with nanocrystals as they do not contain carrier excipient, rendering them superior in terms of drug loading. However, surfactant or a polymer at low concentration is required to stabilize nanocrystals. Nanocrystals are primarily used to increase solubility and dissolution of poorly water-soluble drugs due to increase in surface area-to-volume ratio. Nanocrystals can be either formulated as suspensions (Megace ES®) or incorporated into solid dosage forms, eg, Emend® and Tricor®. The techniques frequently employed to prepare nanocrystals include media milling, high-pressure homogenization, and precipitation (Bobo et al 2016; Chen et al 2017).

*Polymeric nanoparticles:* In polymeric nanoparticles, polymer carrier encapsulates the drug, which can be natural, synthetic, or semisynthetic. The FDA has so far approved only one polymeric nanoparticle dosage form, Abraxane®, which is comprised of nanoparticles of paclitaxel where albumin protein acts as a carrier. The mean particle size of nanoparticles is 130 nm, and the drug is present in both amorphous and crystalline forms. Abraxane demonstrated superiority in terms of therapeutic outcome with significantly lower incidence of adverse events compared to standard paclitaxel treatment. Sponsors can market generic formulation of Abraxane after FDA approval, once the orphan drug exclusivity expires in September 2023. However, it would be challenging to demonstrate the quality sameness and comparable safety and efficacy due to the complex nature of the product. Other challenges include demonstrating content similarity of amorphous and crystalline forms of the drug, stability of amorphous form, particle size of nanoparticles, surface properties, fraction of free and bound paclitaxel, etc (Miele et al 2009).

*Micelles:* Micelles are aggregates of surfactant molecules dispersed in a liquid medium. Surfactant molecules have hydrophilic and hydrophobic regions in their structure, and in an aqueous medium, they dissolve, aggregate, and reorient in such a way that the hydrophilic region is in contact with the aqueous medium while the hydrophobic region is sequestered

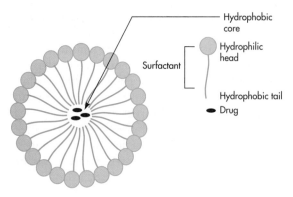

FIGURE 28-6 • Schematic presentation of micelle.

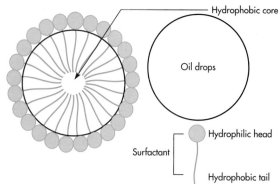

FIGURE 28-7 • Schematic presentation of nanoemulsion.

to minimize contact with the aqueous medium. Basically, the outer shell of micelles is hydrophilic, while the inner core is hydrophobic (Fig. 28-6). However, the orientation of hydrophilic and hydrophobic regions reverses in a non-polar solvent. Micelles are approximately spherical in shape, but other shapes such as ellipsoids, cylinders, and bilayers have also been reported in the literature. The shape and size of micelles depend upon concentration of surfactant and temperature, pH, and ionic strength of the preparation. When a hydrophobic drug is dissolved in the surfactant solution, the drug is encapsulated in the hydrophobic core structure of the micelles structure. This strategy has been utilized to form solution formulations of hydrophobic drugs (Mandal et al 2019). The FDA has approved two micelle products, Taxotere® and Cequa™. Taxotere is an intravenous clear micelle solution of docetaxel with polysorbate 80. Docetaxel is highly lipophilic and practically insoluble in water. Micelle formulation of docetaxel makes it possible to administer docetaxel intravenously without crystallization/precipitation risk. Similarly, the micelle formulation of cyclosporine (Cequa) contains hydrogenated castor oil and Octoxynol-40 surfactants for ophthalmic use.

*Nanoemulsion:* This is a multiphasic colloidal emulsion system comprised of four components: drug, surfactant, oil phase, and aqueous phase. The components are mixed and milled to reduce droplets to nanometer size range (high-shear or high-pressure) (Fig. 28-7). The drug is present in more than one phase of the nanoemulsion, and the relative proportion of drug depends upon the drug's physicochemical properties and formulation

composition. The drug may be present in the nanoemulsion in the following forms: (1) solid particulates (micro/nanoparticles), (2) micelle-associated; (3) oil-associated, and (4) solubilized (in aqueous and/or solvent medium). Examples of FDA-approved nanoemulsions are Xelpros, Restasis®, and Dipirivan®. Nanoemulsion differs from microemulsion in terms of thermodynamic stability. Cosurfactants and surfactants present in microemulsions prevent Ostwald ripening, ie, coalescence of smaller droplets into larger ones that consequently impart thermodynamic stability. On the other hand, a smaller quantity of co-surfactants and surfactants in nanoemulsions renders them susceptible to Ostwald ripening.

*Microemulsion:* These are transparent, monophasic, optically isotropic, and thermodynamically stable colloidal dispersions composed of oil, water, surfactants, and cosurfactants with droplet size in the range of 10–100 nm. Microemulsions are primarily used to improve dissolution and absorption of poorly soluble and permeable drugs. An example of an FDA-approved microemulsion is Neoral®. The active ingredient in this formulation is cyclosporine. It is a BCS class IV (low solubility/low permeability) drug with high intrasubject variability in pharmacokinetics and pharmacodynamics. Solution and capsule forms containing cyclosporine in microemulsion dispersion (Neoral) improved the oral bioavailability and reduced variability in clinical outcome of the drug (Ritschel 1996).

*Nanotube:* Lanreotide acetate self-assembles into hollow monodispersed nanotubes in water (Paternostre 2008). It is approved for the treatment of acromegaly (eg, Somatuline Depot).

*Colloidal iron products*: Colloidal iron products consist of iron oxyhydroxide or iron oxide core and a coat of carbohydrate, with an average particle size ranging from 8 to 24 nm. The carbohydrates used commonly for this purpose are polyglucose, sorbitol carboxymethylether, dextran, sucrose, gluconate, and carboxymaltose. The function of the carbohydrate coat is to stabilize and protect the iron core from hydrolysis, precipitation, and polymerization until delivery of iron to mononuclear phagocyte system (MPS). The other function of a carbohydrate coating is to prevent the release of iron into the systemic circulation before delivery to MPS. The carbohydrate coating indirectly prevents formation of non-transferrin-bound iron and thus reduces oxidative toxicity and inflammation. Low molecular weight and free labile iron compounds are considered impurities (Zhou et al 2017). Commercially available colloidal iron products show differences in size, surface properties, *in-vivo* stability, iron release profile, and content of labile and low-molecular-weight iron species. Colloidal iron products are approved for the treatment of iron deficiency anemia. A generic product of Ferrlecit® is approved; however, the FDA has published a product-specific guidance document to guide sponsors on the data requirements for generic product submissions.

## DRUG–DEVICE COMBINATION PRODUCTS

### Digital Medicines

Digital medicines are oral dosage forms, which combine a medication with an ingestible sensor. The sensor is a part of the digital medication that sends information to wearable mobile and/or web-based application. The sensor can determine whether a patient has taken specific medications at a certain time. One of the objectives of digital medication is to improve patient compliance. Digital medicine is often confused with digital health and digital therapeutics (a subset of digital health). Digital health offers digital technologies to improve human health in some capacities. It includes mobile health, health information technology, wearable devices, telehealth and telemedicine, and personalized medicines. In a broader

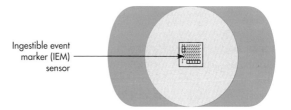

FIGURE 28-8 • Schematic presentation of digital medicine.

sense, digital medicine can be considered part of digital health. In contrast, digital therapeutics are primarily associated with web-based health management tools and stand-alone health applications. Digital therapeutics are used independently or in concert with medications, devices, or other therapy to optimize patient care and health outcomes (Michie et al 2017). The first digital medicine, Abilify Mycite, was approved by the FDA in 2017. Otsuka Pharmaceutical collaborated with Digital Health for its development (Abilify Mycite). It is a drug–device combination product, comprised of the following components (Fig. 28-8):

1. An aripiprazole tablet with an embedded Ingestible Event Marker (IEM, 1 mm in size) sensor. Upon contact with gastric fluid, magnesium and cuprous chloride within the IEM react to activate and power the device. The IEM then communicates to the Mycite patch, to track aripiprazole ingestion.

2. A Mycite patch (a wearable sensor) is designed to detect the ingestion of the Abilify Mycite tablet, record the ingestion of the IEM, and transmit ingestion data to the mobile patient application.

3. A compatible mobile patient application displays this data to allow patients to review their medication ingestion. These data can be shared with healthcare providers and caregivers.

4. The application may have a web-based portal or dashboard for healthcare professionals and caregivers.

   The product is approved for the treatment of schizophrenia, acute treatment of manic and mixed episodes associated with bipolar disorder, and for use as an add-on treatment for depression in adults.

## Drug-Eluting Stents

The first percutaneous coronary intervention (PCI, angioplasty) was performed in 1977. PCI is performed to relieve the symptoms of coronary heart disease or to reduce heart damage after a heart attack. The high incidence of thrombosis, restenosis, and abrupt vessel closure were observed after PCI. These adverse events associated with PCI led to the development of a bare-metal stent (BMS) to scaffold vessels. BMS or stent is a tubular structure placed inside the blood vessels to aid healing or relieve an obstruction (Nakazawa et al 2008). Use of BMS following PCI resulted in significant improvement in the acute clinical outcome, with 20%–30% reduction in restenosis. However, BMS was not totally free of adverse events. Issues reported with BMS are stent-induced vascular injury, neointimal hyperplasia, vascular smooth muscle cell migration, and proliferation, which led to restenosis and need for reintervention in high-risk patients. A drug-eluting stent (DES) was developed to reduce risk of BMS-induced restenosis. DES has shown a decrease in restenosis and need for reintervention by ≥50% when compared to BMS (Lee and Hernandez 2018; Partida and Yeh 2016). FDA has approved a number of DES (Table 28-6), which consist of the following components (Fig. 28-9):

1. Metallic stent platform or scaffold

2. Polymer

3. Antiproliferative drug

*Metallic stent platform or scaffold*: A thicker strut delays full neointimal coverage and increases risk of thrombosis. A thinner strut has better endothelialization and more flexibility. First-generation stents were based on stainless steel, having thick strut and limited compression strength and visibility, whereas newer-generation stents are based on cobalt–chromium or platinum–chromium alloy. New-generation stents have significantly reduced strut thickness, higher yield strength, and modestly higher radiopacity compared with stainless steel. However, stents of stainless steel and cobalt-chromium and platinum–chromium alloy are biocompatible and equivalent in *in vivo* animal models. Strut thickness of commercially available DES varies from 60 to 120 μm.

The stent scaffold consists of two parts: a series of hoops to provide radial strength on expansion, and connectors that join hoops and provide longitudinal strength. Hoops consist of series of Z-shaped structural segments (strut). Hoops are connected in two ways, closed and open-cell designs. Hoops connect every possible segment in a closed-cell configuration, which greatly enhances the radial force and scaffolding uniformity but reduces flexibility and conformability. In the open-cell configuration, some of the internal inflection points of the hoops are joined by bridging connectors. Compared to closed-cell configuration, open-cell provides greater flexibility, adaptability, resistance to fracture, and access to side branches (Fig. 28-10). Furthermore, scaffolds with thinner strut walls and reduced number of hoops improve the device's flexibility and deliverability to target lesions with improved side branch access.

*Polymer coating*: Polymer coating is applied to a metallic stent scaffold, which acts as a carrier for drug. The polymer coating should be thin and biocompatible, with low thrombogenicity. Both non-biodegradable and biodegradable polymers can be used for this purpose. Except for phosphorylcholine, all other polymers used are synthetic, with predictable drug elution pharmacokinetics. Many factors, such as polymer type, molecular weight, drug-to-polymer ratio, coating thickness, etc, affect the drug release profile from the DES. The coating of polymer over the stent can be conformal (inhibiting smooth cell proliferation over the entire surface of the stent) or abluminal (the release of the drug only has an effect on the surface in contact with vessel wall). The advantage of abluminal coating is that it reduces the drug dose and polymer exposure. Coating with PVDF-HFP, a copolymer of vinylidene fluoride and hexafluoropropylene, reduces protein adsorption, platelet adhesion, and thrombus formation. Polylactic acid and PLGA are the most commonly used biodegradable polymers in DES.

*Antiproliferative drug*: Drug embedded in polymer matrix is released locally and enters into blood vessels by passive diffusion. The physicochemical properties and pharmacodynamics of the drug and the type of polymer determine the vascular response and time course of vascular healing. Implantation of a stent induces local mechanical injury to arterial walls and the endothelium, which ultimately leads to smooth muscle cell proliferation and neointimal hyperplasia. Antiproliferative agents reduce the rate of neointimal hyperplasia and restenosis.

## TABLE 28-6 • FDA-Approved Drug Eluting Stents

| Stent Name | Scaffold Alloy | Drug | Release Kinetics | Strut Thickness (µm) | Polymer Thickness (µm) | Polymer | Company | FDA Approval |
|---|---|---|---|---|---|---|---|---|
| TAXUS Liberte | Stainless steel | Paclitaxel | <10% over 10 days 90% unreleased | 97 | 16 | SIBS | Boston Scientific | 2004 |
| TAXUS Element (ION) | Pt-Cr | Paclitaxel | <10% over 10 days 90% unreleased | 81 | 15 | SIBS | Boston Scientific | 2011 |
| Endeavor | Co-Cr | Zotarolimus | 95% over 14 days | 91 | 6 | PC | Medtronic | 2008 |
| Resolute | Co-Cr | Zotarolimus | 80% over 60 days 100% over 6 months | 91 | 6 | BioLinx | Medtronic | 2012 |
| Xience V Xpedition | Co-Cr | Everolimus | 80% over 30 days 100% over 6 months | 81 | 8 | PBMA, PVDF-HFP | Abbott Vascular | 2008 |
| Promus Element | Co-Cr | Everolimus | 80% over 30 days 100% over 6 months | 81 | 8 | PBMA, PVDF-HFP | Boston Scientific | 2008 |
| Promus Premier | Pt-Cr | Everolimus | 80% over 30 days 100% over 6 months | 81 | 8 | PBMA, PVDF-HFP | Boston Scientific | 2013 |
| Synergy | Pt-Cr | Everolimus | 50% over 30 days 80% over 2 months | 74 | 4 | PLGA | Boston Scientific | 2015 |
| Orsiro | Cobalt Chromium | Sirolimus | 120 days | 60-80 | 7 | Polylactide | Biotronik | 2019 |
| BioMatrix Nobor | Stainless steel | Umirolimus (biolimus) | 6–9 months | 120 | 10 | PLA | Biomatrix | |

*HFP, hexafluoropropylene; PBMA, poly(n-butyl methacrylate); PC, phosphorylcholine; PEVA, polyethylene-co-vinyl acetate; PLGA, poly (DL-lactide-co-glycolide); PLA, polylactic acid; PVDF, polyvinylidene fluoride; SIBS, poly(styrene-b-isobutylene-b-styrene)*

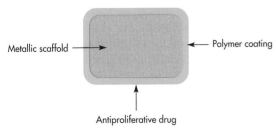

FIGURE 28-9 • Schematic presentation of drug-eluting stents.

Examples of drugs commonly used in DES are paclitaxel, sirolimus, zotarolimus, everolimus, and umirolimus. Paclitaxel acts as a microtubule stabilizing agent to prevent smooth cell proliferation. Sirolimus, zotarolimus, everolimus, and umirolimus bind to FKBP12 receptor to inhibit vascular smooth muscle migration and proliferation. A drug administered through DES implantation results in reduction in systemic exposure and dose, and high localized

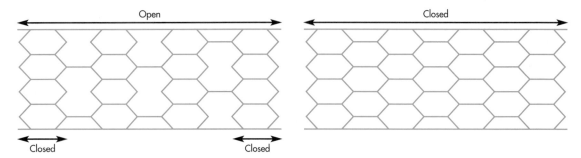

**FIGURE 28-10 •** Schematic presentation of open and closed configuration of stent scaffold (strut).

concentration. For example, the maximum systemic drug concentration observed is typically <2 ng/mL, far below the accepted limits of pharmacological safety for these compounds.

### Intrauterine Devices

Intrauterine devices (IUDs), also known as intrauterine contraceptive devices (IUCDs), are long-acting reversible contraceptive methods of birth control. These are typically T-shaped devices inserted into the uterus to prevent pregnancy. The IUDs may or may not carry the hormonal load. Non-hormonal and hormonal IUDs are copper-containing and progesterone-releasing IUDs, respectively. The two IUDs differ in the duration of contraceptive effect. Non-hormonal IUDs are effective up to 10 years, while the hormonal IUD is effective for a relatively shorter period of time, typically 3–5 years (Table 28-7). Non-biodegradable characteristics of IUDs mandate that they have to be removed after the stated contraceptive period. The T-frame of both types of IUD is typically made of polyethylene and barium sulfate, which aids in detecting the device under x-ray. A monofilament polyethylene or polypropylene thread is tied through the tip, resulting in two white threads, which aid in the detection and removal of the device. Non-hormonal IUDs are based on copper wire coiled along the vertical stem and each side of the horizontal arm of the "T." The total exposed copper surface area is $380 \pm 23$ mm$^2$ (ParaGard® T 380A) (Fig. 28-11). The contraceptive effectiveness of the ParaGard is enhanced by copper, which is continuously released into the uterine cavity. The mechanism(s) by which copper enhances contraceptive efficacy include interference with sperm transport and fertilization of an egg, and possibly prevention of implantation. Hormonal IUDs are similar in design and function to non-hormonal IUDs except they do not contain copper wire. Contraception is achieved by a progestin-releasing drug, normally levonorgestrel. Hormonal IUDs contain a drug reservoir, which is a mixture of hormone and polydimethylsiloxane and a covering of semi-opaque silicone membrane, composed of polydimethylsiloxane and colloidal silica, that controls the rate of drug release besides formulation factors.

### Transdermal Delivery Systems

Transdermal delivery systems (TDS), or patches, deliver drugs through the skin. TDS are an alternative route to oral and parenteral routes with distinct advantages such as bypassing first-pass metabolism, improving patient compliance, reducing dose, dosing frequency, and fluctuation in plasma concentration, minimizing adverse effects, and noninvasive nature. Since the approval of the first patch by the FDA in 1979, the agency has approved TDS for more than a dozen drugs. The main application of TDS is to deliver drugs systemically (Table 28-8). A few TDS products like Flector® Lidoderm, Synera, Qutenza™, and ZTlido™ have also been approved for localizing drug effects, such as to induce local anesthesia, reduce local inflammation, or relieve local pain (Table 28-9). The patch is usually placed for varying durations, from an hour up to 7 days, on the upper outer arm, abdomen, behind the ear, hip area, buttock, back, or in a place where it will not be rubbed by clothing. The patch should not be placed on the breasts, on cut or irritated skin, or at the same location as the previous patch (Valery et al 2012).

## TABLE 28-7 • FDA-Approved Intrauterine Devices

| Brand Name | Drug | Year of Approval | Company | Dimension | Release Rate | Duration |
|---|---|---|---|---|---|---|
| ParaGard® T 380A | Copper, 308 mg | 1984 | CooperSurgical Inc | 32 mm horizontally 36 mm vertically | — | Up to 10 years |
| Mirena | Levonorgestrel, 52 mg | 2000 | Bayer Healthcare Pharmaceuticals Inc | 32 mm horizontally 32 mm vertically | Initial release rate is 20 mcg/day; this rate is reduced by about 50% after 5 years | 5 years |
| Skyla | Levonorgestrel, 13.5 mg | 2013 | Bayer Healthcare Pharmaceuticals Inc | 28 mm horizontally 30 mm vertically | Release rate is 14 mcg/day after 24 days and declines to 5 mcg/day after 3 years | 3 years |
| Kyleena | Levonorgestrel, 19.5 mg | 2016 | Bayer Healthcare Pharmaceuticals Inc | 28 mm horizontally 30 mm vertically | Release rate is 17.5 mcg/day after 24 days and declines to 7.4 mcg/day after 5 years | 5 years |
| Liletta | Levonorgestrel, 52 mg | 2015 | Medicines360 | 32 mm horizontally 32 mm vertically | 19.5 mcg/day and decreases to 17.0 mcg/day at 1 year, 14.8 mcg/day at 2 years, 12.9 mcg/day at 3 years, 11.3 at 4 years, and 9.8 mcg/day at 5 years | 5 years |

Drug is absorbed from TDS via an outer layer of epidermis into dermis followed by systemic distribution. The stratum corneum, the outermost layer of the epidermis, is the major obstacle, and is a rate-limiting step in the drug diffusion through the skin. The drug molecules should be small, non-ionic, and lipophilic in nature to be able to cross the stratum corneum. Large, ionizable, and hydrophilic molecules can be transported across the skin by changing the barrier properties of the skin. The barrier properties can be temporarily and reversibly altered by use of chemical permeation enhancers; eg, alcohols, surfactants, terpenes, fatty acids, etc. The chemical permeation enhancers present in the commercial

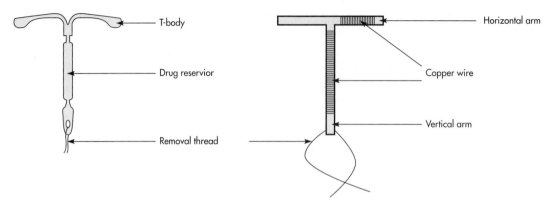

TDS include isopropyl myristate (Duragesic®), oleyl alcohol, dipropylene glycol, propylene glycol (Minivelle® and Vivelle-Dot®), sorbitan monooleate (Alora®), levulinic acid (Butrans®), vitamin E (Execelon and Neupro), oleic acid, and dipropylene glycol (CombiPatch®). The rate of drug diffusion also depends on the size (surface area) of the TDS. TDS of many drugs is available in various sizes to control the rate and extent of drug diffusion. Circular, rectangular, or square-shaped TDS are available.

Commercially available TDS can be broadly classified into three categories—reservoir, matrix, or drug-in-adhesive (DIA)—without rate-controlling membrane, and matrix (matrix diffusion) with rate-controlling membrane. The reservoir type of TDS consists of three components: drug reservoir (drug with excipients), rate-controlling membrane, and adhesive. In the matrix TDS, drug along with excipients is present in adhesive layer. The matrix with rate-controlling membrane contains a membrane sandwiched between layers of the DIA layers (Fig. 28-12). The majority of commercial TDS are based on DIA technology (Table 28-8).

Components of TDS are backing membrane, release liners, rate-controlling membrane, formulation, and adhesive. The ancillary components such as backing membrane and release liners are drug-impermeable layers. The backing layer maintains physical integrity, provides occlusivity, and protects the drug–adhesive/drug–reservoir layer during storage and application. Polymer membranes used as backing layers include polyester/ethylene-vinyl acetate film (Oxytrol®), metalized polyester film

(Neupro, Transderm-Scop®), ethylene-methacrylic acid copolymer/ethylene vinyl acetate (Androderm®), ethylene vinyl acetate/polyethylene terephthalate (Duragesic®), polyolefin (Combipatch), film consisting of ethylene vinyl alcohol copolymer film, a polyurethane film, urethane polymer and epoxy resin (Vivelle®), and polyethylene.

The release liner protects the adhesive layer during storage. Prior to application, the release liner should be peeled off the patch. Some release liners used in TDS are siliconized or fluoropolymer polyester strips (Androderm, Oxytrol, Transderm-Scop) and siliconized polyethylene terephthalate.

The rate-controlling membrane used in a reservoir or matrix-diffusion type TDS is sandwiched between the drug reservoir and adhesive layers. The diffusion properties of membrane make it possible to control delivery of drug to the skin. Microporous polyethylene membrane (Androderm) and microporous polypropylene membrane (Trasderm Scop, Catpress-TTS®) are well-known rate-controlling membranes.

Intimate contact with the skin is essential for a TDS to exert a local or systemic effect. The adhesive layer acts as the bridge between the skin and the TDS by establishing interatomic and intermolecular forces at the interface. The adhesive should deform under pressure and maintain contact with skin even after pressure is removed. Consequently, pressure-sensitive polymers are used as adhesives. The most widely used adhesives are polyisobutylene (Transderm-Scop), acrylics (Oxytrol, Androderm, Exelon), silicone-based adhesive (Neupro), or mixtures of

## TABLE 28-8 • FDA-Approved Transdermal Systems for Systemic Delivery of Drugs

| Brand Name | Drug | Year of Approval | Company | Polymer | Surface Area | Duration | Release Rate | Type |
|---|---|---|---|---|---|---|---|---|
| Transderm-Scop® | Scopolamine | 1979 | GlaxoSmith Kline | Polyisobutylene adhesive | 2.5 cm² | 3 d | 1 mg/3 d | Matrix (DIA) with rate-controlling membrane |
| Catapress-TTS® | Clonidine | 1984 | Boehringer Ingelheim | Polyisobutylene adhesive | 3.5, 7.0, and 10.5 cm² | 7 d | 0.1, 0.2, and 0.3 mg/d | Matrix (DIA) with rate-controlling membrane |
| Nitro-Dur® | Nitroglycerine | 1985 | US Pharma | Acrylic adhesive | 5, 10, 15, 20, 30, and 40 cm² | 12 h | 0.1, 0.2, 0.3, 0.4, 0.6, and 0.8 mg/h | Matrix (DIA) |
| Duragesic® | Fentanyl | 1990 | Janssen Pharma | Polyacrylate adhesive and isopropyl myristate | 5.5, 11, 16.5, 22, 33, and 44 cm² | 3 d | 12, 15, 37.5, 50, 75, 100, 20 µg/h | Matrix (DIA) |
| Habitrol® | Nicotine | 1991 | Dr. Reddys | Acrylate adhesive | — | 24 h | 7, 14, and 21 mg/24 h | — |
| Nicoderm CQ | Nicotine | 1991 | Sanofi Aventis | Polyisobutylene adhesive | — | 24 h | 7, 14, and 21 mg/24 h | — |
| Menostar® | Estradiol | 1994 | Bayer Healthcare | Acrylate adhesive | 3.35 cm² | 7 d | 14 µg/d | Matrix (DIA) |
| Androderm® | Testosterone | 1995 | Allergan | Carbomer copolymer Type B | 6 and 12 cm² | 24 h | 2 and 4 mg/d | Reservoir with rate-controlling membrane |
| Vivelle-Dot® | Estradiol | 1996 | Novartis | Acrylic adhesive and silicone | 2.5, 3.75, 5.0, 7.7, and 10 cm² | 3–4 d | 0.025, 0.050, 0.075, and 0.1 mg/d | Matrix (DIA) |
| Alora® | Estradiol | 1996 | Allergan | Acrylic adhesive | 9, 18, 27, and 36 cm² | 3–4 d | 0.025, 0.050, 0.075, and 0.1 mg/d | Matrix (DIA) |
| Combipatch® | Estradiol/ Norethindrone acetate | 1998 | Novel Pharms Inc | Acrylic adhesive, silicone adhesive, povidone | 9, 16 cm² | 3–4 d | 50 µg/d estradiol 140–250 µg/d levonorgestrel | Matrix (DIA) |
| Vivelle® | Estradiol | 2000 | Novartis | Acrylic adhesive, polyisobutylene, ethylene vinyl acetate copolymer | 7.25, 11.0, 14.5, 22.0, and 29.0 cm² | 3–4 d | 0.025, 0.050, 0.075, and 0.1 mg/d | Matrix (DIA) |
| Oxytrol® | Oxybutynin | 2003 | Allergan | Acrylic adhesive | 39 cm² | 3–4 d | 3.9 mg/d | Matrix (DIA) |
| Climara Pro® | Estradiol/ Levonorgestrel | 2005 | Berlex Lab | acrylate adhesive | 22 cm² | 7 days | 45 µg/d estradiol 15 µg/d lev-onorgestrel | Matrix (DIA) |
| Daytrana® | Methylphenidate | 2006 | Novel Pharms Inc | Acrylic adhesive | 12.5, 18.75, 25, and 37.5 cm² | 9 h | 1.1, 1.6, 2.2, 3.3. mg/h | Matrix (DIA) |

(Continued)

**TABLE 28-8 •** FDA-Approved Transdermal Systems for Systemic Delivery of Drugs (*Continued*)

| Brand Name | Drug | Year of Approval | Company | Polymer | Surface Area | Duration | Release Rate | Type |
|---|---|---|---|---|---|---|---|---|
| Emsam® | Selegiline | 2006 | Somerset | Acrylic adhesive | 20, 30, and 40 cm² | 24 h | 6, 9, and 12 mg/24 h | Matrix (DIA) |
| Exelon | Rivastigemin | 2007 | Novartis | Acrylic copolymer, poly(butylmethacrylate, methylmethacrylate), silicone adhesive | 5, 10, and 15 cm² | 24 h | 4.6 mg/d | Matrix (DIA) |
| Neupro | Rotigotine | 2007 | UCB Inc | Povidone and silicone adhesive | 5, 10, 15, 20, 30, and 40 cm² | 24 h | 1, 2, 3, 4, 6, and 8 mg/d | Matrix (DIA) |
| Sancuso | Granisetron | 2008 | Kyowa Kirin | — | 52 cm² | 7 d | 3.1 mg/day | Matrix |
| Burans® | Buprenorphine | 2010 | Purdue Pharma | Povidone,and polyacrylate | 6.25, 9.375, 12.5, and 18.75 cm² | 7 d | 7.5, 10, 15, and 20 μg/h | Matrix (DIA) |
| Minivelle™ | Estradiol | 2012 | Noven | Acrylic adhesive and silicone adhesive | 2.48, 3.30, 4.95, and 6.6 cm² | 3–4 d | 0.0375, 0.05, 0.075, and 0.1 mg/day | Matrix (DIA) |

acrylic and silicone adhesives (Daytrana®, Combi-Patch, Vivelle-Dot, Minivelle) (Wokovich et al 2006; Van Buskirk et al 2012; Drugs@FDA).

Some of the quality issues observed with the TDS are adhesion failure, residual drug, cold flow, and drug crystallization. These quality defects have prompted recall of many TDS products, such as estradiol (adhesion failure), rotigotine (crystal formation), fentanyl (cold flow or leakage), etc. Adhesion is critical for TDS performance as it is essential for intimate contact between the drug product and skin. Environmental factors such as high humidity may impact the thermodynamics of adhesion between the TDS and the skin. Consequently, a poor clinical outcome may result if TDS fails to adhere during the use period. Inadequate adhesion may also reduce the diffusion surface area. The drug product sponsors need to conduct studies to determine adhesion characteristics of the product and assess if there are any changes in the diffusion surface area as a result.

There is still some drug left in the patch after the intended duration of wear. The amount of drug left in the patch determines safety and efficacy of the TDS. This is potentially dangerous if the patch contains potent drugs such as fentanyl or methylphenidate. Patients throw away the TDS after the period of wear, and it can be chewed by animals or children and consequently expose them to dangerous drugs.

**TABLE 28-9 •** FDA-Approved Transdermal Systems for Local Effects of Drugs

| Brand Name | Drug | Year of Approval | Company | Surface Area | Duration |
|---|---|---|---|---|---|
| Lidoderm | Lidocaine | 1999 | Teikoku Pharma USA | 420 cm² | 12 h |
| Synera | Lidocaine/Tetracaine | 2005 | Galen Speciality | 10 and 50 cm² | 20–30 min |
| Flector® | Diclofenacepolamine | 2007 | Inst Biochem | 140 cm² | 12 h |
| Qutenza™ | Capsaicin | 2009 | Averitas | 280 cm² | 60 min |
| ZTlido™ | Lidocaine topical | 2018 | Scilex Pharmaceiticals | 140 cm² | 12 h |

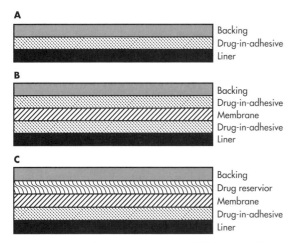

FIGURE 28-12 • Schematic presentation of (**A**) drug-in-adhesive; (**B**) drug-in-adhesive with rate controlling membrane; and **C**, reservoir types of transdermal delivery systems.

The FDA requires data of drug left (residual drug) in the patch after the intended period of wear to determine the safety and efficacy of the product.

To diffuse through the skin, the drug should be in solution form, and TDS must maintain the drug in solution state throughout the product's shelf life. Crystallization of dissolved drug may change the diffusion rate of the drug from the TDS, and potentially make it clinically ineffective. Drug may crystallize in the TDS due to exposure to high temperatures and humidity, formulation change or process, or a combination thereof. Another potential challenge associated with TDS is cold flow, which is the creeping or oozing of the adhesive matrix beyond the perimeter of the backing membrane or through the release liner slit. It is very common in the DIA type of TDS. The propensity of formulations to cold flow needs to be assessed by a combination of methods, as there is no FDA-recommended method.

Barrier properties of the stratum corneum can be modulated by applying external energy, such as iontophoresis, microneedling, electroporation, ultrasound, etc. Iontophoresis involves application of a low-level electric current either directly to the skin or through dosage forms to enhance drug permeation through the skin. Application of low electricity produces changes in the barrier properties of the stratum corneum. This method allows permeation of charged molecules which are difficult to deliver by conventional transdermal methods (passive diffusion). Iontophoresis is affected by electrode type, current intensity, pH of formulation, competitive ion effect, and permeant type. A major limitation of iontophoresis is the possibility of irreversible damage to the skin and failure to significantly improve the delivery of macromolecules of >7000 Da. The FDA has approved two TDS based on iontophoresis—Lidosite® (ephedrine and lidocaine hydrochloride) and Ionsys® (fentanyl hydrochloride). Lidosite consists of a patch and a controller, which is a portable microprocessor-controlled battery-powered DC current ($1.77$ mA/5 cm$^2$). Ionsys applies a low-level current of $62$ μA/cm$^2$. Lidosite and Ionsys contain hydrogel formulation; however, both products have been discontinued.

Microneedling is a mechanical method to overcome the stratum corneum barrier to deliver the drug. It consists of micron size needle that creates microscopic pores in the stratum corneum. There are four different designs of microneedles: biodegradable, that degrade and release the drug after piercing through stratum corneum; solid microneedles coated with drug; hollow microneedles for injection; and solid microneedles to pierce the skin followed by application of drug patch. There is no FDA-approved TDS based on this approach at this time. However, Zosano Pharma submitted an NDA of zolmitriptan (Qtrypta). Qtrypta is a TDS based on microneedles coated with the drug for systemic delivery.

## Nasal Delivery Systems

The nasal route provides an alternative to oral and parenteral routes for systemic delivery of drugs in addition to delivering drugs for symptomatic relief and prevention or treatment of topical conditions of the nasal cavity. The anatomical, physiological, and histological features of the nasal route provide a potential for rapid systemic absorption and quick onset of action. The gastrointestinal and presystemic hepatic metabolism is the hallmark of the oral route, which can be avoided by nasally administered drugs, thus enhancing bioavailability. This route also provides the means to deliver drug directly to the brain by circumventing the blood–brain barrier.

Despite numerous advantages, the nasal route has many limitations. The rate and extent of absorption from the nasal cavity are affected by a variety of physiological and pathological conditions related to nasal mucosa in addition to physicochemical factors of drug and formulations. There is a volume restriction of 100–150 $\mu L$ in the nasal cavity, which limits the dose of drugs. Many enzymes (hydrolases, dehydrogenases, esterases, cytochrome P450 isoenzymes, aminopeptidases, proteases, etc) are present in the nasal cavity, which may cause presystemic metabolism of drugs. Drugs are also cleared by the mucociliary mechanism in the nasal cavity, resulting in short residence time. Many transporters and P-glycoprotein are also present, which may interfere with drug absorption. However, various approaches are reported in the literature to overcome the short residence time, increase permeability, and inhibit or decrease presystemic metabolism. These approaches include incorporating a viscosity-modifying agent to increase residence time and surfactant as a penetration enhancer, using prodrug to modify physiochemical properties or susceptibility to enzymatic metabolism, and use of enzyme inhibitors and novel formulations (mucoadhesive, liposomes, etc).

The FDA has approved a number of nasal delivery systems for localized/topical effects in the nasal cavity and systemic delivery of drugs (Table 28-10). Nasal delivery systems available for topical use are solutions, suspensions, or pressurized aerosol systems applied as drops or spray. Nasal delivery systems also contain devices to form the spray or meter the dose and generate the spray. Suspension or powder formulations may accelerate the mucociliary function of the nasal cavity and hence reduce residence time. Nasal drops are not preferred, as the drug is rapidly cleared by anterior leakage and posterior clearance by the mucociliary mechanism. Application in the form of spray increases nasal residence time by preventing anterior leakage and decreasing posterior clearance. Nasal products are aqueous non-isotonic and non-sterile formulations. They may contain cosolvents to solubilize the drug or other components of formulation, eg, propylene glycol or glycerin. The formulations are buffered for solubility, stability, or absorption (increased proportion of non-ionized form of the drug) purposes. Citrate and phosphate are commonly used buffer systems. Suspending/viscosity-modifying agents used are hydroxypropyl methylcellulose, carboxymethylcellulose, and microcrystalline cellulose. A viscosity-modifying agent is also present in solution formulations to increase nasal residence time. Polysorbate 80 is commonly used in commercial formulations as a surfactant and penetration enhancer. Humectant, such as glycerine, is often added to the formulations to reduce nasal irritation. Additional components present in nasal formulations are chelating agents (edetate disodium), preservatives (benzalkonium chloride and phenethylalchohol), and antioxidants (butylated hydroxyanisole). The formulations may contain sweetener if the drug is bitter, eg, azelastine (Astelin®, Astepro®), beclomethasone dipropionate (Beconase AQ), budesonide (Rhinocort), fluticasone (Flonase® Sensimist™), and triamcinolone acetonide (Nasacort® Allergy). Sweeteners present in FDA-approved formulations are dextrose (Beconase AQ, Flonase, Nasacort Allergy, Xhance™), sorbitol, and sucralose (Astepro). Pressurized aerosol formulations are solution formulations in which propellant or propellant and ethanol act as a solvent system (Zetonna® and Qnasl™) to dissolve the drug. The propellants used in nasal aerosol systems are HFA-134a (1,1,1,2 tetrafluoroethane). Coloring agents are not typically added to nasal formulations; however, there is an exception, cocaine hydrochloride (Goprelto and Numbrino). This formulation is used as a local anesthetic in surgical procedures of the nasal cavity. The probable function of the coloring agent is to mark the area of the nasal cavity that comes in contact with the formulation. The pH of commercial formulations ranges from 4.3 to 6.8.

FDA has approved nasal delivery systems for systemic delivery of drugs which are poorly absorbed, cause irritation, and degrade in the gastrointestinal tract and undergo extensive first-pass metabolism, produce rapid onset of action and reach to brain to some extent (Table 28-11). Dihydroergotamine mesylate (Migranal®) is poorly absorbed by the oral route, and nasal administration resulted in 32% bioavailability. Butorphanol tartrate (Stadol), fentanyl citrate (Lzanda®), esketamine (Spravato™), diazepam (Valtoco®), naloxone hydrochloride (Narcan®), nicotine (Nicotrol® NS), zolmitriptan (Zomig), and midazolam (Nayzilam®) undergo first-pass metabolism. Administering through the nasal route increases the systemic availability of

## TABLE 28-10 • FDA-Approved Nasal Delivery Systems for Localized Effects

| Brand | Drug | Year of Approval | Company | Dosage Form | Strength | Indications |
|-------|------|------------------|---------|-------------|----------|-------------|
| Tyzine® | Tetrazoline hydrochloride | 1979 | Fougera Pharms | Solution and spray solution | 0.05 and 0.1% | Decongestant |
| Beconase AQ | Beclomethasone dipropionate | 1987 | GlaxoSmithKline | Spray suspension | 42 mcg/spray | Allergic conditions |
| Flonase® Sensimist™ | Fluticasone propionate | 1994 | GlaxoSmithKline | Spray suspension | 27.5 mcg/spray | Allergic conditions |
| Astelin® | Azelastine HCl | 1996 | Mylan Speciality LP | Spray solution | 125 mcg/spray | Allergic conditions |
| Nasacort® Allergy 24 hr | Triamcinolone acetonide | 1996 | Sanofi Aventis US | Spray suspension | 55 mcg/spray | Allergic conditions |
| NasalCrom | Cromolyn sodium | 1997 | Blacksmith Brands | Solution | 5.2 mg/spray | Allergic conditions |
| Nasonex | Mometasone furoate | 1997 | Merck Sharp & Dohme | Suspension | 50 mcg/spray | Allergic conditions |
| Rhinocort | Budesonide | 1999 | AstraZeneca | Spray solution | 32 mcg/spray | Allergy conditions |
| Omnaris™ | Ciclesonide | 2007 | Nycomed US Inc | Spray suspension | 50 mcg/spray | Seasonal allergies |
| Astepro® | Azelastine HCl | 2008 | Mylan Speciality LP | Spray solution | 125–187.6 mcg/spray | Allergic conditions |
| Patanase | Olopatadine HCl | 2008 | Novartis | Spray solution | 665 mcg/spray | Allergic conditions |
| Dymista® | Azelastine HCl and fluticasone propionate | 2012 | Mylan Speciality LP | Spray suspension | 137/50 mcg/spray | Allergic conditions |
| Qnasl™ | Beclomethasone dipropionate | 2012 | Teva Branded Pharm | Aerosol, non-aqueous solution | 40–80 mcg/actuation | Allergic conditions |
| Zetonna® | Ciclesonide | 2012 | Covis Pharma BV | Non-aqueous solution, aerosol | 37 mcg/actuation | Seasonal allergies |
| Kovanaze™ | Oxymetazoline HCl and Tetracaine HCl | 2016 | St Renatus | Spray solution | 0.1 mg/ 6 mg/spray | Decongestant |
| Goprelto/ Numbrino | Cocaine HCl | 2017 | Genus Lifesciences | Solution | 4% (160 mg/4 mL) | Local anesthetics |
| Xhance™ | Fluticasone propionate | 2017 | Optinose US Inc | Spray suspension | 93 mcg/spray | Allergic conditions |

drugs. Furthermore, these drugs interact with the receptors or protein present in the brain to elicit a clinical response. It is highly likely that a significant portion of the administered dose reaches the brain directly through the nasal cavity. In some cases, the bioavailability achieved from the nasal delivery system is similar to parenteral route. For example, bioavailability from Valtoco (diazepam) is 97% of the parenterally administered dose. For other drugs, administration from the nasal delivery system reduces the incidence of adverse effects. For example, one of the adverse effects of ketorolac

## TABLE 28-11 • FDA-Approved Nasal Delivery Systems For Systemic Effects

| Brand | Drug | Year of Approval | Company | Dosage Form | Strength/Dose | Indications |
|---|---|---|---|---|---|---|
| DDAVP | Desmopressin acetate | 1978 | Ferring Pharma Inc | Spray solution | 10 µg/spray | Antidiuretic |
| Synarel® | Nafraelin | 1990 | GD Searle LLC | Spray solution | 2 mg/mL, 200 mcg | Precocious puberty |
| Stadol | Butorphanol tartrate | 1991 | Bristol Myers Squibb | Spray solution | 10 mg/mL, 1 mg/spray | Pain management |
| Stimate® | Desmopressin acetate | 1994 | Ferring Pharma Inc | Spray solution | 15 µg/spray | Antidiuretic |
| Nicotrol® NS | Nicotine | 1996 | Pfizer | Spray solution | 10 mg/mL, 0.5 mg/spray | Smoking cessation |
| Imitrex | Sumatriptan | 1997 | GlaxoSmithKline | Spray solution | 5 and 20 mg/spray | Migraine |
| Migranal® | Dihydroergotamine mesylate | 1997 | Bausch | Spray solution | 4 mg/mL, 05 mg/mL | Migraine |
| Minirin | Desmopressin acetate | 2002 | Ferring Pharma Inc | Soar Solution | 10 µg/spray | Antidiuretic |
| Flumist® | Influenza vaccine (Quadrivalent) | 2003 | MedImmune, LLC | Suspension | 0.2 mL/spray | Influenza |
| Zomig | Zolmitriptan | 2003 | AstraZeneca | Spray solution | 2.5 and 5 mg/spray | Migraine |
| Fortical | Calcitonin salmon | 2005 | Upsher Smith Labs | Spray solution | 2200/mL, 200/spray | Osteoporosis |
| Nascobal® | Cyanocobalamin | 2005 | Endo Pharms Inc | Spray solution | 500 mcg/spray | Vitamin B12 deficiency |
| Sprix™ | Ketorolac tromethamine | 2010 | Zyla | Spray solution | 15.75 mg/spray | Moderate to severe pain management |
| Lazanda® | Fentanyl Citrate | 2011 | BTCP Pharm | Spray solution | 100–400 mcg/actuation | Breakthrough pain |
| Natesto | Testosterone | 2014 | Acerus | Metered Gel | 5.5 mg/actuation | Hormonal replacement |
| Narcan® | Naloxone HCl | 2015 | Adapt Pharma | Spray solution | 2–4 mg/0.1 mL | Opioid antagonist |
| Onzetra™ Xsail™ | Sumatriptan succinate | 2016 | Currax | Capsule/Nasal inhalation | 11 mg/nosepiece | Migraine |
| Baqsimi | Glucagon | 2019 | Eli Lilly and Co | Powder | 3 mg | Severe hypoglycemia |
| Nayzilam® | Midazolam | 2019 | UCB Inc | Spray solution | 5 mg/spray | Seizure |
| Spravato™ | Esketamine | 2019 | Janssen Pharm | Spray solution | 28 mg/two sprays | Adjuvant in Depression |
| Tosymra | Sumatriptan | 2019 | Upsher Smith Labs | Spray solution | 10 mg/spray | Migraine |
| Valtoco® | Diazepam | 2020 | Neurelis Inc | Spray solution | 5, 7.5, and 10 mg/spray | Seizure |

tromethamine is irritation and ulcer of gastrointestinal tract. This adverse effect can be avoided by administering through the nasal route. However, administration of ketorolac tromethamine (Sprix™) through the nasal route produces lower bioavailability compared to the oral route. Salmon calcitonin, nafarelin, desmopressin acetate, and glucagon are peptide drugs, which are degraded by enzymes present in gastrointestinal fluid. The nasal route makes it possible to administer peptide drugs for systemic effects. However, systemic bioavailability of these drugs through the nasal route does not increase substantially. For example, systemic bioavailability of salmon calcitonin (Fortical) and nafarelin (Synarel®) is ≤3%, and desmopressin acetate (DDAVP, Minirin, and Stimate®) is >10%. This route also provides opportunity to administer vaccines for systemic protection against disease. The nasal-associated lymphoid tissue (NALT) in the nasal cavity is involved in initiation and execution of immune responses. NALT contains B, T, and dendritic cells, and locally produces immunoglobulin A for defense of the nasal cavity. A commercially available vaccine is Flumist®, which contains four strains of live attenuated influenza virus. Flumist stimulates NALT and delivers vaccine for systemic activation of immune responses to develop specific immunoglobulins against the virus. The nasal delivery systems available for systemic administration of drugs are solution, powder, capsule, and gel. Powder deposition of hydrophobic drugs may stimulate mucous production and enhance mucociliary function for rapid clearance. However, the commercially available nasal delivery system in powder formulation contains a hydrophilic drug, which dissolves in the nasal cavity (glucagon and sumatriptan succinate). Nasal delivery systems intended for systemic effects contain formulation components similar to nasal delivery systems intended for topical effects. They may contain novel surfactants as penetration enhancers such as dodecylphosphocholine, n-dodecyl β-D-maltoside, and oleoyl polyoxylglycerides. Additional components, such as cyclodextrins and flavoring agents, may be used to increase stability (glucagon) and mask unpleasant odor (nicotine) of drugs. Some formulations do not contain any excipients (Onzetra™ Xsail™) at all.

A number of unique nasal drug–device combination products are available for systemic delivery of drugs. These are Onzetra Xsail (sumatriptan succinate) and Baqsimi™ (glucagon). Onzetra Xsail is a capsule that contains sumatriptan succinate without excipients, and the capsule shell is made of hydroxypropyl methylcellulose. It is commercialized as a kit containing a disposable nose piece, which contains the capsule, and a reusable breath-powered delivery device. The device has a port for holding the nose piece, a mechanism to pierce the capsule, and a mouthpiece. The device with the nose piece is inserted into the nose, and the mouthpiece into the mouth. The patient blows forcefully through mouthpiece to deliver the dose to the nasal cavity. The Baqsimi device contains a single dose of glucagon with excipients for severe hypoglycemia. The device contains a tip for insertion into the nostril, and the dose is administered by pressing the plunger (Fig. 28-13). Neither device requires inhalation for dose administration.

## Inhalation Delivery Systems

Lungs can also be used to deliver drugs into the systemic circulation or administer drugs for localized effect. Lungs have unique properties, such as a large surface area for drug absorption (100 m²), a rich blood supply, and relatively low metabolic activity compared to the gastrointestinal tract. The systemic

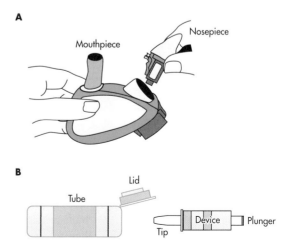

FIGURE 28-13 • Schematic presentation of (A) Onzetra™ Xsail™; and (B) Baqsimi®.

availability of drugs with high first-pass effect, and unstable and proteinous drugs can be increased by administering through the lungs. Similarly, the dose and adverse events can be reduced significantly by localizing the effect of the drugs in the lungs to treat or control symptoms of respiratory diseases such as asthma, pneumonia, influenza virus, infection, etc.

Currently, three drug–device combination products are available that deliver drugs to lungs. These are pressurized metered dose inhalers (pMDIs) with or without spacers, DPIs, and nebulizers. The critical quality attribute affecting their performance is particle size, which is expressed as an aerodynamic diameter (takes into account density and shape). Particle size is expressed as mass median aerodynamic size, which typically varies from 3–4 $\mu$m for commercial inhalation systems. Particle size affects drug deposition in lungs. Drug deposition in lungs occurs by three mechanisms: inertial impaction, gravitational sedimentation, and Brownian diffusion. Drug deposition in the oropharynx region and at the bifurcation of major airways primarily takes place by inertial impaction. In smaller airways and alveoli, the drug is deposited by gravitational sedimentation. Only smaller particles <1 $\mu$m are deposited by Brownian diffusion. In addition to particle size, the patient's inhalation also determines the site of drug deposition. Deep inhalation and breath holding increase gravitational sedimentation, which increases drug deposition in the lung periphery. Inhalation systems are inhaled through a mouthpiece or face mask to avoid drug deposition in nose region.

*Pressurized metered dose inhaler* (pMDI) was first introduced in 1956 by 3M Riker Laboratories. At the time of this writing, 18 pMDIs are available for clinical use. Generic formulations of Proventil® HFA, Ventolin HFA, and Proair HFA are also available. They are widely used in the management of asthma and chronic pulmonary obstructive disease. pMDIs are portable, convenient, and multi-dose devices (Table 28-12). Commercial pMDI products contain 28 (Bevespi Aerosphere™) to 200 (Proventil® HFA) actuations/inhalations. Each actuation delivers 25–100 $\mu$l volume containing a small dose of potent drugs. Some of the products have built-in actuation counters to guide the patient when to discard the pMDI (Qvar® Redihaler™). pMDI is primarily used to deliver potent $\beta$-agonist, anticholinergic,

and glucocorticoid classes of drugs. They are used to deliver one or multiple drugs. The device uses a propellant under pressure to deliver a metered dose in aerosol form. pMDI consists of two components, a formulation and a device (Fig. 28-14). The device consists of a canister, a metering valve, and an actuator. The formulation contains drug either in suspended or dissolved form in a propellant or a mixture of propellants, solvents, and/or other excipients. For the suspension formulation, a suspending agent or a dispersant is required. The suspending agent used in the commercial product is either polymer (povidone K25 in Symbicort®) or surfactant (oleic acid in Proventil® HFA). Suspension formulations also contain lubricants such as oleic acid (Proventil HFA) or polyethylene glycol (Symbicort) to prevent clogging of the valve assembly of the device by the suspended particles as well as to prevent particle growth.

Initially, pMDIs were based on chlorofluorocarbon (CFC) propellants, which have now been replaced by hydrofluoroalkane (HFA) propellants due to the ozone-depleting effects of the CFC. However, some concerns have also been raised over the global warming potential of HFA propellants. The most commonly used HFA propellants in commercial products are HFA-134a (1,1,1,2-tetrafluoroethane) and HFA-127 (1,1,1,2,3,3,3-heptafluoropropane). pMDIs require priming of the device before the first use, which involves shaking well and releasing two to four sprays into the air. Priming is also required if the pMDI has not been used for some time, which varies from product to product. For example, Atrovent® HFA and Xopenex HFA™ require priming of the device if not used for 3 days, while Advair HFA requires priming only if not used for 4 weeks.

Recent developments in inhalation technology have led to the development of low-velocity spray systems, known as soft-mist inhalers. Four soft-mist inhalers have been approved by the FDA (Stiolto® Respimat®, Spiriva® Respimat, Striverdi® Respimat, and Combivent® Respimat·) (Table 28-12). They do not contain propellant, and spray is produced by mechanical energy to generate a slow-moving aerosol. Soft-mist inhalers dispense a very small volume typically 10–11 $\mu$l, and can deliver only solution formulations. The approved formulations are sterile water–based solutions containing antioxidant and preservative. Due to the low speed of spray generated

## TABLE 28-12 • FDA-Approved Pressurized Metered Dose Inhalers

| Brand Name | Drug | Year of Approval | Company | Dose/ Actuation | Propellant | Type | Solvent |
|---|---|---|---|---|---|---|---|
| Proventil® HFA | Albuterol sulfate | 1996 | Merck Sharpe & Dohme | 108 µg | HFA-134a | Suspension | Ethanol |
| Ventolin HFA | Albuterol sulfate | 2001 | GlaxoSmithKline | 108 µg | HFA-134a | Suspension | — |
| Proair HFA | Albuterol sulfate | 2004 | Teva | 108 µg | HFA-134a | Suspension | Ethanol |
| Flovent HFA | Fluticasone propionate | 2004 | GlaxoSmithKline | 44, 110, and 220 µg | HFA-134a | Suspension | — |
| Atrovent® HFA | Ipratropium bromide | 2004 | Boehringer Ingelheim | 21 µg | HFA-134a | Solution | Water and ethanol |
| Xopenex HFA™ | Levalbuterol tartrate | 2005 | Sunovion | 59 µg | HFA-134a | Suspension | Ethanol |
| Symbicort® | Budesonide/Formoterol fumarate | 2006 | AstraZeneca | 91/5.1 and 181/5.1 µg | HFA-227 | Suspension | — |
| Aerospan® | Flunisolide | 2006 | Mylan | 139 µg | HFA-134a | Solution | Ethanol |
| Advair HFA | Fluticasone propionate/ Salmeterol xinafoate | 2006 | GlaxoSmithKline | 45/21, 115/21, and 230/21 µg | HFA-134a | Suspension | — |
| Alvesco® | Ciclesonide | 2008 | Covis Pharm | 80/160 µg | HFA-134a | Solution | Ethanol |
| Dulera® | Formoterol fumarate/ Mometasone furoate | 2010 | Merck Sharpe & Dohme | 100/5 200/5 µg | HFA-227 | Suspension | Ethanol |
| Combivent® Respimat® | Ipratropium bromide/Albuterol sulfate | 2011 | Boehringer Ingelheim | 20/100 µg | — | Liquid solution | Water |
| Asmanex® HFA | Mometasone furoate | 2014 | Merck | 100 and 200 µg | HFA-227 | Suspension | Ethanol |
| Striverdi® Respimat® | Olodaterol hydrochloride | 2014 | Boehringer Ingelheim | 2.5 µg | — | Solution | Water, |
| Spiriva® Respimat® | Tiotropium bromide | 2014 | Boehringer Ingelheim | 1.25/2.5 µg | — | Solution | Water, |
| Stiolto® Respimat® | Olodaterol hydrochloride/ Tiotropium bromide | 2015 | Boehringer Ingelheim | 2.5/2.5 µg | — | Solution | Water, |
| Bevespi Aerosphere™ | Formoterol fumarate/ glycopyrrolate | 2016 | AstraZeneca | 9/4.8 µg | HFA-134a | Suspension | — |
| Qvar® Redihaler™ | Beclomethasone dipropionate | 2017 | Norton Waterford | 40 µg | HFA-134a | Solution | Ethanol |

*HFA-134a-1, 1, 1, 2-tetrafluoroethane; HFA-227-1,1,1,2,3,3,3-heptafluoropropane*

by soft-mist inhalers, drug deposition in lungs is high compared to propellant-based pMDIs.

Both pMDIs and soft-mist inhalers require proper coordination between actuation and inhalation. Poor coordination between the actuation of the device and inspiration through the delivery system may not deliver the required dose to the lung region. This issue can be addressed by using breath-actuated pMDIs or spacer devices. Breath-actuated pMDIs operate on a triggering mechanism provided by the patient's inhalation via a mouthpiece. Qvar® Redihaler™, a recently approved device, is a

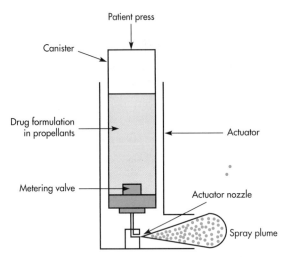

**FIGURE 28-14 •** Schematic presentation of pressurized metered dose inhaler.

breath-actuated pMDI and does not require actuation to deliver the dose. A spacer is an add-on device, extension, or holding chamber which improves efficiency of drug delivery to patients who have difficulty in coordinating inhalation with actuation. Spacers are available in various shapes and sizes, with volume ranging from 50 mL to 750 mL. The spacer is placed between the point at which aerosol is generated and the patient's mouth. This allows propellant to evaporate and slow down rapidly moving aerosol. The typical design of a spacer consists of a one-way valve in the mouthpiece to hold the actuated aerosol, with a brief pause before inhaling the dose. Spacers also reduce drug deposition in the oropharyngeal region and consequently increase lung deposition. Some commercially available products have built-in spacers (Aerospan®).

*Dry powder inhalers (DPIs):* The FDA approved the first DPI in 1969. Since then about 30 products have been approved. However, only the generic formulation of Advair (Diskus) is available (Table 28-13). Unlike pMDIs, DPIs are used for delivering drugs to the lungs for local and systemic effect. This includes drugs for asthma, chronic obstructive pulmonary disease, cystic fibrosis, influenza, psychotic disorders, and Parkinsonism. They are also used for delivering proteinous drugs such as Afrezza® (insulin). DPI products differ considerably from pMDIs. The formulation consists of a

micronized drug along with the larger sized carrier. The carrier improves the flow of the powder and also acts as a diluent. The most commonly used carrier is spray dried lactose monohydrate (Fig. 28-15). The product may contain additional flow promoters such as magnesium stearate (Incruse Ellipta). Moreover, insulin DPI (Afrezza) contains novel excipient, fumaryl diketopiperazine (FDKP). FDKP forms an array of microcrystalline plate structures which then self-assemble into microparticles with large surface areas onto which insulin is adsorbed. The average diameter of FDKP is 2.5 μm. The time to maximum serum insulin concentration from Afrezza ranges from 10 to 20 minutes after oral inhalation. For poorly absorbed drugs, permeation enhancer such as 1,2-dipalmitoyl-sn-glycero-3-phosphocholine can be incorporated into the formulation; eg, tobramycin (Tobi® Podhaler™). Some DPIs such as Adasuve® do not contain excipients. Adasuve is a single-use drug–device combination product that provides rapid systemic delivery of a thermally-generated aerosol of loxapine. The product consists of a thin film of excipient-free loxapine. Controlled rapid heating of the film produces drug vapor which then condenses into aerosol particles that are dispersed into the airstream created by the patient inhaling through the mouthpiece.

DPIs are breath-activated inhaler systems, which do not require inhalation-actuation coordination. The patient's inhalation through the mouthpiece of the device causes the deagglomeration and aerosolization of the drug particles as the formulation moves through the cyclone component of the device (Airduo Respiclick®). This is followed by dispersion into the airstream. The amount of drug delivered to the lung depends on formulation factors, such as particle size and shape, and patient factors, such as inspiratory flow profiles and inspiratory time.

The current design of products includes pre-metered and device-metered DPIs. In pre-metered DPIs, an individual measure of drug formulation is present in the form of a capsule (Tobi Podhaler), blister (Anoro Ellipta), or cartridge (Afrezza). Both gelatin (Arcapta Neohaler®) and hydroxypropyl methylcellulose (Tobi Podhaler) capsules are used. The individual dose, after being placed in the device, is pierced and subsequently aerosolized by the patient. The device meter contains a reservoir of drug powder

## TABLE 28-13 • FDA-Approved Pressurized Dry Powder Inhalers

| Brand Name | Drug | Year of Approval | Company | Dose/Actuation | Carrier | Type | Powder Delivered/ Actuation |
|---|---|---|---|---|---|---|---|
| Serevent Diskus | Salmeterol xinafoate | 1997 | GlaxoSmithKline | 47 $\mu g$ | Lactose | Blister | 12.5 mg |
| Relenza | Zanamivir | 1999 | GlaxoSmithKline | 4 mg | Lactose | Blister | 25 mg |
| Flovent Diskus | Fluticasone propionate | 2000 | GlaxoSmithKline | 46, 94, and 229 $\mu g$ | Lactose | Blister | 12.5 mg |
| Advair Diskus | Fluticasone propionate/ Salmeterol xinafoate | 2000 | GlaxoSmithKline | 93/45, 233/45, and 465/45 $\mu g$ | Lactose | Blister | 12.5 mg |
| Spiriva® Handihaler® | Tiotropium bromide | 2004 | Boehringer Ingelheim | 10.4 $\mu g$ | Lactose | Gelatin capsule | — |
| Asmanex Twisthaler | Mometasone furoate | 2005 | Merck | 100 and 200 $\mu g$ | Lactose | Powder reservoir | 0.75 and 1.5 mg |
| Pulmicort Flexhaler® | Budesonide | 2006 | AstraZeneca | 90 and 180 $\mu g$ | Lactose | Powder reservoir | 1 mg |
| Aridol™ | Mannitol | 2010 | Pharmaxis Ltd | 3.4, 7.7, 16.5, and 34.1 mg | — | Capsule | — |
| Arcapta Neohaler® | Indacaterol maleate | 2011 | Sunovion Pharm | 57 $\mu g$ | Lactose | Gelatin Capsule | 25 mg |
| Tudorza® Pressair® | Aclidinium bromide | 2012 | Circassia | 400 $\mu g$ | Lactose | Powder reservoir | 13 mg |
| Adasuve® | Loxapine | 2012 | Galen | 9.1 mg | — | Thin-film of the drug | 10 mg |
| Breo Ellipta | Fluticasone furoate/ Vilanterol trifenatate | 2013 | GlaxoSmithKline | 92/22 $\mu g$ | Lactose and magnesium stearate | Two blister pack/dose | 12.5 mg |
| Anoro Ellipta | Umeclidinium bromide/ Valanterol trifenatate | 2013 | GlaxoSmithKline | 55/22 $\mu g$ | Lactose and magnesium stearate | Blister | 12.5 mg |
| Tobi Podhaler | Tobramycin | 2013 | Mylan | 102 mg | 1,2-distearoyl-sn-glycero-3-phosphocholine | HPMC capsule | 28 mg |
| Incruse Ellipta | Umeclidinium bromide | 2014 | GlaxoSmithKline | 55 $\mu g$ | Lactose and magnesium stearate | Blister | 12.5 mg |
| Arnuity Ellipta | Fluticasone furoate | 2014 | GlaxoSmithKline | 46, 90, and 192 $\mu g$ | Lactose | Blister | 12.5 mg |
| Afreeza® | Insulin recombinant human | 2014 | Mannkind | — | Fumaryl diketopiperazine and polysorbate 80 | Cartridge | — |
| Proair® Digihaler™ | Albuterol sulfate | 2015 | Teva | 117 mg | Lactose | Powder reservoir | 1 mg |
| Seebri™ Neohaler® | Glycopyrrolate | 2015 | Sunovion Pharm | 13.1 $\mu g$ | Lactose and magnesium stearate | HPMC capsule | 25 mg |

(Continued)

**TABLE 28-13 •** FDA-Approved Pressurized Dry Powder Inhalers (*Continued*)

| Brand Name | Drug | Year of Approval | Company | Dose/Actuation | Carrier | Type | Powder Delivered/ Actuation |
|---|---|---|---|---|---|---|---|
| Utibron® Neohaler® | Indacaterol maleate/ Glycopyrrolate | 2015 | Sunovion Pharm | 20.8/12.8 µg | Lactose and magnesium stearate | HPMC capsule | 25 mg |
| Trelegy Ellipta | Fluticasone Furoate/ Umeclidinium bromide/ Vilanterol trifenatate | 2017 | GlaxoSmithKline | 92/55/22 µg | Lactose and magnesium stearate | Two blister pack/dose | 12.5 mg |
| Armonair Respiclick | Fluticasone propionate | 2017 | Teva | 51, 103, and 210 µg | Lactose | Powder reservoir | 11.5 mg |
| Airduo Respiclick | Fluticasone propionate/ Salmeterol xinafoate | 2017 | Teva | 49/12.75, 100/12.75, and 202/12.75 µg | Lactose | Multi-dose | 5.5 |
| Inbrija™ | Levodopa | 2018 | Acorda | 36.1 mg | 1,2-Dipalmitoyl-sn-glycero-3-phosphocholine | HPMC capsule | 42 mg |
| Duaklir® Pressair® | Aclidinium bromide/ Formoterol fumarate | 2019 | Circassia | 400/12 µg | Lactose | Powder reservoir | 12 mg |

formulation, which is metered by the device. The reservoir may contain 60 (Pulmicort Flexhaler™) to 200 (Proair® Digihaler™) inhalations.

*Nebulizers*: Drug formulations are also delivered to lungs through nebulizers or atomizers. Nebulizers form a spray, which is inhaled by the patient through a mouthpiece or face mask. Unlike pMDIs or DPIs, a nebulizer can be used in relaxed tidal breathing, which means it can be used to deliver drugs to children and elderly patients experiencing

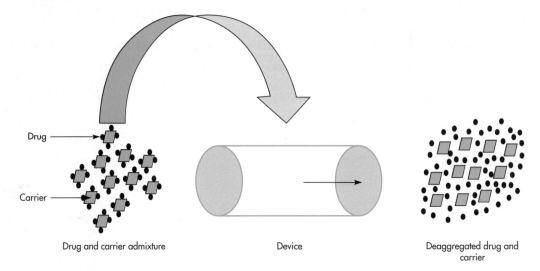

Drug

Carrier

Drug and carrier admixture          Device          Deaggregated drug and carrier

FIGURE 28-15 • Schematic presentation of dry powder inhaler.

asthmatic attacks. The advantage of nebulization over other inhalers is that it can deliver high doses of the drugs (tobramycin, amikacin, and ribavirin) to lung regions without requiring any special provision (Table 28-14). Formulations administered through nebulizers are typically single-dose sterile aqueous solutions, concentrates, suspensions, liposomes, or lyophilized powders. The concentrate solution is

## TABLE 28-14 • FDA-Approved Nebulizers

| Brand Name | Drug | Year of Approval | Company | Dose/ Actuation | Nebulizer Type | Nebulization Time | Dose Delivered | Strength |
|---|---|---|---|---|---|---|---|---|
| Provocholine | Methacholine chloride | 1986 | Methapharm | Powder | — | — | — | 100 mg and 1600 mg |
| Nebupent® | Pentamidine isethionate | 1989 | Fresenius Kabi | Lyophilized | Respirgard® II nebulizer | — | — | 300 mg |
| Xopenex | Levalbuterol hydrochloride | 1999 | Oak Pharm | Solution concentrate | PARI LC® Jet | — | — | 1.25 mg |
| AccuNeb® | Albuterol sulfate | 2001 | Mylan | Solution | PARI LC® Plus (Jet) | 15 min | 39%–43% | 0.75–1.5 mg |
| Pentetate calcium trisodium | Pentetate calcium trisodium | 2004 | Hameln Pharma | Solution | — | — | — | 200 mg |
| Ventavis® | Iloprost | 2004 | Actelion Pharm | Solution | I-neb® AAD® (adaptive aerosol delivery) | — | — | 10 or 20 µg |
| Virazole | Ribavarin | 1985 | Valeant Pharm | Lyophilized powder | Small Particle Aerosol Generator (SPAG®-2) | — | — | 6 gm (20 mg/mL) |
| Brovana® | Arformoterol tartrate | 2006 | Sunovion | Solution | PARI LC® Plus nebulizer (Jet) | 6 min | 27.6% | 22 µg |
| Tobi® | Tobramycin | 1997 | Pulmoflow Inc | Solution | PARI LC Plus nebulizer (Jet) | 15 min | — | 300 mg |
| Perforomist | Formoterol fumarate | 2007 | Mylan | Solution | PARI LC Plus nebulizer (Jet) | 9 min | 37% | 20 µg |
| Tyvaso® | Treprostinil | 2009 | United Therapeutics | Solution | — | 2–3 | — | 1.74 mg |
| Cayston® | Aztreonam | 2010 | Gilead | Lyophilized powder | Altera® Nebulizer System | 2–3 min | — | 75 mg |
| Bethkis | Tobramycin | 2012 | Chiesi USA | Solution | PARI LC Plus nebulizer (Jet) | — | — | 300 mg |
| Kitabis Pak | Tobramycin | 2014 | Pulmoflow Inc | Solution | PARI LC Plus nebulizer (Jet) | 13 | 58% | 300 mg |
| Lonhala Magnair | Glycopyrrolate bromide | 2017 | Sunovion | Solution | MAGNAIR nebulization system | 2–3 | 56.8% | 25 µg |
| Arikayce® | Amikacin sulfate | 2018 | Insmed | Liposomal suspension | Lamira Nebulizer System | — | 53% | 590 mg |
| Yupelri™ | Revefenacin | 2018 | Mylan | Solution | PARI LC Sprint nebulizer | 8 min | 35% | 175 µg |

diluted, whereas lyophilized powder is reconstituted in fluid before atomizing the formulation.

Three types of nebulizers—jet, ultrasonic, and vibrating mesh—are employed to deliver medicines. Jet nebulizers (Pari LC Plus™ and PARI LC® Plus nebulizers) use compressed air or oxygen to generate aerosolized droplets of the liquid formulation. Because they are economical, they are the most commonly used. Typically, a jet nebulizer consists of a venturi through which compressed gas passes to form a jet of air. The liquid formulation and compressed gas interact to form a liquid film, fragmenting into droplets. Only smaller droplets are delivered to patients, and larger ones are prevented from leaving the nebulizer by a baffle and return to the cup holding the formulation. It takes several minutes to aerosolize the entire dose, and a major portion of the dose is left in the device. Jet nebulizers can be used to nebulize solutions as well as micronized suspension formulations. However, they cannot be employed to aerosolize liposome formulations. Ultrasonic nebulizers use a piezoelectric crystal to generate aerosol. They are less popular than jet or vibrating mesh nebulizers owing to the inability of ultrasonic nebulizers to handle suspensions or viscous solutions. In vibrating mesh nebulizers, aerosol is formed by passing liquid formulation through a vibrating mesh or grid of micron-sized holes (I-neb® AAD® and MAGNAIR). They have a short nebulization time and produce high aerosol output. They are compact and portable, and capable of aerosolizing liposome formulations.

## CHAPTER SUMMARY

New and novel dosage forms are developed to improve safety, efficacy, and enhance patient convenience and adherence. Business reasons, such as increasing the life-cycle of exclusivity, patents, and meeting regulatory requirements also provide research interest in their development. Approval of new dosage forms requires submission of an NDA, which can be filed under 505(b)(1) or 505(b)(2) regulatory pathways. 505(b)(1) submissions require exhaustive data to demonstrate safety and efficacy of the dosage form. On the other hand, 505(b)(2) submissions rely on safety data of already approved drug, or literature. The sponsor has to demonstrate efficacy in a bioequivalence study. The regulatory pathway of drug–device combination products is determined by the primary mode of action. The primary mode of action determines which center of the FDA takes the lead in reviewing the drug–device combination product. In the last six decades, the FDA has approved a number of new and novel dosage forms and drug–device combination products, including 3D-printed dosage forms, abuse-deterrent formulations, implants, microparticles/microspheres, vaginal rings, nanomedicines, digital medicines, drug-eluting stents, intrauterine devices, transdermal delivery systems, and inhalation delivery systems. Vaginal rings and intrauterine devices are used primarily for contraceptive application. Implants and microparticles/microspheres are used for localizing or systemic delivery of drugs for a long period of time, typically from days to years. Nanomedicines include nanotechnology-derived products such as liposomes, nanocrystals, microemulsion, nanoemulsion, nanotubes, colloidal iron, polymeric nanoparticles, etc. Inhalation delivery systems are intended for delivering drugs to the lung region for local and systemic effects of drugs. They include pMDIs, dry-powder inhalers, and nebulizers.

## LEARNING QUESTIONS

1. What is the regulatory pathway for approval of new dosage forms of approved drugs?

2. How does the FDA approve drug–device combination products?

3. What is 3D printing? When did the FDA approve the first 3D printed drug product?

4. What is the primary use of abuse deterrent formulations? Explain various approaches to design abuse-deterrent formulations.

5. What are the major differences between pre-formed and *in-situ* implants?

6. What are biodegradable and non-biodegradable polymers and their applications?

7. How does the vaginal contraceptive ring differ from contraceptive implant?

8. What are the different types of FDA-approved nanomedicines?

9. What are the major differences between nano-emulsion and a microemulsion?

10. How do liposomes differ from polymeric nanoparticles?

11. Explain the difference between digital health and digital pills/medicines.

12. Describe the design of drug-eluting stents, their components and applications.

13. What are the different types of transdermal delivery systems? Explain the components of transdermal patch formulations.

14. What issues can be addressed by nasally administered drugs?

15. What are the different types of FDA-approved drug delivery systems?

16. What are the differences between nasal and inhalation delivery systems?

17. What are the different types of FDA-approved inhalation delivery systems?

18. Differentiate among pMDIs dry powder inhalers, and nebulizers.

## ANSWERS

1. 505(b)(1) and 505(b)(2)

2. Primary mode of action, 505(b)(1), 505(b)(2), and 510(k)

3. Manufacturing method of 3D object, 2015.

4. To prevent abuse and misuse of opioid drug products

   Approaches for designing abuse-deterrent products

   a) Physical/chemical barriers

   b) Agonist/antagonist combinations

   c) Aversion

   d) Delivery systems

   e) New molecular entities and prodrugs

   f) Combination of two or more approaches

   g) Novel approaches or technologies

5. Preformed implants physical state is solid prior to administration while in-situ implant is liquid but solidifies after injection.

6. Biodegradable polymers degrade by enzymes present in living beings while non-biodegradable does not degrade by enzyme of living beings. Both biodegradable and non-biodegradable polymers are used in drug delivery systems.

7. A vaginal ring contraceptive is flexible and circular and made of silicone elastomer. It provides contraceptive effect for 3 weeks to 3 months. On the other hand, contraceptive implant (intra-uterine device) is T-shaped and provides contraceptive effect up to years.

8. See Table 28-5.

9. Microemulsion is aerodynamically stable due to presence of large amount of surfactant and co-surfactant in their composition compared to nanoemulsion.

10. Polymeric nanoparticles shapes are both spherical and non-spherical and they can be made of polymers of synthetic or natural origin while liposomes are spherical shape vesicles of phospholipids.

11. Digital medicines/pills are oral dosage forms, which combine a medication with an ingestible sensor. Digital health offers digital technolo¬gies to improve human health in some capacities. It includes mobile health, health information technology, wearable devices, telehealth and tele-medicine, and personalized medicines.

12. Drug-eluting stents consist of following components:

    a) Metallic stent platform or scaffold

    b) Polymer

    c) Antiproliferative drug

Drug-eluting stents are primarily used to relieve symptoms of coronary heart disease or to reduce heart damage after a heart attack.

13. Types of Transdermal delivery systems available in commercial market

a) Drug in adhesive

b) Drug in matrix

c) Drug in reservoir (with rate-controlling membrane)

Following are the components of transdermal delivery systems:

a) Backing membrane

b) Release liner

c) Rate-controlling membrane

d) Formulation

e) Adhesive

14. Nasally administered drug can address following issues

a) Avoid first-pass metabolism

b) Increase local concentration of drug

c) Improve drug penetration to brain

d) Increase systemic bioavailability of the drug

e) Eliminate food effect on drug absorption

f) Can be administered to vomiting/unconscious patients

15. See Tables 28-1 to 28-14

16. Drug is administered through nostrum in nasal delivery systems while drug is administered through oral inhalation for inhalation delivery systems.

17. See Tables 28-12 to Table 28-14

18. Pressurized metered dose inhaler is a multi-dose delivery system. It contains propellant-based solution, suspension, emulsion or semi-solid formulations for oral inhalation delivery of the drugs to lung regions or topical delivery of drug to skin or mucosal membrane. Dry powder is a multidose oral inhalation delivery system consisting primarily of lactose monohydrate and drug in powder form delivered through a device. Nebulizer is a single dose solution/liposome formulation delivered to lung region with a device.

## REFERENCES

Akbarzadeh A, Rezaei-Sadabady R, Davaran S, et al: Liposome: Classification, preparation, and applications. *Nanoscale Res Lett* **8**:102, 2013.

Bayarri L: Drug–device combination products: Regulatory landscape and market growth. *Drugs Today (Barc)* **51**:505–513, 2015.

Bobo D, Robinson KJ, Islam J, Thurecht KJ, Corrie SR: Nanoparticle-based medicines: A review of FDA-approved materials and clinical trials to date. *Pharm Res* **33**:2373-2387, 2016.

Chen V, Faundes A: Contraceptive vaginal rings: A review: *Contraception* **82**:418–427, 2010.

Chen ML, John M, Lee SL, Tyner KM: Development considerations for nanocrystal drug products. *AAPS J* **19**:642–651, 2017.

Columbus L: The state of 3D printing. *Forbes* May 27, 2019.

Cruz CN, Tyner KM, Velazquez L, et al: CDER risk assessment exercise to evaluate potential risks from the use of nanomaterials in drug products. *AAPS J* **15**:623–628, 2013.

Drugs@FDA, https://www.accessdata.fda.gov/scripts/cder/daf/ FDA Guidance: Applications covered by section 505(b)(2), 1999.

Jacobson M: Lessons for medical device manufacturers using 3D printing. Med Device Online, July 18, 2018. Accessed August 22, 2019. https://www.meddeviceonline.com/doc/lessons-for-medical-device-manufacturers-using-d-printing-0001.

Kapoor M, Lee SL, Tyner KM: Liposomal drug product development and quality: Current US experience and perspective. *AAPS J* **19**:632–641, 2017.

Kempe S, Mäder K: In situ forming implants - an attractive formulation principle for parenteral depot formulations. *J Control Release* **161**:668–679, 2012.

Lee DH, Hernandez JMT: The newest generation of drug-eluting stents and beyond. *Eur Cardiol* **13**:54–59, 2018.

Ligon SC, Liska R, Stampfl J, Gurr M, Mülhaupt R: Polymers for 3D printing and customized additive manufacturing. *Chem Rev* **117**:10212–10290, 2017.

Mandal A, Gote V, Pal D, Ogundele A, Mitra AK: Ocular pharmacokinetics of a topical ophthalmic nanomicellar solution of cyclosporine (Cequa®) for dry eye disease. *Pharm Res* **36**:36, 2019.

Mangan D: Economic cost of the opioid crisis: $1 trillion and growing faster. CNBC Feb 13, 2018. https://www.cnbc.com/2018/02/12/economic-cost-of-the-opioid-crisis-1-trillion-and-growing-faster.html.

Michie S, Yardley L, West R, Patrick K, Greaves F: Developing and evaluating digital interventions to promote behavior change in health and health care: recommendations resulting from an international workshop. *J Med Internet Res* **19**:e232, 2017.

Miele E, Spinelli GP, Miele E, Tomao F, Tomao S: Albumin-bound formulation of paclitaxel (Abraxane® ABI-007) in the treatment of breast cancer. *Int J Nanomedicine* **4**:99–105, 2009.

Nakazawa G, Ladich E, Finn AV, Virmani R: Pathophysiology of vascular healing and stent mediated arterial injury. *Euro Intervention* **Suppl C**:C7–10, 2008.

National Institute on Drug Abuse: Opioid overdose crisis, Jan 2019. https://www.drugabuse.gov/drugs-abuse/opioids/opioid-overdose-crisis.

Partida RA, Yeh RW: Contemporary drug-eluting stent platforms: Design, safety, and clinical efficacy. *Interv Cardiol Clin* **5**: 331–347, 2016.

Paternostre M: Molecular origin of the self-assembly of lanreotide into nanotubes: A mutational approach. *Biophys J* **94**:1782–1795, 2008.

Pires A, Fortuna A, Alves G, Falcão A: Intranasal drug delivery: How, why and what for? *J Pharm Pharm Sci* **12**(3):288–311, 2009.

Rahman Z, Barakh Ali SF, Ozkan T, Charoo NA, Reddy IK, Khan MA: Additive manufacturing with 3D printing: Progress from bench to bedside. *AAPS J* **20**:101, 2018.

Rahman Z, Charoo NA, Kuttolamadom M, Asadi, Khan MA: Printing of personalized medication using binder jetting 3D printer. In Faintuch J, Faintuch S (eds). *Precision Medicine for Investigators, Practitioners and Providers.* Elsevier Science, 2019, pp 473–481.

Rahman Z, Siddiqui A, Bykadi S, Khan MA: Determination of tacrolimus crystalline fraction in the commercial immediate release amorphous solid dispersion products by a standardized X-ray powder diffraction method with chemometrics. *Int J Pharm* **475**:462–470, 2014.

Rahman Z, Yang Y, Korang-Yeboah M, et al: Assessing impact of formulation and process variables on in-vitro performance of directly compressed abuse deterrent formulations. *Int J Pharm* **502**:138–150, 2016.

Ritschel WA: Microemulsion technology in the reformulation of cyclosporine: The reason behind the pharmacokinetic properties of Neoral. *Clin Transplant* **10**:364–373, 1996.

Stewart SA, Domínguez-Robles J, Donnelly RF, Larrañeta E: Implantable polymeric drug delivery devices: Classification, manufacture, materials, and clinical applications. *Polymers (Basel)* **10**: 1–24, 2018.

Tyner KM, Zheng N, Choi S, et al: How Has CDER prepared for the nano revolution? Review of risk assessment, regulatory research, and guidance activities. *AAPS J* **19**:1071–1083, 2017.

Valéry C, Pouget E, Pandit A, et al: Passive transdermal systems whitepaper incorporating current chemistry, manufacturing and controls (CMC) development principles. *AAPS PharmSciTech.* **13**:218–230, 2012.

Van Buskirk, G.A., Arsulowicz, D., Basu, P. et al. Passive Transdermal Systems Whitepaper Incorporating Current Chemistry, Manufacturing and Controls (CMC) Development Principles. *AAPS PharmSciTech* **13**, 218–230 (2012). https://doi.org/10.1208/s12249-011-9740-9

Ventola CL: Medical applications for 3D Printing: Current and projected uses. PT **39**:704–711, 2014.

Wieder DR, Pattimakiel L: Examining the efficacy, safety, and patient acceptability of the combined contraceptive vaginal ring (NuvaRing®). *Int J Womens Health* **2**:401–409, 2010.

Wokovich AM, Prodduturi S, Doub WH, Hussain AS, Buhse LF: Transdermal drug delivery system (TDDS) adhesion as a critical safety, efficacy and quality attribute. *Eur J Pharm Biopharm* **64**:1–8, 2006.

Xu X, Siddiqui A, Srinivasan C, et al: Evaluation of abuse-deterrent characteristics of tablets prepared via hot-melt extrusion. *AAPS PharmSciTech* **20**:230, 2019.

Zhong H, Chan G, Hu Y, Hu H, Ouyang D: A comprehensive map of FDA-approved pharmaceutical products. *Pharmaceutics* **10**:E263, 2018.

Zou P, Tyner K, Raw A, Lee S: Physicochemical characterization of iron carbohydrate colloid drug products. *AAPS J* **19**: 1359–1376, 2017.

# 29

# Clinical Development and Therapeutic Equivalence of Generic Drugs and Biosimilar Products

Murray P. Ducharme, and Deniz Ozdin

## CHAPTER OBJECTIVES

- Explain the concepts of interchangeability and bioequivalence for generic drug products in the United States, Canada, and Europe.

- Explain why a generic drug product evaluated to be therapeutically equivalent and interchangeable in one region may not be a therapeutic equivalent in another region.

- Describe what "branded generics" are and why they are more prevalent in developing countries.

- Define the differences between products classified as "AA" versus "AB" in the FDA Orange Book.

- Explain the differences between bioequivalence and a single PK equivalence study.

- List the requirements for clinical generic drug product development for the United States, European, and Canadian markets.

- Define the term biosimilar.

- List the main differences associated with the clinical development of a biosimilar versus that of a generic drug product.

- Describe what are called "locally-acting" drug products by regulators, and explain what particular challenges are associated with their clinical development from a bioequivalence point of view.

## INTRODUCTION

The clinical drug development process involves the scientific investigation of the safety and efficacy of drug products that may receive marketing approval by a regulatory agency. The United States (US), European, and Canadian regulatory agencies are responsible for the US, European, and Canadian drug market. Three highly regulated regions will be the focus of this chapter in terms of generic clinical drug development, and the following (Chapter 30) for new drug clinical development. These agencies regulate the needs in terms of scientific/research testing and minimum equivalence requirements, compliance, and audit. The study requirements for a generic product are much abridged versus those of a new entity because they will rely on the previous safety and effectiveness declaration associated with the latter, so most if not all animal and clinical studies will not need to be repeated. Because of this, generic application/submissions include the term "abbreviated" in the US (Abbreviated New Drug Application [ANDA]) and Canada (Abbreviated New Drug Submission [ANDS]). At the core of generic submissions, the "test" or generic product will need to be shown to be pharmaceutically equivalent (see Chapter 26) and therapeutically equivalent to the marketed "reference" product in the country or region where the generic product will be made available. The establishment of clinical therapeutic equivalence (TE) or bioequivalence (BE) is the focus of this chapter. In general requirements will include both *in vitro* dissolution and *in vivo* PK equivalence studies between the proposed generic and its associated marketed reference product. Once approved and declared to be bioequivalent and interchangeable by the regulators, a generic drug product will be able to be substituted to its associated marketed reference product by the pharmacist, because of its established equivalent safety and efficacy.

In this chapter, the regulatory pathways, scientific policies, and requirements for generic drug products in terms of clinical studies[1] will be explored between the US, Canada, and the European Union (EU) for the clinician. Equivalence metrics between generic drug products (ie, "test" products), and marketed reference products will be explained from a clinical pharmacology perspective. The rationale and methods utilized for the demonstration of BE, and the criteria for interpretation of results will also be discussed. The context of BE assessment for what regulators commonly call "locally-acting" drug products will also be described and explained. The future importance of declaring a unique reference product will be also touched upon to ensure cost- and time-effective generic drug development for the global market.

Some of the information presented in this chapter is a duplication of what has already been discussed in Chapter 8, which focused on *in vivo* drug product performance but only from a US FDA regulatory point of view. Chapter 8 also introduced some *in vitro* dissolution requirements as well as information regarding the Biopharmaceutics Classification System (BCS) and the potential clinical waivers that can be filed. These topics will not be discussed in the current chapter. We will focus on the scientific aspects of clinical equivalence requirements, and present the similarities and differences in the regulatory interpretations of these from not only a US FDA point of view, but also for Health Canada (HC), and the European Medicines Agency (EMA). The reader will notice throughout this and the following chapter that certain concepts, terms, definitions, and approaches may be slightly different between how they are presented regulatory versus scientifically. In addition, the US, EU, and Canadian regulatory agencies may also define or use terms differently between them. Regulatory requirements follow the ever-changing world of science, sometimes with a lag time, explaining in part

some of the different positions. In addition, scientific facts and findings are often not interpretable in a pure "black or white" fashion but instead via different levels of grey. The purpose of this chapter, and the following, is not to criticize any of the US, EU, or Canadian requirements when they are different between them, or with the current level of science as the authors understand and are presenting them. The reader will be informed how scientific facts and findings can be interpreted slightly differently by regulatory scientists, and how certain requirements can be different between agencies while still be reasonable and defendable from a scientific point of view.

## BIOEQUIVALENCE

A generic product is expected to show similar efficacy and safety, and to be available in the same formulation types and strengths as the reference product to which it is BE. The patient should not feel or experience any difference, and the safety and efficacy of their treatment should not be changed whether they are using a generic or the reference product. Although pharmacy laws are different from state to state and from one country to the next, this general consideration of what should be a BE product for a pharmacist is constant. In contrast, BE is not defined in the same manner by the US, Canadian, and European regulatory agencies.

For the FDA, BE is defined in the Code of Federal Regulations (CFR) as "significant difference in the rate and extent to which the active ingredient or active moiety in pharmaceutical equivalents or pharmaceutical alternatives becomes available at the site of drug action when administered at the same molar dose under similar conditions in an appropriately designed study." (US FDA, CDER, 2019). This definition signifies that two products will be bioequivalent if they are pharmaceutical equivalents or alternatives, and if they result in the same concentration time profiles at the site of drug action when administered at the same molar dose. This definition is based on the principle of clinical pharmacology that a given effect is directly related to the concentration of the active ingredient or moiety at the site of activity. This is a scientifically

---

[1]This chapter defines "clinical studies" as any studies that have to be conducted with human subjects.

correct definition that specifies that what is important for safety and efficacy are the concentration time profiles at the site(s) of activity(ies) wherever it is (they are) in the body. In most circumstances, we cannot study concentrations at the site(s) of activity between a generic and its corresponding reference product, and instead, systemic exposures are compared. We will explain later why this is appropriate and in which circumstances this should ensure that concentrations at the site of activity will be equivalent.

HC defines BE as a "high degree of similarity in the bioavailabilities of two pharmaceutical products (of the same active ingredient) from the same molar dose, that is unlikely to produce clinically relevant differences in therapeutic effects, or adverse effects, or both" (Health Canada, 2018a). This definition is slightly different in that it refers to bioavailability, which scientifically refers to systemic exposure, not necessarily exposure at the site of activity.

The EMA states that two medicinal products are bioequivalent if they are "PE or pharmaceutical alternatives, and if their bioavailabilities after administration in the same molar dose are similar to such degree that their effect, with respect to both efficacy and safety, will be essentially the same" (EMA, 2000). This definition is similar to that of HC and would suggest that BE is always equivalent to a systemic PK study.

These three regulatory agencies define BE in a slightly different manner. Some make it clear that only PE products can be bioequivalent between each other, some focus on the comparability of the "bioavailability" of two drug products, suggesting that comparison of systemic exposure is the ultimate endpoint, while the FDA, make it clear that what is important is the exposure of the active ingredient or moiety at the site of drug action. This last definition may be arguably the most appropriate because it links BE to the current major principle of clinical pharmacology (Chapter 22), that efficacy and safety are always related to concentrations of an active moiety at its site(s) of activity(ies). Hence, if two pharmaceutically equivalent products are associated with the same concentration time profile(s) at their site(s) of efficacy and safety, then they will automatically have the same safety and efficacy.

A confusing aspect is that BE is often thought to be just a systemic PK study, where you could then have two products that are not pharmaceutically equivalent "passing" a "BE" study. Therefore considered by some as being BE when they are not (as they are not pharmaceutically equivalent). You could also have the possibility of stating that two "locally-acting" products can be "BE" because of a systemic PK study that passed certain criteria, while they may not be equivalent locally at the site of action and therefore not be associated with the same efficacy.

In order to avoid these conflicting situations, it may be preferable to call the PK comparability studies *PK equivalence studies* instead of "BE studies," and reserve the term *bioequivalence* for regulators who have then verified that ALL criteria for bioequivalence are met and not just those of the comparability PK equivalence studies. In essence, the definition of BE becomes similar to how most scientists view BE, in that the term is used for products that have passed all criteria for equivalence and are substitutable to a reference product. In this regard, the following definition may be useful:

- *Bioequivalence* is the regulatory science of establishing that one product is/should be equivalent to another one in terms of clinical safety and efficacy. Two products that are bioequivalent to each other can be classified as being interchangeable by a regulatory agency because they will/should lead to the same efficacy and safety clinically.

- In its simplest form and for the easiest examples, *bioequivalence* will be established using *in vitro* data only for a product that is pharmaceutically equivalent to a reference marketed product. In the majority of cases, however, one or two equivalence pharmacokinetic (PK) study(ies) where two formulations of the same active ingredient are determined to have the same rate and extent of exposure ($C_{max}$ and $AUC_t$) in healthy volunteers will be needed. Sometimes bioequivalence will need to be established using both equivalence PK and clinical therapeutic equivalence studies.

This chapter will try to avoid calling an individual PK study needed to establish BE as a "BE study" and will call them "PK equivalence" studies. In order for a generic product to be considered bioequivalent and interchangeable with a reference product, it will need to be pharmaceutically equivalent and will need to have passed all the *in vivo* clinical equivalence study requirements that should ensure that it will be associated with the same clinical safety and efficacy.

---

**FREQUENTLY ASKED QUESTION**

▶ What is the relationship between bioequivalence and a PK equivalence or comparative bioavailability study?

---

## INTERCHANGEABILITY, SUBSTITUTION, AND SWITCHABILITY NOTIONS

In North America and other world regions, pharmacists are allowed by law to dispense to a patient a generic product instead of a prescribed innovator /reference product by the physician. Generic substitution is a pharmacy act. The generic product needs, to have been deemed to be *therapeutically equivalent* and *interchangeable* versus the innovator/reference product approved by the regulatory agency.

*Switchability* is, a medical act, in which the physician will modify the drug therapy but for the same therapeutic intent in a patient (also called *therapeutic substitution*). An antidepressant may be switched to another one, for example, in order to improve a patient's response to therapy and/or decrease the likelihood of experiencing side effects. An antibiotic IV treatment can also be switched to an oral treatment after the patient mostly recovers from a severe infection (eg, signs and symptoms of the infection mostly disappear). For example, a patient taking medications at home and having to be urgently hospitalized, after a car accident, may have to be switched from their usual medication to an alternative one, simply because the hospital does not carry all medications that are available on the market. The list of medications that a hospital normally carries is called a *drug formulary*. There is no need for a hospital to carry all the different medications that are part of the same therapeutic class and having similar mechanism of actions. The *Pharmacy and Therapeutics* (P&T) committee in the hospital will decide which drug products will be carried in the institution formulary.

In a hospital setting, the physician can allow other health professionals to "switch" one product for another on his behalf. This act will be described and detailed in a document by the P&T committee. For example, the P&T committee and therefore the physicians of the hospital may allow the pharmacist to "switch" the biologics of a certain class to the only one of these that is carried by the institution.

## DOCUMENTATION SHOWING ESTABLISHMENT OF BIOEQUIVALENCE AND INTERCHANGEABILITY OF GENERIC PRODUCTS

Once a drug product has been considered BE and interchangeable with the reference drug product by the regulatory agency responsible for its market authorization, a pharmacist will be able to substitute the generic drug product for the reference drug product.

In the US, the FDA publishes the Orange Book (which lists all of the US-marketed drug products along with their therapeutic equivalence designations). The Orange Book also defines bioequivalence, therapeutic equivalence, and pharmaceutical equivalence, albeit from a US regulatory perspective. As per the Orange Book, generic drug products are therefore considered to be therapeutic equivalents in the US if they meet the following general criteria:

- They are safe and effective
- They are bioequivalent
- They are pharmaceutical equivalent
- They are adequately labeled
- They are manufactured in compliance with current Good Manufacturing Practice (cGMP) regulations.

The electronically available version on the internet of the Orange Book (http://www.accessdata.fda .gov/scripts/cder/ob/index.cfm) and a mobile app for Apple and Android devices provides critical information for the pharmacist to have up-to-date information on generic and reference drug products. The Orange Book uses the following terminology to classify the therapeutic equivalence evaluations of drug products commercialized in the US:

- The *Reference Listed Drug* (RLD) is the drug identified by FDA as the drug product upon which an applicant relies in seeking approval of its generic application (ie, ANDA, as we will see later on).
- A *Reference Standard* (RS) is the drug product selected by the FDA that an applicant must use for conducting its equivalence studies (eg, *in vitro*, PK, clinical). The RS is normally the RLD, but sometimes they may be different due to market availability. Should the RLD disappear from the market, for example, then the generic product with the largest market share usually (but not always) becomes the RS to which new generic drug products would need to be compared. When an RLD is marketed with different strengths, the FDA will list the strengths that they want applicants to use for the equivalence studies as RS.
- Drug products classified as "AB" are designated to be bioequivalent and interchangeable to the RS and the RLD by the FDA. Should there be more than one RS and RLD on the market (for example, levothyroxine), a number will be added at the end of AB (eg, AB1, AB2, etc.). All products designated as "AB1" will then be interchangeable between each other, but not with AB2 products unless designated as both "AB1, AB2."
- Drug products classified as BX and other letters starting with B (BC, BD, BE, etc) are not interchangeable with the RLD and RS. These are stand-alone products and should not be substituted to the reference product by the pharmacist.
- Drug products classified as "AA" by the FDA are products that the agency considers to be therapeutically equivalent to others typically without the need for PK or clinical equivalence studies, just *in vitro* equivalence. Some products appear in this category, include a limited number of relatively old orally administered products that are immediate-release (IR) formulations. Examples are IR oral formulations of aspirin,

acetaminophen, caffeine, butalbital, codeine, hydrocodone, and oxycodone.

- Drug products classified starting with A, such as AN, AO, AP, or AT are other products for which the FDA considers that there are "no known or suspected BE problems." These are usually solutions. The second letter denotes the route of administration or the dosage form. For example, AN, AO, AP, or AT are solutions that are administered as nasal, ophthalmic, parenteral, or topical products, respectively.

Unfortunately, it is much more difficult for pharmacists in Canada and Europe to know which products are interchangeable between each other, as neither Canada nor Europe provides an equivalent to the Orange Book. The responsibility for declaring a product as interchangeable does not rest with the federal authority but that of the member state or province in Europe and Canada, respectively. In the example of Canada, this means that a product may be accepted as a generic product and declared interchangeable by HC, but a Canadian province may decide that it is not. The reverse is possible as well: HC may accept a stand-alone product (not a generic submission), but a province may decide that it will be the only product reimbursable and therefore artificially "force" interchangeability.

### FREQUENTLY ASKED QUESTIONS

▶ What is the Orange Book?

▶ Are marketed generic and innovator products always interchangeable between each other?

### EXAMPLE ▷ ▷ ▷

A patient comes to the pharmacy with the following prescriptions and accepts to receive generic products when available.
  Prescription:

- Augmentin® 875 BID × 10 days
- Synthroid® 200 mcg die

The pharmacy carries generic products from Hikma and from Mylan. Can they be substituted to the products prescribed?

## Solution

From the Orange Book, the pharmacist will obtain the following information:

The Hickma amoxicillin/clavulanate generic product is rated "AB" versus Augmentin-875, and can be substituted to it. The Mylan levothyroxine sodium product is rated "AB1" and "AB2" (among others) versus Synthroid and can be substituted to it.

| | | | | | | | | | | |
|---|---|---|---|---|---|---|---|---|---|---|
| RX | AMOXICILLIN; CLAVULANATE POTASSIUM | AUGMENTIN '875' | N050720 | TABLET | ORAL | 875MG; EQ 125MG BASE | AB | RLD | | NEOPHARMA INC |
| RX | AMOXICILLIN; CLAVULANATE POTASSIUM | AMOXICILLIN AND CLAVULANATE POTASSIUM | A091568 | TABLET | ORAL | 875MG; EQ 125MG BASE | AB | | | AUROBINDO PHARMA LTD |
| RX | AMOXICILLIN; CLAVULANATE POTASSIUM | AMOXICILLIN AND CLAVULANATE POTASSIUM | A203824 | TABLET | ORAL | 875MG; EQ 125MG BASE | AB | | | HIKMA PHARMA-CEUTICALS |
| RX | AMOXICILLIN; CLAVULANATE POTASSIUM | AMOXICILLIN AND CLAVULANATE POTASSIUM | A204755 | TABLET | ORAL | 875MG; EQ 125MG BASE | AB | | | MICRO LABS LTD INDIA |
| RX | AMOXICILLIN; CLAVULANATE POTASSIUM | AMOXICILLIN AND CLAVULANATE POTASSIUM | A065063 | TABLET | ORAL | 875MG; EQ 125MG BASE | AB | | RS | SANDOZ INC |
| RX | AMOXICILLIN; CLAVULANATE POTASSIUM | AMOXICILLIN AND CLAVULANATE POTASSIUM | A065093 | TABLET | ORAL | 875MG; EQ 125MG BASE | AB | | | SANDOZ INC |
| RX | AMOXICILLIN; CLAVULANATE POTASSIUM | AMOXICILLIN AND CLAVULANATE POTASSIUM | A065096 | TABLET | ORAL | 875MG; EQ 125MG BASE | AB | | | TEVA PHARMA-CEUTICALS USA INC |
| RX | LEVOTHYROXINE SODIUM | EUTHYROX | N021292 | TABLET | ORAL | 0.2MG **See current Annual Edition, 1.8 Description of Special Situations, Levothyroxine Sodium | AB2 | | | PROVELL PHARMACEUTI-CALS LLC |
| RX | LEVOTHYROXINE SODIUM | LEVO-T | N021342 | TABLET | ORAL | 0.2MG **See current Annual Edition, 1.8 Description of Special Situations, Levothyroxine Sodium | AB1,AB2, AB3 | RLD | | CEDIPROF INC |
| RX | LEVOTHYROXINE SODIUM | LEVOTHYROXINE SODIUM | A209713 | TABLET | ORAL | 0.2MG **See current Annual Edition, 1.8 Description of Special Situations, Levothyroxine Sodium | AB1,AB2, AB3 | | | LUPIN ATLANTIS HOLDINGS SA |
| RX | LEVOTHYROXINE SODIUM | LEVOTHYROXINE SODIUM | A076187 | TABLET | ORAL | 0.2MG **See current Annual Edition, 1.8 Description of Special Situations, Levothyroxine Sodium | AB1,AB2, AB3,AB4 | | | MYLAN PHARMA-CEUTICALS INC |
| RX | LEVOTHYROXINE SODIUM | LEVOXYL | N021301 | TABLET | ORAL | 0.2MG **See current Annual Edition, 1.8 Description of Special Situations, Levothyroxine Sodium | AB1,AB3 | RLD | RS | KING PHAR-MACEUTICALS RESEARCH AND DEVELOPMENT LLC |
| RX | LEVOTHYROXINE SODIUM | SYNTHROID | N021402 | TABLET | ORAL | 0.2MG **See current Annual Edition, 1.8 Description of Special Situations, Levothyroxine Sodium | AB1,AB2 | RLD | | ABBVIE INC |
| RX | LEVOTHYROXINE SODIUM | THYRO-TABS | N021116 | TABLET | ORAL | 0.2MG **See current Annual Edition, 1.8 Description of Special Situations, Levothyroxine Sodium | AB2,AB4 | RLD | | ALVOGEN GROUP HOLDINGS 4 LLC |
| RX | LEVOTHYROXINE SODIUM | UNITHROID | N021210 | TABLET | ORAL | 0.2MG **See current Annual Edition, 1.8 Description of Special Situations, Levothyroxine Sodium | AB1,AB2, AB3 | RLD | | JEROME STEVENS PHARMACEUTI-CALS INC |

## APPROVAL OF GENERIC PRODUCTS

A generic product can only appear on the market if it does not infringe on patents, or if patents have expired, and if data and/or market exclusivity have elapsed.

*Patent protection* generally lasts 20 years from the date on which the application for the patent was filed for a specific country or region. Reference drug products are usually covered by multiple patents that are individually filed over many different years. In the US, the FDA publishes the patent information related to each reference product in the Orange Book. A generic product cannot be marketed in the US until all patents have expired, except if the remaining patent(s) are proven to be invalid or not infringed in court.

Regardless of whether the reference product is protected by patents or not, the regulatory agency will grant the reference holder a *marketing exclusivity* for its product after its approval. This marketing exclusivity is 5 years in the US, while it is currently 8 years in Canada and 10 years (eg, 8 years of data exclusivity plus 2 years of market exclusivity) in Europe. The market exclusivity is completely separated from patent protection, can be concurrent, and can therefore last longer or shorter than the patent(s) protection(s) (see Fig. 29-1).

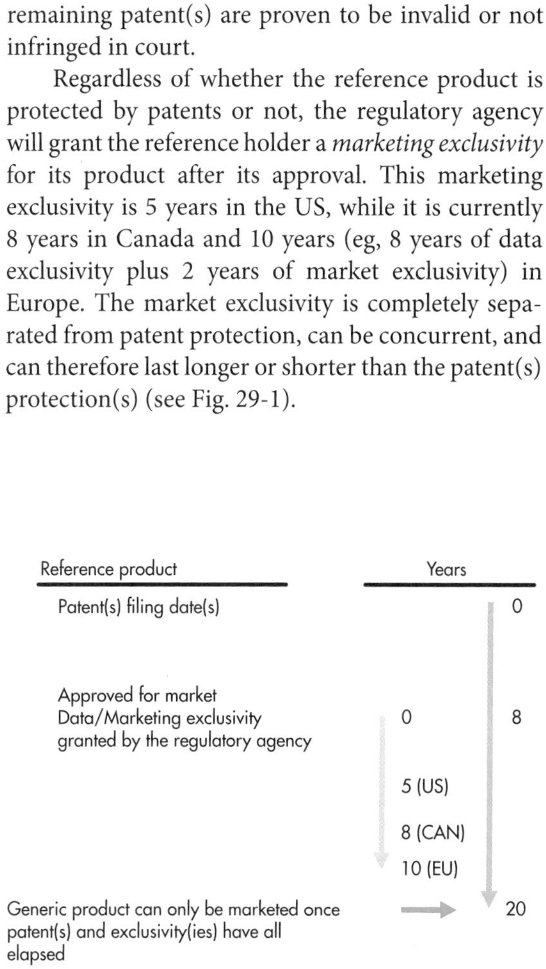

Additional market exclusivity can be given by the regulatory agency for:

- The approval of a supplemental indication necessitating the need for additional clinical trial(s) (3 years additional market exclusivity in the US)
- The approval of pediatric indication(s) after conducting pediatric clinical trials (6 months additional exclusivity in the US, Canada, and Europe)

## FILING OF GENERIC SUBMISSIONS IN THE UNITED STATES, CANADA, AND THE EUROPEAN UNION

The application pathways for the approval and marketing of generic drug products are described for the US, Canadian, and European regulatory agencies.

Section 505 of the Food, Drug, and Cosmetic Act (FD&C Act) of the US FDA addresses the submission of new and generic drugs. A *New Drug Application* (NDA) is submitted under the subsection 505(b) of the Act, while generic drugs are submitted as an *Abbreviated New Drug Application* (ANDA) under the subsection 505(j) of the Act. The statutory generic drug approval process under this subsection was introduced with the Drug Price Competition and Patent Term Restoration Act of 1984, commonly known as the *Hatch–Waxman Act*. With its passage into law, the majority of the costly animal and human studies required for innovator drugs did not need to be repeated for generic drug products based on the premise that the safety and efficacy of the innovator counterpart had already been established through animal and clinical Phase I–III studies. This act was also intended to maintain a balance between innovation and the availability of lower-priced generic drugs for the consumer by ensuring that (1) innovator drug manufacturers would have meaningful patent protection and a period of marketing exclusivity to enable them to recoup their investments in the development of new drugs, and (2) once the patent protection and marketing exclusivity for new drugs had expired, consumers would then benefit from the rapid availability of lower-priced generic versions of these innovator drugs.

| Reference product | Years |
| --- | --- |
| Patent(s) filing date(s) | 0 |
| Approved for market Data/Marketing exclusivity granted by the regulatory agency | 0    8 |
| | 5 (US) |
| | 8 (CAN) |
| | 10 (EU) |
| Generic product can only be marketed once patent(s) and exclusivity(ies) have all elapsed | 20 |

FIGURE 29-1 • Example illustrating how patent protection and data/market exclusivity dictate when generic product can reach the pharmaceutical market.

The timing of an ANDA approval depends partly on patent protections for the innovator drug. As per the FD&C Act, the ANDA applicant must submit one of four specified *paragraph certifications* regarding the patents listed in the Orange Book for the RLD upon which the generic is developed. This certification must state one of the following:

1. That the required patent information relating to such patent has not been filed

2. That such patent has expired

3. That the patent will expire on a particular date

4. That such patent is invalid or will not be infringed by the generic drug for which approval is being sought

Paragraph I or II certification permits the ANDA to be approved immediately, while paragraph III certification indicates that the ANDA may be approved when the patent expires. If an ANDA applicant wishes to seek approval of its ANDA before a listed patent for innovator drug has expired, the applicant must submit a paragraph IV certification to the US FDA by one of the followings:

1. Challenging the validity of one or more patents (eg, invalid or unenforceable)

2. Claiming that the patent would not be infringed upon by the generic drug product proposed in the ANDA

Paragraph IV certification has been very important for consumers and the generic industry in the US, as it has enabled faster availability of generic products that otherwise would have been delayed due to invalid patent protections. Important related items to the industry are the 6-month market exclusivity that the FDA grants as a financial reward to the first company that files a successful generic submission and paragraph IV certification, and the associated 30-month stay to the innovative company. The former is to reward the generic firm because the American public will gain quicker access to the generic product, while the latter is to, in part, allow time for the innovative company to prepare for court litigation. Unfortunately, this has apparently been an incentive for innovative companies to file patent(s) that they suspect may not be enforceable. This is simply because the generic introduction will be delayed by at least this 30-month stay (eg, it can be longer if it takes longer than 30 months to obtain the court decision) if an invalid patent has been filed versus not filed at all. This act of filing invalid or nonenforceable patents by the innovator industry has been called *evergreening* and has been a significant problem as it has been delaying generic competition unfairly and significantly over the last 30 years. Unfortunately, there is no reward in terms of generic exclusivity for a generic marketing holder for fighting a marketed reference product that would have invalid or nonenforceable patent(s) in Europe or Canada.

Approval and marketing authorization of drug products in Canada are regulated under Part C, Division 8, of the Canadian Food and Drug Regulations. Generic drugs are submitted as an ANDS pursuant to Section C.08.002.1. HC is more stringent regarding the identicality of the active pharmaceutical ingredient (API) than the US FDA which often accepts similarity. Certain generic applications in the US will have to be submitted as New Drug Submissions (NDS) in Canada because of the lack of identicality of the API between the test and reference products.

In the EU, new and generic applications are submitted in accordance with the Directive 2001/83/EC and Commission Regulations (EC) No 1084/2003 and 1085/2003. *Generic applications* in the EU are submitted under Article 10(1) of the Directive (EMA 2010; 2019). The EU is also usually more demanding in terms of pharmaceutical equivalence than the US FDA in regard to the API, like Canada. Most products where the API cannot be established as being identical will have to be filed as a *hybrid application* as per Article 10(3) of Directive 2001/83/EC. In addition, non-oral products necessitating a clinical equivalence study or given via alternative routes such as inhalers, and that could be filed as generics in Canada or US, will also be filed as hybrid applications in the EU.

---

## FREQUENTLY ASKED QUESTIONS

▶ What is particular about a generic submission filed with a paragraph IV certification to the US FDA?

▶ What may explain that some products are filed as generics in the US but as hybrid applications in the EU or as New Drug Submissions in Canada?

## THE DIFFERENT "GENERIC" TERMS

Generic drug products are sometimes associated with other names such as "branded generic," "authorized generic," "ultrageneric," "pseudogeneric," and "supergeneric." This last term is not associated with a "true" generic product but to one that represents an improvement over the reference product (eg, given less often, combination product) (Shah et al, 2015). As such, these are stand-alone products on the market and will be submitted as new drug applications or submissions (see Chapter 30). All the other above-specified names are associated with a true generic product, which is therapeutically equivalent to, and therefore substitutable with, its marketed reference product.

Generic drugs are usually marketed using the name of the active ingredient and are not given a proprietary brand name. Nevertheless, some generic drugs are given a brand name and are thus known as *branded generics*. Generics and branded generics have no difference in their quality and performance in highly regulated regions such as Europe, Canada, or the US. Branded generics used to be relatively common on the Canadian and US market many decades ago, but now they are very rare. Companies usually "brand" their generic products to indicate that they are of better or higher quality than other generics, but in Canada and the US, all generic drug products, whether they have a "brand" or not, have to be of the same high quality. So for the US and Canadian market, there is normally no need for a generic to have a "brand" name. In addition, in Canada and the US, branded generics may be confused with the reference drug product by healthcare professionals, and as such, branded generics have diminished greatly over the years to become almost nonexistent in the US and Canada. Branded generics are, however, very common in other countries, where many generics are of questionable quality. In many countries in South America, for example, generics can be put on the market without having to conduct a single PK equivalence study and with a minimal submission package. These generic products are often not comparable to the ones found in Europe, Canada, or the US, which are of equivalent high quality to the reference marketed products and which have been found to result in equivalent efficacy and safety.

A pharmaceutical company wanting to commercialize a high quality generic in these countries will often "brand" it, as to distinguish it from the other generics that are available on the market in terms of quality.

In the US, an *authorized generic* is a product that is made by the same company that markets the associated reference product but that licenses its commercialization, and sometimes manufacture, to a company that will sell it as a generic product (FDA Statement 2019; US FDA, CDER 2019). In that circumstance, the holder of the NDA will simultaneously make its product available as both the reference and as a generic product, although the latter will be marketed by another company. An authorized generic is submitted under 505(j) of the Act for approval in the US like all other generic products. In Canada, these authorized generics are sometimes referred to as *ultragenerics* or *pseudogenerics*. Given the name "ultrageneric," one could interpret it as a "better" or "superior" product to a generic, but it is not as it is subject to the exact same regulations as all other generic products, and so this naming should probably not be encouraged.

> **FREQUENTLY ASKED QUESTION**
>
> ▶ What is an "authorized generic"?

Table 29-1 summarizes the regulatory approval pathways for drug products using "generic" in their names.

## REGULATORY REQUIREMENTS FOR GENERIC SUBMISSIONS IN THE UNITED STATES, CANADA, AND EUROPE

All these regulatory agencies recognize generic products as being therapeutically equivalent and interchangeable with their respective marketed reference products. A generic drug product needs to be identical to its reference product in terms of:

- Pharmaceutical Equivalence (PE, see Chapter 26)
  - Identical (HC and EMA) or Identical/Highly Similar (FDA) active pharmaceutical ingredient (API)
  - Identical formulation type (except for EMA where almost all immediate release formulations are considered similar, eg, tablets and capsules are considered similar)

**TABLE 29-1 • Summary of Regulatory Approval Pathways for Drug Products Using "Generic" in Their Names**

| Application | Approved Product | Substitutability with Reference | FDA Term/Pathway (Regulation) | HC Term/Pathway (Regulation) | EMA Term/Pathway (Regulation) |
|---|---|---|---|---|---|
| New Drug | Innovator/ Reference product | — | NDA 505(b)(1)/ 505(b)(1) (FD&C Act) | NDS/ Section C.08.002 (FDR) | Full application/MAA[†]/ Article 8(3) (Directive 2001/83/EC) |
| | Super-generic | No | NDA 505(b)(1)or (b)(2)/ 505(b)(1) (FD&C Act) | NDS/ Section C.08.002 (FDR) | Hybrid application/ Article 10(3) (Directive 2001/83/EC) |
| Generic Drug | Generic | Yes | ANDA/ 505(j) (FD&C Act) | ANDS/ Section C.08.002.1 (FDR) | Generic application/ Article 10(1) (Directive 2001/83/EC) |
| | Generic products not meeting all requirements | Yes/No* | — | NDS/ Section C.08.002 (FDR) | Hybrid application/ Article 10(3) (Directive 2001/83/EC) |
| | Branded-generic | | Same as generic above | | |
| | Authorized generic[‡]/ Ultrageneric[§]/ Pseudogeneric[§] | | Same as generic above | | |

*Interchangeability is a provincial jurisdiction in Canada and a member state decision in the European Union (EU). Some products may be considered interchangeable in certain provinces in Canada and EU member states even though they were not approved as generic.
[†]MAA: Marketing Authorization Application
[‡]United States
[§]Canada

- Route of administration
- Strength
• Therapeutic Equivalence (efficacy and safety)
• Labeling

A list and a brief description of different terms related to generic applications and submissions to FDA, HC, and EMA is provided in Table 29-2.

One allowed difference between a test (either a generic or a new formulation of the reference product) and its reference product is the composition of the formulation, as excipients can often be qualitatively and quantitatively different. There are exceptions to this, such as for generic products of parenterally administered drug products like IV solutions and suspensions that are directly available ("immediate release"), and for which their formulation needs to be qualitatively (commonly referred to as "Q1"), and quantitatively ("Q2") similar to that of the reference marketed product. Q1/Q2 may not mean pure "identicality" for a regulatory agency, and the FDA, HC, and EMA have allowances for small differences that they have judged unlikely to result in any clinical differences. These were first proposed by the FDA when they elaborated their Scale-Up and Post Approval (SUPAC) guidances, and these rules have also been applied to "preapproval" changes and to generic products even though the guidances were originally not meant for this, simply because it made scientific sense to do so by regulators. For immediate-release (IR) solid oral formulations, the total additive effect of all excipient changes is allowed to be less than or equal to an absolute total of 5% (w/w) of the dosage form weight (Level 1 SUPAC) (US FDA, CDER, 1995). The same extent of changes is allowed for modified-release (MR) solid oral formulations, but only in their inactive ingredients that do not affect the release of drug substance from

**TABLE 29-2 •** Brief Comparison of Stated Regulatory Requirements between the US FDA, HC, and EMA for Generic Dossiers

| Terminology | US FDA | HC | EMA |
|---|---|---|---|
| Pharmaceutical equivalent* | A drug product with:<br><br>– **Identical** dosage form<br>– Identical route(s) of administration<br>– Identical amounts of the identical active drug ingredient(s)[1] | A drug product with:<br><br>– **Comparable** dosage form<br>– Identical route(s) of administration<br>– Identical amounts of the identical medicinal ingredient(s)[1] | A drug product with:<br><br>– **Identical** dosage form<br>– Identical route(s) of administration<br>– Identical amounts of the identical active substance(s)[1] |
| Pharmaceutical alternative* | A drug product with:<br><br>– Comparable dosage form (not necessarily the same dosage form)<br>– Identical therapeutic moiety[2], but not necessarily the same derivatives (eg, salt, ester, etc), and not necessarily in the same amount | No provision for pharmaceutical alternative in Canadian regulations[Ψ] | A drug product with:<br><br>– Comparable dosage form (not necessarily the same dosage form)<br>– Identical active moiety[2], but not necessarily the same derivatives (eg, salt, ester, etc), and not necessarily in the same amount |
| Identical active ingredient(s)* | The same therapeutic moiety in the same chemical form (ie, the same salt, ester, etc) | The same therapeutic moiety in the same chemical form (ie, the same salt, ester, etc) **in the final dosage form** | **Different** salts, esters, ethers, isomers, mixtures of isomers, complexes or derivatives of an active substance (as long as they do not significantly differ in safety and/or efficacy) |
| Reference product for generic submissions | Known as "Reference Listed Drug" (RLD)[3] (US-FDA, CDER, 2019):<br><br>– An innovator product[4] which is approved further to an NDA 505(b)(1)<br>– Another generic product if the innovator product is withdrawn | Known as "Canadian Reference Product" (CRP):<br><br>– Innovative drug[4] which is approved further to an NDS pursuant to Section C.08.002 of FDR (a drug with Notice of Compliance pursuant to C.08.004) and is marketed in Canada<br>– A drug, acceptable to minister, that can be used for the purpose of demonstrating BE when the innovator drugs is no longer marketed in Canada<br>– A foreign-sourced reference product provided that it meets certain criteria for acceptance by the Minister for use as a CRP<br>– For detailed information please refer to the HC Guidance document (Health Canada, 2018c) | Known as "reference medicinal product" (EMA, 2019):<br><br>– An innovator product[4] which has been granted a marketing authorization by a Member State or by the Commission under Article 8(3) of Directive 2001/83/EC |
| Allowable qualitative and quantitative differences in excipients | Oral IR formulations: ≤5% (w/w) of total weight of formulation<br>Oral MR formulations: ≤5% (w/w) of total weight of formulation only in nonrelease-controlling excipients | Oral IR formulations: ≤5% (w/w) of total weight of formulation<br>Oral MR formulations: ≤5% (w/w) of total weight of formulation only in nonrelease-controlling excipients | Oral IR formulations: ≤5% (w/w) of total weight of formulation<br>Oral MR formulations: **No change is allowed** |

formulations (non-release-controlling excipients) (US FDA, CDER, 1997).

Pre- and post-approval allowances are relatively similar between HC or EMA, and FDA for IR products. Minor changes in the composition of generic products are allowed (Health Canada, 1996). Changes in excipients that are not designed to play a role in the drug release mechanism or absorption characteristics such as the color or flavoring agents are generally considered "minor." In addition, the total additive effect of all excipient changes less than or equal to an absolute total of 5% (w/w) of an IR solid oral dosage form weight is considered as a minor change. In Canada, the same extent of changes is allowed for MR solid oral formulations, except for release-controlling excipients, but in contrast, the EMA does not allow any changes for MR products (EMA, 2010).

As stated previously, one difference between the FDA and HC/EMA is in the need for identicality of the API. The US FDA's regulations define pharmaceutical equivalents as drug products, which are of the identical dosage form and route of administration containing identical (same) amounts of the identical active drug ingredient (ie, the same salt or ester of the same therapeutic moiety) (US FDA, CDER, 2019). Under the US FDA's regulations, a drug product which contains the same active moiety as its reference product but differs in chemical form (salt, ester, etc) of that moiety, or two drug products in comparable dosage forms (eg, tablet and capsule), would not be considered PE, and therefore would not be eligible for a generic application. In practice, however, the US FDA will tolerate and allow some differences in the active drug ingredient and relies on "similarity" rather than "identicality" (or "sameness") as long as the difference does not influence the clinical effect and safety profiles. For instance, companies can file generic applications of intravenous formulations of iron with different carbohydrate coatings (eg, dextran, gluconate, or sucrose) in the US, as the FDA will accept similarity in terms of these APIs after extensive specific testing mentioned in these iron individual BE guidances (US FDA, CDER, 2012a; 2013; 2016). In contrast, HC and EMA will not accept generic applications for these iron products because true identicality is not possible, and companies will have to file NDS and hybrid applications, respectively.

## CLINICAL PHARMACOLOGY BASIS LINKING PK EQUIVALENCE STUDIES WITH PRESUMED EQUIVALENT SAFETY AND EFFICACY

A fundamental principle of clinical pharmacology is that the efficacy and safety of an active ingredient are directly related to its exposure at its site(s) of activity. A site of activity is commonly called *biophase*, and its exact location is often unknown and theoretical. The PD relationship between exposure at one theoretical site of action and efficacy or safety is often depicted by an $E_{max}$ curve as shown in Fig. 29-2.

Because of this relationship between concentrations at the biophase and effect (PD), if two formulations of the same API result in the exact same concentrations at the biophase(s), then they will have the same efficacy and safety.

Following the oral administration of most drug products, the active ingredient will start reaching the systemic circulation before or at the same time as it starts reaching its intended site(s) of activity. Under this important assumption, if the PK profiles in the systemic circulation are the same between a generic and the reference product, then they will also have the same exposure at the biophase, because this transfer to the biophase is drug specific and not formulation specific. Hence, they will have the same safety and efficacy. This is highlighted in Fig. 29-3.

Fig. 29-3 shows that the only difference that can exist between a generic formulation and a reference formulation of the same API is in the *formulation*.

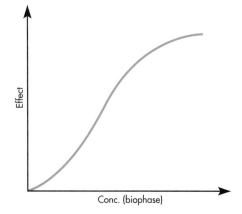

FIGURE 29-2 • Theoretical relationship between the exposure of a drug at the site of action and its effect.

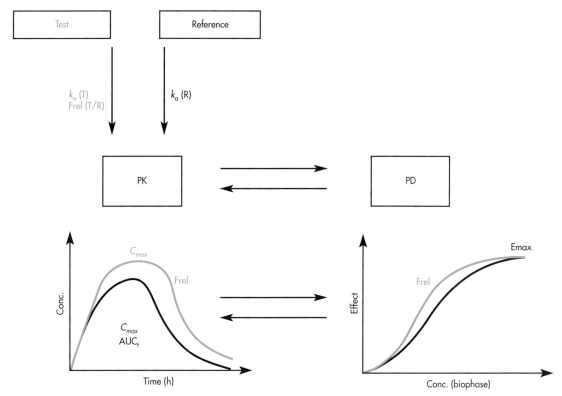

FIGURE 29-3 • PK-PD relationships between a test (blue) and a reference formulation (Ref, in black) when they have different PK profiles within the systemic circulation.

PK parameters that are drug specific ($CL$, $V_{ss}$) will not change between the two products, only those that are formulation specific will ($k_a$, $F$). This explains the old saying that PK "bioequivalence" studies aim at distinguishing the "rate and extent of absorption" of two formulations of the same API. It is preferable nowadays to refer to this as "rate and extent of systemic exposure" or "rate and extent of bioavailability" because absorption ($F_a$), as we have seen in previous chapters, is only one component of bioavailability ($F$), and what we look at in these studies is the difference in systemic exposure, therefore bioavailability, not just absorption.

A bioequivalent generic formulation demonstrates an equivalent systemic exposure profile as that of the reference product. This will ensure equivalent concentrations later on at the site(s) of activity(ies), as the movement of the drug from the systemic circulation to a biophase is drug and not formulation specific, and will therefore ensure that the generic product has equivalent safety and efficacy with the reference product.

What is important in a PK equivalence study is to ensure that the PK profiles between the generic and reference products are equivalent. The maximum exposure ($C_{max}$), and the extent of exposure (AUC), are important metrics for equivalence, for the simple reason that it would be very unlikely for two different formulations of the same API to have a different PK profile if the $C_{max}$ and AUC would be equivalent (because all systemic PK characteristics would be identical). Figure 29-4 illustrates three different scenarios between test and reference formulations, where differences can be seen in the absorption rate constant (panel A), in the relative bioavailability (panel B), or both (panel C). In all cases, the "systemic" PK parameters are constant between the two formulations, and so the terminal elimination phase is similar for all three cases.

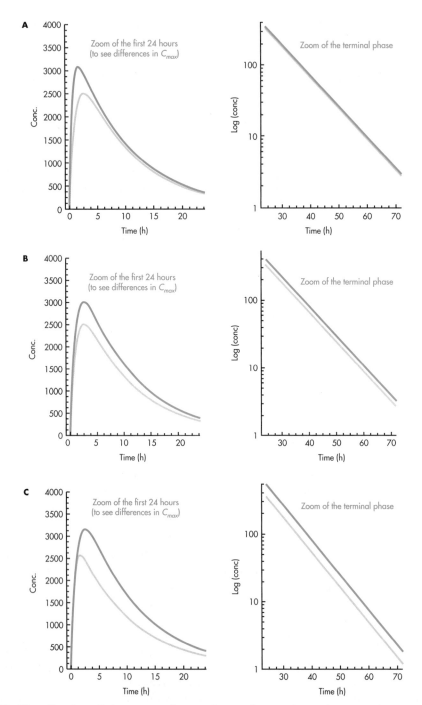

**FIGURE 29-4** • The PK profiles of two IR pharmaceutically equivalent products can be simply compared in terms of $C_{max}$ and AUC because they possess an identical API and thus their systemic PK behavior will be identical while their rate and extent of absorption/exposure ($C_{max}$ and AUC) can be different. Panel A represents a test (in blue) formulation that has only a 20% higher rate of absorption (ie, $C_{max}$ is 20% greater, $T_{max}$ is earlier, and AUC is similar). Panel B shows a test formulation (in blue) that has only a 20% greater bioavailability (ie, $C_{max}$ and AUC are greater by 20% and $T_{max}$ is similar). Panel C illustrates a test formulation (in blue) that has a greater than 30% relative bioavailability (AUC) but with a slower rate of absorption ($T_{max}$ is later).

While similarity of both AUC and $C_{max}$ will result in an overall similar PK profile for IR pharmaceutically equivalent products, this may not suffice in terms of comparison for modified-release products. To illustrate this, we can consider the example of a transdermal product administered once a week versus administering the same API daily orally for 7 days. The two different products could have an overall weekly similar $C_{max}$ and AUC, but the PK profiles for each product may be different leading to safety and efficacy that may greatly vary on a daily basis. To better compare PK profiles, partial AUCs can be used to compare drug exposure after the administration of transdermal, long acting injectables and certain oral MR drug products, such as Concerta (methylphenidate HCI) ER Tablets (Chapter 8). US FDA proposes different metrics for PK equivalence for these types of products in their individual product BE guidances. These metrics are for now only specified in these "product-specific" guidances, the main disadvantage of this being that it is almost impossible for a company developing a new product to predict correctly what the FDA additional metrics may be until a guidance actually becomes available for it. In contrast, the EMA has an overarching BE guideline for MR products, a preferable situation, that either adds the requirement for an additional PK equivalence study to be done at steady state (ie, if there is accumulation potential of more than 10%), or for the single-dose study to pass on two additional partial AUCs (eg, $AUC_{0-midpoint}$ and $AUC_{midpoint-t}$).

### FREQUENTLY ASKED QUESTION

▶ What is the fundamental principle of clinical pharmacology that ensures that an approved interchangeable generic product, based on one or more PK equivalence studies, should have the same efficacy and safety as the reference product?

## STATISTICAL EVALUATION OF BIOEQUIVALENCE METRICS

The preceding section explained how two pharmaceutically equivalent formulations of an identical API will have equivalent clinical safety and efficacy if their systemic PK profiles in humans are similar,

using specific PK metrics, if the API reaches the systemic circulation at the same time or before it reaches its various sites of activity. The current section specifies how these PK metrics are to be shown to be statistically equivalent. Rather than comparing them from a statistical difference viewpoint, statistical clinical equivalence limits of ±20% have been proposed now for many decades. Two PK profiles will typically be determined to be equivalent if the 90% confidence intervals (CI) all of their pivotal PK metrics (eg, minimally $C_{max}$ and $AUC_{0-t}$) are completely within ±20% of the reference product.

### The ±20% Clinical Equivalence Boundary

Asked about what percentage difference in systemic exposure (eg, AUC, $C_{max}$) would lead to a clinical difference prompting the adjustment of dosing regimens, most physicians and pharmacists will argue that nothing less than a doubling or a decrease in half of the systemic exposure will warrant dosing adjustment. Even the most conservative clinician will consider a drug-drug interaction to be clinically relevant only if it results in a ±40% difference in exposure. If ±40% is the minimum difference that would lead to a dosing adjustment clinically, then exposure metrics that are similar at ±20% should ensure clinical equivalence.

### The "Average BE" Approach and the Two-One Sided T-Tests Procedure

The common BE statistical evaluation method is based on the *Two One-Sided T-Tests (TOST) procedure*, developed by the FDA scientist Don Schuirmann in 1987. The TOST procedure resolved issues related to other methods that were used at the time, including the 75/75 rule, power approach, and/or the Hauck–Anderson t-test (Schuirmann, 1987). Since 1992, FDA has recommended that statistical analyses for PK metrics be based on the TOST procedure to determine whether average values selected for the PK metrics of test and reference products are comparable. This method assesses the difference between Test and Ref means, but not their difference in terms of variability. This approach is termed *average BE (ABE)*, and is currently the most common method used for the evaluation of BE worldwide.

The TOST procedure consists of decomposing the interval null hypotheses $H_0$ into two sets of one-sided hypotheses and applying two separate t-tests, in which the null hypothesis, $H_0$, states that test and reference are not equivalent. Alternatively, the hypothesis, $H_1$, states that they are equivalent. Therefore, equivalence of the test and reference can be concluded if and only if the null hypothesis is rejected at a chosen level of significance. By convention, all BE data are expressed as Test to Reference geometric mean ratios for the PK parameters of interest (AUC and $C_{max}$), a statistical significant difference is defined as ±20% change. An absence of a clinical significant difference is defined as less than a +/-20% change on the ln scale, as PK parameters are ln normally distributed. When exponentiated back on the normal scale, the BE limits become 80.0%–125.0% for the 90% confidence intervals (CIs) of all pivotal PK metrics. Because all 90% CIs must be entirely within the 80.0% to 125.0% limits, and each mean of the study data lies in the center of the 90% CI on the logarithmic scale, each geometric mean ratio (ie, the arithmetic mean of the ln-transformed data that has been back exponentiated) of the test to reference (on the normal scale) is usually close to 100% (a test to reference ratio of 1), otherwise, the study sample size would need to be much too large. This is the underlying reason why the TOST procedure normally assures that the actual difference between the reference and the generic product remains small (Kanfer and Shargel, 2007). A 90% CI is used as it allows a statistical α error of 5% at both the lower and upper BE limits. In other words, the 90% CI encompasses the two one-sided tests, each carried out at α = 0.05, which means the maximum probability of incorrectly concluding bioequivalence is 5%. Using this acceptance criteria, it would be difficult for any generic product whose arithmetic mean $C_{max}$ and AUC differ by more than 10% from the reference to meet the CI requirements (Kanfer and Shargel, 2007). The performance of the two one-sided tests for BE assessment was evaluated by Davit et al (2009) through the review of a total of over 2070 single-dose BE studies of orally administered generic drug products approved by the FDA from 1996 to 2007. The mean ± SD of the GMRs from the 2070 studies was 1.00 ± 0.06 for $C_{max}$, and 1.00 ± 0.04 for AUC. It was concluded that while the statistical test analyzed BE from the confidence limits of 80–125%, the actual difference between test

and reference drugs was usually much smaller. This result is due to the fact that the 90% CI for both PK parameters, $C_{max}$ and AUC, must be entirely within the 80%–125% limits. Since the mean of the study data lies in the center of 90% CI in logarithmic scale, the geometric mean ratio of the test to reference (on the normal scale) products is usually close to 100% (a test-to-reference ratio of 1).

A common criticism of generic products is that because they are approved at ±20%, then two generic products may therefore be theoretically ±40% from each other. This is not a valid criticism. Generic products are typically approved with PK equivalence studies indicating a geometric mean ratio difference of less than 5%, otherwise, they would not pass the 90% CI limits of ±20%. In addition, the bioequivalence requirements are the same, for both generic or innovator products. Innovator products are often approved following many formulation or manufacturing changes. The innovator product has to be approved with the same BE requirements versus the previous product that was actually used in the pivotal Phase III studies. If the requirements are stringent enough for the innovator, then they should also be the same for the generic manufacturer (see Fig. 29-5)

The statistical precision depends on the intrasubject variability in the PK metrics of the two products, and on the number of subjects in the study. The width of the 90% CI is proportional to the estimated intrasubject variability of drug (for a crossover design) and inversely proportional to the number of subjects. A test product with no differences in the average response as compared to the reference may still fail to pass the BE criteria if the variability of one or both products is high, and/or if the BE study is not of sufficient statistical

• New Drug Submission
– Phase III pivotal studies (minimum of 2 well controlled, well conducted, successful studies per indication) typically done on one formulation
– BE assessed between the "to be marketed" formulation and the formulation that was used during the pivotal phase III trials

• Generic submission
– BE assessed between the "Reference" formulation and the proposed "Generic" formulation

SAME RULES

FIGURE 29-5 • PK equivalence or bioequivalence requirements are the same, and apply equally for a new drug (eg, innovator) or a generic product.

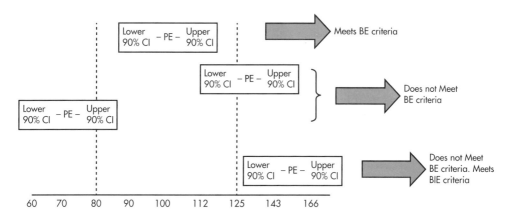

PE: point estimate for the GMR ratio Test/Ref; CI: Confidence interal; BE: Bioequivalence; BIE: Bioinequivalence

FIGURE 29-6 • Examples of PK equivalence study results, and whether or not BE criteria are met.

power (due to insufficient number of subjects). Different scenarios of test-to-reference geometric mean ratios and 90% CIs are presented in Fig. 29-6.

> ### FREQUENTLY ASKED QUESTION
>
> ▶ A common misunderstanding is that if generic products are approved with a ±20% difference to a reference product, then it may mean that two generic products could present a ±40% difference. Explain why this is unlikely to ever occur.

## PK EQUIVALENCE CLINICAL STUDY REQUIREMENTS FOR FDA, HC, AND EMA

Requirements for PK equivalence between generic and reference products have been constantly updated over the last 30 years, because regulatory requirements follow scientific advancements, and science always evolves with time. Despite considerable progress, many topics are still controversial to this day due to conflicting interpretations of what the scientific data suggests. This explains why regulatory agencies such as the FDA, HC, and the EMA are not always aligned in what they require. Interpretation of scientific data and evidence is not always clear. Each regulatory agency has their own scientific reasons and interpretations that help us understand why divergences exist.

### The Choice of the Reference Product

Generic products are approved for marketing in a specific country (eg, US, Canada) or region

(Europe). Regulators demand in the US, Canada, and Europe that every generic product be shown to be bioequivalent to a reference product specifically marketed in that country or region. This results in generic companies developing one generic product for the whole world pharmaceutical market at having to do multiple PK equivalence studies instead of just conducting one fasted and one fed PK equivalence studies for a "global" reference product for all the different countries. Most reference products are identical across countries, as innovative companies also develop products for the whole world pharmaceutical market. This means that generic companies must essentially "duplicate" research work that they have already done for many of the countries in which they wish to market. This results in wasted effort, energy, money, and time. Generic products would be globally more affordable if all these PK equivalence studies would not have to be duplicated unnecessarily. Hopefully in the future, major regulatory agencies will accept a "global" reference product so that all these research studies would not need to be needlessly repeated. The position of the regulatory agencies has been mostly that they do not know for certain that a reference product from one country is identical to the reference product from their own country. A counter-argument to this that is starting to gain traction is simply that most of the time the reference product official monograph or label are listing the exact same pivotal Phase III studies across the different countries. If a reference product from a manufacturer is listing the exact same pivotal efficacy Phase III studies to support its approval in two different countries, then automatically this reference product has to be bioequivalent between the two countries, because they each have to be bioequivalent to the product that was used in the Phase III studies before being approved.

## Main Study Designs for PK Equivalence Studies

Table 29-3 lists the main scientific criteria that need to be addressed in PK equivalence studies between generic and marketed reference products, and highlights some of the similarities and differences between FDA, HC, and EMA regulatory requirements. These requirements are current as of 2020

### TABLE 29-3 • Main Study Design Considerations in PK Equivalence Studies between FDA, HC, and EMA

| | US FDA | HC | EMA |
|---|---|---|---|
| Reference Marketed Product | From US market | From Canadian market Policy allows the use of a foreign reference product under certain circumstances | From EU market |
| Population to be studied | Male and female healthy volunteers preferred (if ethical and safe to do so). | | |
| PK after single-dose and/or steady- state administration | Single-dose conditions are required as they are thought to be more discriminative of formulation performances Steady-state studies are acceptable if single-dose studies cannot be conducted due to ethical and safety reasons (eg, drug product that can only be administered in patients and where treatment cannot be stopped) | | Although single-dose conditions are preferred, steady-state studies are required for certain products (MR leading to more than 10% accumulation in $AUC_{0\text{-}tau}$), and steady-state studies may sometimes replace the need for single dose studies |
| PK under fasting and/or fed conditions | Fasting and Fed conditions (except if label does not mention food at all) | Fasting for IR products Fasting and fed for MR and nonlinear PK drugs | |
| Length of fasting before dosing Volume of water administered with dosing | Min 10 hours fasting 240 mL | Min 10 hours fasting Min 150 mL | Min 8 hours fasting Min 150 mL |
| Population age range | 18 and older If drug is for elderly, should include as many >60 yo as possible | 18 to 55 yo | 18 to 55 or older |
| Strengths to be investigated | In general, the highest | In general, the highest For nonlinear PK drugs, the most discriminative strength should be studied For drugs with solubility issues, the lowest and highest should be studied | |

and can obviously change in the future as regulatory rules continue to evolve.

One large difference in these overall study requirements is that HC allows applicants to file a generic submission where a product has been compared to a non-Canadian Reference Product (CRP). This is called a Foreign Reference Product (FRP), and those marketed in the EU or US can qualify if the following criteria are met (Health Canada, 2018c):

- The FRP has been approved by a regulatory agency with similar criteria as that of HC.
- The FRP is marketed by the same innovator company or corporate entity as the CRP.
- The FRP is pharmaceutically equivalent to the CRP.
- The pharmaceutical ingredient of the CRP/FRP should not be a critical dose drug, and should not require patient monitoring in order to avoid consequences of under- or overtreatment.
- For solid oral and oral suspension IR products, the medicinal ingredient should have "high solubility," and the solid oral FRP and the CRP should have the same color, shape, size, weight, type of coating, and scoring configuration. The non-medicinal ingredients (excipients) should be qualitatively and quantitatively the same between the FRP and the CRP. The FRP and CRP should also pass equivalence dissolution tests.
- Additional criteria also exist for IR orally inhaled and nasal products.

Other notable differences are the need to conduct steady-state PK equivalence studies for EMA on almost any MR products, as most MR products result in a greater than 10% mean accumulation in AUC between the first dosing interval and the one obtained at steady state (eg, by design as they are MR products). This requirement has existed since 2013 when EMA published a draft update to their BE guidance regarding MR products (EMA, 2014). This change in requirements for steady-state studies illustrates how the traditional requirements of $C_{max}$ and AUC for IR after a single dose may not suffice for MR products. Steady-state studies were eliminated as requirements for establishing BE by HC and US FDA approximately 20 years ago, as they were thought to be less discriminative of formulation performance

than single-dose experiments. Since then, however, many "long-acting" MR products have appeared on the market, products that replace many different dosing intervals of IR products, and where one AUC and one $C_{max}$ metrics may not be enough to ensure profile comparability. This explains why EMA has decided to reintroduce the need for steady-state studies in certain circumstances, and why the FDA has been introducing partial AUCs as additional requirements for certain products in the last 10 years in individual product guidances.

One other major difference between these three regulatory agencies is the need to conduct fasted and fed PK equivalence studies for virtually all generic submissions to the FDA (eg, for products where the label discusses food effect, which is a requirement for new drug submissions), while HC and EMA are only asking for fasted studies for IR products, if they do not present nonlinear PK, or are not critical dose drugs.

### Main PK and Statistical Analyses for PK Equivalence Studies

Table 29-4 lists the regulatory requirements in terms of PK and statistical analyses for FDA, HC, and EMA.

Requirements are generally aligned, but some differences are notable. Firstly, HC does not require generic products to pass 90% CIs for $C_{max}$, and only the T/R geometric mean ratios have to be within 80.0 and 125.0%. The rationale for this was to avoid applicants having to conduct overly large studies to establish PK equivalence just because of a highly variable $C_{max}$, and the recognition that safety and efficacy of drugs are mostly related to AUC. Now that there are ways to ensure that highly variable drug products do not necessitate prohibitively large studies, we would argue that this may be a lack of requirement (90% CIs for $C_{max}$) that HC may want to revisit.

A second differentiator between the three regulatory agencies is the lack of guidance at the office of generic drugs of the FDA for nonlinear PK drugs. Both EMA and HC require applicants to conduct their PK equivalence studies on the most discriminative strengths. This means that in the example of Levodopa, a drug used to treat Parkinson disease and that is associated with saturation of its absorption process at high doses, PK equivalence studies should theoretically be conducted on the lowest strength, to

**TABLE 29-4 •** PK and Statistical Requirements for PK Equivalence Studies for FDA, HC, and EMA

| | US FDA | HC | EMA |
|---|---|---|---|
| Analytes to pass on | Parent drug, and active metabolite if formed pre-systemically (for confirmation of equivalence) | Parent drug only | Parent drug only |
| Power and alpha error | 80% power minimum and 5% alpha error maximum | | 80% or greater |
| Geometric mean T/R ratios and 90% CIs | $C_{max}$, $AUC_{0-t}$, and $AUC_{0-inf}$ 90% CIs within 80.0 and 125.0% | $AUC_{0-t}$ 90% CI within 80.0–125.0 $C_{max}$ T/R ratio between 80–125 (except CDD) | $C_{max}$, $AUC_{0-t}$, and $AUC_{inf}$ 90% CIs within 80.00 and 125.00% |
| $AUC_{0-t}/AUC_{inf}$ | 88% or greater | 80% or greater | 80% or greater |
| $K_{el}$ | >3–4 points | >4 points preferable | >3 points |
| Nonlinear PK drugs | | Fed study always required Strengths to pass on has to be discriminative If nonlinearity due to solubility issue, need to pass on lower and higher strengths | |
| Long elimination half-life drugs | $AUC_{0-72}$ allowed instead of $AUC_{0-t}$ and $AUC_{0-inf}$ if $T_{1/2}$ >12 hours | $AUC_{0-72}$ allowed instead of $AUC_{0-t}$ if $T_{1/2}$ >24 hours | $AUC_{0-72}$ allowed instead of $AUC_{0-t}$ and $AUC_{0-inf}$ |
| Critical dose drugs (CDD) | Products called "NTI" "Inverse" scaled ABE needed when intra-CV <22% with a 4-way fully replicated design and minimum of 24 subjects | 90% CI 90–112 for $AUC_{0-t}$ 90% CI 80–125 for $C_{max}$ Fed study always required | Products called "NTID" Some products have 90% CI of 90-111.1 for $AUC_{0-t}$ |
| Highly variable products (intra-CV >30%) | Scaled ABE possible with 3- or 4-way reference replicated designs | Scaling of the 90% CI dependent on the intra-CV of the reference product for $AUC_{0-t}$ until a maximum of 50% (EMA) or 57.4% (HC) | |
| Partial AUC requirements | For mixed IR/ER products, and mesalamine | For early-onset-of-action drugs, and for some multiphasic MR products | For "biphasic" drugs, where both "phases" have to be characterized |

ensure that the study is discriminative of formulation performance.

A third difference is the need to measure and present PK equivalence data for FDA of active metabolites that would have been formed "presystemically;" for example, in the gut wall where newly formed metabolites can undergo an absorption process of their own instead of being formed systemically within the liver after absorption is completed. This is an approach that is in line with the current scientific thinking of the important role of gut wall transporters and metabolism in the bioavailability of drugs, and should also be considered by other regulatory agencies.

All three regulatory agencies propose options for highly variable drug products, those that are associated with intra-CV (ie, the "within" subject CV) of 30% or greater in one or more PK parameters. Fifteen years ago, regular criteria were applied to these drug products and were preventing generic products from being approved on the market because PK equivalence studies were, for monetary reasons, either not conducted at all or were severely underpowered and were thereby failing criteria (Ducharme and Potvin, 2003). The US FDA was the first to propose enlarging criteria based on the variability of the reference product. Reference drug products are only approved for marketing after being established to be safe and effective, despite their within-subject variability. The 90% CI boundaries of ±20% become unecessarily stringent when PK parameters consistently change from one day to the next by more than ±30%. The FDA proposed the Scaled ABE (SABE) criteria, a mixed approach, which meant that PK parameters that were less than 30% variable had to be analyzed by typical ABE, while those that had 30% or greater CV could be analyzed by the SABE. All details concerning the SABE approach are officially listed in the Progesterone Individual BE guidance (US FDA, CDER, 2010a). There are two criteria to be met with the SABE:

- The T/R geometric mean ratio(s) still need(s) to be within 80.0 and 125.0%.
- The 95% upper bound(s) of $(Y_T-Y_R)^2 - \varphi S^2_{wr}$ need(s) to be negative.

The approach proposed by the FDA was welcomed by industry, and the first SABE was submitted in 2007. Applicants need to pre-specify in their protocol that the SABE approach may be used if the intra-CV for the reference product is 30% or greater for a PK parameter, and conduct their PK equivalence studies using either a three-way or a four-way reference replicated study design. The availability of this approach for highly variable drug products enabled the approval of generic versions of several reference products that would have otherwise not been possible (eg, some drug products have intra-CV of 100% or greater like those including mesalamine).

The SABE FDA approach was, however, criticized, most notably by Endrenyi (Endrenyi and Tothfalusi, 2009), as being discontinuous and associated with an enlargement of the alpha error above the 5% limit when the intra-CV% of the reference product is close to the 30% limit. This has been refuted as misunderstanding the approach by officials at FDA

(Schuirmann, 2008), but this criticism has led EMA and HC to propose completely different solutions for highly variable drug products:

- The EMA allows applicants to use an enlargement of the 90% CI up to a maximum of 69.84%–143.19% for a reference product having an intra-CV of 30% or greater, but for $C_{max}$ only (EMA, 2010). The geometric mean ratio still needs to be within 80.00% and 125.00%, though, which theoretically causes part of the discontinuity problem that the FDA was criticized for with their SABE approach. The downsides of the EMA approach are that it does not allow widening of the CI limits for AUC metrics, and that widening of the CI is allowed only until approximately ±30%.

- HC allows applicants to use an enlargement of the 90% CI up to a maximum of 66.7–150.0% for a reference product having an intra-CV of 57.4% or greater for AUC (Health Canada, 2016) (HC does not demand applicants to pass 90% CI for $C_{max}$). The geometric mean ratio still needs to be within 80.0% and 125.0%, also causing discontinuity issues. The enlargement of 90% CIs are not permitted for critical dose drugs, and are only allowed until a maximum of approximately ±35%.

There are many of "narrow therapeutic drugs" (NTD) on the market, with some being more critical than others in terms of their clinical monitoring and dosing requirements. The National Kidney Foundation and later the American Pharmaceutical Association (Alloway et al, 2000) proposed the use of the term "critical dose drugs" (CDD) to denote this special subgroup of NTD that are more "critical." HC was the first regulatory agency to propose tighter criteria for CDDs in a final guidance published in 2006. As of 2018, the list of HC considered CDDs included the following drugs: cyclosporine, digoxin, flecainide, lithium, phenytoin, sirolimus, tacrolimus, theophylline, and warfarin. The tighter equivalence requirements for products that contain these drugs (Health Canada, 2018b) include the necessity of always conducting a fed PK equivalence study, passing the 90% CI 80.0%–125.0% limits for $C_{max}$, and finally passing a restricted 90% CI for $AUC_t$ of 90.0%–112.0%

(approximately ±10%) due to the understanding that the safety and efficacy of drugs are mostly related to AUC.

The US FDA attempted to follow HC's recommendations and the Office of Generic Drugs, OGD proposed the same requirements to their advisory committee in 2010 (US FDA, CDER, 2010b). The committee suggested the term NTD. A subset of the NTDs are considered *critical dose drugs*, CDDs for which many physicians suggested needed for tighter criteria for PK equivalence. OGD later clarified their approach by focusing on the NTDs that have low intra-CV, such that the 90% equivalence limits would be tightened based on the variability of the reference product, in an analogous way to the highly variable drugs but in a "reverse" manner when the intra-CV would be approximately 21% or less. Products having an intra-CV of 5% and 10%, for example, would have to pass 90% CIs of approximately 95%–105% and 90%–111%, respectively. The exact requirements for these products are specified in the warfarin individual drug product guidance (US FDA, CDER, 2012b) and in the scientific literature (Jiang et al, 2015).

The EMA followed US FDA's path and uses the nonspecific term NTD except for the small modification of calling them NTID (for narrow therapeutic "index" drugs). In a similar manner to FDA, the EMA started posting individual product BE guidances on their website, and as of 2020 just a few products characterized as being NTID demand officially the tighter 90.00%–111.11% equivalence criteria for AUC: everolimus, sirolimus, and tacrolimus.

One area of major scientific interest in BE is the necessity of adding partial AUC requirements to the usual $C_{max}$ and AUC metrics to ensure that certain MR generic products have PK profiles equivalent to their reference products (Endrenyi and Tothfalusi, 2010). The US FDA was the first agency to propose additional partial AUC metrics to ensure that generic formulations of methylphenidate products such as Concerta (methylphenidate HCl). Concerta is composed of both IR (22% of the dose) and ER (78% of the dose) components. As such, one dose of Concerta aims at replacing three doses of methylphenidate IR given every 4 hours. Its PK profile

results in two different absorption peaks, one associated with the IR component providing efficacy over the first dosing interval of regular methylphenidate (4 hours), and an ER component ensuring efficacy over the other two dosing intervals. Methylphenidate almost immediate relationship between systemic exposure and activity is analogous to that of caffeine from coffee (eg, three coffees each taken separately by 4 hours will not be "felt" the same for a subject as taking three coffees simultaneously, even though the overall AUC will be identical). If less or more methylphenidate is provided in any one of these three dosing intervals of 4 hours that Concerta replaces, the patient may "feel" a difference between the generic and the reference product. Hence FDA currently demands throughout-the-day additional partial AUC metrics requirements for generic products of Concerta (ie, 0–3, 3–7, and 7–12 h under fasting conditions, and 0–4, 4–8, and 8–12 h under fed conditions) (US FDA, CDER, 2012c). EMA and HC also have special requirements for these types of products (EMA, 2014; Health Canada, 2017). The EMA guideline for MR products states that for "multiphasic MR products additional parameters to be determined include partial AUC, $C_{max}$, and $T_{max}$ in all phases. The time point for truncating the partial AUC should be based on the PK profile for the eg, IR and the MR parts respectively and should be justified and prespecified in the study protocol." For Concerta, for example, it could be separate $C_{max}$ and AUCs for both IR ($C_{max(0-4)}$, $AUC_{0-4}$) and ER components ($C_{max(4-t)}$, $AUC_{4-t}$) (see Fig. 29-7).

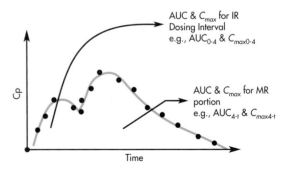

FIGURE 29-7 • The EMA guideline for "mixed" MR products, using Concerta® as an example, stipulates that generic products must pass on both IR and MR components, and not only on one $C_{max}$ and $AUC_{0-t}$.

# EQUIVALENCE REQUIREMENTS FOR PRODUCTS THAT ARE NOT INTENDED TO ACT VIA THE SYSTEMIC CIRCULATION ("LOCALLY ACTING")

We have been discussing so far the scientific /regulatory equivalence requirements for drug products where the drug moiety arrives in the systemic circulation at the same time or before it reaches the various sites of efficacy/safety. For those, as explained earlier, equivalent PK systemic concentration profiles will ensure equivalent safety and efficacy.

Some products, however, result in efficacy well before they reach the systemic circulation. These have been called "locally acting" products by regulators, a misnomer no doubt, as every drug will act locally "somewhere" even if they reach the systemic circulation first. Notwithstanding this, if a product acts well before it reaches the systemic circulation, there can theoretically be a mismatch between its concentrations at the site of activity and its systemic concentrations. Equivalent PK systemic concentration profiles may therefore not ensure equivalent efficacy and safety for these products. Because of this, a proposed generic product must not only show that it has an equivalent PK systemic concentration profile to the reference product (still important as these may be related to safety issues but also efficacy for other types of future indications), it must also show theoretically that it has similar efficacy at the site of activity. In most cases, this will necessitate the need to conduct a clinical equivalence study (often called "therapeutic equivalence [TE] study" or "equivalence study with clinical endpoints [CE]"). Figure 29-8 describes locally acting drug products where their API reaches the site(s) of activity before the systemic circulation

Products considered to be "locally acting," resulting in efficacy before reaching the systemic circulation, include the following examples:

- Topical creams, ointments, and other types of formulations that act locally on the skin; for example for acne, psoriasis, actinic keratosis, among others. These are often referred to as "topicals." Common examples are topical antifungal, antibiotic, or antiviral agents.

- Ophthalmic preparations that act locally in the eye, such as antibiotics, and/or corticosteroid agents.

- Nasal preparations administered via the nose but intended to act locally, such as decongestants and corticosteroids.

Inhalation drug products for asthma and COPD have long been considered to be "acting locally" in the lung before they reach the systemic circulation. This is controversial, and the reader is referred to Al-Numani et al (2015) for more detailed information on this topic. The US FDA still considers Inhalation drug products "locally acting" as of 2020, and thus requires sponsors to conduct a BE study with clinical endpoint for demonstration of efficacy equivalence. Studies for demonstration of efficacy equivalence. In contrast, both EMA and HC have dropped this particular requirement in the recent past, and now allow submissions of generic products ("hybrid" in Europe) without the need to conduct a BE study with clinical endpoint.

Mesalamine delayed and extended release tablets and capsules are other examples of "locally acting" drug products that experienced recent regulatory changes in their BE requirements. These products are given orally for the treatment of ulcerative colitis and/or Crohn's disease where they act locally within the gut. But a mismatch between their "active" local concentrations in the gut and their associated partial systemic exposure is now thought to be unlikely, partly because of the high perfusion nature of the GI tract. FDA now recommends that bioequivalence be established by fasted and fed systemic PK equivalence studies, with the use of specific partial AUC timepoints, instead of a combination of PK and clinical endpoint studies (FDA 2016; FDA 2017; FDA 2019).

# EQUIVALENCE REQUIREMENTS FOR BIOLOGICAL PRODUCTS ("BIOSIMILARS")

Biotechnology-derived products, or *biologics*, are discussed in Chapter 10. The API of a generic *drug* can be chemically synthesized, completely characterized, and can thus be demonstrated to be identical to

**A** Active moiety appears systemically before or at the same time as it reaches the different site (s) of activity

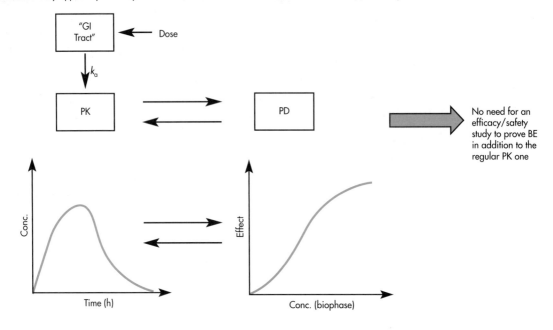

**B** Locally acting compounds

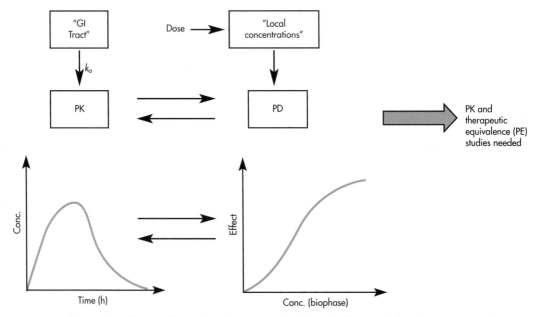

FIGURE 29-8 • "Locally acting" products are those where their API reaches the site(s) of activity before the systemic circulation (eg, an antiviral topical product acting on the skin). Equivalence in terms of systemic PK profile may not suffice to establish bioequivalence, and a therapeutic equivalence study will theoretically be needed.

the API of a reference drug. Biologics, on the other hand, can vary from lot to lot and are not completely identical between lots, and accordingly between a test biologic and a reference biologic product (Weise et al, 2012).

Due to this lack of *identicality* of the API between two products, it is difficult to ensure pharmaceutical equivalence between two biologic products. Regulators have therefore proposed the name *biosimilar* to identify a follow-on biologic that would be as close as possible to a reference biologic, in an almost analogous way that a generic drug is versus a reference drug. A *biosimilar* can be highly similar to the reference biologic product, and its use will result in no clinically meaningful differences in terms of safety, purity, efficacy, and potency of the product. In a similar manner to generic drugs, biosimilars can normally differ in a minor fashion in their clinically inactive components.

The lack of identicality in the API between a test biologic and a reference biologic complicates the development of a biosimilar versus that of a generic drug. Because the APIs are not identical, similarity needs to be established using extensive physicochemical and biological characterizations, preclinical and as clinical comparability. The EMA, FDA, and HC have all issued specific guidances on this topic that highlight the steps needed to establish similarity of the APIs (EMA, 2014; US FDA, 2015; Health Canada, 2017 a and b). Some of the requirements are:

- The amino acid sequence of the protein must be identical.
- The test and reference biologic should be extensively compared using advanced analytical techniques. Major advances have occurred in this regard in the last 20 years, and biosimilars can often now be much better characterized than their reference biologic was able to be when it was accepted for marketing. These advances enable precise physicochemical and functional property assessments and comparability. Not all relevant and functional differences may be able to be characterized, though, and it will be essential for the sponsor to specify to the regulatory agency what the residual uncertainties may be in terms of characterizations.

- The test and reference biological product-related impurities, product-related substances, and process-related impurities should be identified, characterized, quantified, and compared.

Once the test and reference biologics are properly characterized and compared, an assessment of biosimilarity will be conducted by the regulatory agency, who will assist closely every manufacturer that wants to develop a biosimilar. The US FDA, in particular, will assess whether or not the proposed biosimilar has "fingerprint-like" similarity. If it does not, then the preclinical and/or clinical requirements may be much more demanding, the agency may decide that the proposed biosimilar should not be considered for further development (US FDA, 2015).

A proposed biosimilar that has been deemed to be similar enough in terms of its analytical and functional characterizations to a reference biological product will then need to demonstrate similarity regarding the additional following items:

1. Similarity in a nonclinical comparability study using animal species that is/are known to be most appropriate to discriminate the PK or PK/PD of the biologic. This nonclinical study may not have to be conducted if the biosimilar is judged by the regulatory agency (FDA, EMA, or HC) to be highly similar or of "fingerprint-like similarity" to the reference biologic.

2. Equivalence between the test and reference biologic in terms of PK. Because identicality cannot yet be fully established between two biologics, equivalence in humans in terms of PK or of PD only will not suffice to ensure equivalent safety and efficacy. This is illustrated in Fig. 29-9, where equivalent PK may not equal equivalent PD, and vice-versa, because the biological API cannot yet be proven to be identical.

3. Equivalence between the test and reference biologics in terms of efficacy, or in terms of PD when a pivotal PD marker can be used (eg, blood glucose for insulin, absolute neutrophil counts for G-CSF). In the absence of a pivotal PD marker, an efficacy trial typically needs to be conducted in patients for a sensitive indication of the product. Equivalence will need to be demonstrated, and if applicable and appropriate, a placebo group may

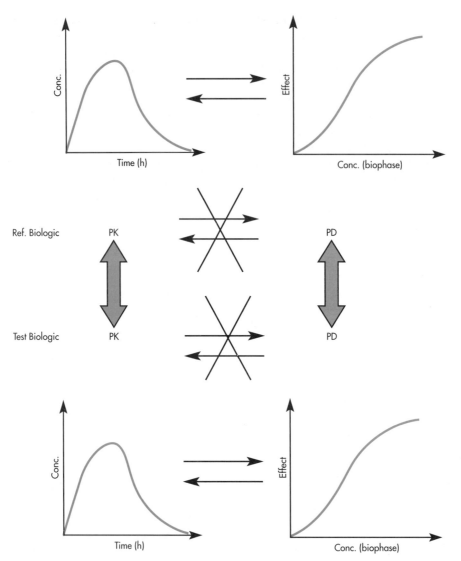

**FIGURE 29-9** • The clinical pharmacology link between exposure and efficacy/safety at the biophase is the same for biologics and for drugs. The impossibility of establishing identicality between two biologics' APIs means that equivalent PK may not be equal to equivalent PD, and vice-versa.

be added to show that the study has enough discriminatory power to show efficacy.

4. Similarity in terms of immunogenicity needs to be established between the test and the reference biological products. This is usually established during a sufficiently long period of time to ensure that significant issues would be identified; for example, over 12 months for an erythropoietin-type product using the route of administration

that has been shown to be associated with greater immunogenicity for the reference product.

PK equivalence between biologics is not the same as between drugs, because two APIs cannot be demonstrated to be identical. Every PK parameter can theoretically be different between two biologics, not just those related to rate and extent of exposure. Equivalence in terms of $C_{max}$ and AUC may therefore not suffice, and other parameters may also need to be compared (eg, half-lives, volumes of distribution).

Principles governing the study designs of PK equivalence studies for drugs should, however, also apply to biosimilars. For example, a subcutaneous solution that is Q1/Q2 versus a reference would not need to be studied if the biologic had already been shown to be similar from a PK point of view after IV administration. Suspensions, on the other hand, should always be studied for SC or IM administrations, as their absorption profile can differ between different formulations.

When all these studies have been successfully conducted and indicate equivalence, the regulatory body may grant a marketing authorization for the biosimilar product. Although the equivalent clinical study will have been conducted in only one patient indication, the other indications of the reference biologic can normally be granted to the biosimilar if they are all resulting from the same mechanism of action.

## Interchangeability Issues

A biosimilar is, by definition, similar and not identical to its reference biological product. As mentioned earlier, even two batches or lots of a reference biologic will not be identical between themselves. In theory, one may therefore expect biologics never to be classified as interchangeable with other products, but in practice, there are specific reasons why some of these products can be treated as interchangeable even though they may not be classified as such.

Many biologics are hospital- or clinic-based products that have to be directly administered by physicians or other healthcare professionals. Hospitals and clinics do not carry every product commercially available. Instead, they only carry products listed in their formulary, as discussed at the beginning of this chapter. Within a formulary, only one biologic per class of similar or alternative agents may be carried. Should the biologic carried be a biosimilar, patients will automatically receive it instead of the reference biologic, in essence "forcing" interchangeability. This phenomenon is occurring in Europe and in Canada, where healthcare is paid for by the government, and the government will only reimburse products that are on its own formulary list, and where acquisition price is a major driving force. Some governments have specifically recommended to physicians to

start all of their new patients on a biosimilar, and to only prescribe reference biologics for patients who are already controlled on them. These steps also "force" interchangeability to a biosimilar in practice, even though regulators may not have classified the biosimilar as interchangeable with its reference biologic. Interchangeability is not under federal jurisdiction in Europe and Canada, contrary to the US. Provinces in Canada, and countries in Europe will decide what is interchangeable or not. Biosimilars may therefore be approved in Europe and Canada as non-interchangeable, but in practice, provinces and/or countries may decide that they are.

Interchangeability is under federal jurisdiction in the US (ie, by the FDA), and healthcare is not a complete public service for its citizens. There is therefore less pressure from a monetary standpoint in the US for the "forced" interchangeability that we sometimes see in practice in Canada and in many European countries. The US FDA has issued a guidance for industry, specifying the types of studies that they would like completed in order to grant interchangeability status (US FDA, CDER and CBER, 2019). Biosimilar products that are officially classified as being interchangeable to a reference biologic will be listed as such in the Purple Book (Purple Book, 2020 US FDA, CDER and CBER, 2020). The Purple Book is the equivalent official document to the Orange Book, but for biologics instead of drugs. The Purple Book therefore provides information about FDA-licensed biological products (approved under the Public Health Service Act) that are regulated by the Center for Biologics Evaluation and Research (CBER), while the Orange Book does the same for FDA-licensed drug products (approved under the CFR) and that are regulated by CDER. The US FDA interchangeability guidance for biosimilars clarifies that data submitted should provide information to show:

- That the biosimilar "can be expected to provide the same clinical result as the reference product in any given patient."
- That "the risk in terms of safety or diminished efficacy of alternating or switching between use of the biological product and the reference product is not greater than the risk of using the reference product without such alternation or switch."

The FDA therefore expects biosimilar applications requesting interchangeability status to include data from at least one switchability study. Not all biosimilar submissions will be treated alike, and the FDA will use a stepwise approach to issue specific recommendations. For example, a biosimilar of a reference biologic associated with high structural complexity and with a history of rare life-threatening adverse events may need reassuring postmarketing data to support the interchangeability status (US FDA, CDER and CBER, 2019).

As with almost every other important biosimilar development topic, the US FDA wants sponsors to meet with them and discuss their strategy and plans for establishing interchangeability before putting them into action. A switchability study supporting interchangeability should include and address the following (US FDA, CDER and CBER, 2019):

- Each product (test and reference) therapy should be given at least twice, indicating that the risk

of switching and alternating between the reference and test biologic should not be greater than just using the reference biologic without any switching.

- The evaluation as to whether "the proposed interchangeable product will affect clinical response in terms of safety or diminished efficacy reflected, in part, through an assessment of whether switching results in differences in immunogenicity and PK and/or PD (if available), as compared to not switching."

In their proposed guidance, the FDA proposes to focus on PK and PD (if available), rather than clinical efficacy endpoint, because they should be more sensitive to detect differences. The FDA also recommends to descriptively assess immunogenicity and safety. Finally, all study samples from switching and non-switching arms should be assessed with the same PK, PD, or immunogenicity assay (US FDA, CDER, and CBER, 2019).

## CHAPTER SUMMARY

The safety and efficacy of generic drug products are strictly regulated under the Food, Drug, and Cosmetic Act in the US, the Food and Drug Regulations in Canada, and the Directive 2001/83/EC in the EU. Generic products are fully substitutable with their reference counterpart and therefore cannot be inferior or better in terms of safety and efficacy. Generic drug products will be approved for marketing only after they have been deemed to be bioequivalent to their reference product through multiple study requirements and criteria. These will differ according to formulation type (IR versus MR), route of administration (oral, inhaled, topical, transdermal, etc), site of action (systemic versus local action), and other characteristics, such as PK non-linearity, solubility, significant presystemic metabolism, intra-individual PK variability, and whether or not they are a CDD. Although a great deal of effort has been spent on regulatory harmonization in the last 30 years, the regulatory agencies of the US FDA, HC, and the EMA still differ significantly regarding their

scientific regulatory advice for a large number of topics and drug products. Among others, the criteria for modified release formulations, nonlinear PK drugs, highly variable drug products, critical dose drugs/narrow therapeutic index drugs, inhaler products, all differ between these regulatory agencies. Generic drug development applies to "drugs," products that contain an active moiety that can be fully characterized and proven to be identical to that of a reference product. In contrast, biosimilar development applies to "biologics," products that contain an active moiety that cannot be at this time fully characterized and established to be identical with that of a reference biological product. Biosimilar development is therefore a much more complicated and lengthy proposal, and in addition to PK equivalence study(s), it will also require extensive comparative characterization of the biologics, preclinical comparative studies, and immunogenicity comparison as well as comparative clinical efficacy and/or PK/PD studies.

# ANSWERS

## Frequently Asked Questions

*What is the relationship between bioequivalence and a PK equivalence or comparative bioavailability study?*

- *Bioequivalence* may be viewed as a regulatory science establishing that one product is/should be equivalent to another one using comparative, in vitro and clinical studies, and ensuring that it should be equivalent in terms of clinical safety and efficacy. The FDA defines Bioequivalence as "the absence of a significant difference in the rate and extent to which the active ingredient or active moiety in pharmaceutical equivalents or pharmaceutical alternatives becomes available at the site of drug action when administered at the same molar dose under similar conditions in an appropriately designed study." (Orange Book) Two pharmaceutically equivalent products that are bioequivalent to each other can be classified as being interchangeable by a regulatory agency because they will/should lead to the same efficacy and safety clinically.

- A PK equivalence study, also called comparative bioavailability study, compares two products typically in terms of their maximum and extent of systemic exposure. PK equivalence studies are often called "bioequivalence studies".

*What is the Orange Book?*

- FDA publishes on-line the Orange Book: Approved Drug Products with Therapeutic Equivalence Evaluations (https://www.accessdata.fda.gov/scripts/cder/ob/index.cfm). The Orange Book lists drug products approved on the basis of safety and effectiveness by the FDA. The Orange Book also contains therapeutic equivalence evaluations for approved multisource prescription drug products so that pharmacists and clinicians know which products are interchangeable.

*Are marketed generic and innovator products always interchangeable?*

- The approved generic drug product must meet all the requirements for therapeutic equivalence to the equivalent brand drug product. FDA believes "that products classified as therapeutically equivalent can be substituted with the full expectation that the substituted product can be expected to have the same clinical effect and safety profile as the prescribed product when administered to patients under the conditions specified in the labeling."

- Therapeutically equivalent products may differ in certain characteristics such as shape, scoring configuration, release mechanisms, packaging, excipients (including colors, flavors, preservatives), expiration date/time, certain aspects of labeling (eg, the presence of specific pharmacokinetic information), and storage conditions. When such differences are important in the care of a particular patient, it may be appropriate for the prescribing physician to require that a specific product be dispensed as a medical necessity.

- Sometimes, certain generic and innovator or reference products will not be interchangeable. This is the case when multiple reference products exist, such as with levothyroxine. As presented in the text, AB1 products will be interchangeable with other AB1, while AB2 products will only be interchangeable with other AB2 products, and so on.

*What is an "authorized generic"?*

- The term "authorized generic" product is most commonly used to describe an approved brand name drug that is marketed without the brand name on its label. Other than the fact that it does not have the brand name on its label, it is the exact same drug product as the branded product. An authorized generic may be marketed by the brand name drug company or by another company with the brand company's permission.

*What is the fundamental principle of clinical pharmacology that ensures that an approved interchangeable generic product, based on one or more PK equivalence studies, should have the same efficacy and safety as the reference product?*

- A fundamental principle of clinical pharmacology is that there is always a relationship between the concentration of the drug at its site(s) of efficacy/safety and efficacy/safety. If a generic product produces an equivalent systemic concentration time profile as that of a reference product, then the concentration profiles at the various sites of efficacy/safety will be the same as the transfer of the drug between the systemic circulation, and the biophase(s) will no longer be dependent on the formulation.

*A common misunderstanding is the belief that if generic products are approved with a ±20% difference to a reference product, then it may mean that two generic products could present a ±40% difference. Explain why this is unlikely to ever occur.*

■ A 90% confidence interval (CI) around the geometric ratio of the test versus the reference product is calculated from the results of a PK equivalence study for each of the pivotal PK metrics. These 90% CIs must completely lie within 80.0%–125.0% for the study to meet the equivalence criteria. Interval estimates are desirable because the estimate of this geometric mean will vary from study to study. Instead of a single estimate for the mean, a 90% CI generates a lower and upper limit for the mean. The 90% CI

estimates give an indication of how much confidence we have that the point estimate values will fall between the upper and lower limits if the procedure or reasearch was to be repeated again and again. The narrower the CI, the more precise is the estimate. CIs become narrower and narrower with increasing study sample sizes. The development cost of a generic drug product directly impacts on its marketed price. The FDA undertook a retrospective analysis of 2070 human studies conducted between 1996 and 2007 that were submitted to them as part of generic applications. The average difference that was found between the generic and the branded drug was only 3.5% (Davit et al, 2009), which supports that most generic products are really identical to the reference product (ie, 5% or less difference in true ratio). Reference product lots are typically marketed with a difference of up to 5% difference in potency from the label claim. Hence it can be argued that there should not be more variability, on average, expected between switching from a reference product to a generic, than switching between different lots of the reference product.

## REFERENCES

Al-Numani D Colucci P, Ducharme MP: Rethinking bioequivalence and equivalence requirements of orally inhaled drug products, *Asian J Pharm Sci* **10**:461–471, 2015.

Alloway R, Barr WH, Flagstad M, Lake K: Substitution of critical dose drugs: Issues, analysis, and decision making. Publication for health care professionals, *American Pharmaceutical Association*: Washington DC, 2000. Pages 1–18.

Davit BM, Nwakama PE, Buehler GJ, et al: Comparing generic and innovator drugs: A review of 12 years of bioequivalence data from the United States Food and Drug Administration. *Ann Pharmacother* **43**:1583–1597, 2009.

Ducharme MP, Potvin D: Understanding bioequivalence: The experience of a global contract research organisation, *Business Briefing: PharmaGenerics* 53–60, Sept 2003.

EMA. Note for Guidance on the Investigation of Bioavailability and Bioequivalence. Last accessed 20 Oct 2019 at: https://www.ema.europa.eu/en/documents/scientific-guideline/draft-note-guidance-investigation-bioavailability-bioequivalence_en.pdf. December 2000.

EMA. Guideline on the Investigation of Bioequivalence. August 2010. Last accessed 20 Oct 2019 at: https://www.ema.europa.eu/en/documents/scientific-guideline/guideline-investigation-bioequivalence-rev1_en.pdf. January 2010.

EMA. Guideline on the pharmacokinetic and clinical evaluation of modified release dosage forms. Last accessed at: https://www.ema.europa.eu/en/documents/scientific-guideline/guideline-pharmacokinetic-clinical-evaluation-modified-release-dosage-forms_en.pdf. November 2014.

EMA. Guideline on similar biological medicinal products. Adopted October 2014. Last accessed 11 Dec 2020 at: https://www.ema.europa.eu/en/documents/scientific-guideline/guideline-similar-biological-medicinal-products-rev1_en.pdf.

EMA. European Medicines Agency procedural advice for users of the centralised procedure for generic/hybrid applications. Last accessed 20 Oct 2019 at: https://www.ema.europa.eu/en/documents/regulatory-procedural-guideline/european-medicines-agency-procedural-advice-users-centralised-procedure-generic/hybrid-applications_en.pdf. August 2019.

Endrenyi L, Tothfalusi L: Regulatory and study conditions for the determination of bioequivalence of highly variable drugs. *J Pharm Pharm Sci* **12**:138–149, 2009.

Endrenyi L, Tothfalusi L: Do regulatory bioequivalence requirements adequately reflect the therapeutic equivalence of modified-release drug products? *J Pharm Pharm Sci* **13**(1):107–113, 2010.

FDA Statement. 2019. Statement from FDA Commissioner Scott Gottlieb, MD, on new agency efforts to shine light on situations where drug makers may be pursuing gaming tactics to delay generic competition. Washington, DC. FDA website. Last accessed at: https://www.fda.gov/NewsEvents/Newsroom/Press Announcements/ucm607930.htm.

Health Canada. Therapeutic Products Directorate Policy: Bioequivalence of Proportional Formulations: Solid Oral Dosage. Last accessed 17 Aug 2019 at: https://www.canada.ca/content/dam/hc-sc/migration/hc-sc/dhp-mps/alt_formats/pdf/prodpharma/applic-demande/pol/bioprop_pol-eng.pdf. Dated March 7, 1996.

Health Canada. Policy on Bioequivalence Standards for Highly Variable Drug Products. Last accessed 27 Oct 2019 at: https://www.canada.ca/en/health-canada/services/drugs-health-products/drug-products/announcements/notice-policy-bioequivalence-standards-highly-variable-drug-products.html. April 188, 2016.

Health Canada. Guidance document, Information and submission requirements for biosimilar biologic drugs. Last revision April 2017. Last accessed 11 Dec 2020 at: https://www.canada.ca/content/dam/hc-sc/migration/hc-sc/dhp-mps/alt_formats/pdf/brgtherap/applic-demande/guides/seb-pbu/seb-p-bu-2016-eng.pdf.

Health Canada. Notice: proposed modification to bioequivalence standards for multiphasic modified-release drug products. Last accessed at: https://www.canada.ca/en/health-canada/services/drugs-health-products/public-involvement-consultations/drug-products/multiphasic-modified-release.html. Dated July 27, 2017.

Health Canada. Guidance Document: Conduct and Analysis of Comparative Bioavailability Studies. Last accessed 25 Oct 2019 at: https://www.canada.ca/content/dam/hc-sc/documents/services/drugs-health-products/drug-products/applications-submissions/guidance-documents/bioavailability-bioequivalence/conduct-analysis-comparative.pdf. June 2018a.

Health Canada. Guidance Document: Comparative Bioavailability Standards: Formulations Used for Systemic Effects. Last accessed 25 Oct 2019 at: https://www.canada.ca/content/dam/hc-sc/migration/hc-sc/dhp-mps/alt_formats/pdf/prodpharma/applic-demande/guide-ld/bio/comparative-bioavailability-standards-formulations-used-systemic-effects.pdf. June 2018b.

Health Canada. Guidance Document: Use of a Foreign-sourced Reference Product as a Canadian Reference Product. Last accessed 15 Sep 2019 at: https://www.canada.ca/content/dam/hc-sc/documents/services/drug-health-product-review-approval/drug-products/guidance-documents/canadian-reference-product-guidance.pdf. July 2018c.

Jiang W, Makhlouf F, Schuirmann DJ et al: A bioequivalence approach for generic narrow therapeutic index drugs: Evaluation of the reference-scaled approach and variability comparison criterion. *AAPS J* **17**:891–901, 2015.

Kanfer I, Shargel L: Introduction - Bioequivalence Issues. In Kanfer I, Shargel L (eds). *Generic Drug Product Development Bioequivalence Issues*, Vol 180. Informa Healthcare United States, 2007.

Orange Book. 2020. Approved drug products with therapeutic equivalence evaluations, 40th edn. U.S. Department of Health and Human Services, Food and Drug Administration, Center for Drug Evaluation and Research, Office of Generic Drugs. Last accessed 7 Jan 2021 at: https://www.fda.gov/media/71474/download.

Purple Book. 2020. Lists of licensed biological products with reference product exclusivity and biosimilarity or interchangeability evaluations. Last accessed 7 Jan 2021 at: https://www.fda.gov/drugs/therapeutic-biologics-applications-bla/purple-book-lists-licensed-biological-products-reference-product-exclusivity-and-biosimilarity-or

Schuirmann DJ: A comparison of the Two One-Sided Tests Procedure and the Power Approach for assessing the equivalence of average bioavailability. *J Pharmacokinet Biopharm* **15**: 657–680, 1987.

Schuirmann DJ: Current issues in Biostatistics. Presentation delivered at the Generic Pharmaceutical Association Fall Technical Conference, Bethesda, MD, October 30, 2008.

Shah DB, Yadav RR, Maheshwari PG: An overview on US FDA 505(b)(2) NDA and EU hybrid medicinal products. *Eur J Pharm Med Res* **2**:88–92, 2015.

US FDA, CDER. Guidance for Industry: Immediate Release Solid Oral Dosage Forms Scale-Up and Postapproval Changes: Chemistry, Manufacturing, and Controls, In Vitro Dissolution Testing, and In Vivo Bioequivalence Documentation. Last accessed 22 Oct 2019 at: https://www.fda.gov/media/70949/download. November 1995.

US FDA, CDER. Guidance for Industry SUPAC-MR: Modified Release Solid Oral Dosage Forms Scale-Up and Postapproval Changes: Chemistry, Manufacturing, and Controls; In Vitro Dissolution Testing and In Vivo Bioequivalence Documentation. Last accessed 22 Oct 2019 at: https://www.fda.gov/media/70956/download. September 1997.

US FDA, CDER. Draft Guidance on Progesterone. Last accessed at: https://www.accessdata.fda.gov/drugsatfda_docs/psg/Progesterone_caps_19781_RC02-11.pdf. Recommended April 2010a.

US FDA, CDER. Briefing Information: FDA Meeting of the Advisory Committee for Pharmaceuticals Science and Clinical Pharmacology. April 13, 2010b.

US FDA, CDER. Draft Guidance on Iron Sucrose, Injectable; Intravenous. Last accessed 1 Dec 2019 at: https://www.accessdata.fda.gov/drugsatfda_docs/psg/Iron_sucrose_inj_21135_RV11-13.pdf. Recommended March 2012a.

US FDA, CDER. Draft Guidance on Warfarin. Last accessed 22 Dec 2019 at: https://www.accessdata.fda.gov/drugsatfda_docs/psg/Warfarin_Sodium_tab_09218_RC12-12.pdf. Recommended December 2012b.

US FDA, CDER. Draft Guidance on Methylphenidate Hydrochloride. Last accessed 22 Dec 2019 at: https://www.accessdata.fda.gov/drugsatfda_docs/psg/Methylphenidate%20Hydrochloride_draft_Oral%20tab%20ER_RLD%2021121_RC07-18.pdf. Recommended Sept 2012c.

US FDA, CDER. Draft Guidance on Sodium Ferric Gluconate Complex, Injectable; Intravenous. Last accessed 1 Dec 2019 at: https://www.accessdata.fda.gov/drugsatfda_docs/psg/Sodium

_ferric_gluconate_complex_inj_20955_RC06-13.pdf. Recommended June 2013.

US FDA, CDER. Draft Guidance on Ferric Carboxymaltose, Injectable; Intravenous. Last accessed 1 Dec 2019 at: https://www.accessdata.fda.gov/drugsatfda_docs/psg/FERRIC%20CARBOXYMALTOSE_injection_RLD%20203565_RC04-16.pdf. Recommended April 2016.

US FDA, CDER. CFR Code of Federal Regulations Title 21 Part 314.3. Definitions. Last accessed at: https://www.ecfr.gov/cgi-bin/text-idx?SID=f0d908c3d43c0ba3c1ff14f093311c7a&mc=true&node=se21.5.314_13&rgn=div8. 2019.

US FDA, CDER and CBER. Guidance for Industry, Quality considerations in demonstrating biosimilarity of a therapeutic protein product to a reference product. Last accessed 11 Dec 2020 at: https://www.fda.gov/media/135612/download.

US FDA, CDER and CBER. Guidance for Industry. Considerations in demonstrating interchangeability with a reference product. Biosimilars. May 2019. Last accessed: Jan 7 2021 at: https://www.fda.gov/media/124907/download.

Weise M, Bielsky MC, De Smet K, et al: Biosimilars: What clinicians should know. *Blood* 120(26):5111–5117, 2012.

## BIBLIOGRAPHY

Benet LZ: Clearance (née Rowland) concepts: A downdate and an update. *J Pharmacokinet Pharmacodyn* 37:529–539, 2010.

Cafruny EJ: Renal tubular handling of drugs. *Am J Med* 62:490–496, 1977.

FDA Draft Guidance on Balsalazide Disodium, 2013.

FDA Guidance on Mesalamine, 2012.

FDA, CDER. Draft guidance on Mesalamine, delayed release 400mg capsule. Revised June 2016. Last accessed 12 Sep 2021 at: https://www.accessdata.fda.gov/drugsatfda_docs/psg/Mesalamine_draft_Oral%20cap%20DR_RLD%20204412_RC06-16.pdf.

FDA, CDER. Draft guidance on Mesalamine, extended release 500mg capsule. Revised Oct. 2017. Last accessed 12 Sep 2021 at: https://www.accessdata.fda.gov/drugsatfda_docs/psg/Mesalamine_draft_Oral%20cap%20ER_RLD%2020049_RC10-17.pdf.

FDA, CDER. Draft guidance on Mesalamine, extended release 375mg capsule. Revised Sept 2019. Last accessed 12 Sep 2021 at: https://www.accessdata.fda.gov/drugsatfda_docs/psg/PSG_022301.pdf

Goldstein A, Aronow L, Kalman SM: *Principles of Drug Action.* New York, Wiley, 1974.

Guyton AC: *Textbook of Medical Physiology*, 8th ed. Philadelphia, Saunders, 1991.

Hewitt WR, Hook JB: The renal excretion of drugs. In Bridges VW, Chasseaud LF (eds). *Progress in Drug Metabolism*, Vol 7. New York, Wiley, 1983, Chap 1.

Holford N, Heo YA, Anderson B: A pharmacokinetic standard for babies and adults. *J Pharm Sci* 102(9):2941–2952, 2013.

Levine RR: *Pharmacology: Drug Actions and Reactions*, 4th ed. Boston, Little, Brown, 1990.

Renkin EM, Robinson RR: Glomerular filtration. *N Engl J Med* 290:785–792, 1974.

Rowland M, Benet LZ, Graham GG: Clearance concepts in pharmacokinetics. *J Pharm Biopharm* 1:123–136, 1973.

Smith H: *The Kidney: Structure and Function in Health and Disease*. New York, Oxford University Press, 1951.

Thomson P, Melmon K, Richardson J, et al: Lidocaine pharmacokinetics in advanced heart failure, liver disease and renal failure in humans. *Ann Intern Med* 78:499–508, 1973.

Tucker GT: Measurement of the renal clearance of drugs. *Br J Clin Pharm* 12:761–770, 1981.

Weiner IM, Mudge GH: Renal tubular mechanisms for excretion and organic acids and bases. *Am J Med* 36:743–762, 1964.

West JB (ed): *Best and Taylor's Physiological Basis of Medical Practice*, 11th ed. Baltimore, Williams & Wilkins, 1985.

Wilkinson GR: Clearance approaches in pharmacology. *Pharmacol Rev* 39:1–47, 1987.

# 30

# Pharmacokinetics and Pharmacodynamics in Clinical Drug Product Development

Murray P. Ducharme, Olga Ponomarchuk, Dana Bakir, Deniz Ozdin, and Leon Shargel

## CHAPTER OBJECTIVES

- To provide a description of the drug development process in the context of PK/PD studies.

- To highlight the main types of regulatory submission pathways and details what is specific to the United States, the European Union, and Canada.

- To give an overview of the critical PK information that is to be presented in the label and/or monograph after appropriately conducting PK/PD study.

- To describe the importance of the relative bioavailability of a drug depending on the different routes of administration.

- To specify the impact of PK nonlinearity on dosing regimen adjustments.

- To describe the objectives of an appropriately conducted single ascending dose (SAD) study and how it relates to multiple ascending dose (MAD) study.

- To describe the objectives of an appropriately conducted SAD study.

- To explain why food effect studies are usually conducted with a high-fat high-calorie breakfast.

- To describe the objectives of a mass balance study.

- To define the relationship between drug clearance, renal clearance, and non-renal clearance in a renal impairment study.

- To describe the importance of measuring unbound concentrations in a liver impairment study.

- To describe the design of a drug–drug interaction study with consideration to induction, irreversible inhibition, or reversible inhibition.

- To describe the importance of assessing QT prolongation for new drug products.

- To describe the importance of conducting population PK/PD studies in all stages of the drug development process.

- To provide a description on how to step-by-step validate a population PK model.

## INTRODUCTION

We have seen throughout the previous chapters that the relationship between pharmacokinetics (PK) and pharmacodynamics (PD) (efficacy and safety) is a fundamental principle of clinical pharmacology. Understanding the PK/PD of a new drug or biological product is therefore essential to its development and to ensure its safe and effective use on the market.

We will see in this chapter what are the necessary requirements in terms of PK/PD that a pharmaceutical company must address for a new drug submission, so that clinicians can better understand how study results relate to the official drug label or monograph.

## OVERVIEW OF THE DRUG DEVELOPMENT PROCESS

The drug development process is planned in different stages, starting with the discovery of new drug molecules and biologics, followed by preclinical[1] testing, initial human (Phase I) studies, followed by clinical safety and efficacy (Phase II and Phase III) studies.

An essential part of drug development is the characterization of the PK and PD of the new drug product and the relationship of PK and PD to safety and efficacy. Estimating, understanding, and predicting the PK and PK/PD of a drug product is an essential part of drug development.

Physiologically-based PK (PBPK) models are more commonly used in the *discovery* phase and nonclinical stages of new molecules in order to better select candidates for preclinical studies. The results of the PBPK studies aid in the selection of drug candidates that have the potential for therapeutic success. Preferred drug candidates are those with higher predicted oral bioavailability, lower risks of associated drug–drug interactions, and those possessing an elimination half-life within a desired range, and these candidates may be prioritized over others.

The *preclinical* phase provides essential safety and PK/PD information about the drug candidates in both animal and *in vitro* models. Results of these studies help both scientists and regulators predict the safest dose to be administered in humans during the first-in-man (FIM) single ascending dose (SAD) Phase I study.

- *Phase I* studies are conducted to explore the safety, the PK, and usually the pharmacological activity of the drug product in humans. As we will see later in this chapter, these studies provide essential PK information that is presented in a product monograph or label (eg, food effect, PK linearity and dose proportionality, and bioequivalence). Phase I studies are most often conducted in healthy volunteers, for ethical and/or safety reasons, but can also be conducted in patients. PK information from these studies in healthy patients include

characterization of the plasma drug concentration versus time profile, PK linearity and dose proportionality, food effect, and bioequivalence. Simple PK methods, such as the noncompartmental (NCPT) approach, are typically used. However, Phase I studies that are conducted in patients with relatively sparse sampling, and with or without PD markers, are better analyzed with population PK methods. Studies that use a PD marker to determine the effectiveness of the drug are often called "proof of concept" (POC) studies.

- *Phase II* studies provide useful PK/PD data to better characterize exposure–effect relationships and validate the clinical activity in people with the disease or condition being studied. Phase II studies investigate the therapeutic effects of the drug. Phase II studies demonstrate the therapeutic effect of the drug in patients with the disease and assist in the selection of the dosing regimen(s) that will be tested in the Phase III pivotal trials. Phase II studies are often called "dose ranging" studies. Population PK/PD methods are particularly useful as they enable scientists to simulate the effects of a multitude of dosing regimens before choosing the final Phase III regimen(s) to study.

- *Phase III* studies, also known as "pivotal efficacy studies," provide PK/PD data in the intended patient population. The data from the population PK/PD analyses provide essential safety and efficacy data that will be used in the drug monograph and/or the approved label. This information may include, but is not limited to, exposure/response relationships, drug–drug interaction information, PK linearity, dosing optimization for the intended population, and/or needed dose adjustments in the presence of renal and/or hepatic impairments.

## OVERVIEW OF THE DRUG SUBMISSION PATHWAYS IN THE UNITED STATES, THE EUROPEAN UNION, AND CANADA

Drug regulatory agencies in Europe (European Medicinal Agency [EMA]), the United States (US) (Food and Drug Administration ([FDA]), and

---

[1]Preclinical studies are sometimes referred to as nonclinical studies and include animal studies and various in vitro drug studies.

**TABLE 30-1 •** Summary of the Different Types of New Drug Submissions to the US Food and Drug Administration (FDA), the European Medicine Agency (EMA), and Health Canada (HC)

| Submission Type | US FDA | EMA | HC | Example |
|---|---|---|---|---|
| **Full submissions** | 505(b)(1) NDA | Full drug application | NDS (can be full or "abridged/ shortened" when referring to a Canadian Reference Product) | New drug product – Complete application contains preclinical and clinical safety and efficacy studies |
| **Abridged" or "shortened" sub-missions, based on an already marketed reference product** | • 505(b)(1) NDA when right of reference to reference product<br>• 505(b)(2) NDA when no right of reference to reference product | Hybrid drug application | | New dosage form of an approved drug product – Application based on PK and clinical study comparisons with the older approved drug product |
| **Abbreviated or generic** | 505(j) ANDA | Generic drug application | ANDS | Generic drug product application contains bioequivalence data and possibly clinical data comparison to a reference listed drug product |

*NDA: New Drug Application; NDS: New Drug Submission; ANDA: Abbreviated New Drug Application; ANDS: Abbreviated New Drug Submission.*

Canada (Health Canada [HC]) have different regulatory requirements for market approval of new and generic drug products.

Pharmaceutical companies commonly submit one of the following three types of drug submissions: (1) a new drug submission, (2) an "abridged" or "shortened" new drug submission that uses prior determination of safety and efficacy from one or more reference marketed products, and (3) an abbreviated or generic product submission (as presented in Chapter 29). Several other types of submissions exist; for example, those that are based on well-established use or bibliographic data; however, the submissions listed above are more common. A summary of the main new drug submission types is presented in Table 30-1.

This chapter will discuss the PK/PD requirements for new drug submissions or applications. The requirements for generic drug product approval were discussed in Chapter 29. As shown in Table 30-1, the regulatory bodies, FDA, HC, and EMA, all accept a "shortened" or "abridged" (not to be confused with the term "abbreviated" which is reserved in Canada and the US for generic submissions) new drug

application/submission based on the known safety and efficacy of a marketed reference product. Even though these submissions will be termed "NDA" and "NDS" for the US and Canada, respectively, they will be "shortened" because what is known about the safety and efficacy of the reference product will not need to be re-established. In Europe, this type of application is called "hybrid."

### New Drug Application Using the FDA 505(b)(2) Pathway

The 505(b)(2) pathway[2] has no direct equivalent in Europe and Canada. The 505(b)(2) pathway allows an applicant to include studies in the application that were conducted by the owner of the marketed reference drug product but that are not publicly available anywhere to the applicant and are therefore only "known" to the US FDA and the company that holds the reference product. The "reference product" is a marketed product, established or considered to be

---

[2]The term 505(b)(2) pathway comes from the U.S. Code of Federal Regulations (CFR) *Section 505 of the US Food, Drug and Cosmetic Act that governs regulatory responsibilities of the U.S. FDA.*

safe and effective for the conditions of use specified in its product label or monograph. If a "shortened" or "abridged" new drug application is filed using the known safety and efficacy of a previously accepted reference product(s), many of the requirements will not need to be re-established for the new drug product. We often refer to these new drug products as "supergeneric." They are considered to be products that display advantage over the reference drug product (eg, once-a-day formulation versus one that is given multiple times per day) and they are not considered generic products as they will be stand-alone on the market.

The 505(b)(2) pathway is often used for the development of new dosage forms of older drugs that have already been approved for marketing in the US. According to the FDA:

*A 505(b)(2) application is an NDA submitted under section 505(b)(1) and approved under section 505(c) of the FD&C Act that contains full reports of investigations of safety and effectiveness, where at least some of the information required for approval comes from studies not conducted by or for the applicant and for which the applicant has not obtained a right of reference or use. (FDA Guidance, 2019)*

## ESSENTIAL PK/PD KNOWLEDGE FOR A NEW DRUG SUBMISSION

A drug product marketed in the US, Canada, or Europe must have demonstrated efficacy and safety in the intended patient population. The associated product label[3] and/or monograph[4] provide the prescriber with essential information on the drug's intended use (indications), summaries of clinical and safety studies, PKPD data, and the recommended dosing regimens.

The suggested dosing regimen(s) in the approved label is developed in patients during the

clinical and safety studies. A major consideration in prescribing the drug is whether the suggested dosing regimen needs to be modified for the individual patient. Some important considerations that need to be detailed in the product label include:

- Should the drug product be taken with food or under fasting conditions? If food impacts the drug product's PK profile, how should the dosing regimen be modified?
- How should the dosing regimen be adjusted if the administration route of this drug product is changed (eg, from IV to oral)?
- How should dosing regimens be adjusted in the presence or addition of a concomitant drug creating a drug–drug interaction?
- Should the dosing regimen be adjusted in a patient with altered kidney or hepatic function or in a special population (eg, elderly, pregnant women, children)?
- If the patient does not respond to the starting dosing regimen, how should it be modified?
- How should the patient be treated in the case of an overdose?

These clinical and scientific queries, among others, are addressed by the results of appropriately conducted PK/PD studies during the drug development process.

A PK study will typically be considered "pivotal" by a regulatory agency such as the FDA, HC, and EMA only if it involves a minimum of 12 subjects or patients. Only two studies are exempted from this minimum requirement—the hepatic impairment and the mass balance.

In the following sections, we will review the main PK studies that have to be conducted during the drug development process, mostly in order of Phase I to Phase III studies, through the specific questions that a clinician would like to have answers to in his review of the product label in order to adequately prescribe a drug product.

### Relative Bioavailability between Administration Routes Should Be Known

The main route of drug administration is decided early in drug development. The clinical decision on which route of administration should be used

---

[3]The product label provides information regarding the official description of the drug product and includes the indicated target population and adverse events as well as safety information for the patient.

[4]The product monograph is a factual scientific document on a drug product that describes the properties, claims, indications, and conditions of use of the drug and contains information required for optimal, safe, and effective use of the drug.

is dependent on many factors, including efficacy, safety, ease of administration, the patient's health, onset of action, and the desired duration of effect.

Biological products, as we have seen in Chapter 10, are mostly administered via the intravenous (IV), subcutaneous (SC), and/or intramuscular route. These last two routes are limited by the volume of the drug product that can be administered. Subcutaneous and intramuscular injections are often limited to a maximum of 1 and 4 mL per site, respectively, in order for patients to tolerate them. The intravenous route does not have such limits. Biologics will often have completely different dosing regimens between routes of administration because of solubility limits.

## PRACTICAL PROBLEM

1. A biological product is being developed but has a solubility limit of 100 mg/mL. A formulation of 100 mg/mL has been developed for IV and SC administrations. Understanding that the predicted efficacious overall exposure ($AUC_{inf}$ or $AUC_{t(ss)}$) has been shown to be 10000 mg.h/L per month (with no safety issues seen with exposures 10 times this amount), the CL is 0.0126 L/h, V is 5 L, the subcutaneous bioavailability is 75% (F), and that the biologic PK profile approximates a one-compartment model, calculate what the dosing regimens may need to be after IV and/or SC administrations.

### Solution

Let us first calculate what the IV dosing regimen may need to be:

- $CL = DOSE/AUC_{inf}$, therefore DOSE $= CL \times AUC_{inf} = 0.0126 \times 10000 = 126$ mg
- $K_{el} = CL/V = 0.0126/5 = 0.00252$ h$^{-1}$
- $T_{1/2} = 0.693/k_{el} = 0.693/0.00252 = 275$ h or 11.5 days
- Administering the biologic every 2.44 half-lives (once every 4 weeks or 672 h, as 672/275 = 2.44) would lead to little accumulation: AR = 1/exp $(-k_{el}*\tau) = 1/\exp(-0.00252 \times 672) = 1.225$.
- With an AR of 1.225, with an $AUC\tau_{(SS)}$ of 10000, the exposure during the first dosing interval would be $AUC\tau_{(SD)} = 10000/1.225 = 8161$ mg.h/L.

- Should we want efficacy during the first dosing interval (first month), we could then administer 155 mg IV every 4 weeks (ie, $126 \times 1.225 \sim 155$), which would translate into an $AUC\tau_{(SS)}$ of 12302 (155/0.0126) and an $AUC\tau_{(SD)}$ of 10040 (12302/1.225).

Let us now estimate what the SC dosing regimen would need to be:

- The maximum dose that can be administered SC is 100 mg/1 mL because of solubility and tolerance issues. A dose of 100 mg SC is only equivalent to 75 mg IV because of the 75% bioavailability. The maximum SC dose that can be administered is only 75/155 = 48.4% of the effective IV monthly dose. The SC dosing regimen will therefore need to be administered much more frequently than once a month, and with a maximum dose that is half of the IV dose, the dosing regimen will need to be associated with an AR of 2 in order to have an equivalent exposure.
- Administering the SC injection every 2 weeks will lead to an AR of 1.75, while administering it every week will lead to an AR of 2.9.
  - AR = 1/exp($-k_{el}*\tau$) = 1/exp ($-0.00252 \times 336$) = 1.75.
  - AR = 1/exp($-k_{el}*\tau$) = 1/exp ($-0.00252 \times 168$) = 2.9.
- With a 100 mg biweekly SC regimen and an accumulation ratio of 1.75, the exposure will be:
  - $AUC\tau_{(SS)} = DOSE/(CL/F) = 100 \times 0.75/0.0126 = 5952.4$ per 2 weeks or 11905 per month.
  - $AUC\tau_{(SD)} = AUC\tau_{(SS)}/AR = 5952.4/1.75 = 2054.5$ during the first 2 weeks.

Administering a SC dose of 100 mg every 2 weeks will result in an efficacious exposure at steady state, similar to the one obtained by giving 155 mg IV every month.

Anti-infective therapy often involves route administration changes, as antimicrobial agents are best administered to severely infected patients by the IV route. This is because severe infections are associated with gastrointestinal disorders, and clinicians cannot risk delaying a potentially life-saving treatment due to inadequate bioavailability. Once the patient has responded to the IV anti-infective therapy and their clinical situation is greatly improved, the therapy may then be changed to the oral route. In situations such as these, knowing the absolute bioavailability of the oral formulation (obtained from the product monograph or label) is essential, as it enables clinicians to continue the anti-infective therapy with an equivalent regimen in terms of safety and efficacy. Finding the absolute bioavailability of an oral formulation is part of the objective of Phase I PK studies.

### Absolute Bioavailability, F

When a drug is given by IV bolus injection or IV infusion, the entire drug dose is given to the patient within the vasculature and therefore "systemic drug absorption" is automatically 100% ($F = 1$). The bioavailability may not be 100% when the same drug is given by a non-IV route of drug administration (eg, oral, intramuscular). The objective of an absolute bioavailability study is to determine what that bioavailability may be compared to the drug administered intravenously.

In an absolute bioavailability study, an IV-administered dose is compared to an oral (or other) formulation of the same drug substance, typically in a crossover design in healthy volunteers. The absolute bioavailability ($F$) will be calculated by dividing the total exposure ($AUC_{inf}$) after oral dosing versus that obtained after IV, multiplied by the ratio of the administered doses (Equation 30.1). This is typically obtained after a single-dose administration study:

$$F = \frac{AUC_{po}}{AUC_{IV}} \times \frac{Dose_{IV}}{Dose_{Po}} \qquad (30.1)$$

An absolute (versus an IV reference) or relative (between different routes of administration) bioavailability study does not have to be conducted if the drug product will never have to be marketed using more than 1 route of administration.

## PRACTICAL PROBLEMS

1. A patient with severe intra-abdominal infection is given an IV infusion of ciprofloxacin 400 mg (Cipro® IV) every 12 hours. Because the signs and symptoms of infection are resolving, the physician wants to switch from IV to oral dosing for better patient compliance and comfort. The drug is supplied as 250-mg and 500-mg Cipro (ciprofloxacin hydrochloride) tablets for oral administration. What would be an appropriate oral dosing regimen that you could recommend?

### Solution

The absolute bioavailability of an oral ciprofloxacin is 70%–80% as per label. In order to achieve the same exposure as its IV administration, we should account for the amount of drug loss when administered orally (PO). Assuming absolute bioavailability is 80% for oral ciprofloxacin tablet, the required dose is calculated as below:

$$F = \frac{AUC_{po}}{AUC_{IV}} \times \frac{Dose_{IV}}{Dose_{Po}}$$

We would desire to have an oral and IV exposure that are exactly the same, therefore,

$$F = \frac{Dose_{IV}}{Dose_{PO}}, \ Dose_{PO} = \frac{400}{0.8} = 500 \text{ mg}$$

The 400 mg IV q12 h therapy can be changed to 500 mg PO q12 h.

2. A patient is hospitalized and being treated for an aspiration pneumonia for which he has been receiving 4 g of ampicillin sodium IV every 6 hours. After 48 hours of sustained clinical improvement, the physician would like to switch to oral therapy. Oral ampicillin is supplied as 250-mg and 500-mg capsules. What would be an appropriate oral dosing regimen?

### Solution

The absolute bioavailability of oral ampicillin is 39%–54%. Assuming an average of 50% oral bioavailability, the equivalent dose to administer would therefore be 8 g PO every 6 hours.

A dose of 8 g of ampicillin cannot be given orally every 6 hours, as it would largely exceed the usually maximum tolerated oral dose of 500 mg every 6 hours. The maximum dose that can be administered PO is therefore 1/16 of the dose that was found to be effective in this patient. An IV to PO switch cannot therefore be done simply with this patient with ampicillin.

Two different alternatives exist. Should the physician believe that the infection is almost completely resolved, then a switch to a lower dose to finish therapy may be considered. This is very unlikely in this case, as the patient has only been treated for 48 hours. The second alternative is to switch to another anti-infective agent that would result in effective concentrations and exposure after oral administration, similar to what is obtained with ampicillin 4 g IV every 6 hours. This is a more complex switch, as it would entail knowing the bacteria causing the infection and making sure that it would be sensitive to the proposed new oral agent.

## Adjustment of Dosing Regimens Over Time

As we have seen in previous chapters, an important attribute of a drug product is its linearity as it regards to both dose and time. Clinicians typically adjust dosing regimens by doubling them in the absence of a sufficient response, or halving them in the presence of safety concerns. This is a simple, yet safe approach to dosing adjustments. But when a drug product is associated with dose nonlinearity, its dosing regimen will have to be modified much more slowly. Should a drug product be associated with nonlinearity over time, then its clearance may increase (eg, due to metabolism induction) or decrease (eg, due to metabolism saturation), resulting in a dosing regimen that may become ineffective or toxic over time. Most drug products that are approved and commercialized display linear pharmacokinetics, but it is essential for a drug product manufacturer to provide this essential PK information in the approved label and/or product monograph so that clinicians know if they can adjust dosing regimens the "typical way" or if they have to be careful and/or follow a particular dosing adjustment algorithm.

A typical example of a drug with nonlinear PK in terms of time is the anticonvulsant agent carbamazepine. Its use induces the expression of CYP3A and P-gp, enzymes and transporter for which carbamazepine is a substrate. Carbamazepine therefore auto-induces its own metabolism and transport such that its dosing regimen in a patient needs to be increased over time as its bioavailability becomes lower (due to increased first-pass metabolism and transport) and its elimination becomes faster

(faster metabolism). Thus, a patient initially dosed with 200 mg BID may need to subsequently receive 200 mg TID, and later 300 mg QID.

PK linearity in terms of dose, commonly called *dose proportionality* by regulators, occurs when exposure increases linearly with dose (Chapter 18). Nonlinearity is usually due to saturation of the elimination processes (eg, phenytoin is a drug example which saturates CYP2C9 enzymes which are responsible for its metabolism). Clearance thereby decreases with increasing plasma concentrations and results in a more than proportional increase in systemic concentrations and exposure with dose. Dose dependence nonlinearity can also be due to other mechanisms, such as saturation of absorption, where a less than proportional increase in concentrations with dose will be observed. Levodopa is a classic example of a drug, which saturates the transporter(s) responsible for its absorption.

Linearity, as it relates to dose and time, will be established within Phase I studies where multiple dosing and range of doses will be studied for their associated safety and pharmacokinetic behavior. The first two studies conducted during Phase I, the FIM SAD and the MAD studies, are described in the next section.

## The First-in-Man Single Ascending Doses Study

The FIM study is traditionally conducted in small single-dose cohorts (eg, four to six healthy volunteers or patients receiving active treatment, and two or three receiving placebo) using a cautious dose escalation scheme. This study is called "SAD" because it tests single doses that are increasing, and will provide essential PK, safety, and tolerability information about the drug.

The starting dose to be given to human subjects is known as the maximum recommended starting dose (MRSD). To establish a safe MRSD, all relevant preclinical results from pharmacology, toxicokinetic studies, and *in vitro* assays and models investigating the drug product have to be considered. Available human experience with other therapies that share the mechanism of action (MOA) should also be considered. The major element in the calculation of the MRSD is the no observed adverse effect levels (NOAELs) which would have been previously obtained in the most appropriate and sensitive species in toxicology studies. The NOAEL is the highest dose level that does not produce a significant increase in adverse effects in comparison to the control group of the tested animal species. The MRSD is most frequently calculated as recommended by the FDA guidance (FDA, 2005) using the following steps:

1. The NOAEL in the most appropriate species is divided by an appropriate conversion factor (scaling factor). This conversion factor (CF) is a unitless number that can convert the animal dose to a human equivalent dose (HED) based on allometric scaling of the average difference in clearance expected. A table is provided in the FDA guidance with recommended CFs.

$$CF = CL \text{ (animal)}/CL \text{ (humans, expected)} \quad (30.2)$$

$$HED = NOAEL \text{ (animal)} \div CF \quad (30.3)$$

2. The MRSD is then obtained by dividing the HED by a safety factor to increase our assurance that the first dose in humans will not cause any significant adverse effects. In general, a safety factor of at least 10 is used.

$$HED \div 10 = MRSD \quad (30.4)$$

## PRACTICAL PROBLEM

The toxicokinetic study results of a new oral drug product indicate the following:

- Sprague Dawley rats receiving single doses of 1, 5, 10, 100, and 1000 mg/kg experienced adverse events at 1000 mg/kg.
- Beagle dogs receiving single doses of 1, 5, 10, 100, and 1000 mg/kg did not experience any adverse events.

What is the MRSD that could be administered in humans in the FIM study?

### Solution

The NOAELs are therefore 100 mg/kg in rats and 1000 mg/kg in dogs (eg, highest dose administered where no effect was seen). The CF proposed in the

US FDA guidance are 6.2 for rats and 1.8 for dogs. The HED are therefore $100/6.2 = 16.13$ mg/kg and $1000/1.8 = 555.55$ mg/kg from the rat and dog NOAELs, respectively. The rat is therefore considered the "sensitive" species, and the HED in humans is therefore 16.13 mg/kg. Using a safety factor of 10, the MRSD in humans is therefore 1.61 mg/kg or 115 mg for a 75 kg person.

Once the starting dose has been determined, it is important to decide what may be the highest dose that will be administered, and how doses will be escalated. The doses studied in the Phase I PK and safety studies should cover the entire range of doses that can be used later during Phase II and III. In addition, what we think may be the therapeutically relevant dose range at that time (which is tentatively determined from *in vitro* and animal disease models) should be covered. A common dose escalation scheme includes five different doses, with what we presume may be the efficacious dose slotted in the middle.

The dose is escalated only if the investigational compound is found to be well tolerated (no serious adverse effect is observed) and the PK data are as expected. Doses are escalated with a difference of approximately 2-fold between each two consecutive ones. In oncology, doses are often increased until the maximum tolerated dose (MTD) is attained, because a lot of oncology agents affect normal cells in addition to cancer cells. The MTD is the highest dose that does not produce unacceptable toxicity (FDA, 2005).

The SAD study is placebo-controlled as well as blinded in order to determine whether the effects observed are due to the study compound or not. The safety and PK results of this study provide an informed decision on dose escalation for investigator review. SAD studies usually include sequential groups (cohorts) in a parallel design, with one cohort for each study dose and the first cohort of subjects receiving the lowest dose (MRSD). For each cohort, sequential dosing entails enrolling two subjects at a 1:1 active-to-placebo ratio followed by the remaining subjects in the respective dose cohort, with an appropriate period of observation between dosing of individual subjects.

There are typically eight to ten subjects per cohort in a SAD study. Within each cohort, subjects receive the same level of dose and each subject receives a single dose. A series of PK samples can be taken to evaluate the PK profiles after the administered dose. In each cohort, subjects are usually randomized in a 3:1 or 4:1 ratio, whereby six to nine subjects receive the active therapy and two to three subjects receive placebo. Therefore, a SAD study with five study doses and eight subjects in each cohort would enroll a total of 40 subjects, with 30 subjects receiving active therapy and the remaining 10 subjects receiving placebo.

The administration of drug in SAD studies is done in a staggered manner with an appropriate period of observation between dosing of individual subjects in a cohort, especially in the early phases. In addition, there is also an observation period between the last dose of a previous cohort and the first dose of the next cohort. After each dosing cohort, safety and tolerability are assessed to determine if the next cohort with a higher dose should be administered or not.

SAD studies are usually conducted in healthy volunteers unless the drug is cytotoxic and has unavoidable toxicity. It is recommended that the healthy volunteers be between 18 and 60 years old to avoid many of the comorbidities or concomitant medications commonly found in the elderly population.

Often when an investigational compound is being dosed in a FIM study, full characterization of its reproductive and embryo/fetal development toxicity has not yet been completed. Therefore, FIM studies are typically conducted in male subjects. Given the gender differences in the PK, safety, and pharmacological response (Liu and Di Pietro Mager, 2016) females of non-childbearing potential (eg, postmenopausal) may be enrolled.

Figure 30-1 illustrates the theoretical mean PK curves, and the associated table shows results for a SAD study involving three different rising doses. From a PK point of view, the objectives of the SAD are to:

1. Investigate what the single dose PK behavior of the drug is, and if it is consistent with the predictions. Should the PK behavior be very different than the predictions in terms of $C_{max}$ and $AUC_{inf}$, then the subsequent planned doses may need to be modified, as the third dose is typically planned to be associated with a target $C_{max}$ and/or $AUC_{inf}$ based on the preclinical and *in vitro* efficacy data.

2. Determine the terminal half-life of the drug, which is used to predict when steady-state conditions may be attained.

3. Determine if the single-dose PK is linear across the dose range studied.

4. Determine the accumulation ratio that should be expected for the future MAD study.

### Multiple Ascending Dose Studies

MAD studies are intended to fully characterize the PK of the investigational compound (and its metabolites if they contribute to the safety and/or efficacy) at steady state. The objectives of the MAD study include the determination of drug accumulation based on a chosen dosing interval, PK behavior (eg, linear or nonlinear PK), and drug safety after repeated dose administration.

Similar to SAD studies, MAD studies are typically conducted in healthy volunteers and include a placebo-controlled cohort. The study design is a single or double blinded parallel design with one cohort for each study dose level and staggered dosing with an appropriate period of observation between two consecutive dose cohorts.

The dose strengths and dosing intervals selected for MAD studies are those that are predicted to be safe (based on SAD study results) while achieving potential therapeutic drug levels. Usually three dose levels at and above what we think may be the expected therapeutic dose level(s) are studied.

In the MAD studies, each dose cohort usually enrolls 6 to 12 subjects randomized in a 3:1 ratio (active treatment: placebo). Each subject receives the same dose multiple times until PK steady-state conditions are achieved. Once steady-state conditions are obtained, systemic PK blood samples are taken to evaluate the PK profiles over the dosing interval at steady state, and the appropriate safety parameters are monitored. Ideally, the PK is also assessed after the first dose, so that PK comparisons in terms of time (single-dose versus steady-state) can be evaluated within individuals. This method is preferred instead of comparing the results of the SAD with the MAD, where different cohorts of subjects are involved.

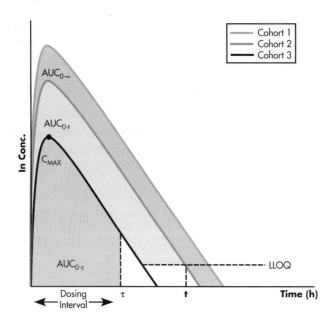

| Cohorts | Dose (mg) | $C_{MAX}$ (mg/L) | $T_{MAX}$(h) | $AUC_{0-\tau}$ (mg.h/L) | $AUC_{0-t}$ (mg.h/L) | $AUC_{0-\infty}$ (mg.h/L) | $t_{1/2}$(h) | CL/F (L/h) |
|---------|-----------|-------|----------|---------|---------|---------|----------|-------|
| 1 | 50 | 10 | 6 | 250 | 350 | 355 | 7 | 0.141 |
| 2 | 150 | 32 | 5.8 | 735 | 980 | 1095 | 7.5 | 0.137 |
| 3 | 300 | 58 | 6.2 | 1652 | 2210 | 2428 | 7.3 | 0.124 |

**These PK parameters should be relatively constants through the different administered doses if the PK is linear**

**These PK parameters should be "dose-proportional" through the different administered doses if the PK is linear**

**FIGURE 30-1 •** Theoretical PK curves and results table for an SAD involving three rising doses.

If the PK is linear, the ratio of $AUC_{0\text{-inf}}/AUC_{0\text{-}\tau}$ or accumulation ratio seen in the SAD will be equal to the ratio of the $AUC_{\tau(ss)}$ seen in the MAD with the $AUC_{0\text{-}\tau}$ seen in the SAD. At steady-state, the $AUC_{0\text{-inf}}$ seen after a single dose in the SAD should be equal to the $AUC_{\tau(ss)}$ that will be seen in the MAD. The therapeutic interval ($\tau$) chosen for the MAD is selected based on the desired accumulation ratio. Figure 30-1 shows a predicted accumulation ratio of ~1.5 with a 12-hour dosing interval from the SAD (ie, $AUC_{0\text{-inf}}/AUC_{0\text{-}\tau}$~1.5). If the drug is very safe and there is no desire for any significant accumulation, the dosing regimen will be designed so that the first

dosing interval is efficacious. It may then be favorable to administer the drug every two half-lives (ie, accumulation ratio of ~1.33) or even less frequently if the minimum effective concentration is very low and allows it. Chapter 12 provides additional details on the clinical utility of the CL and $T_{1/2}$ in selecting dosing regimens. Some antipsychotic drugs give a lot of side effects in the first few doses, with built-up tolerance over time. For these drugs, subjects are given small doses that may not necessarily be efficacious early on, but they increase tolerability. Administering smaller doses more frequently will lead to more drug accumulation (eg, dosing twice every half-life will lead to ~3.4 accumulation), with the goal of having an exposure during the dosing interval at steady state that will be much higher and efficacious. At steady-state conditions with "efficacious" exposure, the subjects will experience fewer side effects due to the slower build-up of drug exposure.

Figure 30-2 illustrates the theoretical mean PK curves and results for the MAD study involving three different rising doses, using the same drug example presented in Fig. 30-1 (SAD). From a PK point of view, the objectives of the MAD are to:

1. Investigate what the steady-state PK profiles of the drug and whether the PK results are consistent with the PK results from the single dose SAD study.

2. Investigate whether the PK is dose proportional (across the different dosing cohorts) and is linear with time (comparing single-dose and steady-state data).

3. Assess the accumulation potential at steady-state with the dosing interval selected, and verify whether

it is consistent with the obtained terminal half-life obtained from the SAD and/or MAD studies.

## PRACTICAL PROBLEM

Based on the following information for each drug to be developed, what dosing regimen do you think may be appropriate for further testing?

Drug A

Safe drug with no significant adverse events,
$CL = 1$ L/h, targeted $AUC_{0-\tau(SS)} = 1000$ mcg*h/L,
$T_{1/2} = 6$ h

Drug B

Drug with significant adverse events that may become better tolerated over time,
$CL = 1$ L/h, targeted $AUC_{0-\tau(SS)} = 1000$ mcg*h/L,
$T_{1/2} = 24$ h

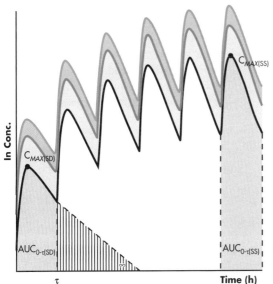

- $AR = C_{MAX(SS)}/C_{MAX(SD)}$
  or
  $AUC_{0-\tau(SS)}/AUC_{0-\tau(SD)}$

- If PK is linear with time
  $AUC_{0-\infty(SD)}=AUC_{0-\tau(SS)}$

| Cohorts | $C_{MAX(SD)}$ (mg/L) | $C_{MAX(SD)}$ (mg/L) | $AR_{(Cmax)}$ | $AUC_{0-\tau}$ (mg.h/L) | $AUC_{0-\tau(SS)}$ (mg.h/L) | $AUC_{0-\infty(SD)}$ (mg.h/L) | $AR_{(AUC)}$ | $T_{1/2(SS)}$ (h) |
|---|---|---|---|---|---|---|---|---|
| 1 | 9.5 | 15 | 1.58 | 237 | 355 | 355 | 1.5 | 8 |
| 2 | 34 | 45 | 1.32 | 842 | 1095 | 1095 | 1.3 | 6.8 |
| 3 | 57 | 85 | 1.49 | 1630 | 2428 | 2428 | 1.49 | 7.5 |

FIGURE 30-2 • Theoretical PK curves and results table for an MAD involving three rising doses.

## Solution

### Drug A

Because the drug is safe, we can take advantage of its tolerability and achieve efficacious exposure during the first dosing interval ($AUC_{0-\tau(SD)}$). We therefore want a dosing interval associated with very little accumulation.

We have seen the accumulation ratio (AR) equation in Chapter 17. Using a dosing interval of two or more half-lives will provide with little accumulation.

With a dosing interval of 12 hours, the AR will be:

$$AR = \frac{1}{1-e^{-\frac{0.693*\Delta t}{T1/2}}} \quad AR = \frac{1}{1-e^{-\frac{0.693*12}{6}}} = 1.33$$

We also know that AR could be calculated as ratio for AUCs:

$$AR = \frac{AUC_{0-\tau(SS)}}{AUC_{0-\tau(SD)}}$$

Hence, with a 12-hour dosing interval, the steady state exposure over the dosing interval will only be 1.33 times higher than the first one:

$$AUC_{0-\tau(SD)} = AUC_{0-\tau(SS)}/1.33 = 1000/1.33 \sim 750$$

### Drug B

Drug B is associated early on with significant adverse events. A dosing regimen can be developed with significant drug accumulation, so that early exposures are smaller, allowing the patient to better tolerate the drug over time.

Using the AR equation in Chapter 17, dosing more frequently than the half-life will lead to accumulation.

With a dosing interval of 12 hours, the AR will be:

$$AR = \frac{1}{1-e^{-\frac{0.693*\Delta t}{T1/2}}} = \frac{1}{1-e^{-\frac{0.693*12}{24}}} = 3.4.$$

Hence the first $AUC_{0-\tau(SD)}$ will be 3.4 times lower than the effective one at steady state. This will mean that efficacy will be delayed in time so that patients can better tolerate the drug.

$$AUC_{0-\tau(SD)} = \frac{AUC_{0-\tau(SS)}}{AR} = \frac{1000}{3.4} = 292.8 \text{ mcg} * \text{h/L}.$$

## Impact of Food on a Drug Product's PK Behavior

We have seen in Chapter 8 how food can affect a drug product in multiple ways. This includes affecting its dissolution and pH stability, delaying gastric emptying time, and possibly affecting the activity of transporters and enzymes within the gut wall. These factors may affect the overall bioavailability of a drug product and the speed at which maximum concentrations are attained ($t_{max}$). The effect of food can be minimal or it can be dramatic, resulting in several-fold increases or decreases in exposure.

The effect of food on BA is evaluated by calculating the geometric mean ratios (GMRs) of exposure measures (AUC and $C_{max}$) under fed versus fasted conditions and the 90% confidence intervals (CIs) around these ratios. An absence of food effect on BA is concluded when the 90% CIs for the GMRs (fed/fasted) of $C_{max}$, $AUC_{0-t}$, and $AUC_{inf}$ are all contained within the considered "clinically equivalent" limits of 80%–125%.

Food effect BA studies are usually conducted in a randomized, balanced, single-dose, two-treatment, two-period, two-sequence crossover design, and in a similar manner to the PK equivalence studies of a generic product under fed conditions (see Chapter 29). The main difference is that in a food effect study we only investigate one drug product but under two conditions. In the fed arm of a food effect study, the drug product is typically administered 30 minutes after the start of a high-caloric, high-fat breakfast that has to be completely ingested within 30 minutes.

Different food regimens can be administered in this food effect study, as long as it is well stated in the product label. As shown in Table 30-2, the FDA final guidance provides an example of a test meal that can be used for such studies. They, and most if not all regulatory agencies, recommend a high-fat (approximately 50% of total caloric content of the meal) and a high-calorie breakfast that is approximately between 800 to 1000 calories (FDA, 2019). As with any PK equivalence study (see Chapter 29), an adequate washout period is required to differentiate the two treatments adequately and to eliminate any possibility of carryover. A rich PK sampling should be used,

## TABLE 30-2 • An Example of a High-Calorie, High-Fat Meal Used in Food Effect Studies

| Food Group | Calories Required | Meal Example |
|---|---|---|
| Carbohydrate | 250 | Two eggs fried in butter, two strips of bacon, two slices of toast with butter, four ounces of hash brown potatoes, and eight ounces of whole milk* |
| Protein | 150 | |
| Fat | 500–600 | |

*Substitutions can be made as long as the meal provides a similar amount of calories from protein, carbohydrate, and fat and has comparable meal volume and viscosity

and the highest drug product strength intended to be marketed is selected unless PK nonlinearity due to food is known (for example, for the EU market), and the most discriminative strength for that condition should then be tested.

Unless safety concerns preclude their enrolment, as is often the case with oncology drugs, the study should be conducted in healthy volunteers. If a significant food effect is expected, then the 90% CI for the GMR (fed/fasted) would not likely fall within the clinical equivalence limits of 80%–125% even when recruiting a large sample of subjects. In those cases, the study will therefore lead to the appropriate conclusion of food effect even when completed with a minimum of 12 subjects. If, however, no significant food effect is expected, then the study will need to be powered correctly (minimum of 80%) to show the absence of food effect on the 90% CIs.

From the generated concentration–time profiles, the PK parameters (particularly $T_{max}$, $C_{max}$, $AUC_{0-t}$, and $AUC_{inf}$) under both fasted and fed conditions should be derived and reported. Population GMR (fed/fasted) of $C_{max}$, $AUC_{0-t}$, and $AUC_{inf}$ and their 90% CIs must then be calculated.

The absence of a food effect allows a manufacturer to report that their drug product can be given with or without food, which in terms of dosing convenience is a very desirable attribute. If a food effect is observed, then the results should be evaluated from a clinical perspective. A difference in the $C_{max}$

fed/fasted ratio of 25% with no concomitant change in AUCs may not be clinically relevant if safety and efficacy are only related to AUCs. The product monograph will need to present the observed results and mention their clinical relevance. Food typically delays stomach emptying and slows the absorption process without affecting its extent. This often results in a $t_{max}$ delay, with up to approximately 20% decrease in $C_{max}$, and without any change in $AUC_{0-t}$ or $AUC_{0-inf}$.

Students and clinicians often question the relevance of the food effect study due to the high-fat, high-caloric content of the meal given. This actual meal is not *meant* to be relevant to what a patient would take in the morning per se. Instead, it is considered to be the "extreme" condition in comparison to fasting. Hence, should a drug product's PK performance be similar under these two extreme conditions (fasted AND high-fat, high-caloric breakfast), it can be assumed that any other type of meal would also be of no PK effect.

### Mass–Balance Study

Mass–balance animal drug studies have to be conducted during the preclinical phase, for example with a radiolabeled drug compound (eg, one or more carbons are labeled with $^{14}C$). That study gives important information on whether or not the drug is completely eliminated from the body, and how. Despite the often very divergent PK characteristics between animal species and humans, there is no strict regulatory requirement for such a study in humans. Feces and urinary excretion data are often collected from the single or multiple ascending dose studies, allowing the estimation of how much drug is eliminated over time and how. For drug products displaying relatively "simple" pharmacokinetics (eg, mostly eliminated unchanged in the urine or metabolized to one main metabolite), the results obtained will be sufficient for deciding if a renal and/or an hepatic impairment study(ies) is(are) needed, and to confirm that the correct analytes are being measured within the pivotal PK studies. As a general rule, a minimum of 80% of the systemic exposure should be characterized. Three hypothetical drug product examples are presented in Table 30-3, showing when a mass–balance study may or may not be needed.

**TABLE 30-3 •** Examples of PK Results for Hypothetical Drug Products from Phase I Studies in Terms of Elimination and Recovery and for Which a Mass Balance Study May Need To Be Conducted

| Drug Product Example | Results of SAD and MAD Studies | Interpretation and Next Steps |
|---|---|---|
| 1 | Dose recovered as 90% of parent drug in the urine | Renal impairment study needed (>20% of elimination through the kidney)<br>No need for hepatic impairment study (<20% of elimination through the liver)<br>No need for mass–balance study (>80% of the dose recovered) |
| 2 | Dose recovered as 20% of parent drug and 70% of active hydroxy-lated metabolite in the urine | Renal *and* hepatic impairment studies needed (>20% of elimination through both kidneys and liver)<br>No need for mass–balance study (>80% of the dose recovered) |
| 3 | Dose recovered as parent drug and inactive metabolite in urine (30%) and feces (10%) | Renal impairment study needed (>20% of elimination through the kidney)<br>Hepatic impairment likely needed (other metabolites must be formed)<br>Mass–balance study should be conducted to better understand the analytes that need to be measured in PK studies to ensure that a minimum of 80% of the exposure and elimination is characterized and understood |

In the mass–balance study, each subject is given a single dose of the drug product that contains a small known amount of radioactivity (micro-curies). Biological samples including blood, urine, and feces are obtained after dosing until the drug product is believed to be at least 90%–95% completely eliminated from the body. All samples are measured in terms of the known analytes (parent and metabolites). The total radioactivity in each sample is assayed and the relationship between what is measured analytically and from a radioactivity point of view is assessed. Because of the complexity of this study, few subjects are enrolled, typically six.

The goal is to make sure that the analytes measured by the analytical method (eg, parent and main metabolite[s]) account for at least 80% of what is measured systemically and what is excreted in the urine and in the feces. This will then suggest that no additional analytes need to be measured. Additional investigations will need to be conducted, such as metabolite profiling, if less than 80% of the total radioactivity is explained by the analytes measured and excreted.

The overall goals of this mass–balance study in humans are:

1. To determine whether additional analytes/metabolites need to be measured and investigated from a PK point of view.

2. To confirm that the drug product is eventually eliminated from the human body.

3. To confirm whether a renal impairment and/or a hepatic impairment study(ies) need(s) to be conducted.

The three goals above are assessed in the following manner:

1. No additional analytes need to be measured in plasma (or serum or blood, depending on the matrix used) if the sum of all of the measured analytes in plasma in terms of $AUC_t$ contribute to at least 80% of the $AUC_t$ of the total plasma radioactivity.

2. A minimum of 80% of the administered dose should be recovered in urine and feces over the studied time interval.

3. If less than 20% of the total radioactivity is recovered in urine, then a renal impairment study would not be needed but a hepatic impairment would be required. Should more than 80% of the total radioactivity be recovered in the urine, then the renal impairment study will be needed, while the hepatic one will not be. Both impairment studies will typically be needed if the recovery in urine ranges between 20% and 80%.

## Renal Impairment Study

Renal drug excretion is one of the principal elimination pathways of the removal of drugs from the body. Impairment of kidney function can therefore affect the PK of drugs by influencing the distribution (changes in protein binding can affect the volumes of distribution) and elimination of drugs. Renal impairment or a decrease in renal function may result in a reduced elimination rate constant (or a longer elimination half-life) resulting in a reduction in the clearance of the drug from the body. Reduced drug clearance can lead to drug accumulation within the body and increased exposure. Patients with impaired renal function may be at significant risk of toxicity or adverse events as a result of the prolonged and/or elevated exposure. Accordingly, if a drug or its major active metabolite(s) is (are) substantially excreted by the kidney, alterations in renal function will impact significantly its (their) exposure(s). Should this be the case, the dosing regimen of the drug product will then need to be adjusted.

The renal clearance of drugs relate to the kidney's glomerular filtration rate, re-absorption, and secretion pathways. As seen in Chapter 25, the overall renal function is typically assessed using the calculated creatinine clearance (CrCL) with the Cockcroft–Gault or the MDRD equations. The majority of renal impairment studies have been so far conducted using the Cockcroft–Gault equation (Cockcroft and Gault, 1976; Equation 30.5):

$$CrCL = \frac{((140 - age) \times weight)}{72 \times Scr} \times 0.85 \text{ (if female)}$$

$$(30.5)$$

CrCL is the estimated creatinine clearance in mL/min, age is the age of the patient in years, weight is the actual body weight in kg, and Scr represents the serum creatinine in mg/dL.

The method used to estimate renal function must be an established method. The approved drug label specifies which equation was used in the renal impairment study so that clinicians can use the same method to adapt the dosing regimen for their patients.

The clearance of drug is composed of the renal $(CL_R)$ and the non-renal $(CL_{NR})$ clearance. The renal clearance will correlate with the renal function as assessed by the creatinine clearance formula used. The non-renal clearance usually stays constant, unless very severe impairment is seen, and during which the hepatic function may also be affected (eg, hepato-renal syndrome). The relationship between these clearances is what the renal impairment study aims to characterize, and is presented for a theoretical drug in Fig. 30-3.

To appropriately determine the relationship between the drug clearance and the calculated creatinine clearance, subjects with varying levels of renal function need to be included in the study. The US FDA guidance on conducting such a study recommends including the groups presented in Table 30-4.

The number of subjects to be enrolled in each group depends on the expected variability in PK. While the EMA suggests six to eight subjects per group (EMA Guidance, 2015), the FDA draft guidance does not provide an exact number of subjects, but specifies that the sample size must be sufficient to detect any meaningful differences in PK between renally impaired patients and control subjects (FDA CDER, 2010). Renal impairment studies are typically conducted as single-dose studies when the drug and active metabolites exhibit linear PK. Multiple-dose studies may be preferred when the PK is nonlinear, and/or when activity is due to metabolites and/or analytes that accumulate over time. For safety purposes, it is recommended to administer the lowest effective dose.

Blood and urine samples should be analyzed for concentrations of the parent drug and the active metabolites in order to estimate the various PK parameters in patients with different stages of renal

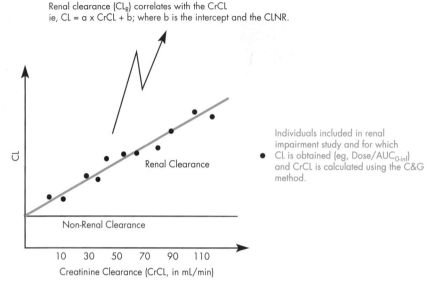

Renal clearance ($CL_R$) correlates with the CrCL
ie, CL = a × CrCL + b; where b is the intercept and the CLNR.

Individuals included in renal
impairment study and for which
CL is obtained (eg, Dose/$AUC_{0-inf}$)
and CrCL is calculated using the C&G
method.

Renal Clearance

Non-Renal Clearance

CL

Creatinine Clearance (CrCL, in mL/min)

10    30    50    70    90    110

**FIGURE 30-3 •** The relationship between drug clearance, renal clearance, and non-renal clearance for a theoretical drug product in a renal impairment study.

impairment. A relationship between the relevant PK parameters and renal function (eg, CrCl or GFR) is then established.

## CLINICAL PROBLEM

A male (70 years old) suffers from a hospital acquired pneumonia due to a suspected strain of *P. aeruginosa*. His level of serum creatinine is 1.1 mg/dL and his actual body weight is 72 kg. What

dosing regimen of imipenem/cilastatin should be administered to the patient based on his apparent renal function?

### Solution

Imipenem/cilastatin is marketed under the trade name Primaxin® by Merck Sharpe and Dohme. According to the approved US FDA drug label, Merck has conducted a renal impairment study for this product which provides the table suggesting the dosing regimens depending on creatine clearance values. On the label, it is clearly stated that the recommendations are based on the use of the Cockroft–Gault equation to calculate the creatinine clearance. The pertinent section of the label is reproduced below and in Table 30-5.

Dosing instructions for Primaxin based on renal impairment study results are presented in the official product label (Merck Sharp & Dohme, 2019).

*Dosage in Adult Patients with Renal Impairment*

*Patients with creatinine clearance less than 90 mL/min require dosage reduction of Primaxin as indicated in Table 30-5. The serum creatinine should represent a steady state of renal function. Use the Cockcroft-Gault method described below to calculate the creatinine clearance.*

**TABLE 30–4 •** Classes of Renal Function Typically Studied in a Renal Impairment Study

| Description of Renal Function | Range of Values for Renal Function (mL/min) |
|---|---|
| Control (normal renal function) | ≥90 |
| Mild impairment in GFR | 60–89 |
| Moderate impairment in GFR | 30–59 |
| Severe impairment in GFR | 15–29 |
| End stage of renal disease (ESRD) | <15 or dialysis patients on non-dialysis days |

**TABLE 30-5** • Dosage of PRIMAXIN˙ for Adult Patients in Various Renal Function Groups Based on Estimated Creatinine Clearance (CLcr), from Primaxin Label

| | Creatinine Clearance (mL/min) | | | |
|---|---|---|---|---|
| | Greater than or equal to 90 | Less than 90 or greater than or equal to 60 | Less than 60 to greater than or equal to 30 | Less than 30 to greater than or equal to 15 |
| Dosage of PRIMAXIN*,† if the infection is suspected or proven to be due to a susceptible bacterial species | 500 mg every 6 hours | 400 mg every 6 hours | 300 mg every 6 hours<br><br>OR | 200 mg every 6 hours |
| | 1000 mg every 8 hours | 500 mg every 6 hours | 500 mg every 8 hours | 500 mg every 12 hours |
| Dosage of PRIMAXIN*,†, if the infection is suspected or proven to be bacterial species with intermediate susceptibility | 1000 mg every 6 hours | 750 mg every 8 hours | 500 mg every 6 hours | 500 mg every 12 hours |

\* Administer doses less than or equal to 500 mg by intravenous infusion over 20–30 minutes. Discard unused portion of the infusion solution.
† Administer doses greater than 500 mg by intravenous infusion over 40–60 minutes. In patients who develop nausea during the infusion, the rate of infusion may be slowed.
Data from Merck Sharp & Dohme: Primaxin®. Highlights of prescribing information, FDA approved label. 2019.

*Males:*

$$CrCL = \frac{((\text{weight in kg}) \times (140 - \text{age in years}))}{72 \times Scr\left(\frac{mg}{100\ mL}\right)}$$

*Females: 0.85 × (value calculated for males)*

Our patient creatinine clearance is:

$$CrCL = (140 - 70) \times 72/(72 \times 1.1) = 63.6\ \text{mL/min}$$

Therefore, the dosing regimen to administer in this patient is 500 mg every 6 hours.

### Hepatic Impairment Study

Hepatic disease can lead to dysfunction of the liver enzymes responsible for drug metabolism. Due to the importance of the liver in removing drugs from the body, its impairment may lead to drug accumulation, failure to form active metabolites, increased bioavailability after oral administration due to lower first-pass metabolism, and other effects such as alterations in drug–protein binding. As a consequence, hepatic dysfunction can alter many aspects of the PK of a drug such as its bioavailability, its elimination, and its volumes of distribution. A drug dosing regimen may therefore need to be adjusted in complicated ways in patients with hepatic impairment.

As mentioned in Chapter 25, there are no known markers at this time that correlate well with hepatic function in a way comparable to creatinine clearance and renal function. Although many techniques, calculations, and nomograms have been proposed and investigated throughout the years, the current method of choice to correlate with hepatic clearance is still the Child–Pugh classification. This method was developed originally to predict the risk of surgery in patients with portal hypertension. This risk was classified as "mild," "moderate," or "severe," and these terms have later been used to classify hepatic function. The Child–Pugh classification (Pugh et al, 1973) is presented in Table 30-6. Other classifications, such as the National Cancer Institute (NCI) index or the model for end-stage liver disease (MELD) score, have been proposed and are sometimes used in hepatic impairment studies, but the Child–Pugh is still currently the method of choice in drug development.

The need to conduct a hepatic impairment study is required when a drug product is eliminated by at least 20% by the liver in a normal adult patient

**TABLE 30-6** • The Child–Pugh (1973) Classification, a Commonly Used Method to Predict Hepatic Impairment in Patients

| Clinical Observation/Situation | Points Scored for Observed Findings | | |
| --- | --- | --- | --- |
| | 1 point | 2 points | 3 points |
| Encephalopathy grade | None | 1–2 | 3–4 |
| Ascites | Absent | Slight | Moderate |
| Bilirubin (mg/dL) | <2 | 2–3 | >3 |
| Albumin (g/dL) | >3.5 | 2.8–3.5 | <2.8 |
| Prothrombin time prolongation (sec) | <4 | 4–6 | >6 |
| Risk of surgery/hepatic function | | | |
| | Mild | Moderate | Severe |
| Total points scored | 5–6 points | 7–9 points | 10–15 points |

or subject. In such a study, patients are recruited so that all three groups are tested ("mild," "moderate," and "severe") often with an additional control group of healthy volunteers. A minimum of six to eight patients in each group is recommended, although in practice the "severe" group is often much smaller (and sometimes absent) due to recruitment difficulties.

In a similar manner to renal impairment studies, the drug product will be studied after single dosing, or multiple dosing should the PK not be linear or the dosing interval associated with significant accumulation of the analytes of interest. As with any other PK studies, the duration of blood sampling should be long enough to characterize the observed AUC (ie, $AUC_{0-t}$) to at least 80% of the total exposure ($AUC_{0-inf}$) of the different analytes. A distinction of the hepatic impairment study is the need to measure free drug concentrations, not only total concentrations, as protein binding is often altered in these patients. As seen in previous chapters, particularly in Chapter 6, the unbound concentrations are the active moiety for the vast majority of drugs, and changes in the percentage of drug unbound ($f_u$) will lead to different interpretation of results for highly versus poorly liver extracted drugs. An example of this is presented in Fig. 30-4 for a theoretical drug only eliminated by the liver (extreme scenario). This figure highlights that, except for the specific case of a high extraction drug administered IV, a liver impairment study

could show a decrease in half of the total exposure ($C_{max}$ and AUC), suggesting erroneously that the dosing regimen would need to be doubled, while in reality, free concentrations would remain unchanged.

Hepatic impairment studies should therefore always include the measurement of free drug concentrations, not only total, to make sure that the correct dosing recommendation be derived and proposed when drugs are bound to plasma proteins.

An example of results and associated proposed dosing regimens is presented in Fig. 30-5. The PK of an anticancer agent, not significantly bound to plasma proteins, and administered in m² of body surface area (BSA) is illustrated.

### Drug–Drug Interaction Studies

Drug–drug interactions (DDIs) may occur when two drugs are concomitantly administered, resulting in potential changes in the efficacy and/or safety of one or both drugs. This change may be due to an alteration in the drug product's local and/or systemic exposure, as well as a direct change in its activity (PD). The PK alterations may occur at many different stages, such as in the absorption, distribution, and/or elimination.

It is essential for the product label to advise clinicians on how to adjust the drug product's dosing regimen for a given patient, when other drugs are concomitantly added or removed. DDIs that should be tested include those involving drugs that

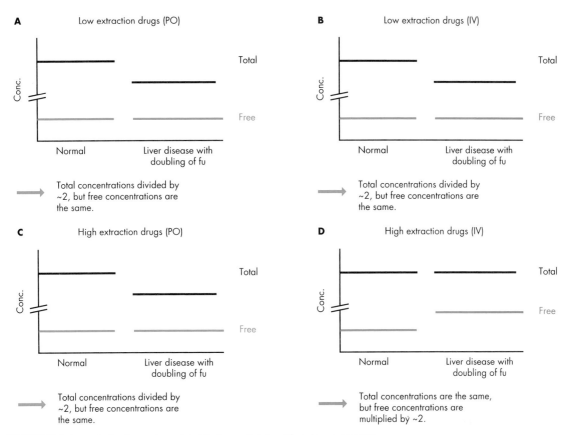

FIGURE 30-4 • Impact of a change in protein binding on total and free drug exposures.

are likely to be coadministered in clinical practice and likely to interact, for example, based on common elimination pathways. Common DDIs involve the induction or inhibition of CYP enzymes which are found in most tissues of the human body, but notably in the liver and the gut wall. Induction of the activity of these enzymes, through the increase of their biosynthesis, will result in an increased metabolism and decreased exposure of their substrates, while inhibition of their activity will lead to decreased elimination and increased exposure of their substrates. DDI knowledge and the understanding of the mechanisms behind their occurrence have become of great interest over the last 30 years. We now know that inhibition or induction of enzymatic and/or transport activity are often responsible for DDIs that originally were thought to be a result of other mechanisms such as plasma protein displacements (eg, warfarin interactions) or changes in the gut bacterial flora (eg, digoxin interactions) (McElnay and D'Arcy, 1983).

Major advances in our knowledge and understanding of drug metabolism and transport have resulted in the conduct of DDI studies that are more focused. Regulatory guidances, especially those of the FDA, are continuously updated as science progresses. In their latest guidance (FDA, 2020), the FDA recommends the use of specific substrates and "index perpetrators" in DDI studies. Substrates are drugs that adequately reflect a metabolic pathway in terms of activity with their own clearance or with a specific metabolite/parent ratio. These are used in *cocktail studies*, experiments where multiple substrates are given together with the drug product, to see if the drug product has the likelihood of interfering with any of these substrates' metabolic pathways.

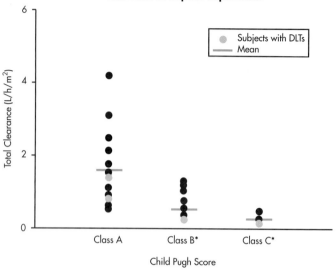

**Relationship between Patient's BSA-adjusted Total Plasma Clearance and Level of Hepatic Impairment**

| PK Parameter | | | Class A (N=16) | Child-Pugh Score Class B (N=13) | Class C (N=4) |
|---|---|---|---|---|---|
| Total CL/BSA (L/h/m²) | Geometric Mean | | 1.320 | 0.421 | 0.245 |
| | | | Statistical Analysis and Interpretation | | |
| | 90% CI | | Class B vs. Class A | Class C vs. Class A | Class C vs. Class B |
| | | | 31.9% (21.2%–47.9%) | 18.6% (10.1%–34.2%) | 58.3% (31.2%–108.8%) |
| | Possible Dosage Adjustment | | Class A | Class B | Class C |
| | | | 1 Dose to be given | 1/3 Dose to be given | 1/5 Dose to be given |

FIGURE 30-5 • Results of a hepatic impairment study for an anticancer agent not significantly bound to plasma proteins.

*Index perpetrators* are the drugs that the FDA recommends to use in DDI studies as inducers or inhibitors of a specific metabolic pathway. The design of a DDI study will be proposed based on the following:

1. The transport and metabolic pathways of the drug product should be known (eg, which CYP, NAT, or UGT enzyme[s], and/or which ABC and/or SLT transporter[s]).

2. Drugs that are likely to be co-administered and which share the same transport and metabolic pathways will be chosen as either substrates

(to see what the effect on them is), or as "DDI-causing drugs," also called index perpetrators (to see the effect they cause on the drug being developed). Some examples can be found in Table 30-7.

3. Drugs that utilize the same enzyme pathway or same transporter will compete competitively or noncompetitively. The result of this competition is that one drug inhibits the metabolism of another drug. Inhibition is usually considered to be "reversible" or "competitive" and will usually be moderate in percentage (40% or lower).

## TABLE 30-7 • Clinical Index Substrates and Perpetrators That Can be Used in DDI Studies

| Enzymes and Transporters | | Index Substrates | Index Perpetrators | |
| --- | --- | --- | --- | --- |
| | | | Inhibitors | Inducers |
| CYP | CYP1A2 | Caffeine<br>Theophylline | Ciprofloxacin<br>Fluvoxamine | Phenobarbital<br>Phenytoin<br>Smoking |
| | CYP2C9 | Tolbutamide<br>S-Warfarin | Fluconazole | Phenobarbital<br>Rifampin |
| | CYP2C19 | Lansoprazole<br>Omeprazole | Fluconazole<br>Fluvoxamine | Rifampin |
| | CYP2D6 | Desipramine<br>Dextromethorphan | Fluoxetine<br>Paroxetine | None known |
| | CYP3A | Midazolam | Clarithromycin<br>Erythromycin<br>Itraconazole<br>Ketoconazole | Carbamazepine<br>Phenobarbital<br>Phenytoin<br>Rifampin |
| NAT | NAT1 | Sulfamethoxazole | | |
| | NAT2 | Caffeine<br>Dapsone<br>Isoniazide<br>Hydralazine<br>Procainamide | | |
| UGT | UGT1A1 | Belinostat<br>Estradiol<br>SN-38 | Indinavir | Phenobarbital<br>Smoking |
| | UGT1A3 | Sulindac sulfone<br>Thyroxine | | |
| | UGT1A4 | Trifluoperazine | | |
| | UGT1A9 | Acetaminophen | | |
| ABC | P-gp (*ABCB1*) | Digoxin<br>Fexofenadine | Cyclosporine<br>Erythromycin<br>Ketoconazole<br>Ritonavir<br>Verapamil | Carbamazepine<br>Phenobarbital<br>Phenytoin<br>Rifampin |
| | MRP2<br>(*ABCC2*) | Indinavir | Cyclosporine | |
| SLC | OATP1B1<br>(*SLCO1B1*) | Pravastatin<br>Rosuvastatin | Cyclosporine | |
| | OAT3<br>(*SLC22A8*) | Methotrexate<br>Pravastatin | Probenecid | |
| | OCT2<br>(*SLC22A2*) | Metformin | Cimetidine | |

*CYP, prefix for CYP enzymes (previously known as P450); NAT, prefix for N-acetyl transferase enzymes; UGT, prefix for UDP-glucuronosyltransferase enzymes; prefix for ABC, prefix for ATP-binding cassette transporters; SLC, prefix for solute carrier transporters.*
*Data from Evans, 1993; Liu et al, 2014; Lv et al, 2019; Drug Development and Drug Interactions. Table of Substrates, Inhibitors and Inducers. U.S. Department of Health and Human Services. Food and Drug Administration.*

4. *Strong* inhibitors, such as ketoconazole for CYP3A or ciprofloxacin for CYP1A2 enzymes, will usually result in a greater than 40% inhibition of the metabolism of substrates for these enzymes.

5. *Strong* inducers of CYP enzymes or of the P-glycoprotein transporter (ABCB1) (eg, phenobarbital, phenytoin, rifampin) will usually result in a greater than 40% increase in metabolism and transport.

The design of the DDI study will be dependent on the suspected mechanism of the interaction. If the DDI study is aimed at looking at the impact of an inducer on the PK of a drug product, then the inducer will normally have to be administered for a minimum of 14 days before co-administering the drug product, because that is the normal time it takes for CYP induction to take place. As seen in Chapter 23, induction in enzymatic activity is due to increased protein synthesis. A certain time period is required for an inducer drug to begin increasing the amount of enzymes or transporters, and to reach the induction "steady state." Withdrawal of the inducer will result in a slow return to the original enzyme concentrations, as a certain number of half-lives of the metabolizing enzymes must elapse in order to return to baseline concentration levels after the inducer has been fully eliminated. Compounds with long half-lives will require a longer period of time for induction to occur and disappear, while it will be shorter for perpetrators with short half-lives. For instance, an inducer drug such as rifampin with a half-life of 2–3 hours can reach maximum levels within 2 days, quicker than the actual time it can take to create the new enzymes (which may take a week or two). Phenobarbital with a half-life of ≈3 days and fluoxetine with a half-life of ≈4 days, may only fully display steady-state levels after weeks of exposure. Therefore, if a patient needs to start phenobarbital (inducer of CYP1A2, CYP2C9, CYP2C19, and CYP3A) and theophylline concomitantly, the full decrease in theophylline concentrations (due to the increased metabolism induced by phenobarbital), may not be observed until 2–3 weeks from the start of the concomitant treatment.

A DDI study looking at inhibition will need to be designed according to the mechanism of the inhibition. Inhibition occurs via three main mechanisms, reversible or competitive, quasi-irreversible, and irreversible. With reversible inhibition, the simplest scenario, the substrate and inhibitor drug products directly compete for binding at the active site of the enzyme or transporter, and therefore the degree of inhibition will be altered by the actual concentration of the inhibitor. Reversible inhibition occurs rapidly with the maximum inhibition seen at the $C_{max}$ of the inhibitor. The minimum of inhibition will be seen at the $C_{min}$ of the inhibitor. The inhibition will completely disappear once the inhibitor has been completely removed from the body (eg, seven terminal half-lives). All inhibitors of CYP enzymes appear to always have the capability of inhibiting substrates of the same enzyme. In contrast, inhibitors of the P-gp transporter do not always inhibit the transport of P-gp substrates. Increased bioavailability of digoxin has been demonstrated when administered with P-gp inhibitors such as clarithromycin or atorvastatin (Boyd et al, 2000; Tanaka et al, 2003), but not every P-gp substrate may interact with digoxin. The current working hypothesis for this is that there are at least two different binding sites on P-gp, and a drug will only interact with another one if they both bind to the exact same site (Aller, 2009; Alam, 2019). With a mechanism of reversible inhibition, the inhibitor perpetrator can be administered 2 or 3 days before the concomitant single dose administration of the drug product in order to make sure that the inhibitor concentrations are high enough to ensure that the interaction will be observed if it exists. The study design will usually be a crossover design study in which the drug product will also be administered as a single dose without the perpetrator. A washout period that is sufficient to ensure the complete disappearance of the drug product and the index perpetrator needs to be included.

Irreversible and quasi-irreversible inhibitors will, in contrast, result in a long-lasting inhibition. Irreversible inhibitors destroy enzymes such that new enzymes have to be synthesized. An example of this is grapefruit juice, which destroys CYP3A enzymes and P-gp transporters in the gut wall, and the overall effect of one glass of grapefruit juice may not completely disappear until 7–14 days have elapsed (Pasternyk Di Marco et al, 2002), which is the time it takes to synthesize new enzymes. Quasi-irreversible inhibitors, while not destroying enzymes, form a complex with the enzyme that results in a long-lasting inhibition that approaches that of irreversible inhibitors. Troleandomycin is a classic example, where its metabolite formed by CYP3A enzymes will create this complex that will result in the long-lasting inhibition of CYP3A activity. The design of a DDI study involving an irreversible or quasi-irreversible inhibition will therefore need to take into account the length it may take before inhibition is seen (eg, immediate with irreversible inhibitors, and delayed with quasi-irreversible inhibitors), and the length of the inhibitory effect. A washout involving seven half-lives of the inhibitor may not suffice, for example, simply because it may take more time for enzymes to be re-synthesized. These concepts are summarized in Table 30-8.

The results of the DDI studies will be included in the product label. Additional information that should be reported include the metabolic and transport pathways, the specific enzymes involved, the relevant metabolites and whether they are active, the nature and degree of the interaction (PK and/or PD), and the recommended dosage adjustments and monitoring recommendations.

## QT Interval Prolongation Study

Torsades de Pointes (TdP), an uncommon but fatal ventricular tachycardia leading to sudden cardiac death, has been linked through diverse studies with QT interval prolongation (Yap and Camm, 2003). Many drugs have the potential to cause QT prolongation and/or TdP, either alone or in a DDI setting. For example, fluoroquinolones (particularly moxifloxacin), antiarrhythmic drugs (flecainide, procainamide, sotalol), and antifungal agents (fluconazole) are currently marketed drugs that are known

## TABLE 30-8 • Design Considerations for DDI Studies

| | Perpetrator | | |
|---|---|---|---|
| | Reversible inhibitors (example, ciprofloxacin on CYP1A2) | Irreversible inhibitors (example, grapefruit juice on CYP3A/PgP) | Inducers (example, phenytoin on CYP3A/PgP) |
| Typical Design | Two-way crossover design, with the drug product given alone or with perpetrator | | |
| Dosage of perpetrator | Recommended daily dosing regimen (when a DDI is expected) or maximum daily dosing regimen (when a DDI is NOT expected and needs to be ruled out) | | |
| Pretreatment Duration of Perpetrator | 2 or 3 days | Until steady state PK conditions of the perpetrator are attained | For a minimum of 10 to 14 days, to ensure that new enzymes or transporters have been synthesized |
| Treatment Duration of Perpetrator | The perpetrator dosing regimen should be continued as long as the PK of the drug product is being investigated through blood sampling | | |
| Drug Product | Drug product needs to be given as a single dose alone in one period, and in the other on the last days of the perpetrator treatment | | |
| Duration of Washout | Minimum of 10 times the average terminal half-lives of both perpetrator and drug product | Minimum of 10 times the average terminal half-lives of both perpetrator and drug product, plus a period of 7 days | Minimum of 10 times the average terminal half-lives of both perpetrator and drug product, plus a period of 10–14 days |
| Sample Size | Minimum of 12 subjects to finish the study if a significant DDI is expected | | |
| | To rule out the presence of a DDI, the sample size should be calculated to ensure that the geometric mean ratios (alone/in combination) and 90% CIs for the PK metrics of interest (eg, $C_{max}$ and AUC) of the drug product are within the usual 80%–125% limits | | |

to prolong QT intervals. Some drugs have been removed from the market after patients died of TdP (ie, terfenadine, astemizole, and cisapride) (Roussel, 1997; FDA Drug Approval package, 2007), while others have had complicated approval (moxifloxacin) or relabeling (thioridazine, droperidol) (Heist and Ruskin, 2005).

The importance of QT prolongation and the necessity of studying this with new drug products was evidenced with the knowledge gained from terfenadine, introduced on the US market as an anti-allergy product in 1985. Terfenadine is a prodrug that needs to be converted to its active metabolite, fexofenadine, in the gut wall and liver via CYP3A enzymes during "first-pass" metabolism. A typical patient taking terfenadine will have minimal systemic exposure from it because of the large first-pass effect, and thereby will show no QT prolongation (fexofenadine has no effect on the QT interval). Reports of TdP associated with its use led the FDA to request a black box warning in 1992. The drug was eventually withdrawn from the market in 1997 after it was hypothesized that the co-administration of terfenadine with strong CYP3A inhibitors may have resulted in up to 125 deaths in the US alone. In patients taking CYP3A inhibitors, terfenadine cannot be metabolized as efficiently via CYP3A enzymes in the gut wall and liver, resulting in a large systemic exposure of the parent drug which then prolongs the QT interval significantly (Schouten, 1991; Finlayson et al, 2004; Kao and Furbee, 2005).

As a result of the market withdrawal of several drugs due to unexpected cases of TdP, regulators proposed to study the QT prolongation in a clinical "thorough QTc study" or "TQT." *Thorough*, so that normal and *supra-therapeutic* doses would have to be studied, so that the impact of renal or hepatic impairment as well as potential DDIs resulting in increased exposure, would be covered. Due to the fact that QT interval determinations are affected by heart rate, studies have to examine the *corrected for heart rate* QT interval, called QTc. The landmark clinical QTc guidance was issued by ICH (E14) and was implemented by the EMA, HC, and the FDA (EMA, 2005; FDA, 2005; HC, 2006).

The guidances call for a TQT study to be conducted before Phase II. A "positive" study showing a significant increase in QTc interval would trigger enhanced QTc monitoring within Phase II and III. Otherwise, normal monitoring would be adequate.

A TQT study is typically designed as a double-blind crossover or parallel study in healthy male and female subjects. In crossover studies, subjects are randomized to one of four treatment sequences and receive each of the following treatments with appropriate wash-out periods:

- Treatment 1: Negative control (placebo)
- Treatment 2: Positive control (most often moxifloxacin)
- Treatment 3: Therapeutic dose of the investigational compound
- Treatment 4: "Supratherapeutic" dose of the investigational compound

To correctly characterize the relationship between the occurrence of QTc prolongation and the drug systemic exposure, the collection of PK samples during the TQT study is essential and should be scheduled in accordance with the timing of the EKG measurements.

An increase in QTc interval of less than 5 msec has been judged unlikely to result in any clinical significance (Shah, 2002). Therefore, if the upper bound of the 95% confidence interval of the placebo corrected maximum increase in QTc does not include 10 msec, the study is then considered "negative." The positive control group should obviously be associated with a positive increase, to show that the study design was planned appropriately.

Recent regulatory proposals recommend investigating the relationship between concentrations and QTc responses in the other usual Phase I studies that are conducted, such as the SAD and MAD, so that a dedicated TQT study would no longer need to be conducted (FDA, 2017; EMA, 2005). For more detailed information, the reader can refer to a recent review article on the topic (Lester et al, 2019).

### Exposure/Effect Relationships and Population PK/PD Studies

#### "Classical" Phase III Population PK/PD Study

Marketed drug products should be characterized in terms of their exposure/effect relationship. In principle, the effective dosing regimen proposed in the product label should be the smallest one possible so that side effects are minimized. Ideally, the PK/PD in the target patient population should be consistent with the PK/PD in healthy volunteers from earlier studies. It is important to conduct population PK/PD studies within the clinical drug development process to better predict the safety and efficacy of the drug in patients after approval for marketing.

The US FDA was instrumental in the use of population PKPD by pharmaceutical companies in the early 1990s. Carl Peck, Thomas Ludden, and others argued eloquently that many unanswered drug development questions could be addressed by conducting a population PK and/or PKPD study within Phase III in addition to simply improving the overall clinical drug development process (Powell, 2007). Lewis Sheiner also confirmed that scientists would make better informed decisions by the information obtained from data through fitting, predictions, and simulations in successive learn-and-confirm cycles through drug development (Sheiner, 1997).

The minimum clinical drug development dossier should include at least one population PK study conducted within Phase III. No ideal set number of patients exist for these studies, but PK studies should never have less than 12 subjects in any given category. If a population PK study is conducted within

Phase III and the PK needs to be characterized in men and women within one disease state, then the study should include at least 12 men and 12 women for the information collected to be considered pivotal. Should the Phase III study involve two different formulations, and/or two different stages of disease or diseases states, and/or combination therapy with another agent versus alone, then ideally a minimum of 12 patients should characterize every situation from a PK perspective in order for the information collected to be considered pivotal from a regulatory point of view.

The objectives of the population PK study are presented in Table 30-9 in order of usual requirements. The main objectives are to confirm the PK behavior observed in previous studies, often conducted in healthy volunteers, and to characterize clinical covariates that influence the PK and therefore dosing regimens (eg, gender, body weight, body surface area, age, and ethnicity). The other objectives aim at filling the eventual knowledge "gaps" of the overall drug submission. These may involve a better characterization of the exposure/effect relationship, a substantiation of the claimed minimum effective dosing regimen, the identification of potential DDIs, the influence of cigarette and/or marijuana smoking, and/or elucidating the relationship between varying

**TABLE 30-9 • Objectives of the Population PK/PD Study Conducted in Phase III**

| | |
|---|---|
| Main objectives | Compare the PK behavior in the target patient population versus that seen in previous studies (most often healthy volunteers). |
| | Investigate the relationship between clinical covariates (demographics, smoking status, etc) and the PK and/or PK/PD of the drug. |
| Additional objectives aimed at filling knowledge gaps before submission | Characterize exposure/response relationship in the target patient population and investigate important covariates such as smoking, age, pathophysiology, etc that influence PK/PD . |
| | Substantiate the minimum effective dosing regimen. |
| | Identify and/or document important clinical DDIs. |
| | Characterize the PK of the drug in patients with varying levels of renal and/or hepatic function. |
| | Demonstrate PK equivalence of a new formulation versus previous ones used in clinical trials or enable the assessment of the PK equivalence of diverse formulations. |
| To answer post-submission queries from regulatory agencies | Answer post-submission questions from regulators using population PK and/or PK/PD techniques. |

degrees of renal or hepatic function and the PK behavior of the drug.

## Modeling and Simulations throughout the Drug Development Process

Population PK/PD analyses have become more popular and utilized by scientists early on during the drug development process (not just in Phase III). By leveraging information from preclinical PK/PD studies, better informed dosing regimens for the SAD and MAD can be proposed.

"Proof of concept" (POC) studies within Phase I can be conducted by fitting PD markers when available, or by using markers that are thought to be related to the mechanism of action of the drug. Careful fitting of all this Phase I data with a mechanistic population PK/PD model allows the simulation of an infinite number of possible dosing regimens. From these simulations, a dosing regimen can be selected for Phase II, and then Phase III studies. A population PK or PK/PD model from Phase I will also enable a better selection of the blood sampling time points for patients participating in Phase II and III studies. Both the number of time points collected and their exact timing can be optimized in order to provide the most informative PK and PK/PD behavior. Optimal sampling strategy techniques such as D-optimality (D'Argenio, 1981) are most often used to achieve this goal.

## Internal Validation of Population PK/PD Models

Population PK analyses are based on fitting of observed data to a model. This is in contrast with noncompartmental PK results, which are mostly "observed" results. When they are well conducted, however, population PK analyses will be the only ones that can yield the information needed for robust exposure/response relationships and characterization of the PK in patient populations.

A population model therefore needs to be internally validated within a research report or scientific article to be deemed trustworthy. Population PK analyses provide two different sets of data: (1) the individual *fit* of the actual observations by the model, and (2) the *predictions* of the population model itself in terms of mean, inter-individual CV, and residual variability. These two sets of results

should be in agreement with each other if the population analysis has been successful and conducted appropriately. Population PK models have to be validated for both components if both sets of results are to be used and trusted. A typical table of results from a population analysis is presented in Table 30-10, and illustrates the two different sets of data results. The individual fits of the observations (individual concentration and/or PD) data are obtained with a Bayesian methodology (eg, maximum a posteriori probability [MAP]) (Seng Yue et al, 2019). These data are relatively independent of the population results if a rich sampling strategy is followed (ie, a minimum of one observation per parameter to fit per subject). The population predictions are usually obtained with a FOCE or an EM approach. The reader is referred to Chapters 19 and 20 for more details.

The quality of the fit of the individual data in a population analysis is an indication of the appropriateness of the *structure* of the model. Figure 30-6 illustrates the fitting results of two different population analyses: one conducted correctly and the other not. The individual fitted data should strictly correlate with the actual dataset if the structure of the retained model is appropriate (Fig. 30-6, panel B).

Once the structure of the model has been found and the graphical representation of the actual versus fitted data is considered to be optimal (see Fig. 30-6), the individual fitted estimates should be compared to the actual data to make sure that both are similar. The data should be separated in all the different studies or subgroups of patients (eg, per dose group, pediatrics versus adults). This approach makes certain that all different studies are correctly fitted by the model, and that the fit is not just good on average when pooling all studies together. This is presented in Fig. 30-7.

The fitted individual results should be compared with the actual data from different studies used in the population analysis, and they should be in agreement for the individual fitted PK parameters to be robust (validation step 2). Once validation steps 1 and 2 have been successfully conducted, the individual PK results arising from the individual fits of the population analysis will be deemed appropriate. They can then be used for reporting of individual PK results.

**TABLE 30-10 •** The Two Components of a Population PK Analysis: An Example of Individual Fitted Results and Population Predicted Values

| PK Parameters | Population Predicted Values | | | Individual Fitted Values | | |
|---|---|---|---|---|---|---|
| | Geometric Mean | Geo CV% | | Geometric Mean | Geo CV% | |
| | Days 1 and 29 | Day 1 | Day 29 | Days 1 and 29 | Day 1 | Day 29 |
| Ka (h⁻¹)* | | | | | | |
| Male | 0.7 | 53.29 | 232.89 | 0.72 | 87.6 | 119.1 |
| Female | 1.8 | | | 2.5 | | |
| tlag (h) | 0.41 | 7.21 | 32.70 | 0.42 | 4.79 | 12.01 |
| CL/F (L/h)** | 11.60 | 39.50 | | 11.28 | 47.26 | |
| Vc/F (L)** | 136.00 | 37.26 | | 145.76 | 51.92 | |
| exponent for Age on Vc/F | 0.95 | — | | — | — | |
| CLd/F (L/h)** | 10.30 | 65.61 | 337.69 | 10.07 | 36.74 | 46.69 |
| Vp/F (L)** | 53.80 | — | | 52.59 | — | |
| **Derived Parameters** | | | | | | |
| Absorption half–life (h) | | | | | | |
| male | 1.05 | — | | 1.02 | — | — |
| female | 0.39 | — | | 0.29 | — | — |
| Elimination half-life (h) | 12.63 | — | | 13.8 | — | — |
| Vss/F (L) | 189.8 | | | 202.5 | | |
| Residual variability in fitted concentrations: | | | 14.3% | | | |

*Centered around the median age (40 years)*
**Centered around the median weight (70 kg)*

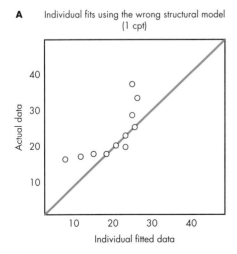

**A**   Individual fits using the wrong structural model (1 cpt)

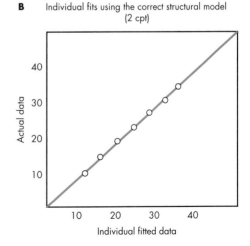

**B**   Individual fits using the correct structural model (2 cpt)

FIGURE 30-6 • The individual fits from a population analysis indicate whether the "structure" of the model is appropriate or not (validation step #1).

| PK Parameter | T/R and 90% CIs | | Agreement |
|---|---|---|---|
| | "Observed" from NCPT | Model "Fitted" | |
| $C_{max}$ | X (Y to Z%) | A (B to C%) | ✓ |
| AUC | X (Y to Z%) | A (B to C%) | ✓ |

FIGURE 30-7 • Individual profiles resulting from the fitted individual results.

The next validation steps are aimed at showing that the second set of results from the population analysis is appropriate, and that the population model could be used for predictions and simulations of new studies. The first step is simply to show that the population results are similar to the individual fitted results, as the latter have already been found to be similar to the actual results of the individual study used in the fitting. An example has already been shown in Table 30-10, where the population results appear to be similar in terms of geometric mean and inter-variability to the individual ones. The next step is to demonstrate that the population model can be used for simulating studies. The population predicted data should correlate well with the actual dataset. An example is shown in Fig. 30-8 where a population model would potentially be appropriate to do simulations (Panel B) while another one would not be (Panel A).

The population analysis indicates whether the model may be appropriate to conduct simulations or not (validation step 3). The inadequate model shown in Panel A (Fig. 30-8) may simply be due to neglecting the inclusion of the actual body weight (ABW) of patients within the model. The population predictions, therefore, cannot inversely fluctuate with changes in body weight (ie, subjects with higher ABW will have lower population predicted concentrations).

The final and fourth step of the internal validation process is through actual simulations. In this step, the patient's data used to create the population model are now completely predicted by the model (not fitted). Through numerous simulations (typically 1000 studies or more), profiles are created with 90% confidence intervals and they are overlayed on the actual data. With a 90% confidence interval, 10% of the actual data are expected to be outside of the boundaries. This is illustrated in Fig. 30-9, and is called a visual predictive check (VPC) representation. The population model will be deemed to be internally validated, and useful for simulations if the results of the VPC graphs are appropriate.

### Bioequivalence of the Proposed Marketed Formulation to the Formulation(s) Used in The Pivotal Phase III Clinical Trials

Two well-conducted and successful Phase III efficacy trials are submitted to establish the efficacy of a drug product for any specific indication. These two

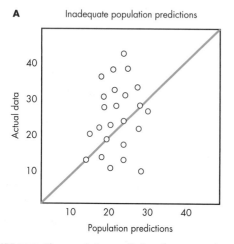

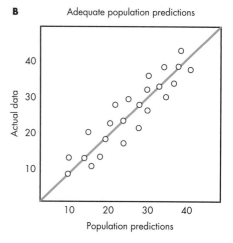

FIGURE 30-8 • The population predictions from a population analysis.

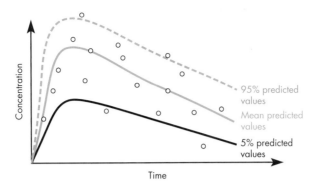

FIGURE 30-9 • An appropriate visual predictive check graph indicates that the population PK model can be used for simulations.

Phase III trials are often conducted with a formulation that is different and/or manufactured at a different location than the formulation intended to be marketed. An essential task of the regulator will be to ensure that the formulation intended *to be marketed* has been established as bioequivalent to the reference product(s) used in the pivotal Phase III clinical trials. The reader is referred to Chapter 29 to better understand how bioequivalence between a test (to be marketed) and a reference (the one used in the Phase III trials) formulation is assessed. Although the rules for bioequivalence for a new drug product should be scientifically the same as those for a generic drug product, in practice, regulatory agencies allow some differences. The US FDA, for instance, is not yet completely aligned in terms of its scientific bioequivalence demands between its Office of New Drugs (OND) and its Office of Generic Drugs (OGD), as each office publishes its own overarching bioavailability/bioequivalence guidance for pharmaceutical companies to follow (US FDA, 2014; FDA, 2021) and they are not in full agreement with one another. In contrast, HC and EMA are more aligned in terms of their scientific demands for bioequivalence, and each of these regulatory agencies has a single overarching guidance that applies to both generic and new drug product submissions.

The main guidance documents that are to be followed for new drugs to establish bioequivalence or PK equivalence between products used in the Phase III studies and the *to-be-marketed* one are what is commonly referred to as the "SUPAC" (Scale-Up and Post-Approval Changes) guidances in the US. Five different SUPAC guidances exist

(immediate release [IR], modified release [MR], semi-solid, Q&A, and manufacturing equipment addendum) and have already been described in greater details in Chapter 26. Although the nomenclature of these guidances suggests they would be for postapproval changes only, they have always been followed for pre-approval changes as well, simply because it makes scientific sense.

Europe and Canada have similar policies and guidances as the US in this regard, despite the fact that they are more restrictive for MR products, where no change is allowed in excipients that may be important to the release characteristics. These policies and guidances for the three regulatory agencies result in two main differences in terms of establishing bioequivalence for pre- and postapproval changes versus those that have been discussed in Chapter 29. First, no clinical PK equivalence study will be needed if the change to the product is a "level 1," meaning that it is a minor change. For example, whether the total change in the excipients is less or more than 5%, a new generic product will always have to be compared to the reference product in a PK equivalence study (except for "AA" products, see Chapter 29, or IR products that are BCS class I, see Chapter 8). For new drugs, a PK equivalence study will not be needed when the total change in excipients is less than 5%. The second major difference is in the types of PK equivalence studies that are required. In Chapter 29, we have seen that in most circumstances both fed and fasted PK equivalence studies are needed for generic products. In contrast, only a fasted single-dose study comparing the new *to-be-marketed* formulation versus the "old/previous" formulation is currently needed for new drugs submissions. This requirement may change in the future as new information is emerging about the importance of conducting food effect PK equivalence trials in addition to fasted ones, even for some small formulation changes and for IR products (Rody, 2019; Tampal, 2019).

### Overdosing and Underdosing Instructions

In clinical practice, the optimal therapeutic effect will be observed when the plasma drug concentrations are within the limits of the *therapeutic window* (above the minimum effective concentration [MEC] but below the minimum toxic concentration [MTC]). It is preferable that the therapeutic window be wide, which suggests a good safety profile for the drug. For some drugs, known as *critical dose drugs* or *narrow therapeutic index* drugs (NTIs) (eg, digoxin, warfarin, phenytoin; see Chapter 29), the therapeutic window is narrow, and a small increase in dosage may cause the patient to display significant adverse events. Specific dosing instructions will need to be specified within the product label for these drugs.

Drug toxicity may also occur in patients inadvertently or purposely. Patients may miss a dose, take a double dose, or may even try to intoxicate themselves. As we have seen in previous chapters, the time it takes for a drug product to be eliminated from the body will depend on its terminal half-life. As such, about 90% of a drug product will be eliminated between three and four half-lives, and 99% after seven half-lives. It is therefore essential that the terminal half-life of any active or potentially toxic analytes associated with the drug product (ie, the parent compound and all its active metabolites) be characterized correctly in PK studies and be reported in the product label. This information will help clinicians know how long it will take for the drug product to be eliminated after overdosing. Local poison control centers can also be contacted for assistance. Patients may also forget to take a required dose at the proper time. Instructions on what needs to be done should be clearly specified in the product label. A drug product with a very short half-life and no significant accumulation with multiple dosing may need to be administered immediately as soon as a patient has realized that they have missed a dose. In contrast, a dose of a drug product with a very long half-life and significant accumulation may

not have to be taken necessarily if a dose is missed, and it may just be less confusing and risky to just continue the therapy at the next regular dose.

## PRE-SUBMISSION SCIENTIFIC MEETINGS WITH REGULATORS

During the new drug development process, the applicant will have meetings with scientists and physicians at the regulatory agency in which the new drug product is to be submitted. The purpose of these meetings is to review all the available data on the drug. The regulatory agency will ascertain that the data and the clinical designs are appropriate for the drug and the sought-after therapeutic indication, and that the drug product is safe. When asked during these pre-submission meetings, the regulatory agency plays a vital role in ensuring that the trial designs are optimal.

## PHASE IV STUDIES

A New drug application or submission should contain all the relevant and necessary information to ensure the safe and efficacious use of the drug product on the market. The regulatory agency may approve the drug product for marketing, but may also feel that some additional data may be necessary to collect or to obtain post marketing. These studies would be requested to the drug company as a postapproval commitment, and are therefore commonly called Phase IV studies. These postapproval commitments used to be relatively common a few decades ago. For example, drug companies were sometimes allowed to do their pediatric, hepatic, or renal impairment PK study postapproval. These postapproval commitments are rare nowadays, as regulatory agencies have frequent pre-submission meetings with pharmaceutical companies, allowing them to request studies to be done before submission.

### Summary of the Minimum PKPD Studies to be Conducted

Table 30-11 summarizes all the minimum studies that have to be conducted to characterize correctly the PK/PD of a new drug product.

## TABLE 30-11 • Summary of Studies That Have to be Conducted to Appropriately Characterize the PK/PD of a New Drug Product

| Studies | Objectives | Designs | Analysis |
|---|---|---|---|
| First in Man/Single Ascending Doses | To obtain general information on PK. To study the toxicity, tolerability and, if appropriate, identify the MTD (eg, for cancer drugs). To investigate dose proportionality. Food, gender, and formulation effect can also be assessed with an adaptive crossover design. To provide single dose PK and dose proportionality information in the label. | Randomized, dose-escalation, double-blind, placebo-controlled, parallel design, single-dose. Healthy volunteers (typically males). $n \approx 4+2$ or $6+3$ per cohort (drug+placebo). Usually 5 or more dose levels with staggered administration to ensure safety and that the PK is as expected. | Safety. Non-compartmental single-dose PK results, and within dose cohorts. |
| Multiple Ascending Doses | To fully characterize the PK at steady state. To investigate dose proportionality and PK linearity. To determine steady-state parameters (accumulation, time-dependency). To determine the safety margin with repeated-dose administration. To provide multiple dose PK, accumulation, dose proportionality, and linearity information in the label. | Randomized, dose-escalation, double-blind, placebo-controlled, parallel design, repeated-dose. Healthy volunteers. $n \approx 6+3$ or more per cohort (drug+placebo). Usually, 3 dose levels at and above the expected therapeutic dose level(s). | Safety Single and multiple dose non-compartmental PK results within dose cohorts, and within periods (single and multiple doses). |
| Food Effect | To investigate the effect of food on the relative bioavailability of the drug product. To provide dosing recommendations as it regards food/meals in the label. | Randomized, balanced, single-dose, two-treatment (fed vs. fasted), two-period, two-sequence crossover design. Healthy volunteers. $n \geq 12$. | Noncompartmental PK analysis with formal "BE" type assessment of the effect of food on at $C_{max}$ and AUCs (90% 80–125 CIs). |
| Mass Balance (Optional if Objectives Obtained from Other Studies) | To assess whether other metabolite(s) need to be assayed besides the parent drug and the other already measured metabolite(s) in other studies. To confirm or assess the percentage of elimination of the important analyte(s) through the hepatic and renal route. To confirm that the percentage recovery of the administered dose is 80% or more with the selected duration of sampling. | Single-dose, intended route of administration as well as IV. Radiolabeled (C14) drug molecule and drug product administrations. Healthy volunteers. $n \approx 6$. Measurement of concentrations of parent and metabolite(s) and determination of the amount of radioactivity in plasma, urine, and feces. | Non-compartmental PK analysis for: Plasma concentrations of parent drug and metabolites Excreted amounts of parent drug and metabolites in the urine and in the feces Total radioactivity in plasma, urine, and feces |
| Renal Impairment | To calculate the impact of varying degrees of renal impairment on the PK of a parent drug and of its active metabolites. To provide dosing recommendations for patients with different levels of renal impairment in the label. | Parallel design, with diverse cohorts of patients with varying levels of renal function, from normal to severely impaired. Males and females. $n \geq 6–8$/group. | Noncompartmental analysis of parent and metabolite: Plasma concentrations Urinary excreted amounts Compartmental analysis of parent and metabolites concentrations and urinary excreted amounts simultaneously with an appropriate PK model. |

*(Continued)*

**TABLE 30-11 •** Summary of Studies That Have to be Conducted to Appropriately Characterize the PK/PD of a New Drug Product (*Continued*)

| Studies | Objectives | Designs | Analysis |
|---|---|---|---|
| **Hepatic Impairment** | To calculate the impact of varying degrees of hepatic impairment on the PK of a parent drug and of its active metabolites.<br>To provide dosing recommendations for patients with different levels of hepatic impairment in the label. | Parallel design, 1 control group and 3 groups with mild, moderate, and severe hepatic impairment as per the Child–Pugh classification.<br>Males and females.<br>n ≥ 4–6 per group. | Noncompartmental analysis of parent and metabolites in terms of total and free (from protein binding) plasma concentrations. |
| **Drug–Drug Interactions** | To calculate the impact of drugs that are likely to be coadministered in the clinic on the investigated drug product, and vice versa.<br>Drugs studied should be chosen based on the known metabolism and transport of the investigated drug.<br>To provide dosing recommendations about drug–drug interactions in the label. | Randomized, single-dose, minimum two-treatments (drug alone or in combination), two-period, two-sequences crossover design.<br>Healthy volunteers.<br>Index perpetrator should be administered for a minimum of 2 (inhibition) to 14 (induction) days before the effect on the single dose of the investigated drug is evaluated.<br>Healthy volunteers. | Noncompartmental PK analysis of parent drugs and active metabolites. |
| **Thorough QTc** | To calculate the potential of the drug product at increasing the QT interval after normal and supratherapeutic doses.<br>To provide information about the potential of the drug to increase the QT interval (with potential risk of *Torsades de Pointes*) in the label. | Double-blind, crossover or parallel, 4 treatment groups (positive control (eg, moxifloxacin), negative control (eg, placebo), normal dose, supratherapeutic dose), randomized design.<br>Healthy volunteers.<br>Multiple EKG measurements taken at the same time as PK samples. | Placebo-matched maximum increase in QTc interval (95% upper bound has to be less than 10 msec).<br>Relationship between QTc changes and PK exposure. |
| **Phase II** | To investigate and find what may be the optimum dosing regimens to study in Phase III.<br>To establish a dose or exposure/response relationship.<br>To estimate the sample size needed for the Phase III studies. | Double-blind, placebo-controlled, parallel, or crossover designs.<br>Efficacy and/or PD markers are collected.<br>Collecting PK samples will allow PK/PD relationships to be estimated. | Compartmental population PK/PD analysis with the use of an appropriate model.<br>Numerous dosing regimens can be simulated using the population model to refine the Phase III sample size and the to be studied dosing regimens. |
| **Population PK (Phase III)** | To assess/confirm the PK behavior in the target patient population.<br>To investigate the relationship between clinical covariates and the PK.<br>To explore the exposure/response relationship in the target patient population. | Population PK is typically done in a subgroup of the Phase III study, usually in a minimum of 50 patients.<br>PK sampling strategy should be based on the PK characteristics of the drug, with a minimum of 1 sample per parameter to fit in the model. | Compartmental population PK/PD analysis with the use of an appropriate model. |

## CHAPTER SUMMARY

Understanding appropriately the PK/PD of a new drug is essential to its safe and effective use on the market. Efficacy of drugs is related to their exposure at the site(s) of activity(ies), which for most will be correlated with systemic exposure. Understanding how clearance may vary between doses (dose proportionality), patient populations (eg, renally or hepatically impaired, elderly, pediatrics), time (linearity), social factors (smoking), and patient characteristics (gender, age, body weight, or body surface area) are critical for dose selection in a given patient. These PK questions are addressed during Phase I, II, and III studies, and the information gained from these studies needs to be summarized in the drug label or monograph in order for clinicians to ensure the safe, effective, and rational use of the drug product.

## REFERENCES

Alam A, Kowal J, Broude E, Roninson I, Locher KP: Structural insight into substrate and inhibitor discrimination by human P-glycoprotein. *Science* **363**(6428):753–756, 2019.

Aller SG, Yu J, Ward A, et al: Structure of P-glycoprotein reveals a molecular basis for poly-specific drug binding. *Science* **323**(5922):1718–1722, 2009.

Boyd RA, et al: Atorvastatin coadministration may increase digoxin concentrations by inhibition of intestinal P-glycoprotein-mediated secretion. *J Clin Pharmacol* **40**(1):91–98, 2000.

Cockcroft DW, Gault WH: Prediction of creatinine clearance from serum creatinine. *Nephron* **16**:31–41, 1976.

D'Argenio DZ: Optimal sampling times for pharmacokinetic experiments. *J Pharmacokinet Biopharm* **9**(6):739–756, 1981.

European Medicines Agency, Committee for Medicinal Products for Human Use (CHMP): Guideline on the evaluation of the pharmacokinetics of medicinal products in patients with decreased renal function. December 2015.

European Medicines Agency: ICH topic E14, the clinical evaluation of QT/QTc interval prolongation and proarrhythmic potential for non-antiarrhythmic drugs. November 2005.

Evans DAP: *Genetic Factors in Drug Therapy: Clinical and Molecular Pharmacogenetics*. Cambridge University Press, 1993.

FDA, CDER. Draft Guidance: Assessing the effects of food on drugs in INDs and NDAs - Clinical pharmacology considerations. Feb 2019. Last accessed Sep 5, 2021 at: https://www.fda.gov/media/121313/download

FDA, CDER. Draft Guidance: Bioequivalence studies with pharmacokinetic endpoints for drugs submitted under an ANDA. August 2021. Last accessed: Sep 5 2021 at: https://www.fda.gov/media/87219/download

FDA, CDER. Draft Guidance: Bioavailability and Bioequivalence studies submitted in NDAs or INDs - General considerations. March 2014. Last accessed: Sep 5 2021 at: https://www.fda.gov/media/88254/download

FDA, CDER. Guidance: E14 Clinical evaluation of QT/QTc interval prolongation and proarrhythmic potential for non-antiarrhythmic drugs, Questions and Answers (R3). June 2017.

FDA, CDER. Guidance for Industry: Determining whether to submit an ANDA or a 505(b)(2) application. May 2019. Last accessed: Sep 4, 2019 at: https://www.fda.gov/media/124848/download

FDA CDER: Guidance for Industry: Pharmacokinetics in patients with impaired renal function - study design, data analysis, and impact on dosing and labeling. March 2010.

FDA: Drug approval package: Prepulsid cisapride monohydrate tablets. May 10, 2007.

FDA Guidance for Industry: Bioequivalence Studies with Pharmacokinetic Endpoints for Drugs Submitted Under an ANDA. December 2013.

FDA Guidance for Industry: Clinical drug interaction studies – Cytochrome P450 enzyme and transporter-mediated drug interactions. January 2020.

FDA Guidance for Industry: E14 clinical evaluation of QT/QTc interval prolongation and proarrhythmic potential for non-antiarrhythmic drugs. October 2005.

FDA Guidance for Industry: Estimating the maximum safe starting dose in initial clinical trials for therapeutics in adult healthy volunteers. July 2005.

FDA Guidance for Industry: Food-Effect Bioavailability and Fed Bioequivalence Studies. December 2002.

Finlayson K, Witchel HJ, McCulloch J, Sharkey: Acquired QT interval prolongation and HERG: Implications for drug discovery and development. *Eur J Pharmacol* **500**(1–3):129–142, 2004.

Health Canada: Guidance for Industry. The clinical evaluation of QT/QTc interval prolongation and proarrhythmic potential for non-antiarrhythmic drugs ICH topic E14. Adopted 05/APR/2006.

Heist EK, Ruskin JN: Drug-induced proarrhythmia and use of QTc-prolonging agents: clues for clinicians. *Heart Rhythm* **2**(11):S1–S8, 2005.

Hoechst MR, Baker Norton Pharmaceuticals: Terfenadine; proposal to withdraw approval of two new drug applications and one abbreviated new drug application; opportunity for a hearing. *Fed Regist* **62**(9):1889–1892, 1997.

Kao LW, Furbee RB: Drug-induced Q–T prolongation. *Med Clin* **89**(6):1125–1144, 2005.

Lester RM, Paglialunga S, Johnson IA: QT assessment in early drug development: The long and the short of it. *Int J Mol Sci* **20**(6):1324, 2019.

Liu K, DiPietro Mager NA: Women's involvement in clinical trials: historical perspective and future implications. *Pharm Pract* **14**(1):708–708, 2016.

Liu W, Ramírez J, Gamazon ER, et al: Genetic factors affecting gene transcription and catalytic activity of UDP-glucuronosyltransferases in human liver. *Hum Mol Gen* **23**(20):5558–5569, 2014.

Lv X, Zhang JB, Hou J, et al: Chemical probes for human UDP-glucuronosyltransferases: A comprehensive review. *Biotechnol J* **14**(1):1800002, 2019.

McElnay JC, D'Arcy PF: Protein binding displacement interactions and their clinical importance. *Drugs* **25**(5):495–513, 1983.

Merck Sharp & Dohme: Primaxin˙. Highlights of prescribing information, FDA approved label. 2019.

Pasternyk Di Marco MP, Edwards DJ, Wainer IW, Ducharme MP: The effect of grapefruit juice and Seville orange juice on the pharmacokinetics of dextromethorphan: The role of gut CYP3A and P-glycoprotein. *Life Sciences* **71**(10):1149–1160, 2002.

Powell JR, Gobburu JVS: Pharmacometrics at FDA: Evolution and Impact on Decisions. *Clinical Pharmacology & Therapeutics* 82(1): 97–102, 2007.

Pugh R, Murray-Lyon IM, Dawson JL, Pietroni MC, Williams R: Transection of the oesophagus for bleeding oesophageal varices. *Br J Surg* 60(8):646–649, 1973.

Rody E: Situation when a fed study is more sensitive to detect formulation differences between IR products, examples from case studies. Presented at the AAPS/EUFEPS Global Bioequivalence Harmonization Initiative 4th International Workshop, Bethesda, MD, December 12–13, 2019.

Sheiner LB: Learning versus confirming in clinical drug development. *Clin Pharmacol Ther* 61(3):275–291, 1997.

Schouten EG, Dekker JM, Meppelink P, Kok FJ, Vandenbroucke JP, Pool J: QT interval prolongation predicts cardiovascular mortality in an apparently healthy population. *Circulation* 84(4):1516–1523, 1991.

Shah RR: Drug-induced prolongation of the QT interval: Why the regulatory concern? *Fundam Clin Pharmacol* 16:147–156, 2002.

Seng Yue C, Ozdin D, Selber-Hnatiw S, Ducharme MP: Opportunities and challenges related to the implementation of model-based bioequivalence criteria. *Clin Pharmacol Ther* 105(2): 350–362, 2019.

Tampal N: Current regulatory approach by US FDA with supporting evidence from case studies. Presented at the AAPS/EUFEPS Global Bioequivalence Harmonization Initiative 4th International Workshop, Bethesda, MD, December 12–13, 2019.

Tanaka H, et al: Effect of clarithromycin on steady-state digoxin concentrations. *Ann Pharmacother* 37(2):178–181, 2003.

Yap YG, Camm AJ: Drug-induced QT prolongation and torsades de pointes. *Heart* 89(11):1363–1372, 2003.

## BIBLIOGRAPHY

Benet LZ: Clearance (née Rowland) concepts: A downdate and an update. *J Pharmacokinet Pharmacodynam* 37:529–539, 2010.

Benet LZ, Hoener BA: Changes in plasma protein binding have little clinical relevance. *Clin Pharmacol Ther* 71(3):115–121, 2002

Cafruny EJ: Renal tubular handling of drugs. *Am J Med* 62: 490–496, 1977.

FDA: Drug Development and Drug Interactions: Table of Substrates, Inhibitors and Inducers. Content current as of 03/10/2020. Last accessed at: https://www.fda.gov/drugs/drug-interactions-labeling/drug-development-and-drug-interactions-table-substrates-inhibitors-and-inducers#table2-1

FDA: E14 Clinical evaluation of QT/QTc interval prolongation and proarrhythmic potential for non-antiarrhythmic drugs, Questions and Answers (R3). June 2017.

FDA Guidance for Industry: Bioavailability and Bioequivalence Studies Submitted in NDAs or INDs - General Considerations. March 2014.

Hewitt WR, Hook JB: The renal excretion of drugs. In Bridges VW, Chasseaud LF (eds). *Progress in Drug Metabolism*, vol. 7. New York, Wiley, 1983, Chap 1.

Holford N, Heo YA, Anderson B: A pharmacokinetic standard for babies and adults. *J Pharm Sci* 102(9):2941–2952, 2013.

Nomeir AA, et al: Estimation of the extent of oral absorption in animals from oral and intravenous pharmacokinetic data in drug discovery. *J Pharm Sci* 98(11):4027–4038, 2009.

Penner N, Xu L, Prakash C: Radiolabeled absorption, distribution, metabolism, and excretion studies in drug development: Why, when, and how? *Chem Res Toxicol* 25(3):513–531, 2012.

Rowland M, Benet LZ, Graham GG: Clearance concepts in pharmacokinetics. *J Pharm Biopharm* 1:123–136, 1973.

# Glossary

| | | | | |
|---|---|---|---|---|
| **$A, B, C$** | Preexponential constants for three-compartment model equation | | **$Ae_{(m)ij}$** | Amount of metabolite excreted from time i to time j (usually in urine or feces) |
| **$\alpha$** | Probability of making a type 1 error | | **ANCOVA** | Analyses of covariance |
| **$\beta$** | Probability of making a type 2 error | | **ANOVA** | Analysis of variance |
| **$\alpha, \beta, \gamma$** | Exponents for three-compartment model equation | | **API** | Active pharmaceutical ingredient |
| **$\lambda_1, \lambda_2, \lambda_{3, \ldots} \lambda_z$** | Exponents for three-compartment-type exponential equation (more terms may be added and indexed numerically with subscripts for multiexponential models), and exponent describing the last terminal phase ($\lambda_z$) regardless of the total number of exponents needed. | | **AR** | Absolute risk |
| | | | **ARI** | Absolute risk increase |
| | | | **AUC** | Area under the concentration–time curve |
| | | | **$AUC_{inf}$, $AUC_{0\text{-}inf}$, $[AUC]_0^\infty$** | Area under the concentration–time curve extrapolated to infinite time |
| **Delta ($\Delta$)** | Delta is sometimes referred to as the "effect size" and is a measure of the degree of difference between tested population samples | | **$AUC_{0\text{-}t}$, $[AUC]_0^t$** | Area under the concentration–time curve from time 0 to the last measurable drug concentration at time $t$ |
| **$\mu_0$** | The null hypothesis value for the mean | | **$AUC_{tau}$, $AUC_\tau$** | Area under the concentration–time curve over the dosing interval |
| **$\mu_a$** | $\mu_a$ is the alternative hypothesis value expected for the mean | | **$AUC_{tau(ss)}$, $AUC_{\tau(ss)}$** | Area under the concentration–time curve at steady state |
| **$\chi^2$** | Chi-square test | | **AUMC** | Area under the (first) moment–time curve |
| **$Ab^\infty$** | Total amount of drug in the body | | **BA** | Bioavailability |
| **ABC** | ATP-binding cassette | | **BCS** | Biopharmaceutics Classification System |
| **ABCB1** | Gene coding for p-Glycoprotein; see also MDR1 | | **BDDCS** | Biopharmaceutics Drug Disposition Classification System |
| **ABW** | Actual body weight | | **BE** | Bioequivalence, Bioequivalent |
| **ADME** | Absorption, distribution, metabolism, and excretion | | **BM** | Biomarker |
| | | | **BMI** | Body mass index |
| **AE** | Adverse event | | **BRCP** | Breast cancer–resistance protein |
| **$Ae_{ij}$** | Amount of drug excreted from time i to time j (usually in urine or feces) | | **BUN** | Blood urea nitrogen |

| | | | |
|---|---|---|---|
| $C$ | Concentration (mass/volume) | $CL_R$ | Renal clearance |
| $C_a$ | Drug concentration in arterial plasma | $CL_u$ | Clearance of unbound drug |
| $C_{av(ss)}, C_{av}^\infty$ | Average steady-state plasma drug concentration | CMC | Chemistry, manufacturing, and control |
| $C_p$ | Concentration of drug in plasma | CRF | Case report form |
| $S_{creat}$ | Serum creatinine concentration, in American units expressed as mg/dL | %CV | Percent coefficient of variation |
| CE | Clinical endpoint | CYP | Prefix of formerly called "cytochrome P-450 enzymes," which are involved in the biotransformation of drugs |
| $C_{eff}$ | Effective drug concentration | | |
| $C_{GI}$ | Concentration of drug in gastrointestinal tract | $D$ | Amount of drug (mass, eg, mg) |
| CI | Confidence interval | $D_A$ | Amount of drug absorbed |
| $C_m$ | Concentration of metabolite | $D_B$ | Amount of drug in body |
| $C_{max}$ | Maximum concentration | $D_{GI}$ | Amount of drug in gastrointestinal tract |
| $C_{max(SS)}, C_{max}^\infty$ | Maximum concentration of drug at steady state | $D_L$ | Loading (initial) dose |
| $C_{min}$ | Minimum concentration of drug | $D_M$ | Maintenance dose |
| $C_{min(SS)}$ | Minimum concentration of drug at steady state | DNA | Deoxyribonucleic acid |
| | | $D_N$ | Normal dose |
| $C_p^0$ | Concentration of drug in plasma at zero time ($t = 0$) (equivalent to $C^0$) | $X_c$ | Amount of drug in central compartment |
| | | $X_t$ | Amount of drug in tissue |
| $C_{ss}, C_p^\infty$ | Steady-state plasma drug concentration | $X_u$ | Amount of drug in urine |
| | | $D_0, D$ | Dose of drug |
| $C_t$ | Concentration of drug in tissue | $D^0$ | Amount of drug at zero time ($t = 0$) |
| CFR | Code of Federal Regulations | E, ER | Extraction ratio |
| cGMP | Current Good Manufacturing Practices | $E_A$ | Absorption extraction ratio |
| CKD | Chronic kidney disease | $E_G$ | Gut extraction ratio |
| CL, $CL_T$ | Total body clearance | $E_H$ | Hepatic extraction ratio |
| $CL_{CR}$ | Creatinine clearance | $E$ | Pharmacological effect |
| $CL_D$ | Distributional clearance | eGFR | Estimate of GFR based on an MDRD equation |
| $CL_{DIAL}$ | Dialysis clearance | | |
| CDD | Critical dose drug | $E_{max}$ | Maximum pharmacologic effect |
| $CL_H$ | Hepatic clearance | $E_0$ | Pharmacologic effect at zero drug concentration |
| $CL_{int}, CL_{int(u)}$ | Intrinsic clearance, unbound intrinsic clearance | $EC_{50}$ | Drug concentration that produces 50% of the maximum pharmacological effect |
| $CL_{(m)}$ | Clearance of metabolite | | |
| $CL_f$ | Formation clearance of parent to a metabolite | EMA | European Medicines Agency |
| | | F | Fraction of dose bioavailable |
| $CL_{NR}$ | Nonrenal clearance | $F_A$ | Fraction of dose absorbed |

| | | | |
|---|---|---|---|
| $F_G$ | Fraction of dose absorbed that is not metabolized in the gut wall | $k_{ij}$ | Rate constant from compartment $i$ to compartment $j$. |
| $F_H$ | Fraction of dose absorbed, that is not metabolized in the gut wall, and that is not metabolized in the liver | $K_I$ | Inhibition constant: $= k_{-1}/k_{1+}$ |
| | | $K_M$ | Michaelis–Menten constant |
| $f_e$ | Fraction of drug excreted unchanged in urine | $k_{(m)}, k_{e(m)}, k_{el(m)}$ | First-order elimination rate constant of a metabolite |
| $f_m$ | Fraction of parent drug converted to a metabolite | $k_R$ | Renal component of the elimination rate constant |
| $f_u$ | Unbound fraction of drug | $k_{NR}$ | Non-renal component of the elimination rate constant |
| FDA | US Food and Drug Administration | $k_o$ | Zero-order absorption rate constant |
| | | LBW | Lean body weight; see also IBW |
| $f(t)$ | Function representing drug elimination over time (time is the independent variable) | MAT | Mean absorption time |
| | | MDR1 | Multidrug-resistance gene, coding for p-Glycoprotein; see also ABCB1 |
| $f'(t)$ | Derivative of $f(t)$ | MDRD | Modification of Diet in Renal Disease; equation used to estimate GFR |
| GFR | Glomerular filtration rate | | |
| GI | Gastrointestinal tract | MDT | Mean dissolution time |
| GMP | Good Manufacturing Practice | MEC | Minimum effective concentration; see also $C_{eff}$ |
| $H_o$ | The null hypothesis | | |
| $H_1$ | The alternative hypothesis | MRP | Multidrug resistance–associated proteins |
| IBW | Ideal body weight, usually calculated by the Dubois & Dubois or the Devine equations; see also LBW | MRT | Mean residence time |
| | | MTC | Minimum toxic concentration |
| | | NDA | New Drug Application |
| ICH | International Council for Harmonisation of technical requirements for pharmaceuticals for human use | NTI | Narrow therapeutic index; see also critical dose drug (CDD) |
| | | Obs | Observed (eg, $C_{max}$ (obs)) |
| IM | Intramuscular | OTC | Over-the-counter [drug] |
| IR | Immediate release | OATP | Organic anion transporting polypeptide |
| IV | Intravenous | | |
| IVIVC | In vitro–in vivo correlation | OAT | Organic anion transporter |
| IVIVR | In vitro–in vivo relationship | PA | Pharmaceutical alternative |
| $k_{10}$ | Rate constant going out from central compartment | PBPK | Physiologically-based pharmacokinetics |
| $K_A$ | Association binding constant | PD | Pharmacodynamics |
| $k_a$ | First-order absorption rate constant | PE | Pharmaceutical equivalent |
| $K_D$ | Dissociation binding constant | PEG | Polyethylene glycol |
| $k, k_e, k_{el}$ | Drug elimination first-order rate constant (eg, $k_{el} = k_R + k_{NR}$) | P-gp | p-Glycoprotein, coded by MDR1 or ABCB1 gene |
| $k_{e0}$ | Transfer rate constant out of the effect compartment | PGt | Pharmacogenetics |
| | | PK | Pharmacokinetics |

**Pred**          Predicted (eg, $C_{max}$ (pred))

**Q**             Blood flow

**$Q_H$**         Hepatic blood flow

**QA**            Quality assurance

**QC**            Quality control

**$R, R_0$**      Infusion rate constant.

**RLD**           Reference-listed drug

**SD**            Standard deviation

**SEM**           Standard error of the mean

**SNP**           Single-nucleotide polymorphism. A DNA sequence variation occurring when a single nucleotide—A, T, C, or G—in the gene (or other shared sequence) is altered.

**SUPAC**         Scale-up and post-approval changes

**t**             Time (hours or minutes)

**TE**            Therapeutic equivalent

**$t_{eff}$**     Duration of pharmacological response to drug

**$t_{inf}$**     Duration of infusion

**$t_{lag}$**     Lag time

**$t_{max}$**     Time of occurrence of maximum (peak) drug concentration

**$t_0$**         Initial or zero time

**$t_{1/2}$**     Half-life

**$T, \tau, tau$** Time interval between doses

**USP**           *United States Pharmacopeia*

**$V, V_D$**      Volume of distribution

**$V_C$**         Volume of central compartment

**$V_{max}$**     Maximum velocity

**$V_p$**         Peripheral volume of distribution

**$V_{(p)}$**     Volume of plasma (central compartment)

**$V_t$**         Volume of tissue compartment

**$V_{ss}, V_{DSS}$** Total volume of distribution

# Index

Page numbers followed by *f* indicate figures; page numbers followed by *t* indicate tables.

## A

AAG. *See* α1-Acid glycoprotein (AAG)
AAV. *See* Adeno-associated virus (AAV)
Abatacept, 704
Abbreviated New Drug Application (ANDA)
   approved, changes to, 839–840
   bioequivalence studies
      description of, 245–246, 265, 278t, 281–282
      waiver, 281–282
   description of, 5, 343, 831
   NDA compared with, 277–278, 278t
   postapproval changes, 867–868
   review of, 277–278, 280f
   submission of, 919
*ABCB1*, 168t
*ABCB4*, 168t
*ABCB11*, 168t
*ABCC1*, 168t
*ABCC2*, 168t
*ABCC3*, 168t
*ABCC4*, 168t
*ABCC5*, 168t
*ABCC6*, 168t
ABCG2, 667
*ABCG2*, 168t
ABC transporters, 666–667
ABE. *See* Average bioequivalence (ABE)
Abelcet, 886t
Abilify. *See* Aripiprazole
Abilify Mycite, 889
Abraxane, 886t
Abscissa, 37
Absolute bioavailability, 36, 246–247, 247f, 950
Absolute risk (AR), 75
Absolute risk increase (ARI), 75

Absolute risk reduction (ARR), 75
Absorption. *See* Drug absorption
Absorption, distribution, metabolism and excretion processes, 162
Absorption rate constant, 509–511, 510f
Absorption window, 106
Abuse-deterrent formulations (ADFs), 878–880
Acceptance criteria, 864
Accumulation, 521–525, 522f, 523t, 525t
Accumulation half-life, 525, 525t
Accumulation ratio, 404–405
Accuracy, 70–71, 724
Acetaminophen, 157t, 165t
Acetylation, 158–159, 160t
Achlorhydric patients, 118
Achromycin V. *See* Tetracycline
Acids. *See* Weak acids
Active pharmaceutical ingredient (API)
   in formulation, 924
   identicality of, 937
   impurities, 862
   manufacturing changes of, 868
   pharmaceutical equivalence of, 834, 835t
   starting materials in synthesis of, 862
Active transport, 94f, 94–95
Active tubular secretion, 176
Acyclovir, 261
ADAPT 5, 621, 623
ADAPT-II, 388, 621, 623
Additive drug effect model, 693–694
Additivity, of clearances, 465–466
Adeno-associated virus (AAV), 364–365
ADFs. *See* Abuse-deterrent formulations
Adjusted body weight (AdjBW), 766–767

ADME processes. *See* Absorption, distribution, metabolism and excretion processes
Administration, routes of
   determination of, 734–735
   drug design considerations, 224, 224f
   extravascular, 497, 499f, 734
   intravenous. *See* Intravenous (IV) bolus administration
   types of, 735f
ADR. *See* Adverse drug reaction
ß-Adrenergic receptors, in older adults, 762–763
Adverse drug reaction (ADR)
   clinical application involving, 504
   with lidocaine, 435
Adverse effects, 868
Adverse events, 727–728
Adverse response, 683–684
Adverse viral drug interactions, 742
Aerosolized drugs, 185
Aerosol therapy, 232
Affinity, 93, 413
Aging. *See* Elderly; Older adults
Akaike information criterion (AIC), 391, 629
Alanine aminotransferase (ALT), 814, 818
Albumin, 148t, 368, 759, 775
Alendronate sodium (Fosamax®), 112
Alkaline ash diet, 176
Alkaline phosphatase, 818
Allometric scaling, 585–589, 586t–587t, 778
Allometry, 585, 589
Alpha, 60, 63t
α1-Acid glycoprotein (AAG), 148, 148t
ALT. *See* Alanine aminotransferase; (ALT)
Alternative testing, 59

AmberLite resins, 812
Ambien. *See* Zolpidem tartrate
AmBisome, 886*t*
Amikacin, 719*t*
Amino acid conjugation, 160*t*
Aminoglycosides, 533–534, 617, 811
Aminotransferase, 818
Amorphous forms, 191
Amphetamine, 157*t*, 177
Amphotericin B, 100
Amylase, 104
Analyses of covariance
    (ANCOVA), 67
Analysis of variance (ANOVA)
    description of, 66–68, 273
    four-way, 67
    repeated measures, 67–68
    three-way, 67
    two-way, 67
Anaphylactic reactions, 683
Anaphylaxis, 683
ANDA. *See* Abbreviated New Drug
    Application
Anhydrous state, 191
Annovera, 885*t*
ANOVA. *See* Analysis of variance
Antacids, 119
Antibiotics. *See also* specific drugs
    elimination half-life, 447
    elimination rate constant and,
        446–447
Antibody-dependent cell-mediated
    cytotoxic effect, 359
Antibody–drug conjugates,
    369–370
Antibody fragments, 361–362
Anticancer drugs, 426. *See also*
    specific drugs
Anticholinergic drugs, 119
Anticholinergics, in older
    adults, 762
Antiepileptic drugs, 224
Antihypertensive drugs. *See* specific
    drugs
Antilogarithm, 38
Antiproliferative drug, 890–891
Anti-therapeutic antibodies
    (ATAs), 377
Antral milling, 103
API. *See* Active pharmaceutical
    ingredient (API)
Apparent clearance, 464

Apparent volume of distribution, 141*f*
    of aminoglycosides, 533–534
    clearance and, 469–471, 479*t*
    definition of, 139–140, 401
    IV infusion for determination of,
        443, 444*f*
    one-compartment open model
        for IV bolus administration,
        401–402
    renal impairment effects on, 788
    in two-compartment model
        central compartment volume,
            422–423
        practical focus, 425–427
        practice problem, 424*f*, 424–425
        tissue compartment volume, 425
        volume by area, 424
Approved Drug Products with
    Therapeutic Equivalence
    Evaluations (Orange Book),
    290–292, 291*t*
*A priori*, 60, 62, 629
AR. *See* Absolute risk (AR)
Arbekacin, 59
Area, volume of distribution by, 424
Area under the curve (AUC),
    15, 15*f*, 28*f*, 29
    definition of, 36, 51, 250, 578
    description of, 57
    in linearity determination,
        568, 568*f*
    partial bioequivalence and,
        273–275, 274*f*
    examples of, 273–275
    of plasma drug concentration
        curve, 273–275, 274*f*, 443, 444*f*
Area under the first moment curve
    (AUMC), 579
Argatroban, 696
ARI. *See* Absolute risk
    increase (ARI)
Aripiprazole (Abilify), 102, 584, 889
Arithmetic mean, 53
ARR. *See* Absolute risk
    reduction (ARR)
Arteriovenous fistula, 808
Arthritis, 707*f*
Artificial membrane
    permeability, 118
Asacol. *See* Mesalamine
Aspartate aminotransferase (AST),
    814, 818

Aspirin
    absorption of, 111*f*
    dissolution rate compared with
        absorption rate of, 193
    enteric coated, 308
    rate of release of, 34, 35*f*
AST. *See* Aspartate
    aminotransferase (AST)
ATAs. *See* Anti-therapeutic
    antibodies (ATAs)
Atorvastatin, 114*t*
ATP-binding cassette (ABC),
    96, 98*t*
ATP binding cassette subfamily B
    member 1, 666–667
AUC. *See* Area under the curve
AUIMC. *See* Area under the first
    moment curve
AUMC. *See* Area under the first
    moment curve (AUMC)
Authorized generic, 921
Auto-induction, 165–167
Auto-inhibition, 165–167
Autoregulation, 174
Average, 53
Average bioequivalence (ABE), 927
Azithromycin (Zithromax),
    431–432, 455
Azone, 335

**B**

Bactrim. *See* Sulfamethoxazole/
    trimethoprim
Balsalazide, 86, 88*t*, 105
Baqsimi, 901, 901*f*
Bare-metal stent (BMS), 890
Base. *See* Weak base
Batch size, 869
Bayesian analysis, 614
Bayesian theory, 742–743
BCRP. *See* Breast cancer resistance
    protein (BCRP)
Beads, 325–327
"Bear," 621
Bell-shaped curve. *See* Normal
    distribution
Benzo[a]pyrene, 157*t*
Benzodiazepines, 762
Berkeley Madonna, 626
Beta, 63*t*
Beta phase. *See* Elimination phase
Bias, 71–72

Biexponential profiles, 418, 433*f*,
    433–434
Bile, 109, 169
Biliary clearance, 170
Biliary excretion
    description of, 171
    inhibition of, 741
Biliary system, 169–171
Bilirubin, 818–819
Bimodal distribution, 52–53
Binding. *See* Protein binding
Bioavailability
    absolute, 36, 246–247,
        247*f*, 950
    absorption versus, 481
    age and, 263
    definition of, 3–4
    drug design considerations,
        222–223
    drug–drug interactions, 223, 262
    excretion and, 481–482
    factors influencing, 260–267
    food effects on, 110*t*, 111*f*, 112
    liver metabolism, 481
    nonlinear pharmacokinetics
        and, 565
    polymorph change effects on, 838
    relative, 4, 36, 243, 244, 246–248,
        948–949
Bioavailability studies
    methods for assessing, 249*t*,
        249–255
        *in vitro*, 255
        *in vivo*, 249, 263
        plasma drug concentration, 249*t*,
            250*f*, 250–251
        urinary drug excretion data,
            249*t*, 251*f*, 251–252
    of MR drug products, 308,
        346–347, 347*f*
    practice problem, new
        investigational drug, 248–249
    purpose of, 243–246
    relative and absolute,
        246–248, 247*f*
    special concerns, 288*t*,
        288–290, 289*t*
    transit time in, 311–312
Biobatch, 205
Bioequivalence
    bases for determining, 269–270
    definition of, 4, 914–915

of drugs with multiple
        indications, 839
    generic products, 265, 914–918
    issues in, 288*t*
    metrics, 927–929
    multiple-dose, 268–269
    proposed market formulation,
        972–974
    redocumentation of, 867
Bioequivalence studies
    for ANDA, 277–278, 280*t*
    clinical endpoints, 249*t*, 253,
        254*t*–255*t*, 255*t*, 269, 270–271
    clinical examples, 270–271
    clinical significance, 287–288
    crossover study designs for,
        265–270
        clinical endpoint, 253,
            254*t*–255*t*, 269
        Latin-square crossover design,
            265–266, 266*t*
        multiple-dose, 268–269, 270*f*
        nonreplicate, parallel, 268
        in patients maintained on
            therapeutic regimen, 269–270
        replicated, 266–267
        scaled average, 267–268
    data evaluation, 272–273
        ANOVA, 273
        partial AUC, 273–275
        pharmacokinetic, 272–273
        purpose of, 243–246
        statistical, 272–273
        two one-sided tests procedure,
            272–273
    description of, 74–75
    design and evaluation of, 256,
        258–264
        analytical methods, 263–264
        objectives, 256
        RLD, 259
        study considerations, 258*t*,
            258–259
    determination of, 256, 269–270
    efflux transporters on, 288
    examples of, 275*t*, 275–277,
        276*f*, 276*t*, 277*f*
    *in vitro*, 249*t*, 255
    *in vitro* approaches, 256
    methods for assessing, 249
    of MR drug products, 347
    multiple endpoints, 256, 257*t*

pharmacodynamic endpoints,
        252–253, 254*t*
    possible surrogate markers for,
        289, 289*t*
    special concerns in, 288*t*,
        288–290
    study designs
        fasting, 264–265
        food intervention, 265
        waivers of, 281–282, 284*t*
Biologics, 935, 939, 949
Biologic specimen sampling, 13
Biologics Price Competition and
    Innovation Act of 2009, 844
Biomarkers
    description of, 684–685, 686*t*
    surrogate, 289, 289*t*
Biopharmaceutical Drug Disposition
    Classification System (BDDCS),
        284–285
Biopharmaceutic Classification
    System (BCS), 283–285, 284*t*
    description of, 117, 220
    dissolution, 284
    drug classification, 172*f*
    drug products where bioavailability
        or bioequivalence may be
        self-evident, 285
    permeability, 283–284
    solubility, 283
Biopharmaceutics. *See also*
    Biotechnology
    basis of, 5
    definition of, 183, 849
    description of, 3–6, 4*f*, 5*t*
    dissolution profile comparisons,
        207–209
    drug design considerations,
        183–186, 189*t*
    drug product performance and,
        851–853
    of MR drug products, 310–313
        large intestine, 312–313
        small intestine transit time,
            311–312
        stomach, 310–311
    pharmacokinetics of, 373–377
    physicochemical properties,
        188–191, 189*t*
    quality by design and, 854
Biopharmaceutics Classification
    System, 283–285, 284*t*

Biopharmaceutics Risk Assessment Roadmap (BioRAM), 852*f*, 857
Biophase, 924
BioRAM. *See* Biopharmaceutics Risk Assessment Roadmap (BioRAM)
Biosignal, 687
Biosimilarity
definition of, 844
interchangeability vs., 286–287, 939
Biosimilars, 844, 935–940
Biotechnology
gene therapy, 362, 363*t*, 364–365
monoclonal antibodies, 359–361, 360*f*
protein drugs, 356, 357*t*–358*t*, 359
Biotransformation
acetylation, 158–159, 160*t*
conjugation reactions, 157–158, 159–160, 160*t*
definition of, 156
enantiomer metabolism, 160–161
glutathione conjugation, 159–160
hepatic enzymes involved in, 153–156, 161–163
pathways of, 156–162
phase II reactions, 156–158, 158*t*
phase I reactions, 156–157, 157*t*–158*t*
reactions, 156
regioselectivity, 161
transporter-mediated drug interactions, 167
Biowaiver, 281–282, 282
Bisphosphonates, 112
Bitolterol mesylate, 327
Bleomycin, 226
Block randomization, 72
Blood
components of, 14*t*, 130
drug concentration measurement of, 13–14, 14*t*, 34
drug interactions with, 130–131
drug movement in, 130*f*, 130–133
Blood–brain barrier, 136, 156
Blood–cerebrospinal fluid barrier, 136
Blood flow
to capillaries, 135
drug distribution facilitated by, 134–135
to GI tract, 108
renal, 173–175
to tissues, 131–133, 135*t*, 413, 414*t*

Blood flow–limited model, 597, 599–600. *See also* Perfusion models
Blood urea nitrogen (BUN), 792
BMI. *See* Body mass index (BMI)
BMS. *See* Bare-metal stent (BMS)
Body clearance, 464
Body mass index (BMI), 735, 765*t*–766*t*
Body surface area (BSA), 766*t*
Body weight, 765–767, 766*t*
Bonferroni correction, 66
Bovine spongiform encephalopathy, 859–860
Bowman's capsule, 173
Branded generics, 921
Breast cancer resistance protein (BCRP), 97, 137
Breast milk, drug distribution in, 138–139
Buccal administration, 87*t*
Buccal tablet, 227
Buffering agents, 226
BUN. *See* Blood urea nitrogen (BUN)
Buprenorphine, 881*t*, 896*t*
Bupropion hydrochloride (Wellbutrin), 308, 538, 841
Busulfan, 777
Butyrylcholinesterase, 664

**C**

Caco-2 cells, 117
Caffeine, 588*f*
Calcium, 119–120
Calcium carbonate, 226
Calculus, 27–29
differential, 27–28
integral, 28*f*, 28–29
Canadian reference product (CRP), 931
Capacity-limited elimination, 552*f*, 552–554, 553*t*
Capacity-limited metabolism, 547–549, 549*f*, 555*f*, 555*t*–556*t*
Capacity-limited pharmacokinetics, 552*f*, 552–554
clearance in, 559–561, 560*f*
clinical focus, 561
determination of Michaelis constant and maximum elimination rate, 554–556, 555*f*, 555*t*–556*t*, 556*f*, 556–558, 557*f*
elimination half-life in, 552–554

interpretation of Michaelis constant and maximum elimination rate, 559, 559*f*
practice problems, 550–551
CAPD. *See* Continuous ambulatory peritoneal dialysis (CAPD)
Capillaries, 135
Carbamazepine, 164, 165*t*, 719*t*
Carboxypeptidase, 104
Carmustine, 881*t*
Carrier-mediated intestinal absorption, 94*f*, 94–98, 95–96, 96*t*, 97*f*
Carriers. *See* Drug carriers
Carryover effects, 266
Cartesian coordinate, 30, 30*f*
CAR-T therapy, 365
Carvedilol, biostatics in interpretation of FDA, 77
Catechol *O*-methyl transferase (COMT), 157
Categorical pharmacodynamic responses, 686
Cationic drugs, 328
Cauchy's method, 592
CAVH. *See* Continuous arteriovenous hemofiltration (CAVH)
$C_{av(ss)}$, 732–733
Cefiderocol (Fetroja), 801, 801*t*
Cefpodoxime, 112
Cefuroxime, 836–837
Celiac disease, 119
Cell membranes, drug passage across
carrier-mediated transport, 94*f*, 94–98, 96*t*, 97*f*
passive diffusion, 90–94, 91*f*, 94*f*
Cellulose acetate, 200
Center for Biologics Evaluation and Research (CBER), 939
Central compartment, 413
volume of distribution in, 422–423
Cephalexin, 119
Cequa, 886*t*
Cerebrospinal fluid–brain barrier, 136
Certolizumab pegol, 361
CFR. *See* Code of Federal Regulations
cGMP. *See* Current Good Manufacturing Practices (cGMP)
Channeling bias, 72
Chemical calibration, 203–205
Chemical purity, 868
Chemistry, manufacturing, and controls, 865, 865*t*

CHF. *See* Congestive heart failure

Child–Pugh score/classification, 814, 817, 817*t*, 961, 962*t*

Children
  absorption in, 774–775
  allometric scaling in, 778
  creatinine clearance calculations in, 794
  CYP enzymes in, 775–776
  distribution in, 775
  dosing in, 735, 773–774, 777–778
  excipient tolerance by, 860–861
  excretion in, 776–777
  formulations for, 860–861
  metabolism in, 775–776
  pharmacodynamics in, 778
  pharmacokinetics in, 774–778
  phase II metabolism in, 776
  phase I metabolism in, 775–776
  subpopulations of, 773, 773*t*

Chirality, 189

Chi-square distribution, 629

Chitosan-coated particle-based system, 312

Chloramphenicol, 191, 191*f*

Cholesteryl ester transfer protein, 684

Cholestyramine, 88*t*, 119

Choroid plexus barrier, 136

Chronic kidney disease, 787–788

Chronic Kidney Disease–Epidemiology Collaboration (CKD-EPI), 796

Chronopharmacokinetics, 563*t*, 563–564
  circadian rhythms and drug exposure, 564
  clinical focus, 564

Chymotrypsin, 104

Cimetidine (Tagamet), 112–113, 165*t*

Circadian rhythms, 564

Clark's rule, 773

Clearance, 463–466. *See also* Creatinine clearance; Hepatic clearance; Renal clearance
  additivity of, 465–466
  body, 464
  calculations, 464–467
  of capacity-limited drug, 559–561, 560*f*
  clinical importance of, 463–464
  compartmental approach to, 466*f*, 466–469, 479
  definition of, 402

distributional, 468

dose adjustments based on, 789–790

first-pass effect, 481

half-life and, 479*t*

hepatic, 484–486

intrinsic, 484–486, 816

IV infusion for determination of, 452–453

liver blood flow and, 485*f*

metabolite, 477–478

"midpoint" method, 477, 792

model-independent approach, 471

models of, 466–469

in multicompartment models, 424*f*, 424–425, 426

noncompartmental approach to, 466*f*, 471–479, 582

non-renal, 959, 960*f*

in older adults, 760

one-compartment model
  description of, 467–468
  IV bolus administration, 402–403

physiologic approach to, 466*f*, 479–488

predictions based on fractions eliminated through kidney and liver, 489

protein binding effects on, 486

rate constants and, 469–471

renal, 470–471, 473–474, 476–477, 489, 959, 960*f*

total body, 464

two-compartment model, 424*f*, 424–425, 468–469

volume of distribution and, 469–471, 479*t*

"well-stirred" model, 479–488, 480*f*, 816

Clearance ratio, 474, 474*t*

Clinical endpoint bioequivalence study, 253, 254*t*–255*t*, 269

Clinically significant differences, 64

Clinical pharmacokinetics
  description of, 7
  software packages, 617

Clinical pharmacokinetic services, 719

Clinical pharmacology, 924

Clinical toxicology, 12

Clonidine, 895*t*

Clopidogrel (Plavix), 101, 162

CMA. *See* Critical material attributes (CMA)

$C_{max(ss)}$, 732–733

CMC. *See* Chemistry, Manufacturing, and Controls

$C_{min(ss)}$, 732–733

CMVs. *See* Critical manufacturing variables (CMVs)

Cocaine, 430*t*, 682

Cockcroft and Gault method, 471, 791, 796–797

Cockcroft–Gault equation
  in adults, 793
  creatinine clearance calculations using, 959
  development of, 796–797
  in obese patients, 770
  in older adults, 761

Cocktail studies, 963

Codeine, 157*t*

Code of Federal Regulations (CFR), 914

Coefficient of variation, 56

Colloidal iron products, 889

Colon, 104–105

Colonic drug delivery, 228

Comparative bioequivalence study, 876

Compartment, 19, 389

Compartmental approach
  to clearance, 466*f*, 466–469, 479
  population, 616
  software packages using, 616–617, 621–625

Compartmental modeling, 595–596

Compartment models, 18*f*, 18–20
  of bolus IV administration determination, 411–412, 412*f*
  mechanistic models, 590–591
  pharmacokinetics/pharmacodynamics, 384–392

Complement-dependent cytotoxic effect (CDC), 359

Complex drug products, 843, 843*t*

Compliance, 313–314

Computers, 31–32. *See also* Software
  pharmacokinetic uses of, 20–21

Concentration. *See* Drug concentration

Concentration-dependent killing activity, 689

Concentration-independent killing activity, 395

Concerta, 274, 927, 934. *See also* Methylphenidate

Confidence intervals, 55–56, 57. *See also* Two one-sided tests procedure

Confounding, 73–74

Congestive heart failure, 118

Conjugation reactions, 157–158, 159–160, 160t. *See also* Phase II reactions

Constant IV infusion, 443, 444f

Continuous ambulatory peritoneal dialysis (CAPD), 807

Continuous arteriovenous hemofiltration (CAVH), 813

Continuous manufacturing, 858t

Continuous pharmacodynamic responses, 686

Continuous renal replacement therapy (CRRT), 812–813

Continuous veno-venous hemofiltration (CVVH), 813

Contraceptive vaginal rings, 883–884, 885t

Controlled porosity osmotic pump (CPOP), 330

Controlled-release drug product, 306

Controlled studies, 72–73

Convective transportation, 374

Cooperativity, 144

Coordinates
    rectangular, 30, 30f, 35, 35f
    semilog, 30, 30f

Core tablets, 328–329

Cortical nephrons, 173, 174f

Corticosteroids, 120

Covariate analyses, 630–631

CPKS. *See* Clinical pharmacokinetic

CPP. *See* Critical process parameters

CQA. *See* Critical quality attributes (CQA)

Creatinine, 760
    definition of, 791
    excretion of, 792
    factors that affect, 796t

Creatinine clearance
    calculation of, 792, 959
    definition of, 792
    description of, 477

elimination rate constants and, 799f

glomerular filtration rate measurement using, 791–792

in obese patients, 771–772

serum creatinine concentration for calculation of, 793–795

in special populations, 792

Creutzfeldt–Jakob disease, 859–860

Critical dose drugs, 718, 933–934, 974. *See also* Narrow therapeutic index (NTI) drugs

Critical manufacturing variables (CMVs), 5, 868

Critical material attributes (CMA), 202

Critical process parameters (CPP)
    description of, 202, 218, 854
    quality by design, 857

Critical quality attributes (CQA)
    description of, 217, 854
    quality by design, 857

Crohn's disease, 104–105, 118–119, 228

Crossover control, 72

Crossover study designs for bioequivalence
    clinical endpoint, 269
    Latin-square crossover designs, 265–266, 266t
    multiple-dose, 268–269
    nonreplicate parallel, 268
    replicated, 266–267
    scaled average, 267–268
    illustration of, 65f

CRP. *See* Canadian reference product (CRP)

CRRT. *See* Continuous renal replacement therapy (CRRT)

Curosurf, 886t

Current Good Manufacturing Practices (cGMP), 850, 863, 864t

Curve fitting, 30

Curve stripping, 385, 418

CVRs. *See* Contraceptive vaginal rings

CVVH. *See* Continuous veno-venous hemofiltration; Continuous veno-venous hemofiltration (CVVH)

Cyclosporine, 767, 876

Cylinder method, 199

CYP1A2, 163, 166t, 662–663, 776

CYP2A6, 663

CYP2B6, 166t

CYP2C9, 166t, 658t, 660t, 663, 768, 776

CYP2C19, 161, 658t, 660t, 663–664, 738

CYP2D6, 163, 166t, 658t, 659, 660t, 662, 776

CYP2E1, 166t, 768

CYP3A4, 101, 166t, 167, 664, 966

CYP3A5, 166t, 664

CYP3A7, 166t, 776

CYP enzymes
    characteristics of, 166t
    description of, 155, 659–665
    genetic variation of, 163–164
    obesity effects on, 768, 772
    in older adults, 759–760
    in pediatric patients, 775–776

Cytochrome P-450 (CYP450), 563

Cytokine release syndrome (CRS), 365

**D**

Data
    ordinal, 52
    parametric vs. nonparametric, 52
    population pharmacokinetic, 744–745

Data analysis
    for linearity determination, 568, 568f, 569t

Daunorubicin, 338

DDIs. *See* Drug–drug interactions (DDIs)

Deconvolution, 211–212

Definite integral, 29

Delayed-release drug products, 306, 307t

DELS. *See* Difference extended least-squares (DELS)

Delta, 62, 63t

Dental implant, 337

Depakene. *See* Valproic acid

Dependent variable, 17, 51

Depocyt, 886t

Dermaflex, 334

DES. *See* Drug-eluting stents (DES)

Design space, 857

Desolvated solvates, 191
Detection bias, 71
Deterrent products, 878–880
Deviation, 31
Dexamethasone, 881t
Dexamethasone/tobramycin, 257t
Dextroamphetamine, 327
Dextromethorphan, 100, 328
Diabetes mellitus, 788t
Diagnostic bias, 71
Dialysance, 809
Dialysis
    definition of, 807
    factors that affect, 808t
    frequency of, 808
    hemodialysis, 807–809, 810t
    peritoneal, 807
    practice problems, 809–812
    vancomycin, 809
Diazepam, 740, 899
Diclofenac, 257t
Didanosine, 262
Diet. See Food
Difference extended least-squares
    (DELS), 745
Difference factor, 208
Differential calculus, 27–28
Differential equations, 389–390, 598
Diffusion
    across cell membranes, 90–94,
        91f, 93f, 93t
    facilitated, 95
    passive, 90–94, 91f, 94f, 131
    schematic diagram of, 134f
Diffusion cells system, 200–201, 201f
Diffusion coefficient, 92
Diffusion-limited model, 598–600
Digestion, 102
Digestive phase, 310
Digital health, 889
Digital medicines, 889, 889f
Digital therapeutics, 889
Digoxin (Lanoxin)
    administration of, 726
    CYP3A4 and, 101
    distribution of, 425–426
    dosage of, 726
    half-lives of, 430t
    hemodialysis removal of, 810t
    loading dose, 425–426
    serum concentrations of, 726–727

therapeutic range for, 719t
two-compartment model for
    distribution of, 420f, 420t,
    420–422, 421t
    in uremic patients, 420
    verapamil and, 741
Dihydropyrimidine dehydrogenase,
    658t, 660t, 664–665
Diprivan, 886t
Dipyridamole, 113
Direct effect model, 696, 696f
Discrete pharmacodynamic
    responses, 686
Discrete variables, 51
Discriminating dissolution test,
    201–202
Disease states
    absorption in, 118–120
    bioavailability in, 263
Disintegrants, 187
Disintegration, 186–187
Dissolution, 187–188
    BCS and, 284
    clinical performance and, 217–218
    excipients and, 192t–193t, 193
    lubricant effect on, 193, 193f
    of MR drug products, 309, 309f
    profile comparisons, 207–209, 208f
    solubility and, 188f
Dissolution in a reactive medium, 193
Dissolution test
    apparatus for, 195, 195t, 198f
    chemical calibration for, 203–205
    development and validation of,
        195–197
    discriminating, 201–202
    of enteric-coated products, 201
    of ER drug products, 309, 344
    mechanical calibration for,
        203–205, 204
    medium for, 196–197
    meeting requirements for,
        205–206
    methods for, 195, 197–201
        cylinder, 195t, 199
        diffusion cell, 195t, 200–201, 201f
        flow-through cell, 195t, 199
        intrinsic dissolution, 200
        paddle, 195t, 197–198, 198f
        paddle-over disk, 195t, 199
        reciprocating cylinder, 195t, 199

        reciprocating disk, 195t, 200
        rotating basket, 195t, 197
        rotating bottle, 195t, 200
    for novel/special dosage forms, 201
    performance verification test,
        203–205
    solid formulations, 206
    variable control problems in,
        206–207
Distributional clearance, 468
Distribution equilibrium, 416
Distribution half-life, 422, 430t
Distribution phase
    length of, 433f
    significance of, 434–435
    in two-compartment open
        model, 415
Divalproex sodium (Depakote®ER), 320
DMF. See Drug master files (DMF)
DNA chip, 655
D-optimality, 970
Dosage
    biopharmaceutic considerations
        for, 221
    drug design considerations,
        223–224
    form, for MR drug products, 313
    in hepatic disease, 814–815, 815t
Dosage intervals, 526, 526t, 527t,
    732–734
Dosage regimens. See also
        Multiple-dosage regimens
    adaptive model for, 729
    adjustment of, 951
    design of, 728–730
    empirical, 730
    fixed model for, 729
    individualization of, 718
    individualized, 729
    nomograms in, 730
    partial pharmacokinetic
        parameters for, 729
    population averages, 729
    population pharmacokinetic
        application to, 742–743
    schedules for, 537f, 537–540
        clinical example, 538
        practice problem, 538–540, 540t
    tabulations in, 730
    therapeutic drug monitoring,
        720–721

Dose
   Cav(ss) in calculations, 732
   determination of, 731–734
   duration of activity and, 680–681
   elimination half-life and, 681
   pharmacologic response and,
      678–680
Dose adjustments
   in hepatic diseases, 819–820
   in renal impairment
      basis for, 798
      limitations of, 806t, 806–807
      nomograms, 798–801
      overview of, 797–798
      tables for, 801–806
Dose-dumping, 111, 314, 343
Dose proportionality, 951
Dosing
   in children, 735, 773–774,
      777–778
   in elderly, 735
   frequency of, 223–224
   in infants, 735
   in obese patients, 769–772
   in pediatric patients, 735, 773–774,
      777–778
   in renal impairment, 789t, 789–791
   in special populations, 735
Double-blind study, 73
Double-dummy study, 73
Double-peak phenomenon, 113
Double reciprocal plot, 145
Doxil, 886t
Doxycycline, 337, 882t
DPIs. See Dry powder inhalers (DPIs)
Drug absorption
   administration route and, 86,
      87t–88t
   bioavailability and, 481, 509–511
   biopharmaceuticals, 373–375
   concentration–time profiles after,
      502–504
   in drug product design, 85–86
   extent of, 36
   first-order
      description of, 501–502
      one-compartment model,
         503–504
      two-compartment model,
         505, 505f
   in GI tract, 105f, 106–114

double-peak phenomenon,
      113, 113f
   emptying time, 106–107, 108f
   food effects on, 109–112,
      110t, 111f
   GI motility, 106, 106f, 107t
   GI perfusion, 108
   inhibition of, 741
   of lipid-soluble drugs, 225–226
   lymphatic system, 108–109
   method for studying, 115–118
   nonlinear elimination with,
      561–562
   obesity effects on, 767
   overview of, 497–498
   particle size and, 190–191
   in pediatric patients, 774–775
   pharmacokinetic calculations
      data fitting, 508
      Wagner-Nelson method, 506f,
         506–508, 507t
   polymorphism, solvates, and drug,
      191, 191f
   processes involved in, 499–500
   rate of, 509–511
   solubility, pH and, 189–190
   stability, pH and, 190
   substance abuse potential, 682
   two-compartment model
      equations, 505
   zero-order
      description of, 500–501
      nonlinear elimination with, 562
      one-compartment model,
         502–503, 503f
Drug accumulation.
      See Accumulation
Drug administration
   frequency of, 733
   route of. See also specific route
      absorption and, 86, 87t–88t, 89
      determination of, 734–735
      intravenous. See Intravenous
         (IV) bolus administration
      types of, 735f
Drug approval
   barriers to, 832f
   pharmacokinetics/
      pharmacodynamics models in,
      706–708
Drug assays, 723–725

Drug carriers
   albumin, 368
   liposomes, 368f, 368–369
   polymeric delivery systems,
      324–325, 340, 341t
   protein drugs, 368
Drug clearance. See Clearance
Drug concentration. See also Plasma
      drug concentration
   drug response and, 8, 12, 12f
   measurement of, 12, 16, 130–131
      biologic specimen sampling, 13
      blood, plasma, or serum
         concentrations, 13–14,
         14f, 16–17
      forensic measurements, 16
      plasma drug concentration time
         curve, 14f, 14–15, 15f
      saliva concentration, 16
      significance of, 16–17
      tissue concentration, 15–16
      units for expressing, 34
      units of expression in, 32–34, 33t
      in urine and feces, 15–16
Drug-concentration effect model,
      690–692
Drug concentration-time curve, 14f,
      14–15, 15f
Drug delivery
   albumin, 368
   colonic, 228
   floating, 332
   of genes, 363t
   imaging-guided system for,
      341–342
   liposomes, 368–369
   osmotic, 323f, 329–330, 331f
   polymeric systems, 324–325, 340
   of protein drugs, 356,
      357t–358t, 359
   rectal, 229
   targeted
      drugs for, 372
      site-specific properties, 372
      target site, 371–372
   transdermal, 121
   vaginal, 229
Drug development
   process of, 674–676, 685,
      913–914, 946, 970
   quality risks in, 862–863

Drug–device combination products
  digital medicines, 889, 889*f*
  drug-eluting stents, 890–892,
    891*f*–892*f*, 891*t*
  inhalation delivery systems,
    901–908
  intrauterine devices, 892, 893*t*, 894*f*
  nasal delivery systems, 897–901,
    899*t*–901*t*
  transdermal delivery systems,
    892–897, 895*t*–896*t*
Drug distribution
  apparent volume of. *See Apparent*
    *volume of distribution*
  barriers that affect, 136
  blood flow-facilitated, 134–135
  in breast milk, 138–139
  description of, 52–53
  extent of, 133–136, 139–141
  factors that affect, 133–136
  lipophilic compound penetration
    of barriers, 136
  measurement of, 139–141
  membrane transporters' effect on,
    136–138
  obesity effects on, 767–768
  in older adults, 759
  overview of, 129–130
  in pediatric patients, 775
  plasma protein binding effects on,
    141–142, 599
  privileged sites of, 136
  rate of, 133–136
  schematic diagram of, 134*f*
  statistical, 52–53
  tissue binding effects on, 140*f*,
    141–142
  volume of. *See Apparent volume*
    *of distribution*
Drug–drug interactions (DDIs),
  962–967, 976*t*
Drug–drug protein binding
  interactions, 149
Drug elimination, 567–568. *See also*
  *Clearance*
  capacity-limited, 552*f*, 552–561,
    553*t*, 555*f*, 555*t*–556*t*, 556*f*,
    559*f*, 560*f*
  definition of, 463
  enzymatic, 550, 550*t*–551*t*
  first-order, 40, 41*t*

  first-pass effects, 169
  kidneys in, 172–178, 177*t*
  liver in, 151–153
  nonlinear, 561–562
  rate of, 550, 550*t*–551*t*
  renal, 172–178, 177*t*
  transporters in, 171–172
  zero-order, 39–40, 42
Drug-eluting stents (DES), 185,
  890–892, 891*f*–892*f*, 891*t*
Drug equilibrium, 132*f*, 599
Drug excretion. *See Excretion*
Drug exposure
  circadian rhythms and, 564
  definition of, 674
  drug response and, 12
  response relationship with, 675
Drug formulary, 720, 916
Drug-in-adhesive, 894, 897*f*
Drug in body
  for capacity-limited drug after IV
    bolus infusion, 552*f*, 552–554
  equilibrium of, 132*f*
  in multiple-dosage regimens,
    526–529, 527*t*
Drug interactions
  adverse viral, 742
  of CYP450 enzymes, 563
  definition of, 735
  drug metabolism and, 164–165
  in GI tract, 100–101
  with grapefruit juice, 100, 120,
    164–165, 165*t*, 742
  pharmaceutical
    compounding of, 736*t*
  pharmacodynamics of, 736*t*
  pharmacokinetics of, 735–739,
    736*t*–737*t*
  protein binding, 149
  screening for, 735, 738
  transporter-mediated, 167
Drug master files (DMF), 835–836
Drug metabolism, 463
  capacity-limited, 547–549, 549*f*
  drug interactions involving,
    164–165
  genetic polymorphisms in,
    657–659
  induction of, 740–741
  inhibition of, 739
  obesity effects on, 768–769, 772

  in older adults, 759–760
  in pediatric patients, 775–776
Drug-metabolizing enzymes, 661*f*
Drug Price Competition and Patent
  Term Restoration Act, 919
Drug product. *See also specific*
  *products*
  "AA," 917
  "AB," 917
  pharmaceutical equivalence of,
    834–835, 835*t*
  pharmacokinetics of, food effects
    on, 956–957
  quality risks in, 855–856, 861–862
Drug product design
  absorption enhancers, 233–234
  absorption in, 85–86, 114–115
  bioavailability for, 222–223,
    246–248, 260–267, 261*t*
  biopharmaceutics for, 221, 233*t*
  colonic drug delivery, 228
  combination drug/medical
    device, 185
  dose considerations for, 223
  dosing frequency considerations
    for, 223–224
  GI side effects, 226–227
  inhalation drug products,
    231–233, 232*t*
  IR and MR drug products, 227
  nasal drug products, 230–231
  parenteral drugs, 229–230, 230*f*
  patient considerations in, 224
  pharmacodynamics for, 221–222
  pharmacokinetics for, 222
  phases in, 674–676, 676*f*
  physicochemical considerations
    for, 188–191, 189*t*
  PK-PD information flow in,
    674–676
  rectal and vaginal drug
    delivery, 229
  route of administration in,
    224, 224*f*
  transdermal products, 233
Drug product development process,
  674–676, 675*f*
Drug product performance
  biopharmaceutics and, 851–853
  definition of, 3, 243, 850
  dissolution and, 217–218

Drug product performance (*Cont.*)
  drug product quality and, 186
  excipient effect on, 192*t*–193*t*,
    192–194, 859
  *in vitro,* 194*t*, 194–195
  *in vivo,* 209–217
Drug product quality
  definition of, 850, 853
  description of, 853
  drug product performance
    and, 186
  factors that affect, 853
Drug–protein binding. *See also*
    Protein binding
  constants, 145–146
  extent of, 142–143
  kinetics of, 143–144
  protein concentration–drug
    concentration relationship
    in, 147
  in renal impairment, 788
  Scatchard plot, 145–146
  sites of, 145–146
Drug recalls, 853, 854*t*
Drug regulatory agencies (DRAs),
    842, 946
Drug release, 184
Drug response, 12
  definition of, 12, 674
  dose relationship with, 347
  drug concentration and, 8, 12, 12*f*
  drug exposure and, 12, 675
  exposure relationship with, 675
  variability in, factors that
    affect, 720*t*
Drug review process, 277–278
  bioequivalence study waiver,
    281–282, 284*t*
  dissolution profile comparison, 282
Drug-specific transporters.
    *See* Transporters
Drug submission
  new, 948–949
  pathways, 946–947
Drug tolerance, 682–683
Drug withdrawals, 853
Dry powder inhalers (DPIs), 904,
    905*t*–906*t*, 906*f*
Duncan method, 68
Dunnett method, 68
Dunn method, 68

Duodenum, 104, 106
Duration of activity (t$_{eff}$)
  dose and, 680–681
  elimination half-life effects on,
    681–682, 682*f*, 682*t*
Duration of drug action, 15
Dynamic range, 724

**E**
Early dose administration, 530
Eculizumab, 361
EDTA, 131
Efavirenz, 262
Effect, 674
Effect compartment model, 696*f*,
    696–699, 700
Effective concentration.
    *See* Minimum effective
    concentration
Effective renal plasma flow, 176
Effect site concentration, 697
Effect size, 62
Efflux transporters, 95, 95*f*, 96–98,
    263, 288
Elderly. *See also* Older adults
  bioequivalence studies in, 287
  dosing in, 735
Elimination half-life, 803*t*–804*t*
  of capacity-limited drug, 552–554
  definition of, 403
  distribution half-life relationship
    with, 422, 430, 431*f*
  dose and, 681
  duration of activity affected by,
    681–682, 682*f*, 682*t*
  infusion method for calculation of,
    447–448
  in multiple-dosage regimens, 525*t*,
    525–526, 526*t*
  one-compartment open model
    for IV bolus administration,
    403–405
Elimination phase
  description of, 499
  in two-compartment open model
    clearance and, 424*f*, 424–425
    of plasma drug concentration-
    time curve, 412, 412*f*, 415
Elimination rate constants
  of aminoglycosides, 533–534
  creatinine clearance and, 799*f*

dose adjustments based on,
    789–790
  for drugs, 800*t*
  one-compartment open model for
    IV bolus administration, 403
  renal, 403
  renal impairment effects on,
    790, 800*t*
EM. *See* Exceptation
    maximization (EM)
Emend, 886*t*
Empirical dosage regimens, 730
Empirical models, 18
  allometric scaling, 585–589,
    586*t*–587*t*
  description of, 584
Emulsions, 835*t*
Enantiomers, 160–161, 161*t*
Endocytosis, 99, 100*f*
Endoplasmic reticulum, 154
Endpoints
  clinical, 253, 254*t*–255*t*
  surrogate, 685, 686*t*
End-stage renal disease (ESRD), 807
Enfortumab vedotin, 369
Enteral administration, 87*t*–88*t*
Enteral system, 102
Enteric-coated products, 306,
    308, 336
  dissolution test of, 201
Enterocytes, 94
Enterohepatic circulation, 170*f*,
    170–171
Enzyme(s). *See also* Capacity-limited
    pharmacokinetics
  hepatic
    in biotransformation, 153–156,
      161–162
    mixed-function oxidases,
      153–156
  saturation of, 550*t*–551*t*, 550–551
Enzyme induction, 164
Enzyme inhibition, 164
Enzyme kinetics. *See*
    Michaelis– Menten kinetics
Equation-based method, 747
Equilibrium dialysis, 142*f*, 143
Ergometrine, 430*t*
ER/MR drug products.
    *See* Extended/modified release
    (EM/MR) products

ERPF. *See* Effective renal plasma flow
Error, 71–72
Erythrocytes, 191*f*
Erythromycin, 111, 111*f*, 165*t*,
    191, 191*f*
Erythropoietin, 359
Esomeprazole (Nexium), 8, 9*t*–11*t*,
    101, 161, 308
Esophagus, 102–103
ESRD. *See* End-stage renal disease;
    End-stage renal disease (ESRD)
Estradiol, 895*t*–896*t*
Estradiol/levonorgestrel, 895*t*
Estring, 885*t*
Ethchlorvynol, 810*t*
Ethinyl estradiol, 114*t*
Etonogestrel, 881*t*
Etoposide, 432–433
European Medicines Agency, 344,
    364, 833, 914–915,
    923*t*, 924, 933
European Union, 920
Evergreening, 920
Exception maximization (EM), 590
Excipients
    description of, 184, 835*t*, 837
    drug product performance effect
        of, 192*t*, 192–194, 859
    in gelatin, 860
    pediatric patient tolerance to,
        860–861
    quality monitoring of, 862
    quantitative changes in, 868–869
Excretion
    biliary, 171
    bioavailability and, 481–482
    description of, 463
    obesity effects on, 769
    in older adults, 760–761
    in pediatric patients, 776–777
    renal drug, 175–178
    renal impairment effects on, 959
Exocytosis, 99–100, 100*f*
Expectation step, 593
Experiment-wise methods, 68
Exploratory data analysis, 628
Exponential functions, 37
Exponents, 37–39
Exposure. *See* Drug exposure
Extended least-squares (ELS),
    591–592, 592*t*

Extended/modified release (EM/MR)
    products
    combination products, 336–337
    core tablets, 328–329
    description of, 186
    drug release from matrix, 318*f*, 320,
        323–324
    gastroretentive system, 332
    gum-type matrix tablets, 324
    implants and inserts, 337
    ion-exchange products, 328
    liposomes, 339*t*
    microencapsulation, 329
    nanotechnology derived, 338
    osmotic drug delivery system,
        323*f*, 329–330, 331*f*, 331*t*
    parenteral dosage forms, 337
    pharmacokinetic simulation of,
        317*f*, 317–318
    plasma drug concentration of,
        317, 317*f*
    polymeric matrix tables,
        324–325, 341*t*
    prolonged-action tablets, 327–328
    slow-release pellets, beads,
        or granules, 325–327, 327*t*
    statistical evaluation of, 347
    transdermal drug delivery system,
        332–335, 333*t*, 334*f*
    types of, 320–342
Extended/modified release (ER/MR)
    products, 205, 208*f*, 227,
        306, 307*t*
    advantages and disadvantages of,
        313–315
    bioavailability study for, 308–309
        pharmacokinetic profile, 346
        rate of drug absorption,
            346–347, 347*f*
        steady-state plasma drug
            concentration, 346
        transit time in, 311–312
    bioequivalence study for, 347
    biopharmaceutic factors of,
        310–313
        large intestine, 312–313
        small intestine, 311–312
        stomach, 310–311
    clinical efficacy and safety of, 342
    clinical example of, 319–320
    dissolution rates of, 309, 309*f*

dosage form selection, 313
evaluation of, 340
    clinical considerations, 345
    dissolution studies, 309*f*
    IVIC, 344
    pharmacodynamic and safety
        considerations, 342–343
    pharmacokinetic studies,
        344–345
examples of, 309
generic substitution of, 345–346
with immediate release
    component, 318
kinetics of, 315–317
Extensive metabolizers, 164
Extent of absorption, 36
External validity, 74, 631–632
Extrapolation, 32
Extravascular drug administration,
    497, 499*f*
Extrusion-spheronization, 326
Ezetimibe, 114*t*

**F**

Facilitated diffusion, 95
Famotidine, 112
Fasting study, for bioequivalence,
    264–265, 275*t*, 275–277,
    276*f*, 276*t*, 277*f*
FDA. *See* Food and Drug
    Administration
Feathering, 418
Feces, 15–16
Femring, 885*t*
Fentanyl, 102, 228, 758, 895*t*
Feraheme, 886*t*
Ferrlecit, 886*t*
Fetroja, 801, 801*t*
Fick's law of diffusion, 33, 91–93, 131
Filtration pressure, 135. *See also*
    Hydrostatic pressure
FIM study. *See* First-in-Man Single
    Ascending Doses Study
First-in-Man Single Ascending Doses
    Study, 951–952, 975*t*
First-order absorption
    description of, 501–502
    nonlinear elimination with, 562
    one-compartment model, 503*f*,
        503–504
    two-compartment model, 505, 505*f*

First-order conditional estimation (FOCE), 590

First-order conditional estimation interaction (FOCEI), 590

First-order elimination, 38–41, 41*f*, 41*t*

First-order half-life, 41*f*, 41*t*

First-order process, 40–41, 41*f*, 41*t*

First-pass effects
  absolute bioavailability, 260–267
  definition of, 169, 481–482

Fisher's exact test, 69

"Fit factors," 208

Fixed model, 729

Flector, 896*t*

Flip-flop pharmacokinetics, 509–511

Floating drug delivery system, 332

Flow-through-cell method, 195*t*, 199

Fluconazole, 229

Fluid-bed coating, 325

Fluid mosaic model, 90

Fluocinolone acetonide, 881*t*

Fluorouracil (FU), 94

Fluoxetine, 164, 165*t*

Fluticasone, 257*t*, 843

Fluvoxamine, 739

FOCE. *See* First-order conditional estimation (FOCE)

FOCEI. *See* First-order conditional estimation interaction (FOCEI)

Food
  drug interactions with, 109, 110*t*, 111*f*, 111–112
  drug product pharmacokinetics affected by, 956–957, 975*t*
  GI absorption and, 109, 111*f*, 111–112
  theophylline and, interactions between, 741–742

Food, Drug, and Cosmetic Act, 919

Food and Drug Administration (FDA). *See also* Abbreviated New Drug Application; New Drug Application
  bioavailability study guidance, 259–260
  505(b)(2) pathway, 947–948
  generic biologics guidance, 287

industry guidance by, 863

Orange Book, 916

Postmarketing Surveillance program, 869–870

Scale-Up and Postapproval Changes guidances, 866

Food-effect bioavailability study, 259

Food intervention study, 265

Foreign reference product (FRP), 931

Forensic drug measurements, 16

Fosamax®. *See* Alendronate sodium

Four-way ANOVA, 67

Fraction of dose in body, 526, 527*t*

Fraction of drug excreted, 803*t*–804*t*

Fraction of drug metabolized, 815

Franz diffusion cell, 200, 201*f*

Free drug hypothesis, 133, 133*f*

FRP. *See* Foreign reference product (FRP)

FU. *See* Fluorouracil

Fumaryl diketopiperazine, 904

## G

Gamma scintigraphy, 115

Gantrisin. *See* Sulfisoxazole

Garamycin. *See* Gentamicin sulfate

Gastrin, 103

Gastrointestinal therapeutic systems (GITs), 323*f*, 329

Gastrointestinal tract
  absorption in, 88*t*, 310–311
  aging effects, 758
  double-peak phenomenon, 113, 113*f*
  emptying time, 116
  food effects on, 109, 110*t*, 111*f*, 111–112
  GI motility and, 106, 106*f*
  GI perfusion, 108
  intestinal motility, 107–108
  in older adults, 758
  anatomic and physiologic considerations, 101–102, 102*f*
  drug interactions in, 100–101
  fluid pH, 103*t*
  side effects involving, 226–227

GastroPlus, 115

Gastroretentive system, 332

Gaussian distribution. *See* Normal distribution

Gauss–Newton method, 592

Gelatin, 859–860

Gemfibrozil, 114*t*

Gemtuzumab ozogamicin, 369

Generic applications, 920

Generic biologics, 285–287

Generic capsules, 841

Generic products
  active pharmaceutical ingredient of, 935
  approval of, 919
  bioequivalence, 265, 914–918
  equivalence requirements, 935–940
  marketing exclusivity, 919
  marketing of, 921, 929
  patent protection, 919
  pharmaceutical equivalence of, 921
  size, shape, and other physical attributes of, 841
  submission of, 921–924
  therapeutic nonequivalence of, 841–842

Generic substitution, 345–346

Generic tablets, 841

Gene therapy, 362, 363*t*, 364–365

Genetic polymorphisms
  definition of, 656
  description of, 163, 656–657
  in drug metabolism, 657–659
  drug-metabolizing enzymes that exhibit, 661*f*
  mutations versus, 656

Genetics. *See* Pharmacogenetics

Gentamicin sulfate (Garamycin), 532–533, 617, 719*t*, 805

Geometric mean, 54

GFR. *See* Glomerular filtration rate

GI tract. *See* Gastrointestinal tract

Givlaari, 371

Glomerular filtration, 175, 474–476

Glomerular filtration rate (GFR)
  age-related changes in, 760–761
  description of, 173, 176
  measurement of, 791–792, 796–797
  Modification of Diet in Renal Disease (MDRD) equation used to estimate, 795–796
  in obese patients, 770, 771*f*

Glomerulus, 173
Glucose 6-phosphate dehydrogenase deficiency, 163
Glucuronidation, 158, 160*t*
Glutathione (GSH), 159–160, 160*t*
Gluten, 119
GMPs. *See* Good Manufacturing Practices (GMPs)
Good Manufacturing Practices (GMPs), 863
Goodness of fit, 69
Goodness-of-fit plots, 631, 631*f*
Goserelin, 881*t*
Gradumet, 324
Granisetron, 896*t*
Granules, 325–327
Grapefruit juice, 100, 120, 164–165, 165*t*, 742, 966
Graphs, 28, 28*f*, 29–31
    curve fitting, 30, 32, 32*f*
    fitting points to, 32, 32*f*
    practice problems, 31–32
    slope determination, 30, 32, 32*f*
Griseofulvin, 111*f*, 190, 226
GSH. *See* Glutathione (GSH)
Gum-type matrix tablets, 324

**H**

Half-life. *See also* Elimination half-life
    accumulation, 525, 525*t*
    distribution, 430, 430*t*
    first-order, 41*f*, 41*t*
    time to reach steady-state drug concentration and, 444*f*, 444–446
    zero-order, 40, 41*t*
Hatch–Waxman Act, 919
Hauck-Anderson t-test, 927
Hazard ratio, 76
Health Canada, 4, 833, 914–915, 924
Heidelberg capsule, 116
*Helicobacter pylori*, 663
Hemodialysis, 807–809, 810*t*
Hemofiltration, 812
Hemoglobin, oxygen binding to, 144
Hemoperfusion, 812
Henderson–Hasselbalch equation, 92–93, 177
Hepatic artery, 152
Hepatic blood flow, 816–817
Hepatic clearance, 484–486

Hepatic diseases
    Child–Pugh score/classification, 814, 817, 817*t*
    dosage considerations in, 814–815, 815*t*
    dose adjustments in, 819–820
    drugs affected by, 818*t*
    fraction of drug metabolized in, 815
    intrinsic clearance, 816
    liver function tests in, 818–819
    metabolites in, 816
    pathophysiologic assessment of, 817–818
    pharmacokinetics affected by, 813–820
    practice problems for, 815–816
    severity classification for, 817*t*
    types of, 813
Hepatic enzymes
    in biotransformation, 153–156, 161–162
    mixed-function oxidases, 153–156
Hepatic impairment study, 961–962, 976*t*
Hepatic portal vein, 154*f*
*HER2*, 684
Hetacillin, 157*t*
High-extracted drugs, 485, 487–488
Higuchi equation, 323
Hill coefficient, 691–692
Hill equation, 691
Historical control studies, 72
Histrelin, 881*t*
HMG-CoA reductase inhibitor, 600
Homeostatic physiologic functions, in regional pharmacokinetics, 748
Housekeeper contractions, 311
Human follicle-stimulating hormone (hFSH), 430
Human growth hormone, 86
Human immunodeficiency virus (HIV), 133, 133*f*
Hyaluronidases, 359
Hydrates, 191
Hydrocodone, 315
Hydrocodone bitartrate, 879*t*
Hydromorphone (Dilaudid) ER, 323*f*, 428*t*, 428–429, 430*t*
Hydrophilic polymers, 325
Hydrostatic pressure, 131–132, 135

Hypersensitivity, 683–684
Hypertension, 788*t*
Hypodermis, 374
Hypothesis testing, 59–63
    with nonparametric data, 69–72
    with parametric data, 62–63
Hypovolemia, 788*t*
Hysteresis loop, 697, 697*f*

**I**

Ibuprofen, 582, 582*t*–583*t*
IBW. *See* Ideal body weight
ICH. *See* International Conference on Harmonisation (ICH)
Ideal body weight (IBW), 766, 766*t*, 792
Ileum, 104
Imaging-guided drug delivery system, 341–342
IM injection. *See* Intramuscular (IM) injection
Immediate-release (IR) drug products, 227, 281, 284*t*
Immunogenicity, 377, 938
Immunotoxins, 370
Implants, 337, 880*f*, 880–883, 881*t*–882*t*
Impurities, 837, 862
Impurities-related therapeutic nonequivalence, 837
Impurity, 864
Incidence rate ratio, 76
Independent samples, 66
Independent variable, 17, 51
Index perpetrators, 964, 965*t*
Indirect response models, 699–704
Individual analyses, 593–594
Infants, dosing in, 735. *See also* Pediatric patients
INFeD, 886*t*
Influx membrane transporters, 137, 137*f*
Infusion. *See* Intravenous (IV) infusion
Inhalation drug delivery, 88*t*, 121, 901–908
Inhalation drug products, 231–233, 835*t*
Inhaled insulin, 89, 121
Initial estimates, 390
Injectafer, 886*t*

Inotuzumab ozogamicin, 369

Inserts, 337

*In silico* screens, 222

*In-situ* implants, 882f, 882–883

Institutional Pharmacy and
    Therapeutic Committee, 720

Institutional Review Board (IRB), 259

Insulin
    inhaled, 89, 121
    oral delivery of, 89

Integral calculus, 28f, 28–29

Integrated equations, 389–390

Interchangeability
    biosimilarity vs., 286–287, 939
    definition of, 916
    federal jurisdiction, 939

Interchangeable biosimilar drug
    products, 844

Interdigestive phase, 310–311

Interferon, 356, 359

Interferon-ß, 740

Interferon-α-2b, 368

Interleukin-6, 706f

Intermittent IV infusion,
    531–532, 532t
    clinical example, 533–534
    superposition of several IV
        infusion doses, 531–532

Internal validity, 74, 631–632,
    970–972

International Conference on
    Harmonisation (ICH),
    844, 850, 864

Interpolation, 32

Interspecies scaling, 585, 586t, 587

Interval data, 52

Intestinal absorption
    transporters in, 95f, 95–98

Intestinal epithelial transporters, 89f

Intestinal motility, 107–108

Intra-arterial injection, 87t

Intradermal injection, 87t

Intrahepatic bile ducts, 169

Intramuscular (IM) injection
    description of, 87t
    design considerations for, 230f
    in older adults, 758–759

Intranasal administration, 88t

Intraperitoneal injection, 87t

Intrathecal injection, 87t

Intrauterine devices (IUDs),
    892, 893t, 894f

Intravenous (IV) bolus
    administration, 87t
    design considerations for,
        229–230, 230f
    disadvantages of, 400
    dose and elimination half-life
        after, 681
    indications for, 734
    multicompartment models,
        411–412, 412f, 413,
        420–422, 434–435
        clinical application of, 425–427
        determination of, 429f, 429–430
    one-compartment open model,
        555f, 556f
        capacity-limited drug elimination,
            552f, 552–554, 555f, 556f
        clearance, 402–403
        disadvantages of, 400
        elimination half-life, 403–405
        elimination rate constant, 403
        example of, 385–387, 386f
        overview of, 399–401
        pharmacokinetics/
            pharmacodynamics model,
            385–387, 386f
        Sawchuk–Zaske method,
            405–406
        volume of distribution, 401–402
    three-compartment open model
        clinical applications, 427f,
            428–429
        description of, 427f, 427–428
    two-compartment open model
        of, 415f, 415–420, 419f, 419t,
            424–425, 430
        apparent volume of distribution
            in, 422, 423–424, 425
        clearance in, 426
        clinical application, 420f, 420t,
            420–422, 421t
        elimination rate constant in, 427
        method of residuals, 418–420,
            419f, 419t
        practical focus, 425–427
        practice problems, 430, 430t
        relation between distribution
            and elimination half-life,
            430, 430t
Intravenous (IV) infusion, 87t, 443
    clearance estimated from, 452–453
    constant, 445

elimination half-life calculated
    from, 447–448
intermittent, 531, 532t
    clinical example of, 533–534
    superposition of several IV
        infusion doses, 531–532
loading dose
    one-compartment open model,
        448–450, 449f–450f
    two-compartment model,
        453f, 453–454
one-compartment model of,
    444–447
    loading dose combined with,
        448–450, 449f–450f
    steady-state drug concentration
        in, 444f, 444–446, 446f
oral dosing and, conversions
    between, 730–731
plasma drug concentration–time
    curve for, 412, 412f
practice problems, 447–448
total body clearance after,
    559–561, 560f
two-compartment model of,
    453–454
    loading dose combined with,
        453f, 453–454
    practical focus, 454–455
    total volume of distribution
        in, 454
Intravenous (IV) injections,
    repetitive, 526–529, 527t
    early or late dose administration
        during, 530
    missed dose during, 529–530
Intrinsic clearance, 484–486, 816
Intrinsic dissolution method, 200
Inulin, 791
Investigator bias, 72
Invirase®. *See* Saquinavir
    mesylate
*In vitro–in vivo* correlation, 209
    definition of, 188, 616
    dissolution and clinical
        performance, 218–220
    failure of, 216–217
    level A correlation, 209–214
    level B correlation, 214–215
    level C correlation, 215
    software packages, 626
    validation of, 215–216

*In vitro–in vivo* relationship (IVIVR), 202
*In vivo* perfusion studies, of GI tract, 116–117
*In-vivo* permeability studies, 116–117
Ion-exchange products, 328
Ionization, 177, 177t
Ion-pair formation, 100
Iontophoresis, 234, 335, 897
IPTC. *See* Institutional Pharmacy and Therapeutic Committee
IRB. *See* Institutional Review Board
Irinotecan, 114t, 666
Irreversible inhibitors, 966
Isoniazid, 159, 666
Isoproterenol hydrochloride, 4–5, 156–157
Isotretinoin, 262
Isozymes, 155
IT2B, 594, 624
IT2S, 594
Iterations, 390
Itraconazole, 118
ITS, 594
IUDs. *See* Intrauterine devices (IUDs)
IV bolus administration. *See* Intravenous (IV) bolus administration
IV infusion. *See* Intravenous (IV) infusion
IV injections. *See* Intravenous (IV) injections
IVIVC. *See* In vitro–in vivo correlation
IVIVR. *See* In vitro–in vivo relationship; *In vitro–in vivo* relationship (IVIVR)

**J**
Jejunum, 104, 117
Jet nebulizers, 908
Juxtamedullary nephrons, 173, 174f

**K**
Ketoconazole, 118
Kidneys
    anatomy of, 172–173
    autoregulation, 174
    blood flow regulation, 173–175
    blood supply to, 173
    cortex of, 172, 173f
    disease of. *See* Renal impairment
    in drug elimination, 172–178
    drug excretion by, 175–178
    elimination rate constant, 403
    failure of, 788t
    functions of, 787
    medulla of, 172, 173f
    nephrons of, 172–173, 173f–174f
    reabsorption alterations in, from urinary pH changes, 741
    urine formation in, 175, 175t
*Klebsiella pneumoniae,* 690
Knowledge sharing, 857
Kurtosis, 53, 54f
Kyleena, 893t

**L**
Labels, 7–8
Lactation, 138
Lactulose, 311
Langmuir adsorption isotherm, 145
Lanoxin. *See* Digoxin
Lanreotide acetate, 888
Lansoprazole (Prevacid), 119, 257t, 841
Laplace transform, 212
Large intestine, 312–313
Late dose administration, 530
Latin-square crossover designs, 265–266, 266t
Law of mass action, 143, 676
Law of parsimony, 32
Layer methods, 68
LBW. *See* Lean body weight (LBW)
Lean body weight (LBW), 766, 766t, 792
Least significance difference, 68
Least-squares method, 30–31, 591–592, 592t, 616
Leuprolide acetate, 882t
Levenberg–Marquardt method, 592
Levodopa, 137, 156, 931
Levonorgestrel implants, 337
Levothyroxine sodium (Levothyroxine, Synthroid), 270–271
Lidocaine
    ADRs involving, 435
    distribution and elimination half-lives of, 430, 430t
    IV infusion of, 453
    patches, 233
    therapeutic range for, 719t
Lidoderm, 896t
Liletta, 893t
Linear concentration effect model, 692
Linearity, 724, 951
    determination of, 568, 568f, 569t
Linear regression, 30–31, 32f
Linezolid, 740
Link model, 696–700
Lipid bilayer theory, 90
Lipid formulation classification system, 225
Lipid-soluble drug absorption, 225–226
Liposomes, 338–340, 368–369, 835t, 886–887, 887f
Lithium, 430t, 719t
Liver
    anatomy of, 151–153
    biliary system of, 169–171
    blood flow to, 482, 485f, 816–817
    diseases of. *See* Hepatic diseases
    drug metabolism in, 153
    extraction ratio for, 482, 483t
    hepatic artery of, 152
    hepatic vein of, 152–153
    impairment study, 961–962
    lobes of, 152
    metabolic markers, 818–819
    physiology of, 151–153
    sinusoids of, 152, 154f
Liver function tests, 818–819
Loading dose
    calculation of, 769
    of digoxin, 425–426
    IV infusion plus
        one-compartment open model of, 448–450, 449f–450f
        practice problem, 450–452
        two-compartment model of, 453f, 453–454
    in multiple-dosage regimens, 536
    in obese patients, 769–770
Locally acting drug, 184
Logarithmic transformation, 54
Log-linear concentration-effect model, 693
Loop of Henle, 173
Loo-Riegelman deconvolution, 212–213, 589
Loperamide (Imodium), 429
Lorazepam, 806

L-Oros Softcap (Alza), 330, 331f
Lovastatin (Mevacor), 162
Low-extracted drugs, 485–488
Lubricant
    absorption effect of, 192
    dissolution effect of, 192, 193f, 193t
Lung perfusion, 598
Lupron® Depot, 340
Lymphatic system, 108–109

## M

mABs. See Monoclonal antibodies
MAC. See Membrane-attack
    complex (MAC)
Macroscopic events, 578
"Mad cow disease," 860
MAD studies. See Multiple ascending
    dose (MAD) studies
Magnesium aluminum hydroxide
    gel, 741
MAM. See Mechanistic absorption
    model (MAM)
Mammillary model, 19, 384–385,
    385f, 414
Manufacturing, quality risks in, 863
MAO. See Monoamine oxidase
MAOIs. See Monoamine oxidase
    inhibitors
Markers. See also Biomarkers
    biomarkers, 684–685, 686t
    surrogate, 289, 289t
Marketing exclusivity, 919
Marqibo, 886t
Mass–balance study,
    957–959, 975t
MAT. See Mean absorption time
Mathematical fundamentals, 27
    calculus
        differential, 27–28
        integral, 28f, 28–29
    exponents, 37–39
    graphs, 28f, 29–31
        curve fitting, 30
        practice problems, 35–37, 37f
        slope determination, 30, 32, 32f
    logarithms, 37–39
    rates and orders of, 39
        first-order reactions, 40–41,
            41f, 41t
        rate constant, 38
        zero-order, 39–40, 41f, 41t

significant figures, 34
spreadsheet use, 31
units, 32–34, 33t
Matrix, drug release from, 320,
    323–324
Matrix tablets, 318f, 324–325
    drug release from, 318f, 320,
        323–324
    gum-type, 324
    polymeric, 324–325
Maximum life-span potential (MLP),
    587–588
Maximum likelihood expectation
    maximization algorithm,
    592, 594
Maximum recommended starting
    dose (MRSD), 675, 951
MDIs. See Metered dose
    inhalers (MDIs)
MDL. See Minimum detectable limit
MDT. See Mean dissolution time
    (MDT); Mean in vivo
    dissolution time (MDT)
Mean, 53–54
Mean absorption time, 580–582
Mean dissolution time (MDT),
    580–582
Mean in vivo dissolution
    time (MDT), 214
Mean residence time (MRT), 214,
    393, 578–579, 583
Mean transit time (MTT), 580–583
Measurement
    significance of, 34
    significant figures, 34
Measures of central tendency, 53–55
MEC. See Minimum effective
    concentration
Mechanical calibration, 204
Mechanistic absorption model
    (MAM), 213
Mechanistic models
    blood flow–limited model, 597,
        599–600
    compartmental models, 590–591,
        595–596, 603–605
    development of, 584–585
    diffusion-limited model, 598–600
    empirical models versus, 584–585
    historical perspective on, 589–590
    individual analyses, 593–594

nonparametric modeling, 594–595
numerical problem solving,
    591–593
parametric modeling, 594–595
physiological approach, 603–605
physiologically-based
    pharmacokinetic model, 596–603
population analyses, 593–594
Median, 54
Medical device, drug designed for use
    with, 185
Medicare Prescription Drug,
    Improvement, and Modernization
    Act of 2003, 717
Medication errors, 849
Medication therapy management,
    717–718
Megace ES, 886t
MELD. See Model for end-stage liver
    disease (MELD)
Membrane-attack complex
    (MAC), 359
Membrane-limited models, 600
Membrane proteins, 90
Membrane transporters
    in cerebral endothelial cells, 137f
    description of, 136
    drug distribution affected by,
        136–138
    influx, 137, 137f
Mercaptopurine (Purinethol),
    oral, 271
Mercapturic acid
    conjugation of, 159–160
    synthesis of, 158
Meropenem, 767
Mesalamine (Asacol), 86, 88t, 105,
    228, 257t, 275t, 935
Mesalamine delayed-R, 312
Metabolic rate, 605, 605f
Metabolite clearance, 477–478
Metallic stent platform or
    scaffold, 890
Metered dose inhalers (MDIs), 902
Method of residuals, 418–420,
    419f, 419t
Methoxypolyethylene glycol
    (MPEG), 338
Methylation, 160t
Methylphenidate (Concerta),
    319, 330, 895t

Metoclopramide, 119
Metoprolol, 104, 560, 560*f*, 861
Mevacor®. *See* Lovastatin
MFOs. *See* Mixed-function
    oxidases
Micafungin, 707–708, 708*f*, 775
Micelles, 887–888, 888*f*
Michaelis constant
    determination of, 554–556, 555*f*,
        555*t*–556*f*, 556*f*, 558
    interpretation of, 559–561
    in one-compartment model with
        IV bolus injection, 552–554
Michaelis–Menten equation, 20
Michaelis–Menten kinetics, 550
    description of, 20–21, 162
    in one-compartment model with
        IV bolus injection, 552–554
    clearance in, 559–561, 560*f*
    clinical focus, 561
    determination of Michaelis
        constant and maximum
        elimination rate, 554–556,
        555*f*, 555*t*–556*t*, 556*f*
    interpretation of Michaelis
        constant and maximum
        elimination rate, 558
Microconstants, 415, 418
Microemulsion, 888
Microencapsulation, 329
Microneedles, 333
Microneedling, 897
Microparticles, 883, 884*t*
Microsome, 155
Microspheres, 883, 884*t*
Microvilli, 105*f*, 106
Midazolam, 698–699, 700*f*
"Midpoint" method, for
    clearance, 477, 792
Migrating motor complex
    (MMC), 106
Milrinone, 430*t*
Minimum detectable limit, 724
Minimum effective
    concentration (MEC)
    definition of, 4, 287
    description of, 14–15, 395
    during multiple-stage
        regimens, 521
    on plasma drug concentration–
        time curve, 14*f*, 14–15, 15*f*

Minimum inhibitory concentration
    (MIC), 538, 690
Minimum objection function
    (MOF), 629
Minimum quantifiable level, 724
Minimum toxic concentration
    (MTC), 7, 14–15, 287, 732–733
    during multiple-dosage
        regimens, 521
    on plasma drug concentration-time
        curve, 14*f*, 14–15, 15*f*
Minimum value of the objective
    function, 391
Mirena, 893*t*
Misclassification bias, 72
Missed dose, 529–530
Mixed drug elimination, 561–562
Mixed-function oxidases
    description of, 153–156
    drug interactions affecting, 165*t*
Mizolastine, 705*f*
MLP. *See* Maximum life-span
    potential
MMC. *See* Migrating motor
    complex (MMC)
Mode, 54
Model discrimination table, 633*f*
Model fitting, 385
Model for end-stage liver disease
    (MELD), 817, 961
Model-independent approach, 471
Models. *See also specific model*
    definition of, 17
    pharmacokinetic, 17–21, 18*f*
Modification of Diet in Renal Disease
    (MDRD) equation
    description of, 796
    development of, 797
    glomerular filtration rate
        estimation using, 795–796
    in obese patients, 771
    in older adults, 761
Modified-release (MR) drug
    products, 227, 275*t*, 305–306,
        321*t*–322t. *See also* Extended/
        modified release (EM/MR)
        products
Modified-release parenteral
    dosage forms, 230
MOF. *See* Minimum objection
    function (MOF)

Moments. *See* Statistical moment
    theory
Mometasone furoate, 881*t*
Monoamine oxidase inhibitors
    (MAOs), 561, 740
Monoclonal antibodies (mAbs), 134,
    359–361, 360*f*
Morphine, 114*t*, 879*t*
Motility
    GI, 106, 107*t*
    intestinal, 107–108
Moxalactam, 423*t*, 430–431, 431*f*
MQL. *See* Minimum quantifiable level
MRA. *See* Multivariate regression
    analysis (MRA)
MRSD. *See* Maximum recommended
    starting dose (MRSD)
MRT. *See* Mean residence time; Mean
    residence time (MRT)
MTC. *See* Minimum toxic
    concentration
MTM. *See* Medication therapy
    management
MTT. *See* Mean transit time (MTT)
Multicompartment models, 392.
    *See also* Three compartment
    open model; Two-compartment
    open model
    for IV bolus administration, 413
    clinical application, 420–422, 435
    practical application, 434*f*,
        434–435
Multidrug-resistance-associated
    proteins, 96, 667
Multidrug-resistance gene, 659*t*
Multidrug-resistance protein 1, 667
Multifactorial ANOVA, 66–67
Multiple ascending dose (MAD)
    studies, 953–956, 975*t*
Multiple comparison methods, 68
Multiple-dosage regimens, 521
    clinical example, 525–526, 538
    drug accumulation in, 521–525,
        522*f*, 523*t*, 525*t*
    intermittent IV infusion,
        531–532, 532*t*
    clinical example, 532–533
    superposition of several IV
        infusion doses, 531–532, 532*t*
    loading dose in, 536
    oral regimens, 534–536

Multiple-dosage regimens (*Cont.*)
  practice problems, 538–540, 540*t*
  repetitive IV injections, 526, 527*t*
    early or late dose administration
      during, 530
    missed dose during, 529–530
  schedules of, 537*f*, 537–540, 540*t*
Multiple-dose bioequivalence,
  268–269, 537*f*, 537–540, 540*t*
Multivariate regression analysis
  (MRA), 74
Mutations, polymorphisms
  versus, 656
Mycophenolate mofetil, 114*t*

**N**

*N*-acetylprocainamide, 158, 798
*N*-acetyltransferase, 658*t*–659*t*,
  660*t*, 666
NADPH, 155
NAFLD. *See* Non-alcoholic fatty liver
  disease (NAFLD)
"Naïve-average data" method, 593
"Naïve-pooled data" approach, 593
Nanocrystals, 887
Nanoemulsion, 888, 888*f*
Nanomedicines, 884–889, 886*t*, 887*f*
Nanosizing, 190
Nanotechnology, 338
Nanotube, 888
Narrow therapeutic index (NTI)
  drugs, 267, 718, 933–934, 974
Nasal drug delivery, 120–121,
  897–901, 899*t*–901*t*
Nasal drug products, 120–121
NASH. *See* Non-alcoholic
  steatohepatitis (NASH)
*NAT1*, 666
*NAT2*, 666
Natural logarithm, 37
NDA. *See* New Drug Application
Nebulizers, 906–908, 907*t*
Negatively skewed data, 54*f*
Negative predictability, 746
Negative skew, 53
Nelder–Mead simplex approach, 592
Nelfinavir, 69
Neophroallergens, 788*t*
Neoral, 886*t*
Nephrons, 172–173, 173*f*–174*f*
Nesiritide, 706–707, 708*f*

Neuroepedyma barrier, 136
New Drug Application (NDA), 5,
  277–278
  ANDA compared with,
    277–278, 278*t*
  approved, changes to, 839–840
  bioequivalence studies in, 245–246
  description of, 7, 831, 876
  FDA 505(b)(2) pathway, 947–948
  goals of, 7
  submission of, 919
New drug development process, 675*f*
Newman-Keuls method, 68
New molecular entity, 675
New/novel dosage forms
  abuse-deterrent formulations,
    878–880
  implants, 880*f*, 880–883, 881*t*–882*t*
  microparticles, 883, 884*t*
  microspheres, 883, 884*t*
  nanomedicines, 884–889,
    886*t*, 887*f*
  regulatory pathway for, 876–877
  3D printed dosage forms,
    877–878, 878*f*
  vaginal rings, 883–884, 885*t*
Nexium. *See* Esomeprazole
Nicotine, 895*t*
Nicotinic acid, 562
Nifedipine (Procardia XL),
  292, 292*t*, 311
Nitazoxanide, 257*t*
Nitrofurantoin, 190
Nitroglycerin, 228, 334, 483
Nitroglycerine, 895*t*
N-methyl pyrrolidone, 883
NNT. *See* Numbers needed to
  treat (NNT)
NOAELs. *See* No observed adverse
  effect levels (NOAELs)
Nominal data, 52
Nomograms, 730, 798–801
Non-alcoholic fatty liver disease
  (NAFLD), 768
Non-alcoholic steatohepatitis
  (NASH), 768
Non-approved indication, 8
Noncompartmental analyses
  description of, 577–578
  mean absorption time, 580–582
  mean dissolution time, 580–582

  mean residence time, 578–579, 583
  mean transit time, 580–583
  pharmacokinetic parameters
    calculated by, 582–584
  software packages, 618–625
  statistical moment theory, 578–579
Noncompartmental analysis, 393
Noncompartmental models
  description of, 393
  pharmacokinetics/pharmacodynamics,
    393, 394*t*, 688–690
Non-endogenous drugs, 151
Nonlinear pharmacokinetics, 13
  bioavailability of drugs with, 565
  chronopharmacokinetics and
    time-dependent pharmacokinetics,
      563*t*, 563–564
    circadian rhythms and drug
      exposure, 564
    clinical focus, 564
  determination of linearity, 568*f*,
    568–569
  dose-dependent, 570
  in one-compartment model
    distribution with nonlinear
      elimination, 561–562
    clinical focus, 562
    first-order absorption with
      nonlinear elimination, 562–563
    mixed drug elimination,
      561–562
    zero-order input and nonlinear
      elimination, 562
  in one-compartment model with
    IV bolus injection, 552*f*,
      552–554
    clinical focus, 561
    interpretation of Michaelis
      constant and maximum
      elimination rate, 558, 559*f*
    practice problems, 550–551, 554
  protein-bound drugs with, 565–567,
    566*f*, 567*f*
    one-compartment model drugs,
      567*f*, 567–568
  saturable enzyme elimination
    processes, 547–549, 549*f*,
      550*t*–551*t*
Nonlinear regressions, 591
NONMEM, 388, 592, 594, 621, 623
Nonparametric modeling, 594–595

Nonpareil seeds, 325
Nonreplicate, parallel bioequivalence
    study, 268
Nonsteroid anti-inflammatory drugs
    (NSAIDs), 111
Non-zero order, 41
No observed adverse effect levels
    (NOAELs), 951–952
Normal distribution, 52–53
Novel constructs, 361–362
Noyes–Whitney equation,
    27, 188, 190
NPAG, 624
NPEM, 624
NPEM2, 624
NSAIDs. See Nonsteroid
    anti-inflammatory drugs
NTI drugs. See Narrow therapeutic
    index (NTI) drugs
Null hypothesis, 59
Numbers needed to treat (NNT), 75
Numerical deconvolution, 214
Numerical problem solving, 591–593
Nutraceuticals, 735
Nutrients, drug absorption
    affected by, 119–120
Nuvaring, 885t

O

OATP. See Organic anion transporting
    polypeptide (OATP)
Obesity/obese patients
    absorption affected by, 767
    blood volume in, 769
    body mass index-based classification
        of, 765t
    body weight descriptors for,
        765–767, 766t
    cardiac output in, 769
    clinical examples of, 771–772
    Cockcroft–Gault equation in, 770
    creatinine clearance estimations in,
        771–772
    CYP enzymes affected by, 768, 772
    definition of, 765
    description of, 735
    distribution affected by, 767–768
    dosing in, 769–772
    excretion in, 769
    glomerular filtration rate in,
        770, 771f

loading dose in, 769–770
maintenance dose in, 770
metabolism affected by,
    768–769, 772
Modification of Diet in Renal
    Disease (MDRD) equation in, 771
pharmacokinetics affected by,
    767–769
physiologic functions
    affected by, 765
renal clearance in, 772
risk factors associated with, 765
summary of, 772
total body weight, 765–766
Objective function, 391
Observer bias, 72
Occupancy time, 347, 347f
Odds ratio, 76
ODTs. See Orally disintegrated
    tablets (ODTs)
Office of Generic Drugs (OGD), 973
Office of New Drugs (OND), 973
Off-label indication, 8
OGD. See Office of Generic
    Drugs (OGD)
Older adults. See also Elderly
    absorption in, 758–760
    ß-adrenergic receptors in, 762–763
    anticholinergics in, 762
    benzodiazepines in, 762
    bioequivalence studies in, 287
    body composition changes in, 759
    cardiovascular drugs in, 762–763
    central nervous system drugs in, 762
    clinical examples of, 763–764
    distribution in, 759
    dosing in, 735
    excretion in, 760–761
    extrahepatic metabolism in, 759–760
    formulations for, 860–861
    gastrointestinal absorption in, 758
    glomerular filtration rate in,
        760–761
    hepatic metabolism in, 759–760
    intramuscular absorption in,
        758–759
    metabolism in, 759–760
    overview of, 757–758
    pharmacodynamics in, 761–762
    pharmacokinetics in, 758–761
    psychotropic drugs in, 762

pulmonary absorption in, 759
QT prolongation drugs in, 763
subcutaneous absorption in,
    758–759
subgroups of, 758
summary of, 764–765
transdermal absorption in, 758
transporters in, 761
warfarin in, 763
Oligonucleotide drugs, 365, 366t, 367
OLS. See Ordinary least-squares
    method
Omeprazole (Prilosec), 101, 119,
    161, 663
OND. See Office of New
    Drugs (OND)
One-compartment open
    model, 18, 18f
    clearance, 467–468
    clinical utility of, 405–406
    definition of, 400
    for distribution, nonlinear
        elimination, combined with,
        561–562
    first-order absorption, 503f,
        503–504
    for IV bolus administration
        capacity-limited drug
            elimination, 555f, 556f
        clearance, 402–403
        disadvantages of, 400
        elimination half-life, 403–405
        elimination rate constant, 403
        example of, 385–387, 386f
        overview of, 399–401
        pharmacokinetics/
            pharmacodynamics model,
            385–387, 386f
        Sawchuk–Zaske method,
            405–406
        volume of distribution, 401–402
    for IV infusion, 444–447
        loading dose combined with,
            448–450, 449f–450f
        steady-state drug concentration
            in, 444f, 444–447, 446f
    of protein-bound drugs, 567f,
        567–568
    Wagner–Nelson method, 506
    zero-order absorption,
        502–503, 503f

One-tailed test, 62, 62*f*, 63*t*
One-way ANOVA, 66
Onset time, 15
Onzetra Xsail, 901, 901*f*
Open system, 19
Opioids, 878–880
Oral absorption
    during drug product development,
        114–115
    GI tract absorption, 101–114, 102*f*,
        105*f*, 106*f*, 107*t*, 108*f*
Oral administration
    absorption and elimination
        processes after, relationship
        between, 498–499
    description of, 497–498
    drug product considerations for,
        86, 230, 230*f*
    of insulin, 89
Oral cavity, 102
Oral dosage
    excipients for, 859*t*
    intravenous infusion and,
        conversions between, 730–731
    regimens, multiple doses, 534–536
Oral drug absorption, 114–115
Orally disintegrated tablets (ODTs),
    102, 306, 721
Orange book. *See* Approved Drug
    Products with Therapeutic
    Equivalence Evaluations
Order of reactions, 41
Ordinal data, 52
Ordinary least-squares
    method, 591, 592*t*
Ordinate, 37
Organic anion transporter
    protein, 659*t*
Organic anion transporting
    polypeptide (OATP), 167,
    600, 667
Organic cation transporter (OCT), 667
Ortho Evra, 501
Osmotic drug delivery system, 323*f*,
    329–330, 331*f*, 331*t*
Osmotic pump systems, 116
OTC drugs. *See* Over-the-counter
    drugs
Overage, 835*t*
Over-discriminating dissolution
    method, 202
Overdosing, 974

Over-the-counter drugs, 718
Overweight, 765
Oxybutynin, 895*t*
Oxycodone hydrochloride, 879*t*
Oxygen, hemoglobin binding of, 144
Oxymorphone ER (Opana ER), 319
Oxytocin, 120

**P**

Paclitaxel (Taxol), 99, 99*f*, 426, 891
Paddle method, 195*t*, 197–198, 198*f*
Paddle-over-disk method, 195*t*, 199
Paired *t*-test, 65
PAMPA. *See* Parallel artificial
    membrane permeability
    assay (PAMPA)
Pan coating, 325–326
Panodermal patch (Elan), 335
Pantoprazole (Pontinex), 119
Paracellular drug absorption, 94
Paracellular drug diffusion, 89, 89*f*
ParaGard, 892, 893*t*
Parallel artificial membrane
    permeability assay (PAMPA), 118
Parametric data, 52, 62–63
Parametric modeling, 594–595
Parametric tests, 65
Parenteral administration
    definition of, 399
    routes of, 86, 87*t*
Parenteral drug products
    description of, 229–230, 230*f*
    modified-release, 230, 337
Paroxetine (Paxil), 525–526, 561
Parsimony, 420
Particle size
    drug absorption and, 121, 190–191
    therapeutic nonequivalence, 839
Partition coefficient, 189
Passive diffusion, 90–94, 91*f*, 94*f*, 131
PAT. *See* Process analytical
    technology (PAT)
Patent protection, 919
Patient package insert (PPI), 7
Paxil. *See* Paroxetine
PBPK. *See* Physiologically-based
    pharmacokinetic model (PBPK)
PDF. *See* Probability density function
Peak drug concentration ($T_{max}$), 184,
    250, 498
Peak plasma drug concentration
    ($C_{max}$), 250

Pediatric patients
    absorption in, 774–775
    allometric scaling in, 778
    creatinine clearance calculations
        in, 794
    CYP enzymes in, 775–776
    distribution in, 775
    dosing in, 773–774, 777–778
    excipient tolerance by, 860–861
    excretion in, 776–777
    formulations for, 860–861
    metabolism in, 775–776
    pharmacodynamics in, 778
    pharmacokinetics in, 774–778
    phase II metabolism in, 776
    phase I metabolism in, 775–776
    subpopulations of, 773, 773*t*
Pediatric Research Equity Act
    (PREA), 223
Peeling, 418. *See also* Method of
    residuals
PEGylated phosphatidyl
    inositol (PI), 338
Pellets, 325–327, 326*f*
Penicillin, 465, 683
Pepcid. *See* Famotidine
Percutaneous coronary
    intervention, 890
Perfusion models, 2*f*, 20, 600
Perfusion of GI tract, 108
Perfusion pressure, 173
Peripheral compartments, 413.
    *See also* Tissue compartment
Peritoneal dialysis, 807
Peritubule capillaries, 173
Permeability, BCS and, 283–284
Permeation enhancers, 233
P-glycoprotein
    age-related changes in, 761
    bioavailability and, 98, 98*t*
    description of, 666–667
    drug removal by, 133
    in older adults, 761
P-glycoprotein transporters, 95,
    96–97, 137, 138*f*
pH
    solubility, drug absorption and,
        189–190
    stability and drug absorption, 190
    urine, renal reabsorption
        alterations caused by
        changes in, 741

Phagocytosis, 99
Pharmaceutical alternatives
    clinical endpoint, 836
    definition of, 836
    excipients, 837
    impurities-related therapeutic
        nonequivalence, 837
    practice problem for, 837–838
    stability-related therapeutic
        nonequivalence, 836
Pharmaceutical compounding, 736t
Pharmaceutical development
    approaches to, 855t
    quality by design in, 217–218,
        853–854, 856t, 856–857
    quality elements of, 856t
Pharmaceutical equivalence
    of active pharmaceutical
        ingredient, 834, 835t
    of drug product, 834–835, 835t
    future of, 842–843
    of generic product, 921
Pharmaceutical equivalents, 833–834,
        837–838, 841
Pharmaceutical inequivalence, 838
Pharmacodynamic models
    exposure-response
        relationships, 675
    software for data fitting, 854
    systems, 704–706
Pharmacodynamic responses
    categorical, 686
    continuous, 686
    definition of, 4
    discrete, 686
Pharmacodynamics
    definition of, 6, 673
    description of, 6–7
    drug design considerations, 221–222
    of ER drug products, 342–343, 343f
    models of, 688
    in older adults, 761–762
    in pediatric patients, 778
    pharmacokinetics and, 673–674
        drug-receptor theory, 677t
Pharmacogenetics
    advances in, 655–656
    definition of, 8, 162–163, 655
    pharmacodynamics application
        of, 656
    pharmacokinetics application
        of, 656

Pharmacogenomics, 8, 655
Pharmacokinetic analysis plan, 628
Pharmacokinetic models
    description of, 17–21, 18f
    selection of, 605–606
Pharmacokinetics. See also Clinical
        pharmacokinetics; Nonlinear
        pharmacokinetics
    absorption, 373–375
    basics of, 18f
    of biopharmaceuticals, 373–377
    capacity-limited, 552f,
        552–554, 553t
        clinical focus, 561
        elimination half-life in, 559
        practice problems, 550–551
    computers in, 20–21
    definition of, 383
    distribution, 375–376
    dose-dependent, 570
    drug design considerations, 222
    drug interactions, 735–739,
        736t–737t
    elimination, 376–377
    experimental approaches, 5
    flip-flop, 509–511
    hepatic disease effects on, 813–820
    metabolism, 376–377
    in older adults, 758–761
    parameters, 17
    population. See Population
        pharmacokinetics
    regional, 570, 748
    renal impairment effects on,
        788–789
    theoretical approaches, 5
    units in, 32–34, 33t
Pharmacokinetics equivalence studies
    designs for, 930t, 930–931
    pharmacokinetic analyses, 931–934
    requirements for, 929–934
    statistical analyses, 931–934
Pharmacokinetics/
        pharmacodynamics
    calculation of, 384
    curve stripping/fitting, 385
    differential equations, 389–390
    drug-receptor theory, 677t
    exposure/effect relationships,
        968–970
    integrated equations, 389–390
    linear processes, 391–392

new drug submission, 948–950
nonlinear processes, 391–392
one-compartment model after
    bolus IV administration,
    385–387
overview of, 383
population, 968–970
receptors for drugs, 676–678, 677t
software packages, 626–635
two-compartment model after IV
    administration, 387
Pharmacokinetics/pharmacodynamics
    models
    compartment, 384–392, 394t,
        595–596
    components of, 686–688, 687f
    development of, 395–396, 674–676,
        675f, 676f
    in drug approval and labeling,
        706–708
    fitting, 385
    multicompartment, 392
    noncompartmental, 393, 394t,
        688–690
Pharmacologic response, 678–680
Pharmacy and Therapeutics (P&T)
    committee, 916
Phase I enzymes, 664–665
Phase I reactions, 156–157,
    157t–158t
Phase I studies, 946
Phase II enzymes
    N-acetyltransferase, 658t–659t,
        660t, 666
    thiopurine methyltransferase,
        659t–660t, 665
    UDP-glucuronosyl-transferase,
        659t–660t, 665–666
Phase III studies, 946
Phase II reactions, 156–158, 158t
Phase II studies, 946, 976t
Phase IV studies, 974
Phenobarbital, 68–69, 157t,
    163, 165t, 740, 810t, 966
Phenothiazine, 119
Phenylbutazone, 157t
Phenytoin
    hemodialysis removal of, 810t
    nonlinear pharmacokinetics of,
        556–558, 557f, 560
    oral, 226
    therapeutic range for, 719t

Phoenix NLME, 624
Phospholipid bilayer, 90
Phospholipids, 886
pH–partition hypothesis, 93
Physical dependency, 683
Physiochemical properties
    drug design considerations, 189t
    particle size and drug absorption, 189t, 190–191
    solubility, pH, an drug absorption, 189t, 190
Physiologic absorption
    administration route and, 86f, 87t–88t
    cell membranes in
        drug passage across, 90–100, 92, 94f, 97f
        nature of, 89f, 89–90
    clinical examples, 98t, 99
    disease states affecting, 118–120
    drug interactions, 100–101, 119
    drug product design and, 114–115
    inhalation drug delivery, 121
    methods for studying
        gamma scintigraphy, 115
        intestinal permeability, 117–118
        in vivo GI perfusion studies, 116–117
        markers, 115–116
        osmotic pump systems, 116
        RDDCs, 116
    nasal drug delivery, 120–121
    nutrients affecting, 119–120
    oral, 101
        anatomic and physiologic considerations, 101–106, 102f
        GI tract absorption, 88t, 96t, 102f, 105f, 110t, 111f
    topical and transdermal drug delivery, 121
Physiological approach, 603–605
Physiologically based biopharmaceutics modeling, 220
Physiologically based mechanistic absorption model, 213
Physiologically-based pharmacokinetic model (PBPK)
    applications of, 602–603
    with binding, 599
    description of, 20, 393–395, 394f, 396f, 596–599, 946

hepatic transporter-mediated clearance incorporated in, 600–602
    limitations of, 602–603
    population pharmacokinetic models versus, 616, 969
    with pravastatin, 600–601, 601f
    software packages, 626
Physiologic models, 2f, 18f, 20
Pia arachnoid barrier, 136
Pinocytosis, 99–100
Pivotal efficacy studies, 946
PK/PD. See Pharmacokinetics/ pharmacodynamics
PK–PD models. See Pharmacokinetics/ pharmacodynamics models
Plasma, 14t
Plasma drug concentration, 12, 12f, 15f, 250f, 250–251. See also Steady-state, drug concentration
    in bioavailability and bioequivalence studies, 250–251
    during multiple-dosage regimens, 522–525, 523t, 526t
        intermittent IV infusion, 531f, 531–533
        repetitive IV injections, 526, 527t
    in saturable enzymatic elimination processes, 549f, 550, 550t–551t
    units of expression for, 34
Plasma drug concentration–time curve, 14f, 14–15, 15f
    AUC of, 273–275, 274f
    enduring saturation, 547–549
    for IV infusion, 444f, 444–446, 445t, 446f
    measurements using, 14f, 14t, 14–15
    of multiple-dosage regimens, 534–536
    of protein-bound drugs with nonlinear pharmacokinetics, 565–567, 566f, 567f
    in two-compartment open model, 415f, 415–420, 419f, 419t
Plasma protein binding, 141–142, 147–149
Plasma pseudocholinesterase, 658t, 660t, 664
Plavix. See Clopidogrel
PLGA. See Polylactide-co-glycolide (PLGA)

pMDIs. See Pressurized metered dose inhalers (pMDIs)
Pmetrics, 624
Polatuzumab vedotin-piiq, 369
Polyethylene glycol (PEG), 367
Polylactide-co-glycolide (PLGA), 882–883
Polymer coating, 890
Polymeric delivery systems, 324–325, 340, 341t
Polymeric matrix tables, 324–325
Polymeric nanoparticles, 887
Polymorphic form-related therapeutic nonequivalence, 838
Polymorphism, 189. See also Genetic polymorphism
Polymorphs, 191, 192t
Polyox, 879
Pooled t-test, 65
Poor metabolizers, 164
PopPK. See Population pharmacokinetics
Population analyses
    compartmental, 605, 605t
    description of, 593–594
    noncompartmental, 605, 605t
Population compartmental approach, 616
Population pharmacokinetics
    Bayesian theory, 742–743
    clinical examples, 745–748
    data analysis, 744–745
    decision analysis involving diagnostic tests, 745, 746t
    definition of, 742
    description of, 729
    features of, 742
    procainamide application of, 745
    summary of, 976t
Pore transport, 100
Portal vein, 154f
Positively skew, 53
Positively skewed data, 54f
Positive predictability, 746
Post absorption, 186
Postapproval changes, 195, 220–221, 245, 840, 866–869
Post hoc tests, 69
Postmarketing surveillance, 869–870
Power, 61
PPI. See Patient package insert (PPI)
Pravastatin, 600–601, 601f

Precision, 724
  accuracy versus, 70–71
  definition of, 70–71
Predicted plasma drug concentration, during multiple dosage regimens, 522, 523t
Prescription drug label, 7–8
Pressurized metered dose inhalers (pMDIs), 902
Presystemic elimination, 169, 481–483
Prilosec. See Omeprazole
PRIMAXIN, 961t
Probability density function, 578
Procainamide, 157t, 158, 666
  multiple-dosage regimens of, 537, 537f
  population pharmacokinetic application to, 745
  renal impairment dose adjustments in, 797–798
  therapeutic range for, 719t
Procardia XL. See Nifedipine
Process analytical technology (PAT), 857–858
Process validation, 866
Prodrugs, 156, 261, 833
Product inhibition, 563
Product label, 948
Product monograph, 948
Product quality, 869, 870t
Prolonged-action drug product, 308, 327–328
Prontosil, 156
Proof of concept studies, 946, 970
Propantheline bromide, 119
Proportional drug effect model, 693, 695f, 695–696
Propranolol, 117, 482–484
Protein binding
  constants for, 145–147
  drug distribution affected by, 133
  drug–drug, 149
  hepatic clearance affected by, 486
  nonlinear pharmacokinetics due to, 565–567, 566f
  one-compartment model drugs, 567f, 567–568
  physiologically-based pharmacokinetic model with, 599

plasma, 141–142, 147–149
  total and free drug exposure affected by, 963f
Protein drugs, 356, 357t–358t, 359, 367–369
Proteresis loop, 698
Prothrombin time, 819
Proton pump inhibitors, 119
Protoporphyrin IX, 155
Prozac. See Paroxetine
Pseudocholinesterase, 658t, 660t, 664
Pseudogenerics, 921
Psychotropic drugs, 762
PT. See Prothrombin time
Pulmonary absorption, 759
Purinethol. See Mercaptopurine
Pyelonephritis, 788t

Q

QA. See Quality assurance; Quality assurance (QA)
QbD. See Quality-by-design (QbD)
QC. See Quality control; Quality control (QC)
Q Guidances, 844
QT interval prolongation
  drugs that cause, 763
  studies of, 967–968
QTPP. See Quality target product profile (QTPP)
Quality
  documents regarding, 856
  drug product. See Drug product quality
  standards of, 863–865
Quality assurance (QA), 861
Quality by design (QbD), 217–218, 853, 856t, 856–857
Quality control (QC), 861
Quality risks
  description of, 855–856
  drug development, 862–863
  manufacturing, 863
  material, 861–862
Quality target product profile (QTPP), 851–853, 857
Quasi-irreversible inhibitors, 966–967
Quinidine, 739
  distribution and elimination half-lives of, 430t
  therapeutic range for, 719t
Qutenza, 896t

R

R, 624
Radioimmunoconjugates, 370
Raloxifene, 114t
Randomization, 72
Random variable, 51
Range, 55
Ranibizumab, 361
Ranitidine (Zantac®), 113, 116
Rate constants. See also Absorption rate constant
  clearance and, 469–471
  definition of, 19
Rate-limiting steps in absorption, 186–188, 187f, 188f
Rate of change of response, 701–702
Rate of drug excretion, 251, 252f
Rate of elimination, 550, 550t–551t
Rate ratio, 76
Ratio scale data, 52
RDDCs. See Remote drug delivery capsules
Reaction order. See Order of reaction
Receptor occupancy theory, 676, 690
Reciprocal plots, 145–146
Reciprocating disk method, 195t, 200
Recombinant drugs, approved, 357t–358t
Recombinant human insulin for inhalation (Exubera), 121
Rectal delivery of drug, 88t
Rectal drug delivery, 229
Rectangular coordinates, 30, 30f, 35, 35f
Rectum, 105–106, 312
Red blood cells. See Erythrocytes
Reference listed drug (RLD), 256, 917
Reference product, 929
Reference standard (RS), 203, 917
Regional pharmacokinetics, 570, 748
Regioselectivity, 161
Regression line, 31–32
Relative bioavailability, 4, 36, 243, 244, 246–248, 948–949
Relative risk (RR), 76
Relative risk increase (RRI), 76
Relative risk reduction (RRR), 76
Release test
  description of, 194t, 194–195
  development and validation of, 195t, 195–197

Remote drug delivery capsules
(RDDCs), 116
Renal artery, 173
Renal clearance
description of, 470–471, 473–474,
476–477
in obese patients, 772
renal impairment effects on, 790
Renal elimination rate constant, 403
Renal impairment
dose adjustments in
basis for, 798
limitations of, 806t, 806–807
nomograms, 798–801
overview of, 797–798
tables for, 801–806
dosing in, 789t, 789–791
excretion affected by, 959
glomerular filtration rate
measurements, 791–792
maintenance dose in, 798
moxalactam disodium response to,
430–431, 431f
overview of, 787–788
pharmacokinetics affected by,
788–789
procainamide dose adjustments in,
797–798
study of, 959–961, 975t
Renal plasma flow (RPF), 173
Repeat-action tablet, 308
Repeated measures ANOVA,
67–68
Repeated measures regression
analysis, 68
Repetitive IV injections,
526–529, 527t
early or late dose administration
during, 530
missed dose during, 529–530
Replicated crossover bioequivalence
study, 266–267
RES. See Reticuloendothelial system
Residence time, 107
Residual sum of squares, 591
Residual variability, 391
Restasis, 886t
Resveratrol, 114t
Reticuloendothelial system, 191
Reye's syndrome, 742
Reynolds number, 206
Rifampin, 165t, 262

Risk, quality
description of, 855–856
drug development, 862–863
manufacturing, 863
material, 861–862
Risk assessment, 853
Risk calculations, 75–77
Risk management, 865–866
Risk ratio, 76
Risperidone, 257t, 882t
Ritonavir, 262
Rivastigmin, 896t
RLD. See Reference listed drug (RLD)
Rotating basket method, 195t, 197
Rotating bottle method, 195t, 200
Route of administration
determination of, 734–735
drug design considerations,
224, 224f
extravascular, 497, 499f, 734
intravenous. See Intravenous (IV)
bolus administration
types of, 735f
RPF. See Renal plasma flow (RPF)
RR. See Relative risk (RR)
RRI. See Relative risk increase (RRI)
RRR. See Relative risk reduction
(RRR)
Ruggedness, 724–725
"Rule of Five," 114

S

SABE. See Scaled average
bioequivalence (SABE)
Sacituzumab govitecan, 369
SAD studies, 952–953
Safety considerations in ER/MR drug
products, 342–343
Salicylic acid
description of, 146f, 810t
pH of, 93t
Saquinavir mesylate (Invirase),
164–165
Saturable enzymatic elimination, 549f,
550t, 550–551. See also Capacity-
limited pharmacokinetics
Saturation, 547–549. See also Capacity-
limited pharmacokinetics
Sawchuk–Zaske method,
405–406
Scaled average bioequivalence
(SABE), 267–268, 933

Scale-up and post-approval changes
(SUPAC), 195, 220–221, 245,
840, 866–869, 922, 973
Scatchard plot, 145–146
Schedules, dosing, 537f, 537–540, 540t
Scheffe method, 68
Scopolamine, 233, 895t
SD. See Standard deviation
Second moment. See Area under the
first moment curve (AUMC)
Selection bias, 71
Selective serotonin reuptake
inhibitors (SSRIs), 561
Selegiline, 896t
Semilog coordinates, 30, 30f
Sensitivity, 746
Sepsis, moxalactam disodium
pharmacokinetics in patients
with, 430–431
Sequential analysis, 629
Serotonin syndrome, 561, 740
Serum, 14t
drug concentrations in, 13–14,
14t, 725t
Serum creatinine concentration
creatinine clearance calculations
from, 793–795
glomerular filtration rate estimations
based on, 796
overview of, 792–793
Side effect, 727, 849. See also Adverse
drug reaction
Sieving coefficient, 813
Significant figures, 34
Sildenafil, 819
Similarity factor, 208, 282
Simple randomization, 72
Single-blind study, 73
Single nucleotide
polymorphisms, 656
Sink conditions, 196
Sinusoids, 152, 154f
Site-specific drug delivery.
See Targeted drug delivery
SITT. See Small intestine transit
time (SITT)
Skewed data, 54f
Skewed distribution, 53
Skyla, 893t
SLC1OA1, 168t
SLCO2B1, 168t
SLCOIB1, 168t

*SLCOIB3,* 168*t*

Slope determination, 30, 31*f*, 32, 32*f*

Slow-erosion core tablet, 3297

Slow-release pellets, beads or granules, 325–327, 327*t*

Small intestine, 311–312, 312*t*

Small intestine transit time (SITT), 102, 108

SNP. *See* Single-nucleotide polymorphism; Single nucleotide polymorphisms

Sodium ferric gluconate complex, 590*f*, 591*t*

Soft-mist inhalers, 903

Software packages and programs
 ADAPT-II, 621, 623
 approaches in, 614–617, 615*t*
 "Bear," 621
 clinical pharmacokinetics, 617
 commercial, 619–621
 compartmental approach, 616–617
 covariate analyses, 630–631
 GastroPlus, 115
 noncompartmental approach, 614–616
 NONMEN, 592, 594, 621, 623
 overview of, 613–614
 pharmacokinetics
  compartmental, 621–625
  description of, 617–618
  noncompartmental, 618–625
 pharmacokinetics/ pharmacodynamics analyses, 626–635
 Phoenix NLME, 624
 Pmetrics, 624
 R, 624
 *in vivo* simulations from *in vitro* data, 626
 WinNonlin, 619, 620*t*–622*t*, 626

Solubility, 187–188
 BCS and, 283
 dissolution and, 187–188
 pH drug absorption and, 189–190

Solubility–pH profile, 189

Solute carrier transporters, 667

Solvates, 191
 absorption and, 191, 191*f*

Somatuline Depot, 886*t*

Sonophoresis, 335

Sorbitrate, 227

Specifications, 864, 866
 clinically relevant, 217–220

Specificity, 746

Spray dry coating, 325

Spreadsheets, 31

Spritam, 341

SSRIs. *See* Selective serotonin reuptake inhibitors

St. John's wort, 735, 740

Stability, 220, 724
 bioavailability and bioequivalence problems, 260
 determination of, 220
 pH, drug absorption and, 190

Stability–pH profile, 190

Stability-related therapeutic nonequivalence, 836

Standard deviation (SD), 56, 62

Standard error of the mean (SEM), 56–57

Standard treatment control, 72–73

Statistical errors, 60

Statistical evaluation
 of bioequivalence, 272, 272*t*
 of ER drug products, 347

Statistical inference study, 69

Statistically significant differences, 64

Statistical moment theory, 393, 578–579

Statistical significance testing, 60

Statistics
 distributions, 52–53
 hypothesis testing, 59–63, 69–72

Steady state
 apparent volume of distribution at, 423–424
 clearance relationship with, 446–447
 drug concentration, 444*f*, 444–445
 during IV infusion, 415–418
  one-compartment model of, 444*f*, 444–446, 445*t*, 446*f*
  two-compartment model of, 453*f*, 453–454
 during loading dose plus IV infusion
  one-compartment model, 448–450, 449*f*–450*f*
  two-compartment model, 415*f*, 415–418

in multiple-dosage regimens, 522, 522*f*, 525, 526*t*

plasma drug concentration, of ER/MR drug products, 444–446, 446*f*

Stents, drug-eluting, 890–892, 891*f*–892*f*, 891*t*

Stereoisomers, 289

Sterile solutions, 835*t*

Stochastic approximation of EM, 624

Stomach, 103–104

Stratification, 74

*Streptococcus pneumoniae,* 689, 689*f*

Student's *t*-test, 65, 70

Study submission, 277–278, 278*t*, 505*t*
 bioequivalence study waiver, 281–282
 dissolution profile comparison, 282

Subcutaneous injection, 86, 87*t*

Sublingual administration, 87*t*

Sublingual tablets, 227–228

Substance abuse potential, 682

Substitution, generic, 290

Sucralfate, 741

Sudlow Site I, 148

Sulfamethoxazole/trimethoprim (Bactrim), 178

Sulfasalazine, 156, 157*t*

Sulfation, 160*t*

Sulfisoxazole (Gantrisin), 178

Sumatriptan, 73, 120

SUPAC. *See* Scale-up and postapproval changes

Superiority trials, 58, 58*f*–60*f*, 61, 61*t*

Superiority trial table, 58*t*

Superposition principle, 522, 523*t*
 for several IV infusion doses, 531–532, 532*t*

Suppositories, 229

Surfactants, dissolution effect, 192

Surgical anesthesia, 129

Surrogate endpoints, 685, 686*t*

Surrogate markers, 289, 289*t*

Switchability, 916

Synera, 896*t*

Synthetic reactions. *See* Phase II reactions

Synthroid. *See* Levothyroxine sodium

Systemic clearance. *See* Clearance

Systems pharmacodynamic models, 704–706

# T

Tabulations, 730
Tachyphylaxis, 683
Tagamet. *See* Cimetidine
Target drug concentration
  during multiple-dosage
    regimens, 521
  steady-state, 445
Targeted drug delivery, 370–373
  drugs for, 372
  general considerations in, 370
  site-specific properties, 372
  targeting modality, 372
  target site, 371–372
Targeted-release products, 306, 308
Target-mediated drug disposition,
    132, 356
Target product profile (TPP), 851
Taxol. *See* Paclitaxel
Taxotree, 886*t*
Taylor series expansion, 592
TBW. *See* Total body weight (TBW)
TCAs. *See* Tricyclic antidepressants
TE. *See* Therapeutic equivalent
Terfenadine, 968
Terminal elimination phase, 509
Testosterone, 895*t*
Tetracycline
  calcium and, 93
  multiple oral-dose regimens, 535
Theophylline, 486
  absorption of, 111, 112*f*
  cimetidine and, 739
  colonic absorption of, 104
  diet and, interactions between,
    741–742
  distribution and elimination
    half-lives of, 430*t*
  extended-release capsules, 282
  IV infusion of, 453, 730–731
  multiple-dosage regimens of, 537
  NONMEM output for, 623, 624*t*
  therapeutic range for, 719*t*, 744
Theranostics, 342
Therapeutic drug monitoring (TDM)
  adverse events, 727–728
  definition of, 719
  description of, 370, 614
  dosage
    adjustment in, 725–726
    forms of, 721
    regimen, 720–721

drug
  assays for, 723–725
  concentration measurements,
    722, 723*t*, 726
  concentrations of, 722
  pharmacokinetics of, 721, 725
  selection of, 720
  functions of, 719–720
  lanoxin, 726–727
  overview of, 718–719
  patient compliance with, 721–722
  patient's response, 722
  serum drug concentrations, 726
  vancomycin, 728, 728*f*
Therapeutic equivalence
  description of, 290–292, 291*t*
  evaluation codes, 290–292, 291*t*
    for nifedipine extended-release
      tablets, 292, 292*t*
  future of, 842–843
Therapeutic equivalent, 832, 841, 916
Therapeutic index (TI), 15, 370
Therapeutic nonequivalence
  of generic products, 841–842
  impurities-related, 837
  particle size-related, 839
  polymorphic form-related, 838
  stability-related, 836
Therapeutic range, 719, 719*t*
Therapeutic substitution, 916
Therapeutic window, 15, 974
Thiopental, 135–136
Thiopurine methyltransferase,
    659*t*–660*t*, 665
Thorough QTc study, 968, 976*t*
3D printed dosage forms,
    877–878, 878*f*
3D printed formulation, 340–341
Three-compartment open model, for
    IV bolus administration, 427*f*,
    427–428
Three-way ANOVA, 67
Ticlopidine (Ticlid®), 112
Tight junctions, 136
Tilting, 206
Time-dependent killing, 689
Time-dependent pharmacokinetics,
    563*t*, 563–564
  circadian rhythms and drug
    exposure, 564
  clinical focus, 564
  description of, 165–167

Time to reach steady-state drug
    concentrations
  in multiple-dosage regimens, 526*t*
  in one-compartment model, 444*f*,
    444–446, 445*t*, 446*f*
Timolol, 560, 560*f*
Tissue(s)
  binding, drug distribution affected
    by, 141–142
  blood flow to, 131–133, 135*t*, 414*t*
  concentration in, 15, 417
  perfusion of, 135
Tissue compartment, 413
TMDD, 376
To-be-marketed formulations, 973
Tobramycin sulfate, 719*t*, 730
Tolerance, drug, 682–683
Top-down approach, 604
Topping, 316, 318
Torsades de pointes, 740, 967
Total body clearance, 32, 464, 788
  after IV bolus infusion,
    559–561, 560*f*
Total body water, 139*f*, 775
Total body weight (TBW), 765–766,
    766*t*, 792
Total predictability, 746
Total time for drug to be excreted,
    251–252, 252*f*
Toxic concentration. *See* Minimum
    toxic concentration
Toxicity, in drug development, 676*f*
Toxicokinetics, 12–13, 585
Toxicology, 12
TPP. *See* Target product profile (TPP)
Transcellular absorption,
    89*f*, 89–90
Transcytosis, 99, 375
Transdermal drug delivery, 88*t*, 233
  description of, 501
  drug product considerations for,
    233, 233*t*
  fentanyl, 758
  in older adults, 758
  systems for, 332–335, 333*t*, 334*f*,
    892–897, 895*t*–896*t*
Transdermal therapeutic systems
    (TTS), 334
Transfer constants, 418
Transit time in absorption
  GI, 311–312, 312*t*
  large intestine, 312–313

Transmissible spongiform encephalopathies (TSE), 859
Transporter-mediated drug interactions, 167
Transporters
ABC, 666–667
age-related changes in, 761
in carrier-mediated intestinal absorption, 94, 95f, 95–98, 96t
dose-dependent pharmacokinetics, 570
in drug elimination, 171–172
efflux, 96–98, 97f
in GI tract, 117
P-gp, 96–97, 98t
solute carrier, 667
Transport protein, 100
Trapezoidal rule, 36, 476, 579
Trastuzumab deruxtecan, 369
Trastuzumab emtansine, 369
Tricor, 886t
Tricyclic antidepressants (TCAs)
absorption of, 118
Trough concentration, 405
Trypsin, 104
TSE. See Transmissible spongiform encephalopathies (TSE)
TTS. See Transdermal Therapeutic Systems
Tubular reabsorption, 176
Tukey method, 68
Two-compartment open model, 18f, 19, 415–427
absorption, 505
clearance, 468–469
curve, 412f, 413
elimination phase in of plasma drug concentration-time curve, 412, 412f
first-order absorption, 505, 505f
for IV bolus administration, 413, 418–423, 420f, 420t, 421t
clinical application, 420f, 420t, 420–422, 421t
method of residuals, 418–420, 419f, 419t
pharmacokinetics/ pharmacodynamics, 387
practical focus, 422–424

practice problems, 424f, 424–425
relation between distribution and elimination half-life, 422, 430, 431f
of IV infusion, 453–454
loading dose combined with, 453f, 453–454
practical focus, 454–455
total volume of distribution in, 454
with nonlinear elimination, 562
Two one-sided tests procedure, 272–273
Two One-Sided T-Tests (TOST), 927–928
Two-tailed test, 62, 62f, 63t
Two-way ANOVA, 67
Two-way repeated measures ANOVA, 68
Type I error, 60–61, 61t
Type II error, 61

U
UDP-glucuronosyl-transferase, 659t–660t, 665–666
Ultrafiltration, 143, 143f
Ultragenerics, 921
Ultrasonic nebulizers, 908
Uncontrolled studies, 72–73
Underdosing, 974
United States Pharmacopeia-National Formulary, 863–864
United States Pharmacopeia (USP), 187
Unit impulse response (UIR), 210–211
Unit membrane theory, 90
Units of measurement, 32, 33t
Un-paired t-test, 65
Uremia, 787, 789
Uridine diphosphate glucuronosyltransferase
in obese patients, 769
in pediatric patients, 776
Uridine diphosphoglucuronic acid (UDPGA), 158
Urinary excretion data, 249t, 251–252, 252f
cumulative amount of drug excreted in urine, 251, 251f
rate of drug excretion, 251, 252f, 475t
total time for drug to be excreted, 251–252, 252f

Urine
drug concentration in, 15–16
pH, renal reabsorption alterations caused by changes in, 741
renal formation of, 175, 175t
Urticaria, 683
USP-NF. See United States Pharmacopeia National Formulary
Ustekinumab, 361

V
Vaginal drug delivery, 229
Vaginal rings, 883–884, 885t
Valacyclovir, 261
Validation, of release test, 195t, 195–197
Validity, 73–74, 631
Valium. See Diazepam
Valproic acid (Depakene), 561, 567, 719t
Vancomycin, 406, 719t, 728, 728f, 809
Variables, 17
nominal-scale type, 52
Variance, 56
Vasa recti, 173
Vasopressin, 120
Vegetable oil, 328
Venofer, 886t
Verapamil, 741
Vesicular transport, 99–100
Viagra. See Sildenafil
Vibrating mesh nebulizers, 908
Vinblastine, 426
Vincristine, 426
Visual predictive check (VPC) figures, 634, 634f
Visudyne, 886t
Vitamin E, 117
Volume of distribution. See Apparent volume of distribution
VPC figures. See Visual predictive check (VPC) figures
Vyxeos, 886t

W
Wagner–Nelson method, 213, 506f, 506–508, 507t, 589
Waivers, of bioequivalence, studies, 281–282
Warfarin, 148–149, 663, 701, 718

Weak acids, 176
  diffusion of, 93
Weak bases, 176
Weighted least-squares method, 591,
  592t, 743
Wellbutrin. *See* Bupropion
  hydrochloride
Welling and Craig nomogram
  method, 799
"Well-stirred" model, of clearance,
  479–488, 480f, 816
WinNonlin, 619, 620t–622t, 626
WLS method. *See* Weighted
  least-squares method

Wobbling, 206

**X**
Xanthine oxidase, 768
Xelpros, 886t
Xenobiotics, 154

**Y**
Young's rule, 773

**Z**
Zantac®. *See* Ranitidine
Zero-order absorption

description of, 500–501
  one-compartment model,
    502–503, 503f
Zero-order elimination,
  39–40, 42
Zero-order half-life, 39–40, 41t
Zero-order process, 39–40
Zero-order reactions, 39–40,
  41f, 41t
Zithromax. *See* Azithromycin
Zolpidem tartrate (Ambien),
  319–320
ZTlido, 896t
Zyvox. *See* Linezolid